Wardlaw-Smith

Contemporary Nutrition: A Functional Approach

ON TRACK . . .

Check out the study tools that best suit your learning style. A variety of interactivities and quizzes keep you motivated and on track to master key concepts.

- **Animations** Access to approximately 75 animations helps you visualize key nutrition concepts and processes. Each animation is accompanied by a quiz to help you test your comprehension.

- **Test Yourself** Prepare for exams by taking a chapter quiz at the *Contemporary Nutrition: A Functional Approach* ARIS site. Use the quiz questions and accompanying feedback for incorrect answers to help you gauge your mastery of the chapter content. You can even e-mail your quiz results to your professor!

- **Learning Activities** Helpful and engaging learning experiences await you at the *Contemporary Nutrition: A Functional Approach* ARIS site. In addition to quizzes and animations, you can study nutrition terminology with flashcards, and you can use links to reliable websites to help you complete assignments.

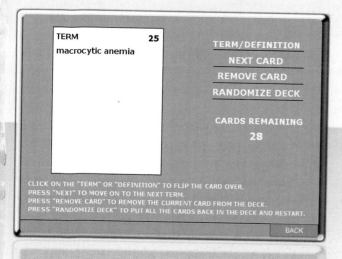

Mc Graw Hill McGraw-Hill Higher Education

Contemporary Nutrition
A Functional Approach

Gordon M. Wardlaw
PH.D.
Formerly of
Department of Human Nutrition,
College of Education and Human Ecology
The Ohio State University

Anne M. Smith
PH.D., R.D., L.D.
Department of Human Nutrition,
College of Education and Human Ecology
The Ohio State University

with contributions of

James W. Bailey
Formerly of University of Tennessee–Knoxville

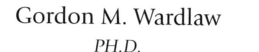

McGraw-Hill Higher Education

Boston   Burr Ridge, IL   Dubuque, IA   New York   San Francisco   St. Louis
Bangkok   Bogotá   Caracas   Kuala Lumpur   Lisbon   London   Madrid   Mexico City
Milan   Montreal   New Delhi   Santiago   Seoul   Singapore   Sydney   Taipei   Toronto

**McGraw-Hill
Higher Education**

CONTEMPORARY NUTRITION: A FUNCTIONAL APPROACH

Published by McGraw-Hill, a business unit of The McGraw-Hill Companies, Inc., 1221 Avenue of the
Americas, New York, NY 10020. Copyright © 2009 by The McGraw-Hill Companies, Inc. All rights reserved.
No part of this publication may be reproduced or distributed in any form or by any means, or stored in a
database or retrieval system, without the prior written consent of The McGraw-Hill Companies, Inc., including,
but not limited to, in any network or other electronic storage or transmission, or broadcast for distance learning.

Some ancillaries, including electronic and print components, may not be available to customers outside the
United States.

This book is printed on recycled, acid-free paper containing 10% postconsumer waste.

1 2 3 4 5 6 7 8 9 0 QPD/QPD 0 9 8

ISBN 978–0–07–337554–0
MHID 0–07–337554–3

Publisher: *Michelle Watnick*
Executive Editor: *Colin H. Wheatley*
Vice-President New Product Launches: *Michael Lange*
Senior Developmental Editor: *Lynne M. Meyers*
Senior Marketing Manager: *Tami Petsche*
Project Manager: *April R. Southwood*
Senior Production Supervisor: *Kara Kudronowicz*
Senior Media Project Manager: *Tammy Juran*
Manager, Creative Services: *Michelle D. Whitaker*
Cover Designer: *Greg Nettles/Squarecrow Design*
Interior Designer: *Ellen Pettengell*
Cover Illustration: *Ellen Pettengell*
(USE) Cover Image: *© Michael Rosenfeld/Getty Images*
Senior Photo Research Coordinator: *John C. Leland*
Photo Research: *Mary Reeg*
Supplement Producer: *Mary Jane Lampe*
Compositor: *S4Carlisle Publishing Services*
Typeface: *10/12 Giovanni Book*
Printer: *Quebecor World Dubuque, IA*

The credits section for this book begins on page 733 and is considered an extension of the copyright page.

Library of Congress Cataloging-in-Publication Data

Wardlaw, Gordon M.
  Contemporary nutrition : a functional approach / Gordon M. Wardlaw, Anne M. Smith.—1st ed.
    p. cm.
  Includes index.
  ISBN 978–0–07–337554–0 — ISBN 0–07–337554–3 (hard copy : alk. paper)
  1. Nutrition. I. Smith, Anne M., Ph.D. II. Title.
  QP141.W377 2009
  613.2—dc22   2008003400

Brief Contents

Contents

Chapter 3 The Human Body: A Nutrition
Perspective 78

Part Two The Energy Nutrients
and Energy Balance 120

Chapter 4 Carbohydrates 120

Part Three Vitamins,
Minerals, and Water 280

Overview of the Micronutrients 280

Chapter 8 Nutrients Involved in Fluid and
          Electrolyte Balance 294

Part Four Nutrition: Beyond the Nutrients 424

Chapter 12 Nutrition: Fitness and Sports 424

Chapter 13 Eating Disorders: Anorexia Nervosa, Bulimia Nervosa, and Other Conditions 462

Part Five Nutrition: A Focus on the Life Stages 554

Chapter 17 Nutrition from Infancy Through Adolescence 592

Preface

INTRODUCING *CONTEMPORARY NUTRITION: A FUNCTIONAL APPROACH*

Teaching nutrition at the college level is a challenging endeavor. Dedicated college instructors strive to provide their students with a positive learning experience that will allow them to master unfamiliar content and to apply sound nutrition principles to their lives. One particular challenge instructors face is the difficult task of effectively teaching the many various aspects of the micronutrients. As we prepared the seventh edition of *Contemporary Nutrition* it became clear that many instructors would like to see an alternate version of our text that presented vitamins and minerals from the perspective of their functions in the body. As a result of this feedback, we enlisted the help of James Bailey to write new micronutrient chapters that are organized in the context of their physiological functions and roles in health and disease. The following pages outline the features and enhancements found in this latest version of *Contemporary Nutrition*.

Our Approach to Teaching Nutrition

If you teach nutrition, you undoubtedly find it a fascinating subject. Nutrition, however, can also be a frustrating subject to teach, for a variety of reasons. The results of new research studies emerge at an incredible pace. Claims and counterclaims abound regarding the need for and benefits of certain constituents in our diets. *Contemporary Nutrition* is designed as a tool to help instructors accurately convey changing and seemingly conflicting messages to introductory nutrition students. Our students commonly have misconceptions about nutrition, and many have not had a college-level biology or chemistry course. *Contemporary Nutrition* conveys complex scientific concepts at a level appropriate for these undergraduate students, in turn helping students meaningfully apply the material we cover in class, to their lives.

Keeping Current

The vast amount of published research is constantly reshaping our knowledge of nutritional science. As authors and teachers, we constantly search the literature to ensure that students' exposure to the study of nutrition in *Contemporary Nutrition* is reliable, accurate, and as up-to-date as this rapidly changing field allows. The seventh edition includes integrated coverage of the 2005 Dietary Guidelines for Americans and the USDA MyPyramid, as well as other recent recommendations and research findings. We are also aware of conflicting opinions in our field and thus draw on many reputable sources to create a balanced resource for nutrition information. Each chapter contains an updated list of "Further Readings" as well as links to reputable nutrition and health information websites. We strive to present an objective approach to newly emerging or controversial topics so that students learn to carefully

scrutinize the nutritional information they read and hear about. To help, several controversial topics are presented in "Making Decisions" boxes within each chapter.

Understanding Our Audience

We have written *Contemporary Nutrition* assuming that our students have a limited background in college-level biology, chemistry, or physiology. We have been careful to include the essential science foundation needed to adequately comprehend certain topics in nutrition, such as the basic discussion of protein synthesis in Chapter 6. These scientific discussions have been written in a simple, straightforward manner.

Students enrolled in an introductory nutrition course often come from a broad range of majors and interests. We address this diversity by incorporating a thorough system of pedagogical tools, such as Critical Thinking questions and Concept Checks, to help them master the material. A variety of applications and case studies are also included to appeal to students whose majors range from business to education.

> "I have just finished my first year of using this textbook, after using another leading nutrition text for almost 15 years, and I am delighted with it as are my students!"
>
> *Karen Schuster, Florida Community College of Jacksonville*

Personalizing Nutrition

A prominent theme in nutrition today is *individuality*. This trait is even incorporated into the name of the most recent USDA food guide: "MyPyramid." Throughout *Contemporary Nutrition* we reinforce that each person responds differently to nutrients. Not all of us, for example, find that saturated fat in our diets raises our blood cholesterol values above recommended standards. The text's discussions do not assume that all students are alike. Chapter content and features, such as "Making Decisions," "Critical Thinking," "Nutrition and Your Health," "Case Studies," and "Rate Your Plate," repeatedly ask students to learn more about themselves and their health status and to use their new knowledge to improve their health.

After reading this textbook, students will be better equipped to understand how the nutrition information coming from all directions—whether on the evening news, on food packages, in popular magazines and newspapers, or from government agencies—applies to them. Our goal is for students to understand that their knowledge of nutrition will allow them to evaluate and personalize nutrition information, rather than follow every guideline issued for an entire population. We emphasize that a population consists of individuals with varying genetic and cultural backgrounds, and these individuals will have varying responses to diet.

As a final note on bringing nutrition down to a personal level, the book covers topics of particular interest to college students such as eating disorders, dietary supplements, vegetarianism, popular weight-loss diets, and sports nutrition. There is even a new section on "Eating Well in College" in Chapter 1. Regardless of topic, the overall emphasis remains the same—the importance of understanding one's food choices and modifying one's diet to best meet personal needs.

A CLOSER LOOK AT *CONTEMPORARY NUTRITION: A FUNCTIONAL APPROACH*

Organizational Changes

Contemporary Nutrition: A Functional Approach is organized into five parts that reflect major topics typically covered in an introductory nutrition course:

Part One	Nutrition: A Key to Health
Part Two	Energy Nutrients and Energy Balance
Part Three	Vitamins, Minerals, and Water
Part Four	Nutrition: Beyond the Nutrients
Part Five	Nutrition: A Focus on Life Stages

Based upon recommendations from a survey of adopters of the text, several modifications to the organization were made:

- Alcohol is no longer the focus of an entire chapter but is now included in the expanded new section, "Nutritional Implications of Alcoholism" in Chapter 18, "Nutrition During Adulthood." Our goal was to make it easier to integrate coverage of this important topic within the typical term of an introductory course.

> "I think this is a great idea. I rarely have time to go over this chapter in length and so try to integrate information on alcohol throughout other chapters."
> *Amy D. Ozier, Northern Illinois University*

- Energy balance and weight maintenance are covered earlier in the text as the topic of Chapter 7, which now more logically follows the energy-yielding nutrient chapters in Part Two.

> "I am strongly in favor of this reorganization….Energy balance fits perfectly after the macronutrients….Of all the changes suggested for the book, this is the one I am most excited to see…."
> *Kevin W. Huggins, Auburn University*

- The discussions of safety of food and water (Ch. 15) and undernutrition throughout the world (Ch. 14), appear earlier in the text within Part Four, "Beyond the Nutrients," as a reflection of the significance and timeliness of these topics.

The book concludes with three chapters in Part Five, "A Focus on Life Stages," to allow flexibility for those schools that offer separate courses on lifecycle nutrition.

Although most frequently used in semester-long courses, the text's organization allows instructors to omit parts or chapters to fit the needs of quarter-length courses. For example, Part Five, "Focus on the Life Stages," can now be easily omitted from an introductory course. In addition each chapter is written in such a way that they can function independently so that instructors can cover the material in the order that best fits their particular course needs.

NUTRITION AND YOUR HEALTH
Eating Well in College

The college years are a leap into adulthood for many young adults. This is a time for freedom and a chance to make personal lifestyle decisions. Studies show that the diets and other health habits of college students are not optimal. Typically, students fall short of recommendations for servings of whole grains, vegetables, fruits, milk, and meat, opting instead to max out on fats, sweets, and alcohol. This information is disturbing from a public health standpoint, because young adulthood is the time when many health behaviors are formed and will likely persist throughout life. With independence comes responsibility, including a responsibility to make smart food choices.

What is it about the college lifestyle that makes it so difficult to build healthy habits? Why do so many young adults gain the dreaded "freshman 15" pounds during the first months of college? How does alcohol consumption affect your waistline and academic performance? What can you do to establish healthful habits to last a lifetime?

WEIGHT CONTROL AND THE "FRESHMAN FIFTEEN"

The college experience is exciting, but stressful. Students face changes in academic requirements, interpersonal relationships, and living environment. These stressful situations contribute to poor health behaviors. For example, take the week of midterms; during this time of writing papers and cramming for exams, balanced meals are all-too-easily replaced by high-fat and high-calorie fast-foods; convenience items; and sugary, caffeinated beverages. Physical activity is sacrificed in favor of study time.

Also consider the university environment. On campus, you are faced with a wide variety of dining choices, some healthy and some not so healthy. Dining halls, fast-food establishments, bars, and vending machines offer food 24 hours per day. While it is certainly possible to make wise food choices at each of these outlets, the temptations of convenience, taste, and value (i.e., oversized portions) may persuade the college student to select unhealthy options.

Eating is about more than just obtaining "fuel." Meals and snacks are times to socialize. You may feel pressured to eat a big lunch at noon without regard to hunger if your peers are meeting in the dining hall to catch up on class work and gossip. While chatting, too, it is easy to lose track of portions and to overeat. In addition, food may be a source of familiarity and comfort in a new and stressful place. Learning to eat based on your body's hunger cues is a great way to avoid weight gain.

▲ Late night pizza can add extra calories to the college student's daily intake.

New Chapter Features

- "Making Decisions" boxes appear throughout each chapter and highlight hot topics or controversial issues in nutrition. Balanced information is provided that can help students make decisions regarding these topics.

MAKING DECISIONS

Trans Fat

Some foods contain *trans* fatty acids, also called *trans* fats. These fats are commonly found in processed foods, and especially deep-fried foods, such as doughnuts and French fries. Large amounts of *trans* fats in the diet pose certain health risks, so intake should be minimized (see Chapter 5 for details). All food labels in the United States and Canada have to list *trans* fat content. Do you still want to eat food rich in *trans* fat?

- The "Nutrition and Your Health" section appears at the end of each chapter and highlights a current health issue or disease related to the chapter topic.

NUTRITION AND YOUR HEALTH
Lipids and Cardiovascular Disease

Cardiovascular disease is the major killer of North Americans. Cardiovascular disease typically involves the coronary arteries and, thus, frequently the term coronary heart disease (CHD) or coronary artery disease (CAD) is used. Each year about 500,000 people die of coronary heart disease in the United States, about 60% more than die of cancer. The figure rises to almost 1 million if strokes and other circulatory diseases are included in the global term *cardiovascular disease*. About 1.5 million people in the United States each year have a heart attack. The overall male-to-female ratio for cardiovascular disease is about 2:1. Women generally lag about 10 years behind men in developing the disease. Still, it eventually kills more women than any other disease—twice as many as does cancer. And, for each person in North America who dies of cardiovascular disease, 20 more (over 13 million people) have symptoms of the disease.

▲ Cardiovascular disease kills more women than any other disease—twice as many as does cancer.

DEVELOPMENT OF CARDIOVASCULAR DISEASE

The symptoms of cardiovascular disease develop over many years and often do not become obvious until old age. Nonetheless, autopsies of young adults under 20 years of age have shown that many of them had atherosclerotic **plaque** in their arteries (Fig. 5-15). This finding indicates that plaque buildup can begin in childhood and continue throughout life, although it usually goes undetected for some time.

The typical forms of cardiovascular disease—coronary heart disease and strokes—are associated with inadequate blood circulation in the heart and brain related to buildup of this plaque. Blood supplies the heart muscle, brain, and other body organs with oxygen and nutrients. When blood flow via the coronary arteries surrounding the heart is interrupted, the heart muscle can be damaged. A heart attack, or **myocardial infarction**, may result (review Fig. 5-15). This may cause the heart to beat irregularly or to stop. About 25% of people do not survive their first heart attack. If blood flow to parts of the brain is interrupted long enough, part of the brain dies, causing a **cerebrovascular accident**, or stroke.

A heart attack can strike with the sudden force of a sledgehammer, with pain radiating up the neck or down the arm. It can sneak up at night, masquerading as indigestion, with slight pain or pressure in the chest. Many times, the symptoms are so subtle in women that death occurs before she or the health professional realizes that a heart attack is taking place. If there is any suspicion at all that a heart attack is taking place, the person should first chew an aspirin (325 milligrams) thoroughly and then call 911. Aspirin helps reduce the blood clotting that leads to a heart attack.

Continuous formation and breakdown of blood clots in the blood vessels is a normal process. However, in areas where plaques build up, blood clots are more

plaque A cholesterol-rich substance[ce depos]ited in the blood vessels; it contains [...] white blood cells, smooth muscle c[ells, vari]ous proteins, cholesterol and other [lipids,] and eventually calcium.

myocardial infarction Death of [part of] the heart muscle. Also termed a *hea[rt attack.]*

cerebrovascular accident (CVA) [Death] of part of the brain tissue due typic[ally to a] blood clot. Also termed a *stroke.*

- Each chapter culminates with a "Case Study" that presents a real-life situation followed by a list of directed questions to assist students in applying the nutrition knowledge from the chapter. Responses to the "Case Study" questions are found in Appendix A.

CASE STUDY

Planning a Training Diet

Michael is training for a 10K run coming up in 3 weeks. He has read a lot about sports nutrition and especially about the importance of eating a high-carbohydrate diet while in training. He also has been struggling to keep his weight in a range that he feels contributes to better speed and endurance. Consequently he is also trying to eat as little fat as possible. Unfortunately, over the past week his workouts in the afternoon have not met his expectations. His run times are slower, and he shows signs of fatigue after just 20 minutes into his training program.

His breakfast yesterday was a large bagel, a small amount of cream cheese, and orange juice. For lunch, he had a small salad with fat-free dressing, a large plate of pasta with marinara sauce and broccoli, and a diet soft drink.

For dinner, he had a small broiled chicken breast, a cup of rice, some carrots, and iced tea. Later, he snacked on fat-free pretzels.

Answer the following questions, and check your responses in Appendix A.

1. Is the low-carbohydrate diet a good idea during Michael's training?
2. Are there any important components missing in Michael's diet? Are missing components contributing to his fatigue?
3. Describe some changes that should be made in Michael's diet including some specific foods that should be included.
4. How should fluid needs be met during workouts?
5. Should Michael focus on fueling his body before, during, or after workouts?

- "Check Your Knowledge" is a new element featuring multiple-choice study questions. These questions are meant to compliment the open-ended "Study Questions" and help students prepare for the type of questions on course examinations. Answers to the "Check Your Knowledge" questions are found in Appendix A.

CHECK YOUR KNOWLEDGE

Answers to the following multiple choice questions are in Appendix A.

1. Vitamins are classified as
   a. organic and inorganic.
   b. fat-soluble and water-soluble.
   c. essential and nonessential.
   d. elements and compounds.

2. Vitamin D is called the sunshine vitamin because
   a. it is available in orange juice.
   b. exposure to sunlight converts a precursor to vitamin D.
   c. it can be destroyed by exposure to sunlight.
   d. All of the above.

3. Vitamin E functions as
   a. a coenzyme.
   b. an antioxidant.
   c. a hormone.
   d. a peroxide.

4. A deficiency of vitamin A can lead to the disease called
   a. xerophthalmia.
   b. osteomalacia.

   c. scurvy.
   d. pellagra.

5. A high intake of vitamin E can
   a. inhibit vitamin K metabolism.
   b. lead to lead poisoning.
   c. inhibit copper absorption.
   d. cause baldness.

6. A vitamin synthesized by bacteria in the intestine is
   a. A.
   b. D.
   c. E.
   d. K

7. Bowed legs, an enlarged and misshapen head, and enlarged knee joints in children are all symptoms of
   a. rickets.
   b. xerophthalmia.
   c. osteoporosis.
   d. vitamin D toxicity.

8. Thiamin, riboflavin, and niacin are called the "energy" vitamins because they

   a. can be broken down to provide energy.
   b. are coenzymes needed for release of energy from carbohydrates, fats, and proteins.
   c. are ingredients in energy drinks such as Powerade.
   d. are needed in large amounts by competitive athletes.

9. A deficient intake of _____ has been shown been shown to increase the risk of having a baby with a neural tube defect such as spina bifida.
   a. vitamin A
   b. vitamin C
   c. vitamin E
   d. folic acid

10. Vitamin C is necessary for the production of
    a. antibodies.
    b. collagen.
    c. hormones.
    d. clotting factors.

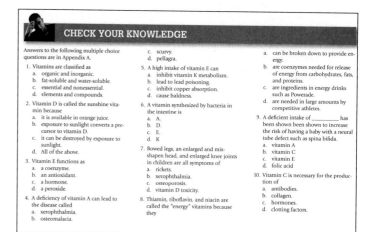

Art and Design Features

The new features and content of this edition were the inspiration for a new look and design. This fresh new look invites students to read and learn about nutrition with an engaging style and presentation. You will find brighter colors, more creative layouts, and exceptional new figures and photos. Each illustration was carefully evaluated for its teaching ability and visual appeal.

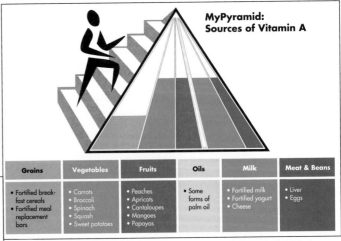

MyPyramid: Sources of Vitamin A

Grains	Vegetables	Fruits	Oils	Milk	Meat & Beans
• Fortified break-fast cereals • Fortified meal replacement bars	• Carrots • Broccoli • Spinach • Squash • Sweet potatoes	• Peaches • Apricots • Cantaloupes • Mangoes • Papayas	• Some forms of palm oil	• Fortified milk • Fortified yogurt • Cheese	• Liver • Eggs

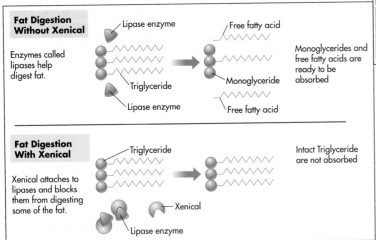

Fat Digestion Without Xenical

Enzymes called lipases help digest fat.

Lipase enzyme — Triglyceride — Lipase enzyme → Free fatty acid — Monoglyceride — Free fatty acid

Monoglycerides and free fatty acids are ready to be absorbed

Fat Digestion With Xenical

Xenical attaches to lipases and blocks them from digesting some of the fat.

Triglyceride — Xenical — Lipase enzyme → Intact Triglyceride are not absorbed

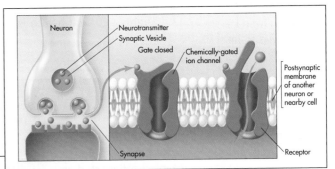

Neuron — Neurotransmitter — Synaptic Vesicle — Gate closed — Chemically-gated ion channel — Postsynaptic membrane of another neuron or nearby cell — Receptor — Synapse

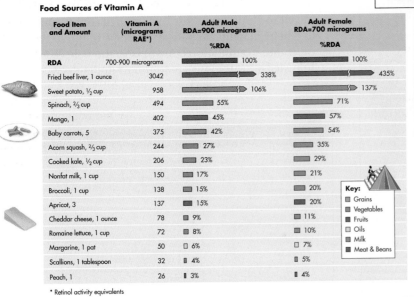

Food Sources of Vitamin A

Food Item and Amount	Vitamin A (micrograms RAE*)	Adult Male RDA=900 micrograms %RDA	Adult Female RDA=700 micrograms %RDA
RDA	700–900 micrograms	100%	100%
Fried beef liver, 1 ounce	3042	338%	435%
Sweet potato, ½ cup	958	106%	137%
Spinach, ⅔ cup	494	55%	71%
Mango, 1	402	45%	57%
Baby carrots, 5	375	42%	54%
Acorn squash, ⅔ cup	244	27%	35%
Cooked kale, ½ cup	206	23%	29%
Nonfat milk, 1 cup	150	17%	21%
Broccoli, 1 cup	138	15%	20%
Apricot, 3	137	15%	20%
Cheddar cheese, 1 ounce	78	9%	11%
Romaine lettuce, 1 cup	72	8%	10%
Margarine, 1 pat	50	6%	7%
Scallions, 1 tablespoon	32	4%	5%
Peach, 1	26	3%	4%

* Retinol activity equivalents

Key:
- Grains
- Vegetables
- Fruits
- Oils
- Milk
- Meat & Beans

Small intestine (duodenal) ulcer — Stomach ulcer — healthy gastric mucosa — ulcer

(a) (b)

Chapter-by-Chapter Highlights

In response to feedback from instructors using the traditionally organized version of *Contemporary Nutrition,* we have stream-lined and refined the content to better meet the needs of today's students. The following list highlights some of the features of *Contemporary Nutrition: A Functional Approach.*

CHAPTER 1: WHAT YOU EAT AND WHY

- Chapter 1 starts with a new focus on the connection be-tween nutrition and good health.
  - See the opening section "Good Health: The Nutrition Connection."
- The introduction to the nutrients and other important chemicals in foods has been streamlined.
  - The chemical structures of the nutrients have been moved to later chapters on each nutrient.
  - Table 1-4 has been enhanced to emphasize good di-etary sources of each nutrient class.
  - The phytochemicals, important chemicals in plants that may contribute to reduced disease risk, are now introduced in Chapter 1.
- Students will relate to the new "Nutrition and Your Health: Eating Well in College." This section is complimented with the new case study on the typical college student.

CHAPTER 2: GUIDELINES FOR DESIGNING A HEALTHY DIET

- Several features have been added to enhance the discus-sion of MyPyramid.
  - The consumer messages graphic from MyPyramid has been added as Figure 2-5.
  - Table 2-4, showing the recommended number of serv-ings, and Table 2-5, showing nutrient contributions, are now color coded using the MyPyramid group colors.

TABLE 2-5 Nutrient Contributions of Groups in the MyPyramid Food Guide Plan

Food Category	Major Nutrient Contributions
Grains	Carbohydrate Vitamins such as thiamin Minerals such as iron Fiber*
Vegetables	Carbohydrate Vitamins such as plant pigments that form vitamin A Minerals such as magnesium Fiber
Fruits	Carbohydrate Vitamins such as folate and vitamin C Minerals such as potassium Fiber
Oils	Fat Essential fatty acids Vitamins such as vitamin E
Milk	Carbohydrate Protein Vitamins such as vitamin D Minerals such as calcium and phosphorus
Meat & Beans	Protein Vitamins such as vitamin B-6 Minerals such as iron and zinc

*Whole-grain varieties

▲ Typical restaurant portions contain numerous servings from the individual groups in MyPyramid.

- Figure 2-7 includes new MyPyramid serving size guides. Each guide is now associated with a food group and is highlighted with MyPyramid colors.
- Presentation of the Dietary Guidelines is now streamlined and more interesting.
- Discussion of the Dietary Reference Intakes is now incor-porated into the body of the chapter.
- The Health Claims Report Card is included to illustrate the FDA regulation process for health information on food labels.
- The chapter culminates with, "Nutrition and Your Health: Evaluating Nutrition Claims and Advice" and the case study on dietary supplements, which both provide sugges-tions for healthful and logical nutrition decisions.

CHAPTER 3: THE HUMAN BODY: A NUTRITION PERSPECTIVE

- A new section on cell metabolism introduces the impor-tance of the nutrients in metabolic reactions in the cell.
- The discussion of bacterial activity in the large intestine has been expanded and the importance of prebiotics and probiotics is introduced.
- "A Closer Look at Genetics and Nutrition" includes an ex-panded discussion of nutrigenomics.
- The chapter concludes with "Nutrition and Your Health: Common Problems with Digestion" and the case study on gastroesophageal reflux disease. The discussion of ulcers has been updated to reflect current theories and treatments.
- Several illustrations have been added or enhanced with new features and more vivid color. More vivid art is used to depict the cell in Figure 3-2; new art illustrates the ac-tion of neurotransmitters in Figure 3-6; the endocrine system is now illustrated in Figure 3-7; phagocytosis is depicted in the new Figure 3-9; the swallowing process is detailed in Figure 3-12; and Figure 3-20 is a new illustra-tion of a stomach and duodenal ulcer.

CHAPTER 4: CARBOHYDRATES

- "Diabetes—When Blood Glucose Regulation Fails" is the focus of "Nutrition and Your Health." This section includes a new box highlighting the symptoms of diabetes. A new section on metabolic syndrome is also featured including an illustration of the metabolic syndrome risk indicators and medical conditions related to metabolic syndrome.
- Several figures have been updated or enhanced with new features and more vivid color.
  - Figure 4-1 features new art better depicting the sun's energy used to produce glucose.
  - Figure 4-6 graphically presents food sources of carbo-hydrates in a new format using the MyPyramid food group colors to depict each food's contribution to the male and female RDA.

- Regulation of blood glucose is now graphically illustrated in Figure 4-9.

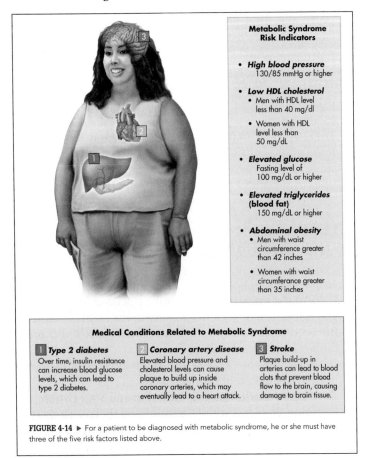

Metabolic Syndrome Risk Indicators

- **High blood pressure**
  130/85 mmHg or higher
- **Low HDL cholesterol**
  - Men with HDL level less than 40 mg/dl
  - Women with HDL level less than 50 mg/dL
- **Elevated glucose**
  Fasting level of 100 mg/dL or higher
- **Elevated triglycerides (blood fat)**
  150 mg/dL or higher
- **Abdominal obesity**
  - Men with waist circumference greater than 42 inches
  - Women with waist circumference greater than 35 inches

Medical Conditions Related to Metabolic Syndrome

1 Type 2 diabetes
Over time, insulin resistance can increase blood glucose levels, which can lead to type 2 diabetes.

2 Coronary artery disease
Elevated blood pressure and cholesterol levels can cause plaque to build up inside coronary arteries, which may eventually lead to a heart attack.

3 Stroke
Plaque build-up in arteries can lead to blood clots that prevent blood flow to the brain, causing damage to brain tissue.

FIGURE 4-14 ▶ For a patient to be diagnosed with metabolic syndrome, he or she must have three of the five risk factors listed above.

CHAPTER 5: LIPIDS

- The discussion of omega-3 fatty acids has been enhanced. This is accompanied by "Making Decisions" boxes on "Mercury in Fish," which highlights the advantages and disadvantages of fish consumption, and on "Flax Seed or Walnuts?," which provides information about plant sources of alpha linolenic acid.
- "Lipids and Cardiovascular Disease" is the focus of "Nutrition and Your Health" and includes several new photos and a margin note listing cardiovascular disease risk factors. "Medical Interventions to Lower Blood Lipids" is updated and appears in this section, followed by the case study on planning a heart healthy diet.
- Several figures and tables have been updated or enhanced with new features and more vivid color.
  - Figure 5-6 graphically presents food sources of fat in a new format using the MyPyramid food group colors to depict each food's contribution to the American Heart Association recommendation.
  - The function of phospholipids in membranes is shown in Figure 5-14.
  - Table 5-4 introduces the American Heart Association 2006 Diet and Lifestyle Goals for Cardiovascular Disease Risk Reduction.

CHAPTER 6: PROTEINS

- Phenylketonuria is presented in a "Making Decisions" box as an illustration of the importance of semiessential amino acids.
- All information related to protein in foods, including "Dietary Considerations—Protein Quality," is found in the major section "Proteins in Foods."
- "Nutrition and Your Health" brings all of the information on vegetarian and plant-based diets together into one section. A new graphic illustrates plant group combinations used in protein complementation. This section is followed by the case study, "Planning a Vegetarian Diet."

CHAPTER 7: ENERGY BALANCE AND WEIGHT CONTROL

- A new section, "Societal Efforts to Reduce Obesity," describes the recent work of many organizations to address obesity.
- The section on surgical treatment of obesity has been expanded and renamed "Bariatric Surgery." Figure 7-18 illustrates new bariatric surgery procedures.
- "Nutrition and Your Health: Popular Diets—Cause for Concern" summarizes diet approaches to weight control and includes a review of the most popular diets. The case study, "Choosing a Weight-Loss Program," follows.

OVERVIEW OF THE MICRONUTRIENTS

- Introduces and explains the classification of vitamins and minerals
- Presents concepts of absorption, storage, toxicity, and preservation.
- Provides the basics needed prior to learning about the specific metabolic roles micronutrients play in the body.

CHAPTER 8: FLUID AND ELECTOROLYTE BALANCE

- The Beverage Guidance System, published in 2005, emphasizes that fluids should not provide a significant amount of energy or nutrients, and is discussed and outlined in Table 8-2.
- All vitamin and mineral Food Source figures have been redesigned and list each food's contribution to the male and female RDA using the MyPyramid food group colors.
- The "Nutrition and Your Health" segment, "Maintaining a Healthy Blood Pressure," includes newly designed figures that diagram the categories of blood pressure (Fig. 8-14) and provides advice on lifestyle and diet habits that can reduce blood pressure (Fig. 8-15).

CHAPTER 9: ANTIOXIDANTS

- Oxidation and reduction are introduced in Figure 9-1.
- Figures 9-3 demonstrates how antioxidants defend against free radicals.
- Figure 9-12 is a new map showing vitamin A deficiencies around the world.
- "Nutrition and Your Health" discusses Nutrient Supplements: Who Needs Them and Why?

CHAPTER 10: BONE HEALTH

- Table 10-1 on biological factors associated with bone status and Table 10-2 on lifestyle factors help students understand the value of applying this important information to their own lives.
- Figure 10-4 illustrates a hip facture caused by osteoporosis.
- Figure 10-7 shows bone density changes due to aging, and Figure 10-8 highlights skeletal regions most susceptible to low-bone density and osteoporosis.
- Figure 10-12 graphically represents how male and female calcium intakes fall below recommended daily intakes in the U.S.

CHAPTER 11: ENERGY METABOLISM AND BLOOD HEALTH

- New Case Study looks at active senior recently diagnosed with anemia.
- New Figure 11-22 presents detailed view of blood components
- Photos of diseases and deficiency conditions include glossitis, pellagra, megaloblastic anemia, spinal bifida, goiter, and zinc deficiency.

CHAPTER 12: FITNESS AND SPORTS NUTRITION

- Aerobic versus anaerobic use of glucose is illustrated in a new diagram in Figure 12-3.
- "A Focus on Fluids Needs" has been reorganized and more strongly emphasizes the American College of Sports Medicine recommendations for appropriate fluid intake before, during, and after physical activity.
- Information regarding popular energy bars and gels has been expanded and completely updated in Table 12-7.
- "Nutrition and Your Health" features "Ergogenic Aids and Athletic Performance." NCAA rulings on supplements are highlighted in a "Making Decisions" box and the case study "Planning a Training Diet" follows.
- Fitness assessments have been added as activities in Rate Your Plate.

CHAPTER 13: EATING DISORDERS: ANOREXIA NERVOSA, BULIMIA NERVOSA, AND OTHER CONDITIONS

- The section on "Other Disordered Eating Patterns" has been updated to include an expanded section on night eating syndrome.
- A discussion of polycystic ovary syndrome and eating disorders has been added in a "Making Decisions" box.

CHAPTER 14: UNDERNUTRITION THROUGHOUT THE WORLD

- Several "Making Decisions" boxes are used to highlight the following topics in Chapter 14:
  - Food insecurity and overweight
  - Benefits of breastfeeding
  - Nutrition and AIDS
  - Sustainable development and the Gender and Development (GAD) Approach
- The impact of AIDS worldwide is now illustrated in Figure 14-4, which depicts the rise in number of cases of HIV.
- The chapter concludes with "Nutrition and Your Health: Undernutrition at Critical Life Stages" and the case study "Undernutrition during Childhood," which highlights the devastating effects of undernutrition on human health. A new figure (14-8) outlines the UNICEF conceptual framework of the causes of malnutrition.

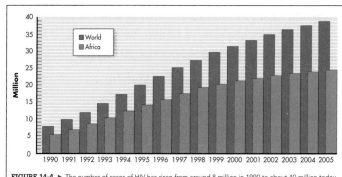

FIGURE 14-4 ▶ The number of cases of HIV has risen from around 8 million in 1990 to about 40 million today. Over 60% of people living with HIV are in sub-Saharan Africa.
Source: UNAIDS/WHO AIDS Epidemic Update, December 2006

CHAPTER 15: SAFETY OF FOOD AND WATER

- The chapter focus has been expanded to include the safety of our water supply.
- The discussion of foodborne infections caused by bacteria and viruses has been expanded to include new information about *E. coli* O157:H7, *Listeria*, and Norovirus.

- Practical tips for safe food handling are consolidated in "Nutrition and Your Health: Preventing Foodborne Illness," followed by the case study on "Preventing Foodborne Illness at Gatherings". The new chart in Figure 15-2 lists the length of time to keep leftovers in the refrigerator.

CHAPTER 16: PREGNANCY AND BREASTFEEDING

- A successful pregnancy is the outcome of interrelated factors. The new section "Success in Pregnancy" discusses these factors:
  - Infant birthweight
  - Prenatal care and counseling
  - Effects of maternal age
  - Closely-spaced and multiple births
  - Smoking, medication use, and drug use
  - Food safety
  - Nutritional status
  - Nutrition assistance for low-income families
- The Dietary Guidelines specific to pregnant and breastfeeding women have been highlighted in margin notes, and key recommendations for this population are listed in Table 16-3.

CHAPTER 17: NUTRITION FROM INFANCY THROUGH ADOLESCENCE

- New growth charts for children released by the World Health Organization in 2006 are discussed and compared to the National Center for Health Statistics growth charts.

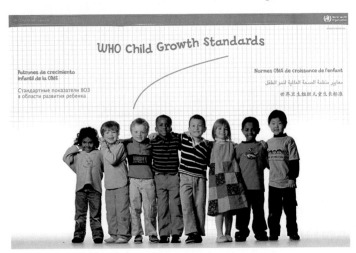

- Information about the dietary intake of infants and toddlers from the recently published "Feeding Infants and Toddlers Study (FITS)" is incorporated in the chapter.
- The most recent guidance from the American Dental Association about the use of fluoridated water during infancy is included.

- New information is presented on the diagnosis and dietary treatment, as well as the prevention of food allergies, in "Nutrition and Your Health: Food Allergies and Intolerances." Figure 17-4 is a new illustration of the percentage of children and adults with various food allergies.

CHAPTER 18: NUTRITION DURING ADULTHOOD

- Strength training recommendations for older adults are highlighted in a "Making Decisions" box.
- Coverage of alcohol has been expanded in the new section, "Nutritional Implications of Alcoholism." This feature includes sections on how alcoholic beverages are produced, absorption and metabolism of alcohol, benefits of moderate alcohol use, risk of alcohol abuse, and guidance regarding alcohol use. Liver cirrhosis is featured in a "Making Decisions" box.
- "Nutrition and Your Health" focuses on nutrition and cancer. The American Institute for Cancer Research Diet and Health Guidelines for Cancer Prevention are included as a margin note.

SPECIAL ACKNOWLEDGMENTS

The functional approach version of *Contemporary Nutrition* would not have been possible without the expertise and talents of Jim Bailey. His years of teaching introductory nutrition provided the insight to expertly reorganize the vitamins and minerals by their functions.

We also thank Angela Collene, M.S., R.D., for her research, editing, and written contributions. She also assisted in the preparation of the Overview of the Micronutrients. Our editors, Colin Wheatley and Lynne Meyers, supported and assisted us through every phase of the revision and facilitated the decisions required to accomplish the enhancements, especially the new design, of this edition. April Southwood and the rest of the McGraw-Hill production staff carefully oversaw the myriad of tasks needed to create a beautiful and precise textbook.

THANK YOU TO REVIEWERS

Our goal is to provide students and educators with the most accurate, up-to-date, and useful textbook possible. As with earlier editions, the quality of the seventh edition of *Contemporary Nutrition* is largely dependent on the meticulous, professional assistance of nutrition educators from academic institutions across the nation. We are indebted to these colleagues who reviewed the sixth edition, evaluated new material for the seventh edition, participated in instructional symposia, and responded to surveys. The advice and suggestions from these colleagues have been used in every chapter and have resulted in a textbook that is current and inviting.

LIST OF REVIEWERS

Valerie K. Adegunleye
Prince George's Community College

James W. Bailey
University of Tennessee

Karyn Baiorunos
Prince George's Community College

Catherine Berry
University of Wisconsin Eau Claire

Michael E. Bizeau
Colorado State University

Ann M. Black
Nevada State College

Brenda Brooks
Arapahoe Community College

Jackie Buell
Ohio State University

Alfred A. Bushway
University of Maine

Patricia A. Chisamore
*SUNY Orange Community
College*

Anne C. Cioffi
*Hudson Valley Community
College*

Margaret C. Craig-Schmidt
Auburn University

Sylvia Crixell
Texas State University - San Marcos

Lisa K. Diewald
Montgomery County Community College

Eugene J. Fenster
Metropolitan Community College

Jennifer L. Fuller
Bluegrass Community & Technical College

Keiko Goto
Shasta College

Nancy Harris
East Carolina University

Beverly W. Henry
Northern Illinois University

Diana Himmel
Tunxis Community College

Kevin W. Huggins
Auburn University

Thunder Jalili
University of Utah

Janine Jensen
Tulsa Community College

Laura J. Kruskall
University of Nevada Las Vegas

Anne B. Marietta
Southeast Missouri State University

Molly Michelman
University of Nevada Las Vegas

Jesse Morrell
University of New Hampshire

Gavin O'Connor
Ozarks Technical Community College

Amy D. Ozier
Northern Illinois University

Jill Patterson
*The Pennsylvania State University –
University Park, PA*

Elizabeth Quintana
West Virginia University School of Medicine

Ruth A. Reilly
University of New Hampshire

Christina Reiter
Metropolitan State College of Denver

Daryl Richter
Tulsa Community College

Rebecca Roach
University of Illinois Urbana Champaign

Joelle E. Romanchik-Cerpovicz
Georgia Southern University

Renee Romig
Western Iowa Tech Community College

Karla Rues
Ozarks Technical Community College

Karen Schuster
Florida Community College of Jacksonville

Padmini Shankar
Georgia Southern University

Lydia Court Steinman
The University of Texas at Austin

Rebecca J. Sullivan
Tunxis Community College

Laurie Ysseldyke Wright
Hillsborough Community College

Gordon M. Wardlaw, Ph.D.
P.O. Box 290
Mendocino, California 95460
Email: gordonmark.wardlaw@gmail.com

Anne M. Smith, Ph.D., R.D., L.D.
Department of Human Nutrition
The Ohio State University
325 Campbell Hall
1787 Neil Avenue, Columbus, Ohio 43210
Email: smith.23@osu.edu

Supplementary Materials

McGraw-Hill offers the following suite of tools and technology products to support *Contemporary Nutrition: A Functional Approach*. Students can order supplemental study materials by contacting their local bookstore or by calling 800-262-4729. Instructors can obtain teaching aids by calling the Customer Service Department at 800-338-3987, visiting the McGraw-Hill website at **www.mhhe.com**, or contacting their McGraw-Hill sales representative.

ARIS with Presentation Center

ARIS.mhhe.com

Assessment, Review, and Instruction System, also known as ARIS, is an electronic homework and course management system designed for greater flexibility, power, and ease of use than any other system. Whether you are looking for a preplanned course or one you can customize to fit your course needs, ARIS is your solution.

Within the ARIS portal, students can access a variety of self-study digital learning objects designed to support the chapter content found in *Contemporary Nutrition: A Functional Approach.*

- Chapter level quizzing
- Animation quizzes
- NBC News nutrition video clips
- Answers to "Critical Thinking Questions"
- Chapter glossaries
- Interactive exercises and more

In addition to having access to all student digital learning objects, ARIS provides instructors with the following tools:

Build Assignments

- Choose from prebuilt assignments or create custom content by importing your own content or editing an existing assignment from the prebuilt assignment.
- Assignments can include quiz questions, animations, and videos—anything found on the website.
- Create announcements and use full course or individual student communication tools.

Track Student Progress

- Assignments are automatically graded
- Gradebook functionality allows full course management including:
    - Dropping the lowest grades
    - Weighting grades/manually adjusting grades
    - Exporting your gradebook to Excel, WebCT, or BlackBoard

Presentation Center

Build instructional materials wherever, whenever, and however you want!

ARIS Presentation Center is an online digital library containing assets such as photos, artwork, animations, PowerPoints, and other media types that can be used to create customized lectures, visually enhanced tests and quizzes, compelling course websites, or attractive printed support materials.

Access to your book, access to all books!
The Presentation Center library includes thousands of assets from many McGraw-Hill titles. This ever-growing resource gives instructors the power to use assets specific to an adopted textbook as well as content from all other books in the library.

Nothing could be easier!
Accessed from the instructor side of your textbook's ARIS website, Presentation Center's dynamic search engine allows you to explore by discipline, course, textbook chapter, asset type, or keyword. Browse, select, and download the files you need to build engaging course materials. All assets are copyright McGraw-Hill Higher Education but can be used by instructors for classroom purposes.

Test Bank

A computerized test bank that uses testing software to quickly create customized exams is available on the ARIS website for this text. The user-friendly program allows instructors to search for questions by topic or format, edit existing questions or add new ones; and scamble questions for multiple versions of the same test. Word files of the test bank questions are provided for those instructors who prefer to work outside the test-generator software.

The Dietary Guidelines for Americans
- Food Groups to Encourage
- Fats
- Carbohydrates
- Sodium and Potassium
- Alcoholic Beverages
- Food Safety

Student Response System

Wireless technology brings interactivity into the classroom or lecture hall. Instructors and students receive immediate feedback through wireless response pads that are easy to use and engage students. This system can be used by instructors to:

- Take attendance
- Administer quizzes and tests
- Create a lecture with intermittent questions
- Manage lectures and student comprehension through the use of the gradebook
- Integrate interactivity into their PowerPoint presentations

NutritionCalc Plus 3.0

CD (Windows only) ISBN: 0-07-332865-0
Online ISBN: 0-07-337552-7

NutritionCalc Plus 3.0 is a suite of powerful dietary self-assessment tools available on CD and online. This newest release features approximately 27,000 foods from the ESHA Research nutrient database and a new user-friendly interface that makes creating a personal diet analysis even easier. Users now have the ability to add up to three profiles and to create recipes. The program functions are supported by detailed "Help" documents and helpful cautionary notes that warn the user of possible entry errors.

Food Composition Table Booklet

This handy printed reference provides data for thirty nutrient categories for approximately 2500 foods. All data is from the ESHA Research nutrient database.

About the Authors

GORDON M. WARDLAW, Ph.D., has taught introductory nutrition courses to students in the Department of Human Nutrition at The Ohio State University, and at other colleges and universities. Dr. Wardlaw is the author of many articles that have appeared in prominent nutrition, biology, physiology, and biochemistry journals and was the 1985 recipient of the American Dietetic Association's Mary P. Huddleson Award. Dr. Wardlaw is a member of the American Society for Nutritional Sciences and is certified as a Specialist in Human Nutrition by the American Board of Nutrition. Dr. Wardlaw is currently retired from academia.

ANNE M. SMITH, PH.D., R.D., L.D. currently teaches nutrition to nutrition majors and nonmajors at The Ohio State University and was the recipient of the 1995 Outstanding Teacher Award from the College of Human Ecology and the 2007 Outstanding Dietetic Educator Award from the Ohio Dietetic Association. Dr. Smith is the Director of the Didactic Program in Dietetics in the Department of Human Nutrition, College of Education and Human Ecology, of The Ohio State University and received the 1998 Emerging Dietetic Leader Award from The American Dietetic Association. Dr. Smith conducts research in the area of vitamin and mineral metabolism and was awarded the 1996 Departmental Research Award from the Ohio Agricultural Research & Development Center. Dr. Smith's research articles have appeared in prominent nutrition journals. She is a member of the American Society for Nutritional Sciences, the American Society for Clinical Nutrition, and the American Dietetic Association.

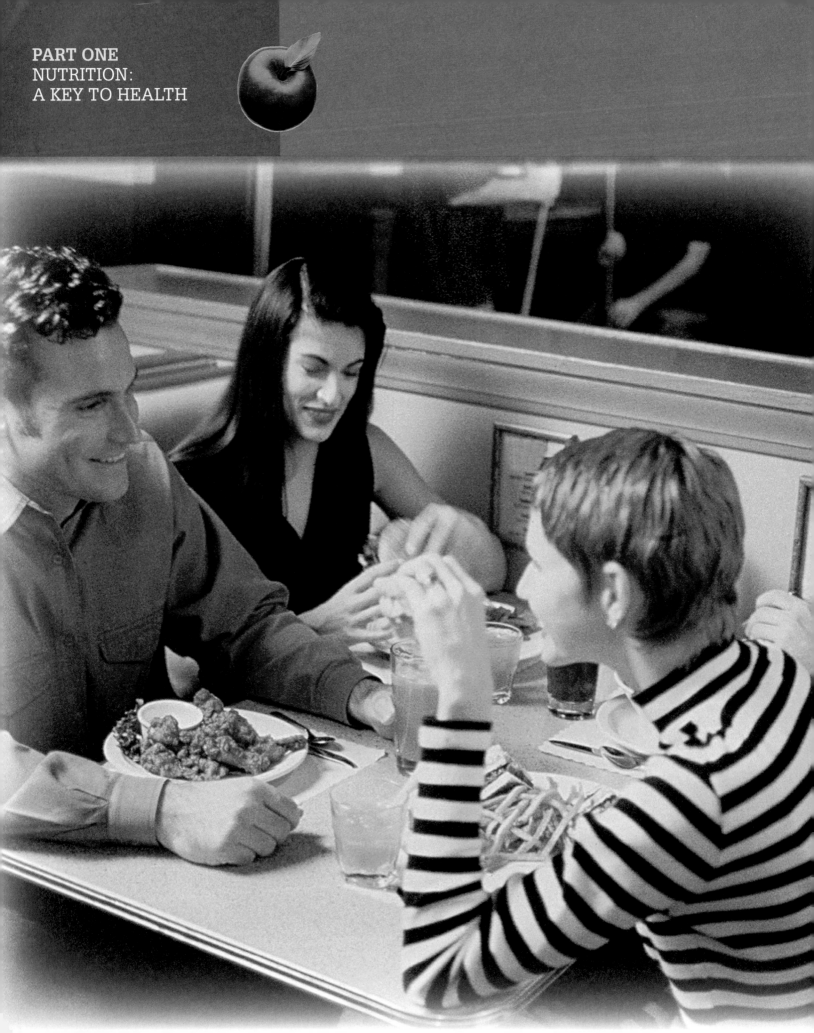

CHAPTER 1 What You Eat and Why

ARE YOU EATING TOO MUCH SATURATED FAT, *TRANS* FAT, AND CHOLESTEROL? Do carbohydrates in our diets cause many of our health problems? Is a high protein diet always safe and foolproof? Are some foods unsafe? Do you need to take a balanced multivitamin and mineral supplement? Should you become a vegetarian? If you have asked yourself any of these questions and are confused about what you should eat, you are not alone. Chapter 1 will help you sort out some of these issues as you are introduced to the science of nutrition.

As you begin this study of nutrition, keep this in mind. Research over the last 40 years has shown that a healthy diet—especially one rich in fruits, vegetables, and whole grains—coupled with regular prolonged, vigorous exercise and some strength-building exercise—can both prevent and treat many age-related diseases. Overall, it is clear that the nutrition aspect of the lifestyles of some (but not all) North Americans are out of balance with their metabolism and physiology. We

3

live longer than our ancestors did, so preventing the diseases that develop during aging is a more important focus today than in the past.

By making optimal dietary choices, we can strive to bring the goal of a long, healthy life within reach. This is the primary theme not just of Chapter 1 but throughout this book.

🕯 Refresh Your Memory

As you begin your study of what you eat and why in Chapter 1, you may want to review:

- The metric system in Appendix I.

GOOD HEALTH: THE NUTRITION CONNECTION

In your lifetime, you will eat about 70,000 meals and 60 tons of food. Chapter 1 will take a close look at the general classes of nutrients supplied by this food, the role research plays in sorting out which food components are essential for the maintenance of health, and the powerful effect of dietary habits in determining overall health. Many factors influence our food choices (see the comic below) and will also be discussed in Chapter 1.

What Is Nutrition?

Nutrition is the science that links foods to health and disease. It includes the processes by which the human organism ingests, digests, absorbs, transports, and excretes food substances.

Nutrients Come from Food

> Some nutrients that perform important functions can be produced by the body if they are missing from the diet. Whether these nutrients are essential is not clear-cut. For example, humans require vitamin D, but the body is capable of synthesizing its own vitamin D upon exposure of the skin to sunlight. This reduces the need for vitamin D from dietary sources among people who experience regular sun exposure (see Chapter 10).

nutrients Chemical substances in food that contribute to health, many of which are essential parts of a diet. Nutrients nourish us by providing calories to fulfill energy needs, materials for building body parts, and factors to regulate necessary chemical processes in the body.

What is the difference between food and **nutrients?** Food provides the energy (in the form of calories) as well as the materials needed to build and maintain all body cells. Nutrients are the substances obtained from food that are vital for growth and maintenance of a healthy body throughout life. For a substance to be considered an **essential nutrient,** three characteristics are needed:

- First, at least one specific biological function of the nutrient in the body must be identified.

What influences daily food choices? How important is taste? Appearance? Nutrition? Convenience? Cost (Value)? Do these daily food choices go on to influence long-term health? If so, to what extent? Chapter 1 provides some answers.

- Second, omission of the nutrient from the diet must lead to a decline in certain biological functions, such as production of blood cells.
- Third, replacing the omitted nutrient in the diet before permanent damage occurs, will restore those normal biological functions.

Why Study Nutrition?

Nutrition is a lifestyle factor that is a key to developing and maintaining an optimal state of health for you. A poor diet and a sedentary lifestyle are known to be **risk factors** for life-threatening **chronic** diseases such as **cardiovascular (heart) disease, hypertension, diabetes,** and some forms of **cancer** (Table 1-1). Together, these and related

TABLE 1-1 Glossary Terms to Aid Your Introduction to Nutrition*

Cancer	A condition characterized by uncontrolled growth of abnormal cells.
Cardiovascular (heart) disease	A general term that refers to any disease of the heart and circulatory system. This disease is generally characterized by the deposition of fatty material in the blood vessels (hardening of the arteries), which in turn can lead to organ damage and death. Also termed coronary heart disease (CHD), as the vessels of the heart are the primary sites of the disease.
Cholesterol	A waxy lipid found in all body cells; it has a structure containing multiple chemical rings. Cholesterol is found only in foods of animal origin.
Chronic	Long-standing, developing over time. When referring to disease, this term indicates that the disease process, once developed, is slow and lasting. A good example is cardiovascular disease.
Diabetes	A group of diseases characterized by high blood **glucose**. Type 1 diabetes involves insufficient or no release of the hormone insulin by the pancreas; requires daily insulin therapy. Type 2 diabetes results from either insufficient release of insulin or general inability of insulin to act on certain body cells, such as muscle cells. Persons with type 2 diabetes may or may not require insulin therapy.
Hypertension	A condition in which blood pressure remains persistently elevated. Obesity, inactivity, alcohol intake, excess salt intake, and genetics may each contribute to the problem.
Kilocalorie (kcal)	Unit that describes the energy content of food. Specifically, a kilocalorie (kcal) is the heat energy needed to raise the temperature of 1000 grams (1 liter) of water 1° Celsius. Kcal is also written as Calorie, with a capital C, signifying a 1000 calorie unit of measurement. The energy content of a food is commonly referred to as calories. It is a familiar term, so we will use it in this book.
Obesity	A condition characterized by excess body fat.
Osteoporosis	Decreased bone mass related to the effects of aging (including estrogen loss during menopause in women), genetic background, and poor diet.
Risk factor	A term used frequently when discussing the factors contributing to the development of a disease. A risk factor is an aspect of our lives—such as heredity, lifestyle choices (e.g., smoking), or nutritional habits.

*All bold terms in the book are defined in the glossary for this book. Many bold terms are also defined in the page margins within each chapter.

▲ The major health problems in North America are largely caused by a poor diet, excessive calorie intake, and not enough physical activity.

glucose A six-carbon sugar that exists in a ring form; found as such in blood, and in table sugar bound to fructose; also known as *dextrose,* it is one of the simple sugars.

▲ Many foods are rich sources of nutrients.

disorders account for two-thirds of all deaths in North America (Table 1-2). Not meeting nutrient needs in younger years makes us more likely to suffer health consequences, such as bone fractures from the disease **osteoporosis**, in later years. At the same time, taking too much of a nutrient—such as vitamin A supplement—can be harmful. Another dietary problem, drinking too much alcohol, is associated with many health problems.

U.S. government scientists have calculated that a poor diet combined with a lack of sufficient physical activity contributes to up to 350,000 fatal cases of cardiovascular disease, cancer, and diabetes each year among adults in the United States. Thus, the combination of poor diet and too little physical activity may be the second leading cause of death in the United States. In addition, **obesity** is considered the second leading cause of preventable death in North America (smoking is the first). Put together, obesity and smoking cause even more health problems. And as you will learn in Chapter 7, surgery to help treat obesity costs about $12,000 to $40,000. Compare that to the low cost of prevention. Obesity and chronic diseases are often preventable. Age fast or age slowly: It is partly your choice.

As you gain understanding about your nutritional habits and increase your knowledge about optimal nutrition, you will have the opportunity to dramatically reduce your risk for many common health problems. For additional help, the U.S. federal government provides two websites that contain links to many sites providing health and nutrition information (www.healthfinder.gov and www.nutrition.gov). Other useful sites are webmd.com and www.eatright.org.

stroke A decrease or loss in blood flow to the brain that results from a blood clot or other change in arteries in the brain. This in turn causes the death of brain tissue. Also called a *cerebrovascular accident.*

TABLE 1-2 Ten Leading Causes of Death in the United States

Rank	Cause of Death	Percent of Total Deaths
	All causes	100
1	Diseases of the heart (primarily coronary heart disease)*†#	29
2	Cancer*‡	23
3	Cerebrovascular diseases (stroke)*†‡#	7
4	Chronic obstructive pulmonary diseases and allied conditions (lung diseases)‡	5
5	Accidents and adverse effects† Motor vehicle accidents All other accidents and adverse effects	4 (2) (2)
6	Diabetes*	3
7	Influenza and pneumonia	3
8	Alzheimer's disease*	2
9	Kidney disease*‡	2
10	Blood-borne infections	1

From Centers for Disease Control and Prevention, *National Vital Statistics Report,* Final Data for 2001, September 18, 2003. Canadian statistics are quite similar.

*Causes of death in which diet plays a part

†Causes of death in which excessive alcohol consumption plays a part

‡Causes of death in which tobacco use plays a part

#Diseases of the heart and cerebrovascular disease are included in the more global term "cardiovascular disease."

CLASSES AND SOURCES OF NUTRIENTS

To begin the study of nutrition, let's start with an overview of the six classes of nutrients. You are probably already familiar with the terms **carbohydrates, lipids** (fats and oils), **proteins, vitamins,** and **minerals**. These, plus **water,** make up the six classes of nutrients found in food (Table 1-3).

Nutrients can then be assigned to three functional categories: (1) those that primarily provide us with calories to meet energy needs (expressed in **kilocalories [kcal]**); (2) those important for growth, development, and maintenance; and (3) those that act to keep body functions running smoothly. Some function overlap exists among these categories. The energy-yielding nutrients make up a major portion of most foods (Table 1-4).

Let's now look more closely at these six classes of nutrients.

Carbohydrates

Chemically, carbohydrates are composed mainly of the **elements** carbon, hydrogen, and oxygen. Carbohydrates provide a major source of calories for the body, on average 4 kcal per gram. Carbohydrates can exist as simple sugars and complex carbohydrates. **Simple sugars,** frequently referred to as *sugars,* are relatively small molecules. The smallest simple sugars consist of a single sugar unit and are called monosaccharides. The sugar in your blood, glucose (also known as *blood sugar* or *dextrose*), is an example of a monosaccharide. Other simple sugars are made by joining two **monosaccharides** to form a **disaccharide.** Table sugar, sucrose, is an example of a disaccharide because it is formed from fructose and glucose (both monosaccharides). Joining many monosaccharides—often found as repeating units—forms **polysaccharides,** also known as **complex carbohydrates.** For example, plants store carbohydrates in the form of **starch,** a polysaccharide made up of hundreds of repeating glucose units.

Aside from enjoying their taste, we need sugars and other carbohydrates in our diets primarily to help satisfy the calorie needs of our body cells. Glucose, a simple sugar that the body can derive from most carbohydrates, is a major source of calories for most cells. When not enough carbohydrate is consumed to supply suffcient glucose, the body is forced to make glucose from proteins—not a healthy change.

During digestion, complex carbohydrates are broken down into single sugar molecules (such as glucose), and absorbed via **cells** lining the small intestine into the bloodstream (see Chapter 3 for more on digestion and absorption). However, the **bonds** between the sugar molecules in certain complex carbohydrates, called **fiber,** cannot be broken down by human digestive processes. Fiber passes through the small intestine undigested to provide bulk for the stool (feces) formed in the large intestine (colon). Chapter 4 focuses on carbohydrates.

Lipids

Lipids (mostly fats and oils) are composed primarily of the elements carbon and hydrogen; they contain fewer oxygen atoms than do carbohydrates. Lipids yield more calories per gram than do carbohydrates—on the average, 9 kcal per gram—because of this difference in composition. Lipids dissolve in certain solvents (e.g., ether and benzene) but not in water.

The basic structure of most lipids is the **triglyceride.** Triglycerides provide a key calorie source (e.g., **fatty acids**) for the body and are the major form of fat in foods. They are also the main form for energy storage in the body. In this book, the more familiar terms *fats* or *fats and oils* will generally be used, rather than lipids or triglycerides. Generally, fats are lipids that are solid at room temperature and oils are lipids that are liquid at room temperature.

carbohydrate A compound containing carbon, hydrogen, and oxygen atoms. Most are known as *sugars, starches,* and *fibers.*

lipid A compound containing much carbon and hydrogen, little oxygen, and sometimes other atoms. Lipids dissolve in ether or benzene, but not in water, and include fats, oils, and cholesterol.

protein Food and body components made of amino acids; proteins contain carbon, hydrogen, oxygen, nitrogen, and sometimes other atoms, in a specific configuration. Proteins contain the form of nitrogen most easily used by the human body.

vitamin Compound needed in very small amounts in the diet to help regulate and support chemical reactions in the body.

mineral Element used in the body to promote chemical reactions and to form body structures.

water The universal solvent; chemically, H_2O. The body is composed of about 60% water. Water (fluid) needs are about 9 (women) or 13 (men) cups per day; needs are greater if one exercises heavily.

atom Smallest combining unit of an element, such as iron or calcium. Atoms consist of protons, neutrons, and electrons.

element A substance that cannot be separated into simpler substances by chemical processes. Common elements in nutrition include carbon, oxygen, hydrogen, nitrogen, calcium, phosphorus, and iron.

macronutrient A nutrient needed in gram quantities in a diet.

micronutrient A nutrient needed in milligram or microgram quantities in a diet.

cell The structural basis of plant and animal organization. In animals it is bounded by a cell membrane. Cells contain both genetic material and systems for synthesizing energy-yielding compounds. Cells have the ability to take up compounds from and excrete compounds into their surroundings.

bond A linkage between two atoms formed by the sharing of electrons, or attractions.

fiber Substances in plant foods not digested by the processes that take place in the human stomach or small intestine. These add bulk to feces. Fiber naturally found in foods is also called dietary fiber.

TABLE 1-3 Essential Nutrients in the Human Diet, Their Classes* and Good Dietary Sources

Class	Energy-Yielding Nutrients			Water	
	Carbohydrate	**Lipids†**	**Protein**		
Essential Nutrients	Glucose (or a carbohydrate that yields glucose)‡	Linoleic acid α-Linolenic acid	Amino acids		
Good Dietary Sources	Breads, starchy vegetables, dairy products, and fruits	Plant oils and animal fats	Meats, eggs, and beans	All beverages and fruits	

triglyceride The major form of lipid in the body and in food. It is composed of three fatty acids bonded to glycerol.

fatty acid Major part of most lipids; primarily composed of a chain of carbons flanked by hydrogen.

saturated fatty acid A fatty acid containing no carbon-carbon double bonds.

unsaturated fatty acid A fatty acid containing one or more carbon-carbon double bonds.

Most lipids can be separated into two basic types—saturated fat and unsaturated fat—based on the chemical structure of their fatty acids. Saturated fats are rich in **saturated fatty acids.** These fatty acids do not contain carbon-carbon double bonds. Unsaturated fats are rich in **unsaturated fatty acids.** These fatty acids contain one or more of carbon-carbon double bonds.

The presence of carbon-carbon double bonds determines whether the lipid is solid or liquid at room temperature. Think of a double bond as a "kink" somewhere along the carbon chain of a fatty acid. Having one or more kinks limits the extent to which fatty acids can pack tightly together, and therefore how solid a mass of fatty acids can be. Plant oils, such as corn oil, tend to contain many unsaturated fatty acids—this makes them liquid at room temperature. Animal fats, such as butter or lard, are often rich in saturated fatty acids—this makes them solid at room temperature. Almost all foods contain a variety of saturated and unsaturated fatty acids. Saturated fat should be limited in our diet because it can raise blood **cholesterol.** High blood cholesterol leads to clogged arteries and can eventually lead to cardiovascular disease (see Chapter 5).

Vita	mins	Min	erals
Water-soluble	**Fat-soluble**	**Major**	**Trace**
Thiamin	A	Calcium	Chromium
Riboflavin	D§	Chloride	Copper
Niacin	E	Magnesium	Fluoride‖
Pantothenic acid	K	Phosphorus	Iodide
Biotin		Potassium	Iron
B-6		Sodium	Manganese
B-12		Sulfur	Molybdenum
Folate			Selenium
C			Zinc

Green leafy vegetables and fruits

Dairy products, breakfast cereals, and oils

Fruits and dairy products

Fish and nuts

*This table includes nutrients for humans that are listed in the current *Dietary Reference Intakes* and related publications. Fiber could be added to the list of essential substances, but it is not a nutrient (see Chapter 4).

†The lipids listed are needed only in small amounts, about 5 to 10% of total calorie needs (see Chapter 5).

‡To prevent ketosis and thus the muscle loss that would occur if protein were used to synthesize carbohydrate (see Chapter 4).

§Sunshine on the skin also allows the body to make vitamin D for itself (see Chapter 10).

‖Primarily for dental health (see Chapter 10).

TABLE 1-4 Major Functions of the Various Classes of Nutrients

Nutrient Classes That Provide Energy	Nutrient Classes That Promote Growth, Development, and Maintenance	Nutrient Classes That Regulate Body Processes
Most carbohydrates	Proteins	Proteins
Proteins	Lipids	Some lipids
Most lipids	Some vitamins	Some vitamins
	Some minerals	Some minerals
	Water	Water

Carbohydrates, proteins, lipids, and water are needed in relatively large amounts, so they are called **macronutrients**. Vitamins and minerals are needed in such small amounts in the diet that they are called **micronutrients**.

▲ Butter is an animal fat made from milk fat and is high in saturated fat.

trans **fatty acids** A form of an unsaturated fatty acid, usually a monounsaturated one when found in food, in which the hydrogens on both carbons forming that double bond lie on opposite sides of that bond, rather than on the same side, as in most natural fats. Stick margarine, shortenings, and deep fat-fried foods in general are rich sources.

enzyme A compound that speeds the rate of a chemical reaction but is not altered by the reaction. Almost all enzymes are proteins (some are made of genetic material).

amino acid The building block for proteins containing a central carbon atom with nitrogen and other atoms attached.

chemical reaction An interaction between two chemicals that changes both chemicals.

MAKING DECISIONS

Trans Fat

Some foods contain **trans fatty acids**, also called *trans* fats. These fats are commonly found in processed foods, and especially deep-fried foods, such as doughnuts and French fries. Large amounts of *trans* fats in the diet pose certain health risks, so intake should be minimized (see Chapter 5 for details). All food labels in the United States and Canada have to list *trans* fat content. Do you still want to eat food rich in *trans* fat?

Certain unsaturated fatty acids are essential nutrients that must come from our diet. These key fatty acids that the body can't produce, called essential fatty acids, perform several important functions in the body: they help regulate blood pressure and play a role in the synthesis and repair of vital cell parts. However, we need only about four tablespoons of a common plant oil (such as the canola or soybean oil) each day to supply these essential fatty acids. A serving of fatty fish, such as salmon or tuna, at least twice a week is another healthy source of essential fatty acids. The unique fatty acids in these fish complement the healthy aspects of common vegetable oils. This will be explained in greater detail in Chapter 5, which focuses on lipids.

Proteins

Like carbohydrates and fats, proteins are composed of the elements carbon, oxygen, and hydrogen. But, unlike the other energy-yielding nutrients, all proteins also contain nitrogen. Proteins are the main structural material in the body. For example, proteins constitute a major part of bone and muscle; they are also important components in blood, body cells, **enzymes,** and immune factors. Proteins can also provide calories for the body—on average, 4 kcal per gram. Typically, however, the body uses little protein for the purpose of meeting daily calorie needs. Proteins are formed when **amino acids** are bonded together. Twenty or so common amino acids are found in food; nine of these are essential nutrients for adults, and one additional amino acid is essential for infants.

Most North Americans eat about one and a half to two times as much protein as the body needs to maintain health. In a person with no evidence of cardiovascular disease, kidney disease, diabetes, or family history of colon cancer or kidney stones, this amount of extra protein in the diet is generally not harmful—it reflects the standard of living and the dietary habits of most North Americans. The excess is used for calorie needs but ultimately can contribute to storage of fat and carbohydrate production. Chapter 6 focuses on proteins.

Vitamins

Vitamins have a variety of chemical structures and can contain the elements carbon, hydrogen, nitrogen, oxygen, phosphorus, sulfur, and others. The main function of vitamins is to enable many **chemical reactions** to occur in the body. Some of these reactions help release the energy trapped in carbohydrates, lipids, and proteins. Remember, however, that vitamins themselves provide no usable calories for the body.

The 13 vitamins are divided into two groups: four are **fat-soluble** in that they dissolve in fat (vitamins A, D, E, and K); nine are **water-soluble** in that they dissolve in water (vitamin C and the B vitamins). The two groups of vitamins often act differently. For example, cooking destroys water-soluble vitamins much more readily than it does fat-soluble vitamins. Water-soluble vitamins are also excreted from the body much more readily than are fat-soluble vitamins. Thus, the fat-soluble vitamins, especially vitamin A, are much more likely to accumulate in excessive amounts in the body, which then can lead to toxicity. Vitamins are the focus of Chapter 8.

Minerals

Minerals are structurally simple, **inorganic** substances, which exist as groups of one or more of the same atoms. All of the nutrients discussed so far are **organic** compounds. These terms, *inorganic* and *organic,* have nothing to do with agriculture but are based on simple chemistry concepts (see Chapter 2 for use of the term organic on food labels). Inorganic substances for the most part do not contain carbon atoms.

Minerals such as sodium and potassium typically function independently in the body, whereas minerals such as calcium and phosphorus function as parts of simple mineral combinations, such as bone mineral. Because of their simple structure, minerals are not destroyed during cooking, but they can still be lost if they dissolve in the water used for cooking and that water is then discarded. Minerals are critical players in nervous system functioning, other cellular processes, water balance, and structural (e.g., skeletal) systems, but yield no calories as such for the body.

The amounts of the 16 or more essential minerals required in the diet for good health vary enormously. Thus, they are divided into two groups: **major minerals** and **trace minerals,** based on dietary needs. If daily needs are less than 100 milligrams, the mineral is classified as a trace mineral, otherwise, it is a major mineral. The dietary requirement for some trace minerals has yet to be determined. Minerals that conduct electricity when dissolved in water are also called **electrolytes;** these include sodium, potassium, and chloride. Minerals are the focus of Chapter 8.

Water

Water makes up the sixth class of nutrients. Although sometimes overlooked as a nutrient, water (chemically, H_2O) has numerous vital functions in the body. It acts as a **solvent** and lubricant, as a vehicle for transporting nutrients and waste, and as a medium for temperature regulation and chemical processes. For these reasons, and because the human body is approximately 60% water, the average man should consume about 3 liters—equivalent to 3000 grams or about 13 cups—of water and/or other fluids containing water every day. Women need closer to 2200 grams or about 9 cups per day.

Water is not only available from the obvious sources, but it is also the major component in some foods, such as many fruits and vegetables (e.g., lettuce, grapes, and melons). The body even makes some water as a by-product of **metabolism.** Water is examined in detail in Chapter 8.

Other Important Components in Food

Another group of compounds in foods, especially within the fruit and vegetable groups, is what scientists call **phytochemicals.** These plant components are not considered essential nutrients in the diet. Still, many of these substances provide significant health benifits. Considerable research attention is focused on various phytochemicals in reducing the risk for certain diseases (e.g., cancer). You can't just buy a bottle of phytochemicals—they are generally available only within whole foods. Table 1-5 lists some noteworthy phytochemicals with their common food sources. Tips for boosting the phytochemical content of your diet will be discussed in Chapter 2.

inorganic Any substance lacking carbon atoms bonded to hydrogen atoms in the chemical structure.

organic Any substance that contains carbon atoms bonded to hydrogen atoms in the chemical structure.

electrolytes Substances that separate into ions in water and, in turn, are able to conduct an electrical current. These include sodium, chloride, and potassium.

solvent A liquid substance in which other substances dissolve.

metabolism Chemical processes in the body by which energy is provided in useful forms and vital activities are sustained.

phytochemical A chemical found in plants. Some phytochemicals may contribute to a reduced risk of cancer or cardiovascular disease in people who consume them regularly.

▲ Fruits, vegetables, beans, and whole-grain breads and cereals are typically rich in phytochemicals.

TABLE 1-5 Food Sources of Some Phytochemical Compounds Under Study

Phytochemical	Food Sources
Allyl sulfides/organosulfurs	Garlic, onions, leeks
Saponins	Garlic, onions, licorice, legumes
Carotenoids (e.g., lycopene)	Orange, red, yellow fruits and vegetables (egg yolks are a source as well)
Monoterpenes	Oranges, lemons, grapefruit
Capsaicin	Chili peppers
Lignans	Flaxseed, berries, whole grains
Indoles	Cruciferous vegetables (broccoli, cabbage, kale)
Isothiocyanates	Cruciferous vegetables, especially broccoli
Phytosterols	Soybeans, other legumes, cucumbers, other fruits and vegetables
Flavonoids	Citrus fruit, onions, apples, grapes, red wine, tea, chocolate, tomatoes
Isoflavones	Soybeans, other legumes
Catechins	Tea
Ellagic acid	Strawberries, raspberries, grapes, apples, bananas, nuts
Anthocyanosides	Red, blue, and purple plants (blueberries, eggplant)
Fructooligosaccharides	Onions, bananas, oranges (small amounts)
Resveratrol	Grapes, peanuts, red wine

Some related compounds under study are found in animal products, such as sphingolipids (meat and dairy products) and conjugated linoleic acid (meat and cheese). These are not phytochemicals per se because they are not from plant sources, but they have been shown to have health benefits.

NUTRIENT COMPOSITION OF DIETS AND THE HUMAN BODY

The quantities of the various nutrients that people consume vary widely, and the nutrient amounts present in different foods also vary a great deal. On a daily basis we consume about 500 grams, or about 1 pound, of protein, fat, and carbohydrate. In contrast, the typical daily mineral intake totals about 20 grams (about 4 teaspoons), and the daily vitamin intake totals less than 300 milligrams (1/15 of a teaspoon). Although we require a gram or so of some minerals, such as calcium and phosphorus, we need only a few milligrams or less of other minerals each day. For example, we need about 10 milligrams of zinc per day, just a few specks of the mineral.

Figure 1-1 contrasts the relative proportions of all the major classes of nutrients in a lean man and a lean woman with the proportions of these nutrients in both a cooked steak and a baked potato. Note how the nutrient composition of the human body differs from the nutritional profiles of the foods we eat. This is because growth, development, and later maintenance of the human body are directed by the genetic

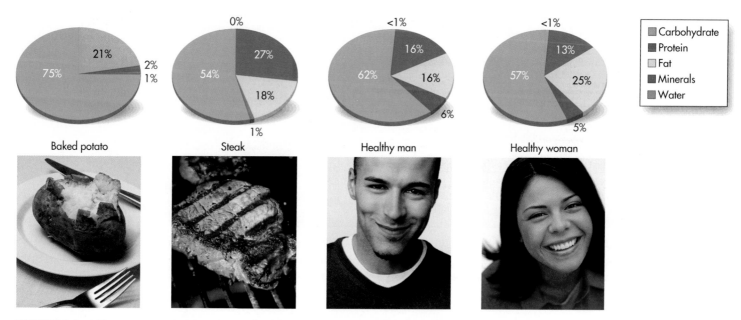

FIGURE 1-1 ▶ The approximate proportions of nutrients in the human body compared to those found in typical foods—animal or vegetable. The amount of vitamins found in the body is negligible, and so is not shown.

material (DNA) inside body cells. This genetic blueprint determines how each cell uses the essential nutrients to perform body functions. These nutrients can come from a variety of sources. Cells are not concerned about whether available amino acids come from animal or plant sources. The carbohydrate glucose can come from sugars or starches. Thus, you really aren't what you eat. Rather, the food that you eat provides cells with basic materials to function according to the directions supplied by the genetic material (**genes**) housed in body cells. Genetics and nutrition will be discussed in Chapter 3.

ENERGY SOURCES AND USES

Humans obtain the energy we need for body functions and to do work from various calorie sources: carbohydrates, fats, and proteins. Foods generally provide more than one calorie source. Plant oils are one exception; these are 100% fat.

Alcohol is also a source of calories for some of us, supplying about 7 kcal per gram. It is not considered an essential nutrient, however, because it has no required function. Still, alcoholic beverages, such as beer—also rich in carbohydrate—are a contributor of calories to the diet of many adults.

The body releases the energy from the chemical bonds in carbohydrate, protein, and fat (and alcohol) into other forms of energy in order to:

- Build new **compounds.**
- Perform muscular movements.
- Promote nerve transmissions.
- Maintain **ion** balance within cells.

Chapters 7 and 12 describe how that energy is released from the chemical bonds in energy-yielding nutrients and then used by body cells to support the processes just described.

You have likely noticed on food labels that the energy in food is often expressed in terms of calories. As defined earlier, a calorie is the amount of heat energy it takes to raise the temperature of 1 gram of water 1 degree Celsius (1°C, centigrade

genes A specific segment on a chromosome. Genes provide the blueprints for the production of all body proteins.

alcohol Ethyl alcohol or ethanol (CH_3CH_2OH) is the compound in alcoholic beverages.

compound A group of different types of atoms bonded together in definite proportion.

ion An atom with an unequal number of electrons and protons. Negative ions have more electrons than protons; positive ions have more protons than electrons.

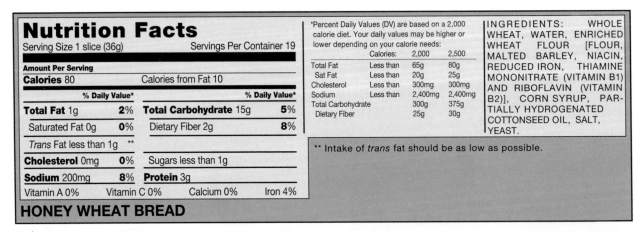

FIGURE 1-2 ▶ Use the nutrient values on the Nutrition Facts label to calculate calorie content of a food. Based on carbohydrate, fat, and protein content, a serving of this food (Honey Wheat Bread) contains 81 kcal ([15 × 4] + [1 × 9] + [3 × 4] = 81). The label lists 80, suggesting that the calorie value was rounded down.

scale). (Chapter 7 has a diagram of the instrument that can be used to measure calories in foods [bomb calorimeter].) A calorie is a tiny measure of heat, so food energy is more conveniently expressed in terms of the kilocalorie (kcal), which equals 1000 calories. (If the "c" in calories is capitalized, this also signifies kilocalories.) A kcal is the amount of heat energy it takes to raise the temperature of 1000 grams (1 liter) of water 1°C. The abbreviation *kcal* is used throughout this book. On food labels, the word *calorie* (without a capital "C") is also used loosely to mean *kilocalorie.* Any values given on food labels in calories are actually in kilocalories (Fig. 1-2). A suggested intake of 2000 calories per day on a food label is technically 2000 kcal.

HELPFUL MATH TOOLS FOR NUTRITION

You will use a few mathematical concepts in studying nutrition. Besides performing addition, subtraction, multiplication, and division, you need to know how to calculate percentages and convert English units of measurement to metric units.

PERCENTAGES

The term percent (%) refers to a part of the total when the total represents 100 parts. For example, if you earn 80% on your first nutrition examination, you will have answered the equivalent of 80 out of 100 questions correctly. This equivalent could be 8 correct answers out of 10; 80% also describes 16 of 20 (16/20 = 0.80 or 80%). The decimal form of percents is based on 100% being equal to 1.00. It is difficult to succeed in a nutrition course unless you know what a percentage means and how to calculate one. Percentages are used frequently when referring to menus and nutrient composition. The best way to master this concept is to calculate some percentages. Some examples follow:

Question	Answer
What is 6% of 45?	6% = 0.06 or 0.06 × 45 = 2.7
What percent of 99 is 3?	3/99 = 0.03 or 3% (0.03 × 100)

Joe ate 15% of the adult Recommended Dietary Allowance (RDA) for iron at lunch. How many milligrams did he eat? (RDA = 8 milligrams)

$$0.15 \times 8 \text{ milligrams} = 1.2 \text{ milligrams}$$

THE METRIC SYSTEM

The basic units of the metric system are the meter, which indicates length; the gram, which indicates weight; and the liter, which indicates volume. Appendix I in this textbook lists conversions from the metric system to the English system (pounds, feet, cups) and vice versa. Here is a brief summary:

A gram (g) is about 1/30 of an ounce (28 grams to the ounce).
5 grams of sugar or salt is about 1 teaspoon.
A pound (lb) weighs 454 grams.
A kilogram (kg) is 1000 grams, equivalent to 2.2 pounds.
To convert your weight to kilograms, divide it by 2.2.
A 154-pound man weighs 70 kilograms (154/2.2 = 70).
A gram can be divided into 1000 milligrams (mg) or 1,000,000 micrograms (µg or mcg).
   10 milligrams of zinc (approximately adult needs) would be a few grains of zinc.
Liters are divided into 1000 units called milliliters (ml).
One teaspoon equals about 5 milliliters (ml), 1 cup is about 240 milliliters, and 1 quart
   (4 cups) equals almost 1 liter (L) (0.946 liter to be exact).

If you plan to work in any scientific field, you will need to learn the metric system. *For now, remember that a kilogram equals 2.2 pounds, an ounce weighs 28 grams, 2.54 centimeters equals 1 inch, and a liter is almost the same as a quart.* In addition, know the fractions that the following prefixes represent: micro (1/1,000,000), milli (1/1000), centi (1/100), and kilo (1000) represent.

Carbohydrate
4 kcal per gram

Protein
4 kcal per gram

Fat
9 kcal per gram

Alcohol
7 kcal per gram

MAKING DECISIONS

Calculating Calories

Use the 4-9-4 estimates for the calorie content of carbohydrate, fat, and protein introduced over the last few pages to determine calorie content of a food. Consider a typical deluxe hamburger sandwich:

Carbohydrate	39 grams × 4 = 156 kcal
Fat	32 grams × 9 = 288 kcal
Protein	30 grams × 4 = <u>120 kcal</u>
Total	564 kcal

You can also use the 4-9-4 estimates to determine what portion of total calorie intake is contributed by the various calorie-yielding nutrients. Assume that one day you consume 290 grams of carbohydrates, 60 grams of fat, and 70 grams of protein. This consumption yields a total of 1980 kcal ([290 × 4] + [60 × 9] + [70 × 4] 5 = 1980). The percentage of your total calorie intake derived from each nutrient can then be determined:

% of kcal as carbohydrate = (290 × 4) ÷ 1980 = 0.59 (× 100 = 59 %)

% of kcal as fat = (60 × 9) ÷ 1980 = 0.27 (× 100 = 27%)

% of kcal as protein = (70 × 4) ÷ 1980 = 0.14 (× 100 = 14%)

Check your calculations by adding the percentages together. Do they total 100?

▲ You can use the steps outlined in the "Making Decisions" section to calculate the total calories, and calories from carbohydrate, fat, and protein in a deluxe hamburger.

CONCEPT CHECK

Nutrition is the study of food and nutrients—their digestion, absorption, and metabolism, and their effect on health and disease. Food contains the vital nutrients essential for good health: carbohydrates, lipids (fats and oils), proteins, vitamins, minerals, and water. Nutrients have three general functions in the body: (1) to provide materials for building and maintaining the body; (2) to act as regulators for key metabolic reactions; and (3) to participate in metabolic reactions that provide the energy necessary to sustain life. A common unit of measurement for this energy is the kilocalorie (kcal). On average, carbohydrates and protein provide 4 kcal per gram of energy to the body, while lipids provide 9 kcal per gram. Although not considered a nutrient, alcohol provides about 7 kcal per gram. The other classes of nutrients do not supply calories but are essential for proper body functioning.

CURRENT STATE OF THE NORTH AMERICAN DIET AND OVERALL HEALTH

▶ The Food and Nutrition Board of the National Academy of Sciences also suggests minimizing saturated fat, *trans* fat, and cholesterol intake when putting their diet guidelines into place (see Chapter 5).

The Food and Nutrition Board (FNB) of the National Academy of Sciences advocates that 10% to 35% of calories come from protein, 45% to 65% from carbohydrate, and 20% to 35% from fat. (These standards apply to both people in the United States and Canada.) If we ignore alcohol, North American adults consume about 16% of their calorie intake as proteins, 50% as carbohydrates, and 33% as fats. These percentages are estimates and vary slightly from year to year and from person to person and fall within the FNB recommendations.

Animal sources supply about two-thirds of protein intake for most North Americans; plant sources supply only about one-third. In many other parts of the world, it is just the opposite: plant proteins—from rice, beans, corn, and other vegetables—dominate protein intake. About half the carbohydrate in North American diets comes from simple sugars; the other half comes from starches (such as in pastas, breads, and potatoes). About 60% of dietary fat comes from animal sources and 40% from plant sources.

Assessing the Current North American Diet

With the aim of finding out what and when North Americans eat, federal agencies conduct surveys to collect data about food and nutrient consumption, as well as connections between diet and health. In the United States, the U.S. Department of Health and Human Services monitors food consumption with the National Health and Nutrition Examination Survey (NHANES). In Canada, this information is gathered by Health Canada in conjunction with Agriculture and Agrifood Canada.

Results from national nutrition surveys and other studies show that North Americans consume a wide variety of foods, but often do not choose the right balance of foods to meet their nutrient needs. Chapter 2 will look at this situation in more detail. For now, more attention should be focused on foods rich in iron, calcium, potassium, magnesium, various B vitamins, vitamin C (especially smokers), vitamin D, vitamin E, and fiber. Daily intake of a balanced multivitamin and mineral supplement is one strategy to help meet nutrient needs, but does not make up for a poor diet, particularly for calcium, potassium, and fiber intake. Also keep in mind that taking numerous dietary supplements can lead to health problems (see Chapter 9).

▲ Taking numerous nutrient supplements can lead to health problems. Chapter 9 will explore the appropriate and safe use of nutrient supplements in detail.

Routinely, experts also recommend that we pay more attention to balancing calorie intake with needs. An excess intake of calories is usually tied to overindulgence in sugar, fat, and alcoholic beverages. African-Americans and Hispanics have a greater chance of developing hypertension than do other ethnic groups in North America and therefore may need to decrease the amount of **salt** (sodium chloride) and alcohol in their diets. These substances are two of the many factors linked to hypertension. Moderation of salt and alcohol intake—along with saturated fat, *trans* fat, cholesterol, and total calorie intake—is a recommended practice for all adults.

Many North Americans would benefit from a healthier balance of food in their diets. Moderation is the key for some foods, such as sugared soft drinks and fried foods. For other foods, such as fruits and vegetables, increased quantity and variety is warranted. Few adults currently meet the "5 to 9 a-day" recommendation promoted for total servings of vegetables and fruits.

Health Objectives for the United States for the Year 2010 Include Numerous Nutrition Objectives

Health promotion and disease prevention have been public health strategies in North America since the late 1970s. One part of this strategy is *Healthy People 2010,* a report issued in 2000 by the U.S. Department of Health and Human Services' Public Health Service. This report outlines health promotion and disease prevention objectives for the nation for the year 2010 and assigns each of the objectives to appropriate U.S. federal agencies to address. Many nutrition-related objectives are part of the overall plan (Table 1-6). The overarching goals of *Healthy People 2010* are to increase quality and years of healthy life and to eliminate health disparities. The following Internet site provides more details on the *Healthy People* program: www.healthypeople.gov.

Another way to promote your health and prevent chronic diseases in the future is to observe the recommendations listed in Table 1-7. In total, these contribute to maximal health and prevention of disease.

▲ Moderation in the intake of some foods, such as sugared soft drinks and fried foods, can lead to a healthier balance of food in the North American diet.

TABLE 1-6 A Sample of Nutrition-Related Objectives from *Healthy People 2010*

	Target	Current Estimate
Increase the proportion of adults at a healthy weight.	60%	42%
Reduce the proportion of overweight or obese children and adolescents.	5%	11%
Increase the proportion of persons age 2 years and older who consume:		
• At least 2 daily servings of fruit.	75%	28%
• At least 3 daily servings of vegetables, with at least one-third being dark green or deep yellow vegetables.	50%	3%
• At least 6 daily servings of grain products, with at least 3 being whole grains (e.g., whole wheat bread and oatmeal).	50%	7%
• Less than 10% of calories from saturated fat.	75%	36%
• Six grams or less of salt (2400 milligrams or less of sodium) daily.	65%	21%
• Enough calcium (see DRI table for elements on inside cover of this book).	74%	45%
Reduce iron deficiency among females of childbearing age.	7%	11%

Note: In later chapters, we will explore additional nutrition-related objectives, such as those addressing osteoporosis, various forms of cancer, diabetes prevention and treatment, food allergies, cardiovascular disease, low birth weight, nutrition during pregnancy, breastfeeding, eating disorders, physical activity, and alcohol use.

▲ Many nutrition-related objectives are part of the *Healthy People 2010* report. The report outlines health promotion and disease prevention objectives for the United States for the year 2010.

TABLE 1-7 Recommendations for Health Promotion and Disease Prevention: What Can Adults Expect from Adequate Nutrition and Good Health Habits?

Diet

Consuming enough essential nutrients, including fiber, while moderating energy, saturated fat, trans fat, cholesterol, and alcohol intake can result in:

- Reduced risk for deficiency diseases, such as cretinism (lack of iodide), scurvy (lack of vitamin C), and anemia (lack of iron, folate, or other nutrients)
- Increased bone mass during childhood and adolescence
- Prevention of some adult bone loss and osteoporosis, especially in older adults
- Fewer dental caries
- Prevention of digestive problems, such as constipation
- Decreased susceptibility to some cancers
- Decreased degradation of the retina (intake of green and orange vegetables in particular)
- Lower risk of obesity and related diseases, such as type 2 diabetes and cardiovascular disease

Physical Activity

Adequate, regular physical activity (at least 30 minutes on most or all days) helps reduce the risk of:

- Obesity
- Type 2 diabetes
- Cardiovascular disease
- Some adult bone loss and loss of muscle tone
- Premature aging
- Certain cancers

Lifestyle

Minimizing alcohol intake (no more than two drinks per day for men and one drink for both women and all adults age 65 years and older) helps prevent:

- Liver disease
- Accidents

Not smoking cigarettes or cigars helps prevent:

- Lung cancer, other lung disease, kidney disease, cardiovascular disease, and degenerative eye diseases

In addition, minimum use of medication, no illicit drug use, adequate sleep (7–8 hours), adequate water and related fluid intake (9–13 cups per day), and a reduction in stress (practice better time management, relax, listen to music, have a massage, and stay physically active) provide a more complete approach to good nutrition and health. Add to this maintaining close relationships with others and a positive outlook on life. Finally, consultation with health-care professionals on a regular basis is important. This is because early diagnosis is especially useful for controlling the damaging effects of many diseases. Prevention of disease is an important investment of one's time, including during the college years.

▲ Regular physical activity complements a healthy diet. Whether it's all at once or in segments throughout the day, ideally incorporate 30 to 60 minutes or more of such activity into your daily routine.

IMPROVING OUR DIETS

Greater efforts are needed by the general public to lower intake of saturated fat, *trans* fat, and cholesterol intake and to improve variety in our diets. However, our cultural diversity, varied cuisines, and generally high nutritional status should be points of pride for North Americans. Today we can choose from a tremendous variety of food products, the result of continual innovation by food manufacturers.

We are eating more breakfast cereals, pizza, pasta entrees, stir-fried meats and vegetables served on rice, salads, tacos, burritos, and fajitas than ever before. Sales of whole milk are down, while in the same period sales of fat-free and 1% low-fat milk have increased. Consumption of frozen vegetables, rather than canned vegetables, is also on the rise.

A dietary objective that deserves more attention is to try to eat with others more often. Mealtime is a key social time of the day. The Japanese are ahead of us in recognizing that food's powers go beyond the realm of nutrition. Their national dietary guidelines stress the importance of eating a variety of foods, maintaining healthy weight, and moderating fat in the diet, but also advise people to make all activities pertaining to food and eating pleasurable.

▲ A healthy diet benefits people of all ages.

Today, North Americans live longer than ever and enjoy better general health. Many also have more money and more diverse food and lifestyle choices to consider. The nutritional consequences of these trends are not fully known. Deaths from various forms of cardiovascular disease, for example, have dropped dramatically since the late 1960s, partly because of better medical care and diets. Still, if affluence leads to sedentary lifestyles and high intakes of saturated fat, *trans* fat, cholesterol, salt, and alcohol, this lifestyle pattern can lead to problems such as cardiovascular disease, hypertension, and obesity. With better technology and greater choices, we can have a much better diet today than ever before—if we know what choices to make.

The goal of this book is to help you find the best path to good nutrition. Nutrition experts generally agree that there are no "good" or "bad" (i.e., "junk") foods, but some foods provide relatively few nutrients in comparison to calorie content. One's total diet is the proper focus in a nutritional evaluation. Chapter 2 will emphasize this point and show you how to balance your diet. As you reexamine your nutritional habits, remember your health is largely your responsibility. Your body has a natural ability to heal itself. Offer it what it needs, and it will serve you well. Confusing and conflicting health messages hinder diet change. Nutrition science does not have all the answers, but as you will see, enough is known to help you (1) set a path to good health and (2) put diet-related recommendations you hear in the future into perspective.

CONCEPT CHECK

Surveys in the United States and Canada show that we generally have a variety of foods available to us. However, some of us could improve our diets by focusing on rich food sources of various vitamins, minerals, and fiber. In addition, many of us should reduce our consumption of calories, sugar, protein, saturated fat, *trans* fat, cholesterol, salt, and alcoholic beverages. These recommendations are consistent with an overall goal to attain and maintain good health.

WHY AM I SO HUNGRY?

Understanding what drives us to eat and what affects food choice will help you understand the complexity of factors that influence eating, especially the effects of ethnicity and societal change. You can then see why foods may have different meanings to different people. In turn, this allows for greater appreciation of food habits that differ from yours.

Two drives, **hunger** and **appetite,** influence our desire to eat. These differ dramatically. Hunger, our primarily physical biological drive to eat, is controlled by internal body mechanisms. For example, as nutrients are processed by the stomach and small intestine, these organs send signals to the liver and brain to reduce further food intake.

hunger The primarily physiological (internal) drive to find and eat food, mostly regulated by innate cues to eating.

appetite The primarily psychological (external) influences that encourage us to find and eat food, often in the absence of obvious hunger.

satiety State in which there is no longer a desire to eat; a feeling of satisfaction.

hypothalamus A region at the base of the brain that contains cells that play a role in the regulation of hunger, respiration, body temperature, and other body functions.

Appetite, our primarily psychological drive to eat, is affected by external food choice mechanisms, such as seeing a tempting dessert or smelling popcorn popping at the movie theater. Fulfilling either or both drives by eating sufficient food normally brings a state of satiety, temporarily halting our desire to continue eating.

The Hypothalamus Contributes to Satiety

The hypothalamus, a region of the brain, helps regulate satiety (Fig. 1-3). Imagine a game of tug-of-war in the brain: two sites in the hypothalamus—the *feeding center* and the *satiety center*—work in opposite ways to promote adequate availability of nutrients at all times. When stimulated, cells in the feeding center of the hypothalamus signal us to eat. As we eat, cells in the satiety center are stimulated, and we stop eating.

What stimulates these two centers of the hypothalamus? The amounts of macronutrients in the blood probably stimulate both the satiety and feeding centers. For example, when we haven't eaten for a while, stimulation of the feeding center signals us to eat. When the macronutrient content in the blood rises after a meal, we no longer have a strong desire to seek food. (Exactly how the two are interrelated is under study.) Certain chemicals, surgery, and some cancers can destroy either center in the hypothalamus. Without satiety center activity, laboratory animals (and humans) eat their way to obesity. Without feeding center activity, the opposite happens and weight is lost.

Admittedly, this concept of a tug-of-war between the feeding and satiety centers is an oversimplification of a complex process. Overall, the entire system depends on the hypothalamus to process the signals generated by nerves throughout the body and influenced in various ways by recent food intake. In reality, the hypothalamus has numerous sites crisscrossed with a network of nerves constantly receiving and passing on information about the body's nutritional state. In addition, the brain's cortex controls conscious thought and can overcome signals from the hypothalamic hunger and satiety centers.

(a)

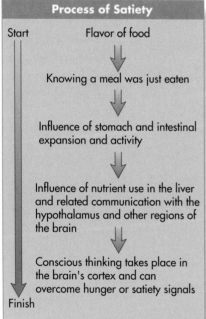

(b)

FIGURE 1-3 ▶ The hypothalamus and satiety. (a) The hypothalamus is one important region in the brain that influences whether we eat or not. (b) The process of satiety starts with eating food and concludes with actions in the hypothalamus and other regions in the brain, such as the cortex.

Meal Size and Composition Affect Satiety

The effects of stomach expansion from food intake combined with the later intestinal absorption of nutrients during a meal likely reduce our desire to eat more food. These actions of the gastrointestinal (GI) tract contribute to a feeling of satiety. In fact, a meal generally ends before significant amounts of nutrients are made available for metabolism and storage. Putting this information into practice, researchers have recently shown that bulky meals (high in fiber and water) produce much more satiety than do more concentrated meals. As the fiber and water content of the foods increase, humans experience increased satiety and thus do not seek another meal as quickly. Consider how satisfied you would feel if you ate five pieces of whole fruit versus a small serving of French fries (each yielding about 380 kcals).

Hormones Affect Satiety

Hormones and hormone-like compounds in our body influence whether we eat. Hormones that increase hunger include endorphins, ghrelin, and neuropeptide Y. Those that cause satiety include leptin (working in conjunction with the hormone insulin), serotonin, and cholecystokinin (CCK). New research has shown how leptin, discovered in 1995, and ghrelin, discovered in 1999, work together to balance our hunger and satiety. Leptin is made by the fat cells, also known as adipose tissue, travels to the brain and stimulates the satiety center and turns off the hunger center. Ghrelin is made by the stomach and travels to the brain where it stimulates the hunger center and turns off the satiety center. High leptin levels also turn off the production of ghrelin. Problems arise when leptin levels are high over a long period, such as in obesity, making the satiety center insensitive to leptin. To add to the confusion, low ghrelin levels make the hunger center sensitive to ghrelin. This situation helps explain why high leptin levels in obese individuals do not decrease hunger. As you can imagine, these hormones and their mechanisms are potential targets for new weight loss drugs.

Does Appetite Affect What We Eat?

Various feeding and satiety messages from body cells do not single-handedly determine what we eat. Almost everyone has encountered a mouthwatering dessert and devoured it, even on a full stomach. Appetite can be affected by a wide variety of external forces, such as environmental and psychological factors as well as social customs (Figure 1-4).

We often eat because food confronts us. It smells good, tastes good, and looks good. We might eat because it is the right time of day, we are celebrating, or we are seeking emotional comfort to overcome the blues. After a meal, memories of pleasant tastes and feelings reinforce appetite. If stress or depression sends you to the refrigerator, you are mostly seeking comfort, not food calories. Appetite may not be a biological process, but it does influence food intake. Table 1-8 lists additional social and other related factors that influence food choices.

MAKING DECISIONS

Satiety

Satiety associated with consuming a meal may actually reside primarily in our psychological frame of mind. We become accustomed to a certain amount of food at a meal. Providing less than that amount leaves us wanting more. One way to put this observation into practice for weight-control purposes is to train your eye to expect less food by slowly decreasing serving sizes to more appropriate amounts (see Figure 2-5 in Chapter 2 for some examples). Your appetites then readjust as you expect less food.

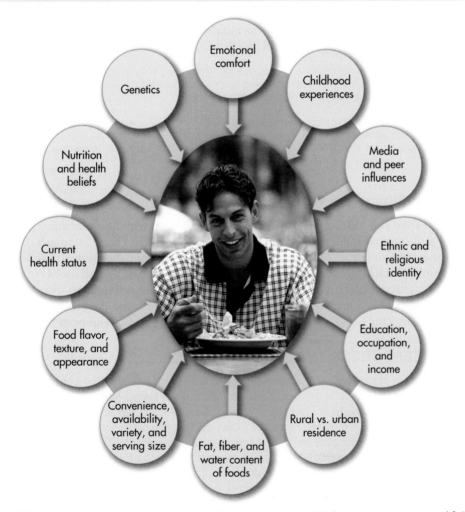

FIGURE 1-4 ▶ Food behavior is influenced by many sources. Which are important in your life?

gastrointestinal (GI) tract The main sites in the body used for digestion and absorption of nutrients. It consists of the mouth, esophagus, stomach, small intestine, large intestine, rectum, and anus. Also called the digestive tract.

hormone A compound secreted into the bloodstream by one type of cell that acts to control the function of another type of cell. For example, certain cells in the pancreas produce insulin, which in turn acts on muscle and other types of cells to promote uptake of nutrients from the blood.

endorphins Natural body tranquilizers that may be involved in the feeding response.

ghrelin A hormone made by the stomach that increases the desire to eat.

neuropeptide Y A chemical substance made in the hypothalamus that stimulates food intake. The hormone leptin inhibits neuropeptide Y production.

leptin A hormone made by **adipose tissue** in proportion to total fat stores in the body that influences long-term regulation of fat mass. Leptin also influences reproductive functions, as well as other body processes, such as release of the hormone insulin.

adipose tissue A group of fat storing cells.

serotonin A neurotransmitter synthesized from the amino acid tryptophan that affects mood (sense of calmness), behavior, and appetite, and induces sleep.

cholecystokinin (CCK) A hormone that participates in enzyme release from the pancreas, bile release from the gallbladder, and hunger regulation.

▲ A market research firm surveyed the eating habits of people in 2000 United States households. The top meal choice was pizza, followed by ham sandwich, hot dog, peanut butter and jelly sandwich, steak, macaroni and cheese, turkey sandwich, cheese sandwich, hamburger on a bun, and spaghetti.

CRITICAL THINKING

Sarah is majoring in nutrition and is well aware of the importance of a healthy diet. She has recently been analyzing her diet and is confused. She notices that she eats a great deal of high-fat foods and few fruits, vegetables, and whole grains. She also has developed a "sweet tooth." What three factors may be influencing Sarah's food choices? What advice would you give her on how to have her diet match her needs?

TABLE 1-8 What Else Influences Our Food Choices?

Food means so much more to us than nourishment—it reflects much of what we think about ourselves. In the course of our lives, we spend the equivalent of 13 to 15 years eating. Beyond simple hunger and emotions, why do we choose what we eat?

- **Flavor, texture, and appearance** are the most important factors determining our food choices. Creating more flavorful foods that are both healthy and profitable is a major focus of the food industry (referred to as "better for you" products).
- **Early influences** that expose us to various people, places, and events have a continuing impact on our food choices. Many ethnic diet patterns begin as we are introduced to foods during childhood.
- **Routines and habits** are tied to some food choices. Food habits, food availability, and convenience strongly influence choices. Most of us eat from a core group of foods: About 100 basic items account for 75% of an individual's total food intake.
- **Nutrition**, or what we think of as "healthy foods," directs our food purchases. North Americans who tend to make health-related food choices are often well-educated, middle-class professionals. These same people are generally health-oriented, have active lifestyles, and focus on weight control.
- **Advertising** is a major media tool for capturing the food interest of the consumer. The food industry in the United States spends well over $33 billion on advertising. Some of this advertising is helpful, as it promotes the importance of food components such as calcium and fiber in our diets. However, the food industry also advertises highly sweetened cereals, cookies, cakes, and soft drinks because they bring in the greatest profits.
- **Restaurants** have long been a growing industry in North America. Today, about 45% of food dollars is spent on meals outside the home. Restaurant food is often calorie-dense and of poorer nutritional quality compared to foods made at home. However, in response to consumer demands, restaurants have placed healthier items on their menus and many are listing nutritional content on their menus.
- **Social changes** are leading to a general time shortage for many of us. This creates the need for convenience. Supermarkets now supply prepared meals, microwavable entrees, and various quick-prep frozen products.
- **Economics** play a minor role in our food choices. The average North American spends only about 12% of after-tax income on food (greater for low-income people). However, as income increases, so do meals eaten away from home.

Overall, daily food intake is a complicated mix of biological and social influences. The first Rate Your Plate activity in Chapter 1 asks you to keep track of what influences your food intake on a daily basis. This assessment is an important part of developing a plan to improve your diet as necessary. How do you compare to the typical North American?

Putting Hunger and Appetite into Perspective

The next time you pick up a candy bar or ask for second helpings, remember the internal and external influences on eating behavior. Body cells (brain, stomach, small intestine, liver, and other organs), macronutrients in the blood, hormones (like leptin and ghrelin), brain chemicals (like serotonin and neuropeptide Y), and social customs all influence food intake. When food is abundant, appetite—not hunger—most likely triggers eating. Keep track of what triggers your eating for a few days. Is it primarily hunger or appetite? Also, satiety regulation is not perfect; body weight can fluctuate.

CONCEPT CHECK

Hunger is the primarily physical or internal desire to find and eat food. Fulfilling it creates satiety—no further desire to eat exists. Satiety is influenced by hunger-related (internal) signals from the brain, gastrointestinal tract, liver, and other organs, as well as fiber and water content of the foods in the meal. Various hormones and hormone-like compounds participate. Food intake is also affected by appetite-related (external) forces like social customs, time of day, flavor, appearance, texture, and being with others. Factors such as health concerns, economics, convenience, seeking emotional comfort, and social changes are also becoming important dietary determinants. North Americans probably respond more to external, appetite-related forces than to hunger-related ones in choosing when and what to eat.

NUTRITION AND YOUR HEALTH
Eating Well in College

The college years are a leap into adulthood for many young adults. This is a time for freedom and a chance to make personal lifestyle decisions. Studies show that the diets and other health habits of college students are not optimal. Typically, students fall short of recommendations for servings of whole grains, vegetables, fruits, milk, and meat, opting instead to max out on fats, sweets, and alcohol. This information is disturbing from a public health standpoint, because young adulthood is the time when many health behaviors are formed and will likely persist throughout life. With independence comes responsibility, including a responsibility to make smart food choices.

What is it about the college lifestyle that makes it so difficult to build healthy habits? Why do so many young adults gain the dreaded "freshman 15" pounds during the first months of college? How does alcohol consumption affect your waistline and academic performance? What can you do to establish healthful habits to last a lifetime?

WEIGHT CONTROL AND THE "FRESHMAN FIFTEEN"

The college experience is exciting, but stressful. Students face changes in academic requirements, interpersonal relationships, and living environment. These stressful situations contribute to poor health behaviors. For example, take the week of midterms; during this time of writing papers and cramming for exams, balanced meals are all-too-easily replaced by high-fat and high-calorie fast-foods; convenience items; and sugary, caffeinated beverages. Physical activity is sacrificed in favor of study time.

Also consider the university environment. On campus, you are faced with a wide variety of dining choices, some healthy and some not so healthy. Dining halls, fast-food establishments, bars, and vending machines offer food 24 hours per day. While it is certainly possible to make wise food choices at each of these outlets, the temptations of convenience, taste, and value (i.e., oversized portions) may persuade the college student to select unhealthy options.

Eating is about more than just obtaining "fuel." Meals and snacks are times to socialize. You may feel pressured to eat a big lunch at noon without regard to hunger if your peers are meeting in the dining hall to catch up on class work and gossip. While chatting, too, it is easy to lose track of portions and to overeat. In addition, food may be a source of familiarity and comfort in a new and stressful place. Learning to eat based on your body's hunger cues is a great way to avoid weight gain.

▲ Late night pizza can add extra calories to the college student's daily intake.

23

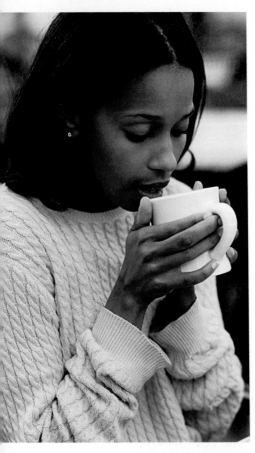

▲ Research has shown that gourmet coffee beverages, such as lattes and cappuccinos, can increase calorie consumption by about 200 kcal per day.

▶ **Five Simple Tips to Avert the Freshman Fifteen**

- Eat a breakfast that includes a source of protein such as an egg or low-fat yogurt, at least one serving of whole grains such as a breakfast cereal, and a fruit such as a banana
- Plan ahead to eat a balanced meal or snack every 3–4 hours
- Drink water instead of high-calorie soft drinks, fruit juice, alcohol, or coffee; if you drink alcohol, limit it to 1 or 2 drinks per day
- Keep a stash of low-calorie, nutritious snacks, such as pretzels, light microwave popcorn, or fruit (fresh, canned, or dried)
- Find a friend to work out with you

There are several health reasons to lose excess weight. Over the long term, risk of chronic diseases goes up as weight increases. In the short term, however, losing excess weight can improve the way you view yourself, how others view you, and how you feel and perform. Detecting "flab" around your midsection or feeling that your clothes are getting tighter are two good indicators that you are carrying excess weight. If you determine that weight loss is necessary, with some knowledge and perseverance, you can safely lose excess pounds.

How do you go about achieving your goal? Behavioral research clearly demonstrates that setting several small, achievable goals will spur motivation. As you will learn in Chapter 7, body weight is a balancing act between calories in and calories burned. Try keeping track of your calorie consumption for several days and comparing that to your energy needs, based on your age, gender, and activity level. You can use one of the equations presented in Chapter 7 or take advantage of the interactive tools on www.mypyramid.gov to estimate your energy needs.

A healthy rate of weight loss is one to two pounds per week. Greater rates of weight loss will not likely be sustained over time. Remember that the numbers on the scale are not as important as your body composition—the amount of fat in relation to lean mass. One pound of weight loss requires a deficit of 3500 kilocalories. Thus, to lose one pound per week, you will need to cut back on food intake and/or increase your exercise routine to shift the energy balance equation by 500 kilocalories per day.

Many students skip breakfast, whether it is to save time, money, or calories. However, breakfast is the *most* important meal of the day. Starting the day off with a fortified, whole-grain breakfast cereal, skim milk, and a serving of fruit puts you on the right path for meeting recommendations for fiber, calcium, and fruit intake. Even though it may seem that a cup of coffee gets your brain going in the morning, your brain is fueled best by carbohydrates, not caffeine. In addition, studies repeatedly show that eating breakfast prevents over-eating later in the day, by preventing hunger from dictating your food choices.

Calories can sneak up on the unsuspecting college student. One of the biggest contributors to weight gain is consuming several hundred calories per day in the form of sugary beverages or alcoholic beverages. One 12-ounce can of regular cola contains about 140 kcal. A 12-ounce can of regular beer has 150 kcal. As one study showed, average calorie consumption goes up by about 200 kilocalories per day among women who consume gourmet coffee beverages, such as lattes and cappuccinos. Even fruit juices, which we perceive to be healthy, have at least 100 kcal per 8-ounce glass. Furthermore, a 24-ounce mug of a soft drink makes you feel no fuller than an equal volume of water, yet the soft drink adds 300 kcal more. A convenient stash of water is the best way to quench your thirst.

Exercise is so important to any weight loss and weight maintenance plan. It's easy to start an exercise routine, but sticking with it is the hard part. When you find yourself short on time, exercise is often the first thing we sacrifice. To ensure your success at boosting daily activity, choose activities you enjoy such as working out with friends at the campus recreation center, participating in intramural sports, or taking an activity class like dancing. Don't forget the brisk walking to and from classes. For more information on planning an exercise program, see Chapter 12.

ALCOHOL AND BINGE DRINKING

Excessive alcohol consumption is a big problem on college campuses. Legal or not, many college students consider drinking alcohol to be a "rite of passage" into adulthood. On campuses, binge drinking—consuming five or more drinks in a row for men, or four drinks or more for women—has become an epidemic.

The statistics on the impact of binge drinking on college campuses are sobering. An estimated two of every five students on college campuses participates in binge drinking. Each year, 1400 college students between the ages of 18 and 24 die from alcohol-related unintentional injuries, including motor vehicle crashes. In addition to deaths and injuries, other problems stemming from binge drinking include unsafe sex and its consequences, long-term health problems, suicides, academic problems, legal troubles, and alcohol abuse or dependence. Thirty one percent of college students meet the criteria for a diagnosis of alcohol abuse and 6% for a diagnosis of alcohol dependence.

In addition to these dire consequences, alcohol consumption definitely contributes to weight gain—by virtue of its own calories and by way of increased food consumption at events where drinking occurs. If you choose to drink alcohol, do so in moderation—no more than two drinks per day for men or no more than one drink per day for women. For your own sake and the safety of your peers, be aware of the warning signs and dangers of alcohol poisoning shown in the margin.

EATING DISORDERS

In college, the stresses of achieving academic and social success put many students, particularly women, at risk. As many as 30% of college students are at risk of developing an eating disorder. As you will learn in Chapter 13, disordered eating is a mild and short-term change in eating patterns that typically occurs in response to life stress, a desire to change appearance, or a bad habit. Sometimes, disordered eating habits may lead to an eating disorder, such as anorexia nervosa, bulimia nervosa, or binge-eating disorder. Chapter 13 also includes advice on what to do if you suspect that your roommate or friend is suffering from an eating disorder.

Starving the body also starves the brain, limiting performance in academics and beyond, and the negative consequences of disordered eating may last a lifetime. Ultimately, eating disorders do not arise from problems with food but rather from problems with self-esteem, control, and abusive relationships. Food happens to be the focus of many emotional issues. Frequently, what begins as a diet spirals into a much larger problem. Eating disorders are not just diets gone bad—they require

professional intervention. Left unchecked, eating disorders lead to serious adverse effects, such as loss of menstrual periods, thinning of bones, gastrointestinal problems, kidney problems, heart abnormalities, and eventually death.

CHOOSING A VEGETARIAN LIFESTYLE

During college, many students experiment with or adopt a vegetarian eating pattern. Interest in plant-based diets has been growing steadily as more research points to their health benefits. While plant-based diets can meet nutrition needs and decrease risk of many chronic diseases, they require appropriate planning at all life stages.

Protein is not typically deficient, even with a vegan diet, which contains no animal products. However, vegetarians, and especially vegans, may be at risk for deficiencies of several vitamins and minerals. Consuming a ready-to-eat breakfast cereal is an easy and inexpensive way to obtain these nutrients. See Chapter 6 for further information on food planning for vegetarians.

▶ **The warning signs and symptoms of alcohol poisoning**
- Semiconsciousness or unconsciousness
- Slow respiration of eight or fewer breaths per minute or lapses between breaths of more than 8 seconds
- Cold, clammy, pale, or bluish skin
- Strong odor of alcohol, which usually accompanies these symptoms

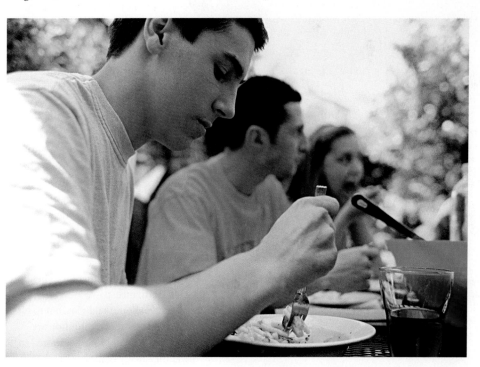

▲ Many students adopt a vegetarian diet during college. Guidelines for planning a nutritious vegetarian diet are presented in Chapter 6.

As interest in vegetarian meals has grown, restaurants and campus dining services have responded by offering a variety of vegetarian options. For optimal health benefits, choose foods that are baked, steamed, or stir-fried rather than deep-fried; select whole grains rather than refined carbohydrates; and consume food fortified with vitamins and minerals. Even if you do not choose to follow a plant-based diet all the time, choosing several plant-based meals each week can help with weight control and boost intake of fiber and many healthy phytochemicals.

FUEL FOR COMPETITION: STUDENT ATHLETES

Students involved in intramural and intercollegiate athletics need to consume more calories and nutrients. Despite an emphasis on a lean physique or a drive to compete at a low weight class, athletes at all levels must take care not to severely restrict calories, as this could impact performance and health. Muscles require adequate carbohydrates for fuel and protein for growth and repair. Fat, as well, is an important source of stored energy for use during exercise. Women who drop to low levels of body fat may become amenorrheic (cease menstruating), a condition costly to long-term bone health.

In addition to fueling the body with calories, fluids are essential for health and performance. Water is adequate for events lasting less than 60 minutes. For longer events, sports drinks are ideal because they also supply carbohydrates to fuel fatigued muscles as well as electrolytes to replenish those lost in perspiration. Induction of fluid losses to "make weight" for a competition are detrimental to health and performance.

Athletes should take care not to be wooed by the supplement industry. The increased food intake required to meet the energy demands of athletic training is usually sufficient to meet vitamin and mineral needs. As an exception, athletes may be at risk for iron-deficiency anemia. Consuming a balanced multivitamin and mineral supplement is adequate for most people, and individual vitamin, mineral, amino acid, or herbal supplements are not advised, in spite of the hype of supplement makers.

TIPS FOR EATING WELL ON A COLLEGE STUDENT'S BUDGET

If you've learned one thing from college, it's that higher education can be hard on the wallet! It is possible to eat well on campus on a budget.

If you live on campus, participate in a prepaid campus meal plan. These are generally designed to offer a great food value with a variety of healthy foods. If you live off campus or have your own kitchen, plan ahead—for the day and for the week. Packing a lunch from home will save a lot of cash compared to grabbing lunch on the run and puts you more in control of healthy choices. For example, preparing a sandwich at home costs less than half as much as purchasing one at a fast-food restaurant or deli.

For those who shop for groceries, never go shopping on an empty stomach—everything will look good and you'll buy more. Also, go to the store with a list in hand and stick to it, because impulse buys tend to drain your wallet. When you shop for foods, buy store-brand foods rather than name-brand items. Make use of canned and frozen fruits and vegetables—they are just as nutritious as fresh fruits and vegetables, particularly if you choose low-sodium and low-sugar varieties. Rather than buying cartons of fruit juice, select cans of fruit juice concentrate and mix with water at home. Likewise, preparing other drinks, such as iced tea, from store-brand powder (look for sugar-free) will save over gallon jugs or vending machine containers of drinks. Canned (fruits, tuna) and dry (oatmeal) foods can be nutritious and last a long time, so you can avoid throwing out spoiled items. Finally, eggs and peanut butter are inexpensive and simple sources of protein.

CASE STUDY

Typical College Student

Andy is like many other college students. He grew up on a quick bowl of cereal and milk for breakfast and a hamburger, French fries, and cola for lunch, either in the school cafeteria or at a local fast-food restaurant. At dinner, he generally avoided eating any of his salad or vegetables, and by 9 o'clock he was deep into bags of chips and cookies. Andy has taken most of these habits to college. He prefers coffee for breakfast and possibly a chocolate bar. Lunch is still mainly a hamburger, French fries, and cola, but pizza and tacos now alternate more frequently than when he was in high school. One thing Andy really likes about the restaurants surrounding campus is that, for just about half a dollar more, he can *supersize* his meal. This helps him stretch his food dollar; searching out value meals for lunch and dinner now has become part of a typical day.

Provide some dietary advice for Andy. Start with his positive habits and then provide some constructive criticism, based on what you now know.

Answer the following questions, and check your response in Appendix A.

1. **Start with Andy's positive habits:** What healthy choices are being made when Andy eats at local restaurants?

2. **Now provide some constructive criticisms:**
   a. What are some of the negative aspects of items available at fast-food restaurants?
   b. Why is supersizing a dangerous habit?
   c. What healthier substitutions could he make at each meal?
   d. List some healthier choices he could make at fast-food restaurants on campus.

SUMMARY

1. Nutrition is the study of the food substances vital for health and the study of how the body uses these substances to promote and support growth, maintenance, and reproduction of cells.

2. Nutrients in foods fall into six classes: (1) carbohydrates, (2) lipids (mostly fats and oils), (3) proteins, (4) vitamins, (5) minerals, and (6) water. The first three, along with alcohol, provide calories for the body to use.

3. The body transforms the energy contained in carbohydrate, protein, and fat into other forms of energy that in turn allow the body to function. Fat provides, on average, 9 kcal per gram, whereas both protein and carbohydrate provide, on average, 4 kcal per gram. Vitamins, minerals, and water do not supply calories to the body but are essential for proper body function.

4. A basic plan for health promotion and disease prevention includes eating a varied diet, performing regular physical activity, not smoking, not abusing nutrient supplements (if used), consuming adequate water and other fluids, getting enough sleep, limiting alcohol intake (if consumed), and limiting or appropriately coping with stress.

5. The primary focus of nutrition planning should be on food, not on dietary supplements. The focus on foods to supply nutrient needs avoids the possibility of severe nutrient imbalances.

6. Results from large nutrition surveys in the United States and Canada suggest that some of us need to concentrate on consuming foods that supply more of certain vitamins, minerals, and fiber. Daily use of a balanced multivitamin and mineral supplement does not substitute for a healthy diet but does provide a strategy to address some dietary shortcomings.

7. Groups of cells in the hypothalamus and other regions in the brain affect hunger, the primarily internal desire to find and eat food. These cells monitor hormonal and nerve signals from digestive organs as well as amounts of nutrients and other substances in the blood to control satiety.

8. A variety of external (appetite-related) forces affect satiety. Hunger cues combine with appetite cues, such as easy availability of food, to promote food intake.

9. The flavor, appearance, and texture of foods primarily influence our food choices. Several other factors also help determine food habits and choices: our upbringing, various social and cultural factors, the image we want to project to others, economics, convenience, emotional state, and concerns about health.

10. There are no true "good" or "bad" foods, but some food choices are healthier than others. The focus should be on balancing a total diet by choosing many nutritious foods.

11. Studies show that the diets and other health habits of college students are not optimal. Students fall short of recommendations for servings of grains, vegetables, fruits, milk, and meat, opting instead to max out on fats, sweets, and alcohol. This information is disturbing from a public health standpoint, because young adulthood is the time when many health behaviors are formed and will likely persist throughout life. Issues of particular importance on college campuses are weight control, making healthy meal choices, alcohol and binge drinking, and eating disorders.

STUDY QUESTIONS

1. Name one chronic disease associated with poor nutrition habits. Now list a few corresponding risk factors.

2. Explain the concept of calories as it relates to foods. What are the values used to calculate kcals from grams of carbohydrate, fat, protein, and alcohol?

3. Identify three ways that water is used in the body.

4. Wendy's Big Bacon Classic contains 44 grams carbohydrate, 36 grams fat, and 37 grams protein. Calculate the percentage of calories derived from fat.

5. Describe two types of fat and explain why the differences are important in terms of overall health.

6. According to national nutrition surveys, which nutrients tend to be underconsumed by many North Americans? Why do you think this is the case?

7. List four health objectives for the United States for the year 2010. How would you rate yourself in each area? Why?

8. Describe the various organs and hormones that control hunger and satiety in the body. List other factors that influence our food patterns.

9. Describe how your food preferences have been shaped by the following factors:
   a. Exposure to foods at an early age
   b. Advertising (what is the newest food you have tried?)
   c. Eating out
   d. Peer pressure
   e. Economic factors

10. What products in your supermarket reflect the consumer demand for healthier foods? For convenience?

CHECK YOUR KNOWLEDGE

Answers to the following multiple choice questions are in Appendix A.

1. Energy-yielding nutrients include
   a. vitamins, minerals, and water.
   b. carbohydrates, proteins, and fats.
   c. trace minerals and fat-soluble vitamins.
   d. iron, vitamin C, and potassium.

2. The *essential* nutrients
   a. must be consumed at every meal.
   b. are required for infants but not adults.
   c. can be made in the body when they are needed.
   d. cannot be made by the body and therefore must be consumed to maintain health.

3. Sugars, starches, and dietary fibers are examples of
   a. proteins.
   b. vitamins.
   c. carbohydrates.
   d. minerals.

4. Which nutrient classes are most important in the regulation of body processes?
   a. vitamins
   b. carbohydrates
   c. minerals
   d. lipids
   e. Both a and c.

5. A kcal is a
   a. measure of heat energy.
   b. measure of fat in food.
   c. heating device.
   d. term used to describe the amount of sugar and fat in foods.

6. A food that contains 10 grams of fat would yield _____ kcal.
   a. 40   c. 90
   b. 70   d. 120

7. If you consume 300 grams of carbohydrate in a day that you consume 2400 kcal, the carbohydrates will provide _____% of your total energy intake.
   a. 12.5   c. 50
   b. 30   d. 60

8. Which of the following is true about the North American diet?
   a. Most of our protein comes from plant sources.
   b. About half of the carbohydrates come from simple sugars.
   c. Most of our fats come from plant sources.
   d. Most of our carbohydrates come from starches.

9. There are _____ grams in on ounce.
   a. 10   c. 28
   b. 16   d. 32

10. The region of the brain that helps regulate hunger is the
    a. cortex.
    b. hypothalamus.
    c. pituitary.
    d. cerebrum.

FURTHER READINGS

1. ADA Reports: Position of the American Dietetic Association and Dietitians of Canada: Nutrition and Women's Health. *Journal of the American Dietetic Association* 104:984, 2004.
   Comprehensive look at health issues related to nutrition that women often face. Diets rich in fruits, vegetables, and whole-grain breads and cereals, with some low-fat dairy and lean meat choices, are widely advocated. Individual nutrients likely to be underconsumed include calcium, iron, vitamin D, vitamin E, and folate.

2. Brown LB and others: College students can benefit by participating in a prepaid meal plan. *Journal of the American Dietetic Association*, 105:445, 2005.
   Participation in a prepaid campus meal plan resulted in modest nutritional benefits to students through an increase in servings of foods from fruit, vegetable, and meat groups.

3. Cotton PA and others: Dietary sources of nutrients among U.S. adults, 1994 to 1996. *Journal of the American Dietetic Association* 104:921, 2004.

The five leading calorie sources for American adults are (in order): yeast bread, beef, cakes/cookies/quick breads/doughnuts, soft drinks/soda, and milk. The cake and so on category also has been moving up in the order compared to the 1980s. Clearly many adults need to improve their dietary choices.

4. Cordain L and others: Origins and evolution of the Western diet: health implications for the 21st century. *American Journal of Clinical Nutrition* 1:341, 2005.

   Throughout human's existence, the number of foods rich in refined sugars, refined flours, salt, and animal fat has increased. This has resulted in a decline in diet quality for many of us in the modern world.

5. de Graaf C and others: Biomarkers of satiation. *American Journal of Clinical Nutrition* 79:946, 2004.

   The feeling of satiety depends on a constellation of factors, such as stomach distention; the action of various hormones, such as ghrelin; and communication between various organs and the brain. This article reviews the latest findings with regard to these and other factors affecting satiety.

6. Food and Nutrition Board: *Dietary reference intakes for energy, carbohydrate, fiber, fat, fatty acids, cholesterol, protein, and amino acids.* Washington DC: The National Academy Press, 2002.

   This report provides the latest guidance for macronutrient intakes. With regard to the amounts of carbohydrate, fat, and protein in a diet, this should be 45% to 65%, 20% to 35%, and 10% to 35%, respectively.

7. Hoffman DY and others: Changes in body weight and fat mass of men and women in the first year of college: A study of the "freshman 15." *Journal of American College of Health.* 55: 41, 2006.

   It is commonly thought that there is a high risk of gaining 15 pounds of weight during freshman year of college. In this study, changes in body weight and percentage of body fat were measured in first-year college students. Body weight increased by an average of almost three pounds (1.3 kilograms) and body fat increased an average of 0.7%. This study, therefore, found that weight and fat gain may occur during the first year of college.

8. How much exercise is enough? *UC Berkeley Wellness Letter,* p. 5, September 2003.

   A minimum amount of physical activity is considered to be 30 minutes at least five times per week. Increasing the amount to 60 minutes per day is even more health-promoting, especially if weight loss/control is an issue. For both recommendations, bouts of physical activity can be broken up into a few sessions in a day.

9. Junk food or junky choices? *Tufts University Health & Nutrition Letter,* p. 3, September 2003.

   Some sweet or high-fat foods can be safely incorporated into an otherwise healthy diet. This healthy diet should be rich in fruits, vegetables, and whole-grain breads and cereals, and contain some low-fat and fat-free dairy choices and lean protein sources. A person's total dietary intake is what determines the quality of a diet.

10. Lichtenstein AH and others: Diet and lifestyle recommendations revision 2006. A scientific statement from the American Heart Association Nutrition Committee. *Circulation* 114:82, 2006.

    The American Heart Association presents recommendations designed to reduce the risk of cardiovascular disease in the general population. Specific goals include consuming an overall healthy diet; aiming for a healthy body weight; achieving healthy targets for blood cholesterol levels, blood pressure, and blood glucose; being physically active; and avoiding the use of and exposure to tobacco products.

11. Litt, AS: *The College Student's Guide to Eating Well on Campus.* Tulip Hill Press, Bethesda, MD, 2000.

    This book provides important information on how to survive and eat well during your college years.

12. Lubin F and others: Lifestyle and ethnicity play a role in all-cause mortality. *Journal of Nutrition* 133:1180, 2003.

    Dietary habits that reduce all-cause mortality include focusing on both high-fiber foods and those low in saturated fat and cholesterol. Positive lifestyle habits include regular physical activity and avoiding smoking and obesity.

13. Mokdad AH and others: Actual causes of death in the United States, 2000. *Journal of the American Medical Association* 291:1238, 2004.

    Smoking is the leading cause of preventable death in the United States, with obesity a close second. A combination of a poor diet and inac-tive lifestyle may account for about one third of deaths in the United States.

14. Olshansky SJ and others: A potential decline in life expectancy in the United States in the 21st century. *The New England Journal of Medicine* 352:1138, 2005.

    The growing problem of overweight and obesity in our society is likely to lead to more overall premature deaths. An alarming concern is that this widespread increase in body weight could result in a life expectancy of fewer years for today's children compared to their parents. Reversing this trend of greater overweight and obesity is crucial.

15. Oz D: *The Dorm Room Diet: The 8-Step Program for Creating a Healthy Lifestyle Plan that Really Works.* Newmarket Press, 2006.

    This book is written to help students stay fit while at college. The 8-step program shows students how to stop eating out of emotional need; navigate the most common danger zones at school for unhealthy eating; get the exercise you need, even in your small dorm room; choose vitamins and supplements wisely and relax and rejuvenate amid the stress of college life.

16. Paeratakul S and others: Fast-food consumption among U.S. adults and children: Dietary and nutrient intake profile. *Journal of the American Dietetic Association* 103:1332, 2003.

    Regular intake of fast-food contributes a lot of fat and calories to a diet. Such foods can also crowd out more healthful foods in a diet. Regular fast-food consumers would be wise to focus on lower-fat items and greatly limit or avoid sugared soft drinks and French fries.

17. Shields DH and others: Gourmet coffee beverage consumption among college women. *Journal of the American Dietetic Association,* 104:650, 2004.

    A significant percentage of college women were shown to consume gourmet coffee beverages which contributed additional calories and fat to their daily dietary intake.

18. Tholin S and others: Genetic and environmental influence on eating behavior: the Swedish Young Male Twins Study. *American Journal of Clinical Nutrition* 81:564, 2005.

    Genetics plays a distinct role in the development of eating habits, such as emotional eating or restrained eating. This may be linked to the amount of various hormones and other physiological factors that can influence eating habits.

▶ ## Check out the **Contemporary Nutrition ARIS site**

www.mhhe.com/wardlawcontfa1 for quizzes, flash cards, other activities, and weblinks designed to further help you learn about what you eat and why.

RATE YOUR PLATE

I. Examine Your Eating Habits More Closely

Choose one day of the week that is typical of your eating pattern. Using the first table found in Appendix E, list all foods and drinks you consumed for 24 hours. In addition, write down the approximate amounts of food you ate in units, such as cups, ounces, teaspoons, and tablespoons. After you record the amount of each food and drink consumed, indicate in the table why you chose to consume the item. Place the corresponding abbreviation in the space provided to indicate why you picked that food or drink.

FLVR	Flavor/texture	ADV	Advertisement	PEER	Peers
CONV	Convenience	WTCL	Weight control	NUTR	Nutritive value
EMO	Emotions	HUNG	Hunger	$	Cost
AVA	Availability	FAM	Family/cultural	HLTH	Health

There can be more than one reason for choosing a particular food or drink.

Application

Ask yourself what your most frequent reason is for eating or drinking. To what degree is health or nutritive value a reason for your food choices? Should you make these higher priorities?

II. Observe the Supermarket Explosion

Today's supermarkets carry up to 60,000 items, compared to 20,000 items 10 years ago. Think about your last grocery shopping trip and the items you purchased to eat. Following is a list of 20 newer food products added to supermarket shelves. Check the items that you have tried. Then use the key from Part I of the Rate Your Plate exercise to identify why you might have chosen these products.

_____ Prepackaged salad greens (variety packs other than iceberg lettuce) _____

_____ Gourmet salad oils (e.g., walnut, almond, olive, or sesame oil) _____

_____ Gourmet vinegars (e.g., balsamic or rice) _____

_____ Prepackaged lunch products (e.g., nacho, pizza, taco, and tortilla Lunchables) _____

_____ Precooked frozen turkey patties _____

_____ Bean soup mixes (e.g., lentil, black bean, combination bean soups) _____

_____ Microwaveable sandwiches (e.g., Hotpockets, frozen sandwiches) _____

_____ Refrigerated, precooked pasta (e.g., tortellini, fettucini) and accompanying sauces (e.g., pesto, tomato basil) _____

_____

_____ Imported grain products (e.g., risotto, farfalline, gnocchi, fusilli) _____

_____ Frozen dinners (list your favorite of any of the wide variety) _____

_____ Imported sauces for food preparation (e.g., hoisin or brown bean sauce; mandarin marinade, sesame, curry, or fire oils)

_____

_____ Bottled waters (flavored or unflavored) _____

_____ Trendy juices (e.g., draft apple cider, hurricane punch) _____

_____ Roasted and/or flavored coffees (e.g., beans, ground, or instant) _____

_____ Gourmet jelly beans and candies (e.g., gummi coca-colas or imported chocolates)_____

_____ Instant hot cereal in a bowl (add water and go!) _____

_____ "Fast-shake" pancake mix (add water, shake, and ready to cook) _____

_____ Breakfast bars (e.g., granola or fruit-flavored bars) _____

_____ Meal replacement/fitness products (e.g., "energy" bars, high-protein bars, sports drinks) _____

_____ Low-carbohydrate meat and pasta dishes _____

Finally, identify three new food products not on this list that you have seen in the past year. Discuss the appeal of these products to the North American consumer.

CHAPTER 2 Guidelines for Designing a Healthy Diet

CHAPTER OBJECTIVES Chapter 2 is designed to allow you to:

1. Develop a healthy eating plan.
2. Outline the ABCDEs of nutrition assessment: anthropometric, *biochemical*, *clinical*, *dietary*, and economic.
3. Describe what the Recommended Dietary Allowances (RDAs) and other dietary standards represent.
4. Learn the food groupings used in MyPyramid.
5. List the Dietary Guidelines and the diseases these guidelines are designed to prevent or minimize.
6. Describe what a nutrition label currently consists of and the various health claims and label descriptors that are allowed.
7. Understand the basis of the scientific method as it is used in developing hypotheses and theories in the field of nutrition.
8. Identify reliable sources of nutrition information.

CHAPTER OUTLINE

HOW MANY TIMES HAVE YOU HEARD WILD CLAIMS ABOUT HOW HEALTHFUL CERTAIN FOODS ARE FOR YOU? As consumers focus more on diet and disease, food manufacturers are asserting that their products have all sorts of health benefits. Supermarket shelves have begun to look like an 1800s medicine show. "Take fish oil capsules to avoid a heart attack." "Eat more olive oil and oat bran to lower blood cholesterol." Hearing these claims, you would think that food manufacturers have solutions to all of our health problems.

Advertising aside, nutrient intakes that are out of balance with our needs—such as excess calories, saturated fat, cholesterol, *trans* fat, salt, alcohol, and sugar intakes—are linked to many leading causes of death in North America, including obesity, hypertension, cardiovascular disease, cancer, liver disease, and type 2 diabetes. Physical inactivity is also too common. In Chapter 2, you will explore the components of a healthy diet and lifestyle—an approach that will minimize your risks of developing nutrition-related diseases. The goal is to provide you with a firm understanding of these concepts before you study the nutrients in detail.

Refresh Your Memory

As you begin your study of diet planning in Chapter 2, you may want to review:

▪ The terms in the margin in Chapter 1 and Table 1-1.

A FOOD PHILOSOPHY THAT WORKS

You may be surprised that what you should eat to minimize the risk of developing the nutrition-related diseases seen in North America is exactly what you've heard many times before: *Consume a variety of foods balanced by a moderate intake of each food.* Health professionals have recommended the same basic diet and health plan for the past 50 years: Control how much you eat, focus on the major food groups, and stay physically active. Whole-grain breads and cereals, fruits, and vegetables have always been among the foods emphasized for our diet for these past 50 years.

It is disappointing, however, that according to a recent survey conducted by the American Dietetic Association, two of five people in the United States believe that following a healthful diet means completely giving up foods they enjoy. To the contrary, a healthful diet requires only some simple planning and doesn't have to mean deprivation and misery. Besides, eliminating favorite foods typically doesn't work for "dieters" in the long run. The best plan, as discussed in the comic in this chapter, consists of learning the basics of a healthful diet—a variety and balance of foods from all food groups and moderate consumption of all foods. Monitoring total calorie intake is also important for many of us, especially if unwanted weight gain is taking place. Let's now fine-tune this advice by focusing on variety, balance, moderation, nutrient density, and energy density.

▲ For the past 50 years, fruits, vegetables, and whole-grain breads and cereals have been among the foods recommended for our diet.

Variety Means Eating Many Different Foods

Variety in your diet means choosing a number of different foods within any given food group rather than eating the "same old thing" day after day. Variety makes meals more interesting and helps ensure that a diet contains sufficient nutrients. A variety

On what do nutrition experts generally agree regarding a healthy food or diet? Why is a diet rich in fiber that includes some fish and is low in fried foods and animal fat emphasized, along with at least 30 minutes or more of physical activity on most or all days of the week? Are North Americans generally following this plan? What are the potential consequences for those who do not? Chapter 2 provides some answers.

STONE SOUP © 2003 Jan Eliot. Reprinted with permission of UNIVERSAL PRESS SYNDICATE. All rights reserved.

of foods is best because no one food meets all your nutrient needs. Meat provides protein and iron but little calcium and no vitamin C. Eggs also provide protein but little calcium because the calcium is mostly in the shell. Cow's milk contains calcium, but very little iron. None of these foods contains fiber. Thus you need a variety of foods in your diet because the required nutrients are scattered among many foods. For example, carrots—a rich source of a pigment that forms vitamin A—may be your favorite vegetable; however, if you choose carrots every day as your only vegetable source, you may miss out on the vitamin folate. Other vegetables, such as broccoli and asparagus, are rich sources of this nutrient. This concept is true of all classes of foods: fruits, vegetables, grains, and so on. Different foods within each class vary somewhat in the nutrients they contain, but they generally provide similar types of nutrients.

An added bonus of variety in the diet, especially within the fruit and vegetable groups, is the inclusion of a rich supply of the **phytochemicals**. Recall from Chapter 1 that the phytochemicals were discussed along with the nutrient classes. Many of these substances provide significant health benefits. Considerable research attention is focused on various phytochemicals in reducing the risk for certain diseases (e.g., cancer). You can't just buy a bottle of phytochemicals—they are generally available only within whole foods. Current multivitamin and mineral supplements contain few or none of these beneficial plant chemicals.

Numerous population studies show reduced cancer risk among people who regularly consume fruits and vegetables. Researchers suspect that some phytochemicals present in the fruits and vegetables block the cancer process. The cancer process and the specific roles of some phytochemicals in this regard are described in the "Nutrition and Your Health" section in Chapter 18. Some phytochemicals also have been linked to a reduced risk of cardiovascular disease. Could it be that, because humans evolved on a wide variety of plant-based foods, the body developed with a need for these phytochemicals, along with the various nutrients present, to maintain optimal health?

It will likely take many years for scientists to unravel the important effects of the myriad of phytochemicals in foods, and it is unlikely that all will ever be available or effective in supplement form. For this reason, leading nutrition and medical experts suggest that a diet rich in fruits, vegetables, and whole-grain breads and cereals is the most reliable way to obtain the potential benefits of phytochemicals. Some research suggests that increasing variety in a diet can lead to overeating. Thus, as one incorporates a wide variety of foods in a diet, attention to total calorie intake is also important to consider. Table 2-1 provides a number of suggestions for including more phytochemicals in your diet, as do the websites www.fruitsandveggiesmorematters. org and www.fruitsandveggiesmatter.gov.

▶ Foods rich in phytochemicals are now part of a family of foods referred to as **functional foods.** A functional food is a food that provides health benefits beyond those supplied by the traditional nutrients it contains. A tomato contains the phytochemical lycopene, so it can be called a functional food. You may hear this term more from the food industry in the future.

Balance Means Not Overconsuming Any Single Type of Food

One way to balance your diet as you consume a variety of foods is to select foods from the six major food groups every day:

- Grains
- Vegetables
- Fruits
- Milk
- Meat & Beans
- Oils

A dinner consisting of a bean burrito, lettuce and tomato salad with oil and vinegar dressing, a glass of milk, and an apple covers all groups.

Moderation Refers Mostly to Portion Size

Although eating moderate (i.e., small) portion sizes is a good practice, eating in moderation also requires planning your entire day's diet so that you don't overconsume any nutrients. For example, if you eat a bacon cheeseburger, relatively high in fat, salt,

▲ Focus on nutrient-rich foods as you strive to meet your nutrient needs. The more colorful your plate, the greater the content of nutrients and phytochemicals.

CRITICAL THINKING

Andy would benefit from more variety in his diet. What are some practical tips he can use to increase his fruit and vegetable intake?

▲ Choosing whole-grain cereals is an excellent way to increase the nutrient content of a diet. Ideally, the cereal should have at least 3 grams of fiber per serving.

TABLE 2-1 Tips for Boosting the Phytochemical Content of a Diet

- Include vegetables in main and side dishes. Add these to rice, omelets, potato salad, and pastas. Try broccoli or cauliflower florets, mushrooms, peas, carrots, corn, or peppers.

- Look for quick-to-fix grain side dishes in the supermarket. Pilafs, couscous, rice mixes, and tabbouleh are just a few that you'll find.

- Choose fruit-filled cookies, such as fig bars, instead of sugar-rich cookies. Use fresh or canned fruit as a topping for puddings, hot or cold cereal, pancakes, and frozen desserts.

- Put raisins, grapes, apple chunks, pineapples, grated carrots, zucchini, or cucumber into coleslaw, chicken salad, or tuna salad.

- Be creative at the salad bar: Try fresh spinach, leaf lettuce, red cabbage, zucchini, yellow squash, cauliflower, peas, mushrooms, or red or yellow peppers.

- Pack fresh or dried fruit for snacks away from home instead of grabbing a candy bar or going hungry.

- Add slices of cucumber, zucchini, spinach, or carrot slivers to the lettuce and tomato on your sandwiches.

- Each week try one or two vegetarian meals, such as beans and rice or pasta; Chinese vegetable stir fry; or spaghetti and tomato sauce.

- If your daily protein intake exceeds the recommended amounts, reduce the meat, fish, or poultry in casseroles, stews, and soups by one-third to one-half and add more vegetables and legumes.

- Keep a bowl of fresh vegetables in the refrigerator for snacks.

- Choose fruit or vegetable juices instead of soft drinks, and preferably 100% juice varieties.

- Substitute tea for coffee or soft drinks on a regular basis.

- Have a bowl of fruit on hand.

- Switch from crisphead lettuce to leaf lettuce, such as romaine.

- Use salsa as a dip for chips in place of creamy dips.

- Choose whole-grain breakfast cereals, breads, and crackers.

- Add flavor to your plate with ginger, rosemary, basil, thyme, garlic, onions, parsley, and chives in place of salt.

- Incorporate soy products, such as tofu, soy milk, soy protein isolate, and roasted soybeans into your meals (see Chapter 6).

and calories, you should eat foods such as fruits and salad greens, that are less concentrated sources of these nutrients at other meals that same day. This helps balance your diet. If you prefer whole milk to low-fat or fat-free milk, reduce the fat elsewhere in your meals. Try low-fat salad dressings, or use jam rather than butter or margarine on toast. Overall, strive to moderate serving sizes of some foods rather than eliminating these foods.

As noted in Chapter 1, many nutrition experts agree that there are no exclusively "good" or "bad" foods. Even so, many North Americans have diets that lack the foundations of a healthy food plan—variety, balance, and moderation. Consuming diets overloaded with foods high in fatty meats, fried foods, sugared soft drinks, and refined starches can result in substantial risk for nutrition-related chronic diseases.

Nutrient Density Focuses on Nutrient Content

The **nutrient density** of a food is a characteristic used to determine its nutritional quality. Nutrient density of a food is determined by comparing its vitamin or mineral content with the amount of calories it provides. A food is said to be nutrient dense if it provides a large amount of a nutrient for a relatively small amount of calories when compared with other food sources. The higher a food's nutrient density, the better it is as a nutrient source. Comparing the nutrient density of different foods is an easy way to estimate their relative nutritional quality. Generally, nutrient density is determined with respect to individual nutrients. For example, many fruits and vegetables have a high content of vitamin C compared with their modest calorie content: That is, they are nutrient-dense foods for vitamin C. Figure 2-1 shows that fat-free milk is much more nutrient dense than sugared soft drinks for many nutrients, especially protein, vitamin A, riboflavin, and calcium.

As noted previously, menu planning should focus mainly on the total diet—not on the selection of one critical food as the key to an adequate diet. Nutrient-dense foods—such as fat-free and low-fat milk, lean meats, legumes (beans), oranges, carrots, broccoli, whole-wheat bread, and whole-grain breakfast cereals—do help balance less nutrient-dense foods—such as cookies and potato chips—which many people like to eat. The latter are often called empty-calorie foods because they tend to be high in sugar and/or fat but few other nutrients.

Eating nutrient-dense foods is especially important for people who tend to consume diets relatively low in calories. This includes some older people and those following weight-loss diets.

nutrient density The ratio derived by dividing a food's nutrient content by its calorie content. When its contribution to our need for that nutrient exceeds its contribution to our calorie need, the food is considered to have a favorable nutrient density.

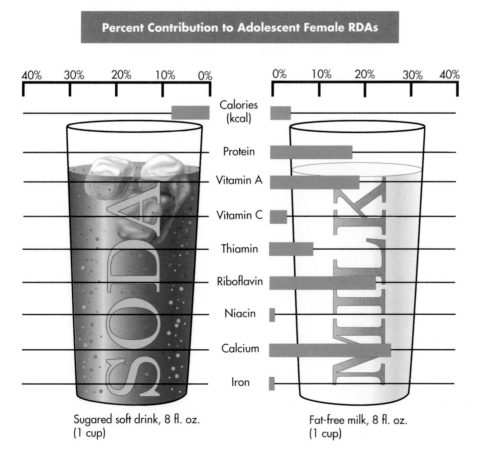

Sugared soft drink, 8 fl. oz. (1 cup)
Fat-free milk, 8 fl. oz. (1 cup)

FIGURE 2-1 ▶ Comparison of the nutrient density of a sugared soft drink with that of fat-free (i.e., nonfat or skim) milk. Choosing a glass of fat-free milk makes a significantly greater contribution to nutrient intake than does a sugared soft drink. An easy way to determine nutrient density from this chart is to compare the lengths of the bars indicating vitamin or mineral contribution with the bar that represents calorie contribution. For the soft drink, no nutrient surpasses calorie content. Fat-free milk, in contrast, has longer nutrient bars for protein, vitamin A, the vitamins thiamin and riboflavin, and the mineral calcium than it does for calories. Including many nutrient-dense foods in your diet is a lower calorie way to meet nutrient needs.

ENERGY (KCAL) DENSITY AFFECTS CALORIE INTAKE

energy density A comparison of the calorie (kcal) content of a food with the weight of the food. An energy-dense food is high in calories but weighs very little (e.g., potato chips), whereas a food low in energy density has few calories but weighs a lot, such as an orange.

MAKING DECISIONS

Some people would like to live mostly on French fries. What is the nutrient content of French fries? Check the food composition supplement for the vitamin C content of French fries. How many servings would you need to eat to meet vitamin C needs (75 to 95 milligrams)?

(Answer: 4 to 5 servings)

Energy density is a measurement that best describes the calorie content of a food. Energy density of a food is determined by comparing the calorie (kcal) content with the weight of food. A food rich in calories but that weighs relatively little is considered energy dense. Examples include nuts; cookies; fried foods in general; and fat-free snacks, such as fat-free pretzels. Foods with low energy density include fruits, vegetables, and any food that incorporates lots of water during cooking, such as oatmeal (Table 2-2).

Researchers have shown that eating a meal with many foods of low energy density promotes satiety without contributing many calories. This is probably because we consume a constant weight of food at a meal, rather than a constant number of calories. How this constant weight of food is regulated is not known, but careful laboratory studies show that people consume fewer calories in a meal if most of the food choices are low in energy density, compared with foods high in energy density. Eating a diet low in energy density can aid in losing (or maintaining) weight.

Overall, foods with lots of water and fiber provide a low-energy-density contribution to a meal and help one feel full, whereas foods with high energy density must be eaten in greater amounts to contribute to fullness. This is one more reason to support a diet rich in fruits, vegetables, and whole-grain breads and cereals, a pattern that also is typical of many ethnic diets throughout rural areas of the world.

Still, favorite foods, even if they are high in energy density, can have a place in your dietary pattern, but you will have to plan for them. For example, chocolate is a very energy-dense food, but a small portion at the end of a meal can supply a satisfying finale. In addition, foods with high energy density can help people with poor appetites, such as some older people, to maintain or gain weight.

TABLE 2-2 Energy Density of Common Foods (Listed in Relative Order)

Very Low Energy Density (less than 0.6 kcal per gram)	Low Energy Density (0.6 to 1.5 kcal per gram)	Medium Energy Density (1.5 to 4 kcal per gram)	High Energy Density (greater than 4 kcal per gram)
Lettuce	Whole milk	Eggs	Graham crackers
Tomatoes	Oatmeal	Ham	Fat-free sandwich cookies
Strawberries	Cottage cheese	Pumpkin pie	Chocolate
Broccoli	Beans	Whole-wheat bread	Chocolate chip cookies
Salsa	Bananas	Bagels	Tortilla chips
Grapefruit	Broiled fish	White bread	Bacon
Fat-free milk	Fat-free yogurt	Raisins	Potato chips
Carrots	Ready-to-eat breakfast cereals with 1% low-fat milk	Cream cheese	Peanuts
Vegetable soup		Cake with frosting	Peanut butter
		Pretzels	Mayonnaise
	Plain baked potato	Rice cakes	Butter or margarine
	Cooked rice		Vegetable oils
	Spaghetti noodles		

Data adapted from Rolls B, Barnett RA: *Volumetrics.* New York: HarperCollins, 2000.

▲ Today, soft drinks are more popular than milk, but not as beneficial to the diet. Soft drinks account for about 10% of the calorie intake of teenagers in North America and in turn contribute to generally poor calcium intakes seen in this age group.

The following sections of Chapter 2 describe various states of nutritional health and provide tools and nutrient guidelines for planning healthy diets to support overall health.

CONCEPT CHECK

Basic diet-planning concepts include consuming a variety of foods, balancing a diet by consuming foods from each of the five food groups, and moderating portion size with each food choice, so that the diet is not excessive in calories. Choosing nutrient-dense foods, such as fat-free milk, fruits, vegetables, and whole-grain breads and cereals, helps supply a diet with many nutrients but not excessive calories. Many of these foods are also rich sources of phytochemicals, supplying an even greater health benefit to the diet. Consuming foods of low energy density, such as fruits and vegetables, may also help in weight control, in that these provide satiety after a meal because of their large weight but relatively few calories.

STATES OF NUTRITIONAL HEALTH

The body's nutritional health is determined by considering the **nutritional state** of each needed nutrient. Three general categories of nutritional status are recognized: desirable nutrition, undernutrition, and overnutrition. The amount of each nutrient needed to maintain a state of desirable nutrition is the basis for published dietary intake recommendations. The diet plans to meet those needs are discussed later in Chapter 2. The common term **malnutrition** can refer to either **overnutrition** or **undernutrition**. Neither state is conducive to good health.

▲ Salads are low in energy density if we limit additional calories from salad dressing and especially minimize bacon bits, cheese crumbles or cubes, and croutons.

Desirable Nutrition

The nutritional state for a particular nutrient is desirable when body tissues have enough of the nutrient to support normal metabolic functions as well as surplus stores that can be used in times of increased need. A desirable nutritional state can be achieved by obtaining essential nutrients from a variety of foods.

Undernutrition

Undernutrition occurs when nutrient intake does not meet nutrient needs. Any surpluses are then put to use and health begins to decline. Many nutrients are in high demand due to the constant cell loss and regeneration in the body, such as in the gastrointestinal tract. For this reason the stores of certain nutrients, including many of the B vitamins, are exhausted rapidly and therefore require a regular intake. In addition, some women in North America do not consume sufficient iron to meet monthly losses and eventually deplete their iron stores (Fig. 2-2).

Once availability of a nutrient falls sufficiently low, biochemical evidence indicates that the body's metabolic processes have slowed or stopped. At this state of deficiency there are no outward **symptoms**, thus it is termed a **subclinical** deficiency. A subclinical deficiency can go on for some time before clinicians are able to detect its effects.

Eventually clinical symptoms will develop. Clinical evidence of a nutritional deficiency; perhaps in the skin, hair, nails, tongue, or eyes, sometimes takes many years. Often, clinicians do not detect a problem until a deficiency produces outward symptoms, such as small areas of bruising on the skin from a vitamin C deficiency.

Overnutrition

Prolonged consumption of more nutrients than the body needs can lead to overnutrition. In the short run (e.g., 1 to 2 weeks), overnutrition may cause only a few symptoms, such as stomach distress from excess iron intake. But if an excess

nutritional state The nutritional health of a person as determined by anthropometric measurements (height, weight, circumferences, and so on), biochemical measurements of nutrients or their by-products in blood and urine, a clinical (physical) examination, a dietary analysis, and economic evaluation; also called nutritional status.

malnutrition Failing health that results from long-standing dietary practices that do not coincide with nutritional needs.

overnutrition A state in which nutritional intake greatly exceeds the body's needs.

undernutrition Failing health that results from a long-standing dietary intake that is not enough to meet nutritional needs.

symptom A change in health status noted by the person with the problem, such as stomach pain.

subclinical Stage of a disease or disorder not severe enough to produce symptoms that can be detected or diagnosed.

FIGURE 2-2 ▶ The general scheme of nutritional status. Green reflects good status, yellow marginal status, and red poor status (undernutrition or overnutrition). This general concept can be applied to all nutrients. Iron was chosen as an example because iron deficiency is the most common nutrient deficiency worldwide.

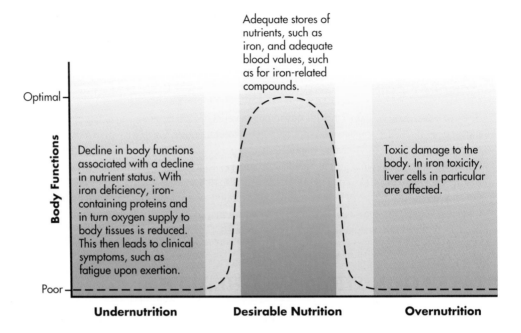

Adequate stores of nutrients, such as iron, and adequate blood values, such as for iron-related compounds.

Decline in body functions associated with a decline in nutrient status. With iron deficiency, iron-containing proteins and in turn oxygen supply to body tissues is reduced. This then leads to clinical symptoms, such as fatigue upon exertion.

Toxic damage to the body. In iron toxicity, liver cells in particular are affected.

Undernutrition   **Desirable Nutrition**   **Overnutrition**

intake continues, some nutrients may accumulate to toxic amounts, which can lead to serious disease. For example, too much vitamin A during pregnancy can cause birth defects.

The most common type of overnutrition in developed nations is an excess intake of calories often leading to obesity. In the long run, outcomes of obesity include other serious diseases, such as type 2 diabetes and certain forms of cancer. Use the website shapeup.org to learn more about the importance of lifelong weight control.

For most vitamins and minerals, the gap between desirable intake and overnutrition is wide. Therefore, even if people take a typical balanced multivitamin and mineral supplement daily, they probably won't receive a harmful dose of any nutrient. The difference between desirable intake and overnutrition is smallest for vitamin A and the minerals calcium, iron, and copper. Thus, if you take nutrient supplements, keep a close eye on your total vitamin and mineral intake from both food and supplements to avoid toxicity (see Chapter 9 for further advice on use of nutrient supplements).

HOW CAN YOUR NUTRITIONAL STATE BE MEASURED?

To find out how nutritionally fit *you* are, a nutritional assessment—either whole or in part—needs to be performed (Table 2-3). Generally, this is performed by a physician, often with the aid of a registered dietitian.

Analyzing Background Factors

Since family health history plays an important role in determining nutritional and health status, it must be carefully recorded and critically analyzed as part of a nutritional assessment. Other related background information includes: (1) a medical history, especially for any disease states or treatments that could decrease nutrient absorption or ultimate use; (2) a list of medications taken; (3) a social history (e.g., marital status, living conditions); (4) level of education to determine the degree of complexity that can be used in written materials and oral discussions; and (5) economic status to determine the ability to purchase, transport, and cook food.

▲ The most common type of overnutrition in North America is the excess intake of calories, which often leads to obesity.

TABLE 2-3 Conducting an Evaluation of Nutritional Health

Parameters	Example
Background	Medical history (e.g., current diseases, past surgeries, current weight, weight history, and current medications)
	Social history (marital status, living conditions)
	Family health history
	Education attainment
	Economic status
Nutritional	Anthropometric assessment: height, weight, skinfold thickness, arm muscle circumference, and other parameters
	Biochemical (laboratory) assessment of blood and urine: enzyme activities, concentrations of nutrients or their by-products
	Clinical assessment (physical examination): general appearance of skin, eyes, and tongue; rapid hair loss; sense of touch; ability to walk
	Dietary assessment: usual intake or record of previous days' meals

Evaluating the ABCDEs

In addition to background factors, four nutritional assessment categories complete the picture of nutritional status. **Anthropometric** measurements of height, weight (and weight changes), skinfold thicknesses, and body circumferences provide information about the current state of nutrition. Measures of body composition are easy to obtain and are generally reliable. However, an in-depth examination of nutritional health is impossible without the more expensive process of **biochemical assessment.** This involves the measurement of the concentrations of nutrients and nutrient by-products in the blood, urine, and feces and of specific blood enzyme activities.

A **clinical assessment** would follow, during which a health professional would search for any physical evidence (e.g., high blood pressure) of diet-related diseases or deficiencies. Then, a close look at the person's diet (**dietary assessment**), including a record of at least the previous few days' food intake, would determine any possible problem areas. Finally, adding the **economic assessment** (from the background analysis) provides further details about the ability to purchase and prepare foods needed to maintain health. Now the true nutritional state of a person emerges. Taken together, these five assessments form the ABCDEs of nutritional assessment: **a**nthropometric, **b**iochemical, **c**linical, **d**ietary, and **e**conomic (Fig. 2-3).

MAKING DECISIONS

Nutritional Assessment

A practical example using the ABCDEs for evaluating nutritional state can be illustrated in a person who chronically abuses alcohol. Upon evaluation, the physician notes:

(A) Low weight-for-height, recent 10 pound weight loss, muscle wasting in the upper body
(B) Low amounts of the vitamins thiamin and folate in the blood
(C) Psychological confusion, facial sores, and uncoordinated movement
(D) Dietary intake of little more than wine and hamburgers for the last week
(E) Currently residing in a homeless shelter; $35.00 in wallet; unemployed

Evaluation: This person needs medical attention, including nutrient repletion.

Recognizing the Limitations of Nutritional Assessment

A long time may elapse between the initial development of poor nutritional health and the first clinical evidence of a problem. Recall that a diet high in saturated (typically solid) fat often increases blood cholesterol, but without producing any

anthropometric assessment Measurement of body weight and the lengths, circumferences, and thicknesses of parts of the body.

biochemical assessment Measurement of biochemical functions (e.g., concentrations of nutrient by-products or enzyme activities in the blood or urine) related to a nutrient's function.

clinical assessment Examination of general appearance of skin, eyes, and tongue; evidence of rapid hair loss; sense of touch; and ability to cough and walk.

dietary assessment Estimation of typical food choices relying mostly on the recounting of one's usual intake or a record of one's previous days' intake.

economic assessment Estimation of the ability of the person to purchase, transport, and cook food. The person's weekly budget for food purchases is also a key factor to consider.

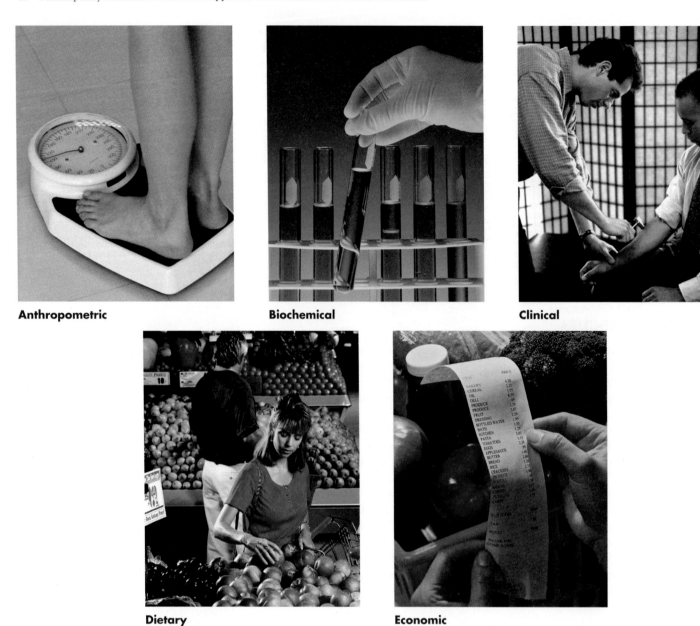

Anthropometric   **Biochemical**   **Clinical**

Dietary   **Economic**

FIGURE 2-3 ▶ Anthropometric, biochemical, clinical, and dietary information help determine a person's nutritional state. Economic status adds further information, rounding out the ABCDEs of nutritional assessment.

heart attack Rapid fall in heart function caused by reduced blood flow through the heart's blood vessels. Often part of the heart dies in the process. Technically called a myocardial infarction.

clinical evidence for years. However, when the blood vessels become sufficiently blocked by cholesterol and other materials, chest pain during physical activity or a **heart attack** may occur. An active area of nutrition research is the development of better methods for early detection of nutrition-related problems such as heart attack risk.

Another example of a serious health condition with delayed symptoms is low bone density resulting from a calcium deficiency—a particularly relevant issue for adolescent and young adult females. Many young women do not consume the needed amount of calcium but suffer no obvious effects in their younger years. However, the bone structures of these women with low calcium intakes do not reach full potential during the years of growth, making osteoporosis more likely later in life.

Furthermore, clinical symptoms of some nutritional deficiencies—diarrhea, an inability to walk normally, and facial sores—are not very specific. These may have different causes. The long time it takes for symptoms to develop and their potential to be vague often make it difficult to establish a link between an individual's current diet and nutritional state.

Concern About the State of Your Nutritional Health Is Important

Table 1-7 in Chapter 1 portrayed the close relationship between nutrition and health. The good news is that people who focus on maintaining nutritional health are apt to enjoy a long, vigorous life. For example, a recent study found that women with a healthy lifestyle had a decreased risk for heart attacks (80% reduction) compared to women without such healthy practices. The healthy habits included:

- Consumed a healthy diet
  - Varied
  - Rich in fiber
  - Included some fish
  - Low in animal fat and *trans* fat
- Maintained a healthy weight
- Occasionally consumed alcohol in small amounts
- Exercised for at least 30 minutes daily
- Avoided use of tobacco

Should all adults follow this example (with optional use of alcohol)?

▲ The first evidence that one's diet is out of balance with one's physiology could be a heart attack. About 25% of heart attack victims do not survive the event.

CONCEPT CHECK

A desirable nutritional state results when the body has enough nutrients to function fully and contains stores to use in times of increased needs. When nutrient intake fails to meet body needs, undernutrition develops. Symptoms of such an inadequate nutrient intake can take months or years to develop. Overloading the body with nutrients, leading to overnutrition, is another potential problem to avoid. Nutritional state can be assessed by using anthropometric, biochemical, clinical, dietary, and economic assessments (ABCDEs).

RECOMMENDATIONS FOR FOOD CHOICE

The following sections of Chapter 2 will describe various guidelines for planning healthy diets.

MyPyramid—A Menu-Planning Tool

Since the early twentieth century, researchers have worked to translate the science of nutrition into practical terms, so that people with no special training could estimate whether their nutritional needs were being met. The United States Department of Agriculture (USDA) simplified the recommendation by the mid-1950s to a four food-group plan: a milk group, a meat group, a fruit and vegetable group, and a bread and cereal group. In 1992 this plan was illustrated using a pyramid shape (i.e., Food Guide Pyramid).

In April 2005, USDA unveiled their latest food guide plan, MyPyramid. Entitled "Steps to a Healthier You," MyPyramid replaces the Food Guide Pyramid and provides a more individualized approach to improving diet and lifestyle than previous food guides. Its goal is to provide advice that will help us live longer, better, and healthier lives.

MyPyramid.gov
STEPS TO A HEALTHIER YOU

▶ Appendix C contains Canada's Food Guide.

discretionary calories The calories allowed in a diet after the person has met overall nutrition needs. This generally small amount of calories gives individuals the flexibility to consume some foods and beverages that may contain alcohol (e.g., beer and wine), added sugars (e.g., soft drinks, candy, and desserts), or added fats that are part of moderate- or high-fat foods (e.g., many snack foods).

▶ What about physical activity as part of MyPyramid? Physical activity is movement of the body that uses energy. Walking, gardening, briskly pushing a baby stroller, climbing the stairs, playing soccer, or dancing the night away are all examples of physical activity. For health benefits, physical activity should be moderate or vigorous and add up to at least 30 minutes on most or all days of the week.

The MyPyramid symbol represents the recommended proportion of foods from each food group to create a healthy diet. Physical activity is a new element in the pyramid. To get the individualized advice that is the hallmark of the plan, however, consumers need to use the website, MyPyramid.gov.

MyPyramid is designed to illustrate personalization, gradual improvement, activity, variety, proportionality, and moderation. These concepts are explained in Figure 2-4. Consumer messages have also been developed to help us navigate MyPyramid (Fig. 2-5).

An innovative aspect of MyPyramid is the interactive technology found on MyPyramid. gov. This includes:

MyPyramid Plan—providing a quick estimate of what and how much food the individual should eat from the different food groups based on age, gender, and activity level.

Inside MyPyramid—providing in-depth information for every food group, including recommended daily amounts in commonly used measures, such as cups and ounces, with examples and everyday tips. The section also includes recommendations for choosing healthy oils, **discretionary calories,** and physical activity. See Making Decisions for an estimation of discretionary calories. This refers to the calories allowed from food choices rich in added sugars or solid fat. The overall intent is not to exceed the discretionary calorie allowance from the combination of calories from foods and beverages with calories from alcohol, added sugars, or added fats. For most of us very few discretionary calories are available in daily diet planning.

MyPyramid Tracker—allows the user to select from 8000 foods and 600 activities and provides more detailed information on diet quality and physical activity status by comparing a day's worth of foods eaten to the guidance provided by MyPyramid. Nutrition and physical activity messages are based on the need to maintain current weight or to lose weight.

Start Today—provides tips and resources that include downloadable suggestions on all the food groups and physical activity and a worksheet to track one's diet.

▲ **Sedentary** means a lifestyle that includes only the light physical activity associated with typical day-to-day life.

MAKING DECISIONS

Discretionary Calories

Discretionary calories are estimated as follows:

Calorie Intake (kcal)	Discretionary Calories (kcal)	Calorie Intake (kcal)	Discretionary Calories (kcal)
1000	165*	2200	290
1200	171*	2400	362
1400	171*	2600	410
1600	132	2800	426
1800	195	3000	512
2000	267	3200	648

*The amount of discretionary calories is higher for 1000–1400 kcal diets than for a 1600 kcal diet because these lower calorie diets are intended for children 2–8 years of age. Adult calorie recommendations typically start at 1600 kcal.

Putting MyPyramid into Action. To put MyPyramid into action, first you need to estimate your calorie needs (the website helps you calculate this). Figure 2-6 provides a rough guide. Overall, MyPyramid translates the latest nutrition advice into twelve separate pyramids based on calorie needs (1000 to 3200 kcal).

Activity
Activity is represented by the steps and the person climbing them, as a reminder of the importance of daily physical activity.

Moderation
Moderation is represented by the narrowing of each food group from bottom to top. The wider base stands for foods with little or no solid fats or added sugars. These should be selected more often. The narrower top area stands for foods containing more added sugars and solid fats. The more active you are, the more of these foods can fit into your diet.

Personalization
Personalization is shown by the person on the steps, the slogan, and the Web site. Find the kinds and amounts of food to eat each day at MyPyramid.gov.

Proportionality
Proportionality is shown by the different widths of the food group bands. The widths suggest how much food a person should choose from each group. The widths are just a general guide, not exact proportions. Check the Web site for how much is right for you.

Variety
Variety is symbolized by the 6 color bands representing the 5 food groups of the Pyramid and oils. This illustrates that foods from all groups are needed each day for good health.

Gradual Improvement
Gradual improvement is encouraged by the slogan. It suggests that individuals can benefit from taking small steps to improve their diet and lifestyle each day.

MyPyramid.gov
STEPS TO A HEALTHIER YOU

| Grains | Vegetables | Fruits | Oils | Milk | Meat & Beans |

FIGURE 2-4 ▶ The anatomy of MyPyramid. USDA's MyPyramid symbolizes a personalized approach to healthy eating and physical activity. The symbol was designed to be simple. It was developed to remind consumers to make healthy food choices and to be active every day. In this figure, the different parts of the symbol are described.

Grains *Make half your grains whole*	Vegetables *Vary your veggies*	Fruits *Focus on fruits*	Milk *Get your calcium-rich foods*	Meat & Beans *Go lean with protein*
Eat at least 3 oz. of whole-grain cereals, breads, crackers, rice, or pasta every day 1 oz. is about 1 slice of bread; about 1 cup of breakfast cereal; or 1/2 cup of cooked rice, cereal, or pasta	Eat more dark-green veggies like broccoli, spinach, and other dark leafy greens Eat more orange vegetables like carrots and sweet potatoes Eat more dry beans and peas like pinto beans, kidney beans, and lentils	Eat a variety of fruit Choose fresh, frozen, canned, or dried fruit Go easy on fruit juices	Go low-fat or fat-free when you choose milk, yogurt, and other milk products If you don't or can't consume milk, choose lactose-free products or other calcium sources such as fortified foods and beverages	Choose low-fat or lean meats and poultry Bake it, broil it, or grill it Vary your protein routine – choose more fish, beans, peas, nuts, and seeds

For a 2,000-calorie diet, you need the amounts below from each food group. To find the amounts that are right for you, go to MyPyramid.gov

| Eat 6 oz. every day | Eat 2 1/2 cups every day | Eat 2 cups every day | Get 3 cups every day; for kids aged 2 to 8, it's 2 | Eat 5 1/2 oz. every day |

Find your balance between food and physical activity
- Be sure to stay within your daily calorie needs.
- Be physically active for at least 30 minutes most days of the week.
- About 60 minutes a day of physical activity may be needed to prevent weight gain.
- For sustaining weight loss, at least 60 to 90 minutes a day of physical activity may be required.
- Children and teenagers should be physically active for 60 minutes every day, or most days.

Know the limits on fats, sugars, and salt (sodium)
- Make most of your fat sources from fish, nuts, and vegetable oils.
- Limit solid fats like butter, stick margarine, shortening, and lard, as well as foods that contain these.
- Check the Nutrition Facts label to keep saturated fats, *trans* fats, and sodium low.
- Choose food and beverages low in added sugars. Added sugars contribute calories with few, if any, nutrients

FIGURE 2-5 ▶ These consumer messages have been developed by the USDA to help you navigate MyPyramid. The amounts shown for each food group are for a 2000 kcal diet. The amounts for other diets are shown in Table 2-4.

Calorie Range (kcal)		
Children	Sedentary ⟶	Active
2–3 years	1000 ⟶	1400
Females		
4–8 years	1200 ⟶	1800
9–13	1600 ⟶	2200
14–18	1800 ⟶	2400
19–30	2000 ⟶	2400
31–50	1800 ⟶	2200
51+	1600 ⟶	2200
Males		
4–8 years	1400 ⟶	2000
9–13	1800 ⟶	2600
14–18	2200 ⟶	3200
19–30	2400 ⟶	3000
31–50	2200 ⟶	3000
51+	2000 ⟶	2800

FIGURE 2-6 ▶ Estimates of calorie needs (kcals) provided by MyPyramid.

Once you have determined the calorie allowance appropriate for you, you can use Table 2-4 to discover how that calorie allowance corresponds to the recommended number of servings from each food group.

What Counts as One Serving?

MyPyramid provides serving sizes of foods for the various food groups in household units. Pay close attention to the stated serving size for each choice when following MyPyramid. This helps control total calorie intake. See Figure 2-7 for a convenient guide to estimating common serving size measurements.

- **Grains:** 1 slice of bread; 1 cup of ready-to-eat breakfast cereal, or ½ cup cooked rice, pasta, or cereal counts as a 1-ounce equivalent.
- **Vegetables:** 1 cup of raw or cooked vegetables or vegetable juice or 2 cups of raw leafy greens.
- **Fruits:** 1 cup of fruit or 100% fruit juice or ½ cup of dried fruit.
- **Milk:** 1 cup of milk or yogurt, 1.5 ounces of natural cheese, or 2 ounces of processed cheese.
- **Meat & Beans:** 1 ounce of meat, poultry, or fish; 1 egg; 1 tablespoon of peanut butter; ¼ cup cooked dry beans, or ½ ounce of nuts or seeds are all 1-ounce equivalents.
- **Oils:** A teaspoon of any oil from plants or fish that is liquid at room temperature counts as a serving, as do such servings of foods rich in oils (e.g., mayonnaise and soft margarine).

TABLE 2-4 MyPyramid Recommendations for Daily Food Consumption Based on Calorie Needs and Resulting in Twelve Separate Pyramids

Daily Amount of Food From Each Group												
Calorie Level	1000	1200	1400	1600	1800	2000	2200	2400	2600	2800	3000	3200
Fruits	1 cup	1 cup	1.5 cups	1.5 cups	1.5 cups	2 cups	2 cups	2 cups	2 cups	2.5 cups	2.5 cups	2.5 cups
Vegetables[1,2]	1 cup	1.5 cups	1.5 cups	2 cups	2.5 cups	2.5 cups	3 cups	3 cups	3.5 cups	3.5 cups	4 cups	4 cups
Grains[3]	3 oz-eq	4 oz-eq	5 oz-eq	5 oz-eq	6 oz-eq	6 oz-eq	7 oz-eq	8 oz-eq	9 oz-eq	10 oz-eq	10 oz-eq	10 oz-eq
Meat & Beans	2 oz-eq	3 oz-eq	4 oz-eq	5 oz-eq	5 oz-eq	5.5 oz-eq	6 oz-eq	6.5 oz-eq	6.5 oz-eq	7 oz-eq	7 oz-eq	7 oz-eq
Milk[4]	2 cups	2 cups	2 cups	3 cups	3 cups	3 cups	3 cups	3 cups	3 cups	3 cups	3 cups	3 cups
Oils[5]	3 tsp	4 tsp	4 tsp	5 tsp	5 tsp	6 tsp	6 tsp	7 tsp	8 tsp	8 tsp	10 tsp	11 tsp
Discretionary calorie allowance[6]	165	171	171	132	195	267	290	362	410	426	512	648

oz-eq stands for ounce equivalent; tsp stands for teaspoon

[1]Vegetables are divided into five subgroups (dark green, orange, legumes, starchy, and other). Over a week's time, a variety of vegetables should be eaten, especially green and orange vegetables.

[2]Dry beans and peas can be counted *either* as vegetables (dry beans and peas subgroup), *or* in the meat & beans group. Generally, individuals who regularly eat meat, poultry, and fish would count dry beans and peas in the vegetable group. Individuals who seldom eat meat, poultry, or fish (vegetarians) would consume more dry beans and peas and count some of them in the meat & beans group until enough servings from that group are chosen for the day.

[3]At least half of the grain servings should be whole-grain varieties.

[4]Most of the milk servings should be fat-free or low-fat.

[5]Limit solid fats such as butter, stick margarine, shortening, and meat fat, as well as foods that contain these.

[6]Discretionary calories refers to food choices rich in added sugars or solid fat.

Grains	1 yo-yo	=	2 ounces	Bagel or English muffin
Vegetables	1 baseball	=	1 cup	Green beans
Fruits	1 tennis ball	=	½ to ⅔ cup	Medium/small apple
Oils	1 golf ball	=	2 tbsp	Salad dressing, peanut butter, margarine, etc.
Milk	4 dice	=	1 ounce	Cheese
Meat & Beans	1 deck of cards	=	3 ounces	Meat, chicken or fish

FIGURE 2-7 ▶ A yo-yo, baseball, tennis ball, golf ball, dice, and deck of cards make convenient guides to judge MyPyramid serving sizes. Additional handy guides include:

Matchbox = 1 oz of meat
Bar of soap = 3 oz of meat
Computer mouse = ½ cup of chopped foods

1 ice cream scoop = ½ cup
Ping-pong ball = 2 tbsp
4 golf balls = 1 cup of dry cereal

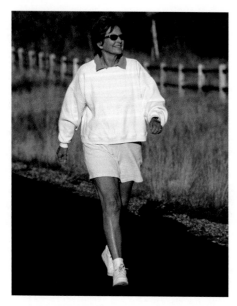

▲ **Active** means a lifestyle that includes physical activity equivalent to walking more than 3 miles per day at 3 to 4 miles per hour, in addition to the light physical activity associated with typical day-to-day life.

Menu Planning with MyPyramid

Remember the following points when using MyPyramid to plan your daily menus:

1. The guide does not apply to infants or children under 2 years of age.
2. No one food is absolutely essential to good nutrition. Each food is rich in some nutrients, but deficient in at least one essential nutrient (Table 2-5).
3. No one food group provides all essential nutrients in adequate amounts. Each food group makes an important, distinctive contribution to nutritional intake.
4. Variety is the key to success of MyPyramid and is first guaranteed by choosing foods from all the groups. Furthermore, one should consume a variety of foods within each group, except possibly in the milk, yogurt, and cheese group.
5. The foods within a group may vary widely with respect to nutrients and calories. For example, the calorie content of 3 ounces of baked potato is 98 kcal, whereas that of 3 ounces of potato chips is 470 kcal. Compare an orange and an apple with respect to vitamin C using the food composition table in the supplement.

Overall, MyPyramid incorporates the foundations of a healthy diet: variety, balance, and moderation. The nutritional adequacy of diets planned using this tool, however, depends on selection of a variety of foods (Table 2-6). In addition, vitamin E, vitamin B-6, magnesium, and zinc are nutrients sometimes low in diets based on this plan. To ensure enough of these nutrients, consider the following advice:

1. Choose primarily low-fat and fat-free items from the milk group. By reducing calorie intake in this way, you can select more items from other food groups. If milk causes intestinal gas and bloating, emphasize yogurt and cheese (see Chapter 4 for details on the problem of lactose maldigestion and lactose intolerance).

▲ Typical restaurant portions contain numerous servings from the individual groups in MyPyramid.

TABLE 2-5 Nutrient Contributions of Groups in the MyPyramid Food Guide Plan

Food Category	Major Nutrient Contributions
Grains	Carbohydrate Vitamins such as thiamin Minerals such as iron Fiber*
Vegetables	Carbohydrate Vitamins such as plant pigments that form vitamin A Minerals such as magnesium Fiber
Fruits	Carbohydrate Vitamins such as folate and vitamin C Minerals such as potassium Fiber
Oils	Fat Essential fatty acids Vitamins such as vitamin E
Milk	Carbohydrate Protein Vitamins such as vitamin D Minerals such as calcium and phosphorus
Meat & Beans	Protein Vitamins such as vitamin B-6 Minerals such as iron and zinc

*Whole-grain varieties

TABLE 2-6 Putting the MyPyramid into Practice. This menu meets nutrient needs for all vitamins and minerals for an average adult that needs 1800 kcal. For adolescents, teenagers, and older adults add one additional serving of milk or other calcium-rich sources.

Meal	Food Group
Breakfast	
1 small orange	Fruits
¾ cup Healthy Choice Low-fat Granola	Grains
with ½ cup fat-free milk	Milk
½ toasted, small raisin bagel	Grains
with 1 tsp soft margarine	Oils
Optional: coffee or tea	
Lunch	
Turkey sandwich	
2 slices whole-wheat bread	Grains
2 oz turkey	Meat & Beans
2 tsp mustard	
1 small apple	Fruits
2 oatmeal-raisin cookies (small)	Discretionary calories
Optional: diet soft drink	
3 P.M. Study Break	
6 whole-wheat crackers	Grains
1 tbsp peanut butter	Meat & Beans
½ cup fat-free milk	Milk
Dinner	
Tossed salad	
1 cup romaine lettuce	Vegetables
½ cup sliced tomatoes	Vegetables
1½ tbsp Italian dressing	Oils
½ carrot, grated	Vegetables
3 oz broiled salmon	Meat & Beans
½ cup rice	Grains
½ cup green beans	Vegetables
with 1 tsp soft margarine	Oils
Optional: coffee or tea	
Late-Night Snack	
1 cup "light" fruit yogurt	Milk
Nutrient Breakdown	
1800 kcal	
Carbohydrate	56% of kcal
Protein	18% of kcal
Fat	26% of kcal

2. Include plant foods that are good sources of proteins, such as beans and nuts, at least several times a week because many are rich in vitamins (such as vitamin E), minerals (such as magnesium), and fiber.

3. For vegetables and fruits, try to include a dark green vegetable for vitamin A and a vitamin C–rich fruit, such as an orange, every day. Don't focus primarily on potatoes (e.g., French fries) for your vegetable choices. Surveys show that fewer than 5% of adults eat a full serving of a dark green vegetable on any given day. Increased consumption of these foods is important because they contribute vitamins, minerals, fiber, and phytochemicals.

4. Choose whole-grain varieties of breads, cereals, rice, and pasta because they contribute vitamin E and fiber. A plate about two-thirds covered by grains, fruits, and vegetables and one-third or less covered by protein-rich foods promotes this diet advice. A daily serving of a whole-grain, ready-to-eat breakfast cereal is an excellent choice because the vitamins (such as vitamin B-6) and minerals (such as zinc) typically added to it, along with fiber, help fill in the potential gaps listed earlier.

5. Include some plant oils on a daily basis, such as those in salad dressing, and eat fish at least twice a week. This supplies you with health-promoting essential fatty acids.

MAKING DECISIONS

Household Units

Common household units are listed here with their metric equivalents. Ounces and fluid ounces differ. Ounces are a measure of weight, while fluid ounces are a measure of volume. Fluid ounces are based on the corresponding volume of water as the standard; 1 ounce of water by weight equals one fluid ounce. Any fluid more or less dense than water will yield a different number of fluid ounces per ounce of material.

3 teaspoons	= 1 tablespoon	= 15 grams
4 tablespoons	= ¼ cup	= 60 grams
5⅓ tablespoons	= ⅓ cup	= 80 grams
8 tablespoons	= ½ cup	= 120 grams
10⅔ tablespoons	= ⅔ cup	= 160 grams
16 tablespoons	= 1 cup	= 240 grams
1 tablespoon	= ½ fluid ounce	= 15 milliliters
1 cup	= 8 fluid ounces	= 240 milliliters
1 cup	= ½ pint	= 240 grams
2 cups	= 1 pint	= 480 grams
4 cups	= 1 quart	= 960 grams = 1 liter
2 pints	= 1 quart	= 960 grams = 1 liter
4 quarts	= 1 gallon	= 3840 grams = 4 liters

How Does Your Current Diet Rate?

Regularly comparing your daily food intake with MyPyramid recommendations for your age, gender, and degree of physical activity, is a relatively simple way to evaluate your overall diet. Strive to meet the recommendations. (The diets of most adults fail in this evaluation, especially with respect to milk, vegetables, fruits, and whole-grain breads and cereals.) If that is not possible, identify the nutrients that are low in your diet based on the nutrients found in each food group (review Table 2-5). For example, if you do not consume enough servings from the milk group, your calcium intake is most likely too low. You need to then find foods that you enjoy that supply calcium, such as calcium-fortified orange juice. Customizing MyPyramid to accommodate your food habits may seem a daunting task, but it is not difficult once you gain some additional nutrition knowledge.

▲ Leafy green vegetables contribute many nutrients to a diet.

Get Going

Start putting MyPyramid into practice and use the MyTracker feature to follow your progress. Implementing even small diet and exercise changes can have positive results. Better health will likely follow as you strive to meet your nutrient needs and balance your physical activity and calorie allowance. In addition, follow the guidance from the **2005 Dietary Guidelines for Americans** regarding alcohol and sodium intake and safe food preparation.

Dietary Guidelines for Americans General goals for nutrient intakes and diet composition set by the USDA and the U.S. Department of Health and Human Services.

CONCEPT CHECK

MyPyramid translates the general needs for carbohydrate, protein, fat, vitamins, and minerals into the recommended number of daily servings from each of five major food groups and oils. It is a convenient and valuable tool for planning daily menus.

Dietary Guidelines—Another Tool for Menu Planning

MyPyramid was designed to help meet nutritional needs for carbohydrate, fat, vitamins, and minerals. However, most of the major chronic "killer" diseases in North America, such as cardiovascular disease, cancer, and alcoholism, are not primarily associated with deficiencies of these nutrients. Deficiency diseases such as scurvy (vitamin C deficiency) and pellagra (niacin deficiency) are no longer common. For many North Americans, the primary dietary culprit is an overconsumption of one or more of the following: calories, saturated fat, cholesterol, *trans* fat, alcohol, and sodium (salt). Underconsumption of calcium, iron, folate and other B-vitamins, vitamin C, vitamin D, vitamin E, potassium, magnesium, and fiber is also a problem for some people.

▶ Appendix C contains nutrient guidelines for Canadians.

In response to concerns regarding these killer disease patterns and poor dietary habits, the USDA and U.S. Department of Health and Human Services (DHHS) have published Dietary Guidelines for Americans (Dietary Guidelines for short) since 1980 to aid diet planning.

▶ A brochure designed for the public based on the 2005 Dietary Guidelines for Americans is entitled "Finding Your Way to a Healthier You." It communicates the major themes of the *2005 Dietary Guidelines for Americans*, but uses simpler messages.

The latest version of the Dietary Guidelines was published in 2005 and compared to past reports, places stronger emphasis on monitoring one's calorie intake and increasing physical activity. This is because more of us are becoming overweight each year.

The 2005 report identifies 41 key recommendations, of which 23 are for the general public and 18 are for special populations. They are grouped into nine general topics:

- Adequate Nutrient Intake Within Calorie Needs
- Weight Management
- Physical Activity
- Specific Food Groups to Encourage
- Fats
- Carbohydrates
- Sodium and Potassium
- Alcoholic Beverages
- Food Safety

Figure 2-8 lists the key recommendations for the general public within each general topic. The advice provided refers to people two years and older.

A basic premise of the Dietary Guidelines is that nutrient needs should be met primarily through consuming foods. Foods provide an array of nutrients and other compounds that may have beneficial effects on health. Fortified foods and dietary supplements, however, are especially important for people whose typical food choices cannot meet one or more nutrient recommendations, such as for vitamin E or calcium. However, dietary supplements are not a substitute for a healthful diet.

Dietary Guidelines
for Americans
2005

ADEQUATE NUTRIENTS WITHIN ENERGY NEEDS

- Consume a variety of nutrient-dense foods and beverages within and among the basic food groups while choosing foods that limit the intake of saturated and *trans* fats, cholesterol, added sugars, salt, and alcohol.

- Meet recommended intakes within energy needs by adopting a balanced eating pattern, such as MyPyramid.

Key Recommendations for Specific Population Groups are listed in Chapters 16 and 18.

WEIGHT MANAGEMENT

- To maintain body weight in a healthy range, balance energy intake from foods and beverages with energy expended.

- To prevent gradual weight gain over time, make small decreases in energy intake from food and beverages and increase physical activity.

Key Recommendations for Specific Population Groups are listed in Chapters 7, 16, 17, and 18.

PHYSICAL ACTIVITY

- Engage in regular physical activity and reduce sedentary activities to promote health, psychological well-being, and a healthy body weight.

- To reduce the risk of chronic disease in adulthood: Engage in at least 30 minutes of moderate-intensity physical activity, above usual activity, at work or home on most days of the week.

- For most people, greater health benefits can be obtained by engaging in physical activity of more vigorous intensity or longer duration.

- To help manage body weight and prevent gradual, unhealthy body weight gain in adulthood: Engage in approximately 60 minutes of moderate- to vigorous-intensity activity on most days of the week while not exceeding energy needs.

- To sustain weight loss in adulthood: Participate in at least 60 to 90 minutes of daily moderate-intensity physical activity while not exceeding energy needs. Some people (men over 40 years of age and women over 50 years of age) may need to consult with a health-care provider before participating in this level of activity.

- Achieve physical fitness by including cardiovascular conditioning, stretching exercises for flexibility, and resistance exercises or calisthenics for muscle strength and endurance.

Key Recommendations for Specific Population Groups are listed in Chapters 16, 17, and 18.

FIGURE 2-8 ▶ Key Recommendations for the general public within each general topic from the latest Dietary Guidelines for Americans.

The 2005 Dietary Guidelines for Americans (and the consumer brochure) are available at www.healthierus.gov/dietaryguidelines. In general the Dietary Guidelines recommend that we:

- Consume a variety of nutrient-dense foods and beverages within and among the basic food groups of MyPyramid, while choosing foods that limit the intake of saturated and *trans* fats, cholesterol, added sugars, salt, and alcohol (if used).

FOOD GROUPS TO ENCOURAGE

- Consume a sufficient amount of fruits and vegetables while staying within energy needs. Two cups of fruit and 2 1/2 cups of vegetables per day are recommended for a reference 2000 kcal intake, with higher or lower amounts depending on one's energy needs.
- Choose a variety of fruits and vegetables each day. In particular, select from all five vegetable subgroups (dark green vegetables, orange vegetables, legumes, starchy vegetables, and other vegetables) several times a week.
- Consume 3 or more ounce-equivalents of whole-grain products per day, with the rest of the recommended grains coming from enriched or whole-grain products. In general, at least half the grains should come from whole grains.
- Consume 3 cups per day of fat-free or low-fat milk or equivalent milk products.

Key Recommendations for Specific Population Groups are listed in Chapter 17.

FATS

- Consume less than 10 percent of energy intake from saturated fatty acids and less than 300 mg per day of cholesterol, and keep *trans* fatty acid consumption as low as possible.
- Keep total fat intake between 20 to 35% of energy intake, with most fats coming from sources of polyunsaturated and monounsaturated fatty acids, such as fish, nuts, and vegetable oils.
- When selecting and preparing meat, poultry, dry beans, and milk or milk products, make choices that are lean, low-fat, or fat-free.
- Limit intake of fats and oils high in saturated and/or *trans* fatty acids, and choose products low in such fats and oils.

Key Recommendations for Specific Population Groups are listed in Chapter 17.

CARBOHYDRATES

- Choose fiber-rich fruits, vegetables, and whole grains often.
- Choose and prepare foods and beverages with little added sugars or caloric sweeteners, such as amounts suggested by MyPyramid.
- Reduce the incidence of dental caries by practicing good oral hygiene and consuming sugar- and starch-containing foods and beverages less frequently.

FIGURE 2-8 ▶ *Continued*

Foods to emphasize are vegetables, fruits, legumes (beans), whole grains, and fat-free or low-fat milk or equivalent milk products.
- Maintain body weight in a healthy range by balancing calorie intake from foods and beverages with calories expended. For the latter, engage in at least 30 minutes of moderate-intensity physical activity, above usual activity, at work or home on most days of the week.
- Practice safe food handling when preparing food. This includes cleaning hands, food contact surfaces, and fruits and vegetables before preparation and cooking foods to a safe temperature to kill microorganisms.

SODIUM AND POTASSIUM

- Consume less than 2300 mg of sodium per day (approximately 1 tsp of salt).

- Choose and prepare foods with little salt. At the same time, consume potassium-rich foods, such as fruits and vegetables.

Key Recommendations for Specific Population Groups are listed in Chapters 8 and 18.

ALCOHOLIC BEVERAGES

- Those who choose to drink alcoholic beverages should do so sensibly and in moderation—defined as the consumption of up to one drink per day for women and up to two drinks per day for men. (12 oz of a regular beer, 5 oz of wine or 1 1/2 oz of 80 proof distilled spirits count as a drink for purposes of explaining moderation.)

- Alcoholic beverages should not be consumed by some individuals, including those who cannot restrict their alcohol intake, women of childbearing age who may become pregnant, pregnant and lactating women, children and adolescents, individuals taking medications that can interact with alcohol, and those with specific medical conditions.

- Alcoholic beverages should be avoided by individuals engaging in activities that require attention, skill, or coordination, such as driving or operating machinery.

FOOD SAFETY

To avoid microbial foodborne illness:

- Clean hands, food contact surfaces, and fruits and vegetables. Meat and poultry should *not* be washed or rinsed to avoid spreading bacteria to other foods.

- Separate raw, cooked, and ready-to-eat foods while shopping, preparing, and storing foods.

- Cook foods to a safe temperature to kill microorganisms.

- Chill (refrigerate) perishable food promptly and defrost foods properly.

- Avoid raw (unpasteurized) milk or any products made from unpasteurized milk, raw or partially cooked eggs or foods containing raw eggs, or raw or undercooked meat and poultry, unpasteurized juices, and raw sprouts.

Key Recommendations for Specific Population Groups are listed in Chapters 16, 17, and 18.

FIGURE 2-8 ▶ *Continued*

CRITICAL THINKING

Shannon has grown up eating the typical American diet. Having recently read and heard many media reports about the relationship between nutrition and health, she is beginning to look critically at her diet and is considering making changes. However, she doesn't know where to begin. What advice would you give her?

Practical Use of the Dietary Guidelines

The Dietary Guidelines are designed to meet nutrient needs while reducing the risk of obesity, hypertension, cardiovascular disease, type 2 diabetes, alcoholism, and foodborne illness.

The Dietary Guidelines are not difficult to implement (Table 2-7). Despite popular misconceptions, this overall diet approach is not especially expensive. Fruits, vegetables, and low-fat and fat-free milk are no more expensive than the chips, cookies, and sugared soft drinks they should in part replace.

Diet recommendations for adults have been issued by other scientific groups, such as the American Heart Association, U.S. Surgeon General, National Academy of Sciences, American Cancer Society, Canadian Ministries of Health (see Appendix C), and

TABLE 2-7 Recommended Diet Changes Based on the Dietary Guidelines

If You Usually Eat This,	Try This Instead	Benefit
White bread	Whole-wheat bread	• Higher nutrient density, due to less processing • More fiber
Sugary breakfast cereal	Low-sugar, high-fiber cereal with fresh fruit	• Higher nutrient density • More fiber • More phytochemicals
Cheeseburger with French fries	Hamburger and baked beans	• Less saturated fat and *trans* fat • Less cholesterol • More fiber • More phytochemicals
Potato salad	Three-bean salad	• More fiber • More phytochemicals
Doughnuts	Bran muffin/bagel with light cream cheese	• More fiber • Less fat
Regular soft drinks	Diet soft drinks	• Fewer calories
Boiled vegetables	Steamed vegetables	• Higher nutrient density, due to reduced loss of water-soluble vitamins
Canned vegetables	Fresh or frozen vegetables	• Higher nutrient density, due to reduced loss of heat-sensitive vitamins • Lower in sodium
Fried meats	Broiled meats	• Less saturated fat
Fatty meats, such as ribs or bacon	Lean meats, such as ground round, chicken, or fish	• Less saturated fat
Whole milk	Low-fat or fat-free milk	• Less saturated fat • Fewer calories • More calcium
Ice cream	Sherbet or frozen yogurt	• Less saturated fat • Fewer calories
Mayonnaise or sour cream salad dressing	Oil and vinegar dressings or light creamy dressings	• Less saturated fat • Less cholesterol • Fewer calories
Cookies	Popcorn (air popped with minimal margarine or butter)	• Fewer calories and *trans* fat
Heavily salted foods	Foods flavored primarily with herbs, spices, lemon juice	• Lower in sodium
Chips	Pretzels	• Less fat

▲ Choose low-sugar, high-fiber cereal with fresh fruit instead of sugary breakfast cereal.

▶ Choose popcorn and pretzels instead of cookies and chips.

▶ Advice from the American Dietetic Association suggests five basic principles with regard to diet and health.

- Be realistic, making small changes over time.
- Be adventurous, trying new foods regularly.
- Be flexible, balancing some sweet and fatty foods with physical activity.
- Be sensible, including favorite foods in smaller portions.
- Finally, be active, including physical activity in daily life.

▶ Although nutrition recommendations are often made for the entire healthy population, each of us have individual needs based on our particular health status and genetic background. It would be more appropriate, but also more expensive, if recommendations were made on an individual basis once a person's health status is known.

World Health Organization. All are consistent with the spirit of the Dietary Guidelines. These groups encourage people to modify their eating behavior in ways that are both healthful and pleasurable.

The Dietary Guidelines and You

When using the Dietary Guidelines, you should consider your state of health. Make specific changes and see whether they are effective. Results are sometimes disappointing, even when you are following a diet change very closely. Some people can eat a lot of saturated fat and still keep blood cholesterol under control. Other people, unfortunately, have high blood cholesterol even if they eat a diet low in saturated fat. Differences in genetic background are a key reason for these different responses, as you will learn in Chapter 3. Thus, we have different individual nutritional needs and risks of developing certain diseases. One's diet should be planned with this individuality in mind, taking into account when possible, one's current health status and family history for specific diseases. However, tailoring a unique nutrition program for every North American citizen is currently unrealistic. MyPyramid and the 2005 Dietary Guidelines provide typical adults with simple advice, which can be actively practiced by anyone willing to take a step toward good health.

There is no "optimal" diet. Instead, there are numerous healthful diets. Visit the website of the International Food Information Council (www.ific.org). This site is a great resource for current nutrition information.

SPECIFIC NUTRIENT STANDARDS AND RECOMMENDATIONS

The overarching goal of any healthy diet plan is to meet nutrient needs. To begin, we must determine what amount of each essential nutrient is needed to maintain health. The standards that have been developed for such nutrient needs—DRI, RDA, AI, EER, and UL—can often seem like an alphabet soup of abbreviations. However, you can more easily sift through these nutrient standards if you have a knowledge base about their development and use (Table 2-8).

▲ Does everyone in this photo have the same nutrient needs?

TABLE 2-8 Recommendations within the Dietary Reference Intakes

RDA	Recommended Dietary Allowance. Use to evaluate your current intake for a specific nutrient. The further you stray above or below this value, the greater your chances of developing nutritional problems.
AI	Adequate Intake. Use to evaluate your current intake of nutrients, but realize that an AI designation implies that further research is required before scientists can establish a more definitive recommendation.
EER	Estimated Energy Requirement. Use to estimate calorie needs of the average person within a specific height, weight, gender, age, and physical activity pattern.
UL	Upper Level. Use to evaluate the highest amount of daily nutrient intake unlikely to cause adverse health effects in the long run in almost all people (97% to 98%) in a population. This number applies to chronic use and is set to protect even very susceptible people in the healthy general population. As intake increases above the Upper Level, the potential for adverse effects generally increases.
DV	Daily Value. Use as a rough guide for comparing the nutrient content of a food to approximate human needs. Typically, the Daily Value used on food labels refers to ages 4 years through adulthood. It is based on a 2000 kcal diet. Some Daily Values also increase slightly with higher calorie intakes (see Fig. 2-12 in the following section on food labeling).

Most of the terms that describe nutrient needs fall under one umbrella term—**Dietary Reference Intakes (DRIs).** The development of DRIs is an ongoing, collaborative effort between the Food and Nutrition Board of the Institute of Medicine in the United States and Health Canada. Included under the DRI umbrella are **Recommended Dietary Allowances (RDAs), Adequate Intakes (AIs), Estimated Energy Requirements (EERs),** and **Tolerable Upper Intake Levels (Upper Levels or ULs).**

RECOMMENDED DIETARY ALLOWANCE

A Recommended Dietary Allowance (RDA) is the recommended amount of a nutrient based on meeting the needs of nearly all individuals (about 97%) in a particular age and gender group. A person can compare his or her individual intake of specific nutrients to the RDA. Although an intake slightly above or below the RDA for a particular nutrient is no reason for concern, a significant deviation below (about 70%) or above (about three times or more for some nutrients) the RDA over an extended time can eventually result in a deficiency or toxicity of that nutrient, respectively.

Adequate Intake

An RDA can be set for a nutrient only if there is sufficient information on the human needs for that particular nutrient. Today, there is not enough information on some nutrients, such as calcium, to set such a precise standard as an RDA. For this and other nutrients, the DRIs include a category called an Adequate Intake (AI). This standard is derived from the dietary intakes of people that appear to be maintaining nutritional health. That amount of intake is assumed to be adequate, as no evidence of a nutritional deficiency is apparent.

Estimated Energy Requirement

For calorie needs, we use the Estimated Energy Requirement (EER) instead of an RDA or AI. As described, the RDAs are set somewhat higher than the average needs for nutrients. This is fine for nutrients rather than calories because a slight excess of vitamins and

▲ With a little bit of study, you can master the alphabet soup of nutrition recommendations.

MAKING DECISIONS

Using Nutrient Recommendations

As nutrient intake increases, the Recommended Dietary Allowance (RDA) for the nutrient, if set, is eventually met and a deficient state is no longer present. An individual's needs most likely will be met since RDAs are set high to include almost all people. Related to the RDA concept of meeting an individual's needs are the standards of Adequate Intake (AI) and the Estimated Energy Requirement (EER). These can be used to estimate an individual's needs for some nutrients and calories, respectively. Still, keep in mind that these standards do not share the same degree of accuracy as the RDA. For example, EER may have to be adjusted upward if the individual is very physically active. Finally, as nutrient intake increases above the Upper Level (UL), poor nutritional health is again likely. However, this poor health is due now to the toxic effects of a nutrient, rather than those of a deficiency.

minerals is not harmful. However, a long-term excess of calories will lead to weight gain. Therefore, the calculation of EER needs to be more specific, taking into account age, gender, height, weight, and physical activity (e.g., sedentary or moderately active). In some cases, the additional calorie needs for growth and lactation are also included (see Chapters 7, 16, and 17 for the specific formulas used). The EER also is based on the "average" person. Thus it can only serve as a starting point for estimating calorie needs.

Tolerable Upper Intake Level

A Tolerable Upper Intake Level (Upper Level or UL) has been set for some vitamins and minerals (see the inside cover). The UL is the highest amount of a nutrient unlikely to cause adverse health effects in the long run. As intake exceeds the UL, the risk of ill effects increases. These amounts generally should not be exceeded day after day, as toxicity could develop. For people eating a varied diet and/or using a balanced multivitamin and mineral supplement, exceeding the UL is unusual. Problems are more likely to arise with diets that promote excessive intakes of a limited variety of foods or with the use of many fortified foods or excessive doses of individual vitamins or minerals.

Daily Value

A nutrition standard more relevant to everyday life is the Daily Value (DV). This is a generic standard used on food labels. It is applicable to both genders from 4 years of age through adulthood, and is based on a 2000 kcal diet. DVs are mostly set at or close to the highest RDA value or related nutrient standard seen in the various age and gender categories for a specific nutrient (see Appendix B). DVs have been set for vitamins, minerals, protein, and other dietary components. DVs allow consumers to compare their intake from a specific food to desirable (or maximum) intakes.

CONCEPT CHECK

Dietary Guidelines for Americans have been set by government organizations. These guidelines are designed to reduce the risk of developing obesity, hypertension, type 2 diabetes, cardiovascular disease, alcoholism, and foodborne illness. In general, they recommend eating a variety of foods, fostered by following MyPyramid. They also recommend performing regular physical activity, aiming for a healthy weight, and moderating total fat, saturated fat, *trans* fat, salt, sugar, and alcohol intake, while focusing more on fruits, vegetables, and whole-grain products in daily menu planning. Safe food preparation and storage are also highlighted. All of the specific dietary standards are included in the broad category of Dietary Reference Intakes (DRIs). The Recommended Dietary Allowances (RDAs) are the amounts of each nutrient that will meet the needs of healthy individuals within specific gender and age categories. If not enough information is available to set an RDA, an Adequate Intake (AI) value is used. Tolerable Upper Intake Levels (ULs) are the highest amounts of a nutrient unlikely to cause adverse health effects. ULs have been set for some vitamins and minerals.

HOW SHOULD THESE NUTRIENT STANDARDS BE USED?

To sum up the acronyms described so far, the type of standard set for nutrients depends on the quality of available evidence. A nutrient recommendation backed by lots of experimental research will have an RDA. For a nutrient that still requires more research, only an AI is presented. We use the EER as a starting point for determining

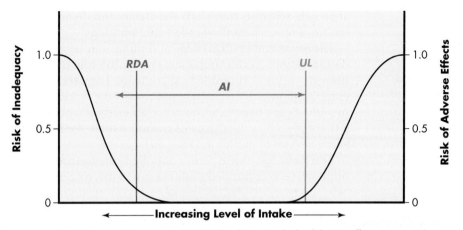

Recommended Dietary Allowance (RDA): The dietary intake level that is sufficient to meet the nutrient requirement of nearly all (97% to 98%) healthy individuals in a particular life stage and gender group. When set for a nutrient, aim for this intake.

Adequate Intake (AI): A recommended intake value based on observed or experimentally determined approximations or estimates of nutrient intake by a group (or groups) of healthy people that is assumed to be adequate — used when an RDA cannot be determined. When set for a nutrient, aim for this intake.

Tolerable Upper Intake Level (Upper Level or UL): The highest level of nutrient intake that is likely to pose no risk of adverse health effects for almost all individuals in the general population. As intake increases above the Upper Level, the risk of adverse effects increases.

FIGURE 2-9 ▶ Dietary Reference Intakes (DRIs). At intakes between the RDA and the UL, the risk of either an inadequate diet or adverse effects from the nutrient in question is close to 0. The UL is then the highest level of nutrient intake likely to pose no risks of adverse health effects to almost all individuals in the general population. At intakes above the UL, the margin of safety to protect against adverse effects is reduced. The AI is set for some nutrients instead of an RDA. In determining the AI for a nutrient, it is expected that the amount exceeds the RDA for that nutrient, if an RDA were known. Thus, the AI should cover the needs of more than 97% to 98% of individuals. The actual degree to which the AI exceeds the RDA is likely to differ among the various nutrients and population groups. The Food and Nutrition Board states that there is no established benefit for healthy individuals if they consume nutrient intakes above the RDA or AI.

calorie needs. Some nutrients also have a UL if information on toxicity is available. Periodically, new DRIs become available as expert committees review and interpret the available research.

RDAs and related standards are intended mainly for diet planning. Specifically, a diet plan should aim to meet the RDA or AI as appropriate and not to exceed the UL over the long term (Fig. 2-9). Specific RDA, AI, EER, and UL standards are printed on the inside cover of this book. To learn more about these nutrient standards, visit the link for the Food and Nutrition Board on the Institute of Medicine's web page (www.iom.edu).

USING THE SCIENTIFIC METHOD TO DETERMINE NUTRIENT NEEDS

How do we know what we know about nutrient needs? In a word, research. Like other sciences, the research that sets the foundation for nutrition knowledge has developed through the use of the *scientific method,* a testing procedure designed to detect and eliminate error.

The first step of the scientific method is the observation of a natural phenomenon. Scientists then suggest possible explanations, called **hypotheses,** about its cause. At times, historical events can provide clues to important relationships in nutrition science, such as the link between vitamin C and **scurvy** (see Chapter 9). In a related

hypotheses Tentative explanations by a scientist to explain a phenomenon.

scurvy The deficiency disease that results after a few weeks to months of consuming a diet that lacks vitamin C; pinpoint sites of bleeding on the skin are an early sign.

epidemiology The study of how disease rates vary among different population groups.

theory An explanation for a phenomenon that has numerous lines of evidence to support it.

approach, scientists may study the dietary and disease patterns among various populations, a research method called **epidemiology**.

Historical and epidemiological findings can *suggest* hypotheses about the role of diet in various health problems. *Proving* the role of particular dietary components, however, requires controlled experiments. The data gathered from experiments may either support or refute each hypothesis. If the results of many experiments support a hypothesis, the hypothesis becomes generally accepted by scientists and can be called a **theory** (such as the theory of gravity). Often, the results from one experiment suggest a new set of questions (Fig 2-10).

The most rigorous type of controlled experiment follows a randomized, double-blind, placebo-controlled study design. In this type of study, a group of participants—

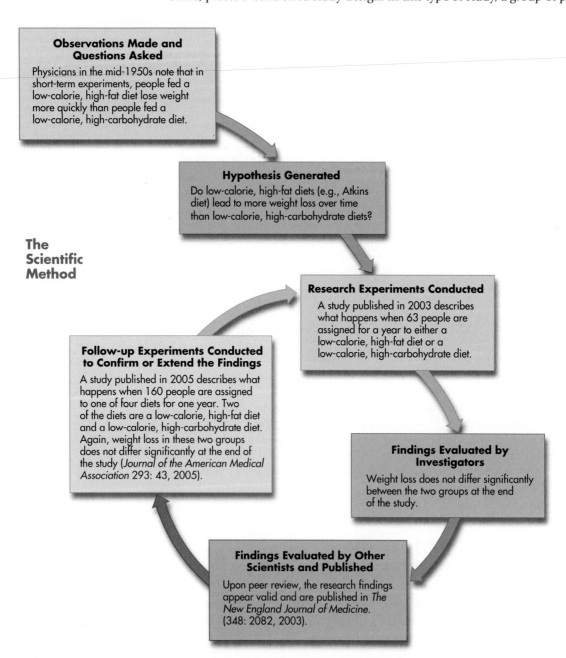

The Scientific Method

Observations Made and Questions Asked

Physicians in the mid-1950s note that in short-term experiments, people fed a low-calorie, high-fat diet lose weight more quickly than people fed a low-calorie, high-carbohydrate diet.

Hypothesis Generated

Do low-calorie, high-fat diets (e.g., Atkins diet) lead to more weight loss over time than low-calorie, high-carbohydrate diets?

Research Experiments Conducted

A study published in 2003 describes what happens when 63 people are assigned for a year to either a low-calorie, high-fat diet or a low-calorie, high-carbohydrate diet.

Follow-up Experiments Conducted to Confirm or Extend the Findings

A study published in 2005 describes what happens when 160 people are assigned to one of four diets for one year. Two of the diets are a low-calorie, high-fat diet and a low-calorie, high-carbohydrate diet. Again, weight loss in these two groups does not differ significantly at the end of the study (*Journal of the American Medical Association* 293: 43, 2005).

Findings Evaluated by Investigators

Weight loss does not differ significantly between the two groups at the end of the study.

Findings Evaluated by Other Scientists and Published

Upon peer review, the research findings appear valid and are published in *The New England Journal of Medicine*. (348: 2082, 2003).

FIGURE 2-10 ▶ Implementing the scientific method using low-calorie, high-fat diets as an example. Scientists consistently follow these steps in conducting scientific research. It is important not to embrace a nutrition or other scientific concept until it has been thoroughly tested using the scientific method. Incidentally, in the final study few people on the low-calorie, high-fat diet were able to follow the guideline of less than 50 grams of carbohydrates per day.

the experimental group—follows a specific protocol (e.g., consuming a certain food or nutrient), and participants in a corresponding **control group** follow their normal habits or consume a **placebo.** People are randomly assigned to each group, such as by the flip of a coin. Scientists then observe the experimental group over time to see if there is any effect not found in the control group.

Human experiments provide the most convincing evidence about relationships between nutrients and health, but they are often not practical or ethical. Thus, much of what we know about human nutritional needs and functions has been generated from animal experiments. The use of animal experiments to study the role of nutrition in certain human diseases depends on the availability of an **animal model**—a disease in laboratory animals that closely mimics a particular human disease. Often, however, if no animal model is available and human experiments are ruled out, scientific knowledge cannot advance beyond what can be learned from epidemiological studies.

Once an experiment is complete, scientists summarize the findings and seek to publish the results in scientific journals. Generally, before articles are published in scientific journals, they are critically reviewed by other scientists familiar with the subject, which helps to ensure that only high-quality, objective research findings are published.

Keep in mind, one experiment is never enough to prove a particular hypothesis or provide a basis for nutritional recommendations. Rather, through follow-up studies, the results obtained in one laboratory must be confirmed by experiments conducted in other laboratories, and possibly under varying circumstances. Only then can we really trust and use the results. The more lines of evidence available to support an idea, the more likely it is to be true (Fig 2-11).

control group Participants in an experiment who are not given the treatment being tested.

placebo Generally a fake medicine used to disguise the treatments given to the participants in an experiment.

animal model Study of disease in animals that duplicates human disease. This can be used to understand more about human disease.

case-control study Individuals who have the condition in question, such as lung cancer, are compared with individuals who do not have the condition.

▲ Scientific research contributes to nutrition knowledge, more so than personal experience.

FIGURE 2-11 ▶ Data from a variety of sources can come together to support a research hypothesis. For example, epidemiological studies show that type 2 diabetes is characteristically found in obese populations, compared with leaner populations. Physicians notice in clinical practice that type 2 diabetes is much more likely in their obese patients, compared with their leaner patients. Laboratory animal studies show that overfeeding that eventually leads to obesity often leads to the development of type 2 diabetes. **Case-control studies** show that obese patients are much more likely to have type 2 diabetes than the leaner comparison group matched for other characteristics. Finally, human intervention trials show that weight loss can correct type 2 diabetes in many people. Laboratory researchers also show that the enlarged adipose cells associated with excess fat deposition and obesity are much less responsive to the hormonal signals involved in blood glucose regulation. All of these lines of data come together with biological plausibility from various laboratory studies to support the research hypothesis that obesity can lead to type 2 diabetes.

ulcer Erosion of the tissue lining, usually in the stomach (gastric ulcer) or the upper small intestine (duodenal ulcer). As a group these are generally referred to as peptic ulcers.

microorganism Bacteria, virus, or other organism invisible to the naked eye, some of which cause diseases. Also called *microbes*.

double-blind study An experimental design in which neither the participants nor the researchers are aware of each participant's assignment (test or placebo) or the outcome of the study until it is completed. An independent third party holds the code and the data until the study has been completed.

MAKING DECISIONS

Research on Stomach Ulcers

Overall, the scientific method requires a skeptical attitude. A recent example of this need for skepticism involves stomach **ulcers.** Not so many years ago, everyone "knew" that stomach ulcers were caused by a stressful lifestyle and a poor diet. Then, in 1983, an Australian physician, Dr. Barry Marshall, reported in a respected medical journal that ulcers are usually caused by a common **microorganism** called *Helicobacter pylori.* Furthermore, he stated that a cure is possible using antibiotics. At first, other physicians were skeptical about this finding and continued to prescribe medications such as antacids that reduce stomach acid. But, as more studies were published demonstrating that patients using antibiotics were cured of ulcers, the medical profession eventually accepted the findings. Today, ulcers are managed for the most part by medications that destroy the microorganism. (We will discuss the treatment of stomach ulcers in more detail in Chapter 3.) Sound scientific discoveries will always be subject to challenge and change.

Epidemiological studies may suggest hypotheses, but controlled experiments are needed to rigorously test hypotheses before nutrition recommendations can be made. Recently, epidemiologists found that smokers who regularly consumed fruits and vegetables had a lower risk for lung cancer than smokers who ate few fruits and vegetables. Some scientists proposed that beta-carotene, a pigment present in many fruits and vegetables, may be responsible for reducing the damage that tobacco smoke creates in the lungs. However, in **double-blind studies** involving heavy smokers, the risk of lung cancer was found to be *higher* for those who took beta-carotene supplements than for those who did not (this is not true for the small amount of beta-carotene found naturally in foods). Soon after these results were reported, the U.S. federal agency supporting two other large ongoing studies that employed beta-carotene supplements called a halt to the research, stating that these supplements are ineffective in preventing both lung cancer and cardiovascular disease.

WHAT DO FOOD LABELS HAVE TO OFFER IN DIET PLANNING?

▲ Use the Nutrition Facts label to learn more about the nutrient content of the foods you eat. Nutrient content is expressed as a percent of Daily Value. Canadian food laws and related food labels have a slightly different format (review Appendix C).

Today, nearly all foods sold in stores must be in a package that has a label containing the following information: the product name, name and address of the manufacturer, amount of product in the package, and ingredients listed in descending order by weight. This food and beverage labeling is monitored in North America by government agencies such as the Food and Drug Administration (FDA) in the United States. The listing of certain food constituents also is required—specifically, on a Nutrition Facts panel (Fig. 2-12). Use the information in the Nutrition Facts panel to learn more about what you eat. The following components must be listed: total calories (kcal), calories from fat, total fat, saturated fat, *trans* fat, cholesterol, sodium, total carbohydrate, fiber, sugars, protein, vitamin A, vitamin C, calcium, and iron. In addition to these required components, manufacturers can choose to list polyunsaturated and monounsaturated fat, potassium, and others. Listing these components becomes *required* if a claim is made about the health benefits of the specific nutrient (see the upcoming section in Chapter 2 entitled "Health Claims on Food Labels") or if the food is fortified with that nutrient.

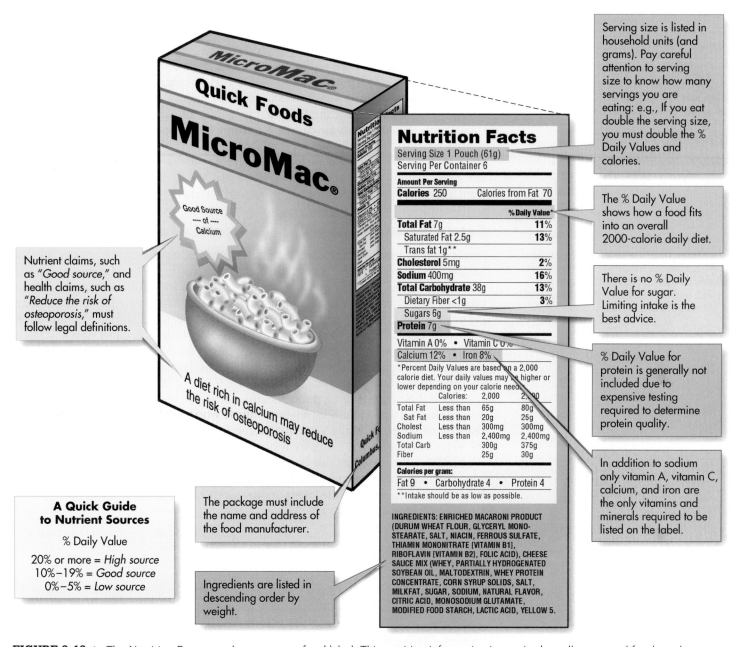

Serving size is listed in household units (and grams). Pay careful attention to serving size to know how many servings you are eating: e.g., If you eat double the serving size, you must double the % Daily Values and calories.

The % Daily Value shows how a food fits into an overall 2000-calorie daily diet.

There is no % Daily Value for sugar. Limiting intake is the best advice.

% Daily Value for protein is generally not included due to expensive testing required to determine protein quality.

In addition to sodium only vitamin A, vitamin C, calcium, and iron are the only vitamins and minerals required to be listed on the label.

Nutrient claims, such as *"Good source,"* and health claims, such as *"Reduce the risk of osteoporosis,"* must follow legal definitions.

A Quick Guide to Nutrient Sources

% Daily Value

20% or more = *High source*
10%–19% = *Good source*
0%–5% = *Low source*

The package must include the name and address of the food manufacturer.

Ingredients are listed in descending order by weight.

Nutrition Facts

Serving Size 1 Pouch (61g)
Serving Per Container 6

Amount Per Serving

Calories 250   Calories from Fat 70

	% Daily Value*
Total Fat 7g	11%
Saturated Fat 2.5g	13%
Trans fat 1g**	
Cholesterol 5mg	2%
Sodium 400mg	16%
Total Carbohydrate 38g	13%
Dietary Fiber <1g	3%
Sugars 6g	
Protein 7g	

Vitamin A 0% • Vitamin C 0%
Calcium 12% • Iron 8%

*Percent Daily Values are based on a 2,000 calorie diet. Your daily values may be higher or lower depending on your calorie needs.

	Calories:	2,000	2,500
Total Fat	Less than	65g	80g
Sat Fat	Less than	20g	25g
Cholest	Less than	300mg	300mg
Sodium	Less than	2,400mg	2,400mg
Total Carb		300g	375g
Fiber		25g	30g

Calories per gram:

Fat 9 • Carbohydrate 4 • Protein 4

**Intake should be as low as possible.

INGREDIENTS: ENRICHED MACARONI PRODUCT (DURUM WHEAT FLOUR, GLYCERYL MONO-STEARATE, SALT, NIACIN, FERROUS SULFATE, THIAMIN MONONITRATE [VITAMIN B1], RIBOFLAVIN [VITAMIN B2], FOLIC ACID), CHEESE SAUCE MIX (WHEY, PARTIALLY HYDROGENATED SOYBEAN OIL, MALTODEXTRIN, WHEY PROTEIN CONCENTRATE, CORN SYRUP SOLIDS, SALT, MILKFAT, SUGAR, SODIUM, NATURAL FLAVOR, CITRIC ACID, MONOSODIUM GLUTAMATE, MODIFIED FOOD STARCH, LACTIC ACID, YELLOW 5.

FIGURE 2-12 ▶ The Nutrition Facts panel on a current food label. This nutrition information is required on all processed food products. The % Daily Value listed on the label is the percentage of the generally accepted amount of a nutrient needed daily present in 1 serving of the product. You can use the % Daily Values to compare your diet with current nutrition recommendations for certain diet components. Let's consider fiber. Assume that you consume 2000 kcal per day, the energy intake for which the % Daily Values listed on labels have been calculated. If the total % Daily Value for dietary fiber in all the foods you eat in one day adds up to 100%, your diet meets the recommendations for fiber. Food labels also contain the name and address of the food manufacturers. This allows consumers to contact the manufacturer if they desire.

Remember that the Daily Value is a generic standard used on the food label. The percentage of the Daily Value (% Daily Value or % DV) is usually given for each nutrient per serving. These percentages are based on a 2000 kcal diet. In other words, they are not as applicable to people who require considerably more or less than 2000 kcal per day with respect to fat and carbohydrate intake. DVs are mostly set at or close to the highest RDA value or related nutrient standard seen in the various age and gender categories for a specific nutrient.

▶ The nutrition label uses the term calorie to express energy content in some cases, but kilocalorie (kcal) values are actually listed.

Serving sizes on the Nutrition Facts panel must be consistent among similar foods. This means that all brands of ice cream, for example, must use the same serving size on their label. (These serving sizes may differ from those of MyPyramid because those of food labels are based on typical serving sizes.) In addition, food claims made on packages must follow legal definitions (Table 2-9). For example, if a product claims to be "low sodium," it must have 140 milligrams of sodium or less per serving.

Many manufacturers list the Daily Values set for dietary components such as fat, cholesterol, and carbohydrate on the Nutrition Facts panel. This can be useful as a reference point. As noted, they are based on 2000 kcal; if the label is large enough, amounts based on 2500 kcal are listed as well for total fat, saturated fat, carbohydrate, and other components. As mentioned, DVs allow consumers to compare their intake from a specific food to desirable (or maximum) intakes.

Exceptions to Food Labeling

▶ Nutrient and herbal supplement labels have a different layout with a "Supplement Facts" heading. The Nutrition and Your Health section at the end of this chapter and Chapter 9 show examples of these labels.

Foods such as fresh fruits and vegetables, fish, meats, and poultry currently are not required to have Nutrition Facts labels. However, many grocers and some meat packers have voluntarily chosen to provide their customers with information about these products. Nutrition Facts labels on meat products will likely be required in the coming years. The next time you are at the grocery store, ask where you might find information on the fresh products that do not have a Nutrition Facts panel. You will likely find a poster or pamphlet near the product; often, these pamphlets contain recipes that use your favorite fruit, vegetable, or cut of meat. They may even assist you in your endeavor to improve your diet.

Protein deficiency is not a public health concern in the United States, so declaration of the % Daily Value for protein is not mandatory on foods for people over 4 years of age. If the % Daily Value for protein is given on a label, FDA requires that the product be analyzed for protein quality. This procedure is expensive and time-consuming, so many companies opt not to list a % Daily Value for protein. However, labels on food for infants and children under 4 years of age must include the % Daily Value for protein, as must the labels on any food carrying a claim about protein content (see Chapter 17).

▲ The nutrition information on the food labels on these three products can be combined to indicate nutrient intake for a peanut butter and jelly sandwich.

TABLE 2-9 Definitions for Comparative and Absolute Nutrient Claims on Food Labels

Sugar

- **Sugar free:** less than 0.5 grams (g) per serving.
- **No added sugar; without added sugar; no sugar added:**
  - No sugars were added during processing or packing, including ingredients that contain sugars (for example, fruit juices, applesauce, or jam).
  - Processing does not increase the sugar content above the amount naturally present in the ingredients. (A functionally insignificant increase in sugars is acceptable for processes used for purposes other than increasing sugar content.)
  - The food that it resembles and for which it substitutes normally contains added sugars.
  - If the food doesn't meet the requirements for a low- or reduced-calorie food, the product bears a statement that the food is not low calorie or calorie reduced and directs consumers' attention to the Nutrition Facts panel for further information on sugars and calorie content.
- **Reduced sugar:** at least 25% less sugar per serving than reference food

Calories

- **Calorie free:** fewer than 5 kcal per serving
- **Low calorie:** 40 kcal or less per serving and, if the serving is 30 g or less or 2 tablespoons or less, per 50 g of the food
- **Reduced or fewer calories:** at least 25% fewer kcal per serving than reference food

Fiber

- **High fiber:** 5 g or more per serving. (Foods making high-fiber claims must meet the definition for low fat, or the level of total fat must appear next to the high-fiber claim.)
- **Good source of fiber:** 2.5 to 4.9 g per serving
- **More or added fiber:** at least 2.5 g more per serving than reference food

Fat

- **Fat free:** less than 0.5 g of fat per serving
- **Saturated fat free:** less than 0.5 g per serving, and the level of *trans* fatty acids does not exceed 0.5 g per serving

- **Low fat:** 3 g or less per serving and, if the serving is 30 g or less or 2 tablespoons or less, per 50 g of the food. 2% milk can no longer be labeled low fat, as it exceeds 3 g per serving. *Reduced fat* will be the term used instead.
- **Low saturated fat:** 1 g or less per serving and not more than 15% of kcal from saturated fatty acids
- **Reduced or less fat:** at least 25% less per serving than reference food
- **Reduced or less saturated fat:** at least 25% less per serving than reference food

Cholesterol

- **Cholesterol free:** less than 2 milligrams (mg) of cholesterol and 2 g or less of saturated fat per serving
- **Low cholesterol:** 20 mg or less cholesterol and 2 g or less of saturated fat per serving and, if the serving is 30 g or less or 2 tablespoons or less, per 50 g of the food
- **Reduced or less cholesterol:** at least 25% less cholesterol and 2 g or less of saturated fat per serving than reference food

Sodium

- **Sodium free:** less than 5 mg per serving
- **Very low sodium:** 35 mg or less per serving and, if the serving is 30 g or less or 2 tablespoons or less, per 50 g of the food
- **Low sodium:** 140 mg or less per serving and, if the serving is 30 g or less or 2 tablespoons or less, per 50 g of the food
- **Light in sodium:** at least 50% less per serving than reference food
- **Reduced or less sodium:** at least 25% less per serving than reference food

Other Terms

- **Fortified or enriched:** Vitamins and/or minerals have been added to the product in amounts in excess of at least 10% of that normally present in the usual product. Enriched generally refers to replacing nutrients lost in processing, whereas fortified refers to adding nutrients not originally present in the specific food.
- **Healthy:** An individual food that is low fat and low saturated fat and has no more than 360 to 480 mg of sodium or 60 mg of cholesterol per serving can be labeled "healthy" if it provides at least 10% of the Daily Value for vitamin A, vitamin C, protein, calcium, iron, or fiber.

- **Light or lite:** The descriptor *light* or *lite* can mean two things: first, that a nutritionally altered product contains one-third fewer kcal or half the fat of reference food (if the food derives 50% or more of its kcal from fat, the reduction must be 50% of the fat) and, second, that the sodium content of a low-calorie, low-fat food has been reduced by 50%. In addition, "light in sodium" may be used for foods in which the sodium content has been reduced by at least 50%. The term *light* may still be used to describe such properties as texture and color, as long as the label explains the intent—for example, "light brown sugar" and "light and fluffy."

Diet: A food may be labeled with terms such as *diet, dietetic, artificially sweetened,* or *sweetened with nonnutritive sweetener* only if the claim is not false or misleading. The food can also be labeled *low calorie* or *reduced calorie.*

Good source: *Good source* means that a serving of the food contains 10% to 19% of the Daily Value for a particular nutrient. If 5% or less it is a **low source.**

High: *High* means that a serving of the food contains 20% or more of the Daily Value for a particular nutrient.

 Organic: Federal standards for organic foods allow claims when much of the ingredients do not use chemical fertilizers or pesticides, genetic engineering, sewage sludge, antibiotics, or irradiation in their production. At least 95% of ingredients (by weight) must meet these guidelines to be labeled "organic" on the front of the package. If the front label instead says "made with organic ingredients," only 70% of the ingredients must be organic. For animal products, the animals must graze outdoors, be fed organic feed, and cannot be exposed to large amounts of antibiotics or growth hormones.

Natural: The food must be free of food colors, synthetic flavors, or any other synthetic substance.

The following terms apply only to meat and poultry products regulated by USDA.

Extra lean: less than 5 g of fat, 2 g of saturated fat, and 95 mg of cholesterol per serving (or 100 g of an individual food)

Lean: less than 10 g of fat, 4.5 g of saturated fat, and 95 mg of cholesterol per serving (or 100 g of an individual food)

Many definitions are from FDA's *Dictionary of Terms,* as established in conjunction with the 1990 Nutrition Education and Labeling Act (NELA).
g = grams; mg = milligrams

Health Claims on Food Labels

As a marketing tool directed toward the health-conscious consumer, food manufacturers like to claim that their products have all sorts of health benefits. The FDA has legal oversight over most food products and permits some health claims with certain restrictions.

Table 2-9 lists the definitions for nutrient claims on food labels. Currently, FDA limits the use of health messages to specific instances in which there is significant scientific agreement that a relationship exists between a nutrient, food, or food constituent and the disease. The claims allowed at this time may show a link between the following:

- A diet with enough calcium and a reduced risk of osteoporosis
- A diet low in total fat and a reduced risk of some cancers
- A diet low in saturated fat and cholesterol and a reduced risk of cardiovascular disease (typically referred to as heart disease on the label)
- A diet rich in fiber—containing grain products, fruits, and vegetables—and a reduced risk of some cancers
- A diet low in sodium and high in potassium and a reduced risk of hypertension and stroke
- A diet rich in fruits and vegetables and a reduced risk of some cancers
- A diet adequate in the synthetic form of the vitamin folate (called folic acid) and a reduced risk of neural tube defects (a type of birth defect) (see Chapter 11)
- Use of sugarless gum and a reduced risk of tooth decay, especially when compared with foods high in sugars and starches
- A diet rich in fruits, vegetables, and grain products that contain fiber and a reduced risk of cardiovascular disease. Oats (oatmeal, oat bran, and oat flour) and psyllium are two fiber-rich ingredients that can be singled out in reducing the risk of cardiovascular disease, as long as the statement also says the diet should also be low in saturated fat and cholesterol.
- A diet rich in whole-grain foods and other plant foods, as well as low in total fat, saturated fat, and cholesterol, and a reduced risk of cardiovascular disease and certain cancers
- A diet low in saturated fat and cholesterol that also includes 25 grams of soy protein and a reduced risk of cardiovascular disease. The statement "one serving of the (name of food) provides _____ grams of soy protein" must also appear as part of the health claim.
- Fatty acids from oils present in fish and a reduced risk of cardiovascular disease
- Margarines containing plant stanols and sterols and a reduced risk of cardiovascular disease (see Chapter 5 for more details on plant stanols and sterols)

A "may" or "might" qualifier must be used in the statement.

In addition, before a health claim can be made for a food product, it must meet two general requirements. First, the food must be a "good source" (before any fortification) of fiber, protein, vitamin A, vitamin C, calcium, or iron. The legal definition of "good source" appears in Table 2-9. Second, a single serving of the food product cannot contain more than 13 grams of fat, 4 grams of saturated fat, 60 milligrams of cholesterol, or 480 milligrams of sodium. If a food exceeds any one of these requirements, no health claim can be made for it, despite its other nutritional qualities. For example, even though whole milk is high in calcium, its label can't make the health claim about calcium and osteoporosis because whole milk contains 5 grams of saturated fat per serving. In another example, a health claim regarding fat and cancer can be made only if the product contains 3 grams or less of fat per serving, the standard for low-fat foods.

Health Claims Report Card

| A | **High**
Significant scientific agreement | 1 |
| B | **Moderate**
Evidence is not conclusive | 2 |
| C | **Low**
Evidence is limited and not conclusive | 3 |
| D | **Extremely Low**
Little scientific evidence supporting this claim | 4 |

▲ In 2003, FDA unveiled a new process to provide more science-based, FDA-regulated health information on food product labels. This new process includes the Health Claims Report card.

MAKING DECISIONS

Health Claims

FDA allows the three preliminary classes of health claims shown on page 66 as long as the label qualifies the food with a disclaimer such as "this evidence is not conclusive." These preliminary health claims haven't shown up on many foods at this time (nuts, such as walnuts, and fish have been some of the first examples). These claims also cannot be used on foods considered unhealthy (review Table 2-9 for the definition of healthy with regard to a food).

Overall, claims on foods fall into one of four categories:

- Health claims—closely regulated by FDA
- Preliminary health claims—regulated by FDA but evidence may be scant for the claim
- Nutrient claims—closely regulated by FDA (review Table 2-9)
- Structure/function claims—as discussed in the Nutrition and Your Health section at the end of this chapter, these are not FDA approved or necessarily valid

CONCEPT CHECK

The Nutrition Facts panel on a food label provides key information for helping track one's food intake. Nutrient quantities are compared with the Daily Values and expressed on a percentage basis (% Daily Value). This information can be used to either increase or reduce intake of specific nutrients. Health and nutrient claims on food labels are closely regulated by FDA. Fruits, vegetables, whole-grain breads and cereals, soy, and good sources of calcium are prominent among the foods that can make specific health claims.

EPILOGUE

The tools discussed in Chapter 2 greatly aid in menu planning. Menu planning can start with MyPyramid. The totality of choices made within the groups can then be evaluated using the Dietary Guidelines. Individual foods that make up a diet can be examined more closely using the Daily Values listed on the Nutrition Facts panel of the product. For the most part, these Daily Values are in line with the Recommended Dietary Allowances and related nutrient standards. The Nutrition Facts panel is especially useful in identifying nutrient-dense foods—foods high in a specific nutrient, such as the vitamin folate, but low in the relative amount of calories provided—and the energy-dense foods—foods that fill you up without providing a lot of calories. Generally speaking, the more you learn about and use these tools, the more they will benefit your diet.

▲ Specific health claims can be made on food labels for whole-grain cereals.

▶ Canadian food labels use a slightly different group of health claims and label descriptors (see Appendix C).

▶ The **Exchange System** is a final menu-planning tool. This tool organizes foods based on calorie, protein, carbohydrate, and fat content. The result is a manageable framework for designing diets, especially for treatment of diabetes. For more information on the Exchange System see Appendix D.

The following suggestions should help you make healthful and logical nutrition decisions:

1. Apply the basic principles of nutrition as outlined in this chapter (along with the 2005 Dietary Guidelines for Americans and related resources in Chapter 2) to any nutrition claim including those on websites. Do you note any inconsistencies? Do reliable references support the claims? Beware of the following:
   • Testimonials about personal experience
   • Disreputable publication sources
   • Dramatic results (rarely true)
   • Lack of evidence from supporting studies made by other scientists

2. Examine the background and scientific credentials of the individual, organizations, or publication making the nutritional claim. Usually, a reputable author is one whose educational background or present affiliation is with a nationally recognized university or medical center that offers programs or courses in the field of nutrition, medicine, or a closely allied specialty.

3. Be wary if the answer is "Yes" to any of the following questions about a health-related nutrition claim:
   • Are only advantages discussed and possible disadvantages ignored?
   • Are claims made about "curing" disease? Do they sound too good to be true?
   • Is extreme bias against the medical community or traditional medical treatments evident? Physicians as a group strive to cure diseases in their patients, using what proven techniques are available. They do not ignore reliable cures.
   • Is the claim touted as a new or secret scientific breakthrough?

4. Note the size and duration of any study cited in support of a nutrition claim. The larger it is and the longer it went on, the more dependable its findings. Also consider the type of study: epidemiology versus case-control versus double-blind. Check out the group studied; a study of men or women in Sweden may be less relevant than one of men or women of Southern European, African, or Hispanic descent, for example. Keep in mind that "contributes to," "is linked to," or "is associated with" does not mean "causes."

5. Beware of press conferences and other hype regarding the latest findings. Much of this will not survive more detailed scientific evaluation.

6. When you meet with a nutrition professional, you should expect that he or she will do the following:
   • Ask questions about your medical history, lifestyle, and current eating habits.
   • Formulate a diet plan tailored to your needs, as opposed to simply tearing a form from a tablet that could apply to almost anyone.
   • Schedule follow-up visits to track your progress, answer any questions, and help keep you motivated.
   • Involve family members in the diet plan, when appropriate.
   • Consult directly with your physician and readily refer you back to your physician for those health problems a nutrition professional is not trained to treat.

7. Avoid practitioners who prescribe **megadoses** of vitamin and mineral supplements for everyone.

8. Examine product labels carefully. Be skeptical of any product promotion not clearly stated on the label. A product is not likely to do something not specifically claimed on its label or package insert (legally part of the label).

megadose intake of a nutrient beyond estimates of needs or what would be found in a balanced diet; 2 to 10 times human needs is a starting point.

▶ Recently major nutrition organizations put together 10 red flags that they consider signals for poor nutrition advice:

1. Recommendations that promise a quick fix
2. Dire warnings of dangers from a single product or regimen
3. Claims that sound too good to be true
4. Simplistic conclusions drawn from a complex study
5. Recommendations based on a single study
6. Dramatic statements refuted by reputable scientific organizations
7. Lists of "good" and "bad" foods
8. Recommendations made to help sell a product
9. Recommendations based on studies published without peer review
10. Recommendations from studies that ignore differences among individuals or groups

▶ FDA can act if evidence accumulates showing that a product is harmful. This has been true for some herbal remedies marketed as dietary supplements, such as ephedra.

Dietary Supplements

This cautious approach to nutrition-related advice and products is even more important today because of sweeping changes in U.S. federal law passed in 1994.

The Dietary Supplement Health and Education Act (DSHEA) of 1994 classified vitamins, minerals, amino acids, and herbal remedies as "foods," effectively restraining the U.S. Food and Drug Administration (FDA) from regulating them as tightly as drugs and food additives. According to this act, rather than the manufacturer having to prove a dietary supplement is safe, FDA must prove it is unsafe before preventing its sale. In contrast, the safety of food additives and drugs must be demonstrated to FDA's satisfaction before they are marketed.

Currently, a dietary supplement (or herbal product) can be marketed in the United States without FDA approval if (1) there is a history of its use or other evidence that it is expected to be reasonably safe when used under the conditions recommended or suggested in its labeling, and (2) the product is labeled as a dietary supplement. It is permissible for the labels on such products to claim a benefit

related to a classic nutrient-deficiency disease, describe how a nutrient affects human body structure or function (called structure/function claims), and claim that general well-being results from consumption of the ingredient(s). Examples could be "maintains bone health" or "improves blood circulation." However, the label of products bearing such claims also must prominently display in boldface type the following disclaimer: "This statement has not been evaluated by the Food and Drug Administration. This product is not intended to diagnose, treat, cure, or prevent disease" (Fig. 2-13). Despite this warning, when consumers find these products on the shelves of supermarkets, health-food stores, and pharmacies, they may mistakenly assume FDA has carefully evaluated the products.

Many of us are willing to try untested nutrition products and believe in their miraculous actions. Popular products claim to increase muscle growth, enhance sexuality, boost energy, reduce body fat, increase strength, supply missing nutrients, increase longevity, and even improve brain function. Clearly, many nutritional products commonly found in stores are not

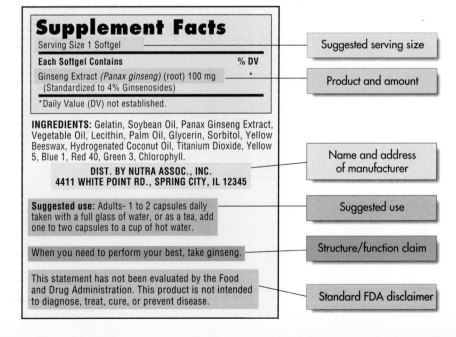

FIGURE 2-13 ▶ Supplement Facts label on an herbal product. Note the structure/function claim and the FDA disclaimer. Any nutrients or other food constituents would also be listed if contained in the product.

strictly regulated in terms of effectiveness and safety. The amount and potency of dietary supplmements have also been in question. In June 2007, FDA issued long-awaited standards that will require supplement manufacturers to test the purity, strength, and composition of all their products. Large companies will be the first to comply (by June 2008), whereas small companies have until 2010. Until then, national brands are more reliable. Supplements are discussed further in the Nutrition and Your Health section in Chapter 9, "Dietary Supplements—Who Needs Them?"

If you embark on a self-cure by means of such products, you will probably waste money and possibly risk ill health. A better approach is to consult a physician or **registered dietitian** first. You can find a registered dietitian in North America by consulting the Yellow Pages in the telephone directory, contacting the local dietetic association, calling the dietary department of a local hospital, or visiting www.eatright.org/find.html or www.dietitians.ca. Make sure the

person has the credentials "R.D." after his/her name ("R.D.N." is also used in Canada). This indicates the person has completed rigorous classroom and clinical training in nutrition and participates in continuing education. Appendix H also lists many reputable sources of nutrition advice for your use. Finally, the following websites can help you evaluate ongoing nutrition and health claims:

http://www.acsh.org/
American Council on Science and Health

http://www.quackwatch.org/
Quackwatch: Your Guide to Quackery, Health Fraud, and Intelligent Decisions

http://www.ncahf.org/
National Council Against Health Fraud

http://dietary-supplements.info.nih.gov/
National Institutes of Health, Office of Dietary Supplements

http://www.fda.gov/
U.S. Food and Drug Administration

Overall, nutrition is a rapidly advancing field and there are always new findings.

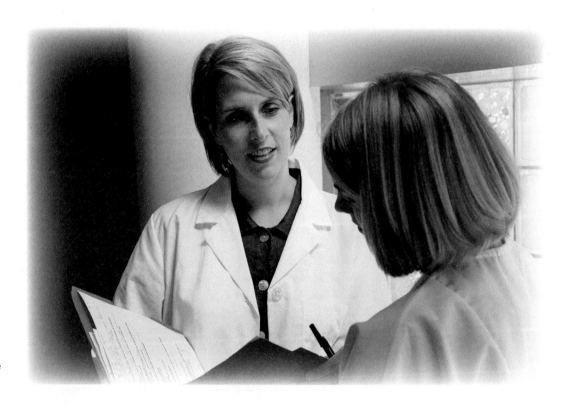

▲ Registered dietitians are a reliable source of nutrition information.

CASE STUDY

Dietary Supplements

While Brenda was driving to campus last week, she heard an advertisement for a supplement containing a plant substance recently imported from China. It supposedly gives people more energy and helps one cope with the stress of daily life. This advertisement caught Brenda's attention because she has been feeling run down lately. She is taking a full-course load and has been working 30 hours a week at a local restaurant to try to make ends meet. Brenda doesn't have a lot of extra money. Still, she likes to try new things and this recent breakthrough from China sounded almost too good to be true. After searching for more information about this supplement on the Internet, she discovered that the recommended dose would cost $60 per month. Because Brenda is looking for some help with her low energy level, she decides to order a 1-month supply.

Answer the following questions, and check your response in Appendix A.

1. Is the advertised supplement regulated by the FDA or other government agency?
2. What type of label claim is the phrase "increases energy," and does it require government approval?
3. Can Brenda feel confident that the supplement is safe and effective?
4. Is the amount of active ingredients in supplements tightly controlled?
5. Does it make sense for Brenda to spend the extra $60 per month for this supplement?
6. What advice would you give Brenda about the fact that she has been feeling run down lately?

▲ Do you agree with Brenda's decision to try this supplement?

SUMMARY

1. *Variety, balance,* and *moderation* are three watchwords of diet planning.

2. Nutrient density is a useful concept. It reflects the nutrient content of a food in relation to its calorie content. Nutrient-dense foods are relatively rich in nutrients, in comparison with calorie content.

3. Energy density of a food is determined by comparing calorie content with the weight of food. A food rich in calories but that weighs relatively very little, such as nuts, cookies, fried foods in general, and most snack foods (including fat-free brands), is considered energy dense. Foods with low energy density include fruits, vegetables, and any food that incorporates lots of water during cooking, such as oatmeal.

4. A person's nutritional state can be categorized as *desirable nutrition,* in which the body has adequate stores for times of increased needs; *undernutrition,* which may be present with or without clinical symptoms; and *overnutrition,* which can lead to vitamin and mineral toxicities and various chronic diseases.

5. Evaluation of nutritional state involves analyzing background factors, as well as anthropometric, biochemical, clinical, dietary, and economic assessments. It is not always possible to detect nutritional inadequacies via nutrition assessment because symptoms of deficiencies are often nonspecific and may not appear for many years.

6. MyPyramid is designed to translate nutrient recommendations into a food plan that exhibits variety, balance, and moderation. The best results are obtained by using low-fat or fat-free dairy products; incorporating some vegetable proteins in the diet in addition to animal-protein foods; including citrus fruits and dark green vegetables; and emphasizing whole-grain breads and cereals.

7. Dietary Guidelines for Americans have been issued to help reduce chronic diseases. The guidelines emphasize eating a variety of foods; performing regular physical activity; maintaining or improving weight; moderating consumption of fat, *trans* fat, cholesterol, sugar, salt, and alcohol; eating plenty of whole-grain products, fruits, and vegetables; and safely preparing and storing foods, especially perishable foods.

8. Recommended Dietary Allowances (RDAs) are set for many nutrients. These amounts yield enough of each nutrient to meet the needs of healthy individuals within specific gender and age categories. Adequate Intake (AI) is the standard used when not enough information is available to set a more specific RDA. Estimated Energy Requirements (EERs) set calorie needs for both genders at various ages and physical activity patterns. Tolerable Upper

Intake Levels (Upper Levels or ULs) for nutrient intake have been set for some vitamins and minerals. All of the many dietary standards fall under the term *Dietary Reference Intakes (DRIs)*. Daily Values are used as a basis for expressing the nutrient content of foods on the Nutrition Facts panel and are based for the most part on the RDAs.

9. The scientific method is the procedure for testing the validity of possible ex-

planations of a phenomenon, called hypotheses. Experiments are conducted to either support or refute a specific hypothesis. Once we have much experimental information that supports a specific hypothesis, it then can be called a theory. All of us need to be skeptical of new ideas in the nutrition field, waiting until many lines of experimental evidence support a concept before adopting any suggested dietary practice.

10. Food labels are a useful tool to track your nutrient intake and learn more about the nutritional characteristics of the foods you eat. Any health claims listed must follow criteria set by FDA.

11. Dietary supplements can be marketed in the United States without FDA approval. Certain health claims can be made on supplement labels, although few have been thoroughly evaluated by reputable scientists.

STUDY QUESTIONS

1. Describe the philosophy underlying the creation of MyPyramid. What dietary changes would you need to make to meet the pyramid guidelines on a regular basis?

2. Trace the progression, in terms of physical results, of a person who went from an overnourished to an undernourished state.

3. How could the nutritional state of the person at each state in question 2 be evaluated?

4. Describe the intent of the Dietary Guidelines for Americans. Point out

one criticism for its general application to all North American adults.

5. Based on the discussion of the Dietary Guidelines for Americans, suggest two key dietary changes the typical North American adult should consider making.

6. How do RDAs and AIs differ from Daily Values in intention and application?

7. How would you explain the concepts of nutrient density and energy density to a fourth grade class?

8. Nutritionists encourage all people to read labels on food packages to learn more about what they eat. What four nutrients could easily be tracked in your diet if you read the Nutrition Facts panels regularly on food products?

9. Explain why consumers can have confidence in FDA-approved health claims on food packages.

10. Relate the importance of variety in a diet, especially with regard to fruit and vegetable choices, to the discovery of various phytochemicals in foods.

CHECK YOUR KNOWLEDGE

Answers to the following multiple choice questions are in Appendix A.

1. Anthropometric measurements include
   a. height, weight, skinfolds, and body circumferences.
   b. blood concentrations of nutrients.
   c. a diet history of the previous days' intake.
   d. blood levels of enzyme activities.

2. Foods with *high* nutrient density offer the _____ nutrients for the _____ calories.
   a. least, lowest
   b. least, most
   c. most, lowest
   d. most, most

3. The steps on the side of the MyPyramid remind us to be physically active at least _____ minutes per day.
   a. 5
   b. 10
   c. 20
   d. 30

4. The Dietary Guidelines for Americans were recently revised in
   a. 2000
   b. 2001
   c. 2003
   d. 2005

5. The term Daily Value is used on
   a. restaurant menus.
   b. food labels.
   c. medical charts.
   d. None of the above.

6. The Tolerable Upper Intake Level, or UL, is to
   a. estimate calorie needs of the average person.
   b. evaluate the highest amount of daily nutrient intake unlikely to cause adverse health effects.
   c. evaluate your current intake for a specific nutrient.
   d. compare the nutrient content of a food to approximate human needs.

7. The current food label must list
   a. a picture of the product.
   b. a uniform and realistic serving size.
   c. the RDA for each age group.
   d. ingredients alphabetically.

8. Dietary supplements are tightly regulated by the
   a. FDA.
   b. USDA.
   c. FTC.
   d. None of the above.

9. The scientific method begins with
   a. a hypothesis.
   b. research experiments.
   c. publication of research findings.
   d. observations made and questions asked.

10. The most common type of malnutrition in industrialized nations, such as the United States, is
    a. anorexia.
    b. protein deficiency.
    c. obesity.
    d. iron deficiency.

FURTHER READINGS

1. ADA Reports: Position of the American Dietetic Association: Fortification and nutritional supplements. *Journal of the American Dietetic Association* 105:1300, 2005.

   Choosing a wide variety of foods is the best strategy for promoting optimal health and reducing the risk of chronic diseases. This paper discusses the benefits of increasing the nutrient density of foods or diets through fortification or supplementation when diets do not contain adequate amounts of vitamins and minerals.

2. ADA Reports: Position of the American Dietetic Association: Food and nutrition misinformation. *Journal of the American Dietetic Association* 106:601, 2006.

   Much food and nutrition misinformation pervades North American society. Individuals should carefully consider the training of those who give such advice and be assured that registered dietitians are a reliable source.

3. Barr SI: Introduction to dietary reference intakes. *Applied Physiology, Nutrition, and Metabolism* 31:61, 2006.

   The development of the dietary reference intakes (DRIs) was a joint initiative by the United States and Canada to update and replace the former Recommended Nutrient Intakes for Canadians and the Recommended Dietary Allowances for Americans. The new DRIs are described.

4. Birt DF: Phytochemicals and cancer prevention: From epidemiology to mechanism of action. *Journal of the American Dietetic Association* 106:20, 2006.

   Studies in laboratory animals and cell cultures indicate a role for many components of fruits and vegetables in cancer prevention. Numerous human case-control studies have suggested that vegetable intake reduces the risk of a variety of cancers. These results have not been demonstrated for fruits. In addition, prospective studies have not supported a relationship between fruit and vegetable intake and cancer prevention. Although the relationship between fruit and vegetable intake and cancer risk is still unclear, a diet rich in fruits and vegetables is still one of the best recommendations to improve health and reduce overall chronic disease.

5. Borra S: Consumer perspectives on food labels. *American Journal of Clinical Nutrition* 83:1235S, 2006.

   An important goal of the nutrition and ingredient information on food labels is to help consumers make nutritious dietary choices. This article summarizes the results of recent quantitative and qualitative research on consumers' use and understanding of the food label information.

6. Drewnowski A: Concept of a nutritious food; toward a nutrient density score. *American Journal of Clinical Nutrition* 82:721, 2005.

   "Naturally nutrient-rich" is a consumer-friendly way to describe naturally nutrient-dense foods. The development of and potential uses for the "naturally nutrient-rich" nutrient density scoring system for foods is outlined in this article.

7. He FJ and others: Fruit and vegetable consumption and stroke: Meta-analysis of cohort studies. *Lancet* 367:320, 2006.

   Increased fruit and vegetable intake was associated with a reduced risk of both ischemic and hemorrhagic stroke. Compared to individuals who had less than 3 servings of fruit and vegetables per day, the risk was reduced for those with 3 to 5 servings per day and even more reduced for those with more than 5 servings per day.

8. Jackson K: Pioneering the frontier of nutrigenomics. *Today's Dietitian*, p. 34, November 2004.

   An exciting development in nutrition will be the ability to use a person's genetic profile to provide more precise nutrition guidance by dietitians and other clinicians. This article discusses this possibility.

9. Johnston CS: Uncle Sam's diet sensation: MyPyramid—an overview and commentary. *Medscape General Medicine* 7:78, 2005.

   This overview of the Internet-based MyPyramid points out several strengths of the new educational tool. These include the focus on reducing calories and increasing physical activity in an effort to address the obesity crisis. In addition, areas that the federal government still needs to address, such as access to this information by the underprivileged, are discussed.

10. Kennedy ET: Evidence for nutritional benefits in prolonging wellness. *American Journal of Clinical Nutrition* 83:410S, 2006.

    The interaction between genes; the environment; and lifestyle factors, especially diet and physical activity, are involved in healthy aging. The need to consider all the lifestyle and environmental factors contributing to suboptimal eating and lifestyle patterns is discussed.

11. Kretser AJ: The new Dietary Reference Intakes in food labeling: The food industry's perspective. *American Journal of Clinical Nutrition* 83:1231S, 2006.

    The food industry is prepared to update food labels using new nutrient recommendations. The Grocery Manufacturers Association welcomes the opportunity to coordinate nutrition information across the Dietary Guidelines for Americans 2005, MyPyramid, and the food label.

12. Meadows M: Healthier eating. *FDA Consumer* p. 10, May-June 2005.

    The latest Dietary Guidelines for Americans (2005) are reviewed. The article provides practical advice to put these guidelines into action—a task too few adults are doing well.

13. Meyer TE and others: Long-term caloric restriction ameliorates the decline in diastolic function in humans. *Journal of the American College of Cardiology* 47:398, 2006.

    Cardiovascular aging is associated with an increased likelihood of developing cardiovascular diseases, such as myocardial infarction (heart attack), stroke, and congestive heart failure. Calorie restriction (1671 kcal vs. 2445 kcal) affected heart functions that typically decline with age. Eating the nutrient-rich diet of less than 2000 kcal slowed the decline in diastolic function, a well-recognized marker of cardiovascular aging in humans. The results suggest that cutting calories will lead to a longer life.

14. Mitka M: Government unveils new food pyramid. *Journal of the American Medical Association* 293:2581, 2005.

    Both the pros and cons of MyPyramid are raised by nutrition and medical experts. The biggest criticism is that the tool is practically useless unless a person logs on to the MyPyramid website to find out the details regarding the diet plan.

15. Pavia M and others: Association between fruit and vegetable consumption and oral cancer: A meta-analysis of observational studies. *American Journal of Clinical Nutrition* 83:1126, 2006.

    Results showed that for each portion of fruit and vegetable consumed per day, the risk of oral cancer was reduced by 49% to 50%. The lower risk of oral cancer associated with fruit consumption was influenced by the type of fruit consumed.

16. Rebuilding the pyramid. *Tufts University Health & Nutrition Letter* p. 1, June 2005.

    The latest nutrition advice from MyPyramid is discussed. How to apply the recommendations to every day life is highlighted.

17. Seal CJ: Whole grains and CVD risk. *Proceedings of the Nutrition Society* 65:24, 2006.

    Evidence from population and epidemiological studies suggest a strong inverse relationship between the consumption of whole-grain foods and the risk of cardiovascular diseases (CVD). This evidence has resulted in recommendations to consume at least 3 servings of whole-grains per day. The mechanisms by which whole-grain foods have this effect on CVD, however, are poorly understood. Intervention studies are needed to support the health claims and promote whole-grain consumption.

18. Uncle Sam's diet book. *Tufts University Health & Nutrition Letter* p. 1, March 2005.

    Implementation of the latest Dietary Guidelines for Americans is discussed. The authors suggest even small changes that conform to this plan provide health benefits.

19. Woolf SH: Weighing the evidence to formulate dietary guidelines. *Journal of the American College of Nutrition* 25:277S, 2006.

    The steps involved in dietary guideline development are discussed. These include some combination of (1) specification of the topic and the guideline development methodology; (2) systematic review of the evidence; (3) consideration of expert opinion; (4) public policy analysis; (5) drafting of the document; and (6) peer review.

20. Zelman K, Kennedy E: Naturally nutrient rich . . . Putting more power on Americans' plates. *Nutrition Today* 40 (2):60, 2005.

    This article provides a review of a symposium that took place in March 2004 where experts discussed the evidence supporting the nutrient density principle and its role in guiding consumer nutrition.

▶ Check out the **Contemporary Nutrition ARIS site**

www.mhhe.com/wardlawcontfa1 for quizzes, flash cards, other activities, and weblinks designed to further help you learn about what you eat and why.

RATE YOUR PLATE

I. Does Your Diet Meet MyPyramid Recommendations?

Using your food-intake record from Chapter 1, place each food item in the appropriate group of the accompanying MyPyramid chart. That is, for each food item, indicate how many servings it contributes to each group based on the amount you ate (see Food Composition Table Supplement for serving sizes). Many of your food choices may contribute to more than one group. For example, toast with soft margarine contributes to two categories: (1) the grains group; and (2) the oils group. After entering all the values, add the number of servings consumed in each group. Finally, compare your total in each food group with the recommended number of servings shown in Table 2-4 or obtained from the www.MyPyramid.gov website. Enter a minus sign (−) if your total falls below the recommendation or a plus sign (+) if it equals or exceeds the recommendation.

Indicate the number of servings from MyPyramid that each food yields:

Food or Beverage	Amount Eaten	Milk	Meat & Beans	Fruits	Vegetables	Grains	Oils
Group totals							
Recommended servings							
Shortages in numbers of servings							

II. Are You Putting the Dietary Guidelines into Practice?

As noted in this chapter, the advice provided by the 2005 Dietary Guidelines for Americans can be summarized into three main points and a number of related activities. Fill out the following inventory to see to what extent you are following the basic intent of the Guidelines.

Food Intake

Do you:

Y	N	Consume a variety of nutrient-dense foods and beverages within and among the basic food groups of MyPryamid?

Choose foods that limit the intake of:

Y	N	Saturated fat
Y	N	*Trans* fat
Y	N	Cholesterol
Y	N	Added sugars
Y	N	Salt
Y	N	Alcohol (if used)

Emphasize in your food choices:

Y	N	Vegetables
Y	N	Fruits
Y	N	Legumes (beans)
Y	N	Whole-grain breads and cereals
Y	N	Fat-free or low-fat milk or equivalent milk products

Body Weight

Y	N	Maintain body weight in a healthy range by balancing energy intake from foods and beverages with energy expended?
Y	N	Engage in at least 30 minutes of moderate-intensity physical activity, above usual activity, at work or home on most days of the week?

Safe Food Handling

Y	N	Clean hands, food contact surfaces, and fruits and vegetables before preparation?
Y	N	Cook foods to a safe temperature to kill microorganisms?

Figure 2-8 points to other health practices that are part of the 2005 Dietary Guidelines for Americans, but this abbreviated list includes the major points to consider.

III. Applying the Nutrition Facts Label to Your Daily Food Choices

Imagine that you are at the supermarket looking for a quick meal before a busy evening. In the frozen food section, you find two brands of frozen cheese manicotti (see labels a and b). Which of the two brands would you choose? What information on the Nutrition Facts label in the figure contributed to this decision?

_____

_____

_____

_____

(a)

Nutrition Facts
Serving Size 1 Package (260g)
Servings Per Container 1

Amount Per Serving

Calories 390   Calories from Fat 160

	% Daily Value*
Total Fat 18g	**27**%
Saturated Fat 9g	**45**%
Trans Fat 2g	**
Cholesterol 45mg	**14**%
Sodium 880mg	**36**%
Total Carbohydrate 38g	**13**%
Dietary Fiber 4g	**15**%
Sugars 12g	
Protein 17g	

Vitamin A 10% • Vitamin C 4%

Calcium 40% • Iron 8%

*Percent Daily Values are based on a 2,000 calorie diet. Your daily values may be higher or lower depending on your calorie needs:

		Calories:	2,000	2,500
Total Fat	Less than		65g	80g
Sat Fat	Less than		20g	25g
Cholesterol	Less than		300mg	300mg
Sodium	Less than		2,400mg	2,400mg
Total Carbohydrate			300g	375g
Dietary Fiber			25g	30g

Calories per gram:
Fat 9 • Carbohydrate 4 • Protein 4

**Intake of *trans* fat should be as low as possible.

(b)

Nutrition Facts
Serving Size 1 Package (260g)
Servings Per Container 1

Amount Per Serving

Calories 230   Calories from Fat 35

	% Daily Value*
Total Fat 4g	**6**%
Saturated Fat 2g	**10**%
Trans Fat 1g	**
Cholesterol 15mg	**4**%
Sodium 590mg	**24**%
Total Carbohydrate 28g	**9**%
Dietary Fiber 3g	**12**%
Sugars 10g	
Protein 19g	

Vitamin A 10% • Vitamin C 10%

Calcium 35% • Iron 4%

*Percent Daily Values are based on a 2,000 calorie diet. Your daily values may be higher or lower depending on your calorie needs:

		Calories:	2,000	2,500
Total Fat	Less than		65g	80g
Sat Fat	Less than		20g	25g
Cholesterol	Less than		300mg	300mg
Sodium	Less than		2,400mg	2,400mg
Potassium			3,500mg	3,500mg
Total Carbohydrate			300g	375g
Dietary Fiber			25g	30g

Calories per gram:
Fat 9 • Carbohydrate 4 • Protein 4

**Intake of *trans* fat should be as low as possible.

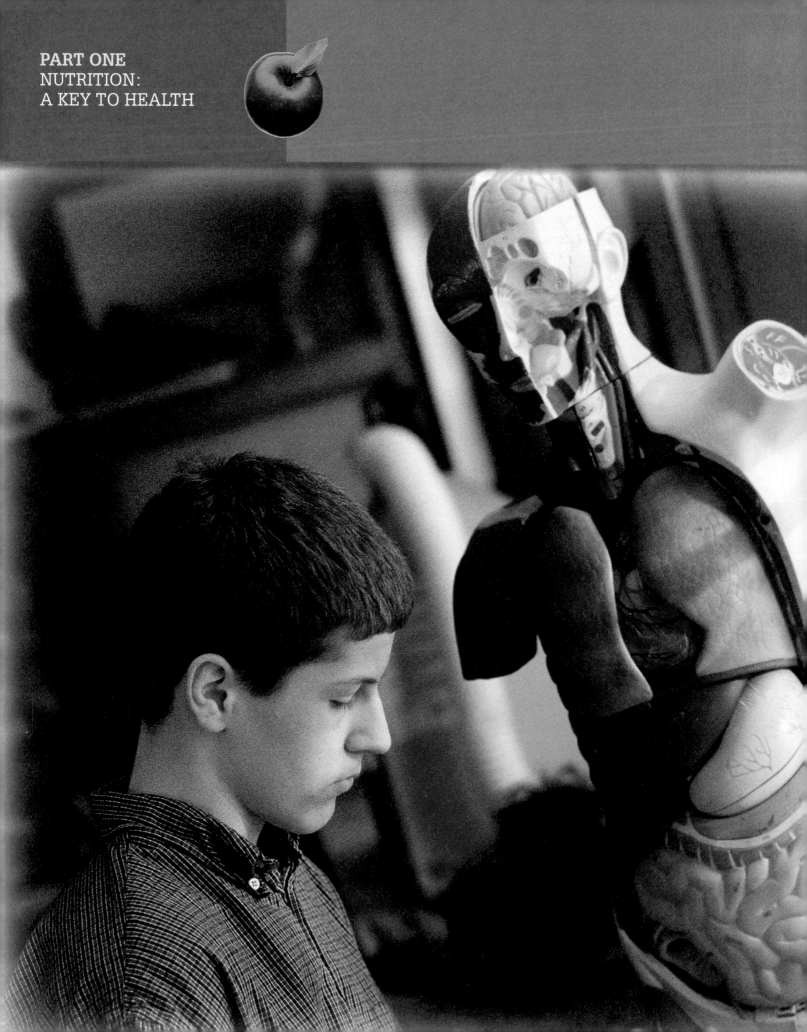

PART ONE
NUTRITION:
A KEY TO HEALTH

CHAPTER 3 The Human Body: A Nutrition Perspective

CHAPTER OBJECTIVES Chapter 3 is designed to allow you to:

1. Identify the functions of the common cellular components.
2. Define tissue, organ, and organ system.
3. List some basic characteristics of the 12 organ systems and outline a role for each related to nutrition.
4. Outline the overall processes of digestion and absorption in the mouth, stomach, small intestine, and large intestine, as well as the roles played by the liver, gallbladder, and pancreas.
5. Become familiar with some specific enzymes and hormones that act in digestion.
6. Understand the role of genetic background in the development of nutrition-related diseases.
7. Identify the major nutrition-related gastrointestinal health problems and approaches to treatment.

CHAPTER OUTLINE

MERELY EATING FOOD WON'T NOURISH YOU. You must first digest the food—break it down into usable forms of the essential nutrients that can be absorbed into the bloodstream. Once nutrients are taken up by the bloodstream, they can be distributed to and used by body cells.

We rarely think about, let alone control, digesting and absorbing foods. Except for a few voluntary responses—such as deciding what and when to eat, how well to chew food, and when to eliminate the remains—most digestion and absorption processes control themselves. As suggested in the comic in this chapter, we don't consciously decide when the pancreas will secrete digestive substances into the small intestine or how quickly foodstuffs will be propelled down the intestinal tract. Various hormones and the nervous system mostly control these functions. Your only awareness of these involuntary responses may be a hunger pang right before lunch or a "full" feeling after eating that last slice of pizza.

Let's examine digestion and absorption as well as other aspects of human physiology that support nutritional health. In the process you will become acquainted with the basic anatomy (structure) and physiology (function) of the circulatory system, nervous system, endocrine system, immune system, digestive system, urinary system, and storage capabilities of the human body.

 Refresh Your Memory

As you begin your study of human physiology in Chapter 3, you may want to review:

- Cell structure and function from previous coursework in university-level biology courses
- Also from any previous biology training, each of the body's organ systems

HUMAN PHYSIOLOGY

The human body is composed of trillions of cells. Each cell is a self-contained, living entity. Cells of the same type normally join together, using intercellular substances to form **tissues,** such as muscle tissue. One, two, or more tissues then combine in a particular way to form more complex structures, called **organs.** All organs contribute to nutritional health, and a person's overall nutritional state determines how well each organ functions. At a still higher level of coordination, several organs can cooperate for a common purpose to form an **organ system,** such as the digestive system. Overall, the human body is a coordinated unit of many highly structured organ systems (Fig. 3-1).

Chemical processes (reactions) occur constantly in every living cell: The production of new substances is balanced by the breaking down of older ones. An example is the constant formation and degradation of bone. For this turnover of substances to occur, cells require a continuous supply of energy in the form of dietary carbohydrate, protein, and/or fat. Cells also need water; building supplies, especially protein and minerals; and chemical regulators, such as the vitamins. Almost all cells also need a steady supply of oxygen. These substances enable the tissues, made from individual cells, to function properly.

tissues Collections of cells adapted to perform a specific function.

organ A group of tissues designed to perform a specific function—for example, the heart, which contains muscle tissue, nerve tissue, and so on.

organ system A collection of organs that work together to perform an overall function.

FRANK & ERNEST® by Bob Thaves

Some popular (fad) diets suggest not combining meat and potatoes to improve digestion and that fruit should only be eaten before noon. These diets might also purport that foods get stuck in the body and in turn putrefy and create toxins. Are there any scientific reasons to suggest that the timing of our food intake should optimize digestion? Do certain food practices improve digestion and subsequent absorption? This chapter provides some answers.

FRANK AND ERNEST reprinted by permission of Newspaper Enterprise Association, Inc.

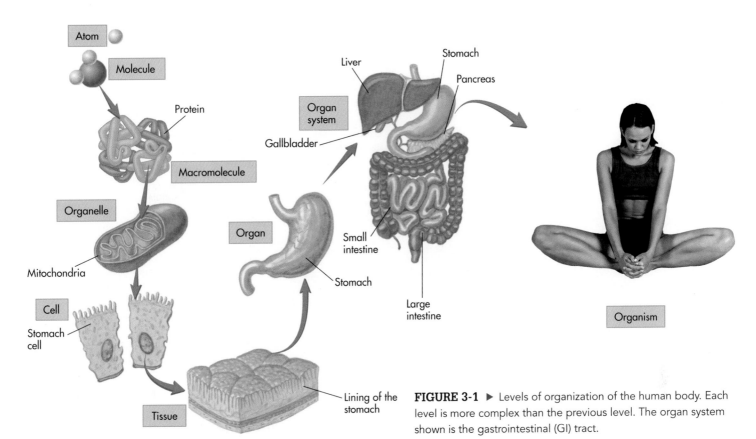

FIGURE 3-1 ▶ Levels of organization of the human body. Each level is more complex than the previous level. The organ system shown is the gastrointestinal (GI) tract.

Getting an adequate supply of all nutrients to the body's cells begins with a healthy diet. To assure optimal use of nutrients, the body's cells, tissues, organs, and organ systems also must work efficiently.

Chapter 3 covers the anatomy and physiology of the cell and major organ systems, especially as they relate to human nutrition. The information you are about to study is limited to the components of the various organ systems specifically influenced by the more than 45 essential nutrients discussed in this text.

THE CELL: STRUCTURE, FUNCTION AND METABOLISM

The cell is the basic structural and functional component of life. Living organisms are made of many different kinds of cells specialized to perform particular functions, and all cells are derived from preexisting cells. In the human body, all cells have certain common features. These cells have compartments and specialized structures that perform particular functions; these components are called **organelles** (Fig. 3-2). There are at least 15 different organelles. Eight of the most important organelles will be discussed. The numbers following the names of the cell structures correspond to the structures illustrated in Figure 3-2. Metabolism, the chemical processes that take place in body cells will also be discussed.

organelles Compartments, particles, or filaments that perform specialized functions within a cell.

Cell (Plasma) Membrane 1

There is an outside and inside to every cell, as defined by the cell (plasma) membrane. This membrane holds the cellular contents together and regulates the direction and flow of substances into and out of the cell. Cell-to-cell communication also occurs by way of this membrane.

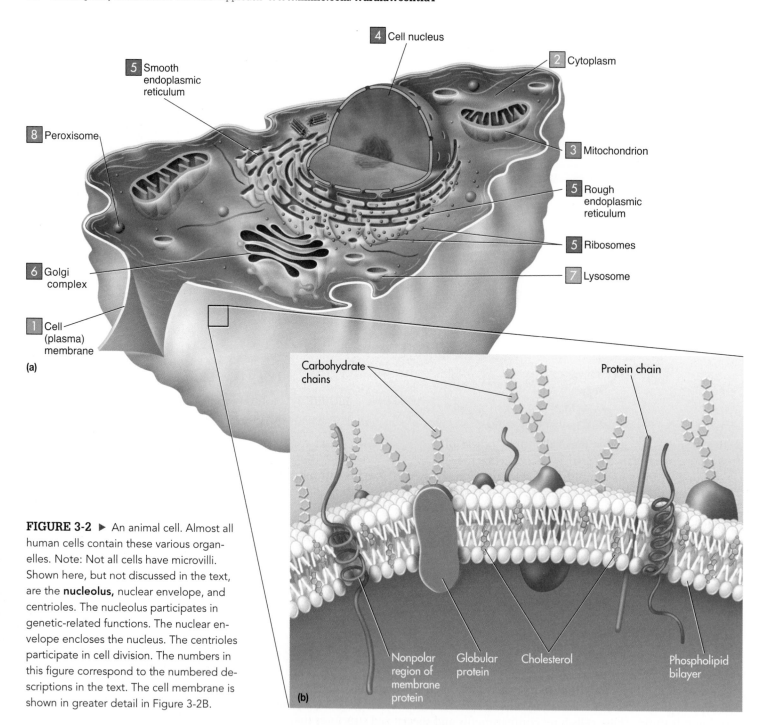

FIGURE 3-2 ▶ An animal cell. Almost all human cells contain these various organelles. Note: Not all cells have microvilli. Shown here, but not discussed in the text, are the **nucleolus,** nuclear envelope, and centrioles. The nucleolus participates in genetic-related functions. The nuclear envelope encloses the nucleus. The centrioles participate in cell division. The numbers in this figure correspond to the numbered descriptions in the text. The cell membrane is shown in greater detail in Figure 3-2B.

phospholipid Any of a class of fat-related substances that contain phosphorus, fatty acids, and a nitrogen-containing component. Phospholipids are an essential part of every cell.

enzyme A compound that speeds the rate of a chemical process but is not altered by that process. Almost all enzymes are proteins.

The cell membrane, illustrated in Figure 3-2(b), is a lipid bilayer (or double membrane) of **phospholipids** with their water-soluble heads facing both the interior of the cell and the exterior of the cell. Their water-insoluble tails are tucked into the center portion of the cell membrane.

Cholesterol is one component of the cell membrane. It is fat soluble, so it is embedded within the bilayer. This cholesterol provides rigidity and thus stability to the membrane.

There are also various proteins embedded in the cell membrane. Proteins provide structural support, act as transport vehicles, and function as **enzymes** that affect chemical processes within the membrane (see the later section on digestion for more about enzymes). Some proteins form open channels that allow water-soluble substances to pass into and out of the cell. Proteins on the outside surface of the membrane act as receptors, snagging essential substances that the cell needs and drawing them into the cell. Other proteins act as gates, opening and closing to control the flow of various particles into and out of the cell.

In addition to the lipid and protein, the membrane also contains carbohydrates that mark the exterior of the cell. These carbohydrates are combined either with protein or fat and provide a delivery service for sending messages to the cell's organelles. These carbohydrate structures also act as identification markers for the cell. In addition, they detect invaders and initiate defensive actions. In sum, these carbohydrates provide tags that are important to cellular identity and interaction.

Cytoplasm 2

The **cytoplasm** is the combination of fluid material and organelles within the cell, not including the nucleus. A small amount of energy for use by the cell can be produced by chemical processes that occur in the cytoplasm. This contributes to the survival of all cells and is the sole source of energy production in red blood cells. This energy production is called **anaerobic** metabolism because it doesn't require oxygen.

Organelles. Included within the cytoplasm are organelles. As described in the next two pages, they carry out vital roles in cell functions.

Mitochondria 3

Mitochondria are sometimes called the "power plants," or the powerhouse of the cell. These organelles are capable of converting the energy in energy-yielding nutrients from food (carbohydrate, protein, and fat) to a form of energy that cells can use. This is an **aerobic** process that uses the oxygen we inhale, as well as water, enzymes, and other compounds (see Chapter 10 for details). With the exception of red blood cells, all cells contain mitochondria; only the size, shape, and quantity vary.

Cell Nucleus 4

With the exception of the red blood cell, all cells have one or more nuclei. The **cell nucleus** is bounded by its own double membrane. The nucleus contains the genetic material responsible for controlling actions that occur in the cell. The genetic material consists of **genes** on **chromosomes** made up of **deoxyribonucleic acid (DNA)**. DNA is the "code book" that contains directions for making substances, specifically proteins, the cell needs. This code book remains in the nucleus of the cell, but sends its information to other cell organelles by way of a similar "messenger" molecule called **ribonucleic acid (RNA)**. The information on the DNA is copied onto the RNA through the process of **transcription** and then moves out to the cytoplasm through pores in the nuclear membrane. The RNA carries the transcribed DNA code to protein-synthesizing sites called **ribosomes**. There, the RNA code is used in the process of **translation** to make a specific protein (see Chapter 6 for details on protein synthesis). This process is also known as **gene expression**.

All of the DNA in a cell is copied during cell replication. DNA is a double-stranded molecule, and when the cell begins to divide, each strand is separated and an identical copy of each is made. Thus, each new DNA contains one new strand of DNA and one strand from the original DNA. In this way, the genetic code is preserved from one cell generation to the next. (The mitochondria contain their own DNA, so they reproduce themselves within a cell independent of action in the cell's nucleus.)

cytoplasm The fluid and organelles (except the nucleus) in a cell.

anaerobic Not requiring oxygen.

mitochondria The main sites of energy production in a cell. They also contain the pathway for oxidizing fat for fuel, among other metabolic pathways.

aerobic Requiring oxygen.

cell nucleus An organelle bound by its own double membrane and containing chromosomes, the genetic information for cell protein synthesis and cell replication.

gene A specific segment on a chromosome. Genes provide the blueprint for the production of cell proteins.

chromosome A single, large DNA molecule and its associated proteins; contains many genes to store and transmit genetic information.

deoxyribonucleic acid (DNA) The site of hereditary information in cells; DNA directs the synthesis of cell proteins.

ribonucleic acid (RNA) The single-stranded nucleic acid involved in the transcription of genetic information and translation of that information into protein structure.

transcription Information on DNA needed to make a protein is copied onto RNA.

▲ Genes are present on DNA—a double helix. The cell nucleus contains most of the DNA in the body.

ribosomes Cytoplasmic particles that mediate the linking together of amino acids to form proteins; may exist freely in the cytoplasm or attached to endoplasmic reticulum.

translation The information contained in RNA is used to determine the amino acids in a protein.

gene expression Use of DNA information on a gene to produce a protein. Thought to be a major determination of cell development.

endoplasmic reticulum (ER) An organelle in the cytoplasm composed of a network of canals running through the cytoplasm. Part of the endoplasmic reticulum contains ribosomes.

Golgi complex The cell organelle near the nucleus that processes newly synthesized protein for secretion or distribution to other organelles.

secretory vesicles Membrane-bound vesicles produced by the Golgi apparatus; contains protein and other compounds to be secreted by the cell.

lysosome A cellular organelle that contains digestive enzymes for use inside the cell for turnover of cell parts.

peroxisome A cell organelle that destroys toxic products within the cell.

adenosine triphosphate (ATP) The main energy currency for cells. ATP energy is used to promote ion pumping, enzyme activity, and muscular contraction.

Endoplasmic Reticulum (ER) 5

The outer membrane of the cell nucleus is continuous with a network of tubes called the **endoplasmic reticulum (ER).** Part of the endoplasmic reticulum (termed the rough [as opposed to smooth] endoplasmic reticulum) contains the ribosomes, where the RNA code is translated into proteins during protein synthesis. Many of these proteins play a central role in human nutrition. Parts of the endoplasmic reticulum also are involved in lipid synthesis, detoxification of toxic substances, and calcium storage and release in the cell.

Golgi Complex 6

The **Golgi complex** is a packaging site for proteins used in the cytoplasm or exported from the cell. It consists of sacs within the cytoplasm in which proteins are "packaged" as **secretory vesicles** for secretion by the cell.

Lysosomes 7

Lysosomes are the cell's digestive system. They are sacs that contain enzymes for the digestion of foreign material. Sometimes known as "suicide bags," they are responsible for digesting worn-out or damaged cell components. Certain cells associated with immune functions contain many lysosomes (see the later section on the immune system).

Peroxisomes 8

Peroxisomes contain enzymes that detoxify harmful chemicals. Peroxisomes get their name from the fact that hydrogen peroxide (H_2O_2) is formed as a result of such enzyme action. Peroxisomes also contain a protective enzyme called *catalase,* which prevents excessive accumulation of hydrogen peroxide in the cell, which would be very damaging. Peroxisomes also play a minor role in metabolizing one possible source of energy for cells—alcohol.

Cell Metabolism

Metabolism refers to the entire network of chemical processes involved in maintaining life. It encompasses all the sequences of chemical reactions that occur in the body's cells. These biochemical reactions take place in the cell cytoplasm and organelles that we have just discussed. They enable us to release and use energy from foods, synthesize one substance from another, and prepare waste products for excretion.

The reactions of metabolism that take place within your body can be categorized into one of two types. One type of reaction, anabolic, puts different molecules together and, therefore, requires energy. The other type of reaction, catabolic, takes molecules apart and, therefore, releases energy. The metabolism of the nutrients, carbohydrates, proteins, and fats are interrelated and yield energy. The other nutrients, vitamins and minerals, contribute to the enzyme activity that supports metabolic reactions in the cell.

As we discussed earlier, the metabolism of energy production begins in the cytoplasm with the initial anaerobic breakdown of glucose. The remaining aerobic steps of energy production take place in the mitochondria. Ultimately the cells of the body use these interconnected processes to convert the energy found in food to energy stored in the high-energy compound, **adenosine triphosphate (ATP).** You will learn more about the metabolism of energy sources in Chapter 12.

CONCEPT CHECK

In Chapter 1, you learned that fat (lipids), protein, and carbohydrate function as fuels. Now you recognize that these organic nutrients also serve as structural materials in the cell membrane. This is typical of many nutrients; they can carry out multiple functions. The cell receives nutrients and other substances through the cell membrane by using various transport systems.

The basic structural unit in the body is the cell. Within the cell are a variety of organelles with unique functions to perform. Although there is no typical cell, virtually all cells have the same organelles, each performing the same essential task.

ORGANIZATION OF THE BODY

As noted earlier, when groups of similar cells work together to accomplish a specialized task, the arrangement is referred to as a tissue. Humans are composed of four primary types of tissue: **epithelial, connective, muscle,** and **nervous.** Epithelial tissue is composed of cells that cover surfaces both inside and outside the body. For example, the lining of the respiratory tract is made up of epithelial cells. These cells of epithelial tissue secrete important substances, absorb nutrients, and excrete waste. Connective tissue supports and protects the body, stores fat, and produces blood cells. Muscle tissue is designed for movement. Nervous tissue found in the brain and spinal cord is designed for communication. These four types of tissues then go on to form various organs, and ultimately, organ systems (Table 3-1).

epithelial tissue The surface cells that line the outside of the body and all external passages within it.

connective tissue Protein tissue that holds different structures in the body together. Some structures are made up of connective tissue— notably, **tendons** and **cartilage.** Connective tissue also forms part of bone and the nonmuscular structures of arteries and veins.

muscle tissue A type of tissue adapted to contract to cause movement.

nervous tissue Tissue composed of highly branched, elongated cells, which transport nerve impulses from one part of the body to another.

TABLE 3-1 Organ Systems of the Body

System	Major Components	Functions Related to Nutrition
Cardiovascular	Heart, blood vessels, and blood	Transports nutrients, waste products, gases, and hormones throughout the body and plays a role in the immune response and the regulation of body temperature
Lymphatic	Lymph vessels, lymph nodes, and other lymph organs	Removes foreign substances from the blood and lymph, combats disease, maintains tissue fluid balance, and aids in fat absorption
Nervous	Brain, spinal cord, nerves, and sensory receptors	A major regulatory system: detects sensation, controls movements, and controls physiological and intellectual functions
Endocrine	Endocrine glands, such as the pituitary, thyroid, and adrenal glands	A major regulatory system: participates in the regulation of metabolism, reproduction, and many other functions through the action of hormones
Immune	White blood cells, lymph vessels and nodes, spleen, thymus gland, and other lymph tissues	Provides defense against foreign invaders; formation of white blood cells
Digestive	Mouth, esophagus, stomach, intestines, and accessory structures (liver, gallbladder, and pancreas)	Performs the mechanical and chemical processes of digestion, absorption of nutrients, and elimination of wastes
Urinary	Kidneys, urinary bladder, and the ducts that carry urine	Removes waste products from the circulatory system and regulates the acidity, chemical composition, and water content of the blood
Integumentary	Skin, hair, nails, and sweat glands	Protects the body, regulates temperature, prevents water loss, and produces a substance that converts to vitamin D upon sun exposure
Skeletal	Bones, associated cartilage, and joints	Supports the body, and allows for body movement, produces blood cells, and stores minerals
Muscular	Smooth, cardiac, and skeletal muscle	Produces body movement, maintains posture, and produces body heat
Respiratory	Lungs and respiratory passages	Exchanges gases (oxygen and carbon dioxide) between the blood and the atmosphere and regulates blood acid-base (pH) balance
Reproductive	Gonads, accessory structures, and genitals of males and females	Performs the processes of reproduction and influences sexual functions and behaviors

Foodstuffs
Water

Digestive System

Unabsorbed
foodstuffs

**Respiratory
System**

Heart

O₂ in
CO₂ out

Organic waste (e.g., **urea**)
Minerals
Water

Cardiovascular System

**Urinary
System**

Blood

Cell

Extracellular
fluid

**Internal
environment**

**External
environment**

FIGURE 3-3 ▶ Exchanges of nutrients occur between our external environment and the internal environment of the circulatory system via the digestive, respiratory, and urinary systems. Overall, the human body is a combination of 12 systems working together to support cell needs.

We will be particularly concerned in Chapter 3 with the digestive system. The nutrients we consume in food are unavailable until such time as they have been processed by the digestive system. This employs chemical and mechanical means to alter food so that the nutrients can be released and absorbed into the body for distribution to body tissues.

Sometimes organs within a system can serve another system. For example, the basic function of the digestive system is to convert the food we eat into absorbable nutrients. At the same time, the digestive system serves the immune system by preventing dangerous pathogens from invading the body and causing illness. As you study nutrition, you will note the multiple roles played by many organs (Fig. 3-3).

The overriding theme of human nutrition is to understand the actions of nutrients as they affect different cells, tissues, organs, and organ systems. Each type of organ system is impacted by nutrient intake and simultaneously determines how each nutrient is used.

Our task now is to explore the key systems in the body as they specifically relate to the study of human nutrition: circulatory (cardiovascular and lymphatic), nervous, endocrine, immune, digestive, and urinary systems. This part of Chapter 3 will set the stage for a more detailed look at these and other organ systems in later chapters covering various aspects of human nutrition.

Also in this chapter, we will also introduce the relatively new area of genetics and nutrition. Throughout this book, discussions will point out how you can personalize nutrition advice based on your genetic background. In this way, you can identify and avoid the "controllable" risk factors that would contribute to development of genetically linked diseases present in your family.

urea Nitrogenous waste product of protein metabolism; major source of nitrogen in the urine.

cardiovascular system The body system consisting of the heart, blood vessels, and blood. This system transports nutrients, waste products, gases, and hormones throughout the body and plays an important role in immune responses and regulation of body temperature.

lymphatic system A system of vessels and lymph that accepts fluid surrounding cells and large particles, such as products of fat absorption. Lymph eventually passes into the bloodstream from the lymphatic system.

CARDIOVASCULAR SYSTEM AND LYMPHATIC SYSTEM

The body has two separate organ systems that circulate fluids in the body: the **cardiovascular system** and the **lymphatic system.** The cardiovascular system consists of the heart and blood vessels. The lymphatic system consists of lymphatic vessels and a number of lymph tissues. Blood flows through the cardiovascular system, while **lymph** flows through the lymphatic system.

Cardiovascular System

The heart is a muscular pump that normally contracts and relaxes 50 to 90 times per minute when the body is at rest. This continual pumping, measured by taking your pulse, keeps blood moving through the blood vessels. The blood that flows through the cardiovascular system is composed of **plasma,** red blood cells, white blood cells, platelets, and many other substances. It travels two basic routes. In the first route, blood circulates from the right side of the heart, through the lungs, and then back to the heart. In the lungs, blood picks up oxygen and releases carbon dioxide. After this exchange of gases has taken place, blood is said to be *oxygenated* and returns to the left side of your heart. In the second route, the oxygenated blood circulates from the left side of the heart to all other body cells, eventually returning back to the right side of the heart (Fig. 3-4). After blood has circulated throughout the body, it is *deoxygenated*. (As you review the cardiovascular system, recall from your previous studies of biology that *left* and *right* designations of the heart refer to the left and right sides of your body, not of the page in your textbook.)

In the cardiovascular system, blood leaves the heart via **arteries,** which branch into **capillaries,** a network of tiny blood vessels. Exchange of nutrients, oxygen, and waste products between the blood and cells occurs through the minute, web-like pores of the capillaries (Fig. 3-5). Capillaries service every region of the body via individual capillary beds only one cell layer thick. The blood then returns to the heart via the **veins.**

The cardiovascular system distributes nutrients absorbed from food and oxygen from the air to all body cells (review Fig. 3-3). Other functions include delivery of hormones to their target cells, maintenance of a constant body temperature, and distribution of white blood cells throughout the body to protect against pathogens as part of the immune system (see the later section, "Immune System").

Portal Circulation in the Gastrointestinal Tract. Water and nutrients are transferred to the circulatory system through capillary beds. Once absorbed through the stomach or intestinal wall, nutrients reach one of two destinations. Some nutrients are taken up by cells in the intestines and portions of the stomach to nourish those organs. Most of the nutrients from recently eaten foods, however, are transferred into **portal circulation.** To enter portal circulation, the nutrients pass from the intestinal capillaries into veins that eventually merge into a very large vein called a **portal vein.** Unlike most veins in the body—which carry blood back to the heart—this portal vein leads directly to the liver. This enables the liver to process absorbed nutrients before they enter the general circulation of the bloodstream. Overall, portal circulation represents a special form of circulation in the cardiovascular system.

Lymphatic System

The **lymphatic system** is also a circulatory system. It consists of a network of lymphatic vessels and the fluid (**lymph**) that moves through them. Lymph is similar to blood, consisting largely of blood plasma that has found its way out of capillaries and into the spaces between cells. It contains a full array of the various white blood cells that play an important role in the immune system. However, neither red blood cells nor platelets are present. Lymph is collected in tiny lymph vessels all over the body and moves through even larger vessels until it eventually enters the cardiovascular system through major veins near the heart. This flow is driven by muscle contractions arising from normal body movements.

▲ The body is made up of numerous organ systems.

plasma The fluid, extracellular portion of the circulating blood. This includes the blood serum plus all blood-clotting factors. In contrast, **serum** is the fluid that remains after clotting factors have been removed from plasma.

artery A blood vessel that carries blood away from the heart.

capillary A microscopic blood vessel that connects the smallest arteries and veins; site of nutrient, oxygen, and waste exchange between body cells and the blood.

vein A blood vessel that carries blood to the heart.

portal circulation The portion of the circulatory system that uses a large vein (portal vein) to carry nutrient-rich blood from capillaries in the intestines and portions of the stomach to the liver.

lymph A clear fluid that flows through lymph vessels; carries most forms of fat after their absorption by the small intestine.

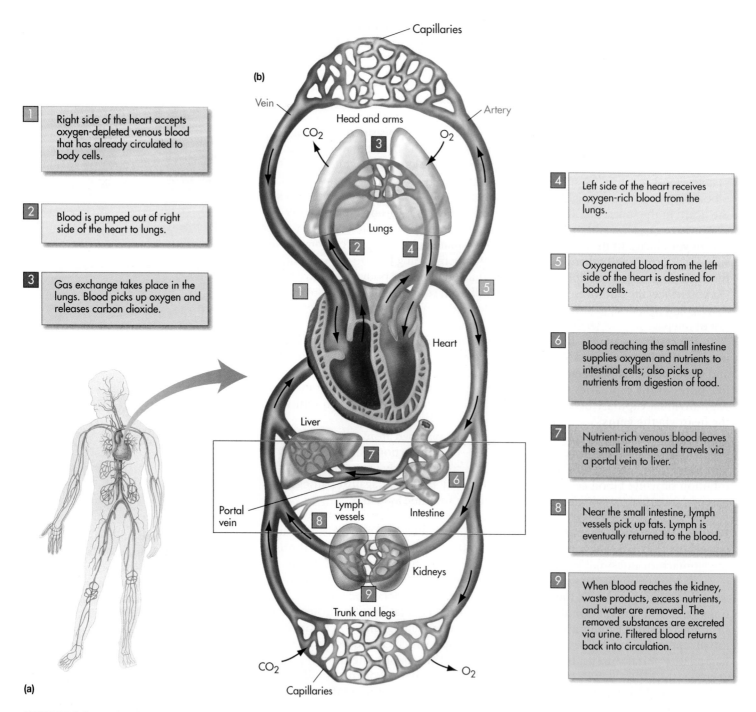

1. Right side of the heart accepts oxygen-depleted venous blood that has already circulated to body cells.

2. Blood is pumped out of right side of the heart to lungs.

3. Gas exchange takes place in the lungs. Blood picks up oxygen and releases carbon dioxide.

4. Left side of the heart receives oxygen-rich blood from the lungs.

5. Oxygenated blood from the left side of the heart is destined for body cells.

6. Blood reaching the small intestine supplies oxygen and nutrients to intestinal cells; also picks up nutrients from digestion of food.

7. Nutrient-rich venous blood leaves the small intestine and travels via a portal vein to liver.

8. Near the small intestine, lymph vessels pick up fats. Lymph is eventually returned to the blood.

9. When blood reaches the kidney, waste products, excess nutrients, and water are removed. The removed substances are excreted via urine. Filtered blood returns back into circulation.

FIGURE 3-4 ▶ Blood circulation through the body. Figure A shows the heart and some examples of the major arteries and veins of the cardiovascular system. Figure B shows the paths that blood takes from the heart to the lungs (1–3), back to the heart (4), and through the rest of the body (5–9). The red color indicates blood richer in oxygen; blue is for blood carrying more carbon dioxide. Keep in mind that arteries and veins go to all parts of the body.

Lymphatic Circulation in the Gastrointestinal Tract. Besides contributing to the defense of the body against invading pathogens, lymphatic vessels that serve the small intestine play an important role in nutrition. These vessels pick up and transport the majority of products of fat digestion and fat absorption. These fat-related products are too large to enter the bloodstream directly and therefore are generally emptied into the bloodstream only after passing through the lymphatic system. The lymph vessels also take up excess fluid that collects between cells and returns it to the bloodstream.

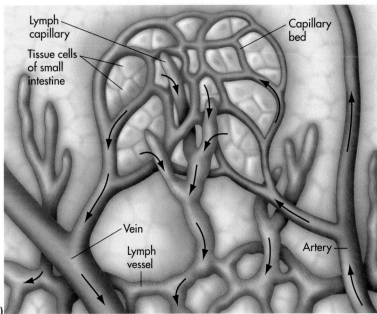

FIGURE 3-5 ▶ Capillary and lymph vessels. (a) Exchange of oxygen (O_2) and nutrients for carbon dioxide (CO_2) and waste products occurs between the capillaries and the surrounding tissue cells. (b) Lymph vessels are also present in capillary beds, such as in the small intestine. Lymph vessels in the small intestine are also called **lacteals.** The lymph vessels have closed ends.

CONCEPT CHECK

Blood is transported from the right side of the heart to the capillaries in the lungs. Carbon dioxide is removed and oxygen is taken up by red blood cells. The oxygenated blood returns to the left side of the heart. Here it is pumped into general circulation. In the capillaries, oxygen is released from the red blood cells and delivered through pores in the capillaries to the surrounding cells. Nutrients also are distributed from the bloodstream to body cells via the capillaries. Carbon dioxide released from cells travels through the capillary pores to the blood.

The lymph system serves several purposes: the transport of absorbed dietary fats, the uptake and return to the bloodstream of excess fluid that collects between cells, and the defense of the body against invading pathogens.

NERVOUS SYSTEM

The **nervous system** is a regulatory system that centrally controls most body functions. The nervous system can detect changes occurring in various organs and the external environment and initiate corrective action when needed to maintain a constant internal environment. The nervous system also regulates activities that change almost instantly, such as muscle contractions and perception of danger. The body has many receptors that receive information about what is happening within the body and in the outside environment. For the most part these receptors are found in our eyes, ears, skin, nose, and stomach. We act on information from these receptors via the nervous system.

The basic structural and functional unit of the nervous system is the **neuron.** These are elongated, highly branched cells. The body contains about 100 billion neurons. Neurons respond to electrical and chemical signals, conduct electrical impulses, and release chemical regulators. Overall, neurons allow us to perceive what is occurring in our environment, engage in learning, store vital information in memory, and control the body's voluntary (and involuntary) actions.

nervous system The body system consisting of the brain, spinal cord, nerves, and sensory receptors. This system detects sensations, directs movements, and controls physiological and intellectual functions.

neuron The structural and functional unit of the nervous system. Consists of a **cell body, dendrites,** and an **axon.**

FIGURE 3-6 ▶ Transmission of a message from one neuron to another neuron or to another type of cell that relies on neurotransmitters. Vesicles containing neurotransmitters, formed within the neuron, fuse with the membrane of the neuron and the neurotransmitter is released into the synapse. The neurotransmitter then binds to the receptors on the nearby neuron (or cell). In this way, the message is transmitted from one neuron to another or to the cell that ultimately performs the action directed by the message.

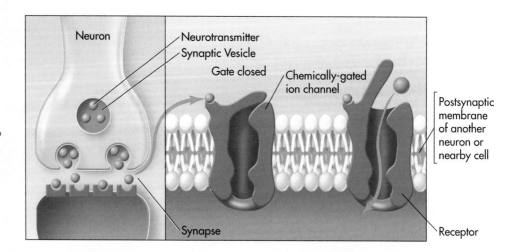

synapse The space between one neuron and another neuron (or cell).

neurotransmitter A compound made by a nerve cell that allows for communication between it and other cells.

norepinephrine A neurotransmitter from nerve endings and and a hormone from the adrenal gland. It is released in times of stress and is involved in hunger regulation, blood glucose regulation, and other body processes.

epinephrine A hormone also known as *adrenaline;* it is released by the adrenal glands (located on each kidney) at times of stress. It acts to increase glycogen breakdown in the liver, among other functions.

myelin sheath A lipid and protein combination (lipoprotein) that covers nerve fibers.

endocrine system The body system consisting of the various glands and the hormones these glands secrete. This system has major regulatory functions in the body, such as reproduction and cell metabolism.

endocrine gland A hormone-producing gland.

The brain stores information, reacts to incoming information, solves problems, and generates thoughts. In addition, the brain plans a course of action based on the other sensory inputs. Responses to the stimuli are carried out mostly through the rest of the nervous system.

Simply put, the nervous system receives information through stimulation of various receptors, processes this information, and sends out signals through its various branches for an action that needs to be taken. Actual transmission of the signal occurs through a change in the sodium and potassium concentration in the neuron. There is an influx of sodium into the neuron and a loss of potassium as the message is sent. Concentrations of these minerals are then restored to normal amounts in the neuron after the signal passes, making it ready to conduct another message.

When the signal must bridge a gap **(synapse)** between the branches of different neurons, the message is generally converted to a chemical signal called a **neurotransmitter.** The neurotransmitter is then released into the gap, and its target may be another neuron or another type of cell, such as a muscle cell (Fig. 3-6). If the signal is sent to another neuron, this allows it to continue on to its final destination. The neurotransmitters used in this process are often made from common nutrients found in foods, such as amino acids. The amino acid tryptophan is converted to the neurotransmitter serotonin, and the amino acid tyrosine is converted to the neurotransmitters **norepinephrine** and **epinephrine** (also called adrenaline).

Other nutrients also play a role in the nervous system. Calcium is needed for the release of neurotransmitters from neurons. Vitamin B-12 plays a role in the formation of the **myelin sheath,** which provides insulation around specific parts of most neurons. Finally, a regular supply of carbohydrate in the form of glucose is important for supplying fuel for the brain. The brain can use other calorie sources, but generally relies on glucose.

ENDOCRINE SYSTEM

The **endocrine system** plays a major role in the regulation of metabolism, reproduction, water balance, and many other functions by producing hormones in the **endocrine glands** of the body and subsequently releasing them into the blood (Fig. 3-7). The term *hormone* comes from the Greek word for "to stir or excite." A true hormone is a regulatory compound that has a specific site of synthesis from which it then enters the bloodstream to reach target cells. Hormones are the messengers of the body. They can be permissive (turn on), antagonistic (turn off), or synergistic (work in cooperation with another hormone) in performing a task. Some compounds must undergo

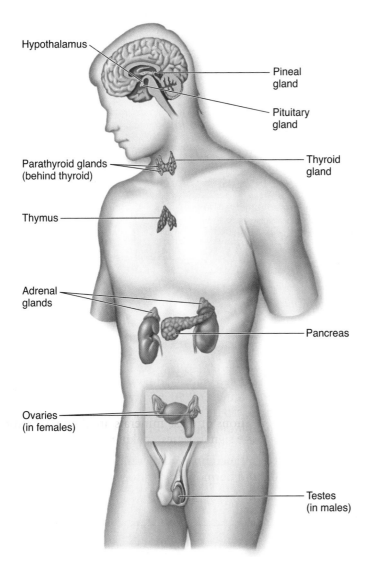

Hypothalamus

Pineal gland

Pituitary gland

Parathyroid glands (behind thyroid)

Thyroid gland

Thymus

Adrenal glands

Pancreas

Ovaries (in females)

Testes (in males)

FIGURE 3-7 ▶ The endocrine system is made up of several glands that act in the regulation of metabolism, reproduction, water balance, and many other functions.

chemical changes before they can function as hormones. For example, vitamin D, synthesized in the skin or obtained from food, is converted into an active hormone by chemical changes made in the liver and kidneys.

The hormone **insulin,** synthesized in and released from the pancreas, helps control the amount of glucose in the blood. Insulin is mostly produced when glucose in the blood rises to a certain level, usually after a meal. At this point, insulin is released and it travels to the muscle, adipose, and liver cells of the body. Among its many functions, insulin allows for the movement of glucose from the blood into muscle and adipose cells. In the liver cells, insulin causes an increase in stored glycogen by stimulating the synthesis of glycogen from glucose. Once a sufficient amount of glucose has been cleared from the blood, the production of insulin lessens. The hormones epinephrine, norepinephrine, glucagon, and growth hormone have just the opposite effect on blood glucose. They all cause an increase in blood glucose through a variety of actions (Table 3-2). **Thyroid hormones,** synthesized in and released from the thyroid gland (Fig. 3-7), help to control the body's rate of metabolism. Other hormones are especially important in regulating digestive processes (see the later section, "Digestive System").

thyroid hormones Hormones produced by the thyroid gland that among their functions increase the rate of overall metabolism in the body.

TABLE 3-2   Some Hormones of the Endocrine System with Nutritional Significance

Hormone	Gland/Organ	Target	Effect	Role in Nutrition
Insulin	Pancreas	Adipose (fat) and muscle cells	Decreased blood glucose	Uptake and storage of glucose, fat, and amino acids by cells
Glucagon	Pancreas	Liver	Increased blood glucose	Release of glucose from liver stores, release of fat from adipose tissue
Epinephrine, Norepinephrine	Adrenal glands	Heart, blood vessels, brain, lungs	Increased body metabolism and blood glucose	Release of glucose and fat into the blood
Growth hormone	Pituitary gland	Most cells	Promotion of amino acid uptake by cells, increased blood glucose	Promotion of protein synthesis and growth, increased fat use for energy
Thyroid hormones	Thyroid gland	Most organs	Increased oxygen consumption, overall growth, brain development of the nervous system	Protein synthesis, increased body metabolism

receptor A site in a cell at which compounds (such as hormones) bind. Cells that contain receptors for a specific compound are partially controlled by that compound.

immune system The body system consisting of white blood cells, lymph glands and vessels, and various other body tissues. The immune system provides defense against foreign invaders, primarily due to the action of various types of white blood cells.

Hormones are not available to all cells in the body, but only those with the correct **receptor** protein. These binding sites are highly specific for a certain hormone. They are generally found on the cell membrane. The hormone attaches to its receptor on the cell membrane. This binding activates additional compounds called second messengers within the cell to carry out the assigned task. This is true of insulin. A few hormones can penetrate the cell membrane and eventually bind to receptors on the DNA in the nucleus (e.g., thyroid hormone and estrogen).

CONCEPT CHECK

The functional unit of the nervous system is the neuron. Communication between neurons themselves, and other types of cells, is via neurotransmitters released into the synapse between the cells.

In the endocrine system, hormones are produced by glands in response to a change in the internal or external environment of the body. The gland secretes the hormone into the blood, and the blood delivers it to target cells. The hormone either attaches to receptors in the cell membrane and, through the action of second messengers, causes changes within the cell, or enters the cell and binds to the DNA in the cell to cause changes within the cell.

IMMUNE SYSTEM

Many types of body cells and body components work in cooperation as part of the **immune system** to maintain a defense against infection (Fig. 3-8). The components that work as part of the immune system include the skin, intestinal cells, and white blood cells. Several nutrients, including protein; minerals iron, copper, and zinc; and vitamins A, B-6, B-12, C, and folate have important roles in the immune system. These nutrients are key factors in the synthesis, growth, development, and activity of immune cells and additional factors that kill pathogens. It is easy to demonstrate the importance of nutritional health for immune function. Early humans were plagued by famine and thus, malnutrition; this contributed to infections, often leading to death. Today, largely because of better nutrition, most of the world avoids that cycle.

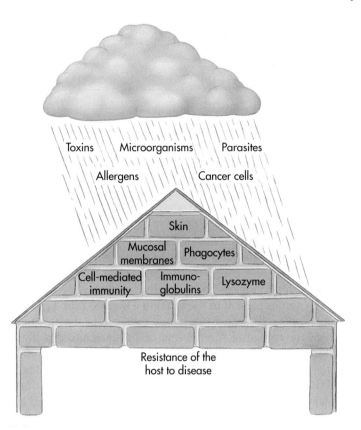

FIGURE 3-8 ▶ Just as the roof and other external structures of a house protect the inside environment from outside elements, host protective factors of the immune system "shelter" humans from threats such as diseases and toxins.

We are born with most aspects of immune function; these are termed **nonspecific** (or innate) because the targets are a variety of microorganisms. In contrast, white blood cells produce **immunoglobulins**, also called antibodies, that target specific organisms or foreign proteins called antigens. These immunoglobulins constitute **specific** (or adaptive) immune function. Once exposed, a memory is created such that a second exposure to the substance will produce a more vigorous and rapid attack.

Skin

The skin is a large component of the immune system, forming an almost continuous barrier surrounding the body. Invading microorganisms have difficulty penetrating the skin. However, if the skin is split by lesions, bacteria can easily penetrate this barrier. Skin health is poor during deficiencies of such nutrients as essential fatty acids, vitamin A, niacin, and zinc. Vitamin A deficiency also decreases gland secretions in the skin that contain the enzyme **lysozyme,** capable of killing bacteria. Bacterial eye infections are common in developing countries, often as a result of a vitamin A deficiency.

Intestinal Cells

The cells of the intestines form an important barrier to invading microorganisms. The cells are packed closely together, producing a physical barrier to microorganisms. In addition, specialized cells that produce immune factors—such as immunoglobulins— are scattered throughout the intestinal tract. These immune factors bind to the invading microorganisms, preventing them from entering the bloodstream. These factors are part of the **mucosal membrane** aspect of immunity.

Nutrient deficiencies can cause the intestinal cells to break down weakening the mucosal membrane so that microorganisms more easily enter the body and cause infections. Thus, two common results of undernutrition related to an impaired immune system are diarrhea and bacterial infections of the bloodstream. To protect the health

immunoglobulins Proteins found in the blood that bind to specific **antigens**; also called **antibodies**. The five major classes of immunoglobulins play different roles in antibody-mediated immunity.

antigen Any substance that induces a state of sensitivity and/or resistance to microorganisms or toxic substances after a lag period; foreign substance that stimulates a specific aspect of the immune system.

antibody Blood protein (immunoglobulin) that binds foreign proteins found in the body. This helps to prevent and control infections.

lysozyme An enzyme produced by a variety of cells; it can destroy bacteria by rupturing their cell membranes.

FIGURE 3-9 ▶ One type of white blood cell, phagocytes, can ingest bacteria, fungi, viruses, and other foreign particles in the process of phagocytosis. An indentation is formed and the particle is engulfed by the cell. The foreign material is eventually digested by lysosomes in the cell.

white blood cells One of the formed elements of the circulating blood system; also called *leukocytes*. White blood cells are able to squeeze through intracellular spaces and migrate. They phagocytize bacteria, fungi, and viruses, as well as detoxify proteins that may result from allergic reactions, cellular injury, and other immune system cells.

phagocytosis A process in which a cell forms an indentation, and particles or fluids entering the indentation are then engulfed by the cell.

cell-mediated immunity A process in which certain white blood cells come in contact with the invading cells to destroy them.

digestive system The body system consisting of the gastrointestinal tract and accessory structures such as the liver, gallbladder, and pancreas. This system performs the mechanical and chemical processes of digestion, absorption of nutrients, and elimination of wastes.

digestion The process by which large ingested molecules are mechanically and chemically broken down to produce basic nutrients that can be absorbed across the wall of the GI tract.

of the intestinal tract, an adequate nutrient intake is necessary—especially of protein, vitamin A, vitamin B-6, vitamin B-12, vitamin C, folate, and zinc.

<u>MAKING **DECISIONS**</u>

Immune Status

Although many studies show that a healthy nutritional state is associated with good immune status, other studies show that an overabundance of certain nutrients can harm the immune system. For example, taking too much zinc may decrease immune function (see Chapter 9).

White Blood Cells

Once a microorganism enters the bloodstream, **white blood cells** move in to attack it. A variety of types of white blood cells participate in this response and function in unique ways. For example, a class called **phagocytes** circulates throughout the circulatory system and ingests and sometimes digests microorganisms and foreign particles (via lysosomes present in the cells) in a process called **phagocytosis** (Fig. 3-9). Other white blood cells participate in **cell-mediated immunity**, achieved when certain immune cells recognize foreign cells or proteins and directly attack and destroy them. Immunoglobulins in their role as antibodies elicit an antibody-antigen response that binds microorganisms and proteins that are foreign to the body and destroys them, and then creates a template (memory) that allows future recognition of the microorganism or foreign protein. Recognition allows more rapid attacks in the future.

Some white blood cells live only a few days. Their constant resynthesis requires steady nutrient intake. The immune system needs (1) iron to produce an important killing factor; (2) copper for the synthesis of a specific type of white blood cell; and (3) adequate amounts of protein, vitamin B-6, vitamin B-12, vitamin C, and folate for general cell synthesis and, later, cell activity. Zinc and vitamin A are also needed for the overall growth and development of immune cells.

<u>CONCEPT **CHECK**</u>

Many types of body cells and body components work in cooperation as part of the immune system to maintain a defense against infection. The skin forms an almost continuous barrier surrounding the body. Cell secretions contain the enzyme lysozyme. Specialized cells in the intestines and certain white blood cells secrete antibodies (immunoglobulins). Phagocytes roam throughout the circulatory system and ingest and sometimes digest microorganisms and foreign particles. Other white blood cells participate in cell-mediated immunity. This occurs when certain immune cells recognize foreign cells and directly attack them. Many nutrients, including protein, iron, copper, zinc, vitamin B-6, B-12, C, and folate, are needed for the overall growth and development of immune cells.

DIGESTIVE SYSTEM

The foods and beverages we consume, for the most part, must undergo extensive alteration by the **digestive system** to provide us with usable nutrients. The processes of **digestion** and **absorption** take place in a long tube that is open at both ends and extends from the mouth to the anus. This tube is called the **gastrointestinal (GI) trac**t (Fig. 3-10). Nutrients from the food we eat must pass through the walls of the GI tract—from the inside to the outside—to be absorbed into the bloodstream. The organs that make up the GI tract, as well as some additional accessory organs located nearby, are collectively known as the digestive system.

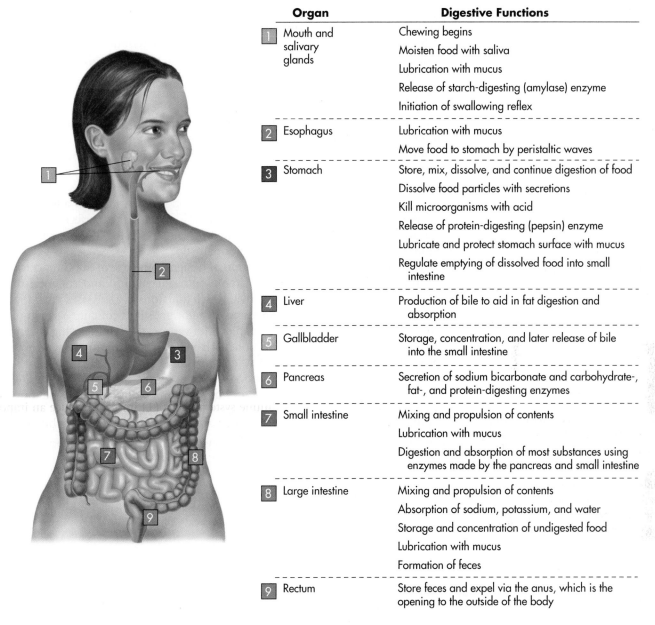

Organ	Digestive Functions
1 Mouth and salivary glands	Chewing begins
	Moisten food with saliva
	Lubrication with mucus
	Release of starch-digesting (amylase) enzyme
	Initiation of swallowing reflex
2 Esophagus	Lubrication with mucus
	Move food to stomach by peristaltic waves
3 Stomach	Store, mix, dissolve, and continue digestion of food
	Dissolve food particles with secretions
	Kill microorganisms with acid
	Release of protein-digesting (pepsin) enzyme
	Lubricate and protect stomach surface with mucus
	Regulate emptying of dissolved food into small intestine
4 Liver	Production of bile to aid in fat digestion and absorption
5 Gallbladder	Storage, concentration, and later release of bile into the small intestine
6 Pancreas	Secretion of sodium bicarbonate and carbohydrate-, fat-, and protein-digesting enzymes
7 Small intestine	Mixing and propulsion of contents
	Lubrication with mucus
	Digestion and absorption of most substances using enzymes made by the pancreas and small intestine
8 Large intestine	Mixing and propulsion of contents
	Absorption of sodium, potassium, and water
	Storage and concentration of undigested food
	Lubrication with mucus
	Formation of feces
9 Rectum	Store feces and expel via the anus, which is the opening to the outside of the body

FIGURE 3-10 ▶ Physiology of the GI tract. Many organs cooperate in a regulated fashion to allow digestion and subsequent absorption of nutrients in foods.

In the digestive system, food is broken down mechanically and chemically. Mechanical digestion takes place as soon as you begin chewing your food and continues as muscular contractions simultaneously mix and move food through the length of the GI tract (as part of a process known as **motility**). Chemical digestion refers to the chemical breakdown of foods by substances secreted into the GI tract. Finally, the digestive system eliminates wastes. In addition to nutrients that arise from digestion of food, the bacteria that live in the large intestine produce vitamin K and the vitamin biotin, some of which we can absorb and use.

Most of the processes of digestion and absorption are under autonomic control; that is, they are involuntary. Almost all of the functions involved in digestion and absorption are controlled by signals from the nervous system, hormones from the endocrine system, and hormone-like compounds. Many common ailments arise from problems with the digestive system. Several of these digestive problems are discussed in the "Nutrition and Your Health" section at the end of this chapter.

absorption The process by which substances are taken up from the GI tract and enter the bloodstream or the lymph.

gastrointestinal (GI) tract The main sites in the body used for digestion and absorption of nutrients. It consists of the mouth, esophagus, stomach, small intestine, large intestine, rectum, and anus. Also called the *digestive tract*.

motility Generally, the ability to move spontaneously. It also refers to movement of food through the GI tract.

GI Tract Flow

Mouth
↓
Esophagus (10 inches long)
↓
Stomach—4-cup (1-liter) capacity. Food remains about 2 to 3 hours, or longer for large meals.
↓
Small intestine—duodenum (10 in long), jejunum (4 ft long), ileum (5 ft long)—about 10 ft (3.1 meters) in total length. Food remains about 3 to 10 hours.
↓
Large intestine (colon)—cecum, ascending colon, transverse colon, descending colon, sigmoid colon—3½ ft (1.1 meters) in total length. Food can remain up to 72 hours.
↓
Rectum
↓
Anus

The digestive system is composed of six separate organs; each organ performs one, or more, specific job(s). Let's look briefly at the role of each organ. These organs are listed in the flow chart on this page. More detailed descriptions of digestive processes will be explained in later chapters as each nutrient is introduced.

Mouth

The mouth performs many functions in the digestion of food. Besides chewing food to reduce it to smaller particles, the mouth also senses the taste of the foods we consume. The tongue, through the use of its taste buds, identifies foods on the basis of their specific flavor(s). Sweet, sour, salty, bitter, and **umami** comprise the primary taste sensations we experience. Surprisingly, the nose and our sense of smell greatly contribute to our ability to sense the taste of food. When we chew a food, chemicals are released that stimulate the nasal passages. Thus, it makes perfect sense that when we have a cold and our noses are stuffed up and congested, even our most favorite foods will not taste as good as they normally do.

The taste of food, or the anticipation of it, signals the rest of the GI tract to prepare for the digestion of food. Once in the mouth, mechanical and chemical digestion begins. Salivary glands produce **saliva,** which functions as a solvent so that food particles can be further separated and tasted. In addition, saliva contains a starch-digesting enzyme, **salivary amylase** (see Chapter 4 for more on starch-digesting enzymes).

Enzymes are a key part of digestion. Each enzyme is specific to one type of chemical process. For example, enzymes that recognize and digest table sugar (sucrose) ignore milk sugar (lactose). Besides working on only specific types of chemicals, enzymes are sensitive to acidic and alkaline conditions, temperature, and the types of vitamins and minerals they require. Digestive enzymes that work in the acidic environment of the stomach do not work well in the alkaline environment of the small intestine. Overall, enzymes work to hasten certain events that take place in the body (Fig. 3-11).

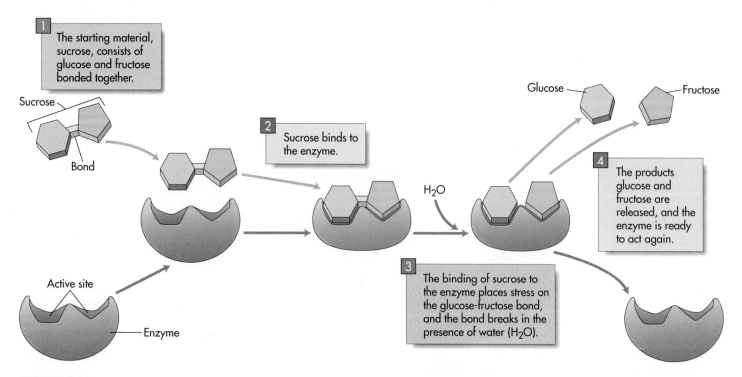

1. The starting material, sucrose, consists of glucose and fructose bonded together.

Sucrose

Bond

Active site

Enzyme

2. Sucrose binds to the enzyme.

H_2O

3. The binding of sucrose to the enzyme places stress on the glucose-fructose bond, and the bond breaks in the presence of water (H_2O).

Glucose   Fructose

4. The products glucose and fructose are released, and the enzyme is ready to act again.

FIGURE 3-11 ▶ A model of enzyme action. Enzymes increase the speed with which chemical reactions occur, but they are not altered themselves as they do so. In the reaction illustrated, an enzyme is splitting the sugar sucrose into two simpler sugars: glucose and fructose. Only these simpler sugars are absorbed from the small intestine to enter the bloodstream. Sometimes energy input is needed to push a reaction along, but not in this case.

The pancreas and the small intestine produce most of the digestive enzymes; however, the mouth and the stomach also contribute their own enzymes to digestion. **Mucus,** another component of saliva, makes it easy to swallow a mouthful of food. The food then travels to the esophagus. The important secretions and products of digestion are listed in Table 3-3.

MAKING DECISIONS

Enzymes and Digestion

The authors of some popular (fad) diet books contend that eating certain combinations of foods, such as meats and fruits together, hinders the digestive process. However, does this make sense in light of our newly gained knowledge about GI tract physiology? The body is able to increase the production of certain digestive enzymes in response to the type of diet consumed. The GI tract can respond to the nutritional makeup and amount of food consumed because of this fine-tuning. Once consumed, foods are attacked by multiple enzymes to release nutrients and other compounds for absorption.

Esophagus

The **esophagus** is a long tube that connects the **pharynx** with the stomach. Near the pharynx is a flap of tissue (called the **epiglottis**) that prevents the **bolus** of swallowed food from entering the trachea (wind pipe) (Fig. 3-12). During swallowing, food lands on the epiglottis, folding it down to cover the opening of the trachea. Breathing also stops automatically. These responses ensure that swallowed food will only travel down the esophagus. If food instead travels down the trachea, choking may occur (the victim will not be able to speak or breathe). A group of techniques to treat such a person are called the Heimlich maneuver (see www.heimlichinstitute.org for details).

umami A brothy, meaty, savory flavor in some foods. Monosodium glutamate enhances this flavor when added to foods.

salivary amylase A starch-digesting enzyme produced by salivary glands.

mucus A thick fluid secreted by many cells throughout the body. It contains a compound that has both carbohydrate and protein parts. It acts as a lubricant and means of protection for cells.

amylase Starch-digesting enzyme produced by the salivary glands and pancreas.

lipase Fat-digesting enzyme produced by the salivary glands, stomach, and pancreas.

protease Protein-digesting enzyme produced by the stomach, small intestine, and pancreas.

esophagus A tube in the GI tract that connects the pharynx with the stomach.

pharynx The organ of the digestive tract and respiratory tract located at the back of the oral and nasal cavities, commonly known as the throat.

epiglottis The flap that folds down over the trachea during swallowing.

bolus A moistened mass of food swallowed from the oral cavity into the pharynx.

TABLE 3-3 Important Secretions and Products of the Digestive Tract

Secretion	Site of Production	Purpose
Saliva	Mouth	Partial starch digestion using **salivary amylase**, lubrication of food for swallowing
Mucus	Mouth, stomach, small intestine, large intestine	Protects GI tract cells, lubricates food as it travels through the GI tract
Enzymes	Mouth, stomach, small intestine, pancreas	Promote digestion of foodstuffs into particles small enough for absorption (Examples: **amylases, lipases, proteases**)
Acid	Stomach	Promotes digestion of protein among other functions
Bile	Liver (stored in gallbladder)	Aids fat digestion in the small intestine by suspending fat in water using **bile acids, cholesterol,** and **lecithin**
Bicarbonate	Pancreas, small intestine	Neutralizes stomach acid when it reaches the small intestine
Hormones	Stomach, small intestine, pancreas	Stimulate production and/or release of acid, enzymes, bile, and bicarbonate; help regulate peristalsis and overall GI tract flow (Examples: **gastrin, secretin, insulin, cholecystokinin, glucagon**)

▲ The body digests the foods as they are presented—the order in which foods are eaten plays no role in digestion.

FIGURE 3-12 ▶ The process of swallowing. (a) During swallowing, food does not normally enter the trachea because the epiglottis closes over the larynx. (b) The closed epiglottis allows food to proceed down the esophagus. When a person chokes, food becomes lodged in the trachea, blocking air flow to the lungs. (c) The food should move down the esophagus.

peristalsis A coordinated muscular contraction used to propel food down the gastrointestinal tract.

lower esophageal sphincter A circular muscle that constricts the opening of the esophagus to the stomach. Also called the *gastroesophageal sphincter.*

 See *Nutrition and Your Health: Common Problems with Digestion* at the end of Chapter 3.

At the top of the esophagus, nerve fibers release signals to tell the GI tract that food has been consumed. This results in an increase in gastrointestinal muscle action, called **peristalsis.** Continual waves of muscle contractions, followed by muscle relaxation, force the food down the digestive tract from the esophagus onward (Fig. 3-13).

At the end of the esophagus is the **lower esophageal sphincter,** a muscle that constricts (closes) after food enters the stomach (Fig. 3-14). The main function of sphincters is to prevent the backflow of GI tract contents. Sphincters respond to various stimuli, such as signals from the nervous system, hormones, acidic versus alkaline conditions, and pressure that builds up around the sphincter. The primary function of the lower esophageal sphincter is to prevent the acidic contents of the stomach from flowing back up into the esophagus—which can cause some of the health problems we will discuss in the "Nutrition and Your Health" section at the end of Chapter 3.

FIGURE 3-13 ▶ Peristalsis. Peristalsis is a progressive type of movement, propelling material from point to point along the GI tract. To begin this, a ring of contraction occurs where the GI wall is stretched, passing the food mass forward. The moving food mass triggers a ring of contraction in the next region, which pushes the food mass even farther along. The result is a ring of contraction that moves like a wave along the GI tract, pushing the food mass down the tract.

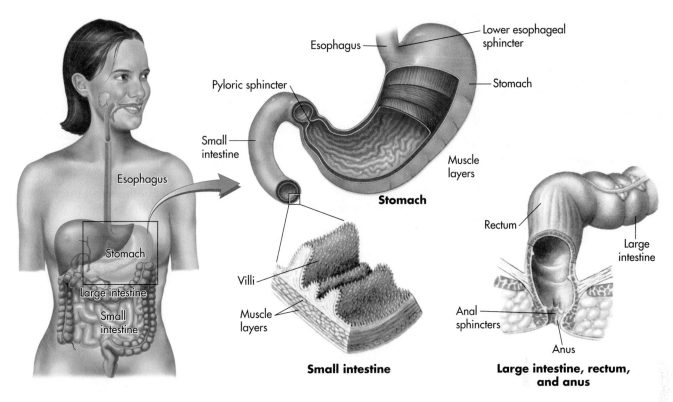

FIGURE 3-14 ▶ A close-up view of the muscles, sphincters, and villi of the GI tract. These features of the GI tract perform key roles in digestion, absorption, and elimination.

Stomach

The stomach is a large sac that can hold up to 4 cups (or 1 quart) of food for several hours until all of the food is able to enter the small intestine. Stomach size varies individually and can be reduced surgically as a radical treatment for obesity (more on this in Chapter 7). While in the stomach, the food is mixed with gastric juice, which contains water, a very strong acid, and enzymes. (Gastric is a term pertaining to the stomach.) The acid in the gastric juice maintains the acidity of the stomach contents and, thereby destroys the biological activity of proteins, converts inactive digestive enzymes to their active form, partially digests food protein, and makes dietary minerals soluble so that they can be absorbed. The mixing that takes place in the stomach produces a watery food mixture, called **chyme,** which slowly leaves the stomach a teaspoon (5 milliliters) at a time and enters the small intestine. Following a meal, the stomach contents are emptied into the small intestine over the course of 1 to 4 hours. The **pyloric sphincter,** located at the base of the stomach, controls the rate at which the chyme is released into the small intestine (review Fig. 3-14). There is very little absorption of nutrients from the stomach, except for some alcohol.

You might wonder how the stomach prevents itself from being digested by the acid and enzymes it produces. First, the stomach has a thick layer of mucus that lines and protects it. The production of acid and enzymes also requires the release of a specific hormone (gastrin). This release happens primarily when we are eating or thinking about eating. Last, as the concentration of acid in the stomach increases, hormonal control causes acid production to taper off.

One other important function of the stomach is the production of a substance called **intrinsic factor.** This vital material is essential for the absorption of vitamin B-12.

chyme A mixture of stomach secretions and partially digested food.

pyloric sphincter The ring of smooth muscle between the stomach and the small intestine.

▲ A close-up view of the fingerlike projections of the intestinal villi.

Small Intestine

The small intestine is about 10 feet (3 meters) long, beginning at the stomach on the "north" and ending at the large intestine (colon) on the "south." The small intestine is considered "small" because of its narrow (1 inch [2.5 centimeters]) diameter. Most of the digestion and absorption of food occurs in the small intestine. The chyme secreted from the stomach is moved through the small intestine by peristaltic contractions so that it can be well mixed with the digestive juices of the small intestine (review Fig. 3-13). These juices contain many enzymes that function in the breakdown of carbohydrates, protein, and fat, as well as in the preparation of vitamins and minerals for absorption.

The physical structure of the small intestine is very important to the body's ability to digest and absorb the nutrients it needs. The lining of the small intestine is called the mucosa and is folded many times; within these folds are fingerlike projections

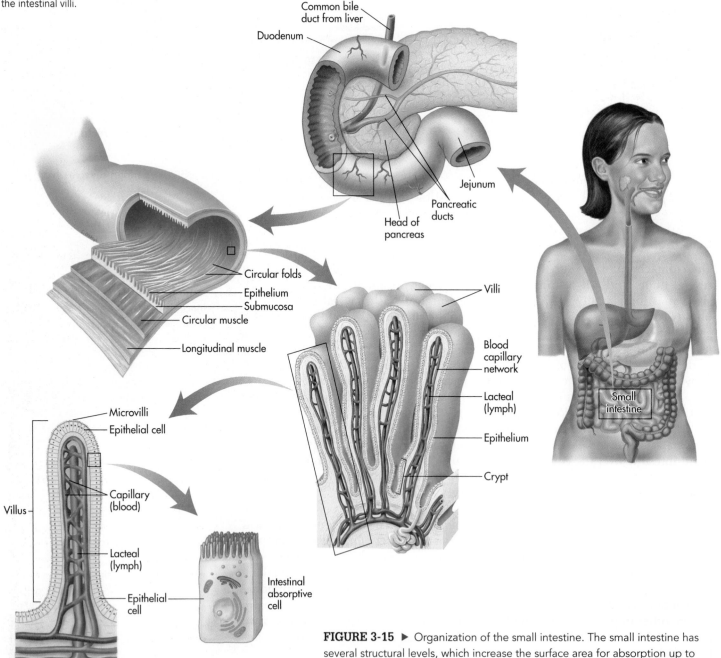

FIGURE 3-15 ▶ Organization of the small intestine. The small intestine has several structural levels, which increase the surface area for absorption up to 600 times that of a simple tube.

called **villi**. These "fingers" are constantly moving, which helps them trap food to enhance absorption. Each individual villus (singular) is made up of many **absorptive cells**, and each of these cells has a highly folded cap. The combined folds, villi, and caps in the small intestine increase its surface area 600 times beyond that of a simple tube (Fig. 3-15).

The absorptive cells have a short life. New intestinal absorptive cells are constantly produced in the crypts of the small intestine (Fig. 3-15) and appear daily along the surface of each villus "finger." This is probably because absorptive cells are subjected to a harsh environment, so renewal of the intestinal cell lining is necessary. This rapid cell turnover leads to high nutrient needs for the small intestine. Fortunately, many of the old cells can be broken down and have their component parts reused. The health of the cells is further enhanced by various hormones and other substances that participate in or are produced as part of the digestive process.

The small intestine absorbs nutrients through the intestinal wall through various means and processes, as illustrated in Figure 3-16:

- **Passive diffusion:** When the nutrient concentration is higher in the cavity (lumen) of the small intestine than in the absorptive cells, the difference in nutrient concentration drives the nutrient into the absorptive cells by diffusion. Fats, water, and some minerals are absorbed by passive diffusion.
- **Facilitated diffusion:** Some compounds require a carrier protein to drive them into absorptive cells. This type of absorption is called faciliated diffusion. Fructose is one example of a compound that makes use of such a carrier to allow for facilitated diffusion.
- **Active absorption:** In addition to the need for a carrier protein, some nutrients also require energy input to move from the lumen of the small intestine into the absorptive cells. This mechanism makes it possible for cells to take up nutrients even when they are consumed in low concentrations. Some sugars, such as glucose, are actively absorbed, as are amino acids.
- **Phagocytosis** and **pinocytosis:** In a further means of active absorption, absorptive cells literally engulf compounds (phagocytosis) or liquids (pinocytosis). As described earlier, a cell membrane can form an indentation of itself so that when particles or fluids move into the indentation, the cell membrane surrounds and engulfs them. This process is used when an infant absorbs immune substances from human milk (see Chapter 16).

villi (singular, **villus**) The fingerlike protrusions into the small intestine that participate in digestion and absorption of food.

absorptive cells The intestinal cells that line the villi; these cells participate in nutrient absorption.

FIGURE 3-16 ▶ Nutrient absorption relies on four major absorptive processes. (A) Passive diffusion is simple diffusion of nutrients across the absorptive cell membranes. (B) Facilitated diffusion uses a carrier protein to move nutrients down a concentration gradient. (C) Active absorption involves a carrier protein as well as energy to move nutrients (against a concentration gradient) into absorptive cells. (D) Pinocytosis and phagocytosis are forms of active absorption in which the absorptive cell membrane engulfs a nutrient to bring it into the cell.

Once absorbed, water-soluble compounds such as glucose and amino acids go to the capillaries and then on to the portal vein. Recall that the liver is the end of this process. Most fats eventually go into the lymph vessels. In doing so, they can eventually enter the bloodstream (see the earlier section on the circulatory system for details; and review Figs. 3-4 and 3-5).

Undigested food cannot be absorbed into cells of the small intestine. Any undigested food that reaches the end of the small intestine must pass through the **ileocecal sphincter** on the way to the large intestine. This sphincter prevents the contents of the large intestine from reentering the small intestine.

ileocecal sphincter The ring of smooth muscle between the end of the small intestine and the large intestine.

Large Intestine

When the contents of the small intestine enter the large intestine, the material left bears little resemblance to the food originally eaten. Under normal circumstances, only a minor amount (5%) of carbohydrate, protein, and fat escape absorption to reach the large intestine (Fig. 3-17).

Physiologically, the large intestine differs from the small intestine in that there are no villi or digestive enzymes. The absence of villi means that little absorption takes place in the large intestine in comparison to the small intestine. Nutrients absorbed from the large intestine include water, some vitamins, some fatty acids, and the minerals sodium and potassium. Unlike the small intestine, the large intestine has a number of mucus-producing cells. The mucus secreted by these cells functions to hold the feces together and to protect the large intestine from the bacterial activity within it. The large intestine is home to a large population of bacteria (over 500 different species). Whereas the stomach and small intes-

FIGURE 3-17 ▶ Major sites of absorption along the GI tract. Some absorption of vitamin K and biotin takes place in the large intestine. With the exception of fat soluble nutrients, most nutrients travel through the portal vein to the liver after their absorption.

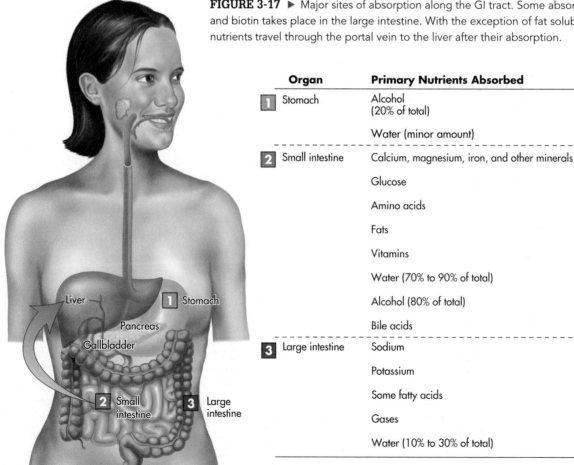

Organ	Primary Nutrients Absorbed
1 Stomach	Alcohol (20% of total)
	Water (minor amount)
2 Small intestine	Calcium, magnesium, iron, and other minerals
	Glucose
	Amino acids
	Fats
	Vitamins
	Water (70% to 90% of total)
	Alcohol (80% of total)
	Bile acids
3 Large intestine	Sodium
	Potassium
	Some fatty acids
	Gases
	Water (10% to 30% of total)

tine have some bacterial activity, the large intestine is the organ most heavily colonized with bacteria. Starting at infancy, the diet plays a major part in determining the type of bacteria in our digestive tracts. The number and type of bacteria in the human colon recently has become of great interest. Research has shown that intestinal bacteria play a significant role in the maintenance of health, especially health of the colon. It is speculated that higher levels of beneficial organisms can reduce the activity of disease-causing bacteria. This is another illustration of the intestinal tract working as important immune organ. The strains *bifidobacteria* and *lactobacilli* are typically associated with health, whereas *clostridia* are considered problematic. These bacteria are able to break down some of the remaining food products that enter the large intestine, such as the milk sugar lactose (in lactose intolerant people), and some components of fiber. The products of bacterial metabolism in the large intestine, which include various acids, can then be absorbed.

Foods containing certain microorganisms such as lactobacilli are getting a lot of attention. The term **probiotic** is used for these microorganisms because once consumed, they take up residence in the large intestine and lead to some health benefits, such as improving intestinal tract health. You can find these probiotic microorganisms in certain forms of fluid milk, fermented milk, and yogurt. They can even be found in pill form. A related term is **prebiotic.** These are substances that increase growth of probiotic microorganisms. One example is fructooligosaccharides (see Table 1-5 in Chapter 1 for dietary sources). The beneficial organisms of the large intestine will be discussed further in Chapter 4 when we explore their use as probiotics.

The small intestine absorbs only 70% to 90% of the fluid it receives, which includes large amounts of GI-tract secretions produced during digestion. Therefore, some water remains in the material that enters the large intestine. The remnants of a meal also contain some minerals and some fiber. Because water is removed from the large intestine, its contents become semisolid by the time they have passed through the first two-thirds of it. What remains in the **feces,** besides water and undigested fiber, is tough connective tissues (from animal foods); bacteria from the large intestine; and some body wastes, such as parts of dead intestinal cells.

Rectum

The feces or stool remains in the last portion of the large intestine, the **rectum**, until muscular movements push it into the **anus** to be eliminated. The presence of feces in the rectum stimulates elimination. The anus contains two **anal sphincters** (internal and external), one of which is under voluntary control (external sphincter). Relaxation of this sphincter allows for elimination.

Accessory Organs

The **liver, gallbladder**, and **pancreas** work with the GI tract and are considered accessory organs to the process of digestion (review Fig. 3-10). These accessory organs are not part of the GI tract through which food passes, but they play necessary roles in the process of digestion. These organs secrete digestive fluids into the GI tract and enable the process of converting food into absorbable nutrients.

The liver produces a substance called **bile.** The bile is stored and concentrated in the gallbladder until the gallbladder receives a hormonal signal to release the bile. This signal is induced by the presence of fat in the small intestine. Bile is released and delivered to the small intestine via a tube called the bile duct.

In action, bile is like soap. Components of the bile enable large portions of fat to break into smaller bits so that they can be suspended in water (Chapter 5 will cover this process in detail). Interestingly, some of the bile constituents can be "recycled" in a process known as **enterohepatic circulation.** These components of bile are reabsorbed from the small intestine, returned to the liver via the portal vein, and reused.

In addition to bile, the liver releases a number of other unwanted substances that travel with the bile to the gallbladder and end up in the small intestine and eventually in

rectum Terminal portion of the large intestine.

anus Last portion of the GI tract; serves as an outlet for that organ.

anal sphincters A group of two sphincters (inner and outer) that help control expulsion of feces from the body.

gallbladder An organ attached to the underside of the liver; site of bile storage, concentration, and eventual secretion.

bile A liver secretion stored in the gallbladder and released through the common bile duct into the first segment of the small intestine. It is essential for the digestion and absorption of fat.

enterohepatic circulation A continual recycling of compounds between the small intestine and the liver; bile acids are one example of a recycled compound.

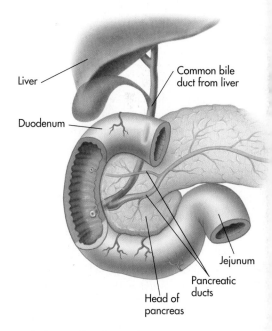

▲ The liver, gallbladder, and pancreas are accessory organs that work with the GI tract. The liver produces bile, stored in the gallbladder and released into the duodenum portion of the small intestine, via the common bile duct, to help digest fat. The pancreas secretes pancreatic juice containing water, bicarbonate, and digestive enzymes into the duodenum via the common bile duct.

the large intestine for excretion. The liver functions in this manner to remove unwanted substances from the blood. (Other byproducts are excreted via the urine; see the next section, "Urinary System.")

The pancreas manufactures hormones and pancreatic juice. The hormones include glucagon and insulin, which as noted earlier function in glucose regulation. Pancreatic juice contains water, bicarbonate, and a variety of digestive enzymes capable of breaking apart carbohydrates, proteins, and fats into small fragments. Bicarbonate is a base that neutralizes the acidity of chyme as it moves from the stomach into the small intestine. Recall that the stomach produces a thick layer of mucus to protect itself from the acid of gastric secretions. The small intestine, however, does not have a protective layer of mucus, because mucus would impede nutrient absorption. Instead, the neutralizing capacity of bicarbonate from the pancreas protects the walls of the small intestine from erosion by acid, which would otherwise lead to formation of an ulcer (see the "Nutrition and Your Health" section at the end of Chapter 3).

 See *Nutrition and Your Health: Common Problems with Digestion* at the end of Chapter 3.

CONCEPT CHECK

Digestion is a mechanical and chemical process mediated by enzymes and coordinated by hormones and nerves. Whereas swallowing and ultimate elimination of feces from the anus are voluntary, the majority of the digestive processes are involuntary. The stomach initiates the process of digestion by mixing food with gastric juice and converting this partially digested food into chyme. The products of digestion are molecules of the original food or beverage small enough to be absorbed into the villi of the small intestine and transferred to the blood or lymph. For the most part, nutrients are absorbed in the small intestine; only a few are absorbed in the large intestine. Any dietary component that escapes digestion by human or bacterial enzymes exits the body as feces.

URINARY SYSTEM

urinary system The body system consisting of the kidneys, urinary bladder, and the ducts that carry urine. This system removes waste products from the circulatory system and regulates blood acid-base balance, overall chemical balance, and water balance in the body.

ureter Tube that transports urine from the kidney to the urinary bladder.

urethra Tube that transports urine from the urinary bladder to the outside of the body.

pH A measure of relative acidity or alkalinity of a solution. The pH scale is 0 to 14. A pH below 7 is acidic; a pH above 7 is alkaline.

erythropoietin A hormone secreted mostly by the kidneys that enhances red blood cell synthesis and stimulates red blood cell release from bone marrow.

The **urinary system** is composed of two kidneys, one on each side of the spinal column. Each kidney is connected to the bladder by a **ureter.** The bladder is emptied by way of the **urethra** (Fig. 3-18). The main function of the kidneys is to remove waste from the body. The kidneys are constantly filtering blood to control its composition. This results in the formation of urine, mostly water, along with dissolved waste products such as urea, and excess and unneeded water-soluble vitamins and various minerals.

Together with the lungs, the kidneys also maintain the acid-base balance (**pH**) of the blood. The kidneys also convert a form of vitamin D into its active hormone form and produce a hormone that stimulates red blood cell synthesis (**erythropoietin;** see Chapter 12 for information on misuse of this hormone by some athletes). During times of fasting, the kidneys even produce glucose from certain amino acids. Thus, the kidneys perform many important functions and are a vital component of the body.

The proper function of the kidneys is closely tied to the strength of the cardiovascular system, particularly its ability to maintain adequate blood pressure, and the consumption of sufficient fluid. Uncontrolled diabetes, hypertension, and drug abuse are harmful to the kidneys.

STORAGE CAPABILITIES

The human body must maintain reserves of nutrients, otherwise we would need to eat continuously. Storage capacity varies for each different nutrient. Most fat is stored in adipose tissue, made up of cells designed specifically for this. Short-term

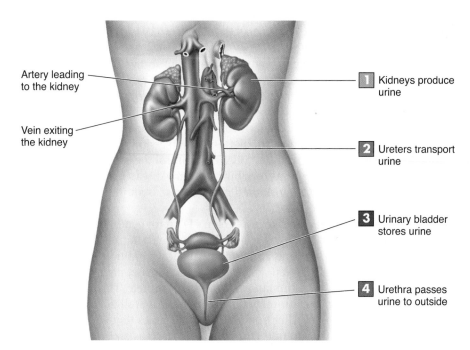

Artery leading
to the kidney

Vein exiting
the kidney

1 Kidneys produce
urine

2 Ureters transport
urine

3 Urinary bladder
stores urine

4 Urethra passes
urine to outside

FIGURE 3-18 ▶ Organs of the urinary system. The kidneys **1** bean-shaped organs located on either side of the spinal column, filter waste from the blood and form urine, which is transported to the bladder by the ureters **2** and stored in the bladder **3** as urine. The urethra **4** transports the urine to outside the body. The urinary system of the female is shown. The male's urinary system is the same, except that the urethra extends through the penis.

storage of carbohydrate occurs in muscle and liver in the form of glygogen. The blood maintains a small reserve of glucose and amino acids. Many vitamins and minerals are stored in the liver, while other nutrient stores are found in other sites in the body.

When people do not meet certain nutrient needs, these nutrients are obtained by breaking down a tissue that contains high concentrations of the nutrient. For example, calcium is taken from bone and protein is taken from muscle. In cases of long-term deficiency, these nutrient losses weaken and harm these tissues.

Many people believe that if too much of a nutrient is obtained—for example, from a vitamin or mineral supplement—only what is needed is stored and the rest is excreted by the body. Though true for some nutrients, such as vitamin C, the large dosages of other nutrients frequently found in supplements, such as vitamin A and iron, can cause harmful side effects because they are not readily excreted. This is one reason why obtaining your nutrients primarily (or exclusively) from a balanced diet is the safest means to acquire the building blocks you need to maintain the good health of all organ systems.

CONCEPT CHECK

The urinary system removes the wastes produced by the body and many nutrients ingested in excess of storage capacity and need. The kidneys maintain the chemical composition and acidity of the blood. In addition, the kidneys help convert vitamin D to its active form and produce a hormone needed for red blood cell synthesis.

In well-nourished individuals, nutrients are constantly present in the blood for immediate use and are stored in the body tissues for later use when sufficient amounts are not consumed from food. However, when the body suffers a nutrient deficiency after an inadequate diet is consumed over a long period, vital tissues will be broken down for their nutrients, which can lead to ill health. Additionally, too much of any nutrient can be detrimental. It's best to focus primarily (or exclusively) on obtaining all essential nutrients from a balanced diet rather than mostly from dietary supplements.

▲ The skeletal system provides a reserve of calcium for day-to-day needs when dietary intake is inadequate. Long-term use of this reserve, however, reduces bone strength.

A CLOSER LOOK AT GENETICS AND NUTRITION

▶ A genetic variation can directly affect the proteins encoded by our genes and result in different:

- nutrient requirements among individuals
- susceptibilities to diseases
- effects of environmental factors (such as our diet) on our genes and their proteins.

Once nutrients and other dietary components are taken up by cells, they may interact with our genes and have an effect on gene expression. The growth, development, and maintenance of cells, and ultimately of the entire organism, are directed by genes present in the cells. Each gene essentially represents a recipe, noting the ingredients (amino acids) and how those ingredients should be put together (to make proteins). The products (proteins) of all the recipes in the cookbook (the human genome) would then make up the human organism. Genes contain the codes that control the expression of individual traits, such as height, eye color, and susceptibility to many diseases. Although it is not the only factor, an individual's genetic risk for a given disease is an important determinant for development of a specific disease.

Soon it will be relatively easy to screen a person's DNA for genes that increase the risk for specific diseases. Genetic screening is a brand new field, but is about to become a significant part of medical practice, as almost every medical condition has a genetic component. Each year, new links between specific genes and diseases are reported.

In 2003, the decoding of the human genome was complete. This information will allow for early detection of health-related genetic risks, as well as tailoring of medical and nutrition therapies. Another hope is to replace genes that encourage diseases, such as cancer, with those that do not. This practice, known as *gene therapy*, has proven to be effective for a few disorders, but is not widely available at this time.

The Emerging Field of Nutrigenomics

In the near future, genetic information will enhance the ability of health professionals to help individuals manage diseases and optimize health. Nutritional genomics or **nutrigenomics** is the study of how food impacts health through its interaction with our genes and its subsequent effect on gene expression. Nutrigenomics includes the study of how genes determine our nutritional requirements. Research in this area highlights the fallacy of a "one-size-fits-all" approach to nutrition interventions for disease prevention and management.

In addition to the direct effect of genes on disease risk, in many cases, genes influence the effect of diet and nutrition on disease development and progression. In some cases, a food component can cause a gene to be turned on or off, thus manipulating the production of proteins that can affect—positively or negatively—development or progression of diseases. With a better understanding of the interactions between genes and our diet, it will not be long before dietary recommendations may be personalized to help those with various genetically-linked diseases.

Nutritional Diseases with a Genetic Link

Studies of families, including those with twins and adopted children, provide strong support for the effects of genetics in various disorders. In fact, family history is considered to be an important risk factor in the development of many nutrition-related diseases.

Cardiovascular Disease. There is strong evidence that cardiovascular disease is the result of gene-environment interactions. About 1 of every 500 people in North America has a defective gene that greatly delays cholesterol removal from the bloodstream. As you saw in Chapter 1, elevated blood cholesterol is one major risk factor for development of cardiovascular disease. The gene-diet interactions being discovered for cardiovascular disease, particularly the cases of high blood lipid levels, will likely be the first to lead to nutrition plans personalized to decrease cardiovascular

▲ Studies of twins have provided strong evidence for the interaction between genes and diet and their combined effects on disease risk.

disease risk. Another type of genetic variation can cause a person to have abnormally high levels of an amino acid called homocysteine, which increases cardiovascular disease risk. Diet changes can help these people, but medications and even surgery are needed to address these problems.

Hypertension. An estimated 10% to 15% of the North American population is sensitive to salt-induced hypertension. Information from the genetic code may one day identify those hypersensitive individuals who have this problem. At present, the only way to determine whether individuals with hypertension are salt sensitive is to place them on a salt-restricted diet and see if their blood pressure falls. Many cases of hypertension are not caused primarily by salt sensitivity, but by other factors, such as obesity and inactivity.

Obesity. Most obese North Americans have at least one obese parent. This strongly suggests a genetic link. Findings from many human studies suggest that a variety of genes (likely 60 or more) are involved in the regulation of body weight. Little is known, however, about the specific nature of these genes in humans or how the actual changes in body metabolism (such as lower calorie-burning in general or fat use in particular) are produced.

Still, although some individuals may be genetically predisposed to store body fat, whether they do so depends on how many calories they consume relative to their needs. A common concept in nutrition is that *nurture*—how people live and the environmental factors that influence them—allows *nature*—each person's genetic potential—to be expressed. Although not every person with a genetic tendency toward obesity becomes obese, those genetically predisposed to weight gain have a higher lifetime risk than individuals without a genetic predisposition to obesity.

Diabetes. Both of the two common types of diabetes—type 1 and type 2—have genetic links. Evidence for these genetic links comes from studies of families and twins and from the high incidence of diabetes among certain population groups (e.g., South Asians or Pima Indians). Only sensitive and expensive testing can determine who is at risk. The most common form of diabetes (90% of all cases), type 2 diabetes, also has a strong link to obesity. Typically a genetic tendency for type 2 diabetes is expressed once a person becomes obese but often not before, again illustrating that nurture affects nature.

Cancer. A few types of cancer (e.g., some forms of colon [*colon* is another name for large intestine] and breast cancer) have a strong genetic link, and genetics may play a role in others, such as **prostate cancer.** Because obesity increases the risk of several forms of cancer, a long-standing excess calorie intake is also a risk factor. Although genes are an important determinant in the development of cancer, environmental and lifestyle factors, such as excessive sun exposure and a poor diet, also contribute significantly to the risk profile.

Your Genetic Profile

From this discussion, you can see that your genes can greatly influence your risk of developing certain diseases. By recognizing your potential for developing a particular disease, you can avoid behavior that further raises your risk. How can you figure out your genetic profile? Many biotechnology companies now offer genetic testing to screen for gene variants known to be associated with disease risk. Currently, hundreds of genetic tests are available, and more are under development. For example, a genetic test is available for a form of breast cancer (abnormal BRCA genes). Although expensive (approximately $2700), as technology advances and evidence of the benefits of genetic testing emerges, such tests will become a routine part of health care.

On the other hand, you can get a good sense of your genetic profile by examining your family history of certain diseases. Put together a family tree of illnesses and deaths by compiling a few key facts on your primary relatives: siblings, parents, aunts

▲ Genetic testing for disease susceptibility will be more common in the future as the genes that increase risk for various diseases are isolated and decoded.

▶ The following weblinks will help you gather more information about genetic conditions and testing:

http://nutrigenomics.ucdavis.edu/
Center for Excellence for Nutritional Genomics. Website dedicated to promoting the new science of nutritional genomics

www.geneticalliance.org
Alliance of Genetic Support Groups

www.kumc.edu/gec/support
Information on genetic and rare conditions

www.cancer.gov/cancertopics/prevention-genetic-causes
Genetics information from the National Cancer Institute

http://www.genome.gov/
National Human Genome Research Institute (at the National Institutes of Health) website. Describes the latest research finding, discusses some ethical issues, and provides a talking glossary.

http://history.nih.gov/exhibits/genetics/
Revolution in Progress: Human Genetics and Medical Research

and uncles, and grandparents, as suggested in the "Rate Your Plate" section. In general, the greater number of your relatives who had a genetically transmitted disease and the closer they are related to you, the greater your risk. If there is a significant family history of a certain disease, lifestyle changes may be appropriate. For example, women with a family history of breast cancer should avoid becoming obese, should minimize alcohol use, and should obtain mammograms regularly.

Figure 3-19 shows an example of a family tree (also called a *genogram*). High-risk conditions include two or more first-degree relatives in a family with a specific disease (first-degree relatives include one's parents, siblings, and offspring). Another sign of risk of inherited disease is development of the disease in a first-degree relative before 50 to 60 years. In the family depicted in Figure 3-19, prostate cancer killed the man's father. Knowing this, the man should be tested regularly for prostate cancer. His sisters should consider frequent mammograms and other preventive practices because their mother died of breast cancer. Because heart attack and stroke are also common in the family, all the children should adopt a lifestyle that minimizes the risk of developing these conditions, such as avoiding excessive animal fat and salt intake. Colon cancer is also evident in the family, so careful screening throughout life is important.

Information about our genetic makeup will increasingly influence our dietary and lifestyle choices. Throughout this book we will discuss "controllable" risk factors that could contribute to development of genetically linked diseases present in your family. This information will help you personalize nutrition advice based on your genetic background and identify and avoid the risk factors that could lead to the diseases present in your family.

This review of human anatomy, physiology and genetics from a nutrition perspective sets the stage for developing a more detailed understanding of the nutrients. Chapters 4, 5, and 6 will build on this information.

FIGURE 3-19 ▶ Example of a family tree for Eugene, designated as "Self" at the trunk of the tree. The gender of each family member is identified by color (blue squares for males, orange circles for females). Dates of birth (b) and death (d) are listed below each family member. If deceased, the cause of death is highlighted using white text against a black background. In addition to causes of death, medical conditions the family members experienced are noted beneath each name. Create your own family tree of frequent diseases using this figure as a guide. Then show your family tree to your physician to get a more complete picture of what the information means for your health.

The fine-tuned organ system we call the digestive system can develop problems. Knowing about these common problems can help you avoid or lessen them. Two common GI tract-related problems are diverticulosis and lactose maldigestion and intolerance. These disorders will be discussed in Chapter 4 after you learn more about carbohydrates.

ULCERS

A peptic **ulcer** can occur when the lining of the esophagus, stomach, or small intestine is eroded by the acid secreted by the stomach cells (Fig. 3-20). As the stomach lining deteriorates in ulcer development, it loses its protective mucus layer, and the acid further erodes the stomach tissue. Acid can also erode the lining of the esophagus and the first part of the small intestine, the duodenum. In young people, most ulcers occur in the small intestine, wheras in older people they occur primarily in the stomach.

Millions of North Americans develop ulcers during their lifetimes. As a result, billions of healthcare dollars are spent annually on the treatment of peptic ulcers and their complications. Fortunately, our understanding of ulcer formation has increased, resulting in a variety of improved treatment options. The typical symptom of an ulcer is pain about 2 hours after eating. Stomach acid acting on a meal irritates the ulcer after most of the meal has moved from the site of the ulcer.

Not long ago, the major cause of ulcer disease was thought to be excess acid. Therefore, neutralizing and curtailing the secretion of stomach acid were the logical treatment choices. Although acid is still a significant player in ulcer formation, the principal causes of ulcer disease are currently thought to be infection of the stomach by the acid-resistant bacteria, *Helicobacter pylori (H. pylori)*; heavy use of nonsteroidal anti-inflammatory drugs **(NSAIDS),** such as aspirin; and disorders that cause excessive acid production in the stomach. Stress is regarded as a predisposing factor for ulcers, especially if the person is infected with *H. pylori* or has certain anxiety disorders. Cigarette smoking is also known to cause ulcers, increase ulcer complications such as bleeding, and lead to ulcer treatment failure.

The *H. pylori* bacteria is common but results in ulcer disease in only 10% to 15% of those infected. The bacteria is found in more than 80% of patients with stomach and duodenal ulcers. Although the mechanism of how *H. pylori* causes ulcers is not well understood, treatment of the infection with antibiotics heals the ulcers and prevents their recurrence. Two Australian physicians were awarded the Nobel Prize in 2005 "for their discovery of the bacterium *Helicobacter pylori* and its role in gastritis and peptic ulcer disease."

NSAIDs are medications for painful inflammatory conditions such as arthritis. Aspirin, ibuprofen, and naproxen are the most commonly used NSAIDs. NSAIDs reduce the mucus secreted by the stomach. Newer medications, called "Cox-2 inhibitors" (e.g., celecoxib [Celebrex]), have been used as a replacement for NSAIDs because they are less likely to cause stomach ulcers. They do offer some advantages over NSAIDs but they may not be totally safe for some people, especially those with a history of cardiovascular disease or strokes.

The primary risk associated with an ulcer is the possibility that it will erode entirely through the stomach or intestinal wall. The GI contents could then spill into the body cavities, causing a massive infection. In addition, an ulcer may erode a blood vessel, leading to substantial blood loss. For these reasons, it is important not to ignore the early warning signs of ulcer development including a persistent gnawing or burning near the stomach that may occur immediately following a meal or awaken you at night. In addition to the pain that may improve with food, other signs and symptoms of ulcers are weight loss, nausea, vomiting, loss of appetite, and abdominal bloating.

ulcer Erosion of the tissue lining, usually in the stomach or the upper small intestine. As a group these are generally referred to as *peptic ulcers.*

NSAIDs Nonsteroidal anti-inflammatory drugs; includes aspirin, ibuprofen (Advil®), and naproxen (Aleve®).

FIGURE 3-20 ▶ (a) A peptic ulcer in the stomach or small intestine. *H. pylori* bacteria and NSAIDs (e.g., aspirin) cause ulcers by impairing mucosal defense, especially in the stomach. In the same way, smoking, genetics, and stress can impair mucosal defense, as well as cause an increase in the release of pepsin and stomach acid. All of these factors can contribute to ulcers. (b) Close-up of a stomach ulcer. This needs to be treated or eventual perforation of the stomach is possible.

proton pump inhibitor A medication that inhibits the ability of gastric cells to secrete hydrogen ions. Low doses of this class of medications are also available without prescription (e.g., omeprazole [Prilosec]).

histamine A breakdown product of the amino acid histidine that stimulates acid secretion by the stomach and has other effects on the body, such as contraction of smooth muscles, increased nasal secretions, relaxation of blood vessels, and changes in relaxation of airways.

▶ When suffering from persistent heartburn or GERD, see a doctor if you have

- Difficulty swallowing or pain when swallowing
- Heartburn that has persisted for more than 10 years
- Initial onset of heartburn after age 50
- Heartburn that resists treatment with medications
- Sudden, unexplained weight loss
- Chest pain
- Blood loss or anemia
- Blood in stool or vomit

In the past, milk and cream therapy was used to help cure ulcers. Clinicians now know that milk and cream are two of the worst foods for an ulcer. The calcium in these foods stimulates stomach acid secretion and actually inhibits ulcer healing.

Today, a combination of approaches is used for ulcer therapy. People infected with *H. pylori* are given antibiotics as well as stomach acid-blocking medications called **proton pump inhibitors** (e.g., omeprazole [Prilosec], esomeprazole [Nexium], and lansoprazole [Prevacid]) and possibly bismuth. (Proton is another name for the hydrogen ion that creates acidity.) In many cases, there is a 90% cure rate for *H. pylori* infections in the first week of this treatment. Recurrence is unlikely if the infection is cured, but an incomplete cure almost certainly leads to repeated ulcer formation.

Antacid medications may also be part of ulcer care, as is a class of medicines called **H₂ blockers.** These include cimetidine (Tagamet), ranitidine (Zantac), nizatidine (Axid), and famotidine (Pepcid), all of which prevent **histamine**-related acid

secretion in the stomach. Medications that coat the ulcer, such as sucralfate (Carafate), are also commonly used.

People with ulcers should refrain from smoking and minimize the use of aspirin and related NSAIDs. These practices reduce the mucus secreted by the stomach. Overall, a combination of lifestyle therapy and medical treatment has so revolutionized ulcer therapy that dietary changes are of minor importance today. Current diet-therapy approaches recommend avoiding foods that increase ulcer symptoms (Table 3-4).

HEARTBURN

About half of North American adults experience occasional **heartburn,** also known as acid reflux. This gnawing pain in the upper chest is caused by the movement of acid from the stomach into the esophagus. The recurrent and therefore more serious form of the problem is called **gastroesophageal reflux disease (GERD).** Unlike the stomach, the esophagus has very little mucus lining to protect it, so acid quickly erodes the lining of the esophagus, causing pain. Symptoms

TABLE 3-4 Recommendations to Prevent Ulcers and Heartburn from Occurring or Recurring

Ulcers
1. Stop smoking if you are now a smoker.
2. Avoid large doses of aspirin, ibuprofen, and other NSAID compounds unless a physician advises otherwise. For people who must use these medications, FDA has approved an NSAID combined with a medication to reduce gastric damage. The medication reduces gastric acid production and enhances mucus secretion.
3. Limit consumption of coffee, tea, and alcohol (especially wine), if this helps.
4. Limit consumption of pepper, chili powder, and other strong spices, if this helps.
5. Eat nutritious meals on a regular schedule; include enough fiber (see Chapter 4 for sources of fiber).
6. Chew foods well.
7. Lose weight if you are currently overweight.

Heartburn
1. Observe the recommendations for ulcer prevention.
2. Wait about 2 hours after a meal before lying down.
3. Don't overeat at mealtime. Smaller meals that are low in fat are advised.
4. Try elevating the head of the bed (6-inch blocks).

may also include nausea, gagging, cough, or hoarseness. GERD is characterized by the occurrence of such symptoms of acid reflux two or more times per week. People who have GERD experience occasional relaxation of the gastroesophageal sphincter. Typically it should be relaxed only during swallowing, but in individuals with GERD it is relaxed at other times as well.

The majority of heartburn sufferers say it significantly affects their quality of life, particularly their enjoyment of many favorite foods. On a more serious note, however, if left untreated, heartburn can, over time, damage the lining of the esophagus, leading to chronic esophageal inflammation and an increased risk of esophageal cancer. Heartburn sufferers should follow the general recommendations given in Table 3-4. For occasional heartburn, quick relief can be found with over-the-counter (OTC) antacids. Taking antacids will reduce the acid in the stomach but will not stop the acid reflux. For more persistent (few days a week or everyday) heartburn or GERD, the H2 blockers or PPIs, discussed in the previous section on ulcers, may be needed. PPIs provide long-lasting relief by reducing stomach acid production and must be taken at

the right time. PPIs should be taken before the first meal of the day because they take longer to work. If the proper medications are not effective at controlling GERD, surgery may be needed to strengthen the weakened esophageal sphincter. A popular theory is that relaxation of the lower esophageal sphincter allows acid and stomach contents to flow back into the esophagus. This situation will be more of a problem when lying down.

Both pregnancy and obesity can lead to heartburn because these conditions result in increased production of estrogen and progesterone. These hormones relax the lower esophageal sphincter, making heartburn more likely. In the case of obesity, adipose tissue turns certain circulating hormones into estrogen; thus, the more adipose tissue one has, the more estrogen produced.

CONSTIPATION AND LAXATIVES

Constipation, difficult or infrequent evacuation of the bowels, is commonly reported by adults. Slow movement of fecal material through the large intestine causes constipation. As fluid is increasingly absorbed during

▲ A number of over-the-counter medications are marketed for heartburn including H_2 blockers as well as proton pump inhibitors. Attention to diet and lifestyle, however, is generally a more important measure to take.

constipation A condition characterized by infrequent bowel movements.

▲ Dried fruits are a natural source of fiber and can help prevent constipation when consumed with an adequate amount of fluid.

laxative A medication or other substance that stimulates evacuation of the intestinal tract.

the extended time the feces stay in the large intestine, they become dry and hard.

Constipation can result when people regularly inhibit their normal bowel reflexes for long periods. People may ignore normal urges when it is inconvenient to interrupt occupational or social activities. Muscle spasms of an irritated large intestine can also slow the movement of feces and contribute to constipation. Calcium, iron supplements, and medications such as antacids can also cause constipation.

Eating foods with plenty of fiber, such as whole-grain breads and cereals, along with drinking adequate fluid to avoid dehydration, is the best method for treating mild cases of constipation. Fiber stimulates peristalsis by drawing water into the large intestine and helping form a bulky, soft fecal output. Dried fruits are a good source of fiber and therefore can also help stimulate the bowel. Additional fluid should be consumed to facilitate fiber's action in the large intestine. In addition, people with constipation may need to develop more regular bowel habits; allowing the same time each day for a bowel movement can help train the large intestine to respond routinely. Finally, relaxation facilitates regular bowel movements, as does regular physical activity.

Laxatives, as well as various other medications, can also lessen constipation. Some laxatives work by irritating the intestinal nerve junctions to stimulate the peristaltic muscles, while others that contain fiber draw water into the intestine to enlarge fecal output. The larger output stretches the peristaltic muscles, making them rebound and then constrict. Regular use of laxatives, however, should be supervised by a physician. Overall the bulk-forming fiber laxatives are the safest to use.

HEMORRHOIDS

Hemorrhoids, also called *piles*, are swollen veins of the rectum and anus. The blood vessels in this area are subject to intense pressure, especially during bowel movements. Added stress to the vessels from pregnancy, obesity, prolonged sitting, violent coughing or sneezing, or straining during bowel movements, particularly with constipation, can lead to a hemorrhoid. Hemorrhoids can develop unnoticed until a strained bowel movement precipitates

symptoms, which may include pain, itching, and bleeding.

Itching, caused by moisture in the anal canal, swelling, or other irritation, is perhaps the most common symptom. Pain, if present, is usually aching and steady. Bleeding may result from a hemorrhoid and appear in the toilet as a bright red streak in the feces. The sensation of a mass in the anal canal after a bowel movement is symptomatic of an internal hemorrhoid that protrudes through the anus.

Anyone can develop a hemorrhoid, and about half of adults over age 50 do. Pressure from prolonged sitting or exertion is often enough to bring on symptoms, although diet, lifestyle, and possibly heredity play a role. For example, a low-fiber diet can lead to hemorrhoids as a result of straining during bowel movements. If you think you have a hemorrhoid, you should consult your physician. Rectal bleeding, although usually caused by hemorrhoids, may also indicate other problems, such as cancer.

A physician may suggest a variety of self-care measures for hemorrhoids. Pain can be lessened by applying warm, soft compresses or sitting in a tub of warm water for 15 to 20 minutes. Dietary recommendations are the same as those for treating constipation, emphasizing the need to consume adequate fiber and fluid. Over-the-counter remedies, such as Preparation H, can also offer relief of symptoms.

IRRITABLE BOWEL SYNDROME

Many adults (25 million or more in the United States alone) have irritable bowel syndrome, noted as a combination of cramps, gassiness, bloating, and irregular bowel function (diarrhea, constipation, or alternating episodes of both). It is more common in younger women than in younger men. In older adults the ratio is closer to 50:50. The disease leads to about 3.5 million visits to physicians in the United States each year.

Symptoms associated with irritable bowel syndrome include visible abdominal distention, pain relief after a bowel movement, increased stool frequency, loose stools with pain onset, mucus in stool, and a feeling of incomplete elimination even after a bowel movement.

The cause is thought to be altered intestinal peristalsis coupled with a decreased pain threshold for abdominal distension—in other words, a minor amount of abdominal bloating causes pain that the average person would not sense. It is also noteworthy that up to 50% of sufferers report a history of verbal or sexual abuse.

Therapy is individualized and can include a trial of high-fiber foods or elimination diets that focus on avoiding dairy products and gas-forming foods, such as legumes, certain vegetables (cabbage, beans, and broccoli), and some fruits (grapes, raisins, cherries, and cantaloupe). This is especially helpful in mild cases of irritable bowel syndrome. The patient should have only moderate caffeine intake or eliminate caffeine-containing foods/beverages altogether. Low-fat and more frequent, small meals may help the patient because large meals can trigger contractions of the large intestine. Other strategies include a reduction in stress, psychological counseling, and certain antidepressant and other medications.

Referral to a registered dietitian can be beneficial, as many patients experience improvement with the elimination of specific problem foods. A good patient/physician relationship is also necessary for the treatment of irritable bowel syndrome; however, before any single treatment is applauded, note that response to placebos alone has been as high as 70% in this population. Although irritable bowel syndrome can be uncomfortable and upsetting, it is harmless as it carries no risk for cancer or other serious digestive problems. The website www.ibsgroup.org provides further information.

DIARRHEA

Diarrhea, a GI tract disease that generally lasts only a few days, is defined as increased fluidity, frequency, or amount of bowel movements compared to a person's usual pattern. Most cases of diarrhea result from infections in the intestines, with bacteria and viruses the usual offending agents. They produce substances that cause the intestinal cells to secrete fluid rather than absorb fluid. Another form of diarrhea can be caused by consumption of substances not readily absorbed, such as the sugar alcohol sorbitol found in sugarless gum (see Chapter 4) or large amounts of a high-fiber source such as bran. When consumed in large amounts, the unabsorbed substance draws much water into the intestines, in turn leading to diarrhea. Treatment of diarrhea generally requires drinking lots of fluid during the affected stage; reduced intake of the poorly absorbed substance also is important if that is a cause. Prompt treatment—within 24 to 48 hours—is especially important for infants and older people, as they are more susceptible to the effects of dehydration associated with diarrhea (see Chapters 17 and 18). Diarrhea that lasts more than 7 days in adults should be investigated by a physician as it can be a symptom of more serious intestinal disease, especially if there is also blood in the stool.

GALLSTONES

Gallstones are a major cause of illness and surgery, affecting 10% to 20% of U.S. adults. Gallstones are pieces of solid material that develop in the gallbladder when substances in the bile—primarily cholesterol (80% of gallstones)—form crystal-like particles. They may be as small as a grain of sand or as large as a golf ball. These stones are caused by a combination of factors, with excess weight being the primary modifiable factor, especially in women 20 to 60 years old. Other factors include genetic background (e.g., Native Americans), advanced age (> 60 years for both women and men), reduced activity of the gallbladder (contracts less than normal), altered bile composition (e.g., too much cholesterol or not enough bile salts), diabetes, and diet (e.g., low-fiber diets). In addition, gallstones may develop during rapid weight loss or prolonged fasting (as the liver metabolizes more fat, it secretes more cholesterol into the bile).

Attacks due to gallstones include intermittent pain in the upper right abdomen, gas and bloating, nausea or vomiting, or other health problems. Surgical removal of the gallbladder is the most common method for treating gallstones (500,000 surgeries per year in the United States).

Prevention of gallstones revolves around avoiding becoming overweight, especially for women. Avoiding rapid weight loss (> 3 lbs. per week), limiting animal protein and focusing more on plant protein intake (especially some nut intake), and following a high-fiber diet can help as well. Regular physical activity is also recommended, as is moderate to no caffeine and alcohol intake.

Less Common Digestive Disorders

In **cystic fibrosis**—an inherited disease of infants, children, and sometimes adults—the pancreas often develops thick mucus that blocks its ducts, and active cells then die. As a result, the pancreas is not able to effectively deliver its digestive enzymes into the small intestine. Digestion of carbohydrate, protein, and—most notably—fat then is impaired. Often the missing enzymes must be ingested in capsule form with meals to aid in digestion. Another intestinal problem gaining attention is **celiac disease.** People with this disease experience an allergic reaction to the protein gluten in certain cereals, such as wheat and rye. This reaction damages the absorptive cells, resulting in a much-reduced surface area due to flattening of the villi. Elimination of wheat, rye, and certain other grains from the diet typically cures the problem.

SUMMARY

Overall, typical medical disorders of the GI tract arise from differences in anatomical features and lifestyle habits among individuals. Because of the importance of various nutrition and lifestyle habits, such as adequate fiber and fluid intake, as well as not smoking or abusing NSAID medications, nutrition and lifestyle therapy is often effective in helping treat GI tract disorders.

▲ Gallbladder and gallstones seen after surgical removal from the body. Size and composition of the stones vary from one case to another.

CASE STUDY

Gastroesophageal Reflux Disease

Caitlin is a 20-year-old college sophomore. Over the last few months, she has been experiencing regular bouts of heartburn. This usually happens after a large lunch or dinner. Occasionally she has even bent down after dinner to pick up something and had some stomach contents travel back up her esophagus and into her mouth. This especially frightened Caitlin, so she visited the University Health Center.

The nurse practitioner at the Center told Caitlin it was good that she came in for a checkup because she suspects Caitlin has a disease called gastroesophageal reflux disease (GERD). She tells Caitlin that this can lead to serious problems, such as a rare form of cancer if not controlled. She provides Caitlin with a pamphlet describing GERD and schedules an appointment with a physician for further evaluation.

Answer the following questions, and check your response in Appendix A.

1. What dietary and lifestyle habits likely contribute to Caitlin's symptoms of GERD?
2. What is the dietary and lifestyle management advice that will help Caitlin cope with this health problem?
3. What types of medications have been especially useful for treating this problem?
4. Overall, how will Caitlin cope with this health problem, and will it ever go away?
5. Why is management of GERD so important?

◄ Caitlin was wise to see a health professional about her persistent heartburn.

SUMMARY

1. The basic structural unit of the human body is the cell. Although almost all cells contain the same collection of organelles (nucleus, mitochondria, endoplasmic reticulum, lysosomes, peroxisomes, and cytoplasm), cell structure varies according to the type of job they must perform.

2. Cells join together to make up tissues, tissues unite to form organs, and organs work together as an organ system.

3. Blood is pumped from the heart to the lungs, picking up oxygen. Then, the blood delivers essential nutrients, oxygen, and water to all body cells. Nutrients and wastes are exchanged between the blood and cells across the cell membrane. This exchange occurs in the capillaries.

4. Water-soluble compounds absorbed by the small intestine cells enter the portal vein and travel to the liver. Fat-soluble compounds enter the lymphatic system, which eventually connects to the bloodstream.

5. The nervous system's neurons are the body's communication network. They control and manage all other organ systems of the body. Neurotransmitters are used to carry the message from one neuron to another (or to another cell).

6. The endocrine system produces hormones, which chemically regulate almost all other cells.

7. The immune system is responsible for protecting the body from invading pathogens. We activate immunity, such as production of antibodies (immunoglobulins), when we come in contact with a pathogen.

8. The gastrointestinal (GI) tract consists of the mouth, esophagus, stomach, small intestine, large intestine (colon), rectum, and anus.

9. Spaced along the GI tract are ring-like valves (sphincters) that regulate the flow of foodstuffs. Muscular contractions, called *peristalsis*, move the foodstuffs down the GI tract. A variety of nerves, hormones, and other substances control the activity of sphincters and peristaltic muscles.

10. Digestive enzymes are secreted by the mouth, stomach, wall of the small intestine, and pancreas. The presence of food in the small intestine stimulates the release of pancreatic enzymes.

11. The major absorptive sites consist of fingerlike projections called *villi*, located in the small intestine. Absorptive cells cover the villi. This intestinal lining is continually renewed. Absorptive cells can perform various forms of passive diffusion and active absorption.

12. Little digestion and absorption occur in the stomach or large intestine, but some protein is digested in the stomach. Some constituents of fiber and undigested starch are broken down by bacteria in the large intestine and some

Chapter 3: The Human Body: A Nutrition Perspective 115

of the products are absorbed; any undigested fiber that remains is eliminated in the feces.

13. Final water and mineral absorption takes place in the large intestine. Products from bacterial breakdown of some fibers and other substances are also absorbed here. The presence of feces in the rectum provides the impetus for elimination.

14. The liver, gallbladder, and pancreas participate in digestion and absorption. Products from these organs, such as enzymes and bile, enter the small intestine and play important roles in digesting protein, fat, and carbohydrate.

15. The urinary system, including the kidneys, is responsible for filtering the blood, removing body wastes, and maintaining the chemical composition of the blood.

16. Limited stores of nutrients are present in the blood for immediate use and stored to a greater or lesser extent in body tissues for later use when sufficient food is unavailable. When the body suffers a nutrient deficiency caused by a poor diet, it breaks down vital tissues for their nutrients, which can lead to ill health.

Additionally, too much of any nutrient can be detrimental.

17. Genetic background influences the risk for many health-related diseases. Examining one's family tree provides clues for an individual to such risks. Preventative measures are then important to implement, especially with respect to diet.

18. Common GI-tract diseases, such as heartburn, constipation, and irritable bowel syndrome, can be treated with diet changes. These can include increasing fiber intake and avoiding large meals high in fat. Medications are also very helpful in many cases.

STUDY QUESTIONS

1. Identify at least one contribution to overall nutrition status provided by each of the 12 organ systems of the body.

2. Draw and label parts of the cell, and explain the function of each organelle discussed in the text as it relates to human nutrition.

3. Trace the flow of blood from the right side of the heart around the body and back to the same site. How is blood routed through the small intestine? Which class of nutrients enters the body via the blood? Via the lymph?

4. Explain why the small intestine is better suited than the other GI tract organs to carry out the absorptive process.

5. Identify the four basic tastes. Give an example of one food that exemplifies each of these basic taste sensations. Why can't you taste food when you have a cold? What is umami?

6. What is one role of acid in the process of digestion? Where is it secreted?

7. Contrast the processes of active absorption and passive diffusion of nutrients.

8. Identify the two accessory organs that empty their contents into the small intestine. How do the digestive substances secreted by these organs contribute to the digestion of food?

9. In which organ systems would the following substances be found?

   chyme
   plasma
   lymph
   urine

10. What is the difference between nature and nurture? Relate these terms to the attempt to prevent three common chronic diseases.

CHECK YOUR KNOWLEDGE

Answers to the following multiple choice questions are in Appendix A.

1. The stomach is protected from digesting itself by producing
   a. bicarbonate only when food is in the stomach.
   b. a thick layer of mucus to coat the lining of the stomach.
   c. hydroxyl ions to neutralize the acid.
   d. antipepsin that destroys digestive substances.

2. The lower esophageal sphincter is located between the
   a. stomach and esophagus.
   b. stomach and duodenum.
   c. ileum and the cecum.
   d. sigmoid colon and the anus.

3. A coordinated muscular contraction that propels food down the GI tract is called
   a. a sphincter.
   b. enterohepatic circulation.
   c. gravitational pull.
   d. peristalsis.

4. Bicarbonate ions (HCO_3^-) from the pancreas
   a. neutralize the acid when it is in the stomach.
   b. are synthesized in the pyloric sphincter.
   c. neutralize the bile in the duodenum.
   d. neutralize the acid contents in the duodenum.

5. Most of the digestive processes occur in the
   a. mouth.
   b. stomach.
   c. small intestine.
   d. large intestine.
   e. colon.

6. Bile is formed in the _____ and stored in the _____.
   a. stomach, pancreas
   b. duodenum, kidney
   c. liver, gallbladder
   d. gallbladder, liver

7. Much of the digestion that occurs in the large intestine is caused by
   a. lipase.
   b. pepsin.
   c. saliva.
   d. bacteria.

8. Nexium ("the purple pill") is a popular drug that acts as a(n)
   a. H2 blocker.
   b. laxative.
   c. analgesic.
   d. proton pump inhibitor.

9. The study of how food impacts health through its interaction with our genes is called
   a. nutrigenomics.
   b. epidemiology.
   c. immunology.
   d. genetics.

10. Energy production that takes place in the cytoplasm is called anaerobic metabolism because it does not require
    a. water.
    b. oxygen.
    c. anabolic steroids.
    d. anaerobic bacteria.

FURTHER READINGS

1. Afman L, Muller M: Nutrigenomics from molecular nutrition to prevention of disease, *Journal of the American Dietetic Association* 106:569, 2006.

   The expanding area of genomics has created new opportunities for increasing our understanding of how nutrients affect gene and protein expression and ultimately metabolism. An overview of nutrigenomics is provided as well as current strategies, future opportunities, and challenges.

2. Against the grain: Who needs to avoid wheat? *Consumer Reports on Health* p. 10, July 2005.

   Although a high-fiber diet leads to many health benefits, using wheat products to achieve such a goal is harmful for people with celiac disease. It is especially important that people who experience flushing, itching, hives, vomitting, or breathing difficulties within two hours of eating wheat be tested for the disease. The article discusses methods of diagnosis and treatment for celiac disease.

3. Andresen V. Camilleri M: Irritable bowel syndrome: Recent and novel therapeutic approaches. *Drugs* 66:1073, 2006.

   Traditional treatment of IBS was mainly symptom oriented and often unsatisfactory. This paper provides an overview of recently approved and novel medications that show promise for the treatment of IBS. The role of probiotics in IBS treatment is summarized.

4. Broekaert IJ, Walker WA: Probiotics and chronic disease. *Journal of Clinical Gastroenterology* 40:270, 2006.

   Probiotic research has suggested several ways that they can be beneficial for the human body. Clinical research has demonstrated its preventive and curative potential in several intestinal diseases. The potential role of probiotics in the prevention and treatment of a wide variety of chronic diseases is reviewed.

5. Camilleri M: Probiotics and irritable bowel syndrome: Rationale, putative mechanisms, and evidence of clinical efficacy. *Journal of Clinical Gastroenterology* 40:264, 2006.

   The evidence that Bifidobacteria or Lactobacilli species alone or in the specific probiotic combination of VSL#3 are beneficial for treatment of symptoms in IBS is discussed.

6. Gropper SS and others: *Advanced nutrition and human metabolism.* 4th ed. Belmont CA: Thomson Wadsworth, 2005.

   Chapter 2 of this textbook provides a detailed description of the digestive processes of the human body. Students seeking more details about digestion and absorption will find this chapter helpful.

7. Heartburn. How to relieve the discomfort. *Mayo Clinic Health Letter* 24: 1, 2006.

   Steps to soothe the fire of heartburn are offered, including foods to limit, medications to take properly, and raising your bed.

8. Jackson K: Pioneering the Frontier of Nutrigenomics. *Today's Dietitian*, p. 34, September 2004.

   The role of the dietitian in analyzing an individual's genetic potential and employing nutrition to optimize the positive genetic influences and reduce the negative through educated lifestyle choices is discussed.

9. Jacobson BC and others: Body-mass index and symptoms of gastroesophageal reflux in women. *New England Journal of Medicine* 354:2340, 2006.

   BMI was associated with symptoms of gastroesophageal reflux disease in 10,545 participants in the Nurses' Health Study. Even moderate weight gain was found to cause or exacerbate symptoms of reflux.

10. Layke JC, Lopez PP: Esophageal cancer. A review and update. *American Family Physician* 73:2187, 2006.

    Esophageal cancer is aggressive and is commonly diagnosed at an advanced stage with a poor prognosis. The associations between the development of esophageal cancer and Helicobacter pylori infection and gastroesophageal reflux disease are discussed along with other factors. Despite the increased use of proton pump inhibitors and the eradication of H. pylori, the number of new cases of esophageal cancer continues to grow.

11. Muller-Lisser and others: Myths and misconceptions about constipation. *American Journal of Gastroenterology* 100:232, 2005.

    Increasing fiber intake and avoiding dehydration often helps in mild cases of constipation. More difficult cases require a careful physician evaluation and likely the use of laxatives and other medications. Often very helpful, the latter are reviewed in the article.

12. Omoruyi O, Holten KB. How should we manage GERD?: *The Journal of Family Practice* 55:410, 2006.

    Guidelines for the use of proton pump inhibitors, histamine type 2 receptor antagonists (H2 blockers), and surgery for the treatment of GERD are presented.

13. Ordovas JM: Nutrigenetics, plasma lipids, and cardiovascular risk. *Journal of the American Dietetic Association* 106:1074, 2006.

    The evidence that gene-environment interactions affect plasma lipid concentrations and potentially cardiovascular disease risk is reviewed. Patients with high blood lipids will likely be the first to benefit from the type of personalized nutrition linked to their genetic information.

14. Pray L: Dieting for the Genome Generation. *The Scientist* 19(1):14, 2005.

    That nutrigenomics has yet to prove its worth is discussed along with the reasons why the public is buying into the idea.

15. Santosa S and others: Probiotics and their potential health claims. *Nutrition Reviews* 64:265, 2006.

This paper reviews evidence of the ability of different probiotic strains to prevent and treat diarrhea, treat irritable bowel syndrome, treat inflammatory bowel disease, and prevent colon cancer. The strongest evidence is related to prevention and treatment of diarrhea and some forms of irritable bowel syndrome.

16. Schardt D: Not everybody must get stones. *Nutrition and Action Healthletter*, p. 89, November 2004.

Excess body weight is the primary modifiable risk factor for developing gallbladder stones. Low-fiber diets are also implicated.

17. Seeley RR and others: *Anatomy and physiology.* 7th ed. Boston: McGraw-Hill, 2006.

This text provides comprehensive coverage of the anatomy and physiology of the gastrointestinal tract, as well as other related body systems.

18. Shanta-Retelny V: Living bacteria: The body's natural defense. *Today's Dietitian*, p. 44, May, 2005.

Evidence that bacteria play an important role in health maintenance is discussed. Many interesting "gut flora" facts are presented. In addition, the idea that probiotics can play a therapeutic role in gut health is introduced. It is speculated that new, well-characterized, scientifically proven probiotic strains with specific health benefits will be developed in the future.

19. Stover PJ: Influence of human genetic variation on nutritional requirements. *American Journal of Clinical Nutrition* 83:436S, 2006.

The complexity of the interaction between genes and diet is discussed as well as the opportunities to reevaluate the criteria used to determine RDAs relative to the contribution of genetic variation to optimal nutrition for individuals.

20. The low-down on hemorrhoids. *UC Berkeley Wellness Letter*, p. 4, July, 2004.

Hemorrhoids are commonly experienced by many adults. Measures to reduce such risk and as well treat the problem are discussed, such as an adequate fluid and fiber intake. Fortunately hemorrhoids rarely lead to serious health problems.

▶ Check out the **Contemporary Nutrition ARIS site**

www.mhhe.com/wardlawcontfa1 for quizzes, flash cards, other activities, and weblinks designed to further help you learn about what you eat and why.

I. Are You Taking Care of Your Digestive Tract?

People need to think about the health of their digestive tracts. There are symptoms we need to notice, as well as habits we need to practice to protect it. The following assessment is designed to help you examine your habits and symptoms associated with the health of your digestive tract. The "Nutrition and Your Health" section explained why these habits are important to examine. Put a Y in the blank to the left of the question to indicate yes and an N to indicate no.

_____ 1. Are you currently experiencing greater than normal stress and tension?

_____ 2. Do you have a family history of digestive tract problems (e.g., ulcers, hemorrhoids, recurrent heartburn, constipation)?

_____ 3. Do you experience pain in your stomach region about 2 hours after you eat?

_____ 4. Do you smoke cigarettes?

_____ 5. Do you take aspirin frequently?

_____ 6. Do you have heartburn at least once per week?

_____ 7. Do you commonly lie down after eating a large meal?

_____ 8. Do you drink alcoholic beverages more than two or three times per day?

_____ 9. Do you experience abdominal pain, bloating, and gas about 30 minutes to 2 hours after consuming milk products?

_____ 10. Do you often have to strain while having a bowel movement?

_____ 11. Do you consume less than 9 (women) or 13 (men) cups of a combination of water and other fluids per day?

_____ 12. Do you perform physical activity for less than 60 minutes or more on most or all days of the week (e.g., jog, swim, walk briskly, row, stair climb)?

_____ 13. Do you eat a diet relatively low in fiber (recall that significant fiber is found in whole fruits, vegetables, legumes, nuts and seeds, whole-grain breads, and whole-grain cereals)?

_____ 14. Do you frequently have diarrhea?

_____ 15. Do you frequently use laxatives or antacids?

Interpretation

Add up the number of yes answers you gave and record the total in the blank to the right. _____

If your score is from 8 to 15, your habits and symptoms put you at risk for experiencing future digestive tract problems. Take particular note of the habits to which you answered yes. Consider trying to cooperate more with your digestive tract.

II. Create Your Family Tree for Health-Related Concerns

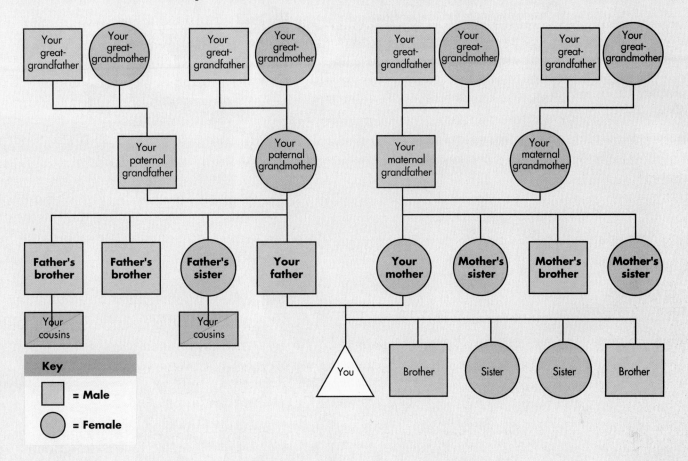

Adapt this diagram to your family tree. Under each heading, list year born, year died (if applicable), major diseases that developed during the person's lifetime, and cause of death (if applicable). Figure 3-19 provides one such example.

You are likely to be at risk for any diseases listed. Creating a plan for preventing such diseases when possible, especially those that developed in your family members before age 50 to 60 years, is advised. Speak with your physician about any concerns arising from this exercise.

CHAPTER 4 Carbohydrates

CHAPTER OBJECTIVES Chapter 4 is designed to allow you to:

1. Identify the basic structures and food sources of the major carbohydrates—monosaccharides, disaccharides, polysaccharides (e.g., starches), and fiber.

2. Describe food sources of carbohydrate and list some alternative sweeteners.

3. Explain how carbohydrates are digested and absorbed, including the consequences of lactose maldigestion (and lactose intolerance).

4. List the functions of carbohydrate in the body and the problems that result from not eating enough carbohydrate.

5. Describe the regulation of blood glucose and discuss how other nutrients can be converted to blood glucose.

6. Outline the beneficial effects of fiber on the body.

7. State the RDA for carbohydrate and various guidelines for carbohydrate intake.

8. Identify the consequences of diabetes, and explain appropriate dietary measures that will reduce the adverse effects of this health problem.

CHAPTER OUTLINE

WHAT DID YOU EAT TO OBTAIN THE ENERGY YOU ARE USING RIGHT NOW? Chapters 4, 5, and 6 will examine this question by focusing on the main nutrients the human body uses for fuel. These nutrients are carbohydrates (on average, 4 kcal per gram) and fats and oils (on average, 9 kcal per gram). Although protein (on average, 4 kcal per gram) *can* be used for energy needs, the body typically reserves this nutrient for other processes. Most people know that potatoes are rich in carbohydrates and steak contains mostly fat and protein, but many people do not know how to use this information.

It is likely that you have recently consumed fruits, vegetables, dairy products, cereal, breads, and pasta. These foods supply carbohydrates. Unfortunately, the benefits of these foods are often underestimated as suggested in the comic in this chapter. Many people think carbohydrate-rich foods are fattening but they are not any more so than fat or protein. In fact, pound for pound, carbohydrates are much less fattening than fats and oils. Furthermore, high-carbohydrate foods, especially fiber-rich foods such as fruits, vegetables, whole-grain breads and cereals, and legumes, provide many important health benefits in addition to the calories they contain. Some people think sugars cause hyperactivity in children—not so, according to well-designed scientific investigations. Almost all carbohydrate-rich foods, except pure sugars, provide several essential nutrients and should generally constitute 45% to 65% of our daily calorie intake. Let's take a closer look at carbohydrates, including why the recent craze of carbohydrate-bashing was misguided.

 Refresh Your Memory

As you begin your study of carbohydrates in Chapter 4, you may want to review:

- The concept of energy density and the health claims for various carbohydrates in Chapter 2
- The processes of digestion and absorption in Chapter 3
- The hormones that regulate blood glucose in Chapter 3

CARBOHYDRATES—AN INTRODUCTION

Carbohydrates are a main fuel source for some cells, especially those in the brain, nervous system, and red blood cells. Muscles also rely on a dependable supply of carbohydrate to fuel intense physical activity. Carbohydrates provide on average 4 kcal per gram and are a readily available fuel for all cells, both in the form of blood glucose and **glycogen** stored in the liver and muscles. The glycogen stored in the liver can be used to maintain blood glucose concentrations in times when you have not eaten for several hours or the diet does not supply enough carbohydrate. Regular intake of carbohydrate is important, because liver glycogen stores are depleted in about 18 hours

glycogen A carbohydrate made of multiple units of glucose with a highly branched structure. It is the storage form of glucose in humans and is synthesized (and stored) in the liver and muscles.

The class of carbohydrate that has gained the most attention recently is fiber. Why is this so? Which health problems typically result from a limited intake of fiber? Which foods are good sources of fiber? How much fiber is enough? Too much? Chapter 4 provides some answers.

if no carbohydrate is consumed. After that point, the body is forced to produce carbohydrate, largely from breakdown of proteins in the body. This eventually leads to health problems including the loss of muscle tissue.

Humans have sensors on our tongues that recognize the sweetness of carbohydrates. Researchers speculate that this sweetness indicated a safe energy source to early humans, and so it became an important energy source.

Despite their important role as a calorie source, some forms of carbohydrate promote health more than others. As you will see in this chapter, whole-grain breads and cereals have greater health benefits than refined and processed forms of carbohydrate. Choosing the healthiest carbohydrate sources most often, while moderating intake of less healthful sources, contributes to a healthy diet. It is difficult to eat so little carbohydrate that body fuel needs are not met, but it is easy to overconsume the simple carbohydrates that can contribute to health problems. Let's explore this concept further as we look at carbohydrates in detail.

Green plants create the carbohydrates in our foods. Leaves capture the sun's solar energy in their cells and transform it to chemical energy. This energy is then stored in the chemical bonds of the carbohydrate glucose as it is produced from carbon dioxide from the air and water from the soil. This complex process is called **photosynthesis** (Fig. 4-1).

▲ Fruits such as peaches are an excellent source of carbohydrate for your diet.

$$6 \text{ carbon dioxide} + 6 \text{ water (solar energy)} \rightarrow \text{glucose} + 6 \text{ oxygen}$$
$$(CO_2) \qquad\qquad (H_2O) \qquad\qquad (C_6H_2O_6) \quad (O_2)$$

Translated into English, this reads: 6 molecules of carbon dioxide combine with 6 molecules of water to form one molecule of **glucose.** Converting solar energy into chemical bonds in the sugar is a key part of the process. Six molecules of oxygen are then released into the air.

SIMPLE CARBOHYDRATES

As the name suggests, most carbohydrate molecules are composed of carbon, hydrogen, and oxygen atoms. Simple forms of carbohydrates are called **sugars.** Larger, more complex forms are primarily called either **starches** or **fibers,** depending on their digestibility by human GI tract enzymes. Starches are the digestible form.

Monosaccharides and disaccharides are often referred to as *simple sugars* because they contain only one or two sugar units. Food labels lump all of these sugars under one category, listing them as "sugars."

Monosaccharides—Glucose, Fructose, and Galactose

Monosaccharides are the simple sugar units (*mono* means one) that serve as the basic unit of all carbohydrate structures. The most common monosaccharides in foods are glucose, fructose, and galactose (Fig. 4-2).

photosynthesis Process by which plants use energy from the sun to synthesize energy-yielding compounds, such as glucose.

glucose A six-carbon monosaccharide that usually exists in a ring form; found as such in blood, and in table sugar bonded to fructose; also known as *dextrose.*

sugar A simple carbohydrate with the chemical composition $(CH_2O)_n$. The basic unit of all sugars is glucose, a six-carbon ring structure. The primary sugar in the diet is sucrose, which is made up of glucose and fructose.

starch A carbohydrate made of multiple units of glucose attached together in a form the body can digest; also known as *complex carbohydrate.*

fiber Substances in plant foods not digested by the processes that take place in the stomach or small intestine. These add bulk to feces. Fibers naturally found in foods are also called dietary fiber.

FIGURE 4-1 ▶ A summary of photosynthesis. Plants use carbon dioxide, water, and energy to produce carbohydrates such as glucose. Glucose is then stored in the leaf but can also undergo further metabolism to form starch and fiber in the plant.

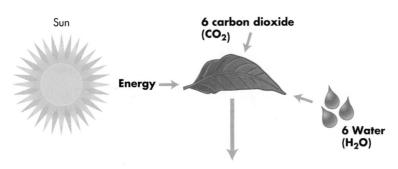

Sun

6 carbon dioxide (CO_2)

Energy →

6 Water (H_2O)

Glucose ($C_6H_{12}O_6$) + 6 Oxygen (O_2)

Monosaccharides

FIGURE 4-2 ▶ Chemical forms of the important monosaccharides.

sucrose Fructose bonded to glucose; table sugar.

fructose A six-carbon monosaccharide that usually exists in a ring form; found in fruits and honey; also known as *fruit sugar.*

galactose A six-carbon monosaccharide that usually exists in a ring form; closely related to glucose.

lactose Glucose bonded to galactose; also known as *milk sugar.*

maltose Glucose bonded to glucose.

Glucose is the major monosaccharide found in the body. Glucose is also known as *dextrose,* and glucose in the bloodstream may be called blood sugar. Glucose is an important source of energy for human cells, although foods contain very little carbohydrate as this single sugar. Most glucose comes from the digestion of starches and **sucrose** (common table sugar) from our food. The latter is made up of the monosaccharides glucose and fructose. For the most part, sugars and other carbohydrates in foods are eventually converted to glucose in the liver. This glucose then goes on to serve as a source of fuel for cells.

Fructose, also called *fruit sugar,* is another common monosaccharide. After it is consumed, fructose is absorbed by the small intestine and then transported to the liver, where it is quickly metabolized. Much is converted to glucose, but the rest goes on to form other compounds, such as fat, if fructose is consumed in very high amounts. Most of the free fructose in our diets comes from the use of **high-fructose corn syrup** in soft drinks, candies, jams, jellies, and many other fruit products and desserts (see the later discussion on nutritive sweeteners). Fructose also is found naturally in fruits and forms half of each sucrose molecule, as previously noted.

The sugar **galactose** has nearly the same structure as glucose. Large quantities of pure galactose do not exist in nature. Instead, galactose is usually found bonded to glucose in **lactose,** a sugar found in milk and other milk products. After lactose is digested and absorbed, galactose arrives in the liver. There it is either transformed into glucose or further metabolized into glycogen.

MAKING DECISIONS

Nutrient Metabolism

Now is a good time to begin emphasizing a key concept in nutrition: the difference between *intake* of a substance and the body's *use* of that substance. The body often does not use all nutrients in their original states. Some of these substances are broken down and later reassembled into the same or a different substance when and where they are needed. For example, much of the galactose in the diet is metabolized to glucose. When later required for the production of milk in the mammary gland of a lactating female, galactose is resynthesized from glucose to help form the milk sugar lactose. Knowing this, do you think it is necessary for a lactating women to drink milk to make milk?

Disaccharides—Sucrose, Lactose, and Maltose

Disaccharides are formed when two monosaccharides combine (*di* means two). The disaccharides in food are sucrose, lactose, and **maltose**. All contain glucose.

Sucrose forms when the two sugars glucose and fructose bond together (Fig. 4-3). Sucrose is found naturally in sugarcane, sugar beets, honey, and maple sugar. These products are processed to varying degrees to make brown, white, and powdered sugars. Animals do not produce sucrose or much of any carbohydrate except glycogen.

Disaccharides

Sucrose: glucose + fructose
Lactose: glucose + galactose
Maltose: glucose + glucose

Sucrose

FIGURE 4-3 ▶ Chemical form of the disaccharide sucrose.

Lactose forms when glucose bonds with galactose during the synthesis of milk. Again, our major food source for lactose is milk products. A later section on lactose maldigestion and lactose intolerance discusses the problems that result when a person can't readily digest lactose.

Maltose results when starch is broken down to just two glucose molecules bonded together. Maltose plays an important role in the beer and liquor industry. In the production of alcoholic beverages, starches in various cereal grains are first converted to simpler carbohydrates by enzymes present in the grains. The products of this step—maltose, glucose, and other sugars—are then mixed with yeast cells in the absence of oxygen. The yeast cells convert most of the sugars to alcohol (ethanol) and carbon dioxide, a process called **fermentation.** Little maltose remains in the final product. Few other food products or beverages contain maltose. In fact, most maltose that we ultimately digest in the small intestine is produced during our own digestion of starch.

COMPLEX CARBOHYDRATES

In many foods, single-sugar units are bonded together to form a chain, known as a polysaccharide (*poly* means many). **Polysaccharides,** also called *complex carbohydrates* or *starch,* may contain 1000 or more glucose units and are found chiefly in grains, vegetables, and fruits. When food labels list "Other Carbohydrates," this primarily refers to starch content.

Plants store carbohydrate in two forms of starch digestible by humans: **amylose** and **amylopectin.** Amylose, a long, straight chain of glucose units, comprises about 20% of the digestible starch found in vegetables, beans, breads, pasta, and rice. Amylopectin is a highly branched chain and makes up the remaining 80% of digestible starches in the diet (Fig. 4-4). Cellulose (a fiber) is another complex carbohydrate in plants. Although similar to amylose, it cannot be digested by humans, as discussed in the next section.

The enzymes that break down starches to glucose and other related sugars act only at the end of a glucose chain. Amylopectin, because it is branched, provides many more sites (ends) for enzyme action. Therefore, amylopectin is digested more rapidly and raises blood glucose much more readily than amylose (see the discussion of glycemic load in a later section of Chapter 4, "Carbohydrates in Foods").

As noted earlier, animals—including humans—store glucose in the form of glycogen. Glycogen consists of a chain of glucose units with many branches, providing even more sites for enzyme action than amylopectin (review Fig. 4-4). Because of its branched structure that can be broken down quickly, glycogen is an ideal storage form of carbohydrate in the body.

The liver and muscles are the major storage sites for glycogen. Because the amount of glucose immediately available in body fluids can provide only about 120 kcal, these glycogen storage sites for carbohydrate energy— amounting to about 1800 kcal—are extremely important. Of this 1800 kcal, liver glycogen (about 400 kcal) can readily contribute to blood glucose. Muscle glycogen stores (about 1400 kcal) cannot raise blood glucose, but instead supply glucose for muscle

Simple	
	Monosaccharides
	Glucose, fructose, galactose
	Disaccharides
	Sucrose, lactose, maltose
	Polysaccharides
	Starches (amylose and amylopectin), glycogen, most fibers
Complex	

fermentation The conversion of carbohydrates to alcohols, acids, and carbon dioxide without the use of oxygen.

polysaccharides Carbohydrates containing many glucose units, from 10 to 1000 or more.

amylose A digestible straight-chain type of starch composed of glucose units.

amylopectin A digestible branched-chain type of starch composed of glucose units.

▲ As plants mature, some sugars are turned into starch.

FIGURE 4-4 ▶ Some common starches and glycogen. We consume essentially no glycogen. All glycogen found in the body is made by our cells, primarily in the liver and muscles.

cellulose An undigestible nonfermentable straight-chain polysaccharide made of glucose molecules.

hemicellulose A nonfermentable fiber containing xylose, galactose, glucose, and other monosaccharides bonded together.

pectin A viscous fiber containing chains of galacturonic acid and other monosaccharides; characteristically found between plant cell walls.

gums A viscous fiber containing chains of galactose, glucuronic acid, and other monosaccharides; characteristically found in exudates from plant stems.

mucilages A viscous fiber consisting of chains of galactose, mannose, and other monosaccharides; characteristically found in seaweed.

lignins A nonfermentable fiber made up of a multiringed alcohol (noncarbohydrate) structure.

dietary fiber Fiber found in food.

whole grains Grains containing the entire seed of the plant, including the bran, germ, and endosperm (starchy interior). Examples are whole wheat and brown rice.

nonfermentable fiber A fiber that is not easily metabolized by intestinal bacteria.

viscous fiber A fiber that is readily fermented by bacteria in the large intestine.

use, especially during high-intensity and endurance exercise (see Chapter 10 for a detailed discussion of carbohydrate use in exercise).

MAKING DECISIONS

Animal Sources of Carbohydrates

If animals store glycogen in their muscles, are meats, fish, and poultry a good source of carbohydrates? No—animal products are not good food sources of this (or any other) carbohydrate because glycogen stores quickly degrade after the animal dies.

FIBER

Fiber as a class is mostly made up of polysaccharides, but they differ from starches insofar as the chemical links that join the individual sugar units cannot be digested by human enzymes in the GI tract. This prevents the small intestine from absorbing the sugars that make up the various fibers. Fiber is not a single substance, but a group of substances with similar characteristics (Table 4-1). The group is comprised of the carbohydrates **cellulose, hemicelluloses, pectins, gums,** and **mucilages,** as well as the noncarbohydrate, **lignin.** In total, these constitute all the nonstarch polysaccharides in foods. Nutrition Facts labels generally do not list these individual forms of fiber, but instead lump them together under the term **dietary fiber.**

Cellulose, hemicelluloses, and lignin form the structural parts of plants. Bran fiber is rich in hemicelluloses and lignin. (The woody fibers in broccoli are partly lignin.) Bran layers form the outer covering of all grains, so **whole grains** (i.e., unrefined) are good sources of bran fiber (Fig. 4-5). Because the majority of these fibers neither readily dissolve in water nor are easily metabolized by intestinal bacteria, they are called **nonfermentable** or insoluble fibers.

Pectins, gums, and mucilages are contained around and inside plant cells. These fibers either dissolve or swell when put into water and are therefore called **viscous** or soluble fibers. They also are readily fermented by bacteria in the large intestine. These fibers are found in salad dressings, some frozen desserts, jams, and jellies as gum arabic, guar gum, locust bean gum, and various pectin forms. Some forms of hemicelluloses also fall into the soluble category.

TABLE 4-1 Classification of Fibers

Type	Component(s)	Physiological Effects	Major Food Sources
Nonfermentable or Insoluble			
Noncarbohydrate form	Lignin	Increases fecal bulk	Whole grains, wheat bran
Carbohydrate form	Cellulose, hemicelluloses	Increases fecal bulk Decreases intestinal transit time	All plants, wheat products Wheat, rye, rice, vegetables
Viscous or Soluble			
Carbohydrate form	Pectins, gums, mucilages, some hemicelluloses	Delays stomach emptying; slows glucose absorption; can lower blood cholesterol	Citrus fruits, apples, bananas, oat products, carrots, barley, beans, thickeners added to foods

Most foods contain mixtures of soluble and insoluble fibers. Food labels do not generally distinguish between the two types, but, manufacturers have the option to do so. Often, if food is listed as a good source of one type of fiber, it usually contains some of the other type of fiber as well. The definition of fiber has recently been expanded to include both the dietary fiber found naturally in foods and additional fiber that is added to foods. This second category is called **functional fiber;** a fiber of this type must show beneficial effects in humans to be included in the category. **Total fiber** (or just the term *fiber*) is then the combination of dietary fiber and functional fiber in the food product. Currently the Nutrition Facts label only includes the category dietary fiber; the label has yet to be updated to reflect the latest definition of fiber.

A newly studied category of functional fiber are the prebiotics. Prebiotics include a group of short-chain carbohydrates or oligosaccharides, resistant to digestion, but fermented by

functional fiber Fiber added to foods that has been shown to provide health benefits.

total fiber Combination of dietary fiber and functional fiber in a food. Also just called *fiber.*

Pectin: viscous fiber

Cellulose in the skin: non-fermentable fiber

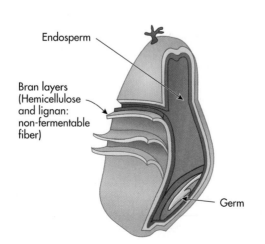

Endosperm

Bran layers (Hemicellulose and lignan: non-fermentable fiber)

Germ

FIGURE 4-5 ▶ Viscous and nonfermentable fiber. (a) The skin of an apple consists of the nonfermentable fiber cellulose, which provides structure for the fruit. The viscous fiber pectin "glues" the fruit cells together. (b) The outside layer of a wheat kernel is made of layers of bran—primarily hemicellulose, a nonfermentable fiber—making this whole grain a good source of fiber. Overall, fruits, vegetables, whole-grain breads and cereals, and beans are rich in fiber.

bacteria in the colon. They are thought to stimulate the growth or activity of beneficial bacteria in the large intestine and therefore promote the host's health.

CONCEPT CHECK

Important monosaccharides in nutrition are glucose, fructose, and galactose. Glucose is a primary energy source for body cells. Disaccharides form when two monosaccharides bond together. Important disaccharides in nutrition are sucrose (glucose + fructose), maltose (glucose + glucose), and lactose (glucose + galactose). Once digested into monosaccharides and absorbed, most carbohydrates are transformed into glucose by the liver.

Amylose, amylopectin, and glycogen are all polysaccharides, which function as storage forms of glucose. Amylose and amylopectin are the major digestible plant polysaccharides and contain multiple glucose units bonded together. Glycogen is a storage form of glucose in our liver and muscle cells.

Fiber is essentially the portion of plant food that remains undigested as it enters the large intestine. There are two general classes of fiber: nonfermentable and viscous. Nonfermentable (insoluble) fibers are mostly made up of cellulose, hemicelluloses, and lignins. Viscous (soluble) fibers are made up mostly of pectins, gums, and mucilages. Both nonfermentable and viscous fibers are resistant to human digestive enzymes, but bacteria in the large intestine can break down viscous fibers.

CARBOHYDRATES IN FOODS

The food components that yield the highest percentage of calories from carbohydrates are table sugar, honey, jam, jelly, fruit, and plain baked potatoes (Fig. 4-6). Corn flakes, rice, bread, and noodles all contain at least 75% of calories as carbohydrates.

FIGURE 4-6 ▶ Food sources of carbohydrates compared to the RDA of 130 grams for carbohydrate.

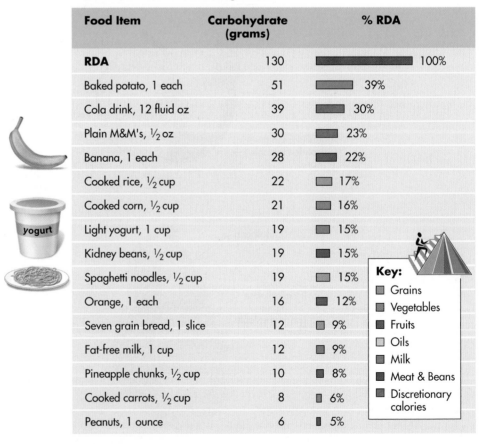

Food Sources of Carbohydrate

Food Item	Carbohydrate (grams)	% RDA
RDA	130	100%
Baked potato, 1 each	51	39%
Cola drink, 12 fluid oz	39	30%
Plain M&M's, 1/2 oz	30	23%
Banana, 1 each	28	22%
Cooked rice, 1/2 cup	22	17%
Cooked corn, 1/2 cup	21	16%
Light yogurt, 1 cup	19	15%
Kidney beans, 1/2 cup	19	15%
Spaghetti noodles, 1/2 cup	19	15%
Orange, 1 each	16	12%
Seven grain bread, 1 slice	12	9%
Fat-free milk, 1 cup	12	9%
Pineapple chunks, 1/2 cup	10	8%
Cooked carrots, 1/2 cup	8	6%
Peanuts, 1 ounce	6	5%

Key:
- Grains
- Vegetables
- Fruits
- Oils
- Milk
- Meat & Beans
- Discretionary calories

Foods with moderate amounts of carbohydrate calories are peas, broccoli, oatmeal, dry beans and other legumes, cream pies, French fries, and fat-free milk. In these foods, the carbohydrate content is diluted either by protein, as in the case of fat-free milk, or by fat, as in the case of a cream pie. Foods with essentially no carbohydrates include beef, eggs, chicken, fish, vegetable oils, butter, and margarine.

The percentage of calories from carbohydrate is more important than the total amount of carbohydrate in a food when planning a healthy high-carbohydrate diet. Figure 4-7 shows that the grain, vegetable, fruit, and milk groups contain the most nutrient-dense sources of carbohydrate. In planning a high-carbohydrate diet, you need to emphasize grains, pasta, fruits, and vegetables. On the other hand, you can't create a diet high in carbohydrate calories from chocolate, potato chips, and French fries because these foods contain too much fat. Currently, the top five carbohydrate sources for U.S. adults are white bread, soft drinks, cookies and cakes (including doughnuts), sugars/syrups/jams, and potatoes. Clearly, many North Americans (teenagers included) should take a closer look at their main carbohydrate sources and strive to improve them from a nutritional standpoint by including more whole grains, fruits, and vegetables.

A Closer Look at Sweeteners

The various substances that impart sweetness to foods fall into two broad classes: nutritive sweeteners, which can provide calories for the body; and alternative sweeteners, which for the most part provide no calories. As shown in Table 4-2, the alternative sweeteners are much sweeter on a per-gram basis than the nutritive

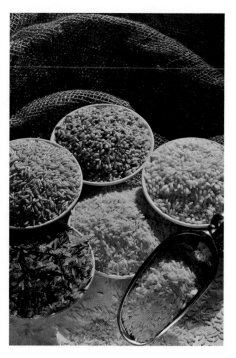

▲ Rice is rich in carbohydrates.

MyPyramid: Sources of Carbohydrates

Food Group	Grains	Vegetables	Fruits	Oils	Milk	Meat & Beans	
Sources of Carbohydrate	• All varieties	• All varieties	• All varieties	• None	• Milk • Yogurt	• Beans	• Nuts
Grams per Serving	15	5	18	0	12	10	4

FIGURE 4-7 ▶ Sources of carbohydrates from MyPyramid. The height of the background color (none, $^1/_3$, $^2/_3$, or completely covered) within each group in the pyramid indicates the average nutrient density for carbohydrate in that group. Overall, the grain group, vegetable group, fruit group, and milk group contain many foods that are nutrient-dense sources of carbohydrate. With regard to physical activity, carbohydrates are a key fuel in most endeavors.

▲ Soft drinks are typical sources of either sugars or alternative sweeteners, depending on the type of soft drink chosen.

TABLE 4-2 The Sweetness of Sugars (Nutritive) and Alternative Sweeteners

Type of Sweetener	Relative Sweetness* (Sucrose = 1)	Typical Sources
Sugars		
Lactose	0.2	Dairy products
Maltose	0.4	Sprouted seeds
Glucose	0.7	Corn syrup
Sucrose	1.0	Table sugar, most sweets
Invert sugar†	1.3	Some candies, honey
Fructose	1.2–1.8	Fruit, honey, some soft drinks
Sugar Alcohols		
Sorbitol	0.6	Dietetic candies, sugarless gum
Mannitol	0.7	Dietetic candies
Xylitol	0.9	Sugarless gum
Maltitol	0.9	Baked goods, chocolate, candies
Alternative Sweeteners		
Tagatose	0.9	Ready-to-eat breakfast cereals, diet soft drinks, meal replacement bars, frozen desserts, candy, frosting
Cyclamate‡	30	Tabletop sweetener, medicines
Aspartame (Equal®)	180	Diet soft drinks, diet fruit drinks, sugarless gum, powdered diet sweetener
Acesulfame-K (Sunette®)	200	Sugarless gum, diet drink mixes, powdered diet sweeteners, puddings, gelatin desserts
Saccharin (sodium salt) (Sweet'N Low®)	300	Diet soft drinks, powdered diet sweetener
Sucralose (Splenda®)	600	Diet soft drinks, powdered diet sweetener, sugarless gums, jams, frozen desserts
Neotame	7000 to 13,000	Powdered diet sweetener, baked goods, frozen desserts, jams

*On a per gram basis.
†Sucrose broken down into glucose and fructose.
‡Not available in the United States, but available in Canada.
From the American Dietetic Association, 2004, and other sources.

sweeteners. The taste and sweetness of sucrose make it the benchmark against which all other sweeteners are measured. Sucrose is obtained from sugar cane and sugar beet plants.

Nutritive Sweeteners

Both sugars and sugar alcohols provide calories along with sweetness. Sugars are found in many different food products, whereas sugar alcohols have rather limited uses.

Sugars

All of the monosaccharides (glucose, fructose, and galactose) and disaccharides (sucrose, lactose, and maltose) discussed earlier are designated *nutritive sweeteners* (Table 4-3). Many forms of sugar are used in food products and result in an intake of about 82 grams or 16 teaspoons of sugar per day.

High-fructose corn syrup, generally 55% fructose, is used extensively in the food industry. High-fructose corn syrup is made by treating cornstarch with acid and en-

TABLE 4-3 Names of Sugars Used in Foods

Sugar	Invert sugar	Honey	Maple syrup
Sucrose	Glucose	Corn syrup or sweeteners	Dextrose
Brown sugar	Sorbitol	High-fructose corn syrup	Fructose
Confectioner's sugar (powdered sugar)	Levulose		Maltodextrins
	Polydextrose	Molasses	Caramel
Turbinado sugar	Lactose	Date sugar	Fruit sugar

▲ There are many forms of sugar on the market. Used in many foods, together they contribute to our daily intake of approximately 82 grams (16 teaspoons) of sugars in our diets.

zymes. This treatment breaks down much of the starch into glucose. Then some of the glucose is converted by enzymes into fructose. The final syrup is usually as sweet as sucrose. Its major advantage is that it is cheaper than sucrose. Also, it doesn't form crystals and it has better freezing properties. High-fructose corn syrups are used in soft drinks, candies, jam, jelly, other fruit products, and desserts (e.g., packaged cookies).

In addition to sucrose and high-fructose corn syrup, brown sugar, turbinado sugar (sold as raw sugar), honey, maple syrup, and other sugars are also added to foods. Brown sugar is essentially sucrose containing some molasses; either the molasses is not totally removed from the sucrose during processing or it is added to the sucrose crystals. Turbinado sugar, a partially refined version of raw sucrose, has a slight molasses flavor.

Maple syrup is made by boiling down and concentrating the sap that runs during the late winter in sugar maple trees. Most pancake syrup sold in supermarkets is not pure maple syrup, which is expensive. Instead, it is primarily corn syrup and high-fructose corn syrup with maple flavor added.

Honey is a product of plant nectar that has been altered by bee enzymes. The enzymes break down much of the nectar's sucrose into fructose and glucose. Honey offers essentially the same nutritional value as other simple sugars—a source of energy and little else. However, honey is not safe to feed to infants because it can contain spores of the bacterium *Clostridium botulinum*. These spores can become the bacteria that cause fatal foodborne illness. Honey does not pose the same threat to adults because the acidic environment of an adult's stomach inhibits the growth of the bacteria. An infant's stomach, however, does not produce much acid, making infants susceptible to the threat that this bacterium poses.

SUGAR ALCOHOLS

Food manufacturers and consumers have numerous options for obtaining sweetness while consuming less sugar and calories. Overall, sugar alcohols and alternative sweeteners enable people with diabetes to enjoy the flavor of sweetness while controlling sugars in their diets; they also provide noncaloric or very-low-calorie sugar substitutes for persons trying to lose (or control) body weight.

Sugar alcohols such as **sorbitol** and **xylitol** are used as nutritive sweeteners. Sugar alcohols contribute fewer calories (about 2.6 kcal per gram) than sugars. They also are absorbed and metabolized to glucose more slowly than are simple sugars. Because of this, they remain in the intestinal tract for a longer time and in large quantities can cause diarrhea. In fact, any products that may be consumed in amounts that may result in a daily ingestion of 50 grams of sugar alcohols, must bear this labeling statement: "Excess consumption may have a laxative effect."

Sugar alcohols are used in sugarless gum, breath mints, and candy. Unlike sucrose, sugar alcohols are not readily metabolized by bacteria to acids in the mouth and thus do not promote tooth decay (see the later section on problems linked to carbohydrate intake).

▲ Sugarless gum is typically sweetened with sugar alcohols.

▶ Sugar alcohols as a class are also called polyols.

Sugar alcohols must be listed on labels. If only one sugar alcohol is used in a product, its name must be listed. However, if two or more are used in one product, they are grouped together under the heading "sugar alcohols." The caloric value of each sugar alcohol used in a food product is calculated so that when one reads the total amount of calories a product provides, it includes the sugar alcohols in the overall amount.

ALTERNATIVE SWEETENERS

Often called artificial sweeteners, alternative sweeteners include **saccharin,** cyclamate, **aspartame, sucralose, neotame,** and **acesulfame-K.** Unlike sugar alcohols, alternative sweeteners yield little or no calories when consumed in amounts typically used in food products. Six are currently available in the United States: saccharin, aspartame, sucralose, neotame, acesulfame-K, and tagatose. Cyclamate was banned for use in the United States in 1970, although it has never been conclusively proven to cause health problems when used appropriately. Cyclamate is used in Canada as a sweetener in medicines and as a tabletop sweetener.

Saccharin

The oldest alternative sweetener, saccharin, was first produced in 1879 and is currently approved for use in more than 90 countries. It represents about half of the alternative sweetener market in North America (typically packaged in pink packets, including Sweet 'N Low®). Based on laboratory animal studies, saccharin was once thought to increase the risk of bladder cancer but it is no longer listed as a potential cause of cancer.

Aspartame

Aspartame is in widespread use throughout the world (typically packaged in blue packets, including Equal®). It has been approved for use by more than 90 countries, and its use has been endorsed by the World Health Organization, the American Medical Association, the American Diabetes Association, and other groups.

▶ Persons with an uncommon disease called **phenylketonuria (PKU),** which interferes with the metabolism of phenylalanine, should avoid aspartame because of its high phenylalanine content. A warning label is required on products containing aspartame, alerting people with PKU that a product with aspartame contains phenylalanine.

The components of aspartame are the amino acids phenylalanine and aspartic acid, along with methanol. Recall that amino acids are the building blocks of proteins, so aspartame is more of a protein than a carbohydrate. Aspartame yields about 4 kcal per gram, but it is about 200 times sweeter than sucrose. Thus, only a small amount of aspartame is needed to obtain the desired sweetness, and the amount of calories added is insignificant unless the product is consumed in unusually high amounts. Aspartame is used in beverages, gelatin desserts, chewing gum, toppings and fillings in precooked bakery goods, and cookies. Aspartame does not cause tooth decay. Like other proteins, however, aspartame is damaged when heated for a long time and thus would lose its sweetness if used in products requiring cooking.

Some complaints have been filed with FDA by people claiming to have had adverse reactions to aspartame: headaches, dizziness, seizures, nausea, and other side effects. It is important for people who are sensitive to aspartame to avoid it, but the percentage of sensitive people is likely to be extremely small.

The acceptable daily intake of aspartame set by FDA is 50 milligrams per kilogram of body weight. This is equivalent to the aspartame in about 14 cans of diet soft drink for an adult or about 80 packets of Equal®. Aspartame appears to be safe for pregnant women and children, but some scientists suggest cautious use by these groups, especially young children, who need ample calories to grow.

INGREDIENTS: SORBITOL, GUM BASE, MANNITOL, GLYCEROL, HYDROGENATED STARCH, XYLITOL, ARTIFICIAL AND NATURAL FLAVORS, ASPARTAME, RED 40, YELLOW 6 AND BHT (TO MAINTAIN FRESHNESS). PHENYLKETONURICS: CONTAINS PHENYLALANINE.

Sugarless Gum

▲ Sugar alcohols and the alternative sweetener aspartame are used to sweeten this product. Note the warning for people with PKU that this product with aspartame contains phenylalanine.

Sucralose

Sucralose (Splenda®) is 600 times sweeter than sucrose. It is made by adding three chlorines to sucrose. Sucralose is approved for use as an additive to foods such as soft drinks, gum, baked goods, syrups, gelatins, frozen dairy desserts such as ice cream, jams, processed fruits and fruit juices, and for tabletop use. Sucralose doesn't break down under high heat conditions and can be used in cooking and baking. It is also excreted as such in the feces. The small amount absorbed is excreted in the urine.

Neotame

Neotame was recently approved by FDA for use as a general-purpose sweetener in a wide variety of food products, other than meat and poultry. Neotame is a nonnutritive, high-intensity sweetener that, depending on its food application, is approximately 7000 to 13,000 times sweeter than table sugar. It has a chemical structure similar to aspartame. Neotame is heat stable and can be used as a tabletop sweetener as well as in cooking applications. Examples of uses for which it has been approved include baked goods, nonalcoholic beverages (including soft drinks), chewing gum, confections and frostings, frozen desserts, gelatins and puddings, jams and jellies, processed fruits and fruit juices, toppings, and syrups. Neotame is safe for use by the general population, including children, pregnant and lactating women, and people with diabetes. In addition, no special labeling for people with phenylketonuria is needed because neotame is not broken down in the body to its amino acid components.

▶ Stevia comes from a South American shrub; it is 100 to 300 times sweeter than sucrose and provides zero calories. It is a sweetener that has been used in small amounts by the Japanese since the 1970s. FDA has not approved the use of stevia in foods, but stevia can be purchased at natural- and health-food stores as a dietary supplement.

Acesulfame-K

The alternative sweetener acesulfame-K (the *K* stands for potassium; Sunette®) was approved by FDA in July 1988. It is approved for use in more than 40 countries and has been in use in Europe since 1983. Acesulfame-K is 200 times sweeter than sucrose. It contributes no calories to the diet because it is not digested by the body, and it does not cause dental caries.

Unlike aspartame, acesulfame-K can be used in baking because it does not lose its sweetness when heated. In the United States, it is currently approved for use in chewing gum, powdered drink mixes, gelatins, puddings, baked goods, tabletop sweeteners, candy, throat lozenges, yogurt, and nondairy creamers; additional uses may soon be approved. One recent trend is to combine it with aspartame in soft drinks.

Tagatose

Tagatose is a slightly altered form of the simple sugar fructose. It is approved for use in ready-to-eat breakfast cereals, diet soft drinks, meal replacement bars, frozen desserts, candy, frosting, and chewing gum. Tagatose is poorly absorbed, so it yields only 1.5 kcal per gram to the body. Use also does not raise the risk for dental caries, nor does it increase blood glucose. Eventual fermentation in the large intestine may even lead to a beneficial effect on that organ (i.e., a prebiotic effect, covered in Chapter 3).

▲ Diet soft drinks are now sweetened with a variety of alternative sweeteners.

CONCEPT CHECK

Table sugar, honey, jam, fruit, and plain baked potatoes contain the highest percentage of calories from carbohydrates. Foods such as cream pies, potato chips, whole milk, and oatmeal contain moderate amounts of carbohydrate. Common nutritive sweeteners added to foods include sucrose, maple sugar, honey, brown sugar, and high-fructose corn syrup. For people who want to limit calories from sugar intake, other sweeteners are available and include the sugar alcohols, saccharin, aspartame, sucralose, neotame, acesulfame-K, and tagatose. Of these, aspartame is the most common alternative sweetener in use.

MAKING CARBOHYDRATES AVAILABLE FOR BODY USE

As discussed in Chapter 3, simply eating a food does not supply nutrients to body cells. Digestion and absorption must occur first.

Digestion

Food preparation can be viewed as the start of carbohydrate digestion because cooking softens tough connective structures in the fibrous parts of plants, such as broccoli stalks. When starches are heated, the starch granules swell as they soak up water, making them much easier to digest. All of these effects of cooking generally make carbohydrate-containing foods easier to chew, swallow, and break down during digestion.

The enzymatic digestion of starch begins in the mouth, when the saliva, which contains an enzyme called salivary **amylase,** mixes with the starchy products during the chewing of the food. This amylase breaks down starch into many smaller units, primarily disaccharides, such as maltose (Fig. 4-8). You can taste this conversion while chewing a saltine cracker. Prolonged chewing of the cracker causes it to taste sweeter as some starch breaks down into the sweeter disaccharides, such as maltose. Still, food

amylase Starch-digesting enzyme from the salivary glands or pancreas.

FIGURE 4-8 ▶ Carbohydrate digestion and absorption. Enzymes made by the mouth, pancreas, and small intestine participate in the process of digestion. Most carbohydrate digestion and absorption takes place in the small intestine. Chapter 3 covered the physiology of digestion and absorption in detail.

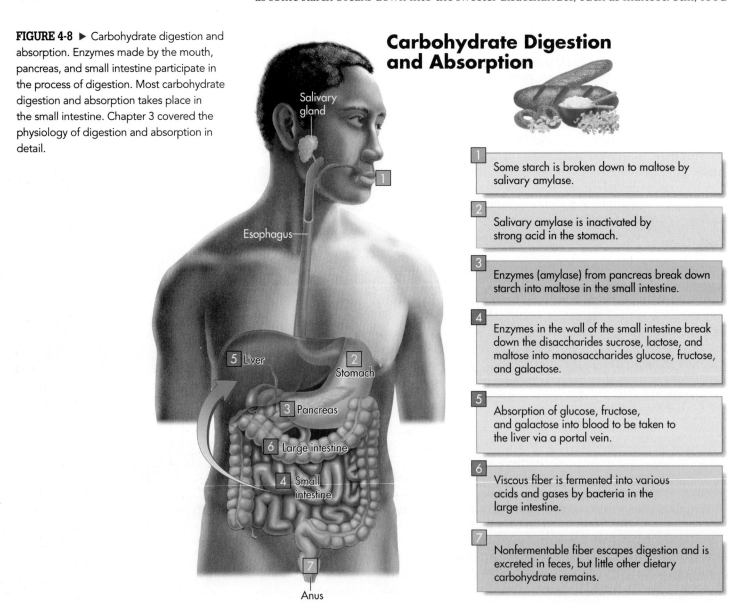

Carbohydrate Digestion and Absorption

1. Some starch is broken down to maltose by salivary amylase.

2. Salivary amylase is inactivated by strong acid in the stomach.

3. Enzymes (amylase) from pancreas break down starch into maltose in the small intestine.

4. Enzymes in the wall of the small intestine break down the disaccharides sucrose, lactose, and maltose into monosaccharides glucose, fructose, and galactose.

5. Absorption of glucose, fructose, and galactose into blood to be taken to the liver via a portal vein.

6. Viscous fiber is fermented into various acids and gases by bacteria in the large intestine.

7. Nonfermentable fiber escapes digestion and is excreted in feces, but little other dietary carbohydrate remains.

is in the mouth for such a short amount of time that this phase of digestion is negligible. In addition, once the food moves down the esophagus and reaches the stomach, the acidic environment inactivates salivary amylase.

When the carbohydrates reach the small intestine, the more alkaline environment of the intestine is better suited for further carbohydrate digestion. The pancreas releases enzymes, such as pancreatic amylase, to aid the last stage of starch digestion. After amylase action, the original carbohydrates in a food are now present in the small intestine as the monosaccharides glucose and fructose, originally present as such in food, and disaccharides (maltose from starch breakdown, lactose mainly from dairy products, and sucrose from food and that added at the table).

The disaccharides are digested to their monosaccharide units once they reach the wall of the small intestine, where the specialized enzymes on the absorptive cells digest each disaccharide into monosaccharides. The enzyme **maltase** acts on maltose to produce two glucose molecules. **Sucrase** acts on sucrose to produce glucose and fructose. **Lactase** acts on lactose to produce glucose and galactose.

Lactose Maldigestion and Lactose Intolerance. **Lactose maldigestion** is a normal pattern of physiology that often begins to develop after early childhood, at about ages 3 to 5 years. It can lead to symptoms of abdominal pain, gas, and diarrhea after consuming lactose, generally when eaten in large amounts. This *primary* form of lactose maldigestion is estimated to be present in about 75% of the world's population, although not all of these individuals experience symptoms. (When significant symptoms develop after lactose intake it is then called **lactose intolerance**.) Another form of the problem, *secondary* lactose maldigestion, is a temporary condition in which lactase production is decreased in response to another condition, such as intestinal diarrhea. The symptoms of lactose intolerance include gas, abdominal bloating, cramps, and diarrhea. The bloating and gas are caused by bacterial fermentation of lactose in the large intestine. The diarrhea is caused by undigested lactose in the large intestine as it draws water from the circulatory system into the large intestine.

In North America, approximately 25% of adults show signs of decreased lactose digestion in the small intestine. Many lactose maldigesters are Asian Americans, African Americans, and Latino/Hispanic Americans, and the occurrence increases as people age. It is hypothesized that approximately 3000 to 5000 years ago, a genetic mutation occurred in regions that relied on milk and dairy foods as a main food source, allowing those individuals (mostly in northern Europe, pastoral tribes in Africa, and the Middle East) to retain the ability to maintain high lactase output for their entire lifetime.

Still, many of these individuals can consume moderate amounts of lactose with minimal or no gastrointestinal discomfort because of eventual lactose breakdown by bacteria in the large intestine. Thus, it is unnecessary for these people to greatly restrict their intake of lactose-containing foods, such as milk and milk products. These calcium-rich food products are important for maintaining bone health. Obtaining enough calcium and vitamin D from the diet is much easier if milk and milk products are included in a diet.

Studies have shown that nearly all individuals with decreased lactase production can tolerate ½ to 1 cup of milk with meals, and that most individuals adapt to intestinal gas production resulting from the fermentation of lactose by bacteria in the large intestine. Combining lactose-containing foods with other foods also helps because certain properties of foods can have positive effects on rates of digestion. For example, fat in a meal slows digestion, leaving more time for lactase action. Hard cheese and yogurt also are more easily tolerated than milk. Much of the lactose is lost in the production of cheese, and the active bacteria cultures in yogurt digest the lactose when these bacteria are broken apart in the small intestine and release their lactase. In addition, an array of products, such as low-lactose milk and lactase pills, are available to assist lactose maldigesters when needed.

Absorption

Monosaccharides found naturally in foods and those formed as by-products of starch and disaccharide digestion in the mouth and small intestine generally follow an active absorption process. Recall from Chapter 3 that this is a process that requires a specific

maltase An enzyme made by absorptive cells of the small intestine; this enzyme digests maltose to two glucoses.

sucrase An enzyme made by absorptive cells of the small intestine; this enzyme digests sucrose to glucose and fructose.

lactase An enzyme made by absorptive cells of the small intestine; this enzyme digests lactose to glucose and galactose.

lactose maldigestion (primary and secondary) Primary lactose maldigestion occurs when production of the enzyme lactase declines for no apparent reason. Secondary lactose maldigestion occurs when a specific cause, such as long-standing diarrhea, results in a decline in lactase production. When significant symptoms develop after lactose intake, it is then called lactose intolerance.

lactose intolerance A condition in which symptoms such as abdominal gas and bloating appear as a result of severe lactose maldigestion.

▲ Use of yogurt helps lactose maldigesters meet calcium needs.

carrier and energy input for the substance to be taken up by the absorptive cells in the small intestine. Glucose and its close relative, galactose, undergo active absorption. They are pumped into the absorptive cells along with sodium.

Fructose is taken up by the absorptive cells via facilitated diffusion. In this case, a carrier is used, but no energy input is needed. This absorptive process is thus slower than that seen with glucose or galactose. So, large doses of fructose are not readily absorbed and can contribute to diarrhea as the monosaccharide remains in the small intestine and attracts water.

Once glucose, galactose, and fructose enter the absorptive cells, some fructose is metabolized into glucose. The single sugars in the absorptive cells are then transferred to the portal vein that goes directly to the liver. The liver then metabolizes those sugars by transforming the monosaccharides galactose and fructose into glucose and:

- Releasing it directly into the bloodstream for transport to organs such as the brain, muscles, kidneys, and adipose tissues
- Producing glycogen for storage of carbohydrate
- Producing fat (minor amount, if any)

Of these three options, producing fat is the least likely, except when carbohydrates are consumed in high amounts and overall calorie needs are exceeded.

Unless an individual has a disease that causes malabsorption, or an intolerance to a carbohydrate such as lactose (or fructose), only a minor amount of some sugars (about 10%) escapes digestion. Any undigested carbohydrate travels to the large intestine and is fermented there by bacteria. The acids and gases produced by bacterial metabolism of the undigested carbohydrate are absorbed into the bloodstream. Scientists suspect that some of these products of bacterial metabolism promote the health of the large intestine by providing it with a source of calories.

MAKING DECISIONS

Fermentable Fiber

Bacteria in the large intestine ferment soluble fibers into such products as acids and gases. The acids, once absorbed, also provide calories for the body. In this way, soluble fibers provide about 1.5 to 2.5 kcal per gram. Although the intestinal gas (flatulence) produced by this bacterial fermentation is not harmful, it can be painful and sometimes embarrassing. Over time, however, the body tends to adapt to a high-fiber intake, eventually producing less gas.

Name some potentially gas-forming foods. Are these foods good sources of soluble fiber?

CONCEPT CHECK

Carbohydrate digestion is the process of breaking down larger carbohydrates into smaller units, and eventually to monosaccharide forms. The enzymatic digestion of starches in the body begins in the mouth with salivary amylase. Enzymes made by the pancreas and small intestine complete the digestion of carbohydrates to single sugars in the small intestine. Lactose maldigestion is a condition that results when cells of the intestine do not make sufficient lactase, the enzyme necessary to digest lactose, resulting in symptoms such as abdominal gas, pain, and diarrhea. Most people with lactose maldigestion can tolerate cheeses and yogurt, as well as moderate amounts of milk. When significant symptoms develop after lactose intake, it is called lactose intolerance. Following primarily an active absorption process, glucose and galactose, (resulting from the digestive process or present in the meal), are taken up by absorptive cells in the intestine. Fructose undergoes facilitated absorption. All of the monosaccharides then enter the portal vein that goes directly to the liver. The liver finally exercises its metabolic options, producing glucose, glycogen, and even fat if carbohydrates are consumed in great excess and overall calorie needs are exceeded.

▲ Beano® is a dietary supplement that contains natural digestive enzymes. Such products can be used to reduce intestinal gas produced by bacterial metabolism of undigested sugars in beans and some vegetables in the large intestine.

PUTTING SIMPLE CARBOHYDRATES TO WORK IN THE BODY

As just discussed, all of the digestible carbohydrate that we eat is eventually converted to glucose. Glucose then is the form of carbohydrate that goes on to function in body metabolism. The other sugars can generally be converted to glucose and the starches are broken down to yield glucose, so the functions described here apply to most carbohydrates. The functions of glucose in the body start with supplying calories to fuel the body.

Yielding Energy

The main function of glucose is to supply calories for use by the body. Certain tissues in the body, such as red blood cells, can use only glucose and other simple carbohydrate forms for fuel. Most parts of the brain and central nervous system also derive energy only from glucose, unless the diet contains almost none. In that case, much of the brain can use partial breakdown products of fat—called **ketone bodies**—for energy needs. Other body cells, including muscle cells, can use simple carbohydrates as fuel but many of these cells can also use fat or protein for energy needs.

Sparing Protein from Use as an Energy Source and Preventing Ketosis

A diet that supplies enough digestible carbohydrates to prevent breakdown of proteins for energy needs is considered *protein sparing*. Under normal circumstances, digestible carbohydrates in the diet mostly end up as blood glucose, and protein is reserved for functions such as building and maintaining muscles and vital organs. However, if you don't eat enough carbohydrates, your body is forced to make glucose from body proteins, draining the pool of amino acids available in cells for other critical functions. During long-term starvation, the continuous withdrawal of proteins from the muscles, heart, liver, kidneys, and other vital organs can result in weakness, poor function, and even failure of body systems.

In addition to the loss of protein, when you don't eat enough carbohydrates, the metabolism of fats is inefficient. In the absence of adequate carbohydrate, fats don't break down completely in metabolism and instead form ketone bodies. This condition, known as **ketosis,** should be avoided because it disturbs the body's normal acid-base balance and leads to other health problems. This is a good reason to question the long-term safety of the low-carbohydrate diets that have been popular.

ketone bodies Partial breakdown products of fat that contain three or four carbons.

ketosis The condition of having a high concentration of ketone bodies and related breakdown products in the bloodstream and tissues.

MAKING DECISIONS

Carbohydrates and Protein Sparing

The wasting of protein that occurs during long-term fasting can be life threatening. This has prompted companies that make formulas for rapid weight loss to include sufficient carbohydrate in the products to decrease protein breakdown and thereby protect vital tissues and organs, including the heart. Most of these very low-calorie products are powders that can be mixed with different types of fluids and are consumed five or six times per day. When considering any weight-loss products, be sure that your total diet provides at least the RDA for carbohydrate.

Regulating Glucose

Under normal circumstances, a person's blood glucose concentration is regulated within a narrow range. Recall from Chapter 3 that when carbohydrates are digested and taken up by the absorptive cells of the small intestine, the resulting monosaccharides are transported directly to the liver. One of the liver's roles, then, is to guard against excess glucose entering the bloodstream after a meal. The liver works in concert with the pancreas to regulate blood glucose.

When the concentration of glucose in the blood is high, such as during and immediately after a meal, the pancreas releases the hormone **insulin** into the bloodstream. Insulin delivers two different messages to various body cells to cause the level of glucose in the blood to fall. First, insulin directs the liver to store the glucose as glycogen. Second, insulin directs muscle, adipose, and other cells to remove glucose from the bloodstream by taking it into those cells. By triggering both glycogen synthesis in the liver and glucose movement out of the bloodstream into certain cells, insulin keeps the concentration of glucose from rising too high in the blood (Fig. 4-9).

On the other hand, when a person has not eaten for a few hours and blood glucose begins to fall, the pancreas releases the hormone **glucagon.** This hormone has the opposite effect of insulin. It prompts the breakdown of liver glycogen into glucose, which is then released into the bloodstream. In this way, glucagon keeps blood glucose from falling too low.

A different mechanism increases blood glucose during times of stress. **Epinephrine** (adrenaline) is the hormone responsible for the "flight or fight" reaction. Epinephrine and a related compound are released in large amounts from the adrenal glands (located on each kidney) and various nerve endings in response to a perceived threat, such as a car approaching head-on. These hormones cause glycogen in the liver to be quickly broken down into glucose. The resulting rapid flood of glucose from the liver into the bloodstream helps promote quick mental and physical reactions.

In essence, the actions of insulin on blood glucose are balanced by the actions of glucagon, epinephrine, and other hormones. If hormonal balance is not maintained, such as during over- or underproduction of insulin or glucagon, major changes in blood glucose concentrations occur. The disease, type 1 diabetes, is an example of the under-production of insulin. To maintain blood glucose within an acceptable range, the body relies on a complex regulatory system. This provides a safeguard against extremely high blood glucose (**hyperglycemia**) or low blood glucose (**hypoglycemia**). The failure of blood glucose regulation will be discussed in the "Nutrition and Your Health" section at the end of this chapter.

insulin A hormone produced by the pancreas. Among other processes, insulin increases the synthesis of glycogen in the liver and the movement of glucose from the bloodstream into body cells.

glucagon A hormone made by the pancreas that stimulates the breakdown of glycogen in the liver into glucose; this ends up increasing blood glucose. Glucagon also performs other functions.

epinephrine A hormone also known as *adrenaline*; it is released by the adrenal glands (located on each kidney) and various nerve endings in the body. It acts to increase glycogen breakdown in the liver, among other functions.

hyperglycemia High blood glucose, above 125 milligrams per 100 milliliters of blood.

hypoglycemia Low blood glucose, below 40 to 50 milligrams per 100 milliliters of blood.

FIGURE 4-9 ▶ Regulation of blood glucose. Insulin and glucagon are key hormones in controlling blood glucose concentration within the normal range of 70 to 99 milligrams per deciliter (mg/dL). Other hormones, such as epinephrine, also contribute to blood glucose regulation. When we eat a meal, insulin is released to promote glucose uptake by cells, thus reversing the increase in blood glucose that results from absorption of various sugars after a meal and in turn restoring the balance. When fasting, blood glucose falls. Glucagon is released to promote glucose release from glycogen stores in the liver. This raises blood glucose, again restoring the balance.

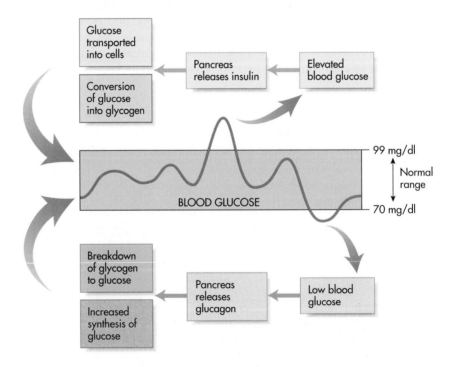

The Glycemic Index and Glycemic Load of Carbohydrate Sources

Our bodies react uniquely to different sources of carbohydrates, such that a serving of a high-fiber food, such as baked beans, results in lower blood glucose levels compared to the same size serving of mashed potatoes. Why are we concerned with the effects of various foods on blood glucose? Foods that result in a high blood glucose elicit a large release of insulin from the pancreas. Chronically high insulin output leads to many deleterious effects on the body: high blood triglycerides, increased fat deposition in the adipose tissue, increased tendency for blood to clot, increased fat synthesis in the liver, and a more rapid return of hunger after a meal (insulin rapidly lowers the macronutrients in the blood as it stimulates their storage, signaling hunger). Over time, this increase in insulin output may cause the muscles to become resistant to the action of insulin, and eventually lead to type 2 diabetes in some people. Two food measurements have been developed that are useful in predicting the blood sugar response to various foods and for planning a diet to avoid hyperglycemia (high blood glucose).

The first of these tools is **glycemic index (GI).** Glycemic index is a ratio of the blood glucose response to a given food compared to a standard (typically, glucose or white bread) (Table 4-4). Glycemic index is influenced by starch structure, fiber content, food processing, physical structure, and other macronutrients in the meal, such as fat. Foods with particularly high glycemic index values are potatoes, especially baking potatoes (due to higher amylopectin content compared to red potatoes), mashed potatoes (due to greater surface area exposed), short grain white rice, honey, and jelly beans. A major shortcoming of glycemic index is that the measurement is based on a serving of food that would provide 50 grams of carbohydrate. As you can imagine, this amount of food may not reflect the amount typically consumed.

Another way of describing how different foods affect blood glucose (and insulin) levels is **glycemic load (GL).** The glycemic load is more useful because it takes into account the glycemic index and the amount of carbohydrate consumed. Glycemic load, therefore, better reflects a food's effect on one's blood glucose than either number alone. To calculate the glycemic load of a food, the amount (in grams) of carbohydrate in a serving of the food is multiplied by the glycemic index of that food, and then divided by 100 (because glycemic index is a percentage). For example, vanilla wafers have a glycemic index of 77, and a small serving contains 15 grams of carbohydrate:

$$(\text{Glycemic Index} \times \text{Grams of Carbohydrate}) \div 100 = \text{Glycemic Load}$$
$$(77 \times 15) \div 100 = 12$$

Even though the glycemic index of vanilla wafers (77) is considered high, the glycemic load calculation shows that the impact of this food on blood glucose levels is fairly low (review Table 4-4).

There are many ways to address this problem of high glycemic load foods. The most important is to not overeat these foods at any one meal. This greatly minimizes their effects on blood glucose and the related increased insulin release. At least once per meal, consider substituting a food that has a low glycemic load for one with a higher value, such as long grain rice or spaghetti for a baked potato. Combining a low glycemic load food, such as an apple, kidney beans, milk, or salad with dressing, with a high glycemic load food also reduces the effect on blood glucose. In addition, maintaining a healthy body weight and performing regular physical activity further reduces the effects of a high glycemic load diet.

Substituting low glycemic load carbohydrates for high glycemic load foods can help in the treatment of diabetes; Chapter 10 discusses the use of foods with different glycemic load values in planning diets for athletes.

 See *Nutrition and Your Health: Diabetes-When Blood Glucose Regulation Fails* at the end of Chapter 4.

▶ The term "net carbs" was popularized a few years ago as a result of the Atkins Diet. This has no legal FDA definition. It is used to describe the content of carbohydrates that increase blood glucose. Fiber and sugar alcohol content are subtracted from total carbohydrate content to yield "net carbs," as these have a negligible effect on blood glucose. Still, sugar alcohols and some fibers do yield calories.

glycemic index (GI) The blood glucose response of a given food, compared to a standard (typically, glucose or white bread). Glycemic index is influenced by starch structure; fiber content; food processing; physical structure; and macronutrients in the meal, such as fat.

glycemic load (GL) The amount of carbohydrate in a serving of food multiplied by the glycemic index of that carbohydrate. The result is then divided by 100.

▲ Carrots, criticized in the popular press for having a high glycemic index (which isn't even true), actually contribute a low glycemic load to a diet.

▲ The glycemic load of breads is due mostly to portion size, not carbohydrate content.

▶ You might wonder why the glycemic index and glycemic load of white bread and whole wheat are similar. This is because whole-wheat flour is typically so finely ground that it is quickly digested. Thus the effect of fiber in slowing digestion and related absorption of glucose is no longer present. Some experts suggest we focus more on minimally processed (e.g., coarsely ground, steel cut, or rolled) grains, such as with whole-wheat flour and oatmeal, to get the full benefits of these fiber sources.

TABLE 4-4 Glycemic Index (GI) and Glycemic Load (GL) of Common Foods

Reference food glucose = 100
Low GI foods—below 55   Low GL foods—below 15
Intermediate GI foods—between 55 and 70   Intermediate GL foods—between 15 and 20
High GI foods—more than 70   High GL foods—more than 20

	Serving Size (grams)	Glycemic Index (GI)	Carbohydrate (grams)	Glycemic Load (GL)
Pastas/Grains				
White, long grain	1 cup	56	45	25
White, short grain	1 cup	72	53	38
Spaghetti	1 cup	41	40	16
Vegetables				
Carrots, boiled	1 cup	49	16	8
Sweet corn	1 cup	55	39	21
Potato, baked	1 cup	85	57	48
Dairy Foods				
Milk, skim	1 cup	32	12	4
Yogurt, low-fat	1 cup	33	17	6
Ice cream	1 cup	61	31	19
Legumes				
Baked beans	1 cup	48	54	26
Kidney beans	1 cup	27	38	10
Navy beans	1 cup	38	54	21
Sugars				
Honey	1 tsp	73	6	4
Sucrose	1 tsp	65	5	3
Fructose	1 tsp	23	5	1
Breads and Muffins				
Bagel	1 small	72	30	22
Whole-wheat bread	1 slice	69	13	9
White bread	1 slice	70	10	7
Fruits				
Apple	1 medium	38	22	8
Banana	1 medium	55	29	16
Orange	1 medium	44	15	7
Beverages				
Orange juice	1 cup	46	26	13
Gatorade	1 cup	78	15	12
Coca-Cola	1 cup	63	26	16
Snack Foods				
Potato chips	1 oz	54	15	8
Vanilla wafers	5 cookies	77	15	12
Jelly beans	1 oz	80	26	21

Source: Foster-Powell K and others: International table of glycemic index and glycemic load. *American Journal of Clinical Nutrition* 76:5, 2002.

CONCEPT CHECK

Carbohydrates provide glucose for the energy needs of red blood cells and parts of the brain and nervous system. Eating too little carbohydrates forces the body to make glucose using primarily amino acids from proteins found in muscles and other vital organs. A low glucose supply in cells also inhibits efficient metabolism of fats. Ketosis can then result.

Blood glucose concentration is maintained within a narrow range. When blood glucose rises after a meal, the hormone insulin is released in great amounts from the pancreas. Insulin acts to lower blood glucose by increasing glucose storage in the liver and glucose uptake by other body cells. If blood glucose falls during fasting, glucagon and other hormones increase the liver's release of glucose into the bloodstream to restore normal blood glucose concentrations. In a similar way, the hormone epinephrine can make more glucose available in response to stress. This balance in hormone activity helps maintain blood glucose within a healthy range.

PUTTING FIBER TO WORK

Fiber supplies mass to the feces, making elimination much easier. This is especially true for insoluble fibers. When enough fiber is consumed, the stool is large and soft because many types of plant fibers attract water. The larger size stimulates the intestinal muscles to contract, which aids elimination. Consequently, less pressure is necessary to expel the stool.

When too little fiber is eaten, the opposite can occur: very little water is present in the feces, making it small and hard. Constipation may result, which forces one to exert excessive pressure in the large intestine during defecation. This high pressure can force parts of the large intestine (colon) wall out from between the surrounding bands of muscle, forming many small pouches called **diverticula** (Fig. 4-10). **Hemorrhoids** may also result from excessive straining during defecation (review Chapter 3).

Diverticula are asymptomatic in about 80% of affected people; that is, they are not noticeable. The asymptomatic form of this disease is called **diverticulosis.** If the diverticula become filled with food particles, such as hulls and seeds, they may eventually become inflamed and painful, a condition known as **diverticulitis.** Surprisingly, intake of fiber then should be reduced to limit further bacterial activity. Once the inflammation subsides, a high-fiber diet is resumed to ease stool elimination and reduce the risk of a future attack.

Aside from its role in maintaining bowel regularity, the consumption of fiber has many additional health benefits. A diet high in fiber likely controls weight and reduces the risk of developing obesity. The bulky nature of high-fiber foods requires more time to chew and fills us up without yielding many calories. Increasing intake of foods rich in fiber is one strategy for feeling satisfied or full after a meal (review the discussion of energy density in Chapter 2). This is still another reason to question the low-carbohydrate diets—where is the whole-grain fiber going to come from?

Over the past 30 years, many population studies have shown a link between increased fiber intake and a decrease in colon cancer development. Most of the research on diet and colon cancer is focusing on the potential preventive effects of fruits, vegetables, whole-grain breads and cereals, and beans (rather than just fiber). Smoking, obesity in men, excessive alcohol use, starch- and sugar-rich foods, and processed meat intake are under study as potential causes of colon cancer. Overall, the health benefits to the colon that stem from a high-fiber diet are partially due to the nutrients that are commonly present in most high-fiber foods, such as vitamins, minerals, phytochemicals, and in some cases essential fatty acids. Thus it is more advisable to increase fiber intake using fiber-rich foods, rather than mostly relying on fiber supplements.

▶ Recall from Chapter 2 that FDA has approved the following claim: "Diets rich in whole-grain foods and other plant foods and low in total fat, saturated fat, and cholesterol may decrease the risk for cardiovascular (heart) disease and certain cancers."

diverticula Pouches that protrude through the exterior wall of the large intestine.

hemorrhoid A pronounced swelling of a large vein, particularly veins found in the anal region.

diverticulosis The condition of having many diverticula in the large intestine.

diverticulitis An inflammation of the diverticula caused by acids produced by bacterial metabolism inside the diverticula.

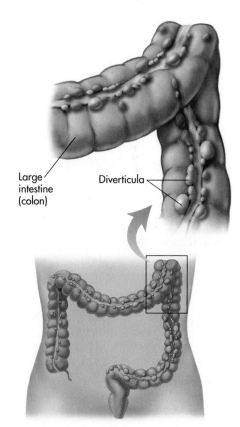

FIGURE 4-10 ▶ Diverticula in the large intestine. A low-fiber diet increases the risk of developing diverticula. About one-third of people over age 45 have diverticulosis, while two-thirds of people over 85 do.

▲ Oatmeal is a rich source of viscous fiber. FDA allows a health claim for the benefits of oatmeal to lower blood cholesterol that arise from the effects of this viscous fiber.

Consuming large amounts of viscous fibers, such as oat fiber, slow glucose absorption from the small intestine, and so contribute to better blood glucose regulation. This effect can be helpful in the treatment of diabetes. In fact, adults whose main carbohydrate source is low-fiber foods are much more likely to develop diabetes than those who have high-fiber diets.

Recall that good sources of viscous fiber are apples, bananas, oranges, carrots, barley, oats, and kidney beans. A high intake of viscous fiber also inhibits absorption of cholesterol and cholesterol-rich bile acids from the small intestine, thereby reducing blood cholesterol and possibly reducing the risk of cardiovascular disease and gallstones. The beneficial bacteria in the large intestine degrade soluble fiber and produce certain fatty acids that probably also reduce cholesterol synthesis in the liver. In addition, the slower glucose absorption that occurs with diets high in viscous fiber is linked to a decrease in insulin release. One of the effects of insulin is to stimulate cholesterol synthesis in the liver, so this reduction in insulin may contribute to the ability of viscous fiber to lower blood cholesterol. Overall, a fiber-rich diet containing fruits, vegetables, beans, and whole-grain breads and cereals (including whole-grain breakfast cereals) is advocated as part of a strategy to reduce cardiovascular disease (coronary heart disease and stroke) risk. And again, this is something that a low-carbohydrate diet can't promise.

CONCEPT CHECK

Fiber forms a vital part of the diet by adding mass to the stool, which eases elimination. Fiber-rich foods also help in weight control and reduce the risk of developing obesity and cardiovascular disease, and possibly colon cancer. Soluble fiber can also be useful for controlling blood glucose in patients with diabetes and in lowering blood cholesterol. Whole-grain breads and cereals, vegetables, beans, and fruits are excellent sources of fiber.

CARBOHYDRATE NEEDS

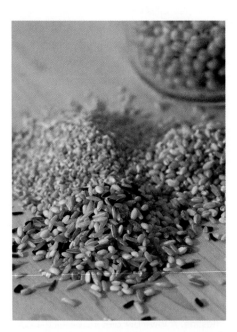

▲ The 2005 Dietary Guidelines define whole grain as the entire grain seed or kernel made of three components: bran, germ, and endosperm.

Currently, recommendations for carbohydrate intake vary widely in the scientific literature and popular press. The RDA for carbohydrates is 130 grams per day for adults. This is based on the amount needed to supply adequate glucose for the brain and nervous system, without having to rely on ketone bodies from incomplete fat breakdown as a calorie source. Somewhat exceeding this amount is fine; the Food and Nutrition Board recommends that carbohydrate intake should range from 45% to 65% of total calorie intake. The Nutrition Facts panel on food labels uses 60% of calorie intake as the standard for recommended carbohydrate intake. This would be 300 grams of carbohydrate when consuming a 2000-calorie diet.

North American adults consume about 180 to 330 grams of carbohydrates per day, which supply about 50% of calorie intake. Worldwide, however, carbohydrates account for about 70% of all calories consumed, and in some countries, up to 80% of the calories consumed. One recommendation on which almost all experts agree is that one's carbohydrate intake should be based primarily on fruits, vegetables, whole-grain breads and cereals, and beans, rather than on refined grains, potatoes, and sugar.

The 2005 Dietary Guidelines for Americans recommend that we choose fiber-rich fruits, vegetables, and whole grains often. More specifically, three or more ounces of grains, roughly one-half of one's grains, should be whole. Remember that the 2005 Dietary Guidelines define whole grain as the entire grain seed or kernel made of three components: the bran, germ, and endosperm, which must be in nearly the same relative proportions as the original grain if cracked, crushed, or flaked.

How Much Fiber Do We Need?

An Adequate Intake for fiber has been set based on the ability of fiber to reduce risk of cardiovascular disease (and likely many cases of diabetes). The Adequate Intake for fiber for adults is 25 grams per day for women and 38 grams per day for men. The goal is to provide at least 14 grams per 1000 kcal in a diet. After age 50, the Adequate Intake falls to 21 grams per day and 30 grams per day, respectively. The Daily Value used for fiber on food and supplement labels is 25 grams for a 2000 kcal diet. In North America, fiber intake averages 13 grams per day for women and 17 grams per day for men and the average whole-grain intake is less than one serving per day. This low intake is attributed to the lack of knowledge on the benefits of whole grains, and the inability to recognize whole-grain products at the time of purchase. Thus, most of us should increase our fiber intake. At least three servings of whole grains per day is recommended. Eating a high-fiber cereal (at least 3 grams of fiber per serving) for breakfast is one easy way to increase fiber intake (Fig. 4-11).

The "Rate Your Plate" exercise shows a diet containing 25 or 38 grams of fiber within moderate calorie intakes. Diets to meet the fiber recommendations are possible and enjoyable if you incorporate plenty of whole-wheat bread, fruits, vegetables, and beans. Use the "Rate Your Plate" exercise to estimate the fiber content of your diet. What is *your* fiber score?

▲ Look for the term "whole-grain" or "whole-wheat" flour on the label for breads that are an excellent source of fiber.

MAKING DECISIONS

Whole Grains

When buying bread, if you see the name "wheat bread" on the label, do you think you are buying a whole-wheat product? Most people do. The flour is from the wheat plant, so manufacturers correctly list enriched white (refined) flour as wheat flour on food labels. However, if the label does not list "whole-wheat flour" first, then the product is not primarily a whole-wheat bread and thus does not contain as much fiber as it could. Careful reading of labels is important in the search for more fiber. Look especially for the term whole grains on the food label to ensure that you are getting a good source of natural fiber.

In the final analysis, keep in mind that any nutrient can lead to health problems when consumed in excess. High carbohydrate, high fiber, and low fat does not mean zero calories. Carbohydrates help moderate calorie intake in comparison with fats, but high-carbohydrate foods also contribute to total calorie intake.

HEALTH CONCERNS RELATED TO CARBOHYDRATE INTAKE

Aside from the health risks related to ketosis, both excessive fiber and sugar intakes can pose health problems. Too much lactose in the diet is also a problem for some people.

Problems with High-Fiber Diets

Very high intakes of fiber—for example, 60 grams per day—can pose some health risks and therefore should be followed only under the guidance of a physician. Increased fluid intake is extremely important with a high-fiber diet. Inadequate fluid intake can leave the stool very hard and painful to eliminate. In more severe cases, the combination of excess fiber and insufficient fluid may contribute to blockages in the intestine, which may require surgery.

Aside from problems with the passage of materials through the GI tract, a high-fiber diet may also decrease the availability of nutrients. Certain components of fiber

▶ The 2005 Dietary Guidelines for Americans provide the following advice regarding carbohydrate intake:

- Choose fiber-rich fruits, vegetables, and whole grains often. (In general, at least half of one's intake of grains [3 ounces or more] should come from whole grains.)

- Choose and prepare foods and beverages with little added sugars or caloric sweeteners, such as in amounts suggested by MyPyramid.

- Reduce the incidence of dental caries by practicing good oral hygiene and consuming sugar- and starch-containing foods and beverages less frequently.

FIGURE 4-11 ▶ Reading the Nutrition Facts on food labels helps us choose more nutritious foods. Based on the information from these nutrition labels, which cereal is the better choice for breakfast? Consider the amount of fiber in each cereal. Did the ingredient lists give you any clues? (Note: Ingredients are always listed in descending order by weight on a label.) When choosing a breakfast cereal, it is generally wise to focus on those that are rich sources of fiber. Sugar content can also be used for evaluation. However, sometimes this number does not reflect added sugar but simply the addition of fruits, such as raisins, complicating the evaluation.

▲ Whole-grain foods, such as granola, are excellent sources of fiber.

Nutrition Facts

Serving Size: 1 cup (55g/2.0 oz.)
Servings Per Container: 10

Amount Per Serving	Cereal	Cereal with ½ Cup Vitamins A & D Skim Milk
Calories	170	210
Calories from Fat	10	10
	% Daily Value**	
Total Fat 1.0g*	**2%**	**2%**
Sat. Fat 0g	**0%**	**0%**
Trans Fat 0g		*
Cholesterol 0mg	**0%**	**0%**
Sodium 300mg	**13%**	**15%**
Potassium 340mg	**10%**	**16%**
Total Carbohydrate 43g	**14%**	**16%**
Dietary Fiber 7g	**28%**	**28%**
Sugars 16g		
Other Carbohydrate 20g		
Protein 4g		
Vitamin A	15%	20%
Vitamin C	20%	22%
Calcium	2%	15%
Iron	65%	65%
Vitamin D	10%	25%
Thiamin	25%	30%
Riboflavin	25%	35%
Niacin	25%	25%
Vitamin B$_6$	25%	25%
Folic acid	30%	30%
Vitamin B$_{12}$	25%	35%
Phosphorus	20%	30%
Magnesium	20%	25%
Zinc	25%	25%
Copper	10%	10%

*Amount in cereal. One half cup skim milk contributes an additional 40 calories, 65mg sodium, 6g total carbohydrate (6g sugars), and 4g protein.
**Percent Daily Values are based on a 2,000 calorie diet. Your daily values may be higher or lower depending on your calorie needs:

		Calories:	2,000	2,500
Total Fat	Less than		65g	80g
Sat Fat	Less than		20g	25g
Cholesterol	Less than		300mg	300mg
Sodium	Less than		2,400mg	2,400mg
Potassium			3,500mg	3,500mg
Total Carbohydrate			300g	375g
Dietary Fiber			25g	30g

Calories per gram:
Fat 9 • Carbohydrate 4 • Protein 4

*Intake of *trans* fat should be as low as possible.

Ingredients: Wheat bran with other parts of wheat, raisins, sugar, corn syrup, salt, malt flavoring, glycerin, iron, niacinamide, zinc oxide, pyridoxine hydrochloride (vitamin B$_6$), riboflavin (vitamin B$_2$), vitamin A palmitate, thiamin hydrochloride (vitamin B$_1$), folic acid, vitamin B$_{12}$, and vitamin D.

Nutrition Facts

Serving Size: ¾ Cup (30g)
Servings Per Package: About 17

Amount Per Serving	Cereal	Cereal With ½ Cup Skim Milk
Calories	170	210
Calories from Fat	0	5
	%Daily Value**	
Total Fat 0g*	**0%**	**1%**
Saturated Fat 0g	**0%**	**1%**
Trans Fat 0g		*
Cholesterol 0mg	**0%**	**1%**
Sodium 60mg	**2%**	**4%**
Potassium 80mg	**2%**	**8%**
Total Carbohydrate 35g	**9%**	**11%**
Dietary Fiber 1g	**4%**	**4%**
Sugars 20g		
Other Carbohydrate 13g		
Protein 3g		
Vitamin A	25%	30%
Vitamin C	0%	2%
Calcium	0%	15%
Iron	10%	10%
Vitamin D	10%	20%
Thiamin	25%	25%
Riboflavin	25%	35%
Niacin	25%	25%
Vitamin B$_6$	25%	25%
Folic acid	25%	25%
Vitamin B$_{12}$	25%	30%
Phosphorus	4%	15%
Magnesium	4%	8%
Zinc	10%	10%
Copper	2%	2%

*Amount in Cereal. One-half cup skim milk contributes an additional 65mg sodium, 6g total carbohydrate (6g sugars), and 4g protein.
**Percent Daily Values are based on a 2,000 calorie diet. Your daily values may be higher or lower depending on your calorie needs:

		Calories:	2,000	2,500
Total Fat	Less than		65g	80g
Sat. Fat	Less than		20g	25g
Cholesterol	Less than		300mg	300mg
Sodium	Less than		2,400mg	2,400mg
Potassium			3,500mg	3,500mg
Total Carbohydrate			300g	375g
Dietary Fiber			25g	30g

Calories per gram:
Fat 9 • Carbohydrate 4 • Protein 4

*Intake of *trans* fat should be as low as possible.

Ingredients: Wheat, Sugar, Corn Syrup, Honey, Caramel Color, Partially Hydrogenated Soybean Oil, Salt, Ferric Phosphate, Niacinamide (Niacin), Zinc Oxide, Vitamin A (Palmitate), Pyridoxine Hydrochloride (Vitamin B6), Riboflavin, Thiamin Mononitrate, Folic Acid (Folate), Vitamin B12 and Vitamin D.

may bind to essential minerals, keeping them from being absorbed. For example, when fiber is consumed in large amounts, zinc and iron absorption may be hindered. In children, a very high fiber intake may reduce overall calorie intake, because fiber can quickly fill a child's small stomach before food intake meets energy needs.

Problems with High-Sugar Diets

The main problems with consuming an excess amount of sugar are that it provides empty calories and increases the risk for dental decay.

Diet Quality Declines When Sugar Intake Is Excessive. Overcrowding the diet with sweet treats can leave little room for important, nutrient-dense foods, such as fruits and vegetables. Children and teenagers are at the highest risk for overconsuming empty calories in place of nutrients essential for growth. Many children and teenagers are drinking an excess of sugared soft drinks and other sugar-containing beverages and much less milk than ever before. This exchange of soft drinks for milk can compromise bone health because milk contains calcium and vitamin D, both essential for bone health.

▶ An excess intake of sugared soft drinks has recently been linked to a risk for both weight gain and type 2 diabetes in adults.

Supersizing sugar-rich beverages is also a growing problem; for example, in the 1950s a typical serving size of a soft drink was a 6½ ounce bottle, and now a 20 ounce plastic bottle is a typical serving. This one change in serving size contributes 170 extra kcal of sugars to the diet. Most convenience stores now offer cups that will hold 64 ounces of soft drinks. Filling up on sugared soft drinks in place of foods is not a healthy practice, but enjoying an occasional soft drink or limiting intake to one 12 ounce serving a day is generally fine. Switching to diet soft drinks would spare the simple sugar calories, but still lacks nutritional value, except for the fluid.

The sugar found in cakes, cookies, and ice cream also supplies many extra calories that promote weight gain, unless an individual is physically active. Today's low-fat and fat-free snack products usually contain lots of added sugar to produce a product with an acceptable taste. The result is to produce a high-calorie food equal to or greater in calorie content than the high-fat food product it was designed to replace.

With regard to sugar intake, an upper limit of 25% of total calorie intake from "added sugars" has been set by the Food and Nutrition Board (sugars added to foods during processing and preparation). Diets that go beyond this upper limit are likely to be deficient in vitamins and minerals. The World Health Organization suggests that added sugars provide no more than 10% of total daily calorie intake.

A moderate intake of about 10% of calorie intake corresponds to a maximum of approximately 50 grams (or 12 tsp) of sugars per day, based on a 2000 kcal diet. Most of the sugars we eat come from foods and beverages to which sugar has been added during processing and/or manufacture. On average, North Americans eat about 82 grams of added sugars daily, amounting to about 16% of calorie intake. Major sources of added sugars include soft drinks; cakes; cookies; fruit punch; and dairy desserts, such as ice cream. Following the recommendation of having no more than 10% of added calories from sugars is easier if sweet desserts such as cakes, cookies, and ice cream (full and reduced fat) are consumed sparingly (Table 4-5).

MAKING DECISIONS

Sugar and Hyperactivity

There is a widespread notion that high sugar intake by children causes hyperactivity, typically part of the syndrome called *attention deficit hyperactivity disorder (ADHD)*. However, most researchers find that sucrose may have the opposite effect. A high-carbohydrate meal, if also low in protein and fat, has a calming effect and induces sleep; this effect may be linked to changes in the synthesis of certain neurotransmitters in the brain, such as serotonin. If there is a problem, it is probably the excitement or tension in situations in which high sugar-rich foods are served, such as at birthday parties and on Halloween.

FIGURE 4-12 ▶ Dental caries. Bacteria can collect in various areas on a tooth. Using simple sugars such as sucrose, bacteria then create acids that can dissolve tooth enamel, leading to caries. If the caries process progresses and enters the pulp cavity, damage to the nerve and resulting pain are likely. The bacteria also produce plaque whereby they adhere to the tooth surface.

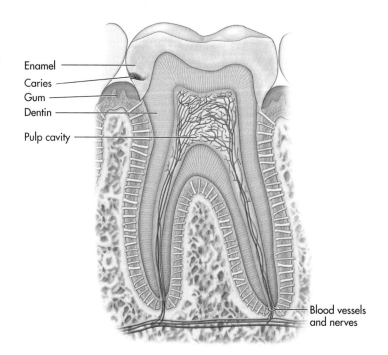

Enamel

Caries

Gum

Dentin

Pulp cavity

Blood vessels and nerves

dental caries Erosions in the surface of a tooth caused by acids made by bacteria as they metabolize sugars.

Dental Caries

Sugars in the diet (and starches readily fermented in the mouth, such as crackers and white bread) also increase the risk of developing **dental caries.** Recall that caries, also known as cavities, are formed when sugars and other carbohydrates are metabolized into acids by bacteria that live in the mouth (Fig. 4-12). These acids dissolve the tooth enamel and underlying structure. Bacteria also use the sugars to make plaque, a sticky substance that both adheres acid-producing bacteria to teeth and diminishes the acid-neutralizing effect of saliva.

The worst offenders in terms of promoting dental caries are sticky and gummy foods high in sugars, such as caramel, because they stick to the teeth and supply the bacteria with a long-lived carbohydrate source. Frequent consumption of liquid sugar sources (e.g., fruit juices) can also cause dental caries. Snacking regularly on sugary foods is also likely to cause caries because it gives the bacteria on the teeth a steady source of carbohydrate from which to continually make acid. Sugared gum chewed between meals is a prime example of a poor dental habit. Still, sugar-containing foods are not the only foods that promote acid production by bacteria in the mouth. As mentioned, if starch-containing foods (e.g., crackers and bread) are held in the mouth for a long time, the starch will be broken down to sugars by enzymes in the mouth; bacteria can then produce acid from these sugars. Overall, the sugar and starch content of a food and its ability to remain in the mouth largely determine its potential to cause caries.

Fluoridated water and toothpaste have contributed to fewer dental caries in North American children over the past 20 years due to fluoride's tooth-strengthening effect (see Chapter 10). Research has also indicated that certain foods—such as cheese, peanuts, and sugar-free chewing gum—can help reduce the amount of acid on teeth. In addition, rinsing the mouth after meals and snacks reduces the acidity in the mouth. Certainly, good nutrition, habits that do not present an overwhelming challenge to oral health (e.g., chewing sugar-free gum), and routine visits to the dentist all contribute to improved dental health.

CRITICAL THINKING

John and Mike are identical twins who like the same games, sports, and foods. However, John likes to chew sugar-free gum and Mike doesn't. At their last dental visit, John had no cavities, but Mike had two. Mike wants to know why John, who chews gum after eating, doesn't have cavities and he does. How would you explain this to him?

TABLE 4-5 Suggestions for Reducing Simple-Sugar Intake

At the Supermarket

- Read ingredient labels. Identify all the added sugars in a product. Select items lower in total sugar when possible.
- Buy fresh fruits or fruits packed in water, juice, or light syrup, rather than those packed in heavy syrup.
- Buy fewer foods high in sugar, such as prepared baked goods, candies, sugared cereals, sweet desserts, soft drinks, and fruit-flavored punches. Substitute vanilla wafers, graham crackers, bagels, English muffins, and diet soft drinks, for example.
- For snacks, buy reduced-fat microwave popcorn to replace candy.

In the Kitchen

- Reduce the sugar in foods prepared at home. Try new low-sugar recipes or adjust your own. Start by reducing the sugar gradually until you've decreased it by one-third or more. Consider using Splenda to substitute for some sugar.
- Experiment with spices such as cinnamon, cardamom, coriander, nutmeg, ginger, and mace to enhance the flavor of foods.
- Use home-prepared items (with less sugar) instead of commercially prepared ones higher in sugar.

At the Table

- Use less of all sugars. This includes white and brown sugars, honey, molasses, syrups, jams, and jellies.
- Choose fewer foods high in sugar, such as prepared baked goods, candies, and sweet desserts.
- Reach for fresh fruit instead of cookies or candy for dessert or between-meal snacks.
- Add less sugar to foods—coffee, tea, cereal, and fruit. Get used to using half as much; then see if you can cut back even more.
- Cut back on the number of sugared soft drinks, punches, and fruit juices you drink. Substitute water, diet soft drinks, and whole fruits rather than fruit juice.

Modified from USDA *Home and Garden Bulletin* No. 232-5, 1986.

▲ Many foods we enjoy are sweet. These should be eaten in moderation.

CONCEPT CHECK

The RDA for carbohydrate is 130 grams per day. The typical North American diet provides 180 to 330 grams per day. A reasonable goal is to have about half of our calorie intake coming from starch and our total carbohydrate intake making up about 60% of our calorie intake, with a range of 45% to 65%. This should allow for the recommended intake of 25 to 38 grams of fiber per day for women and men, respectively. High-fiber diets must be accompanied by adequate fluid intakes to avoid constipation and should be followed only under a physician's guidance.

North Americans eat about 82 grams of sugars added to foods each day. Most of these sugars are added to foods and beverages in processing. To reduce consumption of sugars, one must reduce consumption of items with added sugars, such as some baked goods, sweetened beverages, and presweetened ready-to-eat breakfast cereals. This is one practice that can help reduce the development of dental caries and likely improve diet quality and various aspects of health.

Improper regulation of blood glucose results in either hyperglycemia (high blood glucose) or hypoglycemia (low blood glucose) as noted in this chapter. High blood glucose is most commonly associated with diabetes (technically, *diabetes mellitus*), a disease that affects 6.5% of the North American population. Of these, it is estimated one-third to one-half of these people do not know that they have the disease. Diabetes leads to about 200,000 deaths each year in North America. Diabetes is currently increasing in epidemic proportions in North America. New recommendations promote testing fasting blood glucose in adults over age 45 every 3 years to help diagnose the problem. Diabetes is diagnosed when one's fasting blood glucose is 126 milligrams per 100 milliliters of blood or greater. In contrast, low blood glucose is a much rarer condition.

DIABETES

There are two major forms of diabetes: **type 1** (formerly called insulin-dependent or juvenile-onset diabetes), and **type 2 diabetes** (formerly called non–insulin-dependent or adult-onset diabetes) (Table 4-6). The change in names to type 1 and type 2 diabetes stems from the fact that many type 2 diabetics eventually must also rely on insulin injections as a part of their treatment. In addition, many children today have type 2 diabetes. A third form, called gestational diabetes, occurs in some pregnant women (see Chapter 14). It is usually treated with an insulin regimen and diet and resolves after delivery of the baby. However, women who have gestational diabetes during pregnancy are at high risk for developing type 2 diabetes later in life.

type 1 diabetes A form of diabetes prone to ketosis and that requires insulin therapy.

type 2 diabetes A form of diabetes characterized by insulin resistance and often associated with obesity. Insulin therapy can be used but is often not required.

TABLE 4-6 Comparing and Contrasting Type 1 and Type 2 Diabetes

	Type 1 Diabetes	Type 2 Diabetes
Occurrence	5%–10% of cases of diabetes	90% of cases of diabetes
Cause	Immune system attack of the pancreas	Insulin resistance
Risk Factors	Moderate genetic predisposition	Strong genetic predisposition Obesity Sedentary lifestyle Ethnicity
Characteristics	Distinct symptoms (frequent thirst, hunger, and urination) Ketosis	Mild symptoms, especially in early phases of the disease (fatigue and nighttime urination)
Cell Response to Insulin	Normal	Resistant
Treatment	Diet Exercise Insulin Aspirin Medications to lower blood cholesterol	Diet Exercise Oral medications Insulin (in advanced cases) Aspirin Medications to lower blood cholesterol
Complications*	Cardiovascular disease Kidney disease Nerve damage Blindness	Cardiovascular disease Kidney disease Nerve damage Blindness

*In both cases maintaining a healthy blood lipid profile and normal blood pressure is vital to avoid these complications (see Chapters 5 and 9 for strategies).

Traditional symptoms of diabetes are excessive urination, excessive thirst, and excessive hunger. No one symptom is diagnostic of diabetes, and other symptoms—such as unexplained weight loss, exhaustion, blurred vision, tingling in hands and feet, frequent infections, poor wound healing, and impotence—often accompany traditional symptoms.

TYPE 1 DIABETES

Type 1 diabetes often begins in late childhood, around the age of 8 to 12 years, but can occur at any age. The disease runs in certain families, indicating a clear genetic link. Children usually are admitted to the hospital with abnormally high blood glucose after eating, as well as evidence of ketosis.

The onset of type 1 diabetes is generally associated with decreased release of insulin from the pancreas. As insulin in the blood declines, blood glucose increases, especially after eating. Figure 4-13 shows a typical glucose tolerance curve observed in a patient with this form of diabetes after consuming about 75 grams of glucose. When blood glucose levels are high, the kidneys let excess glucose spill into the urine, resulting in frequent urination of urine high in sugar.

A common clinical method to determine a person's success in controlling blood glucose is to measure glycated (also termed glycosylated) hemoglobin (hemoglobin A1c). Over time, blood glucose attaches to (glycates) hemoglobin in red blood cells and more so when blood glucose remains elevated. A hemoglobin A1c value of over 7% indicates poor blood glucose control. An acceptable value is 6% or less. Maintaining near-normal hemoglobin A1c levels greatly reduces the risk of death and developing other diseases in people with diabetes. Elevated blood glucose also leads to glycation of other proteins and fats in the body, forming what are called advanced glycation endproducts (AGEs). These have been shown to be toxic to cells, especially those of the immune system and kidneys.

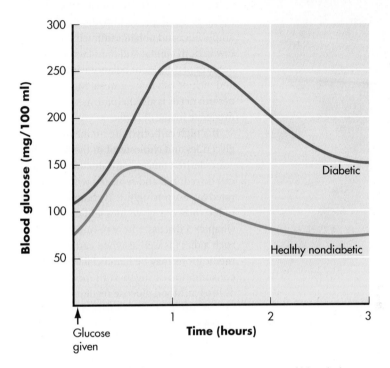

FIGURE 4-13 ▶ Glucose tolerance test. A comparison of blood glucose concentrations in untreated diabetic and healthy (normal) persons after consuming a load of glucose (about 75 grams).

Most cases of type 1 diabetes begin with an immune system disorder, which causes destruction of the insulin-producing cells in the pancreas. Most likely, a virus or protein foreign to the body sets off the destruction. In response to their damage, the affected pancreatic cells release other proteins, which stimulate a more furious attack. Eventually, the pancreas loses its ability to synthesize insulin, and the clinical stage of the disease begins. Consequently, early treatment to stop the immune-linked destruction in children may be important. Research into this area is ongoing.

Type 1 diabetes is treated primarily by insulin therapy, either with injections two to six times per day or with an insulin pump. The pump dispenses insulin at a steady rate into the body, with greater amounts delivered after each meal. Inhaled forms of insulin also are available. Dietary therapy includes three regular meals and one or more snacks (including one at bedtime) and having a regulated ratio of carbohydrate: protein:fat to maximize insulin action and

Symptoms of Diabetes

The symptoms of diabetes may occur suddenly, and include one or more of the following:

- Extreme thirst
- Frequent urination
- Drowsiness, lethargy
- Sudden vision changes
- Increased appetite
- Sudden weight loss
- Sugar in urine
- Fruity, sweet, or winelike odor on breath
- Heavy, labored breathing
- Stupor, unconsciousness

▲ Regularly checking blood glucose is part of diabetes therapy.

minimize swings in blood glucose. If one does not eat often enough, the injected insulin can cause a severe drop in blood glucose or hypoglycemia, because it acts on whatever glucose is available. The diet should be moderate in simple carbohydrates, include ample fiber and polyunsaturated fat, but be low in both animal and *trans* fats, supply an amount of calories in balance with needs, and include fish twice a week. Meeting magnesium needs is also helpful, as well as a moderate intake of coffee.

If a high carbohydrate intake raises triglycerides and cholesterol in the blood beyond desired ranges, carbohydrate intake can be reduced and replaced with unsaturated fat. Surprisingly, this change tends to reduce blood triglycerides and cholesterol. Chapter 5 discusses how to implement such a diet (as well as when certain related medications may be beneficial). Some consumption of sugars with meals is fine, as long as blood glucose regulation is preserved and the sugars replace other carbohydrates in the meal, so that undesirable weight gain does not take place.

The latest evidence suggests that diabetes essentially guarantees development of cardiovascular disease. Because people with diabetes (type 1, as well as type 2) are at a high risk for cardiovascular disease and related heart attacks, they should take an aspirin each day (generally 80 to 160 milligrams per day) if their physicians find no reason not to do so. Blood cholesterol lowering medications also may be prescribed. As discussed in Chapter 5, these practices reduce the risk of heart attack.

The hormone imbalances that occur in people with untreated type 1 diabetes—chiefly, not enough insulin—lead to mobilization of body fat, taken up by liver cells. Ketosis is the result because the fat is partially broken down to ketone bodies. Ketone bodies can rise excessively in the blood, eventually forcing ketone bodies into the urine. These pull sodium and potassium ions and water with them into the urine. This series of events also causes frequent urination and can contribute to a chain reaction that eventually leads to dehydration; ion imbalance; coma; and even death, especially in patients with poorly controlled type 1 diabetes. Treatment includes provision of insulin, fluids, and minerals such as sodium and potassium.

In addition to cardiovascular disease, other degenerative complications that result from poor blood glucose regulation, specifically long-term hyperglycemia, include blindness, kidney disease, and deterioration of nerves. The high blood sugar concentration physically deteriorates small blood vessels (capillaries) and nerves. When improper nerve stimulation occurs in the intestinal tract, intermittent diarrhea and constipation result. Because of nerve deterioration in the extremities, many people with diabetes lose the sensation of pain associated with injuries or infections. They do not have as much pain, so they often delay treatment of hand or foot problems. This delay, combined with a rich environment for bacterial growth (bacteria thrive on glucose) sets the stage for damage and death of tissues in the extremities, sometimes leading to the need for amputation of feet and legs. Current research has shown that the development of blood vessel and nerve complications of diabetes can be slowed with aggressive treatment directed at keeping blood glucose within the normal range. The therapy poses some risks of its own, such as hypoglycemia, so it must be implemented under the close supervision of a physician.

A person with diabetes generally must work closely with a physician and registered dietitian to make the correct alterations in diet and medications and to perform physical activity safely. Physical activity enhances glucose uptake by muscles independent of insulin action, which in turn can lower blood glucose. This outcome is beneficial, but people with type 1 diabetes need to be aware of their blood glucose response to physical activity and compensate appropriately.

TYPE 2 DIABETES

Type 2 diabetes usually begins after age 40. This is the most common type of diabetes, accounting for about 90% of the cases diagnosed in North America. Minority populations such as Latino/Hispanic Americans, African Americans, Asian Americans, Native Americans, and those from Pacific Islands are at particular risk. As noted in the introduction, the overall number of people affected also is on the rise, primarily because of widespread inactivity and obesity in our population. There has been a substantial increase in type 2 diabetes in children, due mostly to an increase in overweight in this population (coupled with limited physical activity). Type 2 diabetes is also genetically linked, so family history is an important risk factor. However, the initial problem is not with the insulin-secreting cells of the pancreas. Instead, type 2 diabetes arises when the insulin receptors on the cell surfaces of certain body tissues, especially muscle tissue, become insulin resistant. In this case, blood glucose is not readily transferred into cells, so the person develops high blood glucose as a result of the glucose remaining in the bloodstream. The pancreas attempts to increase insulin output to compensate, but there is a limit to its ability to do this. Thus, rather than insufficient insulin production, there is an abundance of insulin, particularly during the onset of the disease. As the disease develops, pancreatic function can fail, leading to reduced insulin output. Because of the genetic link for type 2 diabetes, those who have a family history should schedule regular blood glucose tests and be careful to avoid risk factors such as obesity, inactivity, a diet rich in animal and *trans* fats, and simple carbohydrates.

Many cases of type 2 diabetes (about 80%) are associated with obesity (especially with fat located in the abdominal region), but high blood glucose is not directly caused by the obesity. In fact, some lean people also develop this type of diabetes. Obesity associated with oversized adipose cells increases the risk for insulin resistance by the body as more fat is added to these cells during weight gain.

Type 2 diabetes linked to obesity often disappears if the obesity is corrected. Achieving a healthy weight therefore should be a primary goal of treatment, but even limited weight loss can lead to better blood glucose regulation. Although many cases of type 2 diabetes can be relieved by reducing excess adipose tissue stores, many people are not able to lose weight. They remain affected with diabetes and may experience the degenerative complications seen in the type 1 form of the disease. Ketosis, however, is not usually seen in type 2 diabetes. Certain oral medications can also help control blood glucose. Adequate chro-

▲ Regular exercise is a key part of a plan to prevent (and control) type 2 diabetes.

mium intake is also important for blood glucose regulation (see Chapter 11). Patients with type 2 diabetes may experience decreased effectiveness of their treatments over time resulting in spikes in blood glucose after meals and weight gain. New classes of drugs that mimic gut hormones are helping diabetic patients overcome the chronic problems that conventional treatments alone have been unable to control.

Sometimes it may be necessary to provide insulin injections in type 2 diabetes because nothing else is able to control the disease. (This eventually becomes true in about half of all cases of type 2 diabetes.) Regular physical activity also helps the muscles take up more glucose. And regular meal patterns, with an emphasis on control of calorie intake and consumption of mostly fiber-rich carbohydrates, as well as regular fish intake, is important therapy. Nuts help fulfill the goal of increased fiber consumption. (An almost daily intake of nuts was even shown to reduce the risk of developing type 2 diabetes in one study.) Some sugar consumption is fine with meals, but again these must be substituted for other carbohydrates, not simply added to the meal plan. Distributing carbohydrates throughout the day is also important, as this helps minimize the high and low swings in blood glucose concentrations. Moderate alcohol use is acceptable (1 serving per day) and has been shown

► For more information on diabetes, consult the following websites: www.diabetes.org and ndep.nih.gov.

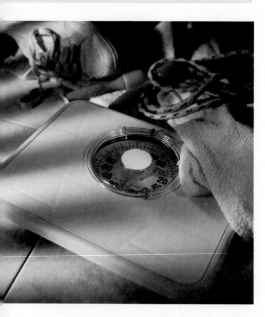

▲ Decreasing body weight and increasing physical activity are interventions to help prevent the metabolic syndrome.

to substantially reduce heart attack risk in people with type 2 diabetes. Still, the person must be warned that alcohol can lead to hypoglycemia and that regular testing for this possibility is necessary. And, as mentioned before, meeting magnesium needs and moderate coffee intake are also helpful.

People with type 2 diabetes who have high blood triglycerides should moderate their carbohydrate intake and increase their intake of unsaturated fat and fiber, as noted earlier for people with type 1 diabetes.

HYPOGLYCEMIA

As noted earlier, people with diabetes who are taking insulin sometimes have hypoglycemia if they don't eat frequently enough. Hypoglycemia can also develop in nondiabetic individuals. The two common forms of nondiabetic hypoglycemia are termed *reactive* and *fasting*.

Reactive hypoglycemia occurs 2 to 4 hours after eating a meal, especially a meal high in simple sugars. It results in irritability, nervousness, headache, sweating, and confusion. The cause of reactive hypoglycemia is unclear, but it may be overproduction of insulin by the pancreas in response to rising blood glucose. In **fasting hypoglycemia,** blood glucose falls to low concentrations after fasting for about 8 hours to 1 day. It usually is caused by pancreatic cancer, which may lead to excessive insulin secretion. This form of hypoglycemia is rare.

The diagnosis of hypoglycemia requires the simultaneous presence of low blood glucose and the typical hypoglycemic symptoms. Blood glucose of 40 to 50 milligrams per 100 milliliters is suggestive, but just having low blood glucose after eating is not enough evidence to make the diagnosis of hypoglycemia. Although many people think they have hypoglycemia, few actually do.

It is normal for healthy people to have some hypoglycemic symptoms, such as irritability, headache, and shakiness, if they have not eaten for a prolonged period. If you sometimes have symptoms of hypoglycemia, you need to eat regular meals, make sure you have some protein and fat in each meal, and eat complex carbohydrates with ample soluble fiber. Avoid meals or snacks

that contain little more than simple carbohydrates. This standard nutrition therapy is one we all could follow. If symptoms continue, try small protein-containing snacks or fruits and juice between meals. Fat, protein, and viscous fiber in the diet tend to moderate swings in blood glucose. Last, moderate caffeine and alcohol intake.

METABOLIC SYNDROME

Metabolic syndrome, also known as Syndrome X, is characterized by the occurrence of several risk factors for diabetes and cardiovascular disease. The precise definition and criteria for diagnosis have recently been debated by health scholars. A person with metabolic syndrome has several or all of the following conditions: abdominal obesity (accumulation of fat around and within the midsection), high blood triglycerides, low HDL or "good" cholesterol, hypertension, high fasting blood glucose, increased blood clotting, and increased inflammation (Fig. 4-14). Each aspect of metabolic syndrome is a unique health problem with its own treatment. In metabolic syndrome, however, these risk factors are clustered together, making a person twice as likely to develop cardiovascular disease and five times more likely to develop diabetes.

It is generally accepted that one key element unifies all the aspects of metabolic syndrome: *insulin resistance.* As you learned in this chapter, insulin is a hormone that directs tissues to pull glucose out of the blood and into cells for storage or fuel. With insulin resistance, the pancreas produces plenty of insulin, but the cells of the body do not respond to it effectively. Instead, excess glucose stays in the bloodstream. For a while the pancreas may be able to compensate for the resistance of cells to insulin by overproducing insulin. Over time, however, the pancreas is unable to keep up the accelerated insulin production and blood glucose levels remain elevated. With metabolic syndrome, blood glucose is not high enough to be classified as diabetes (≥126 milligrams per deciliter), but without intervention, it is likely to get worse and eventually lead to diabetes.

Genetics and aging contribute to the development of insulin resistance and the

Metabolic Syndrome Risk Indicators

- **High blood pressure**
  130/85 mmHg or higher

- **Low HDL cholesterol**
  - Men with HDL level less than 40 mg/dl
  - Women with HDL level less than 50 mg/dL

- **Elevated glucose**
  Fasting level of 100 mg/dL or higher

- **Elevated triglycerides (blood fat)**
  150 mg/dL or higher

- **Abdominal obesity**
  - Men with waist circumference greater than 42 inches
  - Women with waist circumferance greater than 35 inches

Medical Conditions Related to Metabolic Syndrome

1 Type 2 diabetes
Over time, insulin resistance can increase blood glucose levels, which can lead to type 2 diabetes.

2 Coronary artery disease
Elevated blood pressure and cholesterol levels can cause plaque to build up inside coronary arteries, which may eventually lead to a heart attack.

3 Stroke
Plaque build-up in arteries can lead to blood clots that prevent blood flow to the brain, causing damage to brain tissue.

FIGURE 4-14 ▶ For a patient to be diagnosed with metabolic syndrome, he or she must have three of the five risk factors listed above.

other elements of metabolic syndrome, but environmental factors such as diet and activity play an important role. Obesity, particularly abdominal obesity, is highly related to insulin resistance. More than half of adults in the United States are overweight, 30% are obese, and these numbers continue to climb year after year. Increases in body weight among children and adolescents are of great concern because it places them at high risk for these health problems. This increase in body weight

has precipitated a dramatic surge in cardiovascular disease and diabetes risk—an estimated 50 million Americans now have metabolic syndrome.

There is controversy among health professionals, over whether to treat each risk factor uniquely or to attempt to integrate therapies to treat all the risk factors simultaneously. For example, the chief culprits contributing to the high blood triglycerides of metabolic syndrome are excessively large meals full of foods rich in simple sug-

ars and refined starches and low in fiber, coupled with little physical activity. Nutrition and lifestyle changes are key strategies in addressing all of the unhealthy conditions of metabolic syndrome as a whole. Suggested interventions include:

- Decrease body weight. Even small improvements (e.g., 5% weight loss) for overweight and obese individuals can lessen disease risk. The most successful weight loss and weight maintenance programs include moderate dietary restriction combined with physical activity.
- Increase physical activity. To alleviate risks for chronic diseases, the Dietary Guidelines for Americans include a recommendation for at least 30 minutes of moderate-intensity physical activity on most days of the week.
- Choose healthy fats. Limiting intakes of total fat, saturated fat, and *trans* fat are generally recommended for improving blood lipids. Including omega-3 fats, such as those found in fish and nuts, is another way to combat chronic disease.
- For those with particularly high risk for cardiovascular disease, medications may be warranted.

CASE STUDY

Problems with Milk Intake

Myeshia is a 19-year-old African-American female who recently read about the health benefits of calcium and decided to increase her intake of dairy products. To start, she drank a cup of 1% milk at lunch. Not long afterward, she experienced bloating, cramping, and increased gas production. She suspected that the culprit of this pain was the milk she consumed, especially because her parents and her sister complain of the same problem. She wanted to determine if other milk products were, in fact, the cause of her discomfort so the next day she substituted a cup of yogurt for the glass of milk at lunch. Subsequently, she did not have any pain.

Answer the following questions, and check your response in Appendix A.

1. Why did Myeshia believe that she was sensitive to milk?

2. What component of milk is likely causing the problems that Myeshia experiences after drinking milk?

3. Why does this component cause intestinal discomfort in some individuals?

4. What is the name of this condition?

5. What groups of people are most likely to experience this condition?

6. Why did consuming yogurt not cause the same effects for Myeshia?

7. Are there any other products on the market that can replace regular milk or otherwise alleviate symptoms for individuals with this problem?

8. Can people with this condition ever drink regular milk?

9. What nutrients may be inadequate in the diet if dairy products are not consumed?

10. Why do some individuals have trouble tolerating milk products during or immediately after an intestinal viral infection?

SUMMARY

1. The common monosaccharides in food are glucose, fructose, and galactose. Once these are absorbed from the small intestine and delivered to the liver, much of the fructose and galactose is converted to glucose.

2. The major disaccharides are sucrose (glucose + fructose), maltose (glucose + glucose), and lactose (glucose + galactose). When digested, these yield their component monosaccharides.

3. One major group of polysaccharides consists of storage forms of glucose: starches in plants and glycogen in humans. These can be broken down by human digestive enzymes, releasing the glucose units. The main plant starches—straight-chain amylose and branched-chain amylopectin—are digested by enzymes in the mouth and small intestine. In humans, glycogen is synthesized in the liver and muscle tissue from glucose. Under the influence of hormones, liver glycogen is readily broken down to glucose, which can enter the bloodstream.

4. Fiber is composed primarily of the polysaccharides cellulose, hemicellulose, pectin, gum, and mucilage, as well as the noncarbohydrate lignins. These substances are not broken down by human digestive enzymes. However, soluble (also called viscous) fiber is fermented by bacteria in the large intestine.

5. Table sugar, honey, jelly, fruit, and plain baked potatoes are some of the most concentrated sources of carbohydrates. Other high-carbohydrate foods, such as pie and fat-free milk, are diluted by either fat or protein. Nutritive sweeteners in food include sucrose, high-fructose corn syrup, brown sugar, and maple syrup. Several alternative sweeteners are approved for use by FDA: saccharin, aspartame, sucralose, neotame, acesulfame-K, and tagatose.

6. Some starch digestion occurs in the mouth. Carbohydrate digestion is completed in the small intestine. Some plant fibers are digested by the bacteria present in the large intestine; undigested plant fibers become part of the feces. Monosaccharides in the intestinal contents mostly follow an active absorption process. They are then transported via the portal vein that leads directly to the liver.

7. The ability to digest large amounts of lactose often diminishes with age. People in some ethnic groups are especially affected. This condition often develops early in childhood and is referred to as *lactose maldigestion.* Undigested lactose travels to the large intestine, resulting in such symptoms as abdominal gas, pain, and diarrhea. Most people with lactose maldigestion can tolerate cheese, yogurt, and moderate amounts of milk.

8. Carbohydrates provide calories (on average, 4 kcal per gram), protect against wasteful breakdown of food and body protein, and prevent ketosis. The RDA for carbohydrate is 130 grams per day. If carbohydrate intake is inadequate for the body's needs, protein is metabolized to provide glucose for energy needs. However, the price is loss of body protein, ketosis, and eventually a general body weakening. For this reason, low-carbohydrate diets are not recommended for extended periods.

9. Insoluble (also called nonfermentable) fiber provides mass to the feces, thus easing elimination. In high doses, soluble fiber can help control blood glucose in diabetic people and lower blood cholesterol.

10. Diets high in complex carbohydrates are encouraged as a replacement for high-fat diets. A goal of about half of calories as complex carbohydrates is a good one, with about 45% to 65% of total calories com-

ing from carbohydrates in general. Foods to consume are whole-grain cereal products, pasta, legumes, fruits, and vegetables. Many of these foods are rich in fiber.

11. Moderating sugar intake, especially between meals, reduces the risk of dental

caries. Alternative sweeteners, such as aspartame, aid in reducing intake of sugars.

12. Diabetes is characterized by a persistent high blood glucose concentration. A healthy diet and regular physical activ-

ity are helpful in treating both type 1 and type 2 diabetes. Insulin is the main medication employed—it is required in type 1 diabetes and may be used in type 2 diabetes.

STUDY QUESTIONS

1. Outline the basic steps in blood glucose regulation, including the roles of insulin and glucagon.

2. What are the three major monosaccharides and the three major disaccharides? Describe how each plays a part in the human diet.

3. Why are some foods that are high in carbohydrates, such as cookies and fat-

free milk, not considered to be concentrated sources of carbohydrates?

4. Describe the digestion of the various types of carbohydrates in the body.

5. Describe the reason why some people are unable to tolerate high intakes of milk.

6. What are the important roles that fiber plays in the diet?

7. What, if any, are the proven ill effects of sugar in the diet?

8. Why do we need carbohydrates in the diet?

9. Summarize current carbohydrate intake recommendations.

10. List three alternatives to simple sugars for adding sweetness to the diet.

CHECK YOUR KNOWLEDGE

Answers to the following multiple choice questions are in Appendix A.

1. Dietary fiber
   a. raises blood cholesterol levels.
   b. speeds up transit time for food through the digestive tract.
   c. causes diverticulosis.
   d. causes constipation.

2. When the pancreas detects excess glucose, it releases the
   a. enzyme amylase.
   b. monosaccharide glucose.
   c. hormone insulin.
   d. hormone glucagon.

3. Cellulose is a(n)
   a. indigestible fiber.
   b. simple carbohydrate.
   c. energy-yielding nutrient.
   d. animal polysaccharide.

4. Digested white sugar is broken into
   _____ and _____.

   a. glucose, lactose
   b. glucose, fructose
   c. sucrose, maltose
   d. fructose, sucrose

5. Starch is a
   a. complex carbohydrate.
   b. fiber.
   c. simple carbohydrate.
   d. gluten.

6. Fiber content of the diet can be increased by adding
   a. fresh fruits.
   b. fish and poultry.
   c. eggs.
   d. whole grains and cereals.
   e. Both a and d.

7. Which form of diabetes is most common?
   a. type 1
   b. type 2
   c. type 3
   d. gestational

8. The recommended daily intake for fiber is approximately _____ grams.
   a. 5
   b. 30
   c. 100
   d. 450

9. Glucose, galactose, and fructose are
   a. disaccharides.
   b. sugar alcohols.
   c. monosaccharides.
   d. polysaccharides

10. One of the components of metabolic syndrome is
    a. obesity.
    b. diabetes.
    c. low blood sugar.
    d. low blood pressure.

FURTHER READINGS

1. ADA Reports: Position of the American Dietetic Association: Use of nutritive and nonnutritive sweeteners. *Journal of the American Dietetic Association* 104:225, 2004.

   When currently recommended diet practices are met, such as the Dietary Guidelines for Americans, use of some nutritive and nonnutritive

   sweeteners is acceptable. The text of the article explores in detail both classes of sweeteners, in turn supporting this overall conclusion.

2. American Diabetes Association: Nutrition recommendations and interventions for diabetes: A position statement of the American Diabetes Association. *Diabetes Care* 30:548, 2007.

   This article provides a comprehensive look at the treatment of diabetes. Goals for therapy and medical tools to help reach those goals are highlighted.

3. Artificial Sweeteners: No calories…Sweet! *FDA Consumer* 40(4):406, 2006.

   This article is an update on the artificial sweeteners approved by the FDA. To date, five artificial sweeteners are approved by the FDA: aspartame, saccharin, acesulfame-K, neotame, and sucralose. The typical amount of each of these sweeteners used by U.S. consumers is well within designated levels that can be consumed safely every day over a lifetime. The article provides a detailed look at each of the sweeteners.

4. Carey RE: Full speed ahead: Progressing toward better diabetes management. *Today's Dietitian* 8(7):26, 2006.

The understanding of diabetes has increased greatly over the past 10 years. Along with this better understanding have come new products and treatment options. These new products include new insulin analogues, inhaled insulin, and new therapies that mimic other factors that work alongside insulin (glucagonlike peptide 1 and amylin). These therapies are welcome because they provide great promise for increasing numbers of people with diabetes.

5. Cowie CC and others: Prevalence of diabetes and impaired fasting glucose in adults in the U.S. population. *Diabetes Care* 29:1263, 2006.

The results of this study of the National Health And Nutrition Examination Survey (NHANES) suggest that 73 million Americans have diabetes or are at risk based on higher-than-normal blood glucose levels. The prevalence of diagnosed diabetes increased significantly over the last decade, and minority groups remain disproportionately affected. The overall prevalence of total diabetes in 1999–2002 was 9.3% (19.3 million), consisting of 6.5% diagnosed and 2.8% undiagnosed. The prevalence of diagnosed diabetes rose from 5.1% in 1988–1994 to 6.5% in 1999–2002. The prevalence of total diabetes was much greater (21.6%) in older individuals aged ≥65 years. Diagnosed diabetes was twice as prevalent in non-Hispanic blacks and Mexican-Americans compared with non-Hispanic whites.

6. Diverticular disease: The importance of getting enough fiber. *Mayo Clinic Health Letter* 23(2): 1, 2005.

Meeting one's fiber needs is very important for preventing diverticular disease. To do so, eat plenty of fruits, vegetables, and whole grain products. Regular physical activity also helps prevent the problem.

7. Ebbeling CB and others: Effects of decreasing sugar-sweetened beverage consumption on body weight in adolescents: A randomized, controlled pilot study. *Pediatrics* 117:673, 2006.

The consumption of sugar-sweetened drinks by children has increased dramatically over the past 20 years right along with the rise in childhood obesity. A new intervention aimed at limiting consumption of sugary drinks had a beneficial effect on weight loss in teens. The intervention was the home delivery of noncaloric beverages (water and artificially sweetened drinks) to displace sugar-sweetened beverages. The teens were also instructed on how to choose noncaloric drinks outside the home. The intervention decreased con-

sumption of sugary drinks by 82%. The heavier the teen, the greater was the effect on body weight. The authors calculate that a single 12-ounce sugar-sweetened beverage per day results in about 1 pound of weight gain over 3 to 4 weeks.

8. Food and Nutrition Board: *Dietary reference intakes for energy, carbohydrate, fiber, fat, fatty acids, cholesterol, protein, and amino acids.* Washington, DC: National Academy Press, 2002.

This report provides the latest guidance for macronutrient intakes. With regard to carbohydrate, the RDA has been set at 130 grams per day. Carbohydrate intake should range from 45% to 65% of calorie intake. Sugars added to foods should constitute no more than 25% of calorie intake.

9. Grundy SM: Does a diagnosis of metabolic syndrome have a value in clinical practice? *American Journal of Clinical Nutrition* 83:1248, 2006.

The metabolic syndrome concept has led to the development of clinical guidelines by the World Health Organization and the National Cholesterol Education Program. These guidelines have been well accepted by medical professionals. This article reviews the new diagnosis of metabolic syndrome and discusses why organizations including the American Diabetes Association and many diabetes specialists have not embraced the clustering of its risk factors.

10. McMillan-Price J and others: Comparison of 4 diets of varying glycemic load on weight loss and cardiovascular risk reduction in overweight and obese young adults. *Archives of Internal Medicine* 166:1466, 2006.

In this study of 128 overweight or obese young adults, both high-protein and low-glycemic index diets increased body fat loss. Cardiovascular disease risk was decreased best with a high-carbohydrate, low-glycemic index diet.

11. Park Y and others: Dietary fiber intake and risk of colorectal cancer. *Journal of the American Medical Association* 294:2849, 2005.

In this large analysis of pooled data from 13 prospective studies, dietary fiber was inversely associated with risk of colorectal cancer when data were adjusted for age. However, when other dietary risk factors (red meat, total milk, and alcohol intake) were accounted for, high-dietary fiber intake was not associated with a decreased risk of colorectal cancer. The authors conclude that a diet high in dietary fiber from whole plant foods can still be advised because this has been related to lower risks of other chronic conditions, including heart disease and diabetes.

12. Pastors JG: Metabolic syndrome—is obesity the culprit? *Today's Dietitian* 8(3):12, 2006.

Metabolic syndrome, especially its link to obesity, has become better understood in recent years. This article reviews the role of obesity, the dilemmas of diagnosis, new diet and activity guidelines, and the need for a combination of therapeutic approaches for metabolic syndrome.

13. Riddle MC, Drucker DJ: Emerging therapies mimicking the effects of amylin and glucagon-like peptide 1. *Diabetes Care* 29:435, 2006.

Patients with diabetes, especially type 2 diabetes, experience spikes in blood glucose after meals, weight gain, and decreased effectiveness of their treatments over time. New classes of diabetes drugs that mimic gut hormones are helping diabetic patients overcome the chronic problems that conventional treatments alone have been unable to control. Some new drugs are already available and others are under development.

14. Savaiano DA and others: Lactose intolerance symptoms assessed by meta-analysis: A grain of truth that leads to exaggeration. *Journal of Nutrition* 136: 1107, 2006.

An analysis of the results of 21 studies of lactose intolerance revealed that lactose is not a major cause of symptoms for lactose maldigesters after a moderate intake of dairy foods equaling about 1 cup.

15. Swann L: Educate your brain about whole grain. *Today's Dietitian* 8(6):36, 2006.

The 2005 Dietary Guidelines recommend 3 or more ounces of whole-grain products per day. This equals about one-half of one's intake from the grain group. Recent surveys, however, have found that only 5% of American adults eat one-half of their grains as whole grains. This article discusses the need to better educate consumers about whole grain including better definitions and ways of measuring these foods.

16. Sweeteners can sour your health. *Consumer Reports on Health* p. 8, January 2005.

Limiting simple sugars in a diet is important to lessen the risk of developing obesity, diabetes, and dental caries, as well as increasing diet quality. Moderate use of the alternative sweeteners listed in the article helps one meet that goal.

17. The whole grain story. *Tufts University Health & Nutrition Letter* p. 4, July 2005.

Regular whole-grain consumption may help prevent cardiovascular disease, unnecessary weight gain, and the metabolic syndrome. This is easier to do today because many whole-grain products are available.

18. Wang Y and others: Comparison of abdominal adiposity and overall obesity in predicting risk of type 2 diabetes in men. *American Journal of Clinical Nutrition* 81:555, 2005.

Obesity and excess upper body fat stores are both risk factors for developing type 2 diabetes. Avoiding both conditions is important, especially excess upper body fat distribution.

19. Warshaw HS: FAQs about polyols. *Today's Dietitian* p. 37, April 2004.

Polyols (i.e., sugar alcohols) yield from 0.2– 3.0 kcal per gram, so still need to be considered when calculating the calorie content of a diet. A major attribute of these products is that they do not increase the risk for dental caries.

▶ Check out the **Contemporary Nutrition ARIS site**

www.mhhe.com/wardlawcontfa1 for quizzes, flash cards, other activities, and weblinks designed to further help you learn about what you eat and why.

I. Estimate Your Fiber Intake

Review the sample menus shown in Table 4-7. The first menu contains 1600 kcal and 25 grams of fiber (AI for women); the second menu contains 2100 kcal and 38 grams of fiber (AI for men).

TABLE 4-7 Sample of Menus Containing 1600 kcal and 25 grams of Fiber, and 2000 kcal and 38 grams of Fiber*

Menu	25 grams Fiber			38 grams Fiber		
	Serving Size	Carbohydrate Content (grams)	Fiber Content (grams)	Serving Size	Carbohydrate Content (grams)	Fiber Content (grams)
Breakfast						
Orange juice (with pulp)	1 cup	28	0.5	1 cup	28	0.5
Wheaties	¾ cup	17	2	¾ cup	17	2
2% milk	½ cup	6	—	½ cup	6	—
Whole-wheat toast	1 slice	13	2	1 slice	13	2
Margarine	1 tsp	—	—	1 tsp	—	—
Coffee	1 cup	1	—		1	—
Lunch						
Lean ham	2 oz	—	—	2 oz	—	—
Whole-wheat bread	2 slices	26	4	2 slices	26	4
Mayonnaise	2 tsp	2	—	2 tsp	2	—
Lettuce	¼ cup	—	0.2	¼ cup	—	0.2
Cooked white beans	⅓ cup	15	4	1 cup	45	12
Pear (with skin)	½	12	2	1	25	4
1% milk	½ cup	6	—	½ cup	6	—
Snack						
Carrot (as carrot sticks)	1	8	2	1	8	2
Dinner						
Broiled chicken (no skin)	3 oz	—	—	3 oz	—	—
Baked potato (large, with skin)	½	15	1.5	1	30	3
Margarine	1½ tsp	—	—	1½ tsp	—	—
Cooked green beans	1 cup	10	4	1 cup	10	4
Margarine	½ tsp	—	—	½ tsp	—	—
1% milk	1 cup	12	—	1 cup	12	—
Apple (with peel)	½	16	1.8	1	32	3.7
Snack						
Raisin bagel	1	39	1.2	1	39	1.2
Total		226 grams	25 grams		300 grams	38 grams

*The overall diet pattern is based on MyPyramid. Breakdown of approximate calorie content: carbohydrate, 55%; protein, 20%; fat, 25%.

To roughly estimate your daily fiber consumption, determine the number of servings that you ate yesterday from each food category listed here. If you are not meeting your needs, how could you do so? Multiply the serving amount by the value listed and then add up the total amount of fiber.

Food	Servings	Grams
Vegetables		
(serving size: 1 cup raw leafy greens or 1/2 cup other vegetables)	_____ ×2	_____
Fruits		
(serving size: 1 whole fruit; 1/2 grapefruit; 1/2 cup berries or cubed fruit; 1/4 cup dried fruit)	_____ ×2.5	_____
Beans, lentils, split peas		
(serving size: 1/2 cup cooked)	_____ ×7	_____
Nuts, seeds		
(serving size: 1/4 cup; 2 tbsp peanut butter)	_____ ×2.5	_____
Whole grains		
(serving size: 1 slice whole-wheat bread; 1/2 cup whole-wheat pasta, brown rice, or other whole grain; 1/2 each bran or whole-grain muffin)	_____ ×2.5	_____
Refined grains		
(serving size: 1 slice bread, 1/2 cup pasta, rice, or other processed grains; and 1/2 each refined bagels or muffins)	_____ ×1	_____
Breakfast cereals		
(serving size: check package for serving size and amount of fiber per serving)	_____ × grams of fiber per serving	_____
Total Grams of Fiber =		_____

Adapted from Fiber: Strands of protection. *Consumer Reports on Health*, p. 1, August 1999.

How does your total fiber intake for yesterday compare with the general recommendation of 25 to 38 g of fiber per day for women and men, respectively? If you are not meeting your needs, how could you do so?

II. Can You Choose the Sandwich with the Most Fiber?

Assume the sandwiches on this blackboard are available at your local deli and sandwich shop. All of the sandwiches provide about 350 kcal. The fiber content ranges from about 1 gram to about 7.5 grams. Rank the sandwiches from highest amount of fiber to lowest amount; then check your answers at the bottom of the page.

Deli   Specials

Turkey & Swiss on Rye
Served with tomato slices, sliced cucumbers, romaine lettuce, and mustard

Ham & Swiss on Sourdough
Extra-lean ham served with mayonnaise

Tuna Salad on Whole Wheat
Our tuna salad contains tuna, grated carrots, onions, and mayonnaise, and is served with alfalfa sprouts, romaine lettuce, and cucumber slices

Hot Dog
Served on a white bun with relish, mustard, and catsup

Soyburger
Served on a whole-wheat English muffin with tomato and pickle slices, romaine lettuce, and mayonnaise

PB & J
Soft white bread with strawberry jelly and smooth peanut butter

Answer Key:
1. Soyburger: 7.5 grams
2. Tuna Salad on Whole Wheat: 7 grams
3. Turkey & Swiss on Rye: 4 grams
4. PB & J: 3 grams
5. Ham & Swiss on Sourdough: 1.5 grams
6. Hot Dog: 1 gram

159

CHAPTER 5 Lipids

CHAPTER OBJECTIVES Chapter 5 is designed to allow you to:

1. List four classes of lipids (fats) and the role of each in nutritional health.

2. Distinguish between fatty acids and triglycerides.

3. Differentiate among saturated, monounsaturated, and polyunsaturated fatty acids in terms of structure and food sources.

4. Explain how lipids are digested and absorbed.

5. Name the classes of lipoproteins and classify them according to their functions.

6. List the function of lipids, including the two essential fatty acids.

7. Discuss the implications of various fats, including omega-3 fatty acids, with respect to cardiovascular disease.

8. Characterize the symptoms of cardiovascular disease and highlight some known risk factors.

CHAPTER OUTLINE

YOUR BILL FROM A MEDICAL LABORATORY READS "BLOOD LIPID PROFILE— $95." Your doctor informs you that your "triglycerides are too high." A health-food advertisement suggests using Benecol margarine to lower blood cholesterol. Advertisers plug foods "lowest in saturated fat." All of these substances—triglycerides, cholesterol, and saturated fat—are lipids, a collective term referring to fats and oils.

Lipids contain more than twice the calories per gram (on average, 9 kcal) as proteins and carbohydrates (on average, 4 kcal each). Consumption of common saturated fatty acids also contributes to the risk of cardiovascular disease. As the comic in this chapter suggests, for these reasons, some concern about certain lipids is warranted, but lipids also play vital roles both in the body and in foods. Their presence in the diet is essential to good health, and in general, lipids such as those found in vegetable oils should comprise 20% to 35% of an adult's total calorie intake.

Let's look at lipids in detail—their forms, functions, metabolism, and food sources. Chapter 5 will also look at the link between various lipids and the major "killer" disease in North America: cardiovascular disease, which involves the heart, including the coronary arteries (coronary heart disease), as well as other arteries in the body.

Refresh Your Memory

As you begin your study of lipids in Chapter 5, you may want to review:

- Legal definitions for various label descriptors, such as low-fat and fat-free in Chapter 2
- The concept of energy density in Chapter 2
- The processes of digestion and absorption in Chapter 3
- The metabolic syndrome in Chapter 4

LIPIDS: COMMON PROPERTIES

Humans need very little fat in their diet to maintain health. In fact, the body's need for the essential fatty acids can be met by daily consumption of about 2 to 4 tablespoons of plant oil incorporated into foods and consumption of fatty fish such as salmon or tuna at least twice weekly. If fish is not consumed, the essential fatty acids in canola oil, soybean oil, and walnuts contribute much of the same health benefits as those found in fish. Thus, one could follow a purely vegetarian diet containing about 10% of calories from fat and still maintain health. However, as long as saturated fat, cholesterol, and partially-hydrogenated fat (which contains *trans* fat) is minimized, fat intake can safely be higher than that 10% allotment. The Food and Nutrition Board suggests that fat intake can be as high as 35% of calories consumed for an adult. Some experts sug-

FUNKY WINKERBEAN

High fat, low fat, no fat—which is best? And why is there such a debate? Would it be easier just to avoid fat altogether? Doesn't a high-fat diet lead to obesity? To cardiovascular disease? Overall, which are the "best" fats, and why are French fries, doughnuts, stick margarine, and crackers getting such a bad rap? Chapter 5 provides some answers.

gest that an intake as high as 40% of calories is appropriate. After learning more about lipids—fats, oils, and related compounds—in Chapter 5, you can decide for yourself how much fat you want to consume, as well as how to track your daily intake.

Lipids are a diverse group of chemical compounds. They share one main characteristic: They do not readily dissolve in water. Think of an oil and vinegar salad dressing. The oil is not soluble in the water-based vinegar; on standing, the two separate into distinct layers, with oil on top and vinegar on the bottom.

LIPIDS: MAIN TYPES

The chemical structure of lipids is diverse. **Triglycerides** are the most common type of lipid found in the body and in foods. Each triglyceride molecule consists of three fatty acids bonded to **glycerol. Phospholipids** and **sterols**, including **cholesterol,** are also classified as lipids, although their structures can be quite different from the structure of triglycerides. All of these lipid compounds are described in Chapter 5.

Food experts, such as chefs, call lipids that are solid at room temperature *fats,* and lipids that are liquid *oils.* Most people use the word *fat* to refer to all lipids because they don't realize there is a difference. However, *lipid* is a generic term that includes triglycerides and many other substances. To simplify our discussion, Chapter 5 primarily uses the term *fat.* When necessary for clarity, the name of a specific lipid, such as cholesterol, will be used. This word use is consistent with the way many people use these terms.

Fatty Acids: The Simplest Form of Lipids

In the body and in foods, fatty acids are found in the main form of lipids, triglycerides. A fatty acid is basically a long chain of carbons bonded together and flanked by hydrogens. At one end of the molecule (the alpha end), is an acid group. At the other end (the omega end), is a methyl group (Fig. 5-1).

Fats in foods are not composed of a single type of fatty acid. Rather, each dietary fat, or triglyceride, is a complex mixture of many different fatty acids, the combination of which provides each food its unique taste and smell.

Recall from Chapter 1 that fatty acids can be saturated or unsaturated. Chemically speaking, a carbon atom can form four bonds. Within the carbon chain of a fatty acid, the carbons bond to other carbons and to hydrogens. The carbons that make up the chain of a **saturated fatty acid** are all connected to each other by single bonds. This allows for the maximum number of hydrogens to be bound. Just as a sponge can be saturated (full) with water, a saturated fatty acid such as stearic acid is saturated with hydrogen (Fig. 5-1a).

As noted earlier, most fats high in saturated fatty acids, such as animal fats, remain solid at room temperature. A good example is the solid fat surrounding a piece of uncooked steak. Chicken fat, semisolid at room temperature, contains less saturated fat than beef fat. However, in some foods, saturated fats are suspended in liquid, such as the butterfat in whole milk, so the solid nature of these fats at room temperature is less apparent.

If the carbon chain of a fatty acid contains a double bond, those carbons in the chain have fewer bonds to share with hydrogen, and the chain is said to be *unsaturated.* A fatty acid with only one double bond is **monounsaturated** (Fig. 5-1b). Canola and olive oils contain a high percentage of monounsaturated fatty acids. Likewise, if two or more of the bonds between the carbons are double bonds, the fatty acid is even less saturated with hydrogens, and so it is **polyunsaturated** (Fig. 5-1c, d). Corn, soybean, sunflower, and safflower oils are rich in polyunsaturated fatty acids.

Unsaturated fatty acids can exist in two different structural forms, the *cis* and *trans* forms. The form of fatty acids known as *trans* fatty acids was briefly described

acid group

$$-\overset{\displaystyle \overset{O}{\|}}{\underset{\displaystyle |}{C}}-OH$$

methyl group $-CH_3$

FIGURE 5-1 ▶ Chemical forms of saturated, monounsaturated, and polyunsaturated fatty acids. Each of the depicted fatty acids contains 18 carbons, but they differ from each other in the number and location of double bonds. The linear shape of saturated fatty acids, as shown in (a), allows them to pack tightly together and so form a solid at room temperature. In contrast, unsaturated fatty acids have "kinks" where double bonds interrupt the carbon chain (see Figure 5-2). Thus, unsaturated fatty acids pack together only loosely, and are usually liquid at room temperature.

in Chapter 1. In their natural form, monounsaturated and polyunsaturated fatty acids usually are in the *cis* form (Fig. 5-2). By definition, the resulting *cis* **fatty acid** has the hydrogens on the same side of the carbon-carbon double bond. During certain types of food processing (discussed later in this chapter), some hydrogens are transferred to opposite sides of the carbon-carbon double bond, creating the *trans* form, or a *trans* **fatty acid**. As seen in Figure 5-2, the *cis* bond causes the fatty acid backbone to bend, whereas the *trans* bond allows the backbone to remain straighter. This makes it similar to the shape of a saturated fatty acid. The Food and Nutrition Board suggests limiting intake of *trans* fatty acids in processed foods (also referred to as *trans* fats) as much as possible. Later you will see why.

You may be surprised to learn that some *trans* fatty acids, known as conjugated linoleic acid (CLA), occur naturally. CLA is a family of derivatives of the fatty acid linoleic acid. The bacteria that live in the rumens of some animals (cows, sheep, and goats, for example) produce *trans* fatty acids that eventually appear in foods such as beef, milk, and butter. These naturally occurring *trans* fats are currently under study for possible health benefits, including prevention of cancer, decreasing body fat, and improvement in insulin levels in diabetics. About 20% of *trans* fatty acids in our diets come from this source. Dietary supplements of CLA are available but are highly variable in their quality.

Overall, a fat or an oil is classified as saturated, monounsaturated, or polyunsaturated based on the type of fatty acids present in the greatest concentra-

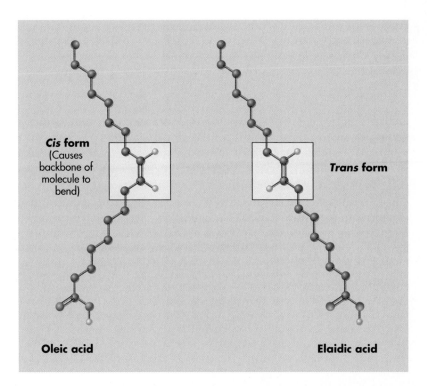

FIGURE 5-2 ▶ *Cis* and *trans* fatty acids. In the *cis* form at carbon-carbon double bonds in a fatty acid, the hydrogens (in blue) lie on the same side of the double bond. This causes a "kink" at that point in the fatty acid, typical of unsaturated fatty acids in nature. In contrast, in the *trans* form at carbon-carbon double bonds in a fatty acid, the hydrogens lie across from each other at the double bond. This causes the fatty acid to exist in a linear form, like a saturated fatty acid. *Cis* fatty acids are much more common in foods than *trans* fatty acids. The latter are primarily found in foods containing partially-hydrogenated fats, notably stick margarine, shortening, and deep-fat fried foods.

cis **fatty acid** A form of an unsaturated fatty acid that has the hydrogens lying on the same side of the carbon-carbon double bond.

trans **fatty acid** A form of an unsaturated fatty acid, usually a monounsaturated one when found in food, in which the hydrogens on both carbons forming the double bond lie on opposite sides of that bond.

long-chain fatty acid A fatty acid that contains 12 or more carbons.

omega-3 (ω-3) fatty acid An unsaturated fatty acid with the first double bond on the third carbon from the methyl end ($-CH_3$).

omega-6 (ω-6) fatty acid An unsaturated fatty acid with the first double bond on the sixth carbon from the methyl end ($-CH_3$).

alpha-linolenic acid An essential omega-3 fatty acid with 18 carbons and three double bonds.

linoleic acid An essential omega-6 fatty acid with 18 carbons and two double bonds.

essential fatty acids Fatty acids that must be supplied by the diet to maintain health. Currently, only linoleic acid and alpha-linolenic acid are classified as essential.

oleic acid An omega-9 fatty acid with 18 carbons and one double bond.

tion (Fig. 5-3). Fats in foods that contain primarily saturated fatty acids are solid at room temperature, especially if the fatty acids have long carbon chains (i.e., a **long-chain fatty acid**), as opposed to shorter versions. In contrast, fats containing primarily polyunsaturated or monounsaturated fatty acids (long chain or shorter) are usually liquid at room temperature. Almost all fatty acids in the body and in foods are long-chain varieties.

An important characteristic of unsaturated fatty acids is the location of the double bonds. If the first double bond starts three carbons from the methyl (omega) end of the fatty acid, it is an **omega-3 (ω-3) fatty acid** (review Fig. 5-1c). If the first double bond is located six carbons from the omega end, it is an **omega-6 (ω-6) fatty acid** (review Fig. 5-1d). Following this scheme, an omega-9 fatty acid has its first double bond starting at the ninth carbon from the methyl end (review Fig. 5-1b). In foods, **alpha-linolenic acid** is the major omega-3 fatty acid; **linoleic acid** is the major omega-6 fatty acid. These are also the **essential fatty acids** we need to consume (more on this in the later section on putting lipids to work in the body). **Oleic acid** is the major omega-9 fatty acid.

Triglycerides

Fats and oils in foods are mostly in the form of triglycerides. The same is true for fats found in body structures. Although some fatty acids are transported in the bloodstream attached to proteins, most fatty acids are formed into triglycerides by cells in the body.

▲ Plant oils vary in their content of specific fatty acids. Oils similar in appearance may vary significantly in fatty acid composition. Olive and canola oils are rich in monounsaturated fat; olive oil has been awarded much attention in recent years. Canola oil, however, is a much less expensive choice of monounsaturated fat. Safflower oil is rich in polyunsaturated fat.

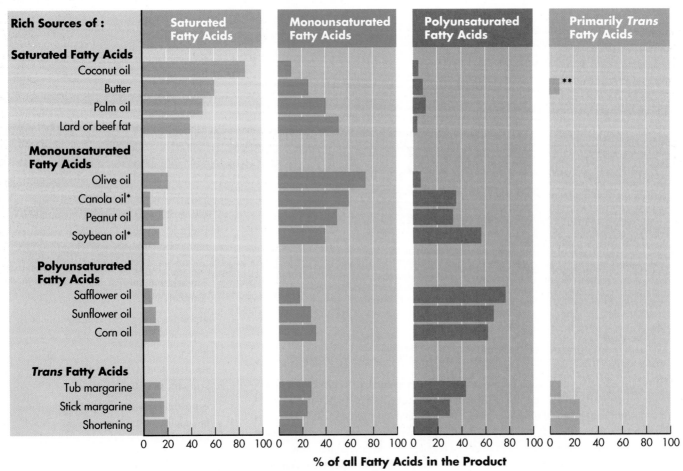

*Rich source of the omega-3 fatty acid alpha-linolenic acid (7% and 12% of total fatty acid for soybean oil and canola oil, respectively).
**The natural *trans* fatty acids in butter are not harmful and may even have health-promoting properties, such as preventing certain forms of cancer.

FIGURE 5-3 ▶ Saturated, monounsaturated, polyunsaturated, and *trans* fatty acid composition of common fats and oils (expressed as % of all fatty acids in the product).

As noted before, triglycerides contain a simple three-carbon alcohol, glycerol, which serves as a backbone for the three attached fatty acids (Fig. 5-4a). Removing one fatty acid from a triglyceride forms a **diglyceride**. Removing two fatty acids from a triglyceride forms a **monoglyceride.** Later you will see that before most dietary fats are absorbed in the small intestine, the two outer fatty acids are typically removed from the triglyceride. This produces a mixture of fatty acids and monoglycerides, absorbed into the intestinal cells. After absorption, the fatty acids and monoglycerides are mostly re-formed into triglycerides.

diglyceride A breakdown product of a triglyceride consisting of two fatty acids bonded to a glycerol backbone.

monoglyceride A breakdown product of a triglyceride consisting of one fatty acid attached to a glycerol backbone.

lecithin A group of compounds that are major components of cell membranes.

Phospholipids

Phospholipids are another class of lipid. Like triglycerides, they are built on a backbone of glycerol. However, at least one fatty acid is replaced with a compound containing phosphorus (and often other elements, such as nitrogen) (Fig. 5-4b). Many types of phospholipids exist in the body, especially in the brain. They form important parts of cell membranes. **Lecithin** is a common example of a phospholipid. Various forms are found in body cells and they participate in fat digestion in the small intes-

FIGURE 5-4 ▶ Chemical forms of common lipids: (a) triglyceride, (b) phospholipid (in this case, lecithin), and (c) sterol (in this case, cholesterol).

tine. The body is able to produce all the phospholipids it needs. Even though lecithin is sold as a dietary supplement and is present as an additive in many foods, phospholipids such as this one are not essential components of the diet.

Sterols

Sterols are the last class of lipids Chapter 5 covers. Their characteristic multi-ringed structure makes them different from the other lipids already discussed (Fig. 5-4c). The most common example of a sterol is cholesterol. This waxy substance doesn't look like a triglyceride—it doesn't have a glycerol backbone or any fatty acids. Still, because it doesn't readily dissolve in water, it is a lipid. Among other functions, cholesterol is used to form certain hormones and bile acids and is incorporated into cell structures. The body can make all the cholesterol it needs.

CONCEPT CHECK

Lipids are a group of compounds that do not dissolve readily in water. Included in this group are fatty acids, triglycerides, phospholipids, and sterols. Fatty acids can be distinguished from one another by the length of the carbon skeleton and the number and position of double bonds along that skeleton. Saturated fatty acids contain no double bonds within their carbon skeleton; that is, they are fully saturated with hydrogens. Monounsaturated fatty acids contain one carbon-carbon double bond, and polyunsaturated fatty acids contain two or more of these bonds. Certain omega-3 and omega-6 fatty acids are essential in the human diet.

Triglycerides are the major form of fat in the body and in foods. These consist of three fatty acids bonded to a glycerol backbone. Phospholipids are similar to triglycerides in structure, but at least one fatty acid is replaced by another compound containing phosphorus. Phospholipids play an important structural role in cell membranes. Sterols, another class of lipids, do not resemble either triglycerides or phospholipids, but instead have a multi-ringed structure. Cholesterol, one example of a sterol, forms parts of cells, some hormones, and bile acids. Whereas certain essential fatty acids (as components of triglycerides) are needed in the diet, the body produces all the triglycerides, phospholipids, and cholesterol it needs. Next we will discuss the sources of fat in foods (Fig. 5-5).

MyPyramid: Sources of Fats

Food Group	Grains	Vegetables	Fruits	Oils	Milk	Meat & Beans
Sources of Fat	• Crackers • Pasta dishes with added fat	• French fried potatoes	• Fruit pies • Avocados	• All	• Whole milk • Some yogurts • Many cheeses • Premium ice cream	• Marbled meat • Bacon • Poultry (skin) • Deep-fat fried meat • Nuts
Grams per Serving	0–18	0–27	0–11	12–14	0–10	7–17

FIGURE 5-5 ▶ Sources of fats from MyPyramid. The height of the background color (none, ⅓, ⅔, or completely covered) within each group in the pyramid indicates the average nutrient density for fat in that group. The fruit group and vegetable groups are generally low in fat. In the other groups, both high-fat and low-fat choices are available. Careful reading of food labels can help you choose lower-fat versions of some foods. In general, any type of frying adds significant amounts of fat to a product, as with French fries and fried chicken. With regard to physical activity, fats are a key fuel in prolonged events, such as long-distance cycling, long-distance running, and prolonged slow to brisk walking.

FATS AND OILS IN FOODS

Lipids in the form of triglycerides are abundant in the North American diet. The foods highest in fat (and therefore energy dense) include salad oils and spreads such as butter, margarine, and mayonnaise. All of these foods contain close to 100% of calories as fat. In reduced-fat margarines, water replaces some of the fat. Whereas regular margarines are 80% fat by weight (11 grams per tablespoon), some reduced-fat margarines are as low as 30% fat by weight (4 grams per table-spoon). When used in recipes, the extra water added to these margarines can cause texture and volume changes in the finished product. Cookbooks can pro-vide guidance for appropriate use of these products by suggesting alterations in recipes to compensate for the increased water content.

Still considering the overall fat content, whole foods highest in fat include nuts, bologna, avocados, and bacon, which have about 80% of calories as fat. Next, pea-nut butter and cheddar cheese have about 75%. Marbled steak and hamburgers (ground chuck) have about 60%, and chocolate bars, ice cream, doughnuts, and whole milk have about 50% of calories as fat. Eggs, pumpkin pie, and cupcakes have 35%, as do lean cuts of meat, such as top round (and ground round) and sirloin. Bread contains about 15%. Finally, foods such as cornflakes, sugar, and fat-free milk have essentially no fat. Careful label reading is necessary to determine the true fat content of food—these are only rough guidelines (Fig. 5-6).

▲ The North American diet contains many high-fat foods—including typical cookie choices. Portion control with these foods is thus important, especially if one is trying to control calorie intake.

Food Sources of Fat

FIGURE 5-6 ▶ Food sources of fat compared to the American Heart Association (AHA) recommendation of 70 grams per day, or 30% of calories from fat for a 2100 kcal diet.

Food Item	Fat (grams)	Calories from Fat %	% AHA Recommendation
AHA Recommendation	70	30%	100%
T-bone steak, 3 ounces	17	66%	24%
Mixed nuts, 1 ounce	16	78%	23%
Canola oil, 1 tablespoon	14	100%	20%
Hamburger with bun, 1 each	12	39%	17%
Margarine, 1 tablespoon	12	100%	17%
Avocado, ½ cup	11	86%	16%
Cheddar cheese, 1 ounce	10	74%	14%
Whole milk, 1 cup	8	49%	11%
Chicken breast with skin, 3 ounces	7	36%	10%
Whole milk yogurt, 8 ounces	7	28%	10%
Snack crackers, 1 ounce	7	45%	10%
Baked beans, ½ cup	7	31%	10%
M&M chocolate candies, 1 ounce	6	39%	9%
Flax seeds, 1 tablespoon	3	62%	4%
Fig Newton cookies, 2 each	3	23%	4%

Key:
- Grains
- Vegetables
- Fruits
- Oil
- Milk
- Meat & Beans
- Discretionary calories

▲ Peanuts are a source of lecithins, as are wheat germ and egg yolks.

emulsifier A compound that can suspend fat in water by isolating individual fat droplets, using a shell of water molecules or other substances to prevent the fat from coalescing.

The type of fat in food is important to consider along with the total amount of fat. Animal fats are the chief contributors of saturated fatty acids to the North American diet. About 40% to 60% of total fat in dairy and meat products is in the form of saturated fatty acids. In contrast, plant oils contain mostly unsaturated fatty acids, ranging from 73% to 94% of total fat. A moderate to high proportion of total fat (49% to 77%) is supplied by monounsaturated fatty acids in canola oil, olive oil, and peanut oil. Some animal fats are also good sources of monounsaturated fatty acids (30% to 47%) (review Fig. 5-3). Corn, cottonseed, sunflower, soybean, and safflower oils contain mostly polyunsaturated fatty acids (54% to 77%). These plant oils supply the majority of the linoleic and alpha-linolenic acid in the North American food supply.

Wheat germ, peanuts, egg yolk, soy beans, and organ meats are rich sources of phospholipids. Phospholipids such as lecithin, a component of egg yolks, are often added to salad dressing. Lecithin is used as an **emulsifier** in these and other products because of its ability to keep mixtures of lipids and water from separating (see Fig. 5-7). Emulsifiers are added to salad dressings to keep the vegetable oil suspended in water. Eggs added to cake batters likewise emulsify the fat with the milk.

Cholesterol is found only in animal foods (Table 5-1). An egg yolk contains about 210 milligrams of cholesterol. Eggs are our main dietary source of cholesterol, along with meats and whole milk. Manufacturers who advertise their brand of peanut butter, vegetable shortening, margarines, and vegetable oils as "cholesterol-free" are taking advantage of uninformed consumers—all of these products are naturally cholesterol-free. Some plants contain other sterols similar to cholesterol, but they do not pose the heart health risks associated with cholesterol. In fact, some plant sterols have blood cholesterol-lowering properties (see the later section on medical interventions to lower blood lipids).

Fat Is Hidden in Some Foods

Some fat discussed so far is obvious: butter on bread, mayonnaise in potato salad, and marbling in raw meat. Fat is harder to detect in other foods that also contribute significant amounts of fat to our diets. Foods that contain hidden fat include whole milk, pastries, cookies, cake, cheese, hot dogs, crackers, French fries, and ice cream.

FIGURE 5-7 ▶ Emulsifiers in action. Emulsifiers prevent many brands of salad dressings and other condiments from separating into layers of water and fat. Emulsifiers attract fatty acids inside and have a water-attracting group on the outside. Add them to salad dressing, shake well, and they hold the oil in the dressing away from the water. Emulsification is important in both food production and fat digestion/absorption.

Emulsifiers and Agitation in Salad Dressing

Oil

Water

Water

Emulsified fat

Oil droplet attracted to fatty acid core

Water attracted to shell

Phospholipid acting as an emulsifier

TABLE 5-1 Cholesterol Content of Selected Foods in Ascending Order

Food	Amount	Cholesterol in Milligrams	Food	Amount	Cholesterol in Milligrams
Skim milk	1 cup	4	Oysters, salmon	3 ounces	40
Mayonnaise	1 tablespoon	10	Clams, halibut, tuna	3 ounces	55
Butter	1 pat	11	Chicken, turkey* (white meat)	3 ounces	70
Lard	1 tablespoon	12	Beef,* pork	3 ounces	75
Cottage cheese	½ cup	15	Lamb, crab	3 ounces	85
Low-fat milk (2%)	1 cup	22	Shrimp, lobster	3 ounces	110
Half-and-half	¼ cup	23	Heart (beef)	3 ounces	165
Hot dog*	1	29	Egg (egg yolk)*†	1	210
Ice cream, ~10% fat	½ cup	30	Liver (beef)	3 ounces	410
Cheese, cheddar	1 ounce	30	Kidney	3 ounces	540
Whole milk	1 cup	34	Brains	3 ounces	2640

*Leading contributors of cholesterol to the North American diet.

†Egg whites are cholesterol-free.

When we try to cut down on fat intake, hidden fats need to be considered, along with the more obvious sources.

A place to begin searching for hidden fat is on the Nutrition Facts labels of foods you buy. Some signals from the ingredient list that can alert you to the presence of fat are animal fats, such as bacon, beef, ham, lamb, pork, chicken, and turkey fats; lard; vegetable oils; nuts; dairy fats, such as butter and cream; egg and egg-yolk solids; and partially-hydrogenated shortening or vegetable oil. Conveniently, the label lists ingredients by order of weight in the product. If fat is one of the first ingredients listed, you are probably looking at a high-fat product. Use food labels to learn more about the fat content of the foods you eat (Fig. 5-8).

FIGURE 5-8 ▶ Reading labels helps locate hidden fat. Who would think that wieners (hot dogs) can contain about 85% of food calories as fat? Looking at the hot dog does not suggest that almost all of its food calories comes from fat, but the label shows otherwise. Let's do the math: 13 grams total fat × 9 kcal per gram of fat = 120 kcal from fat; 120 kcal/140 kcal per link = 0.84 or 84% kcal from fat.

Definitions for Nutrient Claims About Fat and Cholesterol on Food Labels

Fat

- **Fat free:** less than 0.5 g of fat per serving
- **Saturated fat free:** less than 0.5 g per serving, and the level of *trans* fatty acids does not exceed 0.5 g per serving
- **Low fat:** 3 g or less per serving and, if the serving is 30 g or less or 2 tablespoons or less, per 50 g of the food. 2% milk can no longer be labeled low fat, as it exceeds 3 g per serving. *Reduced fat* will be the term used instead.
- **Low saturated fat:** 1 g or less per serving and not more than 15% of kcal from saturated fatty acids
- **Reduced or less fat:** at least 25% less per serving than reference food
- **Reduced or less saturated fat:** at least 25% less per serving than reference food

Cholesterol

- **Cholesterol free:** less than 2 milligrams (mg) of cholesterol and 2 g or less of saturated fat per serving
- **Low cholesterol:** 20 mg or less cholesterol and 2 g or less of saturated fat per serving and, if the serving is 30 g or less or 2 tablespoons or less, per 50 g of the food
- **Reduced or less cholesterol:** at least 25% less cholesterol and 2 g or less of saturated fat per serving than reference food

The definitions for various fat descriptors on food labels, such as "low-fat," "fat-free," and "reduced-fat," were listed in Table 2-9 in Chapter 2 and are reprinted in the margin here. Recall that "low-fat" indicates, in most cases, that a product contains no more than 3 grams of fat per serving. Products marketed as "fat-free" must have less than one-half of a gram of fat per serving. A claim of "reduced-fat" means the product has at least 25% less fat than is usually found in that type of food. When there is no Nutrition Facts label to inspect, controlling portion size is a good way to control fat intake.

When many North Americans think of a low-fat diet, they include reduced-fat versions of pastries, cookies, and cakes. When health professionals refer to a low-fat diet, they often have a different plan in mind: focusing primarily on fruits, vegetables, and whole-grain breads and cereals. Whether to choose a fat-rich food should depend on how much fat you have eaten or will eat during that particular day. So, if you plan to eat high-fat foods at your evening meal, you could reduce your fat intake at a previous meal to balance overall fat intake for the day.

Fat in Food Provides Some Satiety, Flavor, and Texture

Fat in foods has generally been considered to be the most satiating of all the macronutrients. However, studies show that protein and carbohydrate probably lead to the most satiety (gram for gram). High-fat meals do provide satiety, but primarily because one consumes a lot of calories in the process. A high-fat meal is likely to be a high-calorie meal.

Various fats play important roles in foods, so much ingenuity must go into the production of reduced-fat products to preserve flavor and texture. In some cases, "fat-free" also means tasteless. Fat components in foods provide important textures and carry flavors. If you've ever eaten a high-fat yellow cheese or cream cheese, you probably agree that fat melting on the tongue feels good. The fat in reduced-fat and whole milk also gives body, which fat-free milk lacks. The most tender cuts of meat are high in fat, visible as the marbling of meat. In addition, many flavorings dissolve in fat. Heating spices in oil intensifies the flavors of an Indian curry or a Mexican dish, carried to the sensory cells that discriminate taste and smell in the mouth.

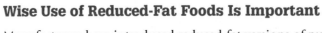

MAKING DECISIONS

Low-Fat Diets

A person who has been following a typical North American diet will probably need some time to adjust to the taste of a lower-fat diet. Emphasizing flavorful fruits, vegetables, and whole grains will help one to adapt to a low-fat diet. Interestingly, after an adjustment period, higher-fat foods may not be as palatable or may lead to gastrointestinal discomfort. For example, after switching from whole to 1% low-fat milk for a few weeks, whole milk begins to taste more like cream than milk. It is certainly possible to make the change from a higher-fat diet to a lower-fat diet. The benefits of weight control and reduced risk for several chronic diseases make the adjustment worth the effort.

Wise Use of Reduced-Fat Foods Is Important

Manufacturers have introduced reduced-fat versions of numerous food products. The fat content of these alternatives ranges from 0% in fat-free Fig Newtons to about 75% of the original fat content in other products. However, the total calorie content of most fat-reduced products is not substantially lower than that of their conventional versions. Generally, when fat is removed from a product, something must be added—commonly, sugars—in its place. It is difficult to reduce both the fat and sugar contents of a product at the same time and maintain flavor and texture. For this reason, many reduced-fat products (e.g., cakes and cookies) are still energy dense. Use the Nutrition Facts label to choose the portion size with the desired calories.

▲ Fat is an important component of the flavor and overall appeal of cheese.

Fat Replacement Strategies for Foods

Five types of fat replacements are available to food manufacturers. Addition of these substances during manufacturing yields products that, to varying degrees, satisfy consumers' desire for reduced-fat products that are still tasty.

Water, Starch Derivatives, and Fibers. The simplest fat replacement is water. The addition of water yields a product, such as diet margarine, with less fat per serving than the normal product. Starch derivatives that bind water to form a gel are a second type of fat replacement. The resulting gel replaces some of the mouth feel lost by the removal of fat. Starch derivatives are made from the hulls or bran of various plants, including oats, peas, soybeans, rice, corn, and wheat. Starch derivatives commonly used by food manufacturers include the fiber cellulose, Maltrin, Stellar, Z-trim, and Oatrim. These substances are used in a variety of foods, including luncheon meats, salad dressings, frozen desserts, table spreads, dips, baked goods, and candies. Most starch derivatives contain some calories, but at least half the amount in fat. These starch derivatives cannot be used in fried foods.

Gum fiber extracted from plants can also be used to replace fat. This thickens a product and replaces some of the body that fat provides. Diet salad dressings and fat-reduced ice cream have gums added for this reason.

Protein-Derived Fat Replacements. Both egg and milk proteins can be used as fat replacements. These proteins are treated to produce microscopic, mistlike protein globules. When these substances replace fat in a food product, they feel like fat in the mouth, although the product does not contain any fatty acids. These proteins are used in milk and other dairy products, baked goods, frostings, salad dressings, and mayonnaise-type products. Such fat replacements yield some calories—but only about 1 to 2 kcal per gram. They have this low-calorie value for two reasons: Proteins contain only 4 kcal per gram, and the products have a high water content.

Engineered Fats and Related Products. The newest form of fat replacement is engineered fat. This type of product is synthesized in the laboratory from various food constituents. Olestra (Olean) is a good example. It is made by chemically bonding fatty acids to sucrose (table sugar). The resulting product cannot be digested by either the human digestive enzymes or bacteria that live in the intestinal tract. Therefore, olestra cannot be absorbed and so provides no calories for the body.

Olestra can replace much of the fat in salad dressing and cakes. It was the first fat replacement that could function like fat in fried foods. Olestra is approved by FDA for use in fried snack foods, such as potato chips.

The major problem associated with the use of olestra is that it binds the fat-soluble vitamins A, D, E, and K, and other fat-soluble phytochemicals such as the carotenoids, thus reducing their absorption. To compensate, food manufacturers add these vitamins to food products containing olestra. Other suspected problems, such as GI tract discomfort, have not been supported by careful research. Thus, warnings about use of olestra and GI tract disturbances, which used to be required on labels for olestra-containing foods, are no longer mandatory.

Food manufacturers are working on other types of engineered fats, which either wholly or partially escape absorption by the body. One example is salatrim, marketed under the name Benefat, which yields only about 5 kcal per gram. It is composed of some saturated fatty acids poorly absorbed by the body. This product has been used in reduced-fat chocolate.

So far, fat replacements have had little impact on our diets, partly because the approved forms either are not very versatile or have not been used extensively by manufacturers. The public has shown little interest in the use of fat replacers, such as olestra. In addition, fat replacements are not practical to use in the foods that contribute the greatest quantity of fat to our diets—beef, cheese, whole and reduced-fat milk, and pastries.

The main benefit of fat replacements will be in helping us cut some fat and calories from our diets. The reduction in overall calorie intake, however, will probably be small because we tend to compensate for the fewer calories per serving by eating more servings.

CRITICAL THINKING

Allison has decided to start eating a low-fat diet. Allison has mentioned to you that all she needs to do is add less butter, oil, or margarine to her foods and she will dramatically lower her fat intake. How can you explain to Allison that she needs to be aware of the hidden fats in her diet as well?

▲ Fat replacements such as gum fiber are typically seen in soft serve ice cream.

▶ Canada has not approved the use of olestra in food products; the United States is the sole country that permits the use of this fat substitute in foods.

CONCEPT CHECK

Fat-dense foods—those with more than 60% of total calories as fat—include plant oils, butter, margarine, mayonnaise, nuts, bacon, avocados, peanut butter, cheddar cheese, steak, and hamburger. Of the foods we typically eat, cholesterol is found naturally only in those of animal origin, with eggs being a primary source. Emulsifiers, such as the phospholipids, lecithins, are added to salad dressings and other fat-rich products to keep the vegetable oils and other fats suspended in the water. Hidden fat exists in foods such as whole milk, pastries, cookies, cake, cheese, hot dogs, crackers, French fries, and ice cream. Fat has a variety of roles in foods, including that of contributing to flavor and texture. Fat also provides the pleasurable mouth feel of many of our favorite foods, intensifies the taste of many spices, and tenderizes many popular cuts of meat. Fat free doesn't mean calorie free; moderation in the use of reduced-fat products is still important.

Fat Rancidity Limits Shelf Life of Foods

Decomposing oils emit a disagreeable odor and taste sour and stale. Stale potato chips are a good example. The double bonds in unsaturated fatty acids break down, producing rancid by-products. Ultraviolet light, oxygen, and certain procedures can break double bonds and, in turn, destroy the structure of polyunsaturated fatty acids. Saturated fats and *trans* fats can much more readily resist these effects because they contain fewer carbon-carbon double bonds.

Rancidity is not a major problem for consumers because the odor and taste generally discourage us from eating enough to become sick. However, rancidity is a problem for manufacturers because it reduces a product's shelf life. To increase shelf life, manufacturers often add partially-hydrogenated plant oils to products. Foods most likely to become rancid are deep-fried foods and foods with a large amount of exposed surface. The fat in fish is also susceptible to rancidity because it is highly polyunsaturated.

Antioxidants such as vitamin E help protect foods against rancidity by guarding against fat breakdown. The vitamin E naturally occuring in plant oils reduces the breakdown of double bonds in fatty acids. When food manufacturers want to prevent rancidity in polyunsaturated fats, they often add the synthetic antioxidants **BHA** and **BHT** or vitamin C to products that contain fat such as salad dressings and cake mixes. Manufacturers also tightly seal products and use other methods to reduce oxygen levels inside packages.

Hydrogenation of Fatty Acids in Food Production Increases *Trans* Fatty Acid Content

As mentioned previously, most fats with long-chain saturated fatty acids are solid at room temperature, and those with unsaturated fatty acids are liquid at room temperature. In some kinds of food production, solid fats work better than liquid oils. In pie crust, for example, solid fats yield a flaky product, whereas crusts made with liquid oils tend to be greasy and more crumbly. If oils with unsaturated fatty acids are used to replace solid fats, they often must be made more saturated (with hydrogen), as this solidifies the vegetable oils into shortenings and margarines. Hydrogen is added by bubbling hydrogen gas under pressure into liquid vegetable oils in a process called **hydrogenation** (Fig. 5-9). The fatty acids aren't fully hydrogenated to the saturated fatty acid form, as this would make the product too hard and brittle. Partial hydrogenation—leaving some monounsaturated fatty acids—creates a semisolid product.

The process of hydrogenation produces *trans* fatty acids as was described earlier in this chapter. Most natural monounsaturated and polyunsaturated fatty acids exist in the *cis* form, causing a bend in the carbon chain, whereas the straighter carbon forms of *trans* fat more closely resemble saturated fatty acids. This may be

BHA, BHT Butylated hydroxyanisole and butylated hydroxytoluene—two common synthetic antioxidants added to foods.

hydrogenation The addition of hydrogen to a carbon-carbon double bond, producing a single carbon-carbon bond with two hydrogens attached to each carbon. Hydrogenation of unsaturated fatty acids in a vegetable oil increases its hardness, so this process is used to convert liquid oils into more solid fats, used in making margarine and shortening. *Trans* fatty acids are a by-product of hydrogenation of vegetable oils.

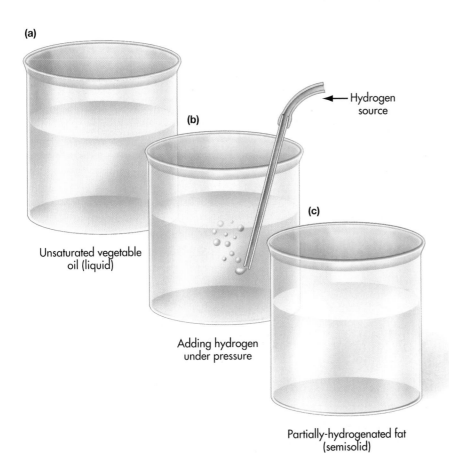

FIGURE 5-9 ▶ How liquid oils become solid fats. (a) Unsaturated fatty acids are present in liquid form. (b) Hydrogens are added (hydrogenation), changing some carbon-carbon double bonds to single bonds and producing some *trans* fatty acids. (c) The partially-hydrogenated product is likely to be used in margarine, shortening, or for deep-fat frying.

the mechanism whereby *trans* fat increases the risk for heart disease. Studies also indicate that *trans* fats increase overall inflammation in the body, which is not healthful. Thus, people should limit intake of partially-hydrogenated fat and thus *trans* fat. This may not be such a concern for the average person, as long as *trans* fat intake is not excessive and the diet is adequate in polyunsaturated fat. However, because *trans* fatty acids serve no particular role in maintaining body health, the latest Dietary Guidelines for Americans, the American Heart Association, and the Food and Nutrition Board each recommend minimal *trans* fat intake.

Not so long ago, public pressure persuaded manufacturers to eliminate the tropical oils rich in saturated fat (palm, palm olein, and coconut) from food processing. Partially-hydrogenated soybean oil—rich in *trans* fat—became the major replacement. Currently, *trans* fat intake in North America is estimated to contribute about 3% to 4% of total calories, amounting to 10 grams per day, on average. Table 5-2 lists typical sources.

FDA is now requiring the *trans* fat content of foods on food labels (review Fig 5-8). The food labels in Canada also must list *trans* fat content. FDA hopes to make consumers more aware of the amounts of *trans* fat in foods as well as the negative health consequences associated with their excessive consumption. North American companies are already responding to this issue by creating products free of *trans* fat. For example, Promise, Smart Beat, and some Fleischmann's margarines are lower in or free of *trans* fat (less than 0.5 grams per serving) compared to typical margarines.

This addition of the *trans* fat listing on labels helps consumers at the supermarket, but when dining out, consumers are "left in the dark" as to which foods contain *trans* fat. Knowing which foods are low in *trans* fat when ordering at a restaurant is difficult because information about preparation methods and precise fat composition is rarely available. To minimize *trans* fat intake, a general guideline is to limit consumption of

▲ Tub margarine is much lower in *trans* fat than stick margarine or shortenings. Some brands of tub margarines are even free of *trans* fatty acids.

TABLE 5-2 Total Fat, Saturated Fat, and *Trans* Fat Content of Typical Sources of *Trans* Fat (in descending order of *trans* fat)

Food Item	Serving Size	Kcal	Fat (grams)	Saturated Fat (grams)	*Trans* Fat (grams)
French fried potatoes (fast-food variety)	Medium size	540	26.9	6.7	7.8
Doughnut	1	330	18.2	4.7	5.0
Cake, pound	1 slice	290	16.4	3.4	4.3
Shortening	1 tbsp	110	13.0	3.4	4.2
Potato chips	Small bag	170	11.2	1.9	3.2
Margarine, stick	1 tbsp	100	11.0	2.1	2.8
Cookies (cream-filled)	3	150	6.1	1.2	1.9
Margarine, tub	1 tbsp	60	6.7	1.2	0.6
Butter	1 tbsp	100	10.8	7.2	0.3
Milk, whole	1 cup	140	6.6	4.3	0.2
Mayonnaise (soybean oil)	1 tbsp	100	10.8	1.6	0

The five major sources of *trans* fat are (in order); cakes, cookies, crackers, pies, and bread; margarine; fried potatoes; potato chips, corn chips, and popcorn; and shortening used in the home.

Source: http://www.cfsan.fda.gov/~dms/qatrans2.html

▲ French fries and other fried foods are a common source of fat and *trans* fatty acids for many adults. For those who choose to consume these products on a regular basis, a small serving size is recommended, especially if a person has elevated blood lipids.

fried (especially deep-fat fried) food items, any pastries or flaky bread products (such as pie crusts, crackers, croissants, and biscuits), and cookies.

Until all foods are labeled with *trans* fat content, consumers can also make educated guesses on the *trans* fat content of foods by examining the list of ingredients on the food label. If partially-hydrogenated vegetable oil is one of the first three ingredients on the label, you can assume there is a significant amount of *trans* fat in the product.

Limiting *trans* fat at home is a much easier task. Most importantly, use little or no stick margarine or shortening. Instead, substitute vegetable oils and softer tub margarines (whose labels list vegetable oil or water as the first ingredient). Avoid deep-fat frying any food in shortening. Substitute baking, panfrying, broiling, steaming, grilling, or deep-fat frying in unhydrogenated vegetable oils. Replace nondairy creamers with reduced-fat or fat-free milk, since most nondairy creamers are rich in partially-hydrogenated vegetable oils. Finally, read the ingredients on food labels, using the previous tips to estimate *trans* fat content.

CONCEPT CHECK

Hydrogenation of unsaturated fatty acids is the process of adding hydrogen to carbon-carbon double bonds to produce single bonds. This results in the creation of some *trans* fatty acids. Hydrogenation changes vegetable oil to solid fat. It is wise to monitor *trans* fat intake, as this form of fat increases the risk for heart disease.

The carbon-carbon double bonds in polyunsaturated fatty acids are easily broken, yielding products responsible for rancidity. The presence of antioxidants, such as vitamin E in oils, naturally protects unsaturated fatty acids against oxidative destruction. Manufacturers can use hydrogenated fats and add natural or synthetic antioxidants to reduce the likelihood of rancidity.

MAKING LIPIDS AVAILABLE FOR BODY USE

It's no secret that fats and oils make foods more appealing. Their presence in foods adds flavor, lubrication, and texture. What happens to lipids once they are eaten? Let's take a closer look at the digestion, absorption, and physiological roles of lipids in the body.

Digestion

In the first phase of fat digestion, the stomach (and salivary glands to some extent) secretes **lipase.** This enzyme acts primarily on triglycerides that have fatty acids with short chain lengths, such as those found in butterfat. The action of salivary and stomach lipase, however, is usually dwarfed by that of the lipase enzyme released from the pancreas and active in the small intestine. Triglycerides and other lipids found in common vegetable oils and meats have longer chain lengths and are generally not digested until they reach the small intestine (Fig. 5-10).

> **lipase** Fat-digesting enzyme produced by the salivary glands, stomach, and pancreas.

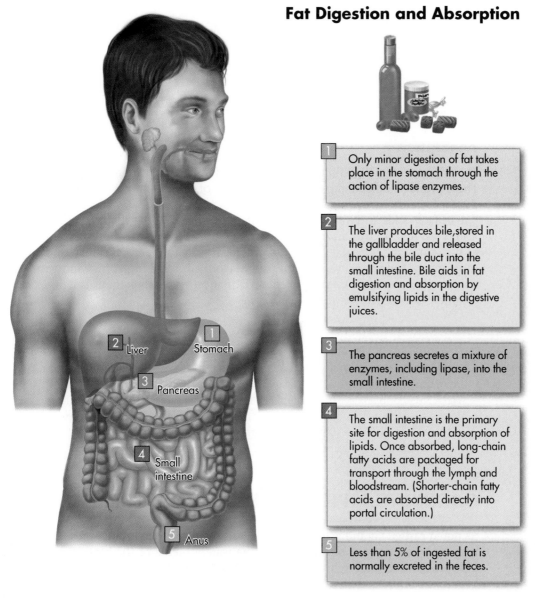

Fat Digestion and Absorption

1. Only minor digestion of fat takes place in the stomach through the action of lipase enzymes.

2. The liver produces bile, stored in the gallbladder and released through the bile duct into the small intestine. Bile aids in fat digestion and absorption by emulsifying lipids in the digestive juices.

3. The pancreas secretes a mixture of enzymes, including lipase, into the small intestine.

4. The small intestine is the primary site for digestion and absorption of lipids. Once absorbed, long-chain fatty acids are packaged for transport through the lymph and bloodstream. (Shorter-chain fatty acids are absorbed directly into portal circulation.)

5. Less than 5% of ingested fat is normally excreted in the feces.

Labels on figure: 2 Liver, 1 Stomach, 3 Pancreas, 4 Small intestine, 5 Anus

FIGURE 5-10 ▶ A summary of fat digestion and absorption. Chapter 3 covered general aspects of this process.

In the small intestine, triglycerides are broken down by lipase into smaller products, namely monoglycerides (glycerol backbones with a single fatty acid attached) and fatty acids. Under the right circumstances, digestion is rapid and thorough. The "right" circumstances include the presence of bile from the gallbladder. Bile acids present in the bile act as emulsifiers on the digestive products of lipase action, suspending the monoglycerides and fatty acids in the watery digestive juices. This emulsification improves digestion and absorption because as large fat globules are broken down into smaller ones, the total surface area for lipase action increases.

With regard to phospholipid digestion, certain enzymes from the pancreas and cells in the wall of the small intestine digest phospholipids. The eventual products are glycerol, fatty acids, and remaining parts. With regard to cholesterol digestion, any cholesterol with a fatty acid attached is broken down to free cholesterol and fatty acids by certain enzymes released from the pancreas.

▶ If the gall bladder is surgically removed (e.g., in cases of gall stone formation), bile will enter the small intestine directly from the liver.

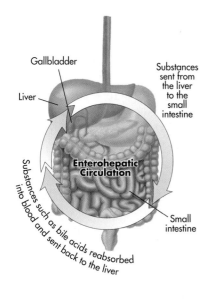

MAKING DECISIONS

Bile Acids

During meals, bile acids circulate in a path that begins in the liver, goes on to the gallbladder, and then moves to the small intestine. After participating in fat digestion, most bile acids are absorbed and end up back at the liver. Approximately 98% of the bile acids are recycled. Only 1% to 2% ends up in the large intestine to be eliminated in the feces. Using medicines that block some of this reabsorption of bile acids is one way to treat high blood cholesterol. The liver takes cholesterol from the bloodstream to form replacement bile acids. Viscous fiber in the diet can also bind to bile acids to produce the same effect (see a later section on medical interventions related to cardiovascular disease for details).

Absorption

The products of fat digestion in the small intestine are fatty acids and monoglycerides. These products diffuse into the absorptive cells of the small intestine. About 95% of dietary fat is absorbed in this way. The chain length of fatty acids affects the ultimate fate of fatty acids and monoglycerides after absorption. If the chain length of a fatty acid is less than 12 carbon atoms, it is water soluble and will therefore probably travel as such through the portal vein that connects directly to the liver. If the fatty acid is a more typical long-chain variety, it must be reformed into a triglyceride in the intestinal absorptive cell and eventually enter circulation via the lymphatic system (review Chapter 3 for an overview of this process).

CONCEPT CHECK

In the small intestine, a lipase enzyme released from the pancreas digests dietary triglycerides into monoglycerides (glycerol backbones with single fatty acids attached) and fatty acids. These breakdown products then diffuse into the absorptive cells of the small intestine. Long-chain fatty acids are transported through the lymphatic system, whereas fatty acids with shorter carbon chains are absorbed directly into the portal vein that connects directly to the liver. Other lipids are prepared for absorption by different enzymes.

CARRYING LIPIDS IN THE BLOODSTREAM

lipoprotein A compound found in the bloodstream containing a core of lipids with a shell composed of protein, phospholipid, and cholesterol.

As noted earlier, fat and water don't mix easily. This incompatibility presents a challenge for the transport of fats through the watery media of the blood and lymph. **Lipoproteins** serve as vehicles for transport of lipids from the small intestine and liver to the body tissues (Table 5-3).

TABLE 5-3 Composition and Roles of the Major Lipoproteins in the Blood

Lipoprotein	Primary Component	Key Role
Chylomicron	Triglyceride	Carries dietary fat from the small intestine to cells
VLDL	Triglyceride	Carries lipids made and taken up by the liver to cells
LDL	Cholesterol	Carries cholesterol made by the liver and from other sources to cells
HDL	Protein	Contributes to cholesterol removal from cells and, in turn, excretion of it from the body

Lipoproteins are classified into four groups—chylomicrons, VLDL, LDL, and HDL–based on their densities. Lipids are less dense than proteins. Therefore, lipoproteins that contain a large percentage of lipids in comparison to protein are less dense than those depleted of lipids.

Dietary Fats Are Carried by Chylomicrons

As you learned in the previous section, digestion of dietary fats results in a mixture of glycerol, monoglycerides, and fatty acids. Once these products are absorbed by the cells of the small intestine, they are reassembled into triglycerides. Then, the intestinal cells package the triglycerides into **chylomicrons,** which enter the lymphatic system and eventually the bloodstream (review Fig. 3-5 in Chapter 3 for a depiction of lymphatic circulation). Chylomicrons contain dietary fat and originate only from the intestinal cells. Like the other lipoproteins described in the next section, chylomicrons are composed of large droplets of lipid surrounded by a thin, water-soluble shell of phospholipids, cholesterol, and protein (Fig. 5-11). The water-soluble shell around a chylomicron allows the lipid to float freely in the water-based blood. Some of the proteins present may also help other cells identify the lipoprotein as a chylomicron.

Once a chylomicron enters the bloodstream, the triglycerides in its core are broken down into fatty acids and glycerol by an enzyme called **lipoprotein lipase,** attached to the inside walls of the blood vessels (Fig. 5-12). As soon as the fatty acids

chylomicron Lipoprotein made of dietary fats surrounded by a shell of cholesterol, phospholipids, and protein. Chylomicrons are formed in the absorptive cells of the small intestine after fat absorption and travel through the lymphatic system to the bloodstream.

lipoprotein lipase An enzyme attached to the cells that form the inner lining of blood vessels; it breaks down triglycerides into free fatty acids and glycerol.

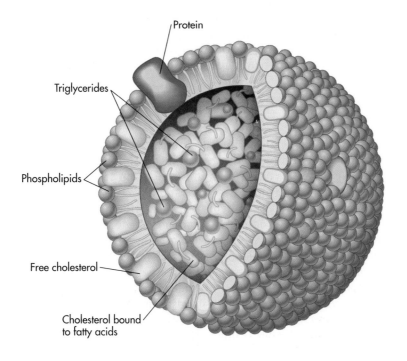

Protein

Triglycerides

Phospholipids

Free cholesterol

Cholesterol bound to fatty acids

FIGURE 5-11 ▶ The structure of a lipoprotein, in this case an LDL. This structure allows fats to circulate in the water-based bloodstream. Various lipoproteins are found in the bloodstream. The primary component of LDL is cholesterol.

Source of Fat	Various fats in a meal	Various lipids collected (or made) by the liver	Cholesterol that arises from dying cells or during lipoprotein metabolism
Lipoprotein Production	Packaged into chylomicrons in the intestine	Packaged into VLDL by the liver	HDL made by the liver and intestine
Lipoprotein Function	The chylomicrons deliver fatty acids to cells.	The VLDL deliver fatty acids to cells	HDL pick up these lipids and transfer them to other lipoproteins or to the liver.
Ultimate LDL Production		LDL arise from the VLDL particle as the fatty acids are removed.	
LDL Function		LDL deliver primarily cholesterol to cells.*	

* Cholesterol not taken up by body cells can be taken up by scavenger cells in the arteries. The eventual cholesterol buildup leads to atherosclerosis.
VLDL: Very-Low-Density Lipoprotein   LDL: Low-Density Lipoproteinn   HDL: High-Density Lipoprotein

FIGURE 5-12 ▶ Lipoprotein production and function. Chylomicrons carry absorbed fat to body cells. VLDL carries fat taken up from the bloodstream by the liver, as well as any fat made by the liver, to body cells. LDL arises from VLDL and carries mostly cholesterol to cells. HDL arises mostly from the liver and intestine. HDL carries cholesterol from cells to other lipoproteins and to the liver for excretion.

are released to the bloodstream, they are absorbed by cells in the vicinity, while much of the glycerol circulates back to the liver. Muscle cells can immediately use the absorbed fatty acids for fuel. Adipose cells, on the other hand, tend to re-form the fatty acids into triglycerides for storage. After triglycerides have been removed, a chylomicron remnant remains. Chylomicron remnants are removed from circulation by the liver and their components are recycled to make other lipoproteins and bile acids.

Other Lipoproteins Transport Lipids from the Liver to the Body Cells

The liver takes up various lipids from the blood. The liver also is the manufacturing site for lipids and cholesterol. The raw materials for lipid and cholesterol synthesis include free fatty acids taken up from the bloodstream, as well as carbon and hydrogen derived from carbohydrates, protein, and alcohol. The liver then must package these synthesized lipids as lipoproteins for transport in the blood to body tissues.

First in our discussion of lipoproteins made by the liver are **very-low-density lipoproteins (VLDL).** These particles are composed of cholesterol and triglycerides surrounded by a water-soluble shell. VLDLs are rich in triglycerides and thus are very low in density. Once in the bloodstream, lipoprotein lipase on the inner surface of the blood vessels breaks down the triglyceride in the VLDL into fatty acids and glycerol. Fatty acids and glycerol are released into the bloodstream and taken up by the body cells.

As its triglycerides are released, the VLDL becomes proportionately denser. Much of what eventually remains of the VLDL fraction is then called **low-density lipoprotein**

very-low-density lipoprotein (VLDL) The lipoprotein created in the liver that carries cholesterol and lipids that have been taken up or newly synthesized by the liver.

low-density lipoprotein (LDL) The lipoprotein in the blood containing primarily cholesterol; elevated LDL is strongly linked to cardiovascular disease risk.

(LDL); this is composed primarily of the remaining cholesterol. The primary function of LDL is to transport cholesterol to tissues. LDL particles are taken up from the bloodstream by specific receptors on cells, especially liver cells, and are then broken down. The cholesterol and protein components of LDL provide some of the building blocks necessary for cell growth and development, such as synthesis of cell membranes and hormones.

The final group of lipoproteins, **high-density lipoproteins (HDL),** is a critical and beneficial participant in this process of lipid transport. Its high proportion of protein makes it the densest lipoprotein. The liver and intestine produce most of the HDL in the blood. It roams the bloodstream, picking up cholesterol from dying cells and other sources. HDL donates the cholesterol primarily to other lipoproteins for transport back to the liver to be excreted. Some HDL travels directly back to the liver.

"Good" and "Bad" Cholesterol in the Bloodstream

HDL and LDL are often described as "good" and "bad" cholesterol, respectively. Many studies demonstrate that the amount of HDL in the bloodstream can closely predict the risk for cardiovascular disease. Risk increases with low HDL because little cholesterol is transported back to the liver and excreted. Women tend to have high amounts of HDL, especially before **menopause,** compared to men. High amounts of HDL slow the development of cardiovascular disease, so any cholesterol carried by HDL can be considered "good" cholesterol.

On the other hand, LDL is sometimes considered "bad" cholesterol. In our discussion of LDL, you learned that LDL is taken up by receptors on various cells. If LDL is not readily cleared from the bloodstream, **scavenger cells** in the arteries take up the lipoprotein, leading to a buildup of cholesterol in the blood vessels. This buildup, known as **atherosclerosis,** greatly increases the risk for cardiovascular disease (see the following "Nutrition and Your Health" section). LDL is only a problem when it is too high in the bloodstream because low amounts are needed as part of routine body functions.

MAKING DECISIONS

LDL Cholesterol

The cholesterol in foods is not designated as "good" or "bad." It is only after cholesterol has been made or processed by the liver that it shows up in the bloodstream as LDL or HDL. Dietary patterns can affect the metabolism of cholesterol, however. Diets low in saturated fat, *trans* fat, and cholesterol encourage the uptake of LDL by the liver, thereby removing LDL from the bloodstream and decreasing the ability of scavenger cells to form atherosclerotic plaques in the blood vessels. Likewise, diets high in saturated fat, *trans* fat, and cholesterol reduce the uptake of LDL by the liver, increasing cholesterol in the blood and the risk for cardiovascular disease. What foods in your diet are high in saturated fat, *trans* fat, or cholesterol?

CONCEPT CHECK

Lipids generally move through the bloodstream as part of lipoproteins. Dietary fats absorbed from the small intestine are packaged and transported as chylomicrons, whereas lipids synthesized in the liver are packaged as very-low-density lipoproteins (VLDL). Lipoprotein lipase removes triglycerides from the interiors of both chylomicrons and VLDL, breaking the triglycerides down into glycerol and fatty acids, which are taken up by tissues for energy needs or storage. What remains after the action of lipoprotein lipase are chylomicron remnants (from chylomicrons), the components of which are recycled by the liver, or low-density lipoproteins (LDL, from VLDL), rich in cholesterol. LDL is picked up by receptors on body cells, especially liver cells. Scavenger cells in the arteries may do the same, speeding the development of atherosclerosis. High-density lipoprotein (HDL), also produced in part by the liver, picks up cholesterol from cells and transports it primarily to other lipoproteins for eventual transport back to the liver. Risk factors for cardiovascular disease include an elevated level of LDL and/or low amounts of HDL in the blood.

---

high-density lipoprotein (HDL) The lipoprotein in the blood that picks up cholesterol from dying cells and other sources and transfers it to the other lipoproteins in the bloodstream, as well as directly to the liver; low HDL increases the risk for cardiovascular disease.

menopause The cessation of the menstrual cycle in women, usually beginning at about 50 years of age.

scavenger cells Specific form of white blood cells that can bury themselves in the artery wall and accumulate LDL. As these cells take up LDL, they contribute to the development of atherosclerosis.

atherosclerosis A buildup of fatty material (plaque) in the arteries, including those surrounding the heart.

 See *Nutrition and Your Health: Lipids and Cardiovascular Disease* at the end of Chapter 5.

▶ It appears that saturated fatty acids promote an increase in the amount of free cholesterol (not attached to fatty acids) in the liver, whereas unsaturated fatty acids do the opposite. As free cholesterol in the liver increases, it causes the liver to reduce cholesterol uptake from the bloodstream, contributing to elevated LDL in the blood. (*Trans* fatty acids are thought to act in the same ways as saturated fatty acids.)

Omega-3 Fatty Acids in Fish (grams per 3 ounce serving)	
Atlantic salmon	1.8
Anchovy	1.7
Sardines	1.4
Rainbow trout	1.0
Coho salmon	0.9
Bluefish	0.8
Striped bass	0.8
Tuna, white, canned	0.7
Halibut	0.4
Catfish, channel	0.2

Recommended omega-3 fatty acid (alpha-linolenic acid) intake per day:	
Men	1.6 grams
Women	1.1 grams

eicosapentaenoic acid (EPA) An omega-3 fatty acid with 20 carbons and five carbon-carbon double bonds. It is present in large amounts in fatty fish and is slowly synthesized in the body from alpha-linolenic acid.

docosahexaenoic acid (DHA) An omega-3 fatty acid with 22 carbons and six carbon-carbon double bonds. It is present in large amounts in fatty fish and is slowly synthesized in the body from alpha-linolenic acid. DHA is especially present in the retina and brain.

arachidonic acid An omega-6 fatty acid made from linoleic acid with 20 carbon atoms and 4 carbon-carbon double bonds.

▲ The American Heart Association recommends eating fatty fish such as salmon at least twice a week. As a source of omega-3 fatty acids, fish is a heart-healthy alternative to other animal sources of protein, which can be high in saturated fat and cholesterol.

ESSENTIAL FUNCTIONS OF FATTY ACIDS

The various classes of lipids have diverse functions in the body. All are necessary for health, but, as mentioned earlier, many can be made by the body and therefore are not needed in our diet. Of all the classes of lipids, only certain polyunsaturated fatty acids are essential parts of a diet.

The Essential Fatty Acids

We must obtain linoleic acid (an omega-6 fatty acid) and alpha-linolenic acid (an omega-3 fatty acid) from foods to maintain health, so they are called *essential* fatty acids (Fig. 5-13). These omega-6 and omega-3 fatty acids form parts of vital body structures, perform important roles in immune system function and vision, help form cell membranes, and produce hormone-like compounds. Omega-6 and omega-3 fatty acids must be obtained through the diet because human cells lack the enzymes needed to produce these fatty acids. Other fatty acids, such as omega-9 fatty acids, can be synthesized in the body, and therefore are not essential components of the diet.

Still, we need to consume only about 5% of our total calories per day from essential fatty acids. That corresponds to about 2 to 4 tablespoons of plant oil each day. We can easily get that much—from mayonnaise, salad dressings, and other foods—without much effort. Regular consumption of vegetables and whole-grain breads and cereals also helps to supply enough essential fatty acids.

Research also suggests that we include a regular intake of the omega-3 fatty acids, **eicosapentaenoic acid (EPA)** and **docosahexaenoic acid (DHA),** which can be made from alpha-linolenic acid. EPA and DHA are naturally high in fatty fish such as salmon, tuna, sardines, anchovies, striped bass, catfish, herring, mackerel, trout, or halibut. Consumption of one or more of these fish at least twice a week is recommended to obtain EPA and DHA. Additional sources of omega-3 fatty acids include canola and soybean oils, walnuts, flax seeds, mussels, crab, and shrimp.

MAKING DECISIONS

Mercury in Fish

Consumption of fatty fish at least twice a week is recommended as a good source of the omega-3 fatty acids. Some fish can be a source of mercury, toxic in high amounts, especially swordfish, shark, king mackerel, and tile fish (see Chapter 13). Albacore tuna also is a potential source, while other forms of tuna are much lower in mercury. Those fish low in mercury are salmon, sardines, bluefish, and herring. Shrimp is also low in mercury. For others, varying your choices rather than always eating the same species of fish and limiting overall intake to 12 ounces per week (on average 2 to 3 meals of fish or shellfish per week) is recommended to reduce mercury exposure, especially for pregnant women and children. Existing research indicates that the benefits of fish intake, especially in reducing the risk of cardiovascular disease, outweigh the possible risks of mercury contamination.

The recommendation to consume omega-3 fatty acids stems from the observation that compounds made from omega-3 fatty acids tend to decrease blood clotting and inflammatory processes in the body. The omega-6 fatty acids, notably **arachidonic acid** made from linoleic acid, generally increase clotting and inflammation, and saturated fatty acids also increase blood clotting.

Some studies show that people who eat fish at least twice a week (total weekly intake: 8 ounces [240 grams]) run lower risks for heart attack than do people who rarely eat fish. In these cases, the omega-3 fatty acids in fish oil are probably acting to reduce blood clotting. As will be covered in detail in the "Nutrition and Your Health"

FIGURE 5-13 ▶ The essential fatty acid (EFA) family. All these fatty acids are available from dietary sources; linoleic acid and alpha-linolenic acid must be consumed as body synthesis does not take place. These are the essential fatty acids. The other fatty acids in this figure can be synthesized from the essential fatty acids.

section, blood clots are part of the heart attack process. In addition, these omega-3 fatty acids have a favorable effect on heart rhythm. Consequently, the risk of heart attack decreases with the consumption of omega-3 fatty acids from fish, especially for people already at high risk.

We need to remember, however, that blood clotting is a normal body process. Certain groups of people, such as Eskimos in Greenland, eat so much seafood that their normal blood-clotting ability can be impaired. An excess of omega-3 fatty acid intake can allow uncontrolled bleeding and may cause **hemorrhagic stroke.** However, no increase in risk of stroke has been observed in studies using moderate amounts of omega-3 fatty acids.

Studies also have shown that large amounts of omega-3 fatty acids from fish (2 to 4 grams per day) can lower blood triglycerides in people with high triglyceride concentrations. In addition, these omega-3 fatty acids are suspected to be helpful in managing the pain of inflammation associated with rheumatoid arthritis by suppressing immune system responses. This may also help with certain behavioral disorders and cases of mild depression.

In some instances, fish oil capsules can be safely substituted for fish consumption if a person does not like fish. Generally, about 1 gram of omega-3 fatty acids (about three capsules) from fish oil per day is recommended, especially for people with evidence of cardiovascular disease. (Freezing fish oil capsules before consumption or using enteric coated capsules will reduce the fishy aftertaste.) The American Heart Association also recently suggested that fish oil supplements (providing 2 to 4 grams of omega-3 fatty acids per day) could be employed to treat elevated blood triglycerides, as previously noted. However, fish oil capsules should be limited for individuals who have bleeding disorders, take anticoagulant medications, or anticipate surgery, because they may increase risk of uncontrollable bleeding and hemorrhagic stroke. Thus for fish oil capsules, as well as other dietary supplements, it is important to follow a physician's recommendations. Remember that fish oil supplements are not regulated by the FDA. The quality of these supplements, therefore, is not standardized, and contaminants naturally present in the fish oil may not have been removed.

In summary, the regular consumption of fatty fish is advised. Consuming whole fish is thought to have greater benefits and be safer than using fish oil supplements. Fish is not only a rich source of omega-3 fatty acids, but is also a valuable source of protein and trace elements that may also provide protective effects for the cardiovascular system. Broiled or baked fish is recommended rather than fried fish because frying may decrease the ratio of omega-3 to omega-6 fatty acids and may produce *trans* fatty acids and oxidized lipid products that may increase cardiovascular disease risk.

 See *Nutrition and Your Health: Lipids and Cardiovascular Disease* at the end of Chapter 5.

hemorrhagic stroke Damage to part of the brain resulting from rupture of a blood vessel and subsequent bleeding within or over the internal surface of the brain.

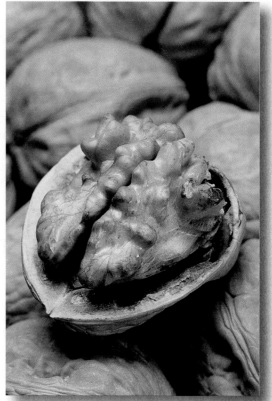

▲ Walnuts are one of the richest plant sources of the omega-3 fatty acid, alpha-linolenic acid, and are also a good source of plant sterols.

CRITICAL THINKING

Advertisements often claim that fats are bad. Your classmate Mike asks, "If fats are so bad for us, why do we need to have any in our diets?" How would you answer him?

rancid Containing products of decomposed fatty acids that have an unpleasant flavor and odor.

total parenteral nutrition The intravenous feeding of all necessary nutrients, including the most basic forms of protein, carbohydrates, lipids, vitamins, minerals, and electrolytes.

▲ When at rest or during light activity, the body uses mostly fatty acids for fuel.

MAKING DECISIONS

Flax Seeds or Walnuts?

Flax seeds and walnuts are getting attention today because they are rich vegetable sources of the omega-3 alpha-linolenic acid. About 2 tablespoons per day is typically recommended if used as an omega-3 fatty acid source. Flax seeds can be purchased in many natural food stores rather inexpensively. These need to be chewed thoroughly or they will pass through the GI tract undigested. Many people find it easier to grind them in a coffee grinder before eating them. Flax seed oil is also available, but it turns **rancid** very quickly, especially if not refrigerated. Compared to other nuts and seeds, walnuts are one of the richest sources of alpha-linolenic acid (2.6 grams per 1-ounce serving or 14 walnut halves). The DRI for alpha-linolenic acid is 1.6 grams/day for men and 1.1 grams/day for women. In addition, walnuts are a rich source of plant sterols known to inhibit intestinal absorption of cholesterol.

Effects of a Deficiency of Essential Fatty Acids

If humans fail to consume enough essential fatty acids, their skin becomes flaky and itchy, and diarrhea and other symptoms such as infections often are seen. Growth and wound healing may be restricted. These signs of deficiency have been seen in people fed intravenously by **total parenteral nutrition** containing little or no fat for 2 to 3 weeks, as well as in infants receiving formulas low in fat. However, because our bodies need the equivalent of only about 2 to 4 tablespoons of plant oils a day, even a low-fat diet will provide enough essential fatty acids if it follows a balanced plan such as MyPyramid and includes a serving of fatty fish at least twice a week.

CONCEPT CHECK

Because humans can't make either omega-3 or omega-6 fatty acids, which perform vital functions in the body, they must be obtained from the diet and therefore are called essential fatty acids. Plant oils are generally rich in omega-6 fatty acids. Eating fatty fish at least twice a week is a good way to meet omega-3 fatty acid needs. Fish oil supplementation (about 1 gram per day of the related omega-3 fatty acids) is generally acceptable under a physician's guidance if a person does not like fish; however, people with certain medical conditions (e.g., taking anticoagulant medications) should be cautious with use of fish oil supplements due to increased risk of hemorrhagic stroke. Essential fatty acid deficiency can occur after 2 to 3 weeks if fat is omitted from total parenteral nutrition solutions, which in turn can lead to skin disorders, diarrhea, and other health problems.

BROADER ROLES FOR FATTY ACIDS AND TRIGLYCERIDES IN THE BODY

Many key functions of fat in the body require the use of fatty acids in the form of triglycerides. Triglycerides are used for energy storage, insulation, and transportation of fat-soluble vitamins.

Providing Energy

Triglycerides contained in the diet and stored in adipose tissue provide the fatty acids that are the main fuel for muscles while at rest and during light activity. Muscles use carbohydrate for fuel in addition to fatty acids supplied by triglycerides only in endurance exercise, such as long-distance running and cycling, or in short bursts of intense activity, such as a 200-meter run. Other body tissues also use fatty acids for energy needs. Overall, about half of the energy used by the entire body at rest and during light activity comes from fatty acids. When considering the whole-body, the use of fatty acids by skeletal and heart muscle is balanced by the use of glucose by the nervous system and red blood cells. Recall from Chapter 4 that cells need a supply of carbohydrate to efficiently process fatty acids for fuel. The details about how we burn fat as a fuel will be discussed in Chapter 7.

Storing Energy for Later Use

We store energy mainly in the form of triglycerides. The body's ability to store fat is essentially limitless. Its fat storage sites, adipose cells, can increase about 50 times in weight. If the amount of fat to be stored exceeds the ability of the existing cells to expand, the body can form new adipose cells.

An important advantage of using triglycerides to store energy in the body is that they are energy dense. Recall that these yield, on average, 9 kcal per gram, whereas proteins and carbohydrates yield only about 4 kcal per gram. In addition, triglycerides are chemically stable, so they are not likely to react with other cell constituents, making them a safe form for storing energy. Finally, when we store triglycerides in adipose cells, we store little else, especially water. Adipose cells contain about 80% lipid and only 20% water and protein. In contrast, imagine if we were to store energy as muscle tissue, which is about 73% water. Body weight linked to energy storage would increase dramatically. The same would be true if we stored energy primarily as glycogen, as about 3 grams of water are stored for every gram of glycogen.

Adipose cell

Insulating and Protecting the Body

The insulating layer of fat just beneath the skin is made mostly of triglycerides. Fat tissue also surrounds and protects some organs—kidneys, for example—from injury. We usually don't notice the important insulating function of fat tissue, because we wear clothes and add more as needed. A layer of insulating fat is important in animals living in cold climates. Polar bears, walruses, and whales all build a thick layer of fat tissue around themselves to insulate against cold-weather environments. The extra fat also provides energy storage for times when food is scarce.

Transporting Fat-Soluble Vitamins

Triglycerides and other fats in food carry fat-soluble vitamins to the small intestine and aid their absorption. People who absorb fat poorly, such as those with the disease cystic fibrosis, are at risk for deficiencies of fat-soluble vitamins, especially vitamin K. A similar risk comes from taking mineral oil as a laxative at mealtimes. The body cannot digest or absorb mineral oil, so the undigested oil carries the fat-soluble vitamins from the meal into the feces, where they are eliminated. Unabsorbed fatty acids can bind minerals, such as calcium and magnesium, and draw them into the stool for elimination. This can harm mineral status (see Chapter 10). Recall that the main problem with the fat replacer, olestra, is that it can bind the fat-soluble vitamins and reduce their absorption.

PHOSPHOLIPIDS IN THE BODY

Many types of phospholipids exist in the body, especially in the brain. They form important parts of cell membranes. Phospholipids are found in body cells, and they participate in fat digestion in the intestine. Recall that the various forms of lecithin (discussed earlier) are common examples of phospholipids (review Fig. 5-4b).

Cell membranes are composed primarily of phospholipids. A cell membrane looks much like a sea of phospholipids with protein "islands" (Fig. 5-14). The proteins

FIGURE 5-14 ▶ Phospholipids are the main components of cell membranes, forming a double or bilayer of lipid.

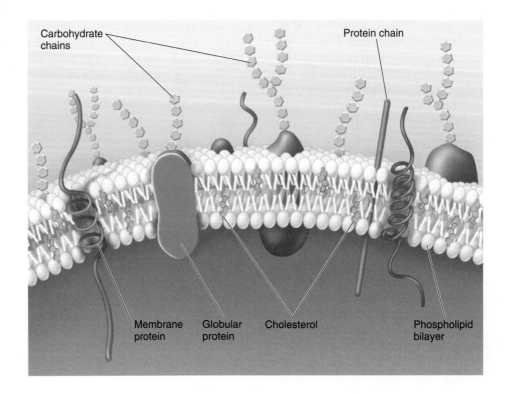

form receptors for hormones, function as enzymes, and act as transporters for nutrients. The fatty acids on the phospholipids serve as a source of essential fatty acids for the cell. Some cholesterol is also present in the membrane.

In some foods, phospholipids function as emulsifiers (as covered earlier) allowing fat and water to mix. By breaking fat globules into small droplets, emulsifiers enable a fat to be suspended in water. They act as bridges between the oil and water that in turn lead to the formation of tiny oil droplets surrounded by thin shells of water. In an emulsified solution, such as salad dressing or mayonnaise, millions of tiny oil droplets are separated by shells of water (review Fig. 5-7).

The body's main emulsifiers are the lecithins and bile acids, produced by the liver and released into the small intestine via the gallbladder during digestion.

CHOLESTEROL IN THE BODY

Cholesterol plays many vital roles in the body. It forms part of some important hormones, such as estrogen, testosterone, and a form of the active vitamin D hormone. Cholesterol is also the building block of bile acids, needed for fat digestion. Finally, cholesterol is an essential structural component of cells and the outer layer of the lipoprotein particles that transport lipids in the blood. The cholesterol content of the heart, liver, kidney, and brain is high, reflecting its critical role in these organs.

About two-thirds of the cholesterol circulating through your body is made by body cells; the remaining one-third is consumed in the diet. Each day, our cells produce approximately 875 milligrams of cholesterol. Of the 875 milligrams of cholesterol made by the body, about 400 milligrams are used to make new bile acids to replenish those lost in the feces, and about 50 milligrams are used to make hormones. In addition to all the cholesterol cells make, we consume about 180 to 325 milligrams of cholesterol per day from animal-derived food products, with men consuming the higher amount compared to women. Absorption of cholesterol from food ranges from about 40% to 65%. The effect of blood cholesterol, especially LDL cholesterol, on cardiovascular disease risk will be discussed in the "Nutrition and Your Health" section.

See Nutrition and Your Health: Lipids and Cardiovascular Disease at the end of Chapter 5.

CONCEPT CHECK

Triglycerides are the major form of fat in the body. They are used for energy and stored in adipose tissue, they insulate and protect body organs, and they transport fat-soluble vitamins. Phospholipids are emulsifiers—compounds that can suspend fat in water. Phospholipids also form parts of cell membranes and various compounds in the body. Cholesterol, a sterol, forms part of cell membranes, hormones, and bile acids. If sufficient amounts are not consumed, the body makes what phospholipids and cholesterol it needs.

RECOMMENDATIONS FOR FAT INTAKE

There is no RDA for total fat intake for adults, although there is an Adequate Intake set for total fat for infants (see Chapter 17). The 2005 Dietary Guidelines for Americans recommend that total fat intake should not exceed 20% to 35% of total calories, which equates to 44 to 78 grams per day for a person who consumes 2000 kcal daily. The most specific recommendations for fat intake come from the American Heart Association (AHA). Many North Americans are at risk for developing cardiovascular disease, so AHA promotes dietary and lifestyle goals aimed at reducing this risk. The AHA diet and lifestyle goals for cardiovascular disease risk reduction for the general public are presented in Table 5-4. These goals include aiming for an overall healthy eating pattern; appropriate body weight; and a desirable blood cholesterol profile, blood pressure, and blood glucose level. In Table 5-5, a more detailed list of recommendations is provided for those who currently are at high risk or have cardiovascular disease.

To reduce risk for cardiovascular disease, the AHA recommends that no more than 7% of total calories come from saturated fat and no more than 1% from *trans* fat. These are the primary fatty acids that raise LDL. In addition, cholesterol should amount to a maximum of 300 mg per day. This often happens along with the reduction in saturated fat and *trans* fat intake. Table 5-6 is an example of a diet that adheres to 20% or 30% of calories as fat. Compare these recommendations to the actual dietary intake patterns of these fats by North Americans: 33% of calories from total fat, about 13% of calories from saturated fat, and 180 to 320 milligrams of cholesterol each day.

Both the National Cholesterol Education Program (NCEP) and the Food and Nutrition Board are in agreement with the advice of the AHA. One exception in the

▲ Trim the fat from meats before cooking to help reduce your saturated fat intake. Also, limit use of meat that is highly marbled with fat (seen as streaks of fat).

▶ One goal of *Healthy People 2010* is to increase the proportion of persons age 2 years and older who consume less than 10% of calorie intake from saturated fat.

TABLE 5-4 American Heart Association 2006 Diet and Lifestyle Goals for Cardiovascular Disease Risk Reduction

- Consume an overall healthy diet.

- Aim for a healthy body weight.

- Aim for recommended levels of low-density lipoprotein (LDL) cholesterol, high-density lipoprotein (HDL) cholesterol, and triglycerides.

- Aim for a normal blood pressure.

- Aim for a normal blood glucose level.

- Be physically active.

- Avoid use of and exposure to tobacco products.

From: Lichtenstein AH et al: Diet and lifestyle recommendations revision 2006. A scientific statement from the American Heart Association Nutrition Committee. *Circulation* 114:82, 2006.

▶ Some advice regarding fat intake from the 2005 Dietary Guidelines:

- Limit intake of fats and oils high in saturated and/or *trans* fatty acids, and choose products low in such fats and oils.

- Consume fats high in polyunsaturated and monounsaturated fatty acids, such as from fish, nuts, and vegetable oils.

- When selecting and preparing meat, poultry, dry beans, and milk or milk products, make choices that are lean, low-fat, or fat-free.

TABLE 5-5 American Heart Association 2006 Diet and Lifestyle Recommendations for Cardiovascular Disease Risk Reduction

- Balance calorie intake and physical activity to achieve or maintain a healthy body weight.

- Consume a diet rich in vegetables and fruits.

- Choose whole-grain, high-fiber foods.

- Consume fish, especially oily fish, at least twice a week.

- Limit your intake of saturated fat to less than 7% of energy, *trans* fat to less than 1% of energy, and cholesterol to less than 300 milligrams per day by
  — choosing lean meats and vegetable alternatives;
  — selecting fat-free (skim), 1%-fat, and low-fat dairy products; and
  — minimizing intake of partially hydrogenated fats.

- Minimize your intake of beverages and foods with added sugars.

- Choose and prepare foods with little or no salt.

- If you consume alcohol, do so in moderation.

- When you eat food prepared outside of the home, follow the AHA Diet and Lifestyle Recommendations.

From: Lichtenstein AH and others: Diet and lifestyle recommendations revision 2006. A scientific statement from the American Heart Association Nutrition Committee. *Circulation* 114:82, 2006.

TABLE 5-6 Daily Menu Examples Containing 2000 kcal and 30% or 20% of Calories as Fat

30% of Calories as Fat		20% of Calories as Fat	
Food	**Fat (grams)**	**Food**	**Fat (grams)**
Breakfast			
Orange juice, 1 cup	0.5	Same	0.5
Shredded wheat, ¾ cup	0.5	Shredded wheat, 1 cup	0.7
Toasted bagel	1.1	Same	1.1
Tub margarine, 3 teaspoons	11.4	Tub margarine, 2 teaspoons	7.6
1% low-fat milk, 1 cup	2.5	Fat-free milk, 1 cup	0.6
Lunch			
Whole-wheat bread, 2 slices	2.4	Same	2.4
Roast beef, 2 ounces	4.9	Light turkey roll, 2 ounces	0.9
Mayonnaise, 3 teaspoons	11.0	Mayonnaise, 2 teaspoons	7.3
Lettuce	—	Same	—
Tomato	—	Same	—
Oatmeal cookie, 1	3.3	Oatmeal cookie, 2	6.6
Snack			
Apple	—	Same	—
Dinner			
Chicken tenders frozen meal	18.0	Fat-free chicken tenders	—
Carrots, ½ cup	—	Same	—
Dinner roll, 1	2.0	Same	2.0
Margarine, 1 teaspoon	3.8	Same	3.8
Banana	0.6	Same	0.6
1% low-fat milk, 1 cup	2.5	Fat-free milk, 1 cup	0.6
Snack			
Raisins, 2 teaspoons	—	Raisins, ½ cup	—
Air-popped popcorn, 3 cups	1.0	Air-popped popcorn, 6 cups	2.0
Margarine, 2 teaspoons	7.6	Same	7.6
Totals	**73.1**		**44.3**

▲ **Whole grains** (shredded wheat, whole-wheat bread, oatmeal cookies, popcorn), **fruits** (orange juice, apple, banana, raisins), **vegetables** (carrots, lettuce, tomato), **lean meats** (roast beef, turkey, chicken), and **fat-free milk** are the primary components of the low-fat menus in Table 5-6.

TABLE 5-7 Food and Nutrition Board Recommendations for Omega-6 and Omega-3 Fatty Acids per Day

	Men (grams per day)	Women (grams per day)
Linoleic acid (omega-6)	17	12
Alpha-linolenic acid (omega-3)	1.6	1.1

latest guidelines from the NCEP is that fat intake could be as high as 35% of total calories as long as intakes of saturated fat, cholesterol, and *trans* fat are minimized. The Food and Nutrition Board combines the AHA and NCEP recommendations, suggesting that fat provide a range of 20% to 35% of calories. The 2005 Dietary Guidelines also support this advice. In addition to fat intake, controlling total calorie intake is also significant, as weight control is a vital component of cardiovascular disease prevention.

Regarding essential fatty acids, the Food and Nutrition Board has issued recommendations for both omega-6 and omega-3 fatty acids. The amounts listed in Table 5-7 work out to about 5% of calorie intake for the total of both essential fatty acids. Infants and children have lower needs (again, see Chapter 17). Consumption of fish at least twice a week is one step toward meeting requirements for essential fatty acids.

The typical North American diet derives about 7% of calories from polyunsaturated fatty acids, and thus meets essential fatty acid needs. An upper limit of 10% of calorie intake as polyunsaturated fatty acids is often recommended, in part because the breakdown (oxidation) of those present in lipoproteins is linked to increased cholesterol deposition in the arteries (see the "Nutrition and Your Health" section in this chapter). Depression of immune function is also suspected to be caused by an excessive intake of polyunsaturated fatty acids.

In recent years, the Mediterranean diet has attracted a lot of attention as a result of lower rates of chronic diseases seen in people following such a diet plan. The major sources of fat in the Mediterranean diet include liberal amounts of olive oil compared to a small amount of animal fat (from animal flesh and dairy products). In contrast, major sources of fat in the typical North American diet include animal flesh, whole milk, pastries, cheese, margarine, and mayonnaise. While dietary fat sources definitely play a role in prevention of chronic disease, it is important to remember that other aspects of one's lifestyle also contribute to disease risk. People who follow a Mediterranean diet also tend to consume moderate alcohol (usually in the form of red wine, which contains many antioxidants), eat plenty of whole grains and few refined carbohydrates, and are also more physically active than typical North Americans.

An alternative plan for reduction of cardiovascular disease is Dr. Dean Ornish's purely vegetarian (**vegan**) diet plan. This diet is very low in fat, including only a scant quantity of vegetable oil used in cooking and the small amount of oils present in plant foods. Individuals restricting fat intake to 20% of calories should be monitored by a physician, as the resulting increase in carbohydrate intake can increase blood triglycerides in some people, which is not a healthful change. Over time, however, the initial problem of high blood triglycerides on a low-fat diet may self-correct. Among people following the Ornish plan, blood triglycerides initially increased, but within a year, fell to normal values as long as they emphasized high-fiber carbohydrate sources, controlled (or improved) body weight, and followed a regular exercise program.

▶ The advice to consume 20% to 35% of calories as fat does not apply to infants and toddlers below the age of 2 years. These youngsters are forming new tissue that requires fat, especially in the brain, so their intake of fat and cholesterol should not be greatly restricted.

▲ If you are looking to decrease the amount of saturated and *trans* fats in your diet, it is a good idea to opt for lower-fat substitutes for some of your current high-fat food choices. How do you think this meal compares with the chicken nuggets and French fries meal on p. 176.

vegan A person who eats only plant foods.

To avoid too much saturated fat and cholesterol, for breakfast eat fewer foods like bacon, sausage, and whole eggs and more foods like whole-grain waffles and fresh fruit.

TABLE 5-8 Tips for Avoiding Too Much Fat, Saturated Fat, Cholesterol, and *Trans* Fat

	Eat Less of These Foods	Eat More of These Foods
Grains	• Pasta dishes with cheese or cream sauces • Croissants • Pastries • Doughnuts • Pie crust	• Whole-grain breads • Whole-grain pasta • Brown rice • Angel food cake • Animal or graham crackers • Air-popped popcorn
Vegetables	• French fries • Potato chips • Vegetables cooked in butter, cheese, or cream sauces	• Fresh, frozen, baked, or steamed vegetables
Fruit	• Fruit pies	• Fresh, frozen, or canned fruits
Milk	• Whole milk • Ice cream • High-fat cheese • Cheesecake	• Fat-free and reduced-fat milk • Low-fat frozen desserts (e.g., yogurt, sherbet, ice milk) • Reduced-fat/part-skim cheese
Meat and beans	• Bacon • Sausage • Organ meats (e.g., liver) • Egg yolks	• Fish • Skinless poultry • Lean cuts of meat (with fat trimmed away) • Soy products • Egg whites/egg substitutes
Oils	• Butter and stick margarine	• Canola oil or olive oil • Tub or liquid margarine (in small amounts)

In summary, the general consensus among nutrition experts suggests that limitation of saturated fat, cholesterol, and *trans* fat intake should be the primary focus, and that the diet needs to contain some omega-3 and omega-6 fatty acids (Table 5-8). Furthermore, if fat intake exceeds 30% of total calories, the extra fat should come from monounsaturated fat.

CONCEPT CHECK

There is no RDA for fat. We need about 5% of total calorie intake from plant oils to obtain the needed essential fatty acids. Eating fatty fish at least twice a week is also advised to supply omega-3 fatty acids. Many health-related agencies recommend a diet containing no more than 35% of calorie intake as fat, with no more than 7% to 10% of calorie intake as a combination of saturated fat and *trans* fat for the general public. Cholesterol intake should be limited to 200 to 300 milligrams per day. These practices help maintain a normal LDL value in the blood. The North American diet contains about 33% of calories as fat, with about 13% of calories as saturated fat and about 3% as *trans* fatty acids. Cholesterol intake varies from about 200 to 400 milligrams per day.

Cardiovascular disease is the major killer of North Americans. Cardiovascular disease typically involves the coronary arteries and, thus, frequently the term coronary heart disease (CHD) or coronary artery disease (CAD) is used. Each year about 500,000 people die of coronary heart disease in the United States, about 60% more than die of cancer. The figure rises to almost 1 million if strokes and other circulatory diseases are included in the global term *cardiovascular disease*. About 1.5 million people in the United States each year have a heart attack. The overall male-to-female ratio for cardiovascular disease is about 2:1. Women generally lag about 10 years behind men in developing the disease. Still, it eventually kills more women than any other disease—twice as many as does cancer. And, for each person in North America who dies of cardiovascular disease, 20 more (over 13 million people) have symptoms of the disease.

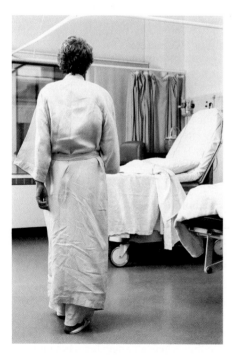

▲ Cardiovascular disease kills more women than any other disease—twice as many as does cancer.

DEVELOPMENT OF CARDIOVASCULAR DISEASE

The symptoms of cardiovascular disease develop over many years and often do not become obvious until old age. Nonetheless, autopsies of young adults under 20 years of age have shown that many of them had atherosclerotic **plaque** in their arteries (Fig. 5-15). This finding indicates that plaque buildup can begin in childhood and continue throughout life, although it usually goes undetected for some time.

The typical forms of cardiovascular disease—coronary heart disease and strokes—are associated with inadequate blood circulation in the heart and brain related to buildup of this plaque. Blood supplies the heart muscle, brain, and other body organs with oxygen and nutrients. When blood flow via the coronary arteries surrounding the heart is interrupted, the heart muscle can be damaged. A heart attack, or **myocardial infarction,** may result (review Fig. 5-15). This may cause the heart to beat irregularly or to stop. About 25% of people do not survive their first heart attack. If blood flow to parts of the brain is interrupted long enough, part of the brain dies, causing a **cerebrovascular accident,** or stroke.

A heart attack can strike with the sudden force of a sledgehammer, with pain radiating up the neck or down the arm. It can sneak up at night, masquerading as indigestion, with slight pain or pressure in the chest. Many times, the symptoms are so subtle in women that death occurs before she or the health professional realizes that a heart attack is taking place. If there is any suspicion at all that a heart attack is taking place, the person should first chew an aspirin (325 milligrams) thoroughly and then call 911. Aspirin helps reduce the blood clotting that leads to a heart attack.

Continuous formation and breakdown of blood clots in the blood vessels is a normal process. However, in areas where plaques build up, blood clots are more

plaque A cholesterol-rich substance deposited in the blood vessels; it contains various white blood cells, smooth muscle cells, various proteins, cholesterol and other lipids, and eventually calcium.

myocardial infarction Death of part of the heart muscle. Also termed a *heart attack*.

cerebrovascular accident (CVA) Death of part of the brain tissue due typically to a blood clot. Also termed a *stroke*.

▶ Typical warning signs of a heart attack are:

- Intense, prolonged chest pain or pressure, sometimes radiating to other parts of the upper body (men and women)
- Shortness of breath (men and women)
- Sweating (men and women)
- Nausea and vomiting (especially women)
- Dizziness (especially women)
- Weakness (men and women)
- Jaw, neck, and shoulder pain (especially women)
- Irregular heartbeat (men and women)

▲ At the first sign of a possible heart attack, the person should first thoroughly chew an aspirin and then call 911.

▶ *Healthy People 2010* has set a goal of reducing death from coronary heart disease by 30%, compared with today's incidence.

homocysteine An amino acid not used in protein synthesis, but instead arises during metabolism of the amino acid methionine. Homocysteine is likely toxic to many cells, such as those lining the blood vessels.

FIGURE 5-15 ▶ The road to a heart attack. Injury to an artery wall begins the process. This is followed by a progressive buildup of plaque in the artery walls. The heart attack represents the terminal phase of the process. Blockage of the left coronary artery by a blood clot is evident. The heart muscle served by the portion of the coronary artery beyond the point of blockage lacks oxygen and nutrients and is damaged and may die. This damage can lead to a significant drop in heart function and often total heart failure.

likely to remain intact and then lead to a blockage, cutting off or diminishing the supply of blood to the heart (via the coronary arteries) or brain (via the carotid arteries). More than 95% of heart attacks are caused by such blood clots. Heart attacks generally are caused by total blockage of the coronary arteries due to a blood clot forming in an area of the artery already partially blocked by plaque. Disruption of the plaque may even lead to eventual clot formation.

Atherosclerosis probably first develops to repair damage in a vessel lining. The damage that starts this process can be caused by smoking, diabetes, hyperten-

sion, **homocysteine** (likely, but not a major factor), LDL, and viral and bacterial infection. Ongoing inflammation in the blood vessel is also suspected to cause blood vessel damage. (A laboratory test for c-reactive protein in the blood is used to assess if inflammation is present.) Atherosclerosis can be seen in arteries throughout the body. The damage develops especially at points where an artery branches into two smaller vessels. A great deal of stress is placed on the vessel walls at these points due to changes in blood flow.

Once blood vessel damage has occurred, the next step in the development of atherosclerosis is the progression phase. This step is characterized by deposition of plaque at the site of initial damage. The rate of plaque buildup during the progression phase is directly related to the amount of LDL in the blood. The form of LDL that contributes to atherosclerosis is **oxidized** LDL. This form is preferentially taken up by scavenger cells in the arterial wall. Nutrients and phytochemicals that have **antioxidant** properties may reduce LDL oxidation. Fruits and vegetables are particularly rich in these compounds. Eating fruits and vegetables regularly is one positive step we can make to reduce plaque buildup and slow the progression of cardiovascular disease. Some fruits and vegetables particularly helpful in this regard include legumes (beans), nuts, dried plums (prunes), raisins, berries, plums, apples, cherries, oranges, grapes, spinach, broccoli, red bell peppers, potatoes, and onions. Tea and coffee are also sources of antioxidants.

As plaque accumulates, arteries harden, narrow, and lose their elasticity. Affected arteries become further damaged as blood pumps through them and pressure increases. Finally, in the terminal phase, a clot or spasm in a plaque-clogged artery leads to a heart attack.

Factors that typically bring on a heart attack in a person already at risk include dehydration; acute emotional stress (such as firing an employee); strenuous physical activity when not otherwise physically fit (shoveling snow, for example); waking during the night or getting up in the morning (linked to an abrupt increase in stress); and consuming large, high-fat meals (increases blood clotting).

RISK FACTORS FOR CARDIOVASCULAR DISEASE

Many of us are free of the risk factors that contribute to rapid development of atherosclerosis. If so, the advice of health experts is to consume a balanced diet, perform regular physical activity, have a complete fasting lipoprotein analysis performed at age 20 or beyond, and reevaluate risk factors every 5 years.

For most people, however, the most likely risk factors are:

- **Total blood cholesterol over 200 milligrams per 100 milliliters of blood**

(mg/dl; dl is short for deciliter or 100 milliliters). Risk is especially high when total cholesterol is at or over 240 mg/dl and LDL-cholesterol readings are over 130 to 160 mg/dl. (The terms LDL-cholesterol and HDL-cholesterol are used when expressing the blood concentration because it is the cholesterol content of these lipoproteins that is measured.)

- **Smoking.** Smoking is the main cause of about 20% of cardiovascular disease deaths and generally negates the female advantage of later occurrence of the disease. A combination of smoking and oral contraceptive use increases the risk of cardiovascular disease in women even more. Smoking greatly increases the expression of a person's genetically linked risk for cardiovascular disease, even if one's blood lipids are low. Smoking also makes blood more likely to clot. Even secondhand smoke has been implicated as a risk factor.
- **Hypertension. Systolic blood pressure** over 139 (millimeters of mercury) and **diastolic blood pressure** over 89 indicate hypertension. Healthy blood pressure values are less than 120 and 80, respectively. (Treatment of hypertension is reviewed in Chapter 8.)
- **Diabetes.** Diabetes virtually guarantees development of cardiovascular disease, and so puts a person with diabetes in the high-risk group. Insulin increases

oxidize In the most basic sense, the loss of an electron or gain of an oxygen by a chemical substance. This change typically alters the shape and/or function of the substance.

antioxidant Generally a compound that stops the damaging effects of reactive substances seeking an electron (i.e., oxidizing agents). This prevents breakdown (oxidizing) of substances in foods or the body, particularly lipids.

systolic blood pressure The pressure in the arterial blood vessels associated with the pumping of blood from the heart.

diastolic blood pressure The pressure in the arterial blood vessels when the heart is between beats.

▲ Smoking is one of the four major risk factors for developing cardiovascular disease.

MAKING DECISIONS

Antioxidant Supplements and Cardiovascular Disease

Are large doses of antioxidant vitamin supplements a reliable way to reduce LDL oxidation, and thereby prevent cardiovascular disease? Controversy about such dietary supplementation exists among the experts, as will be detailed in Chapter 9. The American Heart Association does not support use of antioxidant supplements (such as vitamin E) to reduce cardiovascular disease risk. This is because large-scale studies have shown no decrease in cardiovascular disease risk with use of antioxidant supplements. One study even showed a modest increase for heart failure in people with diabetes or otherwise at high risk for cardiovascular disease after taking antioxidant supplements. However, further trials of antioxidant supplementation (e.g., 600 IU of vitamin E every other day) for prevention of heart disease in men are ongoing. With regard to women, 600 IU of natural-source vitamin E taken every other day provided no overall benefit for major cardiovascular events (or cancer). More research is warranted, however, as a decrease in sudden cardiac death was seen in a subset of older women in this study. Some experts suggest daily vitamin E supplementation (100 IU to 400 IU) may be helpful for *preventing* cardiovascular disease, while other experts recommend against the practice. One thing is certain: any supplementation of vitamin E should be taken only under the guidance of a physician, because of interactions with vitamin K and anticlotting medications (and possibly high-dose aspirin use).

▶ For more information on cardiovascular disease, see the website of the American Heart Association at www.americanheart.org or the heart disease section of Healthfinder at www.healthfinder.gov/tours/heart.htm. This is a site created by the U.S. government for consumers. In addition, visit the website www.nhlbi.nih.gov/.

▶ *Healthy People 2010* has set a goal of reducing total blood cholesterol among adults from the average of 206 mg/dl to 199 mg/dl, as well as reducing the percentage of adults with high blood cholesterol from 21% to 17%.

▶ Cardiovascular Disease Risk Factors

- Total blood cholesterol >200 mg/dl
- Smoking
- Hypertension
- Diabetes
- HDL cholesterol < 40 mg/dl
- Age: Men >45 yr; Women > 55 yr
- Family history of cardiovascular disease
- Blood triglycerides > 200 mg/dl
- Obesity
- Inactivity

▶ Two approaches have been shown to cause reversal of atherosclerosis in the body. One employs a vegan diet and other lifestyle changes that are part of the Dr. Dean Ornish program. The other employs aggressive LDL lowering with medications.

▶ As noted earlier, aspirin in small doses reduces blood clotting. It is often used under a physician's guidance to treat people at risk for heart attack or stroke, especially if one has already occurred. About 80 to 160 milligrams per day is needed for such benefits. Individuals who may especially benefit from aspirin therapy are men over 40, smokers, postmenopausal women, and people with diabetes, hypertension, or a family history of cardiovascular disease.

cholesterol synthesis in the liver, in turn increasing LDL in the bloodstream. This disease negates any female advantage.

Together, the previous four risk factors explain most cases of cardiovascular disease. Other risk factors to consider:

- HDL-cholesterol under 40 mg/dl, especially when the ratio of total cholesterol to HDL-cholesterol is greater than 4:1 (3.5:1 or less is optimal). Women often have high values for HDL-cholesterol, and therefore it is important for this to be measured in women to establish cardiovascular disease risk. A value of 60 mg/dl or more is especially protective. Exercising for at least 45 minutes four times a week can increase HDL by about 5 mg/dl. Losing excess weight (especially around the waist) and avoiding smoking and overeating also help maintain or raise HDL, as does moderate alcohol consumption.
- Age. Men over 45 years and women over 55 years.
- Family history of cardiovascular disease, especially before age 50.
- Blood triglycerides 200 mg/dl or greater in the fasting state (less than 100 mg/dl is optimal).
- Obesity (especially fat accumulation in the waist). Typical weight gain seen in adults is a chief contributor to the increase in LDL seen with aging. Obesity also typically leads to insulin resistance, creating a diabetes-like state, and ultimately the disease itself. It also increases overall inflamation throughout the body.
- Inactivity. Exercise conditions the arteries to adapt to physical stress. Regular exercise also improves insulin action in the body. The corresponding reduction in insulin output leads to a reduction in lipoprotein synthesis in the liver. Both regular aerobic exercise and resistance exercise are recommended. A person with existing cardiovascular disease should seek physician approval before starting such a program, as should older adults.

Researchers are trying to unravel and quantify numerous other factors that may be linked to premature cardiovascular disease, such as the connection between inad-

equate intake of vitamin B-6, folate, and vitamin B-12, which can lead to increased homocysteine in the blood. As noted, homocysteine may damage the cells lining the blood vessels, in turn promoting atherosclerosis. Studies show that supplementation with folic acid and B vitamins does not reduce risk of recurrent cardiovascular disease in patients that had previous heart attacks or had existing vascular diseases.

The term *risk factor* is not equivalent to cause of disease; nevertheless, the more of these risk factors one has, the greater the chances of ultimately developing cardiovascular disease. A good example is the **metabolic syndrome** (also called *Syndrome X*) discussed in Chapter 4. A person with the metabolic syndrome would have abdominal obesity, high blood triglycerides, low HDL-cholesterol, hypertension, poor blood glucose regulation (i.e., high fasting blood glucose), and increased blood clotting. This profile raises the risk for cardiovascular disease considerably. On a positive note, cardiovascular disease is rare in populations who have low LDL-cholesterol, normal blood pressure, and do not smoke or have diabetes. By minimizing these risk factors, as well as following the dietary recommendations of the American Heart Association on page 188 and staying physically active, one will most likely reduce many of the other controllable risk factors listed. In other words, develop and follow a total lifestyle plan. Medications may also be added to lower blood lipids, as discussed next. Finally, if a person has a family history of cardiovascular disease but the usual risk factors aren't present, a rarer defect might be the cause. In this case, having a detailed physical examination for other potential causes is advised.

MEDICAL INTERVENTIONS TO LOWER BLOOD LIPIDS

Some people need even more aggressive therapy added to their regimen of a diet and lifestyle overhaul to treat elevated blood lipids. The clearest indication for this more aggressive approach is in people who already have had a heart attack or have cardiovascular disease symptoms or diabetes.

Medications are the cornerstone of this more aggressive therapy. The National Cholesterol Education Program in the United States has developed a formula based on age, total blood cholesterol, HDL-cholesterol, smoking history, and blood pressure to determine who needs such medications. Check out this formula at http://hp2010.nhlbihin.net/atpiii/calculator.asp?usertype=pub. This formula provides an estimate for having a heart attack in the next 10 years.

Medications work to lower LDL in one of two ways. Some reduce cholesterol synthesis in the liver. Such medicines are known as "statins" (e.g., atorvistatin [Lipitor]). The cost of treatment with one of these drugs can be from $1,600 or more per year, depending on the dose needed. These medications lead to problems in some people, and so require physician monitoring, especially of liver function. Another group of medications binds bile acids or the cholesterol that is part of bile secreted into the small intestine. This binding leads to their elimination in the feces and so requires the liver to synthesize new bile acids and/or cholesterol. The liver removes LDL from the blood to do this. Some of these medications taste gritty and therefore are not popular.

The current therapeutic goal for people with (or at high risk for) cardiovascular disease (Table 5-9) is to drive LDL down to less than 70 mg/dl.

The statin drug simvastatin (Zocor) has been combined with another drug (ezetimibe) and is marketed as Vytorin, a drug that will treat the two sources of cholesterol, "food and family." While the statin reduces the cholesterol made by the liver, the ezetimibe helps block the absorption of cholesterol from food.

A third group of drugs can be used to lower blood triglycerides by decreasing the triglyceride production of the liver. These include gemfibrozil (Lopid) and megadoses of the vitamin nicotinic acid. The use of nicotinic acid does result in pesky side effects, however, but these are typically manageable.

Other Possible Medical Therapies for Cardiovascular Disease

FDA has approved two margarines that have positive effects on blood cholesterol levels—Benecol and Take Control. These margarines contain plant stanols/sterols. The plant stanols/sterols, also called phytosterols, work by reducing cholesterol absorption in the small intestine and lowering its return to the liver. The liver responds by taking up more cholesterol from the blood so it can continue to make bile acids. The studies done on the cholesterol-lowering effect of these margarines have found that 2 to 5 grams of plant stanols/sterols per day reduces total blood cholesterol by 8% to 10% and LDL-cholesterol by 9% to 14% (similar to what is seen with some cholesterol-lowering drugs).

Benecol is made from plant stanols extracted from wood pulp. This product is sold as margarine and has been added to salad dressings. Take Control is made from plant sterols isolated from soybeans. The recommended amount for both is about 2 to 3 grams per day as part of at least two meals; this works out to about 1 tablespoon of Benecol or 2 tablespoons of Take Control per day. Use would cost about $1.00 per day, as these margarines are more expensive than regular margarines.

In people who have borderline high total blood cholesterol (between 200 and 239 mg/dl), these margarines can be helpful in avoiding future drug therapy. Plant stanols/sterols have been made available in pill form as well. Remember that plant sterols are naturally present in nuts in high concentrations. Wheat germ, sesame seeds, pistachios, and sunflower seeds are some of the richest sources.

The two most common surgical treatments for coronary artery blockage are percutaneous transluminal coronary angioplasty (PTCA) and coronary artery bypass graft (CABG). PTCA involves the insertion of a balloon catheter into an artery. Once it is advanced to the area of the lesion, the balloon is expanded to crush the lesion. This method works best when only one vessel is blocked, and it may be held open with metal mesh, called a stent. CABG involves the removal and use of a saphenous vein, a large vein in the leg, or use of a mammary artery. The relocated vein is sewn to the main heart vessel (aorta) and then used to bypass the blocked artery. The procedure can be performed on one or more blockages.

▲ Benecol and Take Control are margarines that are examples of "functional foods" because they contain added cholesterol-lowering plant stanols/sterols.

TABLE 5-9 Sorting Out One's Goals for Cardiovascular Disease Prevention/Treatment

Risk Class	This Is You If . . .	Your LDL (mg/dl) goal
Very high	You have cardiovascular disease and other risk factors such as diabetes, obesity, smoking	Below 70
High	You have cardiovascular disease or diabetes or two or more risk factors for cardiovascular disease (e.g., smoking, hypertension)	Below 100
Moderately high	You have cardiovascular disease risks and an increased 10-year risk of developing a heart attack	100–130
Moderate	You have 2 or more risk factors and a marginal chance of developing cardiovascular disease in the next 10 years.	Below 130
Low	You have few or no cardiovascular disease risk factors	Below 160

CASE STUDY

Planning a Heart Healthy Diet

Jackie is a 21-year-old health-conscious individual majoring in business. She recently learned that a diet high in saturated fat can contribute to high blood cholesterol and that exercise is beneficial for the heart. Jackie now takes a brisk 30-minute walk each morning before going to class, and she has started to cut as much fat out of her diet as she can, replacing it mostly with carbohydrates. A typical day for Jackie now begins with a bowl of Fruity Pebbles with 1 cup of skim milk and ½ cup of apple juice. For lunch, she might pack a turkey sandwich on white bread with lettuce, tomato, and mustard; a small package of fat-free pretzels; and a handful of reduced-fat vanilla wafers. Dinner could be a large portion of pasta with some olive oil and garlic mixed in, and a small iceberg lettuce salad with lemon juice squeezed over it. Her snacks are usually baked chips, low-fat cookies, fat-free frozen yogurt, or fat-free pretzels. She drinks diet soft drinks throughout the day as her main beverage.

▲ Are there important food groups missing from Jackie's new diet plan?

Answer the following questions, and check your response in Appendix A.

1. Has Jackie made the best diet changes with regard to lowering blood cholesterol and maintaining heart health?
2. Is there much fat left in Jackie's new diet plan? Is it necessary for her to drastically lower her fat intake?
3. What types of fat should Jackie try to consume? Why are these types of fat the most desirable?
4. What types of foods has Jackie used to replace the fat in her diet?
5. What food groups are missing from her new diet plan? How many servings should she be including from these food groups?
6. Is Jackie's new exercise routine appropriate?

SUMMARY

1. Compared with carbohydrates and proteins, lipids are a group of relatively oxygen-poor compounds that do not dissolve in water. Saturated fatty acids contain no carbon-carbon double bonds, monounsaturated fatty acids contain one carbon-carbon double bond, and polyunsaturated fatty acids contain two or more carbon-carbon double bonds in the carbon chain.

2. In omega-3 polyunsaturated fatty acids, the first of the carbon-carbon double bonds is located three carbons from the methyl end of the carbon chain. In omega-6 polyunsaturated fatty acids, the first carbon-carbon double bond counting from the methyl end occurs at the sixth carbon. Both omega-3 and omega-6 fatty acids are essential fatty acids; these must be included in the diet to maintain health.

3. Triglycerides are formed from a glycerol backbone with three fatty acids. Triglycerides rich in long-chain saturated fatty acids tend to be solid at room temperature, whereas those rich in mono-unsaturated and polyunsaturated fatty acids are liquid at room temperature. Triglyceride is the major form of fat in both food and the body. It allows for efficient energy storage, protects certain organs, transports fat-soluble vitamins, and helps insulate the body.

4. Phospholipids are derivatives of triglycerides in which one or two of the fatty acids are replaced by phosphorus-containing compounds. Phospholipids are important parts of cell membranes, and some act as efficient emulsifiers.

5. Cholesterol forms vital biological compounds, such as hormones, components of cell membranes, and bile acids. Cells in the body make cholesterol whether we eat it or not. It is not a necessary part of an adult's diet.

6. Body cells can synthesize hormone-like compounds from both omega-3 and omega-6 fatty acids. The compounds produced from omega-3 fatty acids tend to reduce blood clotting, blood pressure, and inflammatory responses in the body. Those produced from omega-6 fatty acids tend to increase blood clotting.

7. Foods rich in fat include salad oils, butter, margarine, and mayonnaise. Nuts, bologna, avocados, and bacon are also high in fat, as are peanut butter and cheddar cheese. Steak and hamburger are moderate in fat content, as is whole milk. Many grain products, and fruits and vegetables in general, are low in fat.

8. Fats and oils have several functions as components of foods. Fats add flavor and texture to foods and provide some satiety after meals. Some phospholipids are used in foods as emulsifiers, which suspend fat in water. When fatty acids break down, food becomes rancid, resulting in a foul odor and unpleasant flavor.

9. Hydrogenation is the process of converting carbon-carbon double bonds into single bonds by adding hydrogen at the point of unsaturation. The

partial-hydrogenation of fatty acids in vegetable oils changes the oils to semisolid fats and helps in food formulation and reduces rancidity. Hydrogenation also increases *trans* fatty acid content. High amounts of *trans* fat in the diet are discouraged, as these increase LDL and reduce HDL.

10. Fat digestion takes place primarily in the small intestine. Lipase enzyme released from the pancreas digests long-chain triglycerides into smaller breakdown products—namely, monoglycerides (glycerol backbones with single fatty acids attached) and fatty acids. The breakdown products are then taken up by the absorptive cells of the small intestine. These products are mostly remade into triglycerides and eventually enter the lymphatic system, in turn passing into the bloodstream.

11. Lipids are carried in the bloodstream by various lipoproteins, which consist of a central triglyceride core encased in a shell of protein, cholesterol, and phospholipid. Chylomicrons are released from intestinal cells and carry lipids arising from dietary intake. Very-low-density lipoprotein (VLDL) and low-density lipoprotein (LDL) carry lipids both taken up by and synthesized in the liver. High-density lipoprotein (HDL) picks up cholesterol from cells and facilitates its transport back to the liver.

12. There is currently no RDA for fat for adults. Plant oils should contribute about 5% of total calories to achieve the Adequate Intakes proposed for essential fatty acids (linoleic acid and alpha-linolenic acid). Fatty fish are a rich source of omega-3 fatty acids and should be consumed at least twice a week.

13. Many health agencies and scientific groups suggest a fat intake of no more than 30% to 35% of total calories. Some health experts advocate an even further reduction to 20% of calorie intake for some people to maintain a normal LDL value, but such a diet requires professional guidance. Medications such as "statins" may be added also to lower LDL. If fat intake exceeds 30% of total calories, the diet should emphasize monounsaturated fat. The typical North American diet contains about 33% of total calories as fat.

14. In the blood, elevated amounts of LDL and low amounts of HDL are strong predictors of the risk for cardiovascular disease. Additional risk factors for the disease are smoking, hypertension, diabetes, obesity, and inactivity.

STUDY QUESTIONS

1. Describe the chemical structures of saturated and polyunsaturated fatty acids and their different effects in both food and the human body.

2. Relate the need for omega-3 fatty acids in the diet to the recommendation to consume fatty fish at least twice a week.

3. Describe the structures, origins, and roles of the four major blood lipoproteins.

4. What are the recommendations from various health-care organizations

regarding fat intake? What does this mean in terms of food choices?

5. What are two important attributes of fat in food? How are these different from the general functions of lipids in the human body?

6. Describe the significance of and possible uses for reduced-fat foods.

7. Does the total cholesterol concentration in the bloodstream tell the whole

story with respect to cardiovascular disease risk?

8. List the four main risk factors for the development of cardiovascular disease.

9. What three lifestyle factors decrease the risk of cardiovascular disease development?

10. When are medications most needed in cardiovascular disease therapy, and how in general do the various classes of medications operate to reduce risk?

CHECK YOUR KNOWLEDGE

Answers to the following multiple choice questions are in Appendix A.

1. Margarine usually is made by a process called _____, in which hydrogen atoms are added to carbon-carbon double bonds in the polyunsaturated fatty acids found in vegetable oils.
   a. saturation
   b. esterification
   c. isomerization
   d. hydrogenation

2. Essential fatty acids that cause a decrease in blood clotting are
   a. omega-3.
   b. omega-6.
   c. omega-9.
   d. prostacyclins.

3. Cholesterol is
   a. a dietary essential; the human body cannot synthesize it.
   b. found in foods of plant origin.

   c. an important part of human cell membranes and necessary to make some hormones.
   d. All of the above.

4. Which of the following groups of foods would be important sources of saturated fatty acids?
   a. olive oil, peanut oil, canola oil
   b. palm oil, palm kernel oil, coconut oil
   c. safflower oil, corn oil, soybean oil
   d. All of the above.

5. Lipoproteins are important for
   a. transport of fats in the blood and lymphatic system.
   b. synthesis of triglycerides.
   c. synthesis of adipose tissue.
   d. enzyme production.

6. Which of the following foods is the best source of omega-3 fatty acids?
   a. fatty fish
   b. peanut butter and jelly
   c. lard and shortenings
   d. beef and other red meats

7. Immediately after a meal, newly digested and absorbed dietary fats appear in the lymph, and then blood, as part of which of the following?
   a. LDL
   b. HDL
   c. chylomicrons
   d. cholesterol

8. High blood concentrations of _____ decrease the risk for cardiovascular disease.
   a. low-density lipoproteins
   b. chylomicrons
   c. high-density lipoproteins
   d. cholesterol

9. Phospholipids such as lecithin are used extensively in food preparation because they
   a. provide the agreeable feel of fat melting on the tongue.
   b. are excellent emulsifiers.
   c. provide important textural features.
   d. impart delicate flavors.

10. The main form of lipid found in the food we eat is
    a. cholesterol.
    b. phospholipids.
    c. triglycerides.
    d. plant sterols

FURTHER READINGS

1. ADA Reports: Position of the American Dietetic Association: Fat replacers. *Journal of the American Dietetic Association* 105:266, 2005.

   The majority of fat replacers, when used in moderation by adults, can be safe and useful adjuncts to lowering the fat content of foods and may play a role in decreasing total calorie and fat intake. Still, consumers should not be led to believe that fat and calorie-reduced products can be consumed in unlimited amounts

2. Bønaa KH and others: Homocysteine lowering and cardiovascular events after acute myocardial infarction. *The New England Journal of Medicine* 354:1578, 2006.

   The risk of recurrent cardiovascular disease after acute myocardial infarction was not lowered by treatment with folic acid, vitamin B-12, or vitamin B-6. A trend toward an increased risk suggested a harmful effect of the combined B vitamin treatment. Treatment with these B vitamins is therefore not recommended.

3. Diercks DB and others: The obesity paradox in non–ST-segment elevation acute coronary syndromes. *American Heart Journal* 152:140, 2006.

   This study discovered that although obese individuals are at increased risk of suffering a heart attack, their outcomes are better because they are treated more aggressively. Overweight and obese patients were more likely than normal-weight patients to receive medications and to have invasive cardiac procedures.

4. Fisler JS, Warden CH: Dietary fat and genotype: Toward individualized prescriptions for lifestyle changes. *American Journal of Clinical Nutrition* 81:1255, 2005.

   There is great variation in the effect of dietary fat on blood lipids. At least part of that variation is due to genetics. This article discusses the challenges involved in identifying the interactive effects of nutrients and genes in the area of lipids, cholesterol, and coronary artery disease.

5. Fletcher B and others: Managing abnormal blood lipids: A collaborative approach. *Circulation* 112:3184, 2005.

   The treatment of abnormal blood lipids is complex and therefore requires involvement of various types of healthcare professionals, including dietitians. This paper describes a model multidisciplinary case management approach for patients with abnormal blood lipids. The model includes both primary and secondary prevention across the lifespan and incorporates nutritional and exercise intervention.

6. Grundy SM and others: Diagnosis and management of the metabolic syndrome. *Circulation* 112: 1350, 2005.

   The constellation of metabolic risk factors known as metabolic syndrome consists of many factors, including elevated blood triglycerides, low HDL cholesterol concentrations, elevated blood pressure, elevated blood glucose, increased blood clotting, and an inflammatory state in the body. The most important of these underlying risk factors are abdominal obesity and insulin resistance. Other associated conditions include physical inactivity, aging, hormonal imbalance, and genetic or ethnic predisposition.

7. Hansson GK: Inflammation, atherosclerosis, and coronary artery disease. *The New England Journal of Medicine* 352:1685, 2005.

   Excellent review of the role of inflammation in causing cardiovascular disease. Identifying atherosclerosis as an inflammatory disease offers new opportunities for the prevention and treatment of coronary artery disease.

8. He KA, Daviglus ML: A few more thoughts about fish and fish oil. *Journal of the American Dietetic Association* 105:428, 2005.

   Fish consumption has been shown to have beneficial effects on cardiovascular disease. Consuming whole fish is thought to have greater benefits and be safer than using fish oil supplements. Fish is not only a rich source of omega-3 fatty acids, but is also a valuable source of protein and trace elements that may also provide protective effects for the cardiovascular system. Broiled or baked fish is recommended rather than fried fish because frying may decrease the ratio of omega-3 to omega-6 fatty acids and may produce trans *fatty acids and oxidized lipid products that may increase cardiovascular disease risk.*

9. Kuller LH: Nutrition, lipids, and cardiovascular disease. *Nutrition Reviews* 64:S15, 2006.

   The development of coronary heart disease is discussed as an epidemic due to increased consumption of saturated fat and cholesterol, low intakes of polyunsaturated fat, and obesity. The risk of the disease is increased by hypertension, smoking, and diabetes. The careful monitoring and prevention of this disease beginning in young adults is important but expensive.

10. Lau VWY and others: Plant sterols are efficacious in lowering plasma LDL and non-HDL cholesterol in hypercholesterolemic type 2 diabetic and nondiabetic persons. *American Journal of Clinical Nutrition* 81:1351, 2005.

    Incorporation of plant sterols into a low-saturated-fat and low-cholesterol diet for persons at increased risk of CVD mortality could have a positive effect on reducing the mortality rate, including in those people with type 2 diabetes.

11. Lee I and others: Vitamin E in the primary prevention of cardiovascular disease and cancer: The women's health study: A randomized controlled trial. *Journal of the American Medical Association* 294:56, 2005.

The data from this large trial indicated that 600 IU of natural-source vitamin E taken every other day provided no overall benefit for major cardiovascular events or cancer. These data do not support recommending vitamin E supplementation for cardiovascular disease or cancer prevention among healthy women, but more research is warranted, as a decrease in sudden cardiac death was seen in a subset of older women in this study.

12. Lewis NM and others: The walnut: A nutritional nut case. *Today's Dietitian* 6(8):36, 2004.

Compared to other nuts and seeds, walnuts are one of the richest sources of alpha-linolenic acid (2.6 grams per 1-ounce serving or 14 walnut halves). The DRI for alpha-linolenic acid is 1.6 grams/day for men and 1.1 grams/day for women. In addition, walnuts are a rich source of plant sterols known to inhibit intestinal absorption of cholesterol.

13. Lichtenstein AH and others: Diet and lifestyle recommendations revision 2006. A scientific statement from the American Heart Association Nutrition Committee. *Circulation* 114:82, 2006.

The American Heart Association presents recommendations designed to reduce the risk of cardiovascular disease risk reduction in the general population. Specific goals are presented and include consuming an overall healthy diet; to aim for a healthy body weight, recommended levels of low-density lipoprotein cholesterol, high-density lipoprotein cholesterol, and triglycerides; normal blood pressure; normal blood glucose level; being physically active; and avoiding the use of and exposure to tobacco products.

14. Lonn E and others: Effects of long-term vitamin E supplementation on cardiovascular events and cancer: A randomized controlled trial. *Journal of the American Medical Association* 293:1338, 2005.

No significant differences were noted between the vitamin E supplementation group and the control group in the incidence of cancer or deaths related to cancer. There also were no differences in the main composite of cardiovascular outcomes including death or rehospitalization. A significant increased risk in heart failure and related complications occurred in the vitamin E group.

15. Lukaczer D and others: Effect of a low glycemic index diet with soy protein and phytosterols on CVD risk factors in postmenopausal women. *Nutrition* 22(2):104, 2006.

Women in this 12-week study showed decreases in total cholesterol, LDL cholesterol, and triglycerides after consuming a low-glycemic index diet with a functional food delivering 30 grams of soy protein and 4 grams of phytosterols per day.

16. Meisinger C and others: Plasma oxidized low-density lipoprotein, a strong predictor for acute coronary heart disease events in apparently healthy, middle-aged men from the general population. *Circulation* 112:651, 2005.

Elevated concentrations of oxidized low-density lipoprotein are predictive of future coronary heart disease events in apparently healthy men. Thus, oxidized LDL may represent a promising risk marker for clinical coronary heart disease complications and should be evaluated in further studies.

17. Ohr LM: The (heart) beat goes on. *Food Technology* 60(6):87, 2006.

Research and ingredient innovations in the food industry related to the heart-health field are described. Ingredients that have the advantage of a heart-health claim include omega-3 fatty acids and plant sterols. Also discussed are dietary fiber and grains, soy, antioxidants, and nuts.

18. Phillips KM and others: Phytosterol composition of nuts and seeds commonly consumed in the United States. *Journal of Agriculture and Food Chemistry* 53:9436, 2005.

This study set out to find the nuts and seeds that could provide the most heart-protective benefits. Of the 27 nuts and seeds analyzed, wheat germ and sesame seeds had the greatest concentration of phytosterols and Brazil nuts and walnuts ranked the lowest. Pistachio and sunflower seeds were the richest sources of phytosterols for products typically consumed as snack foods.

19. Reese MATB: Beyond the headlines: The lowdown on low-fat diets. *Today's Dietitian* 8(6):32, 2006.

Results of the 8-year Women's Health Initiative study showed that a reduction in dietary fat had almost no effect on the incidence of heart attacks and strokes or breast and colon cancer. This article explains some of the study characteristics that most likely contributed to the unexpected results. Most important to consider is that the subjects were all postmenopausal women who had all been on a high-fat diet. The results suggest that starting a low-fat diet at 50 to 79 years may be too late to see extraordinary benefits.

20. Wang C and others: n-3 fatty acids from fish or fish-oil supplements, but not alpha-linolenic acid, benefit cardiovascular disease outcomes in primary- and secondary-prevention studies: A systematic review. *American Journal of Clinical Nutrition* 84:5, 2006.

This review of previous studies found that consumption of omega-3 fatty acids from fish or fish oil but not alpha-linolenic acid, significantly reduced all-cause mortality, myocardial infarction, cardiac and sudden death, or stroke.

▶ Check out the **Contemporary Nutrition ARIS site**
www.mhhe.com/wardlawcontfa1 for quizzes, flash cards, other activities, and weblinks designed to further help you learn about what you eat and why.

I. Are You Eating a Diet That Includes Many Saturated Fat and *Trans* Fatty Acid Sources?

Instructions: In each row of the following list, circle your typical food selection from either column A or B.

Column A		Column B
Bacon and eggs	*or*	Ready-to-eat whole-grain breakfast cereal
Doughnut or sweet roll	*or*	Whole-wheat roll, bagel, or bread
Breakfast sausage	*or*	Fruit
Whole milk	*or*	Reduced-fat, low-fat, or fat-free milk
Cheeseburger	*or*	Turkey sandwich, no cheese
French fries	*or*	Plain baked potato with salsa
Ground chuck	*or*	Ground round
Soup with cream base	*or*	Soup with broth base
Macaroni and cheese	*or*	Macaroni with marinara sauce
Cream/fruit pie	*or*	Graham crackers
Ice cream	*or*	Frozen yogurt, sherbet, or reduced-fat ice cream
Butter or stick margarine	*or*	Vegetable oils or soft margarine in a tub

Interpretation

The foods listed in column A tend to be high in saturated fat, *trans* fatty acids, cholesterol, and total fat. Those in column B generally are low in these dietary components. If you want to help reduce your risk of cardiovascular disease, choose more foods from column B and fewer from column A.

II. Applying the Nutrition Facts Label to Your Daily Food Choices

Imagine that you are at the supermarket looking for a quick snack to help you keep your energy up during afternoons. In the snack section, you settle on two choices (see labels a and b). Evaluate the products using the table on the left.

Compare the nutrients in each product by completing this list. For each serving, which product is lower in each of the following?

Calories	(a)	(b)	no difference
Calories from Fat	(a)	(b)	no difference
Total Fat	(a)	(b)	no difference
Saturated Fat	(a)	(b)	no difference
Trans Fat	(a)	(b)	no difference
Cholesterol	(a)	(b)	no difference
Sodium	(a)	(b)	no difference
Total Carbohydrates	(a)	(b)	no difference
Dietary Fiber	(a)	(b)	no difference
Sugars	(a)	(b)	no difference
Protein	(a)	(b)	no difference
Iron	(a)	(b)	no difference

Which package has more servings per container?
(a) (b) no difference

Which of the two brands would you choose?
(a) (b) neither

What information on the Nutrition Facts labels contributed to your decision?

Nutrition Facts

Serving Size: 2 bars (42g)
Servings Per Container: 6

Amount Per Serving	2 bars
Calories 180	Calories from Fat 50

	% Daily Value*
Total Fat 6g	9%
Saturated Fat 0.5g	3%
Trans fat 0g	**
Cholesterol 0mg	0%
Sodium 160mg	7%
Total Carbohydrates 29g	10%
Dietary Fiber 2g	8%
Sugars 11g	
Protein 4g	
Iron	6%

Not a significant source of Vitamin A, Vitamin C, and calcium.

** Intake of *trans* fat should be as low as possible.

* Daily values are based on a 2,000 calorie diet. Your daily values may be higher or lower depending on your calorie needs:

** Intake should be as low as possible.	Calories	2,000	2,500
Total Fat	Less than	65g	80g
Saturated Fat	Less than	20g	25g
Cholesterol	Less than	300mg	300mg
Sodium	Less than	2,400mg	2,400mg
Total Carbohydrates		300g	375g
Dietary Fiber		25g	30g

INGREDIENTS: WHOLE GRAIN ROLLED OATS, SUGAR, CANOLA OIL, CRISP RICE WITH SOY PROTEIN (RICE FLOUR, SOY PROTEIN CONCENTRATE, SUGAR, MALT, SALT), HONEY, BROWN SUGAR SYRUP, HIGH FRUCTOSE CORN SYRUP, SALT, SOY LECITHIN, BAKING SODA, NATURAL FLAVOR, PEANUT FLOUR, ALMOND FLOUR, HAZELNUT FLOUR, WALNUT FLOUR, PECAN FLOUR.

Nutrition Facts

Serving Size: 2 cookies (38g)
Servings Per Container: about 12

Amount Per Serving	
Calories 180	Calories from Fat 70

	% Daily Value*
Total Fat 7g	11%
Saturated Fat 2g	10%
Trans fat 2g	**
Cholesterol 0mg	0%
Sodium 100mg	4%
Total Carbohydrate 26g	9%
Dietary Fiber 1g	4%
Sugars 12g	
Protein 2g	

Vitamin A 0%	•	Vitamin C 0%
Calcium 0%	•	Iron 2%

** Intake of *trans* fat should be as low as possible.

* Daily values are based on a 2,000 calorie diet. Your daily values may be higher or lower depending on your calorie needs:

** Intake should be as low as possible.	Calories	2,000	2,500
Total Fat	Less than	65g	80g
Saturated Fat	Less than	20g	25g
Cholesterol	Less than	300mg	300mg
Sodium	Less than	2,400mg	2,400mg
Total Carbohydrates		300g	375g
Dietary Fiber		25g	30g

Calories per gram: • Fat 9 • Carbohydrate 4 • Protein 4

INGREDIENTS: ENRICHED FLOUR (WHEAT FLOUR, NIACIN, REDUCED IRON, THIAMINE MONONITRATE, RIBOFLAVIN, FOLIC ACID), SUGAR, VEGETABLE OIL SHORTENING (PARTIALLY HYDROGENATED SOYBEAN, COCONUT, COTTONSEED, CORN AND/OR SAFFLOWER AND/OR CANOLA OIL), CORN SYRUP, HIGH FRUCTOSE CORN SYRUP, WHEY (A MILK INGREDIENT), CORN STARCH, SALT, SKIM MILK, LEAVENING (BAKING SODA, AMMONIUM BICARBONATE), ARTIFICIAL FLAVOR, SOYBEAN LECITHIN, COLOR (CONTAINING FD&C YELLOW #5 LAKE).

CHAPTER 6 Proteins

CHAPTER OBJECTIVES Chapter 6 is designed to allow you to:

1. Describe how amino acids make up proteins.
2. Distinguish between essential and nonessential amino acids.
3. Explain why adequate amounts of each of the essential amino acids are required for protein synthesis.
4. List the primary functions of protein in the body.
5. Calculate the RDA for protein for an adult when a healthy weight is given.
6. Describe what is meant by positive protein balance, negative protein balance, and protein equilibrium.
7. Distinguish between high-quality and low-quality proteins, identify examples of each, and describe the concept of complementary proteins.
8. Describe how protein-calorie malnutrition eventually can lead to disease in the body.
9. Develop vegetarian diet plans that meet the body's nutritional needs.

CHAPTER OUTLINE

CONSUMING ENOUGH PROTEIN IS VITAL FOR MAINTAINING HEALTH. Proteins form important structures in the body, make up a key part of the blood, help regulate many body functions, and can fuel body cells.

North Americans generally eat more protein than is needed to maintain health. Our daily protein intake comes mostly from animal sources such as meat, poultry, fish, eggs, milk, and cheese. In contrast, in the developing world, diets can be deficient in protein. High-protein diets have come and gone over the past 30 years. Recently, these have become popular as weight-loss diets, with some containing about 35% of calories as protein. This figure falls within the latest advice for protein intake from the Food and Nutrition Board (10% to 35% of calorie intake), so in general these diets are appropriate if otherwise nutritionally sound (e.g., they follow MyPyramid).

Diets that are mostly vegetarian still predominate in much of Asia and areas of Africa, and some North Americans are currently adopting the practice. Plant sources of protein are worthy of more attention from North Americans. In the early 1900s, plant sources of proteins—nuts, seeds, and legumes—were consumed just as often as animal proteins. Over the years, though, plant proteins have been sidelined by meats. During this time, nuts have been viewed as high-fat foods, and beans have gotten the inferior reputation of "the poor man's meat." Contrary to these popular misconceptions, sources of plant proteins offer a wealth of nutritional benefits—from lowering blood cholesterol to preventing certain forms of cancer.

We could benefit from eating more plant sources of proteins. As shown in the comic in this chapter, it takes some knowledge to do so. It is possible—and desirable—to enjoy the benefits of animal and plant protein as we work toward the goal of meeting protein needs. This chapter takes a close look at protein, including the benefits of plant proteins in a diet. It will also examine vegetarian diets: their benefits and their risks, if not properly planned. Let's see why a detailed study of protein is worth your attention.

 Refresh Your Memory

As you begin your study of proteins in Chapter 6, you may want to review:

- Organization of the cell in Chapter 3
- The processes of digestion and absorption in Chapter 3
- The nervous system and immune system in Chapter 3
- The role of carbohydrates in preventing ketosis in Chapter 4

PROTEIN—AN INTRODUCTION

Diets in the developed parts of the world, such as the United States and Canada, are typically rich in protein, and therefore a specific focus on eating enough protein is generally not needed. In the developing world, however, it is important to focus on protein in diet planning because diets in those areas of the world can be deficient in protein.

FRANK & ERNEST® by Bob Thaves

Can a vegetarian diet provide enough protein? What is prompting the growing interest in various forms of vegetarian diets? Why are plant protein sources, especially soy and nuts, gaining more attention? Should meat-eaters abandon that dietary practice? Chapter 6 provides some answers.

High-protein diets have recently been popular as weight-loss diets. The latest advice from the Food and Nutrition Board allows for up to 35% of total calorie intake to be supplied by protein, so in general these diets are appropriate if otherwise nutritionally sound, especially with regard to being moderate in fat and having enough fiber. Still, as discussed in Chapter 7, these types of diets are hardly a magic wand for weight loss.

Thousands of substances in the body are made of proteins. Aside from water, proteins form the major part of lean body tissue, totaling about 17% of body weight. Amino acids—the building blocks for proteins—are unique in that they contain nitrogen bonded to carbon. Plants combine nitrogen from the soil with carbon and other elements to form amino acids. They then link these amino acids together to make proteins. We get the nitrogen we need by consuming dietary proteins. Proteins are thus an essential part of a diet because they supply nitrogen in a form we can readily use—namely, amino acids. Using simpler forms of nitrogen is, for the most part, impossible for humans.

Proteins are crucial to the regulation and maintenance of the body. Body functions such as blood clotting, fluid balance, hormone and enzyme production, visual processes, transport of many substances in the bloodstream, and cell repair require specific proteins. The body makes proteins in many configurations and sizes so that they can serve these greatly varied functions. Formation of these body proteins begins with amino acids from both the protein-containing foods we eat and those synthesized from other compounds within the body. Proteins can also be broken down to supply energy for the body—on average, 4 kcal per gram.

If you fail to consume an adequate amount of protein for weeks at a time, many metabolic processes slow down. This is because the body does not have enough amino acids available to build the proteins it needs. For example, the immune system no longer functions efficiently when it lacks key proteins, thereby increasing the risk of infections, disease, and death.

Amino Acids

Amino acids—the building blocks of proteins—are formed mostly of carbon, hydrogen, oxygen, and nitrogen. The following diagram shows the structure of a generic amino acid and also what one of the specific amino acids, glutamic acid, looks like. The amino acids have different chemical makeups, but all are slight variations of the generic amino acid pictured (see Appendix F). Each amino acid has an "acid" group; an "amino" group; and a "side" or R group specific to the amino acid.

The R group on some amino acids has a branched shape, like a tree. These so-called **branched-chain amino acids** are leucine, isoleucine, and valine (see Appendix F for the chemical structures of the amino acids). The branched-chain amino acids are the primary amino acids used by muscles for energy needs. This is one reason why proteins from milk (e.g., whey proteins) are popular with strength-training athletes (see Chapter 10 for details).

Acid group - - - - - - - - -

Side group - - - - - - - -

Amino group - - - - - - - - -

"Generic" amino acid. The R signifies another chemical group that would be present.

One example of an R group | Part of generic amino acid foundation

Glutamic acid

branched-chain amino acids Amino acids with a branching carbon backbone; these are leucine, isoleucine, and valine. All are essential amino acids.

nonessential amino acids Amino acids that can be synthesized by a healthy body in sufficient amounts; there are 11 nonessential amino acids. These are also called *dispensable amino acids.*

Your body needs to use 20 different amino acids to function (Table 6-1). Although all these commonly found amino acids are important, 11 are considered **nonessential** (also called *dispensable*) with respect to our diets. Human cells can produce these certain amino acids as long as the right ingredients are present—the key factor being

semiessential amino acids Amino acids that, when consumed, spare the need to use an essential amino acid for their synthesis. Tyrosine in the diet, for example, spares the need to use phenylalanine for tyrosine synthesis. Also called *conditionally essential amino acids.*

essential amino acids The amino acids that cannot be synthesized by humans in sufficient amounts or at all and therefore must be included in the diet; there are nine essential amino acids. These are also called *indispensable amino acids.*

limiting amino acid The essential amino acid in lowest concentration in a food or diet relative to body needs.

TABLE 6-1 Classification of Amino Acids

Essential Amino Acids	Nonessential Amino Acids
Histidine	Alanine
Isoleucine*	Arginine†
Leucine*	Asparagine
Lysine	Aspartic acid
Methionine	Cysteine†
Phenylalanine	Glutamic acid
Threonine	Glutamine†
Tryptophan	Glycine†
Valine*	Proline†
	Serine
	Tyrosine†

*A branched-chain amino acid

†These amino acids are also classed as **semiessential** (or conditionally essential). This means they must be made from essential amino acids if insufficient amounts are eaten.

nitrogen that is already part of another amino acid. Therefore it is not essential that these amino acids be in our diet.

The nine amino acids the body cannot make in sufficient amounts or at all are known as **essential** (also called *indispensable*)—they must be obtained from foods. This is because body cells either cannot make the needed carbon-based foundation of the amino acid, cannot put a nitrogen group on the needed carbon-based foundation, or just cannot do the whole process fast enough to meet body needs.

Eating a balanced diet can supply us with both the essential and nonessential amino-acid building blocks needed to maintain good health. Both nonessential and essential amino acids are present in foods that contain protein. If you don't eat enough essential amino acids, your body first struggles to conserve what essential amino acids it can. However, eventually your body progressively slows production of new proteins until at some point you will break protein down faster than you can make it. When that happens, health deteriorates.

The essential amino acid in smallest supply in a food or diet in relation to body needs becomes the limiting factor (called the **limiting amino acid**) because it limits the amount of protein the body can synthesize. For example, assume the letters of the alphabet represent the 20 or so different amino acids we consume. If *A* represents an essential amino acid, we need three of these letters to spell the hypothetical protein *BANANA*. If the body had a *B*, two *N*s, but only two *A*s, the "synthesis" of *BANANA* would not be possible. *A* would then be seen as the limiting amino acid.

Adults need only about 11% of their total protein requirement to be supplied by essential amino acids. Typical diets supply an average of 50% of protein as essential amino acids.

The estimated needs for essential amino acids for infants and preschool children are 40% of total protein intake; however, in later childhood the need drops to 20%. Diets designed for infants and young children need to take this into account to make sure enough proteins are present to yield a high-quality protein intake. Including some animal products in the diet, such as human milk or formula for infants, or cow's milk for children, helps

▲ When combined with vegetables, high-protein foods such as meats also help balance the amino acid content of the diet.

MAKING DECISIONS

Phenylketonuria

Some of the nonessential amino acids are also classed as **semiessential** (or conditionally essential). This means they must be made from essential amino acids if insufficient amounts are eaten. When that occurs, the body's supply of certain essential amino acids is depleted. Tyrosine is an example of a semiessential amino acid that can be made from the essential amino acid phenylalanine.

The disease phenylketonuria (PKU) illustrates the importance of phenylalanine to make tyrosine. Recall from Chapter 4 that a person with PKU has a limited ability to metabolize the essential amino acid phenylalanine. Normally, the body uses an enzyme to convert much of our dietary phenylalanine intake into tyrosine.

In PKU-diagnosed persons, the activity of the enzyme used in processing phenylalanine to tyrosine is insufficient. When the enzyme cannot synthesize enough tyrosine, both amino acids must be derived from foods. The point is that phenylalanine and tyrosine become *essential* in terms of dietary needs because the body can't produce enough tyrosine from phenylalanine. Phenylalanine levels in the blood increase because it is not converted to tyrosine. PKU is treated by limiting the consumption of phenylalanine with a special diet so that phenylalanine and its by-products do not rise to toxic concentrations in the body and cause the severe mental retardation seen in untreated PKU cases.

Rina is 7 months pregnant and has read about various tests that her baby will undergo when he or she is born. How can you explain to Rina the purpose and significance of one of those tests, the one that screens for PKU?

▲ Within the first few days of life all newborns are tested for phenylketonuria.

ensure this. Otherwise, complementary amino acids from plant proteins should be consumed in each meal or within two subsequent meals. A major health risk for infants and children occurs in famine situations in which only one type of cereal grain is available, increasing the probability that one or more of the nine essential amino acids is lacking in the total diet. This is discussed further in a later section on protein-calorie malnutrition.

CONCEPT CHECK

The human body uses 20 different amino acids from protein-containing foods. A healthy body can synthesize 11 of the amino acids, so it is not necessary to obtain all amino acids from foods—only nine of these must come from the diet and are therefore termed *essential (indispensable) amino acids*. The essential amino acid in smallest supply in a food in relation to body needs is called the limiting amino acid because it limits the amount of protein the body can synthesize.

PROTEINS—AMINO ACIDS BONDED TOGETHER

Amino acids are linked together by chemical bonds—technically called **peptide bonds**—to form proteins. Although these bonds are difficult to break, acids, enzymes, and other agents are able to do so—for example, during digestion.

The body can synthesize many different proteins by linking together the 20 common types of amino acids with peptide bonds.

peptide bond   A chemical bond formed between amino acids in a protein.

Protein Synthesis

Our discussion of protein synthesis, begins with DNA. DNA is present in the nucleus of the cell and contains coded instructions for protein synthesis (i.e., which specific amino acids are to be placed in a protein and in which order). Recall from Chapter 3 that DNA is a double-stranded molecule.

Protein synthesis in a cell, however, takes place in the cytoplasm, not in the nucleus. Thus, the DNA code used for synthesis of a specific protein must be transferred from the

polypeptide   A group of amino acids bonded together, from 50 to 2000 or more.

▲ Genes are present on DNA—a double-stranded helix. The cell nucleus contains most of the DNA in the body.

1 DNA contains the information necessary to produce proteins.

2 Transcription or copying of a segment of DNA results in mRNA, a copy of the information in DNA needed to make a protein.

3 The mRNA leaves the nucleus and goes to a ribosome.

4 Amino acids, the building blocks of proteins, are carried to the ribosome by tRNAs containing the code that matches that on the mRNA.

5 In the process of translation, the information contained in mRNA is used to determine the number, types, and arrangement of amino acids in the protein.

nucleus to the cytoplasm to allow for protein synthesis. This transfer is the job of messenger RNA (mRNA). Enzymes in the nucleus read the code on one segment (a gene) of one strand of the DNA and *transcribe* that information into a single-stranded mRNA molecule (Fig. 6-1). This mRNA undergoes processing and then it is ready to leave the nucleus.

Once in the cytoplasm, mRNA travels to the ribosomes. The ribosomes read the mRNA code and *translate* those instructions to produce a specific protein. Amino acids are added one at a time to the growing **polypeptide** chain according to the instructions on the mRNA. Another key participant in protein synthesis, transfer RNA (tRNA), is responsible for bringing the specific amino acids to the ribosomes as needed during protein synthesis (review Fig. 6-1). Energy input is required to add each amino acid to the chain, making protein synthesis "costly" in terms of calorie use.

Once synthesis of a polypeptide is complete, it twists and folds into the appropriate three-dimensional structure of the intended protein. These structural changes occur based on specific interactions between the amino acids that make up the polypeptide chain (see the next section on protein organization for details). Some polypeptides, such as the hormone insulin, also undergo further changes in the cell before they are functional.

The important message in this discussion is the relationship between DNA and the proteins eventually produced by a cell. If the DNA code contains errors, an incorrect mRNA will be produced. The ribosomes will then read this incorrect message and an incorrect amino acid will be added and an incorrect polypeptide chain will be produced. As discussed in Chapter 3, genetic engineering may ultimately be able to correct many gene defects in humans, by placing the correct DNA code in the nucleus, so that the correct protein can be made by the ribosomes.

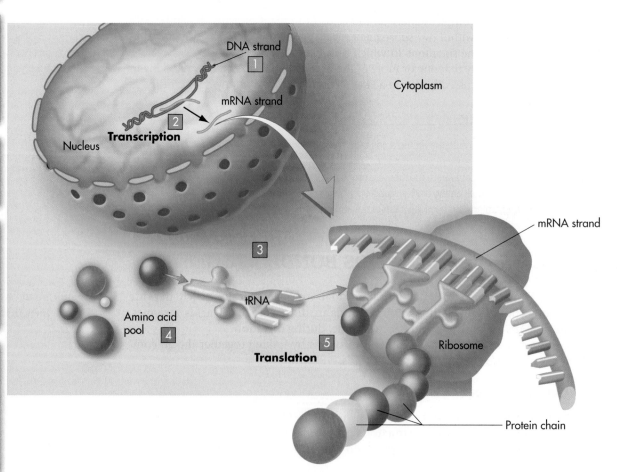

DNA strand

mRNA strand

Cytoplasm

Transcription

Nucleus

mRNA strand

tRNA

Amino acid pool

Translation

Ribosome

Protein chain

FIGURE 6-1 ▶ Protein synthesis (simplified). Once the mRNA is fully read, the amino acids have been connected into the polypeptide which is released into the cytoplasm. It generally is then processed further to become a cell protein.

Protein Organization

As noted before, by bonding together various combinations of the 20 common types of amino acids, the body synthesizes thousands of different proteins. The sequential order of the amino acids then ultimately determines the protein's shape. The main point is that only correctly positioned amino acids can interact and fold properly to form the intended shape for the protein. The resulting unique, three-dimensional form goes on to dictate the function of each particular protein (Fig. 6-2). If it lacks the proper structure, a protein cannot function.

Sickle cell disease (also called **sickle cell anemia**) is one example of what happens when amino acids are out of order on a protein. North Americans of African descent are especially prone to this genetic disease. It occurs because of defects in the structure of the protein chains of hemoglobin, a protein that carries oxygen in red blood cells. In two of its four protein chains, an error in the amino-acid order occurs. This error produces a profound change in hemoglobin structure. It can no longer form the shape needed to carry oxygen efficiently inside the red blood cell. Instead of forming normal circular disks, the red blood cells collapse into crescent (or sickle) shapes (Fig. 6-3). Health deteriorates, and eventually episodes of severe pain in the bones and joints, abdominal pain, headaches, convulsions, and paralysis may occur.

These life-threatening symptoms are caused by a minute, but critical, error in the hemoglobin amino-acid order. Why does this error happen? It results from a defect in a person's genetic blueprint, DNA, inherited through one's parents. A defect in the DNA can dictate that a wrong amino acid will be built into the sequence of the body proteins. Many diseases, including cancer, stem from errors in the DNA code.

Denaturation of Proteins

Exposure to acid or alkaline substances, heat, or agitation can alter a protein's structure, leaving it unraveled or otherwise deformed. This process of altering the three-dimensional structure of a protein is called **denaturation** (see Fig. 6-7 on p. 213). Changing a protein's shape often destroys its ability to function normally, such that it loses its biological activity.

Denaturation of proteins is useful for some body processes, especially digestion. The heat produced during cooking denatures some proteins. After food is ingested, the secretion of stomach acid denatures some bacterial proteins, plant hormones, many active enzymes, and other forms of proteins in foods, making it safer to eat. Digestion is also enhanced by denaturation because the unraveling increases exposure of the polypeptide chain to digestive enzymes. Denaturing proteins in some foods can also reduce their tendencies to cause allergic reactions.

FIGURE 6-2 ▶ Protein organization. Proteins often form a coiled shape, as shown by this drawing of the blood protein hemoglobin. This shape is dictated by the order of the amino acids in the protein chain. To get an idea of its size, consider that each teaspoon (5 milliliters) of blood contains about 10^{18} hemoglobin molecules. One billion is 10^9.

sickle cell disease (sickle cell anemia) An illness that results from a malformation of the red blood cell because of an incorrect structure in part of its hemoglobin protein chains. The disease can lead to episodes of severe bone and joint pain, abdominal pain, headache, convulsions, paralysis, and even death.

denaturation Alteration of a protein's three-dimensional structure, usually because of treatment by heat, enzymes, acid or alkaline solutions, or agitation.

(a)

(b)

FIGURE 6-3 ▶ An example of the consequences of errors in DNA coding of proteins. (a) Normal red cell, (b) red blood cells from a person with sickle cell disease. Note the abnormal crescent (sickle-like) shape of the red blood cell near the center that reduces the ability of the cell to carry oxygen.

Recall that we need the essential amino acids that the proteins in the diet supply—not the proteins themselves. We dismantle ingested dietary proteins and use the amino acid building blocks to assemble the proteins we need.

CONCEPT CHECK

Amino acids are bonded together in specific sequences to form distinct proteins. DNA provides the directions for synthesizing these new proteins. Specifically, DNA directs the order of the amino acids on the protein. The amino acid order within a protein determines its ultimate shape and function. Destroying the shape of a protein denatures it. Stomach acid, heat, and other factors can denature proteins, causing them to lose their biological activity. Proteins must be denatured during digestion so that amino acids are available for absorption.

PROTEIN IN FOODS

Of the typical foods we eat, about 70% of our protein comes from animal sources (Fig. 6-4). The most nutrient-dense source of protein is water-packed tuna, which has 87% of calories as protein (Fig. 6-5). The top five contributors of protein to the North

MyPyramid: Food Sources of Protein

Food Group	Grains	Vegetables	Fruits	Oils	Milk	Meat & Beans
Sources of Protein	• Bread • Breakfast cereals • Rice • Noodles	• Carrots • Corn • Broccoli	• Apples • Oranges • Bananas	• None	• Milk • Yogurt • Cheese	• Meat • Eggs • Fish • Dry beans • Nuts
Grams per Serving	2–3	2–3	<1	<1	8–10	7

FIGURE 6-4 ▶ Sources of protein from MyPyramid. The height of the background color (none, 1/3, 2/3, or completely covered) within each group in the pyramid indicates the average nutrient density for protein in that group. Overall, the milk group and the meat & beans group contain many foods that are nutrient-dense sources of protein. Based on serving sizes listed for MyPyramid, the fruits group and oils group provide little or no protein (less than 1 gram per serving). Food choices from the vegetables group and grains group provide moderate amounts of protein (2 to 3 grams per serving). The milk group provides much protein (8 to 10 grams per serving), as does the meat & beans group (7 grams per serving). With regard to physical activity, proteins are a minor source of fuel for most endeavors, but can become somewhat important during endurance activities.

Food Sources of Protein

Food Item and Amount	Protein (grams)	% RDA
RDA	56*	100%
Canned tuna, 3 ounces	21.6	38.6%
Broiled chicken, 3 ounces	21.3	38%
Beef chuck, 3 ounces	15.3	27%
Yogurt, 1 cup	10.6	19%
Kidney beans, ½ cup	8.1	14.5%
1% low-fat milk, 1 cup	8.0	14%
Peanuts, 1 ounce	7.3	13%
Cheddar cheese, 1 ounce	7.0	12.5%
Egg, 1	5.5	10%
Cooked corn, ½ cup	2.7	5%
Seven grain bread, 1 slice	2.6	4.6%
White rice, ½ cup	2.1	4%
Pasta, 1 ounce	1.2	2%
Banana, 1	1.2	2%
* for 70 kg man		

Key:
- Grains
- Vegetables
- Fruits
- Oils
- Milk
- Meat & Beans

FIGURE 6-5 ▶ Food sources of protein compared to the RDA of 56 grams for a 70 kg man.

American diet are beef, poultry, milk, white bread, and cheese. In North America, meat and poultry consumption amounts to about 150 pounds per person per year. Worldwide, 35% of protein comes from animal sources. In Africa and East Asia, only about 20% of the protein eaten comes from animal sources.

Protein Quality of Foods

Animal and plant proteins can differ greatly in their proportions of essential and nonessential amino acids. Animal proteins contain ample amounts of all nine essential amino acids. (Gelatin—made from the animal protein collagen—is an exception because it loses one essential amino acid during processing and is low in other essential amino acids.) With the exception of soy protein, plant proteins don't match our need for essential amino acids as precisely as animal proteins. Many plant proteins, especially those found in grains, are low in one or more of the nine essential amino acids.

As you might expect, human tissue composition resembles animal tissue more than it does plant tissue. The similarities enable us to use proteins from any single animal source more efficiently to support human growth and maintenance than we do those from any single plant source. For this reason, animal proteins, except gelatin, are considered **high-quality** (also called **complete**) **proteins**, which contain the nine essential amino acids we need in sufficient amounts. Individual plant sources of proteins, except for soy beans, are considered **lower-quality** (also called **incomplete**) **proteins** because their amino-acid patterns can be quite different from ours. Thus, a single plant protein source, such as corn alone, cannot easily support body growth and maintenance. To obtain a sufficient amount of essential amino acids, a variety of plant proteins need to be consumed because each plant protein lacks adequate amounts of one or more essential amino acids.

When only lower-quality protein foods are consumed, enough of the essential amino acids needed for protein synthesis may not be obtained. Therefore, when compared to

▲ Small amounts of animal protein in a meal easily add up to meet daily protein needs.

high-quality (complete) proteins
Dietary proteins that contain ample amounts of all nine essential amino acids.

lower-quality (incomplete) proteins
Dietary proteins that are low in or lack one or more essential amino acids.

high-quality proteins, a greater amount of lower-quality protein is needed to meet the needs of protein synthesis. Moreover, once any of the nine essential amino acids in the plant protein we have eaten is used up, further protein synthesis becomes impossible. Because the depletion of just one of the essential amino acids prevents protein synthesis, the process illustrates the *all-or-none principle:* Either all essential amino acids are available or none can be used. The remaining amino acids would then be used for energy needs, or converted to carbohydrate or fat.

When two or more proteins combine to compensate for deficiencies in essential amino acid content in each protein, the proteins are called **complementary proteins.** Mixed diets generally provide high-quality protein because a complementary protein pattern results. Therefore, healthy adults should have little concern about balancing foods to yield the proteins needed to obtain enough of all nine essential amino acids. Even on plant-based diets, complementary proteins need not be consumed at the same meal by adults. Meeting amino-acid needs over the course of a day is a reasonable goal because there is a ready supply of amino acids from those present in body cells and in the blood (see Fig. 6-10 on page 217).

In general, plant sources of protein deserve more attention and use than they currently receive from many North Americans. Plant foods contribute fewer calories to the diet than most animal products and they supply an ample amount of protein, plus magnesium, plenty of fiber, and several other nutritional benefits (Fig. 6-6). The vegetable proteins we eat are a heart-healthy alternative to animal proteins because they contain no cholesterol and little saturated fat, aside from that added during processing or cooking. Legumes and nut sources of protein especially have received a lot of recent attention.

complementary proteins Two food protein sources that make up for each other's inadequate supply of specific essential amino acids; together they yield a sufficient amount of all nine and, so provide high-quality (complete) protein for the diet.

CRITICAL THINKING

Leon, a vegetarian, has heard of the "all-or-none principle" of protein synthesis but doesn't understand how this principle applies to protein synthesis in the body. He asks you, "How important is this nutritional concept for diet planning?" How would you answer his question?

A Closer Look at Plant Sources of Proteins

In proportion to the amount of calories they supply, plant foods provide not only protein, but also magnesium, fiber, folate, vitamin E, iron (absorption is increased by the vitamin C also present), zinc, and some calcium. In addition, phytochemicals from these foods are implicated in prevention of a wide variety of chronic diseases.

Nuts have a hard shell surrounding an edible kernel. Almonds, pistachios, walnuts, and pecans are some common examples. The defining characteristic of a nut is that it grows on a tree. (Peanuts, because they grow underground, are legumes.) Seeds (such as pumpkin, sesame, and sunflower seeds) differ from nuts in that seeds grow on vegetable or flowering plants, but they are similar to nuts in nutrient composition. In general, nuts and seeds supply 160 to 190 kcal, 6 to 10 grams of protein, and 14 to 19 grams of fat per 1 ounce serving. Although they are a dense source of calories, nuts and seeds make a powerful contribution to health when consumed in moderation.

Legumes are a plant family with pods that contain a single row of seeds. Besides peanuts, examples include garden and black-eyed peas, kidney beans, great northern beans, lentils, and soy beans. Dried varieties of the mature legume seeds—what we know as beans— also make an impressive contribution to the protein, vitamin, mineral, and fiber content of a meal. A one-half cup serving of legumes provides 100 to 150 kcal, 5 to 10 grams of protein, less than one gram of fat, and about 5 grams of fiber. Recall from Chapter 4 that consumption of beans can lead to intestinal gas because our bodies lack the enzymes to break down certain carbohydrates that beans contain. An over-the counter preparation called Beano® can greatly lessen symptoms if taken right before the meal. It is also helpful to soak dry beans in water, which leaches the indigestible carbohydrates into the water so they can be disposed. However, intestinal gas is not harmful. In fact, fermentation products of ingestible carbohydrates promote the health of your colon (review Chapter 3 for more information on probiotics and prebiotics).

DARK RED
Kidney Beans

Nutrition Facts
Serving Size 1/2 cup (180g)
Servings Per Container about 3.5

Amount Per Serving

Calories 130	Calories from Fat 5

	% Daily Value*
Total Fat 0.5g	**1%**
Saturated Fat 0g	**0%**
Trans Fat 0g	***
Cholesterol 0mg	**0%**
Sodium 530mg	**22%**
Total Carbohydrate 23g	**8%**
Dietary Fiber 9g	**36%**
Sugars 3g	
Protein 6g	

Vitamin A 4%	•	Vitamin C**
Calcium 6%	•	Iron 10%

** Contains less than 2 percent of the Daily Value of this nutrient.
Percent Daily Values are based on a 2,000 calorie diet. Your daily values may be higher or lower depending on your calorie needs.

	Calories	2,000	2,500
Total Fat	Less than	65g	80g
Saturated Fat	Less than	20g	25g
Cholesterol	Less than	300mg	300mg
Sodium	Less than	2,400mg	2,400mg
Total Carbohydrate		300g	375g
Dietary Fiber		25g	30g

*** Intake from *trans* fat should be as low as possible.

FIGURE 6-6 ▶ Legumes are rich sources of protein. One-half cup meets about 10% of protein needs, but contributes only about 5% of energy needs.

The impact of plant proteins on health will be discussed in the "Nutrition and Your Health" section at the end of this chapter.

▲ Rich sources of plant proteins add much nutritional value to a diet.

MAKING DECISIONS

Soy and Nut Allergies

For some of us, food allergies from soy, peanuts and tree nuts (e.g., almonds and walnuts), and wheat are a concern. Overall, food allergies occur in up to 8% of children 4 years of age or younger and in up to 2% of adults. Eight foods account for 90% of food-related allergies; soy, peanuts, tree nuts, and wheat are four of these foods. (The other foods are milk, egg, fish, and shellfish.) The allergic reactions can range from a mild intolerance to fatal allergic rections (see Chapter 15 for details). Current guidelines regarding plant sources of allergens advise that infants not be fed wheat products before 6 months of age. Children less than 3 years of age should not eat peanuts or tree nuts. In addition, any of the plant sources of allergens need to be avoided in children and adults who continue to experience such allergies.

In sum, plant proteins are a nutritious alternative to animal proteins. They are inexpensive, versatile, tasty, add color to your plate, and benefit health beyond their contribution of protein to the diet. Simply adding these foods to your diet can lead to weight gain, but learning to substitute plant proteins in place of other less healthy foods is one way to reduce your risk for many diseases. Watch for news about additional research progress into this area.

See *Nutrition and Your Health: Vegetarian and Plant-Based Diets* at the end of Chapter 6.

PROTEIN DIGESTION AND ABSORPTION

As with carbohydrate digestion, protein digestion begins with the cooking of food. Cooking unfolds (denatures) proteins (Fig. 6-7) and softens tough connective tissue in meat. Cooking also makes many protein-rich foods easier to chew and swallow, and facilitates their breakdown during later digestion and absorption. As you will see in Chapter 15, cooking also makes many protein-rich foods, such as meats, eggs, fish, and poultry, much safer to eat.

(a)

Heat /Acid

(b)

FIGURE 6-7 ▶ Denaturation. (a) Protein showing typical coiled state. (b) Protein is now partly uncoiled. This uncoiling can reduce biological activity and allow digestive enzymes to act on peptide bonds.

Digestion

The enzymatic digestion of protein begins in the stomach (Fig. 6-8). Proteins are first denatured by stomach acid. **Pepsin,** a major stomach enzyme for digesting proteins, then goes to work on the unraveled polypeptide chains. Pepsin breaks the polypeptide into shorter chains of amino acids because it can break only a few of the many peptide bonds found in these large molecules. The release of pepsin is controlled by the hormone gastrin. Thinking about food or chewing food stimulates gastrin release in the stomach. Gastrin also strongly stimulates the stomach to produce acid.

The partially-digested proteins move from the stomach into the small intestine along with the rest of the nutrients and other substances in a meal (chyme). Once in the small intestine, the partially-digested proteins (and any fats accompanying them) trigger the release of the hormone cholecystokinin (CCK) from the walls of the small intestine. CCK, in turn, travels through the bloodstream to the pancreas where it causes the pancreas to release protein-splitting enzymes, such as **trypsin.** These digestive enzymes further divide the chains of amino acids into segments of two to three amino acids and some individual amino acids. Eventually, this mixture is digested into amino acids, using other enzymes from the lining of the small intestine and enzymes present in the absorptive cells themselves.

Absorption

The short chains of amino acids and any individual amino acids in the small intestine are taken up by active transport into the absorptive cells lining the small intestine. Any remaining peptide bonds are broken down to yield individual amino acids inside the intestinal

pepsin A protein-digesting enzyme produced by the stomach.

trypsin A protein-digesting enzyme secreted by the pancreas to act in the small intestine.

FIGURE 6-8 ▶ A summary of protein digestion and absorption. Enzymatic protein digestion begins in the stomach and ends in the absorptive cells of the small intestine, where any remaining short groupings of amino acids are broken down into single amino acids. Stomach acid and enzymes contribute to protein digestion. Absorption from the intestinal lumen into the absorptive cells requires energy input.

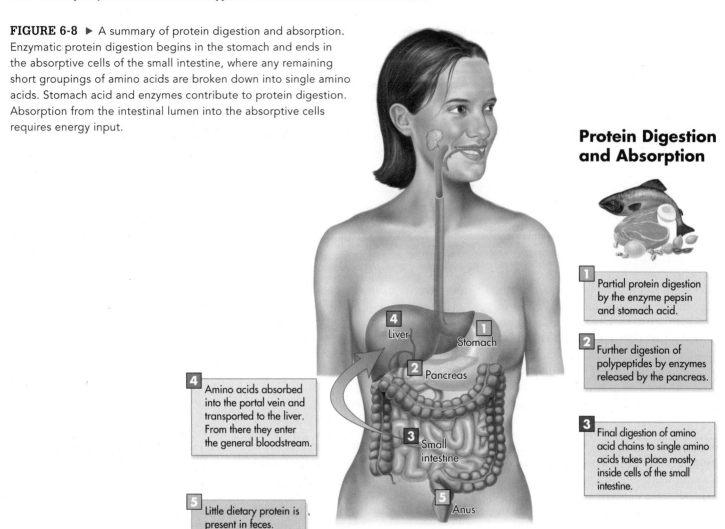

Protein Digestion and Absorption

1 Partial protein digestion by the enzyme pepsin and stomach acid.

2 Further digestion of polypeptides by enzymes released by the pancreas.

3 Final digestion of amino acid chains to single amino acids takes place mostly inside cells of the small intestine.

4 Amino acids absorbed into the portal vein and transported to the liver. From there they enter the general bloodstream.

5 Little dietary protein is present in feces.

Liver
Stomach
Pancreas
Small intestine
Anus

cells. They are water-soluble, so the amino acids travel to the liver via the portal vein, which drains absorbed nutrients from the intestinal tract. In the liver, individual amino acids can undergo several modifications, depending on the needs of the body. Individual amino acids may be combined into the proteins needed by the body; broken down for energy needs; released into the bloodstream; or converted to nonessential amino acids, glucose, or fat. With excess protein intake, amino acids are converted to fat as a last resort.

Except during infancy, it is uncommon for intact proteins to be absorbed from the digestive tract. In infants up to 4 to 5 months of age, the gastrointestinal tract is somewhat permeable to small proteins, so some whole proteins can be absorbed. Because proteins from some foods (e.g., cow's milk and egg whites) may predispose an infant to food allergies, pediatricians and registered dietitians recommend waiting until an infant is at least 6 to 12 months of age before introducing commonly allergenic foods (see Chapter 17 for details).

CONCEPT CHECK

Protein digestion begins with cooking, as proteins are denatured by heat. Once protein reaches the stomach, enzymes cleave proteins into smaller segments of amino acids. As food travels through the small intestine, protein breakdown products formed in the stomach are broken down further to individual amino acids or short segments of amino acids and taken up into the absorptive cells of the small intestine where final breakdown into amino acids occurs. The amino acids then travel to the liver via the portal vein.

PUTTING PROTEINS TO WORK IN THE BODY

Proteins function in many crucial ways in human metabolism and in the formation of body structures. We rely on foods to supply the amino acids needed to form these proteins. However, only when we also eat enough carbohydrate and fat can food proteins be used most efficiently. If we don't consume enough calories to meet needs, some amino acids from proteins are broken down to produce energy, rendering them unavailable to build body proteins.

Producing Vital Body Structures

Every cell contains protein. Muscles, connective tissue, mucus, blood-clotting factors, transport proteins in the bloodstream, lipoproteins, enzymes, immune antibodies, some hormones, visual pigments, and the support structure inside bones are primarily made of protein. Excess protein in the diet doesn't enhance the synthesis of these body components, but eating too little protein can prevent it.

Most vital body proteins are in a constant state of breakdown, rebuilding, and repair. For example, the intestinal tract lining is constantly sloughed off. The digestive tract treats sloughed cells just like food particles, digesting them and absorbing their amino acids. In fact, most of the amino acids released throughout the body can be recycled to become part of the pool of amino acids available for synthesis of future proteins. Overall, **protein turnover** is a process by which a cell can respond to its changing environment by producing proteins that are needed and disassembling proteins that are not needed.

During any day, an adult makes and degrades about 250 grams of protein, recycling many of the amino acids. Relative to the 65 to 100 grams of protein typically consumed by adults in North America, recycled amino acids make an important contribution to total protein metabolism.

If a person's diet is low in protein for a long period, the processes of rebuilding and repairing body proteins will slow down. Over time, skeletal muscles; blood proteins; and vital organs, such as the heart and liver, will decrease in size or volume. Only the brain resists protein breakdown.

Maintaining Fluid Balance

Blood proteins help maintain body fluid balance. Normal blood pressure in the arteries forces blood into capillary beds. The blood fluid then moves from the **capillary beds** into the spaces between nearby cells (**extracellular spaces**) to provide nutrients to those cells (Fig. 6-9). Proteins in the bloodstream are too large however, to move out of the capillary beds into the tissues. The presence of these proteins in the capillary beds attracts the proper amount of fluid back to the blood, partially counteracting the force of blood pressure.

With an inadequate consumption of protein, the concentration of proteins in the bloodstream drops below normal. Excessive fluid then builds up in the surrounding tissues because the counteracting force produced by the smaller amount of blood proteins is too weak to pull enough of the fluid back from the tissues into the bloodstream. As fluids accumulate in the tissues, the tissues swell, causing **edema.** Edema may be a symptom of a variety of medical problems, so its cause must be identified. An important step in diagnosing the cause is to measure the concentration of blood proteins.

Contributing to Acid-Base Balance

Proteins help regulate acid-base balance in the blood. Proteins located in cell membranes pump chemical ions in and out of cells. The ion concentration that results from the pumping action, among other factors, keeps the blood slightly alkaline. In addition, some blood proteins are especially good **buffers** for the body. Buffers are compounds that maintain acid-base conditions within a narrow range.

▲ Protein contributes to the structure and function of muscle.

protein turnover   The process by which cells break down old proteins and resynthesize new proteins. In this way the cell will have the proteins it needs to function at that time.

capillary bed   Network of one-cell thick vessels that create a junction between arterial and venous circulation. It is here that gas and nutrient exchange occurs between body cells and the blood.

extracellular space   The space outside cells; represents one-third of body fluid.

edema   The buildup of excess fluid in extracellular spaces.

buffers   Compounds that cause a solution to resist changes in acid-base conditions.

FIGURE 6-9 ▶ Blood proteins in relation to fluid balance. (a) Blood proteins are important for maintaining the body's fluid balance. (b) Without sufficient protein in the bloodstream, edema develops.

Forming Hormones and Enzymes

Amino acids are required for the synthesis of many hormones—our internal body messengers. Some hormones, such as the thyroid hormones, are made from only one type of amino acid, tyrosine. Insulin, on the other hand, is a hormone composed of 51 total amino acids. Almost all enzymes are proteins or have a protein component.

Contributing to Immune Function

Proteins are a key component of the cells within the immune system. An example is the antibodies, proteins produced by one type of white blood cell. These antibodies can bind to foreign proteins in the body, an important step in removing invaders from the body. Without sufficient dietary protein, the immune system lacks the materials needed to function properly. For example, a low protein status can turn measles into a fatal disease for a malnourished child.

▶ Neurotransmitters, released by nerve endings, are often derivatives of amino acids. This is true for dopamine and norepinephrine (both synthesized from the amino acid tyrosine), and serotonin (synthesized from the amino acid tryptophan).

Forming Glucose

In Chapter 4 you learned that the body must maintain a fairly constant concentration of blood glucose to supply energy for the brain, red blood cells, and nervous tissue. At rest, the brain uses about 19% of the body's energy requirements, and it gets most of that energy from glucose. If you don't consume enough carbohydrate to supply the glucose, your liver (and kidneys, to a lesser extent) will be forced to make glucose from amino acids present in body tissues (Fig. 6-10).

Making some glucose from amino acids is normal. For example, when you skip breakfast and haven't eaten since 7 P.M. the preceding evening, glucose must be manufactured. In an extreme situation, however, such as in starvation, amino acids from muscle tissue are converted into glucose, which wastes muscle tissue and can produce edema.

Providing Energy

Proteins supply little energy for a weight-stable person. Two situations in which a person does use protein to meet energy needs are during prolonged exercise (see Chapter 12 for information about the use of amino acids for energy needs during

▶ The vitamin niacin can be made from the amino acid tryptophan, illustrating another role of proteins.

FIGURE 6-10 ▶ Amino acid metabolism. The amino acid **pool** in a cell can be used to form body proteins, as well as a variety of other possible products. When the **carbon skeletons** of amino acids are metabolized to produce glucose or fat, ammonia (NH_3) is a resulting waste product. The ammonia is converted to **urea** and excreted in the urine.

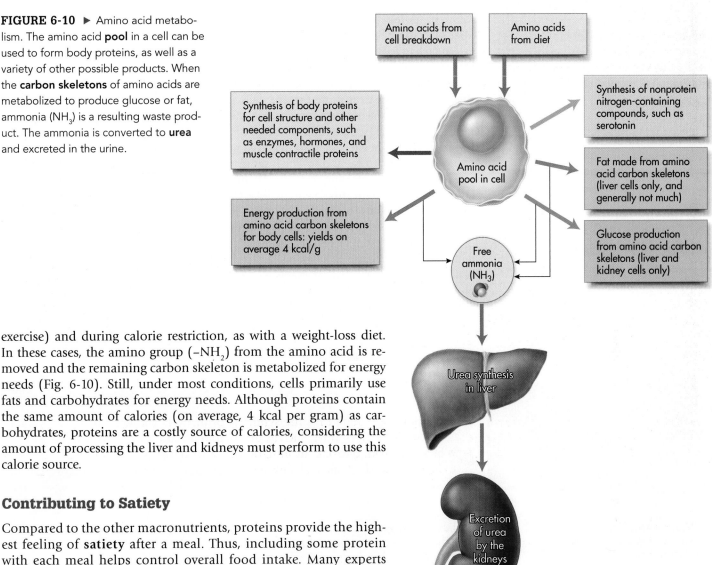

exercise) and during calorie restriction, as with a weight-loss diet. In these cases, the amino group ($-NH_2$) from the amino acid is removed and the remaining carbon skeleton is metabolized for energy needs (Fig. 6-10). Still, under most conditions, cells primarily use fats and carbohydrates for energy needs. Although proteins contain the same amount of calories (on average, 4 kcal per gram) as carbohydrates, proteins are a costly source of calories, considering the amount of processing the liver and kidneys must perform to use this calorie source.

Contributing to Satiety

Compared to the other macronutrients, proteins provide the highest feeling of **satiety** after a meal. Thus, including some protein with each meal helps control overall food intake. Many experts warn against skimping on protein when trying to reduce energy intake to lose weight. Meeting protein needs is still important and exceeding needs somewhat may provide an additional benefit when dieting to lose weight.

CONCEPT CHECK

Vital body constituents—such as muscle, connective tissue, blood transport proteins, enzymes, hormones, buffers, and immune factors—are mainly proteins. The degradation of existing proteins and synthesis of new proteins takes place constantly, amounting to a turnover rate of about 250 grams a day for the entire human body. Proteins can also be used for glucose and other fuel production and contributes to satiety.

PROTEIN NEEDS

How much protein (actually, amino acids) do we need to eat each day? People who aren't growing need to eat only enough protein to match whatever they lose daily from protein breakdown. The amount of breakdown can be determined by measuring the amount of urea and other nitrogen-containing compounds in the urine, as well as

pool The amount of a nutrient stored within the body that can be mobilized when needed.

carbon skeleton Amino acid structure that remains after the amino group ($-NH_2$) has been removed.

urea Nitrogenous waste product of protein metabolism; major source of nitrogen in the urine, chemically $NH_2-\overset{\overset{\text{O}}{\|}}{C}-NH_2$.

satiety A state in which there is no longer a desire to eat; a feeling of satisfaction.

protein equilibrium A state in which protein intake is equal to related protein losses; the person is said to be in protein balance.

positive protein balance A state in which protein intake exceeds related protein losses, as is needed during times of growth.

negative protein balance A state in which protein intake is less than related protein losses, such as often seen during acute illness.

losses of protein from feces, skin, hair, nails, and so on. In short, people need to balance protein intake with such losses to maintain a state of **protein equilibrium,** also called *protein balance* (Fig. 6-11).

When a body is growing or recovering from an illness or injury, it needs a **positive protein balance** to supply the raw materials required to build new tissues. To achieve this, a person must eat more protein daily than he or she loses. In addition, the hormones insulin, growth hormone, and testosterone all stimulate positive protein balance. Resistance exercise (weight training) also enhances positive protein balance. Consuming less protein than needed leads to **negative protein balance,** such as when acute illness reduces the desire to eat and so one loses more protein than consumed.

For healthy people, the amount of dietary protein needed to maintain protein equilibrium (wherein intake equals losses) can be determined by increasing protein intake until it equals losses of protein and its related breakdown products (e.g., urea). Calorie needs must also be met so that amino acids are not diverted for such use.

Today, the best estimate for the amount of protein required for nearly all adults to maintain protein equilibrium is 0.8 grams of protein per kilogram of healthy body weight. This is the RDA for protein. Requirements are higher during periods of growth, such as pregnancy and infancy (see Chapters 16 and 17 for specific values for pregnant women, infants, and children). Healthy weight is used as a reference in the determination of protein needs

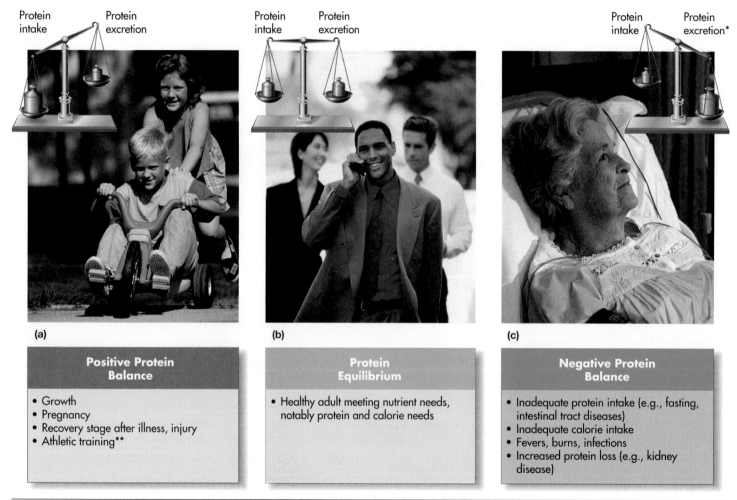

Positive Protein Balance

- Growth
- Pregnancy
- Recovery stage after illness, injury
- Athletic training**

Protein Equilibrium

- Healthy adult meeting nutrient needs, notably protein and calorie needs

Negative Protein Balance

- Inadequate protein intake (e.g., fasting, intestinal tract diseases)
- Inadequate calorie intake
- Fevers, burns, infections
- Increased protein loss (e.g., kidney disease)

*Based on losses of urea and other nitrogen-containing compounds in the urine, as well as protein lost from feces, skin, hair, nails, and other minor routes.

**Only when additional lean body mass is being gained. Nevertheless, the athlete is probably already eating enough protein to support this extra protein synthesis; protein supplements are not needed.

FIGURE 6-11 ▶ Protein balance in practical terms: (a) positive protein balance; (b) protein equilibrium; (c) negative protein balance.

because excess fat storage doesn't contribute much to protein needs (see Chapter 7 for insight into the concept of healthy weight). Calculations using this RDA are shown in the margin and estimate a requirement of about 56 grams of protein daily for a typical 70-kilogram (154-pound) man and about 46 grams of protein daily for a typical 57-kilogram (125-pound) woman.

The RDA for protein translates into about 10% of total calories. Many experts recommend up to 15% of total calories to provide more flexibility in diet planning, in turn allowing for the variety of protein-rich foods North Americans typically consume. As noted earlier, the Food and Nutrition Board has set an upper range for protein intake at 35% of calories consumed. It is easy to meet currently suggested daily protein needs (Table 6-2). On a daily basis, typical North American protein intakes are about 100 grams of protein for men and 65 grams for women. Thus, most of us consume much more protein than the RDA recommends because we like many high-protein foods and can afford to buy them. Our bodies cannot store excess protein once it is consumed, so the excess amino acids are converted to carbon skeletons that are turned into glucose or fat and then stored as fat or metabolized for energy needs (review Fig. 6-10).

Mental stress, physical labor, and recreational weekend sports activities do not require an increase in the protein RDA. For some highly trained athletes, such as those participating in endurance or strength training, protein consumption may need to exceed the RDA. This is an area of debate in sports nutrition: the Food and Nutrition Board does not support an increased need, but some experts suggest an increase to about 1.7 grams per kilogram. Many North Americans already consume that much protein, especially men.

Convert weight from pounds to kilograms:

$$\frac{154 \text{ pounds}}{2.2 \text{ pounds/kilogram}} = 70 \text{ kilograms}$$

$$\frac{125 \text{ pounds}}{2.2 \text{ pounds/kilogram}} = 57 \text{ kilograms}$$

Calculate protein RDA:

$$70 \text{ kilograms} \times \frac{0.8 \text{ grams protein}}{\text{kilogram body weight}} = 56 \text{ grams}$$

$$57 \text{ kilograms} \times \frac{0.8 \text{ grams protein}}{\text{kilogram body weight}} = 46 \text{ grams}$$

TABLE 6-2 The Protein Contents of a Typical 1600 kcal Diet and a 2400 kcal Diet*

1600 kcal Diet	Protein (grams)	2400 kcal Diet	Protein (grams)
Breakfast			
1% milk, 1 cup	8	2% reduced-fat milk, 1 cup	8
Cheerios, 1 cup	2	Cheerios, 1 cup	2
Orange	1	Eggs, hard boiled, 2	12
		Orange	1
Lunch			
Whole-wheat bread, 2 slices	5	Whole-wheat bread, 2 slices	5
Chicken breast, 2 ounces	17	Chicken breast, 2 ounces	17
Mayonnaise, 1 teaspoon	—	Provolone cheese, 2 ounces	15
Tomato slices, 2	—	Tomato slices, 2	—
Carrot sticks, 1 cup	1	Mayonnaise, 1 teaspoon	—
Oatmeal raisin cookie, 1	2		
Fig, 1 large	0.5	Oatmeal-raisin cookies, 2	4
Diet soft drink	—	Figs, 2	1
		Diet soft drink	—
Dinner			
Mixed green salad, 1 cup	—	Mixed green salad, ½ cup	—
Italian dressing, 2 teaspoons	—	Italian dressing, 2 teaspoons	—
Beef tenderloin, 3 ounces	21	Beef tenderloin, 4 ounces	28
Spinach pasta, 1 cup, with garlic butter, 1 teaspoon	7	Spinach pasta, 1 cup, with garlic butter, 1 teaspoon	7
Zucchini, ½ cup, sauteed in oil, 1 teaspoon	0.5	Zucchini, ½ cup, sauteed in oil, 1 teaspoon	0.5
1% milk, 1 cup	8	Carrot sticks, ½ cup	0.5
		2% reduced-fat milk, 1 cup	8
Snack			
Bagel, toasted, ½ of a 3½-inch bagel	4	Bagel, toasted, ½ of a 3½-inch bagel	4
Jam, 2 teaspoons	—	Jam, 2 teaspoons	—
Fruited yogurt, 1 cup	10	Fruited yogurt, 1 cup	10
TOTAL	87		124

*This table illustrates how few calories need be consumed while still meeting the RDA for protein. It also shows how much protein we eat when we consume typical calorie intakes.

DOES EATING A HIGH-PROTEIN DIET HARM YOU?

▲ Animal protein foods are typically our main sources of protein in the North American diet.

People frequently ask about the potential harm of protein intakes in excess of the RDA. Problems with diets that are high in protein foods primarily stem from the fact that they typically rely on animal sources of protein. Diets rich in animal products will most likely be simultaneously low in the beneficial substances found in plant sources, including fiber, some vitamins (e.g., folate), some minerals (e.g., magnesium), as well as phytochemicals, and high in substances such as saturated fat and cholesterol. A high animal-protein diet, therefore, is unlikely to follow the recommendations of the Dietary Guidelines for Americans or the Food and Nutrition Board in terms of reducing risk for cardiovascular disease.

Some, but not all, studies show that high-protein diets can increase calcium losses in urine. For people with adequate calcium intakes, little concern about this relationship is warranted, but keep in mind that calcium is commonly deficient in North American diets.

Meat is one of the richest sources of protein. Excessive intake of red meat, however, especially processed forms, is linked to colon cancer in population studies. There are several possible explanations for this connection. The curing agents used to process meats such as ham and salami may cause cancer. Substances that form during cooking of red meat at high temperatures may also cause cancer. The excessive fat or low-fiber contents of diets rich in red meat may also be a contributing factor. Because of these concerns, some nutrition experts suggest we focus more on poultry, fish, nuts, legumes, and seeds to meet protein needs. In addition, any red or other type of meat should be trimmed of all visible fat before grilling.

Some researchers have expressed concern that a high-protein intake may overburden the kidneys by forcing them to excrete the extra nitrogen as urea. Additionally, animal proteins may contribute to kidney stone formation in certain individuals. There is some support for limiting protein intake for people in the early stages of kidney disease, because low-protein diets somewhat slow the decline in kidney function. Laboratory animal studies show that moderate protein intakes that just meet nutritional needs preserve kidney function over time better than high-protein diets. Preserving kidney function is especially important for those who have diabetes, early signs of kidney disease, or only one functioning kidney, so a high-protein diet is not recommended for these people. High-protein diets increase urine output, in turn posing a risk for dehydration. This is a special concern for athletes (see Chapter 12).

MAKING DECISIONS

Amino Acid Supplements

Protein and amino acid supplements are used primarily by athletes and dieters. Athletes use them hoping they will help build muscle. The branched-chain amino acids described earlier are especially popular with athletes looking to enhance their performance. Dieters have turned to these supplements hoping they will increase their weight loss. Although the right amount of protein in the diet will aid athletic performance and help in weight control, consuming this protein in the form of amino acid supplements cannot be considered safe.

Earlier in this chapter, you learned that the body is designed to handle whole proteins as a dietary source of amino acids. When individual amino acid supplements are taken, they can overwhelm the absorptive mechanisms in the small intestine, triggering amino acid imbalances in the body. Imbalances occur because groups of chemically similar amino acids compete for absorption sites in the absorptive cells. For example, lysine and arginine are absorbed by the same transporter, so an excess of lysine can impair absorption of arginine. The amino acids most likely to cause toxicity when consumed in large amounts are methionine, cysteine, and histidine. Due to the potential for imbalances and toxicities of individual amino acids, the best advice to ensure adequacy is to stick to whole foods rather than supplements as sources of amino acids. Amino acids as such also have a disagreeable odor and flavor and are also much more expensive than food protein. In Canada the sale of individual amino acids to consumers is banned.

CONCEPT CHECK

The Recommended Dietary Allowance (RDA) for adults is 0.8 grams of protein per kilogram of healthy body weight. This is approximately 56 grams of protein daily for a 70-kilogram (156-pound) person. The average North American man consumes about 100 grams of protein daily, and a woman consumes about 65 grams. Thus, typically we eat more than enough protein to meet our needs. This even includes well-balanced vegetarian diets. Diets high in protein can compromise kidney health in people with diabetes and those with kidney disease, and animal protein sources likely increase cardiovascular disease and kidney stone risk when consumed in high amounts.

PROTEIN-CALORIE MALNUTRITION

Protein deficiency is rarely an isolated condition and usually accompanies a deficiency of calories and other nutrients resulting from insufficient food intake. In the developed world, alcoholism can lead to cases of protein deficiency because of the low protein content of alcoholic beverages. In developing areas of the world, people often have diets low in calories and also in protein. This state of undernutrition stunts the growth of children and makes them more susceptible to disease throughout life. (Undernutrition is a main focus of Chapter 14.) People who consume too little protein calories can eventually develop **protein-calorie malnutrition (PCM)**, also referred to as *protein-energy malnutrition (PEM)*. In its milder form, it is difficult to tell if a person with PCM is consuming too little calories or protein, or both. When an inadequate intake of nutrients, including protein, is combined with an already existing disease, especially an infection, a form of malnutrition called **kwashiorkor** can develop. But if the nutrient deficiency—especially for calories—becomes severe, a deficiency disease called **marasmus** can result. Both conditions are seen primarily in children, but also may develop in adults, even in those hospitalized in North America. These two conditions form the tip of the iceberg with respect to states of undernutrition, and symptoms of these two conditions can even be present in the same person (Fig. 6-12).

Kwashiorkor

Kwashiorkor is a word from Ghana that means "the disease that the first child gets when the new child comes." From birth, an infant in developing areas of the world is usually breastfed. Often by the time the child reaches 1 to 1.5 years of age, the mother is pregnant or has already given birth again, and the new child gets preference for breastfeeding. The older child's diet then abruptly changes from nutritious human milk to starchy roots and **gruels.** These foods have low-protein densities, compared with total energy. Additionally, the foods are usually full of plant fibers, often bulky, making it difficult for the child to consume enough to meet calorie needs. The child generally also has infections, which acutely raise calorie and protein needs. For these reasons, calorie needs of these children are met just barely, at best, and their protein consumption is grossly inadequate, especially in view of the increased amount needed to combat infections. Many vitamin and mineral needs are also far from being fulfilled. Famine victims face similar problems.

The major symptoms of kwashiorkor are apathy, diarrhea, listlessness, failure to grow and gain weight, and withdrawal from the environment. These

protein-calorie malnutrition (PCM) A condition resulting from regularly consuming insufficient amounts of calories and protein. The deficiency eventually results in body wasting, primarily of lean tissue, and an increased susceptibility to infections.

kwashiorkor A disease occurring primarily in young children who have an existing disease and consume a marginal amount of calories and insufficient protein in relation to needs. The child generally suffers from infections and exhibits edema, poor growth, weakness, and an increased susceptibility to further illness.

marasmus A disease resulting from consuming a grossly insufficient amount of protein and calories; one of the diseases classed as protein-calorie malnutrition. Victims have little or no fat stores, little muscle mass, and poor strength. Death from infections is common.

gruels A thin mixture of grains or legumes in milk or water.

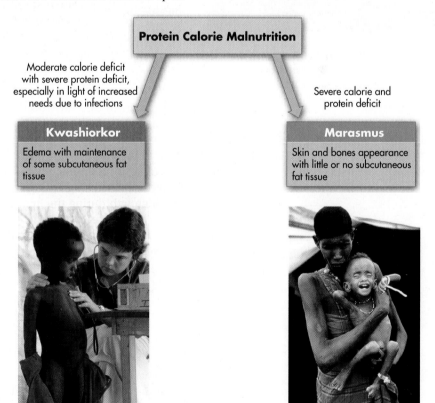

FIGURE 6-12 ▶ Schema for classifying undernutrition in children. The presence of subcutaneous fat (directly underneath the skin) is a diagnostic key for distinguishing kwashiorkor from marasmus.

▶ Toxic products in moldy grains may also contribute to kwashiorkor.

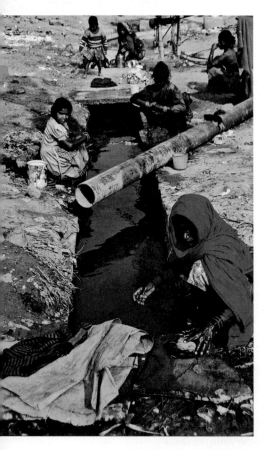

▲ Unsafe water supplies in developing countries contribute to the incidence of marasmus, particularly in bottle-fed infants.

preterm An infant born before 37 weeks of gestation; also referred to as premature.

symptoms complicate other diseases present. For example, a condition such as measles, a disease that normally makes a healthy child ill for only a week or so, can become severely debilitating and even fatal. Further symptoms of kwashiorkor are changes in hair color, potassium deficiency, flaky skin, fatty liver, reduced muscle mass, and massive edema in the abdomen and legs. The presence of edema in a child who has some subcutaneous fat (i.e., directly under the skin) is the hallmark of kwashiorkor (review Fig. 6-12). In addition, these children seldom move. If you pick them up, they don't cry. When you hold them, you feel the plumpness of edema, not muscle and fat tissue.

Many symptoms of kwashiorkor can be explained based on what we know about proteins. Proteins play important roles in fluid balance, lipoprotein transport, immune function, and production of tissues, such as skin, cells lining the GI tract, and hair. Children with an insufficient protein intake do not grow and mature normally.

If children with kwashiorkor are helped in time—if infections are treated and a diet ample in protein, calories, and other essential nutrients is provided—the disease process reverses. They begin to grow again and may even show no signs of their previous condition, except perhaps shortness of stature. Unfortunately, by the time many of these children reach a hospital or care center, they already have severe infections. Despite the best care, they still die. Or, if they survive, they return home only to become ill again.

Marasmus

Marasmus typically occurs as an infant slowly starves to death. It is caused by diets containing minimal amounts of calories, as well as too little protein and other nutrients. As previously noted, the condition is also commonly referred to as *protein-calorie malnutrition*, especially when experienced by older children and adults. The word *marasmus* means "to waste away," in Greek. Victims have a "skin-and-bones" appearance, with little or no subcutaneous fat (review Fig. 6-12).

Marasmus commonly develops in infants who either are not breastfed or have stopped breastfeeding in the early months. Often the weaning formula used is improperly prepared because of unsafe water and because the parents cannot afford sufficient infant formula for the child's needs. The latter problem may lead the parents to dilute the formula to provide more feedings, not realizing that this provides only more water for the infant.

Marasmus in infants commonly occurs in the large cities of poverty-stricken countries. When people are poor and sanitation is lacking, bottle feeding often leads to marasmus. In the cities, bottle feeding is often necessary because the infant must be cared for by others when the mother is working or away from home. An infant with marasmus requires large amounts of calories and protein—like a **preterm** infant—and, unless the child receives them, full recovery from the disease may never occur. The majority of brain growth occurs between conception and the child's first birthday. In fact, the brain is growing at its highest rate after birth. If the diet does not support brain growth during the first months of life, the brain may not grow to its full adult size. This reduced or retarded brain growth may lead to diminished intellectual function. Both kwashiorkor and marasmus plague infants and children; mortality rates in developing countries are often 10 to 20 times higher than in North America.

CONCEPT CHECK

Most undernutrition consists of mild deficits in calories, protein, and often other nutrients. If a person needs more nutrients because of disease and infection but does not consume enough calories and protein, a condition known as kwashiorkor can develop. The person suffers from edema and weakness. Children around age 2 are especially susceptible to kwashiorkor, particularly if they already have other diseases. Famine situations in which only starchy root products are available to eat contribute to this problem. Marasmus is a condition wherein people—infants, especially—starve to death. Symptoms include muscle wasting, absence of fat stores, and weakness. Both an adequate diet and the treatment of concurrent diseases must be promoted to regain and then maintain nutritional health.

NUTRITION AND YOUR HEALTH
Vegetarian and Plant-Based Diets

Vegetarianism has evolved over the centuries from a necessity into an option. Historically, vegetarianism was linked with specific philosophies and religions or with science. Today, about 1 in 40 adults in the United States (and about 1 in 25 in Canada) is a vegetarian. Vegetarian diets have evolved to include such new products as soy-based sloppy joes, chili, tacos, burgers, and more. In addition, cookbooks that feature the use of a variety of fruits, vegetables, and seasonings are enhancing food selection for vegetarians of all degrees.

Vegetarianism is popular among college students. Fifteen percent of college students in one survey said they select vegetarian options at lunch or dinner on any given day. In response, dining services offer vegetarian options at every meal, such as pastas with meatless sauce and pizza. Many teenagers are also turning to vegetarianism. In addition, a survey by the National Restaurant Association found that 20% of its customers want a vegetarian option when they eat out. Many customers cite health and taste as reasons for choosing vegetarian meals.

As nutrition science has grown, new information has enabled the design of nutritionally adequate vegetarian diets. It is important for vegetarians to take advantage of this information because a diet of only plant-based foods has the potential to promote various nutrient deficiencies and substantial growth retardation in infants and children. People who choose a vegetarian diet can meet their nutritional needs by following a few basic rules and knowledgeably planning their diets.

Studies show that death rates from some chronic diseases, such as certain forms of cardiovascular disease, hypertention, many forms of cancer, type 2 diabetes, and obesity, are lower for vegetarians than for nonvegetarians. Vegetarians often live longer, as shown in religious groups that practice vegetarianism. Other aspects of healthful lifestyles, such as not smoking, abstaining from alcohol and drugs, and regular physical activity often go along with vegetarianism and probably partially account for the lower risks of chronic disease and longer lives seen in this population.

As you learned in Chapter 2, MyPyramid and the 2005 Dietary Guidelines for Americans emphasize a plant-based diet of whole-grain breads and cereals, fruits, and vegetables. In addition, the American Institute for Cancer Research promotes "The New American Plate," which includes plant-based foods covering two-thirds (or more) of the plate and meat, fish, poultry, or low-fat dairy covering only one-third (or less) of the plate. Although these recommendations do allow the inclusion of animal products, they are definitely more "vegetarian-like" than typical North American diets.

▲ Recipes for vegetarian and plant-based foods are widely available today.

The New American Plate

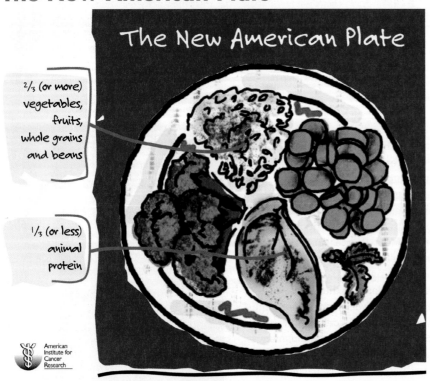

The New American Plate

²/₃ (or more) vegetables, fruits, whole grains and beans

¹/₃ (or less) animal protein

American Institute for Cancer Research

▲ Plant proteins, like those in walnuts, can be incorporated into one's diet in numerous ways, such as adding them to banana bread.

WHY DO PEOPLE BECOME VEGETARIANS?

People choose vegetarianism for a variety of reasons including ethics, religion, economics, and health. Some believe that killing animals for food is unethical. Hindus and Trappist monks eat vegetarian meals as a practice of their religion. In North America, many Seventh Day Adventists base their practice of vegetarianism on biblical texts and believe it is a more healthful way to live.

Some advocates of vegetarianism base their food preference upon the inefficient use of animals as a source of protein. Forty percent of the world's grain production is used to raise meat-producing animals. Although animals that humans eat sometimes eat grasses that humans cannot digest, many also eat grains that humans can eat.

People might also practice vegetarianism because it limits saturated fat and cholesterol intake, while encouraging a high intake of complex carbohydrates, vitamins A, E, and C, carotenoids, magnesium, and fiber.

GOOD FOR YOUR HEART

Plant sources of proteins can positively impact heart health in several ways. First, the plant foods we eat contain no cholesterol nor *trans* fat and little saturated fat. The major type of fats in plant foods are monounsaturated and polyunsaturated fats. Nuts in particular are high in monounsaturated fat, which helps to keep blood cholesterol low.

Beans and nuts contain soluble fiber, which binds to cholesterol in the small intestine and prevents it from being absorbed by the body. Also, due to the activity of some phytochemicals, foods made from soybeans can lower production of cholesterol by the body. The effect is modest (about a 2% to 6% drop). In 1999, the Food and Drug Administration allowed health claims for the cholesterol-lowering properties of soy foods, and in 2000, the American Heart Association recommended inclusion of some soy protein in the diets of people with high blood cholesterol. As noted in Chapter 2, to list a health claim for soy on the label, a food product must have at least 6.25 grams of soy protein and

less than 3 grams of fat, 1 gram of saturated fat, and 20 milligrams of cholesterol per serving.

There are several other compounds in plant foods under study for their heart-protective roles. Some of the phytochemicals may help to prevent blood clots and relax the blood vessels. Nuts are an especially good source of nutrients implicated in heart health, including vitamin E, folate, magnesium, and copper. Frequent consumption of nuts (about 1 ounce of nuts five times per week) is associated with a decreased risk of cardiovascular disease. Recall from Chapter 2 that FDA also allows a provisional health claim to link nuts with a reduced risk of developing cardiovascular disease. As noted in Chapter 5, a vegan diet coupled with regular exercise and other lifestyle changes can lead to a reversal of atherosclerotic plaque in various arteries in the body.

CANCER-FIGHTING AGENTS

The numerous phytochemicals in plant foods are thought to aid in preventing cancers of the breast, prostate, and colon. Many of the proposed anti-cancer effects of foods containing plant protein are through antioxidant mechanisms.

Consumption of plant sources of proteins can aid in prevention of cardiovascular disease and cancer, but there are also other areas for future study. Some studies show that replacing animal proteins with plant proteins is beneficial for kidney health. However, because plant foods such as soy are high in oxalates, people with a history of kidney stones should probably limit intake of soy. Plants may be particularly good sources of protein for people with diabetes or impaired glucose tolerance because the high fiber content of plant foods leads to a slower increase in blood glucose (review Chapter 4 for a discussion of glycemic load). Frequent nut consumption may even reduce the risk of developing gallstones; a reduced risk for obesity and type 2 diabetes is also likely. Much of the excitement surrounding the ability of soy to combat a host of medical problems has waned. Several studies have shown little benefit of soy in preventing many forms of cancer, in lowering blood cholesterol, contributing to bone maintenance in women after menopause, and in treating menopausal symptoms in women. A recent review of eighteen studies, however, concluded that soy consumption was associated with a 14% reduction in breast cancer risk.

INCREASING PLANT PROTEINS IN YOUR DIET

Now that you've seen how much you can benefit from including plant proteins in your diet, here are some suggestions for putting the theory onto your plate:

- At your next cookout, try a veggie burger instead of a hamburger. These are usually made from beans and are available in the frozen foods section of the grocery store and come in a variety of delicious flavors. Many restaurants have added veggie burgers to their menus.
- Sprinkle sunflower seeds or chopped almonds on top of your salad to add taste and texture.
- Mix chopped walnuts into the batter of your banana bread to boost your intake of monounsaturated fats.
- Eat soy nuts (oil-roasted soybeans) as a great snack.

- Spread some peanut butter on your bagel instead of butter or cream cheese.
- Instead of having beef or chicken tacos for dinner, heat up a can of great northern beans in your skillet with one half of a packet of taco seasoning and chopped tomatoes. Use this as a filling in a tortilla shell.
- Consider using soy milk, especially if you have lactose malabsorption or lactose intolerance. Look for varieties fortified with calcium.

FOOD PLANNING FOR VEGETARIANS

There are a variety of vegetarian diet styles. **Vegans,** or "total vegetarians," eat only plant foods (and do not use animal products for other purposes, such as leather shoes or feather pillows). **Fruitarians** primarily eat fruits, nuts, honey, and vegetable oils. This plan is not recommended because it can lead to nutrient deficiencies in people of all ages. **Lactovegetarians** modify vegetarianism a bit—they include dairy products in their plant-based diet. **Lactoovovegetarians** modify the diet even further and eat dairy products and eggs, as well as plant foods. Including these animal products makes food planning easier because they are rich in some nutrients that are missing or minimal in plants, such as vitamin B-12 and calcium. The more variety in the diet, the easier it is to meet nutritional needs. Thus, the practice of eating no animal sources of food significantly separates the vegans and fruitarians from all other semivegetarian styles.

Most people who call themselves vegetarians consume at least some dairy products, if not all dairy products and eggs. A food-group plan has been developed for lactovegetarians and vegans (Table 6-3). This plan includes servings of nuts, grains, legumes, and seeds to help meet protein needs. There is also a vegetable group, a fruit group, and a milk group.

VEGAN DIET PLANNING

Planning a vegan diet requires knowledge and creativity to yield high-quality protein and other key nutrients without animal products. Earlier in this chapter, you

▶ American Institute for Cancer Research Diet and Health Guidelines for Cancer Prevention

1. Choose a diet rich in a variety of plant-based foods.
2. Eat plenty of vegetables and fruit.
3. Maintain a healthy weight and be physically active
4. Drink alcohol only in moderation, if at all.
5. Select foods low in fat and salt.
6. Prepare and store food safely.

And always remember...

Do not use tobacco in any form.

vegan A person who eats only plant foods.

fruitarian A person who primarily eats fruits, nuts, honey, and vegetable oils.

lactovegetarian A person who consumes plant products and dairy products.

lactoovovegetarian A person who consumes plant products, dairy products, and eggs.

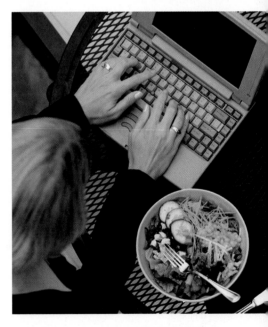

▲ A salad containing numerous types of vegetables and legumes is a healthy vegetarian choice.

TABLE 6-3 Food-Group Plan for Lactovegetarians and Vegans, Which Also Follows MyPyramid[§]

| Group[†] | Servings | | Key Nutrients Supplied |
	Lactovegetarian[‡]	Vegan[§‖]	
Grains[¶]	6–11	8–11	Protein, thiamin, niacin, folate, vitamin E, zinc, phosphorus, magnesium, iron, and fiber
Legumes	2–3	3	Protein, vitamin B-6, zinc, phosphorus, magnesium, and fiber
Nuts, seeds	2–3	3	Protein, vitamin E, and magnesium
Vegetables	3–5 (include one dark green or leafy variety daily)	4–6 (include one dark green or leafy variety daily)	Vitamin A, vitamin C, and folate
Fruits	2–4	4	Vitamin A, vitamin C, and folate
Milk	3	—	Protein, riboflavin, vitamin D, vitamin B-12, calcium, and phosphorus

[†]Base serving size on those listed for MyPyramid (see Chapter 2). This plan yields about 1600 to 1800 kcal. Increase the number of servings, or add other foods to meet higher calorie needs.

[‡]Contains about 75 grams of protein in 1650 kcal.

[§]A calcium-fortified food, such as orange juice or soy milk, is needed unless a calcium supplement is used. In addition, use of or foods fortified with vitamin B-12 or a supplemental source of vitamin B-12 is a must. Use of iodized salt is also important.

[‖]Contains about 79 grams of protein in 1800 kcal.

[¶]One serving of vitamin- and mineral-enriched breakfast cereal is recommended. Alternately, a balanced multivitamin and mineral supplement can be used to help close possible nutrient gaps.

learned about complementing proteins, whereby the essential amino acids deficient in one protein source are supplied by those of another consumed at the same meal or the next (Fig. 6-13). Many legumes are deficient in the essential amino acid methionine, while cereals are limited in lysine. Eating a combination of legumes and cereals, such as beans and rice, will supply the body with adequate amounts of all essential amino acids (Figure 6-13). As for any diet, variety is an especially important characteristic of a nutritious vegan diet.

Aside from amino acids, low intakes of certain micronutrients can be a problem for the vegan. At the forefront of nutritional concerns are riboflavin, vitamins D and B-12, iron, zinc, iodide, and calcium. The following dietary advice should be implemented. In addition, use of a balanced multivitamin and mineral supplement can help as well.

Riboflavin can be obtained from green leafy vegetables, whole grains, yeast, and legumes—components of most vegan diets. Alternate sources of vitamin D include fortified foods (e.g., margarine), as well as regular sun exposure (see Chapter 10).

Vitamin B-12 only occurs naturally in animal foods. Plants can contain soil or microbial contaminants that provide trace amounts of vitamin B-12, but these are negligible sources of the vitamin. Because the body can store vitamin B-12 for about 4 years, it may take a long time after removal of animal foods from the diet for a vitamin B-12 deficiency to surface. If dietary B-12 inadequacy persists, deficiency can lead to a form of anemia, nerve damage, and mental dysfunction. These deficiency consequences have been noted in the infants of vegetarian mothers whose breast milk was low in vitamin B-12. Vegans can prevent a vitamin B-12 deficiency by finding a reliable source of vitamin B-12, such as fortified soybean milk, ready-to-eat breakfast cereals, and special yeast grown on media rich in vitamin B-12.

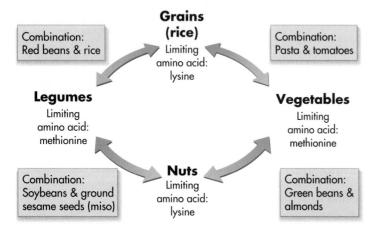

FIGURE 6-13 ▶ Plant group combinations in which the proteins complement each other in a meal based on their limiting amino acids.

▲ Keep in mind that amino acids in vegetables are best used when a combination of sources is consumed.

For iron, the vegan can consume whole grains (especially ready-to-eat breakfast cereals), dried fruits and nuts, and legumes. The iron in these foods is not absorbed as well as iron in animal foods. A good source of vitamin C helps with the absorption of iron so it is recommended that vitamin C be consumed with every meal that contains iron-rich plant foods. Cooking in iron pots and skillets can also add iron to the diet (see Chapter 11).

The vegan can find zinc in whole grains (especially ready-to-eat breakfast cereals), nuts, and legumes, but phytic acid and other substances in these foods limit zinc absorption. Breads are a good source of zinc because the leavening process (rising of the bread dough) reduces the influence of phytic acid. Iodized salt is a reliable source of iodide. It should be used instead of plain salt, both of which are found in U.S. supermarkets.

Of all nutrients, calcium is the most difficult to consume in sufficient quantities for vegans. Fortified foods including fortified soy milk, fortified orange juice, calcium-rich tofu (check the label), as well as certain ready-to-eat breakfast cereals and snacks are the vegan's best option for obtaining calcium. Green leafy vegetables and nuts also contain calcium, but the mineral is either not well absorbed or not very plentiful from these sources. Calcium supplements are another option (see Chapter 10). Special diet planning is always required, because even a multivitamin and mineral supplement will not supply enough calcium to meet the needs of the body.

Consuming adequate quantities of omega-3 fatty acids is yet another nutritional concern for vegetarians, especially vegans. Fish and fish oils, abundant sources of these heart-healthy fats, are omitted from many types of vegetarian diets. Alternative plant sources of

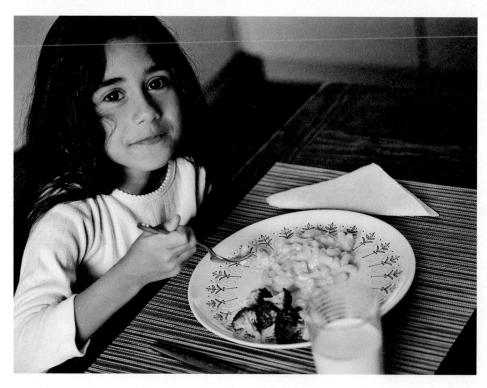

▲ Children can safely enjoy vegetarian and vegan diets as long as certain adjustments are made to meet their age-specific nutritional needs.

omega-3 fatty acids include canola oil, soybean oil, seaweed, microalgae, flax seeds, and walnuts.

SPECIAL CONCERNS FOR INFANTS AND CHILDREN

Infants and children, notoriously picky eaters in the first place, are at highest risk for nutrient deficiencies as a result of improperly planned vegetarian and vegan diets. With the use of complementary proteins and good sources of problem nutrients just discussed, the calorie, protein, vitamin, and mineral needs of vegetarian and vegan infants and children can be met. The most common nutritional concerns for infants and children following vegetar-

ian and vegan diets are deficiencies of iron, vitamin B-12, vitamin D, and calcium.

Vegetarian and vegan diets tend to be high in bulky, high-fiber, low-calorie foods that cause a feeling of fullness. While this is a welcome advantage for adults, children have small stomach volume and relatively high nutrient needs compared to their size, and therefore may feel full before their calorie needs are met. For this reason, the fiber content of a child's diet may need to be decreased by replacing high-fiber sources with some refined grain products, fruit juices, and peeled fruit. Other concentrated sources of calories for vegetarian and vegan children include fortified soy milk, nuts, dried fruits, avocados, and cookies made with vegetable oils or tub margarine.

CASE STUDY

Planning a Vegetarian Diet

Jordan is a freshman in college. He lives in a campus residence hall and teaches martial arts in the afternoon. He eats two or three meals a day at the residence hall cafeteria and snacks between meals. Jordan and his roommate both decided to become vegetarians because they recently read a magazine article describing the health benefits of a vegetarian diet. Yesterday Jordan's vegetarian diet consisted of a Danish pastry for breakfast and a tomato-rice dish (no meat) with pretzels and a diet soft drink for lunch. In the afternoon, after his martial arts class, he had a milk shake and two cookies. At dinnertime he had a vegetarian sub sandwich consisting of lettuce, sprouts, tomatoes, cucumbers, and cheese, with two glasses of fruit punch. In the evening, he had a bowl of popcorn.

Answer the following questions, and check your response in Appendix A.

1. What type of health benefits can Jordan expect from following a well-planned vegetarian diet?
2. What is missing from Jordan's current diet plan in terms of foods that should be emphasized in a vegetarian diet?
3. Which nutrients are missing in this current diet plan?
4. Are there any food components in the current diet plan that should be minimized or avoided?
5. How could he improve his new diet at each meal and snack to meet his nutritional needs and avoid undesirable food components?

▲ Has Jordan planned a healthy and nutritious vegetarian diet?

SUMMARY

1. Amino acids, the building blocks of proteins, contain a very usable form of nitrogen for humans. Of the 20 common types of amino acids found in food, nine must be consumed in food (essential) and the rest can be synthesized by the body (nonessential).

2. Individual amino acids are bonded together to form proteins. The sequential order of amino acids determines the protein's ultimate shape and function. This order is directed by DNA in the cell nucleus. Diseases such as sickle cell anemia can occur if the amino acids are incorrect on a polypeptide chain. When the three-dimensional shape of a protein is unfolded—denatured— by treatment with heat, acid or alkaline solutions, or other processes, the protein also loses its biological activity.

3. Almost all animal products are nutrient-dense sources of protein. The high quality of these proteins means that they can be easily converted into body proteins. Rich plant sources of protein, such as beans, are also available.

4. High-quality (complete) protein foods contain ample amounts of all nine essential amino acids. Furthermore, foods derived from animal sources provide high biological value protein. Lower-quality (incomplete) protein foods lack sufficient amounts of one or more essential amino acids. This is typical of plant foods, especially cereal grains. Different types of plant foods eaten together often complement each other's amino-acid deficits, thereby providing high-quality protein in the diet.

5. Protein digestion begins in the stomach, dividing the proteins into breakdown products containing shorter polypeptide chains of amino acids. In the small intestine, these polypeptide chains eventually separate into amino acids in the absorptive cells. The free amino acids then travel via the portal vein that connects to the liver. Some then enter the bloodstream.

6. Important body components—such as muscles, connective tissue, transport proteins in the bloodstream, visual pigments, enzymes, some hormones, and immune cells—are made of proteins. These proteins are in a state of constant turnover. The carbon chains of proteins may be used to produce glucose (or fat) when necessary.

7. The protein RDA for adults is 0.8 grams per kilogram of healthy body weight. For a typical 70-kilogram (154-pound) person, this corresponds to 56 grams of protein daily; for a 57-kilogram (125-pound) person, this corresponds to 46 grams per day. The North American diet generally supplies plenty of protein. Men typically consume about 100 grams of protein daily, and women consume closer to 65 grams. These usual protein intakes are also of sufficient quality to support body functions. This is even true for well-balanced vegetarian diets.

8. Undernutrition can lead to protein-calorie malnutrition in the form of kwashiorkor or marasmus. Kwashiorkor results primarily from an inadequate calorie and protein intake in comparison with body needs, which

often increase with concurrent disease and infection. Kwashiorkor often occurs when a child is weaned from human milk and fed mostly starchy gruels. Marasmus results from extreme starvation—a negligible intake of both protein and calories. Marasmus commonly occurs during famine, especially in infants.

9. Consumption of vegetarian and other plant-based diets provides many health benefits, including lower risks of chronic diseases including cardiovascular disease, diabetes, and certain cancers. The benefits associated with the plant-based diets appear to stem from the lower content of saturated fat and cholesterol and the higher amount of fiber, vitamins, minerals, and phytochemicals.

STUDY QUESTIONS

1. Discuss the relative importance of essential and nonessential amino acids in the diet. Why is it important for essential amino acids lost from the body to be replaced in the diet?

2. Describe the concept of complementary proteins.

3. What is a limiting amino acid? Explain why this concept is a concern in a vegetarian diet. How can a vegetarian compensate for limiting amino acids in specific foods?

4. Briefly describe the organization of proteins. How can this organization be altered or damaged? What might be a result of damaged protein organization?

5. Describe four functions of proteins. Provide an example of how the structure of a protein relates to its function.

6. How are DNA and protein synthesis related?

7. What would be one health benefit of reducing high-protein intake(s) to RDA amounts for some people?

8. What characteristics of vegetable proteins could improve the North American diet? What foods would you include to provide a diet that has ample protein from both plant and animal sources but is moderate in fat?

9. Outline the major differences between kwashiorkor and marasmus.

10. What are the possible long-term effects of an inadequate intake of dietary protein among children between the ages of 6 months and 4 years?

CHECK YOUR KNOWLEDGE

Answers to the following multiple choice questions are in Appendix A.

1. The "instructions" for making proteins are located in the
   a. cell membrane.
   b. DNA and RNA genetic material.
   c. stomach.
   d. small intestine.

2. A nutrient that could easily be deficient in the diet of a vegan would be
   a. vitamin C.
   b. folic acid.
   c. calcium.
   d. All of the above.

3. If an essential amino acid is unavailable for protein synthesis, the
   a. cell will make the amino acid.
   b. synthesis of the protein will stop.
   c. cell will continue to attach amino acids to the protein.
   d. partially completed protein will be stored for later completion.

4. An example of protein complementation used in vegetarian diet planning would be the combination of

   a. cereal and milk.
   b. bacon and eggs.
   c. rice and beans.
   d. macaroni and cheese.

5. An individual who eats only plant food is referred to as a
   a. planetarium.
   b. vegan.
   c. lactovegetarian.
   d. ovovegetarian.

6. Which of the following groups accounts for the differences among amino acids?
   a. amine group
   b. side chain
   c. acid group
   d. keto group

7. Absorption of amino acids takes place in the
   a. stomach.
   b. liver.
   c. small intestine.
   d. large intestine.

8. Jack is not an athlete and weighs 176 pounds (80 kilograms). His RDA for protein would be _____ grams.
   a. 32
   b. 40
   c. 64
   d. 80

9. Which of the following is true about protein intake of people in the United States?
   a. Most do not consume enough protein.
   b. Most consume approximately the amount needed to balance losses.
   c. Athletes generally do not get enough protein without supplementation.
   d. Most consume more than is needed.

10. The basic building block of a protein is called a(n)
   a. fatty acid.
   b. monosaccharide.
   c. amino acid.
   d. gene.

FURTHER READINGS

1. ADA Reports: Position of the American Dietetic Association and Dietitians of Canada: vegetarian diets. *Journal of the American Dietetic Association* 103:748, 2003.

   It is the position of the American Dietetic Association and Dietitians of Canada that appropriately planned vegetarian diets are healthful, nutritionally adequate, and provide health benefits in the prevention and treatment of certain diseases. In some cases, however, use of fortified foods or a multivitamin and mineral supplement may be needed to meet recommendations for individual nutrients.

2. Antony AC: Vegetarianism and vitamin B-12 (colbalamin) deficiency. *American Journal of Clinical Nutrition* 78:3, 2003.

   It is vital that a vegetarian focus on meeting vitamin B-12 needs. Use of vitamin B-12-fortified foods or a vitamin and mineral supplement are two options.

3. Aronson D: Vegetarian nutrition. *Today's Dietitian* p. 3, March 2005.

   This article summarizes the possible nutrient deficiencies that can result from a vegetarian diet. Plant food sources to counteract these risks are reviewed, such as rich sources of calcium.

4. Barnard ND and others: A low-fat vegan diet improves glycemic control and cardiovascular risk factors in a randomized clinical trial in individuals with type 2 diabetes. *Diabetes Care* 29:1777, 2006.

   Improvements in glycemic (decreased hemoglobin A1C) and lipid (decreased LDL cholesterol) control were greater in type 2 diabetic patients that followed a low-fat vegan diet compared to a diet based on American Diabetes Association guidelines. In the vegan group, 43% of the subjects reduced their diabetes medications compared to 26% of the subjects on the ADA diet.

5. Berkow SE, Barnard ND: Blood pressure regulation and vegetarian diets. *Nutrition Reviews* 63:1, 2005.

   Vegetarian diets are associated with lower blood pressure. It is likely that the fruit, vegetables, legumes, and nuts in such a diet lead to this health benefit.

6. Chao A and others: Meat consumption and colorectal cancer. *Journal of the American Medical Association* 293:172, 2005.

   Diets rich in red meat, especially processed meat, increase the risk of colon cancer. Protein from poultry and fish, in contrast, does not pose the same risk.

7. Dunn-Emke SR and others: Nutrient adequacy of a very low-fat vegan diet. *Journal of the American Dietetic Association* 105:1442, 2005.

   Men with early stage prostate cancer followed a very low-fat (10%) vegan diet that also included a fortified soy protein beverage. The study found that a very low-fat vegan diet, along with comprehensive nutrition education that emphasized nutrient-fortified plant foods, was nutritionally adequate, with the exception of vitamin D. Vitamin D supplementation, especially for individuals with limited sun exposure, is recommended for those following a very low-fat vegan diet.

8. Food and Nutrition Board: *Dietary reference intakes for energy, carbohydrate, fiber, fat, fatty acids, cholesterol, protein, and amino acids.* Washington DC: The National Academy Press, 2002.

   This report provides the latest guidance for macronutrient intakes. With regard to protein intake, the RDA has been set at 0.8 grams per kilogram per day. Protein intake can range from 10% to 35% of calorie intake. The 10% allotment approximates the RDA, based on typical calorie intakes.

9. Garlick PJ: The nature of human hazards associated with excessive intakes of amino acids. *Journal of Nutrition* 134:1633S, 2004.

   The most toxic amino acids are methionine, cysteine, and histidine. Possible health risks from excessive intakes of other amino acids are also reviewed. These risks are seen with amino acid supplements, not whole food sources.

10. Gardner CD and others: The effect of a plant-based diet on plasma lipids in hypercholesterolemic adults. *Annals of Internal Medicine* 142:725, 2005.

    Adding plant proteins to a diet already low in saturated fat and cholesterol provides additional benefits regarding lowering blood cholesterol. The authors emphasize the importance of including fruits, vegetables, legumes, and whole grains in a diet.

11. Key TJ and others: Health effects of vegetarian and vegan diets. *Proceedings of the Nutrition Society* 65:35, 2006.

    This study reviewed recent findings from large studies and summarizes the latest understanding of the health effects of vegetarian and vegan diets. Results indicated that vegetarians have a lower BMI and lower obesity rates than comparable nonvegetarians; total plasma cholesterol is lower in vegetarians that nonvegetarians; between vegetarians and nonvegetarians there is no significant differences in blood pressure; studies of vegetarians indicate a moderate reduction in mortality from ischemic heart disease; and studies showed no differences between vegetarians and nonvegetarians for colorectal cancer, breast cancer, prostate cancer, or total mortality.

12. Leitzmann C: Vegetarian diets: What are the advantages? *Forum of Nutrition* 57:147, 2005.

    The benefits of a vegetarian diet are a lower intake of saturated fat, cholesterol, and animal protein, as well as a higher intake of complex carbohydrates, fiber, magnesium, folate, vitamin C, vitamin E, carotenoids, and other phytochemicals. Well-balanced vegetarian diets are appropriate for all stages of the life cycle. The article provides evidence to support these statements, as well as reviews other possible health benefits.

13. Lejeune MP and others: Additional protein intake limits weight regain after weight loss in humans. *British Journal of Nutrition* 93: 281, 2005.

    Adding 30 grams of protein per day to their usual diets helped people in this study limit weight regain after weight loss. The diet ended up 18% of calorie intake as protein, compared to 15% in the control group. This protein intake in the experimental group would not be considered excessive given an upper limit of 35% of calorie intake set by the Food and Nutrition Board.

14. Mangels R: Weight control the vegan way. *Vegetarian Journal* XXV (1), 2006.

    This article provides suggestions for vegans, or people interested in following a vegan diet, who want to lose weight. Two eating plans are included that were developed for people who are moderately active, spending 30-60 minutes daily in moderate physical activity. The first eating plan has approximately 1500 calories and is designed for women who want to lose 1–2 pounds per week. The second has about 1900 calories and is designed for men who want to lose 1–2 pounds per week. Protein foods include kidney beans, chickpeas, and other beans; tofu; lite or plain soymilk; nuts and nut butters; seitan (say-than, wheat meat); and meat analogs. Recipes are also included.

15. Newby PK: Risk of overweight and obesity among semivegetarian, lactovegetarian, and vegan women. *American Journal of Clinical Nutrition* 81:1267, 2005.

    Semivegetarian women in this study were less likely to be overweight and obese compared to omnivorous women. Consuming more plant foods and less animal products may help individuals control their weight.

16. Rosell MS and others: Long-chain n–3 polyunsaturated fatty acids in plasma in British meat-eating, vegetarian, and vegan men. *American Journal of Clinical Nutrition* 82:327, 2005.

    The plasma composition of the long-chain omega-3 fatty acids was compared among meat-eaters, vegetarians, and vegans. The proportions of the omega-3 fatty acids in the plasma were not affected by the consumption of a vegetarian or vegan diet. The authors conclude that when animal foods are excluded from the diet, the omega-3 fatty acids will be produced endogenously, resulting in a low but stable plasma concentration.

17. Sabate J: The contribution of vegetarian diets to human health. *Forum of Nutrition* 56:218, 2005.

    Components of a healthy vegetarian diet include a variety of vegetables, fruits, whole-grain breads and cereals, legumes, and nuts. Such a diet contributes to overall health and increased longevity when these foods are emphasized.

18. Sacks FM and others: Soy protein, isoflavones, and cardiovascular health. An American Heart Association Science Advisory for Professionals From the Nutrition Committee, *Circulation* 113:1034, 2006.

    This scientific advisory evaluates recent work published on soy protein and its component isoflavones and their potential role in improving risk factors for cardiovascular disease. In the majority of studies, soy protein with isoflavones, as compared with milk or other proteins, decreased LDL cholesterol concentrations; the average effect was ~3% and no significant effects on HDL cholesterol, triglycerides, lipoprotein(a), or blood pressure were evident. The authors conclude that soy products should be beneficial to cardiovascular and overall health because of their high content of polyunsaturated fats, fiber, vitamins, and minerals and low content of saturated fat.

19. Taylor SL: Estimating prevalence of soy protein allergy. *The Soy Connection* 14 (2):1, 2006.

    This article discusses the issue of soy protein allergy. Although soy protein has been designated one of the major allergens by the U.S. Food and Drug Administration, rigorous prevalence data for this allergy are not available, and indirect evidence suggests it occurs less frequently than other common allergens including shellfish, peanuts, tree nuts, and fish.

20. Trock BJ and others: Meta-analysis of soy intake and breast cancer risk. *Journal of the National Cancer Institute*, 98 (7):459, 2006.

    This study analyzed data from 18 previously published studies and concludes that consumption of soy foods among healthy women was associated with a significant reduction (14%) in breast cancer risk.

▶ Check out the **Contemporary Nutrition ARIS site**

www.mhhe.com/wardlawcontfa1 for quizzes, flash cards, other activities, and weblinks designed to further help you learn about what you eat and why.

I. Protein and the Vegetarian

Alana is excited about all the health benefits that might accompany a vegetarian diet. However, she is concerned that she will not consume enough protein to meet her needs. She is also concerned about possible vitamin and mineral deficiencies. Use NutritionCalc Plus or Appendix N to calculate her protein intake and see if her concerns are valid.

	Protein (g)
Breakfast Calcium fortified orange juice, 1 cup Soy milk, 1 cup Fortified bran flakes, 1 cup Banana, medium	
Snack Calcium-enriched granola bar	
Lunch GardenBurger, 4 oz Whole-wheat bun Mustard, 1 tbsp Soy cheese, 1 oz Apple, medium Green leaf lettuce, 1 ½ cups Peanuts, 1 oz Sunflower seeds, 1/4 cup Tomato slices, 2 Mushrooms, 3 Vinaigrette salad dressing, 2 tbsp Iced tea	
Dinner Kidney beans, ½ cup Brown rice, 3/4 cup Fortified margarine, 2 tbsp Mixed vegetables, 1/4 cup Hot tea	
Dessert Strawberries, ½ cup Angel food cake, 1 small slice Soy milk, ½ cup	
	TOTAL PROTEIN (grams) _____

Alana's diet contained 2150 kcal, with _____ grams (you fill in) of protein (Is this plenty for her?), 360 grams of carbohydrate, 57 grams of total dietary fat (only 9 grams of which came from saturated fat), and 50 grams of fiber. Her vitamin and mineral intake with respect to those of concern to vegetarians—vitamin B-12, vitamin D, calcium, iron, and zinc—met her needs.

II. Meeting Protein Needs When Dieting to Lose Weight

Your father has been steadily gaining weight for the last 30 years and now has developed hypertension and type 2 diabetes as a result. His physician recommends that he lose some weight by following an 1800 kcal diet. You know that it will be important for your father to meet protein needs as he tries to lose weight. Design a 1-day diet for him that contains about 20% of calorie intake as protein. Table 6-2 will provide some help. Will this diet meet his protein RDA? Does the diet look like a plan you could also follow?

CHAPTER 7 Energy Balance and Weight Control

CHAPTER OBJECTIVES Chapter 7 is designed to allow you to:

1. Describe the uses of energy by the body and what constitutes energy balance.

2. Describe various ways to diagnose overweight and obesity.

3. Outline the risks to health posed by overweight and obesity.

4. List and discuss factors affecting energy balance, and describe the concept of set point.

5. Describe why and how reduced calorie intake, behavior modification, and increased physical activity fit into a weight-loss plan.

6. Outline the benefits and hazards of various weight-loss methods for severe obesity.

7. Evaluate popular weight-reduction diets and determine which are unsafe, doomed to fail, or both.

CHAPTER OUTLINE

OF PEOPLE YOU SEE ON THE STREET, 29% OF THE MEN AND 44% OF THE WOMEN ARE TRYING TO LOSE WEIGHT. Still, despite all their efforts, the ranks of the obese in North America and worldwide are growing. Recall from Chapter 1 that an estimated 1 billion people in the world are overweight. This problem is increasing not only in the United States but also globally among affluent peoples in Brazil, China, India, Russia, the United Kingdom, and Germany. Excess weight increases the likelihood of many health problems, such as cardiovascular disease, cancer, hypertension, strokes, certain bone and joint disorders, and type 2 diabetes, especially if a person performs minimal physical activity.

Currently, most weight-reduction efforts fizzle before bodies fall into a healthy weight range. Typical popular ("fad") diets are generally monotonous, ineffective, and confusing. They may even endanger some populations, such as children, teenagers, pregnant women, and people with various health disorders. A more logical approach to weight loss is straightforward: (1) eat less; (2) increase physical activity; and (3) change problematic eating behaviors.

A national commitment has begun from a variety of groups, including government agencies, the food industry, health professionals, and communities, to address the growing weight problem in North America. It has become obvious that, without this national effort to promote weight maintenance and effective new approaches to making our social environment more favorable to maintaining healthy weight, the current trends will not be reversed. Chapter 7 discusses these recommendations to help you understand obesity's causes, consequences, and potential treatments.

Refresh Your Memory

As you begin your study of weight control in Chapter 7, you may want to review:

- Biological and social dimensions of food intake in Chapter 1
- The concept of energy density and appropriate single serving sizes for foods in Chapter 2
- The causes and consequences of ketosis in Chapter 4
- The fat content of various foods in Chapter 5
- The long-term risks of high-protein diets in Chapter 6

What components make up a successful diet plan? What constitutes a "fad" diet? Why is overweight and obesity a growing problem worldwide? What might be the future consequences of this trend? Chapter 7 provides some answers.

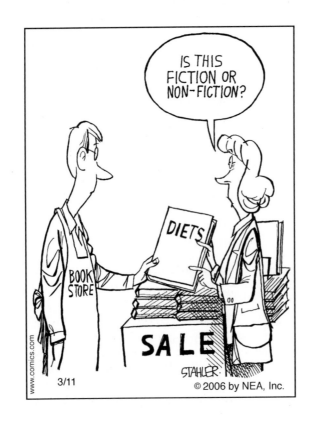

ENERGY BALANCE

We begin this chapter with some good news and some bad news. The good news is that if you stay at a healthy body weight, you increase your chances of living a long and healthy life. The bad news is that currently 65% of all North American adults are overweight, significantly more than in the 1980s. Of those, about 45% (30% of the total population) are obese. There is a good chance that any of us could become part of those statistics if we do not pay attention to the prevention of significant weight gain in adulthood. Gaining more than 10 pounds or 2 inches in waist circumference are signals that a re-evaluation of diet and lifestyle is in order.

There is no quick cure for overweight, despite what the advertisements claim. Successful weight loss comes from hard work and commitment. A combination of decreased calorie intake, increased physical activity, and behavior modification is considered to be the most reliable treatment for the overweight condition. And without a doubt, the prevention of the overweight condition in the first place is the most successful approach.

The Growing Overweight/ Obesity Problem

Adults 20 to 74 who are overweight or obese:

1960–1962	**45%**
1971–1974	**47%**
1976–1980	**47%**
1988–1994	**56%**
1999–today	**64.5%**

Positive and Negative Energy Balance

A healthy weight can result from paying more attention to the important concept of **energy balance.** Think of energy balance as an equation:

$$\text{Energy Input} = \text{Energy Output}$$
$$\text{(calories from food intake)} = \text{(metabolism; digestion, absorption, and transport of nutrients; physical activity)}$$

The balance of calories (measured in kcals) on the two sides of this equation can influence energy stores, especially the amount of triglyceride stored in adipose tissue (Fig. 7-1). When energy input is greater than energy output, the result is **positive energy balance.** The excess calories consumed are stored, which results in weight gain. There are some situations in which positive energy balance is normal and healthy. During pregnancy, a surplus of calories supports the developing fetus. Infants and children require a positive energy balance for growth and development. In adults, however, even a small positive energy balance is usually in the form of fat storage rather than muscle and bone and, over time, can cause body weight to climb.

On the other hand, if energy input is less than energy output, there is a calorie deficit and **negative energy balance** results. A negative energy balance is necessary for successful weight loss. It is important to realize that during negative energy balance, weight loss involves a reduction in both lean and adipose tissue, not just "fat."

The maintenance of energy balance substantially contributes to health and well-being in adults by minimizing the risk of developing many common health problems. Adulthood is often a time of subtle increases in weight gain, which eventually turns into obesity if left unchecked. The process of aging does not cause weight gain; rather the problem stems from a pattern of excess food intake coupled with limited physical activity and slower metabolism. Let's look in detail at the factors that affect the energy balance equation.

energy balance   The state in which energy intake, in the form of food and beverages, matches the energy expended, primarily through basal metabolism and physical activity.

positive energy balance   The state in which energy intake is greater than energy expended, generally resulting in weight gain.

negative energy balance   The state in which energy intake is less than energy expended, resulting in weight loss.

CRITICAL THINKING

A 26-year-old classmate of yours has been thinking about the process of aging. One of the things she fears most as she gets older is gaining weight. How would you explain energy balance to her?

Energy Intake

Energy needs are met by food intake, represented by the number of calories eaten each day. Determining the appropriate amount and type of food to match our energy needs is a challenge for many of us. Our desire to consume food and the ability of our bodies to use it efficiently are survival mechanisms that have evolved with humans. However, because of current North American food supplies and accessibility, many of us are now too successful in obtaining food energy. The abundant food supply has essentially replaced the need to store body fat. Given the wide availability of food in vending machines, drive-up windows, social gatherings, and fast-food restaurants—combined with *supersized* portions—it is no wonder that the average adult is 8 pounds heavier than just 10 years ago. In response to this cultural trend of food being widely available, "defensive

FIGURE 7-1 ▶ A model for energy balance—input vs. output. This figure depicts energy balance in practical terms.

eating" (i.e., making careful and conscious food choices, especially in regard to portion size,) on a continual basis is important for many of us.

bomb calorimeter An instrument used to determine the calorie content of a food.

The number of calories in a food is determined with an instrument called a **bomb calorimeter.** This calorie determination is described in Figure 7-2. The bomb calorimeter measures the amount of calories coming from carbohydrate, fat, protein, and alcohol. Recall that carbohydrates yield about 4 kcal per gram, proteins yield about 4 kcal per gram, fats yield about 9 kcal per gram, and alcohol yields 7 kcal per gram. These energy figures have been adjusted for (1) our ability to digest the food and (2) substances in food, such as fibrous plant parts that burn in the bomb calorimeter but do not provide calories to the human body. The figures are then rounded to whole numbers. However, today it is also possible and more common to determine the calo-

Thermometer

Wire to ignite food

Insulation around chamber

Chamber for food

Air space

Water

FIGURE 7-2 ▶ Cross-section of a bomb calorimeter. A dried portion of food is burned inside a chamber containing oxygen and surrounded by water to determine energy content. As the food is burned, it gives off heat, which raises the temperature of the water surrounding the chamber. The increase in water temperature indicates the number of kcal contained in the food, because 1 kcal equals the amount of heat needed to raise the temperature of 1 kilogram of water 1 degree Celsius.

rie content of a food by quantifying its carbohydrate, protein, and fat (and possibly alcohol) content. Then the kcal per gram factors listed previously are used to calculate the total kcals. (Recall that Chapter 1 showed how to do this calculation.)

Energy Output

So far, some factors concerning energy intake have been discussed. Now let's look at the other side of the equation—energy output.

The body uses energy for three general purposes: basal metabolism; physical activity; and digestion, absorption, and processing of ingested nutrients. A fourth minor form of energy output, known as thermogenesis, refers to energy expended during fidgeting or shivering in response to cold (Fig. 7-3).

Basal Metabolism. Basal metabolism is expressed as basal metabolic rate (BMR) and represents the minimal amount of calories expended in a fasting state (for 12 hours or more) to keep a resting, awake body alive in a warm, quiet environment. For a sedentary person, basal metabolism accounts for about 60% to 70% of total energy use by the body. Some of the processes involved include the beating of the heart, respiration by the lungs, and the activity of other organs such as the liver, brain, and kidney. It does not include energy used for physical activity or digestion, absorption, and processing of recently consumed nutrients. If the person is not fasting or completely rested, the term **resting metabolism** is used and expressed as resting metabolic rate (RMR). An individual's RMR is typically 6% higher than his or her BMR.

To see how basal metabolism contributes to energy needs, consider a 130-pound woman. First, knowing that there are 2.2 pounds for every kilogram, convert her weight into metric units:

$$130 \text{ lbs} \div 2.2 \text{ lbs/kilograms} = 59 \text{ kilograms}$$

▲ The cultural trend of serving large quantities can easily lead to positive energy balance. Sharing your meal with another person is a good way to avoid overeating when served large portions.

basal metabolism   The minimal amount of calories the body uses to support itself in a fasting state when resting (e.g., 12 hours for both) and awake in a warm, quiet environment. It amounts to roughly 1 kcal per kilogram per hour for men and 0.9 kcal per kilogram per hour for women; these values are often referred to as *basal metabolic rate (BMR)*.

resting metabolism   The amount of calories the body uses when the person has not eaten in 4 hours and is resting (e.g., 15 to 30 minutes) and awake in a warm, quiet environment. It is roughly 6% higher than basal metabolism due to the less strict criteria for the test; often referred to as *resting metabolic rate (RMR)*.

FIGURE 7-3 ▶ The components of energy intake and expenditure. This figure incorporates the major variables that influence energy balance. *Remember that alcohol is an additional source of energy for some of us.* The size of each component shows the relative contribution of that component to energy balance.

lean body mass Body weight minus fat storage weight equals lean body mass. This includes organs such as the brain, muscles, and liver, as well as bone and blood and other body fluids.

▶ While a person is resting, the percentage of total energy use and corresponding energy use by various organs is approximately as follows:

Brain	19%	265 kcal/day
Skeletal muscle	18%	250 kcal/day
Liver	27%	380 kcal/day
Kidney	10%	140 kcal/day
Heart	7%	100 kcal/day
Other	19%	265 kcal/day

Then, using a rough estimate of basal metabolic rate of 0.9 kcal per kilogram per hour for an average female (1.0 kcal per kilogram per hour is used for an average male), calculate her basal metabolic rate:

$$59 \text{ kg} \times 0.9 \text{ kcal/kg} = 53 \text{ kcal per hour}$$

Finally, use this hourly basal metabolic rate to find her basal metabolic rate for an entire day:

$$53 \text{ kcal/hr} \times 24 \text{ hrs} = 1272 \text{ kcal}$$

These calculations give us only an estimate of actual basal metabolism, as it can vary 25% to 30% among individuals. Factors that increase a person's basal metabolism include:

- Greater **lean body mass**
- Larger body surface area
- Male gender (caused by greater lean body mass)
- Body temperature (fever or cold environmental conditions)
- Thyroid hormones
- Aspects of nervous system activity (release of norepinephrine)
- Pregnancy
- Caffeine and tobacco use. (Using the practice of smoking to control body weight is not recommended as too many health risks are increased.)

Of those factors, the amount of lean body mass a person has is the most important one.

In contrast to factors that increase basal metabolism, a low calorie intake, such as that during an extreme diet regime, decreases basal metabolism by about 10% to 20% (about 150 to 300 kcal per day) as the body shifts into a conservation mode. This is a barrier to sustained weight loss during dieting that involves extremely low calorie diets. In addition, the effects of aging make weight maintenance a challenge. As lean body mass slowly and steadily decreases, basal metabolism declines 1% to 2% for each decade past the age of 30. However, because physical activity aids in maintenance of lean body mass, remaining active as one ages helps to preserve a high basal metabolism and, in turn, aids in weight control.

Energy for Physical Activity. Physical activity increases energy expenditure above and beyond basal energy needs by as much as 25% to 40%. In choosing to be active or inactive, we determine much of our total calorie expenditure for a day. Calorie expenditure from physical activity varies widely among people. For example, climbing stairs rather than riding the elevator, walking rather than driving to the store, and standing in a bus rather than sitting increase physical activity and, hence, energy use. The alarming incidence of and recent increase in obesity in North America are partially the result of our inactivity. Jobs demand less physical activity, and leisure time is often spent in front of a television or computer.

Thermic Effect of Food (TEF). In addition to basal metabolism and physical activity, the body uses energy to digest food, and absorb and further process the nutrients recently consumed. Energy used for these tasks is referred to as the **thermic effect of food (TEF).** TEF is similar to a sales tax—it is like being charged about 5% to 10% for the total amount of calories you eat to cover the cost of processing that food eaten. We may even recognize this increase in metabolism as a warming of the body during and right after a meal. Because of this "tax," you must eat between 105 and 110 kcal for every 100 kcal needed for basal metabolism and physical activity. If your daily calorie intake was 3000 kcal, TEF would account for 150 to 300 kcal. As with other components of energy output, the total amount can vary somewhat among individuals.

Food composition influences TEF. For example, the TEF value for a protein-rich meal is 20% to 30% of the calories consumed and is higher than that of a carbohydrate-rich (5% to 10%) or fat-rich (0% to 3%) meal. This is because it takes more energy to metabolize amino acids into fat than to convert glucose into glycogen or transfer absorbed fat into adipose stores. In addition, large meals result in higher TEF values than the same amount of food eaten over many hours.

Thermogenesis. **Thermogenesis** represents the increase in nonvoluntary physical activity triggered by cold conditions or overeating. Some examples of nonvoluntary activities include shivering when cold, fidgeting, maintenance of muscle tone, and maintaining body posture when not lying down. Studies have shown that some people are able to resist weight gain from overfeeding by inducing thermogenesis, while others are not able to do so to a great extent.

The contribution of thermogenesis to overall calorie output is fairly small. The combination of basal metabolism and TEF accounts for 70% to 80% of energy used by a sedentary person. The remaining 20% to 30% is used mostly for physical activity, with a small amount used for thermogenesis.

Brown adipose tissue is a specialized form of adipose tissue that participates in thermogenesis. It is found in small amounts in infants. The brown appearance results from its rich blood flow. Brown adipose tissue contributes to thermogenesis by releasing some of the energy from energy-yielding nutrients into the environment as heat. In infants, brown adipose tissue contributes as much as 5% of body weight and is thought to be important for heat regulation. Hibernating animals also use brown adipose tissue to generate heat to withstand a long winter. Adults have very little brown adipose tissue, and its role in adulthood is unknown.

▲ Classwork leads to mental stress but puts little physical stress on the body. Hence, energy needs are only about 1.5 kcal per minute.

▶ The TEF value for alcohol is 20%.

thermic effect of food (TEF) The increase in metabolism that occurs during the digestion, absorption, and metabolism of energy-yielding nutrients. This represents 5% to 10% of calories consumed.

thermogenesis This term encompasses the ability of humans to regulate body temperature within narrow limits (thermoregulation). Two visible examples of thermogenesis are fidgeting and shivering when cold.

brown adipose tissue A specialized form of adipose tissue that produces large amounts of heat by metabolizing energy-yielding nutrients without synthesizing much useful energy for the body. The unused energy is released as heat.

CONCEPT CHECK

Energy balance involves matching energy intake with energy output. Energy content of food is expressed in kcals and can be determined using a bomb calorimeter. This analysis yields the 4-9-4-7 estimates for the kcals in a gram of carbohydrate, fat, protein, and alcohol, respectively.

The body uses energy for four main purposes:

1. Basal metabolism (60% to 70% of total energy output) represents the minimal amount of calories needed to maintain the body at rest. Primary determinants of basal metabolic rate include quantity of lean body mass, amount of body surface, and thyroid hormone concentrations in the bloodstream.
2. Physical activity calorie expenditure (20% to 30% of total energy output) represents calorie use for total body cell metabolism above what is needed during rest.
3. Thermic effect of food (5% to 10% of total energy output) represents the calories needed to digest food and absorb and process nutrients recently consumed.
4. Thermogenesis (small, variable percentage of total energy output) includes nonvoluntary, heat-producing activities, such as fidgeting, as well as shivering when cold.

DETERMINATION OF ENERGY USE BY THE BODY

The amount of energy a body uses can be measured by both direct and indirect calorimetry or can be estimated based on height, weight, degree of physical activity, and age.

Direct and Indirect Calorimetry

Direct calorimetry measures the amount of body heat released by a person. The subject is put into an insulated chamber, often the size of a small bedroom, and body heat released raises the temperature of a layer of water surrounding the chamber. A kcal, as you recall, is related to the amount of heat required to raise the temperature of water. By measuring the water temperature in the direct calorimeter before and after the body releases heat, scientists can determine the energy expended.

Direct calorimetry works because almost all the energy used by the body eventually leaves as heat. However, few studies use direct calorimetry, mostly because of its expense and complexity.

The most commonly used method of **indirect calorimetry** measures the amount of oxygen a person consumes instead of measuring heat output (Fig. 7-4). A predictable relationship exists between the body's use of energy and oxygen. For example, when metabolizing a typical mixed diet of the energy-yielding nutrients, carbohydrate, fat, and protein, the human body uses 1 liter of oxygen to yield about 4.85 kcal of energy.

Instruments to measure oxygen consumption for indirect calorimetry are widely used. They can be mounted on carts and rolled up to a hospital bed or carried in backpacks while a person plays tennis or jogs. There are even newly developed handheld instruments (Body Gem). Tables showing energy costs of various forms of exercises rely on information gained from indirect calorimetry studies.

Estimates of Energy Needs

As covered in Chapter 2, the Food and Nutrition Board has published a number of formulas to estimate energy needs, called Estimated Energy Requirements (EER). Those for adults are shown here (remember to do multiplication and division before addition and subtraction). (Formulas for pregnant women, lactating women, children, and teenagers, are listed in Chapters 16 and 17.) The calories used for basal metabolism are already factored into these formulas.

Estimated Energy Requirement Calculation for Men 19 years and older

$$\text{EER} = 662 - (9.53 \times \text{AGE}) + \text{PA} \times (15.91 \times \text{WT} + 539.6 \times \text{HT})$$

Estimated Energy Requirement Calculation for Women 19 years and older

$$\text{EER} = 354 - (6.91 \times \text{AGE}) + \text{PA} \times (9.36 \times \text{WT} + 726 \times \text{HT})$$

The variables in the formulas correspond to the following:

EER = Estimated Energy Requirement
AGE = age in years
PA = Physical Activity Estimate (see following table)
WT = weight in kilograms (pounds ÷ 2.2)
HT = height in meters (inches ÷ 39.4)

Physical Activity (PA) Estimates

Activity Level	PA (Men)	PA (Women)
Sedentary (e.g., no exercise)	1.00	1.00
Low activity (e.g., walks the equivalent of 2 miles per day at 3 to 4 mph)	1.11	1.12
Active (e.g., walks the equivalent of 7 miles per day at 3 to 4 mph)	1.25	1.27
Very active (e.g., walks the equivalent of 17 miles per day at 3 to 4 mph)	1.48	1.45

FIGURE 7-4 ▶ Indirect calorimetry. Measurements of oxygen use and carbon dioxide output can be used to determine calorie use during daily activities.

direct calorimetry A method of determining a body's energy use by measuring heat released from the body. An insulated chamber is usually used.

indirect calorimetry A method to measure energy use by the body by measuring oxygen uptake. Formulas are then used to convert this gas exchange value into energy use.

The following is a sample calculation for a man who is 25 years old, 5 feet, 9 inches (1.75 meters), 154 pounds (70 kilograms), and has an active lifestyle. His EER is:

$$EER = 662 - (9.53 \times 25) + 1.25 \times (15.91 \times 70 + 539.6 \times 1.75) = 2997 \text{ kcal}$$

The next equation is a sample calculation for a woman who is 25 years old, 5 feet, 4 inches (1.62 meters), 120 pounds (54.5 kilograms), and has an active lifestyle. Her EER is:

$$EER = 354 - (6.91 \times 25) + 1.27 \times (9.36 \times 54.5 + 726 \times 1.62) = 2323 \text{ kcal}$$

You have determined the man's EER to be about 3000 kcal and the woman's EER to be about 2300 kcal per day. Remember that this is only an estimate; many other factors, such as genetics and hormones, can affect actual energy needs.

A simple method of tracking your energy expenditure, and thus your energy needs, is to use the forms in Appendix E. Begin by taking an entire 24-hour period and listing all activities performed, including sleep. Record the number of minutes spent in each activity; the total should equal 1440 minutes (24 hours). Next record the energy cost for each activity in kcal per minute following the directions in Appendix E. Multiply the energy cost by the minutes. This gives the energy expended for each activity. Total all the kcal values. This gives your estimated energy expenditure for the day.

CONCEPT CHECK

Energy use by the body can be measured as heat given off by direct calorimetry or as oxygen used by indirect calorimetry. A person's Estimated Energy Requirement can be calculated based on the following factors: gender, height, weight, age, and amount of physical activity.

MyPyramid Calorie Guidelines

Children	Sedentary →	Active
2–3 years	1000	1400

Females	Sedentary →	Active
4–8 years	1200	1800
9–13	1600	2200
14–18	1800	2400
19–30	2000	2400
31–50	1800	2200
51+	1600	2200

Males	Sedentary →	Active
4–8 years	1200	2000
9–13	1800	2600
14–18	2200	3200
19–30	2400	3000
31–50	2200	3000
51+	2000	2800

ESTIMATION OF A HEALTHY WEIGHT

Numerous methods are used to establish what body weight should be, typically called *healthy weight*. Healthy weight is currently the preferred term to use for weight recommendations. Older terms, such as *ideal weight* and *desirable weight*, are subjective and are no longer used in medical literature. Several tables exist, generally based on weight-for-height. These tables arise from studies of large population groups. When applied to a population, they provide good estimates of weight associated with health and longevity. However, they do not necessarily indicate the healthiest body weight for each individual. For example, *athletes with large, lean body mass but low-fat content will have greater healthy weights than sedentary individuals.*

Overall, the individual, under a physician's guidance, should establish a "personal" healthy weight (or need for weight reduction) based on weight history, fat distribution patterns, family history of weight-related disease, and current health status. Evidence of the following weight-related conditions is important:

- Hypertension
- Elevated LDL-cholesterol
- Family history of obesity, cardiovascular disease, or certain forms of cancer (e.g., uterus, colon)
- Pattern of fat distribution in the body
- Elevated blood glucose

This assessment points out how well the person is tolerating any existing excess weight. Thus, current height/weight standards are only a rough guide. On a more practical note, other questions can be pertinent: What is the least one has weighed as an adult for at least a year? What is the largest size clothing one would be happy with? What weight has one been able to maintain during previous diets without feeling constantly hungry? Furthermore, a healthy lifestyle may make a more important contribution to a person's health status than the number on the scale. Fit and overweight

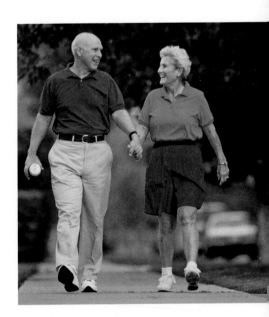

▲ Physical activity, such as walking, is an important component of our energy expenditure.

are not necessarily mutually exclusive (although not often seen together), and neither is thin synonymous with healthy if the person is not also physically active.

Using Body Mass Index (BMI) to Set Healthy Weight

For the past 50 years, weight-for-height tables issued by the Metropolitan Life Insurance Company have been the typical way healthy weight was established. These tables are organized by gender and frame size, predicting the weight range at a specific height that was associated with the greatest longevity. The latest table (issued in 1983) and methods for determining frame size can be found in Appendix G.

Currently **body mass index (BMI)** is the preferred weight-for-height standard because it is the clinical measurement most closely related to body fat content (Fig. 7-5).

Body mass index is calculated as

$$\frac{\text{body weight (in kilograms)}}{\text{height}^2 \text{ (in meters)}}$$

An alternate method for calculating BMI is

$$\frac{\text{weight (pounds)} \times 703}{\text{height}^2 \text{ (inches)}}$$

Figure 7-6 lists the BMI for various heights and weights. A healthy weight-for-height is a BMI between 18.5 to 24.9. Health risks from excess weight may begin when the body mass index is 25 or more. What is your BMI? How much would your weight need to change to yield a BMI of 25? 30? These are general cut-off values for the presence of overweight and obesity, respectively. BMI offers another way to define obesity (Fig. 7-6).

30–39.9	Obese	Increased health risk
40 or greater	Severely obese	Major health risk. The number of North Americans falling into this category is increasing rapidly.

The concept of body mass index is convenient to use because the values apply to both men and women (i.e., gender neutral). However, any weight-for-height standard is a crude measure. Keep in mind, also, that a BMI of 25 to 29.9 is a marker of *overweight* (compared to a standard population) and not necessarily a marker of *overfat*. Many men (especially athletes) have a BMI greater than 25 because of extra muscle tissue. Also, very short adults (under 5 feet tall) may have high BMIs that may not reflect overweight or fatness. For this reason, BMI should be used only as a screening test for overweight or obesity. Even agreed upon weight standards for BMI are not for everyone. Adult BMIs should not be applied to children, still growing adolescents, frail older people, pregnant and lactating women, and highly muscular individuals. Pregnant women and children have unique BMI standards (see Chapters 16 and 17).

Still, overfat and overweight conditions generally appear together. The focus is on BMI in clinical settings mainly because this is easier to measure than total body fat.

Putting Healthy Weight into Perspective

Listening to the body for hunger cues, regularly eating a healthy diet, and remaining physically active (not to be overlooked) eventually helps one maintain an appropriate height/weight value. This concept will be further addressed in the upcoming discussion on treatment for obesity. Another school of thought is to let nature take its course with regard to body weight. Support for this proposal is that after weight is lost during dieting, people often regain their original weight plus more. The clearest idea regarding a healthy weight is that it is personal. Weight has to be considered in terms of health, not a mathematical calculation.

▶ One BMI unit = 6–7 pounds

body mass index (BMI) Weight (in kilograms) divided by height (in meters) squared; a value of 25 and above indicates overweight and a value of 30 and above indicates obesity.

Women Men

BMI 20

BMI 25

BMI 30

FIGURE 7-5 ▶ Estimates of body shapes at different BMI values.

Weight in pounds

Height	120	130	140	150	160	170	180	190	200	210	220	230	240	250
4'6"	29	31	34	36	39	41	43	46	48	51	53	56	58	60
4'8"	27	29	31	34	36	38	40	43	45	47	49	52	51	56
4'10"	25	27	29	31	34	36	38	40	42	44	46	48	50	52
5'0"	23	25	27	29	31	33	35	37	39	41	43	45	47	49
5'2"	22	24	26	27	29	31	33	35	37	38	40	42	44	46
5'4"	21	22	24	26	28	29	31	33	34	36	38	40	41	43
5'6"	19	21	23	24	26	27	29	31	32	34	36	37	39	40
5'8"	18	20	21	23	24	26	27	29	30	32	34	35	37	38
5'10"	17	19	20	22	23	24	26	27	29	30	32	33	35	36
6'0"	16	18	19	20	22	23	24	26	27	28	30	31	33	34
6'2"	15	17	18	19	21	22	23	24	26	27	28	30	31	32
6'4"	15	16	17	18	20	21	22	23	24	26	27	28	29	30
6'6"	14	15	16	17	19	20	21	22	23	24	25	27	28	29
6'8"	13	14	15	17	18	19	20	21	22	23	24	26	26	28

Height in feet and inches

⬜ Healthy weight   ⬜ Overweight   ⬜ Obese

Developed by the National Center for Health Statistics in collaboration with the National Center for Chronic Disease Prevention and Health Promotion

FIGURE 7-6 ▶ Convenient height/weight table based on BMI. A healthy weight for height generally falls within a BMI range of 18.5–24.9 kilograms/meters^2.

ENERGY IMBALANCE

If calorie intake exceeds output over time, overweight (and often obesity) is a likely result. Often, health problems eventually follow (Table 7-1). As just discussed, BMI values can be used as a convenient clinical tool to estimate overweight (BMI ≥ 25), obesity (BMI ≥ 30), and severe obesity (BMI ≥ 40) in individuals greater than 20 years of age. Medical experts, however, recommend that an individual's diagnosis of obesity should not be based primarily on body weight but, rather, on the total amount of fat in the body, the location of body fat, and the presence or absence of weight-related medical problems.

Estimating Body Fat Content and Diagnosing Obesity

Body fat varies widely among individuals and can range from 2% to 70% of body weight. Desirable amounts of body fat are about 8% to 24% for men and 21% to 35% for women. Men with over 24% body fat and women with over about 35% body fat are considered obese. Women need the higher percentage of body fat compared to men because fat is a source of sex hormones, including estrogen, that are necessary for reproductive functions.

To measure body fat content accurately using typical methods, both body weight and body volume of the person must be known. Body weight is easy to measure on a conventional scale. Of the typical methods used to estimate body volume, **underwater weighing**

▲ A high BMI may not reflect overweight or fatness. Extra muscle tissue can result in a BMI greater than 25.

underwater weighing A method of estimating total body fat by weighing the individual on a standard scale and then weighing him or her again submerged in water. The difference between the two weights is used to estimate total body volume.

TABLE 7-1 Health Problems Associated with Excess Body Fat

Health Problem	Partially Attributable To
Surgical risk	Increased anesthesia needs, as well as greater risk of wound infections (the latter is linked to a decrease in immune function)
Pulmonary disease and sleep disorders	Excess weight over lungs and pharynx
Type 2 diabetes	Enlarged adipose cells, which poorly bind insulin and poorly respond to the message insulin sends to the cell; less synthesis of factors that aid insulin action, and greater synthesis of factors by adipose cells that lessen insulin action
Hypertension	Increased miles of blood vessels found in the adipose tissue, increased blood volume, and increased resistance to blood flow related to hormones made by adipose cells
Cardiovascular disease (e.g., coronary heart disease and stroke)	Increases in LDL-cholesterol and triglyceride values, low HDL-cholesterol, decreased physical activity, and increased synthesis of blood clotting and inflamatory factors by enlarged adipose cells. A greater risk for heart failure is also seen, due in part to altered heart rhythm.
Bone and joint disorders (including gout)	Excess pressure put on knee, ankle, and hip joints
Gallstones	Increased cholesterol content of bile
Skin disorders	Trapping of moisture and microorganisms in tissue folds
Various cancers, such as in the kidney, gallbladder, colon and rectum, uterus (women), and prostate gland (men)	Estrogen production by adipose cells; animal studies suggest excess calorie intake encourages tumor development
Shorter stature (in some forms of obesity)	Earlier onset of puberty
Pregnancy risks	More difficult delivery, increased number of birth defects, and increased needs for anesthesia
Reduced physical agility and increased risk of accidents and falls	Excess weight that impairs movement
Menstrual irregularities and infertility	Hormones produced by adipose cells, such as estrogen
Vision problems	Cataracts and other eye disorders are more often present
Premature death	A variety of risk factors for disease listed in this table
Infections	Reduced immune system activity
Liver damage and eventual failure	Excess fat accumulation in the liver
Erectile dysfunction in men	Low-grade inflammation caused by excess fat mass and reduced function of the cells lining the blood vessels associated with being overweight

The greater the degree of obesity, the more likely and the more serious these health problems generally become. They are much more likely to appear in people who show an upper-body fat distribution pattern and/or are greater than twice healthy body weight.

air displacement A method for estimating body composition that makes use of the volume of space taken up by a body inside a small chamber.

is the most accurate. This technique determines body volume using the difference between conventional body weight and body weight under water, along with the relative densities of fat tissue and lean tissue, and a specific mathematical formula. This procedure requires that an individual be totally submerged in a tank of water, with a trained technician directing the procedure (Fig. 7-7). **Air displacement** is another method of determining body volume. Body volume is quantified by measuring the space a person takes up inside a measurement chamber, such as the BodPod (Fig. 7-8). A less accurate method to measure body volume is to submerge a person in a tank and observe the level of the water before and after submersion. The volume of the displaced water is then calculated.

FIGURE 7-7 ▶ Underwater weighing. In this technique the subject exhales as much air as possible and then holds his or her breath and bends over at the waist. Once the subject is totally submerged, the underwater weight is recorded. Using this value, body volume can be calculated.

FIGURE 7-8 ▶ BodPod. This device determines body volume based on the volume of displaced air, measured as a person sits in a sealed chamber for a few minutes.

Once body volume is known, it can be used along with body weight in the following equation to calculate body density. Then using body density, body fat content finally can be determined.

$$\text{Body density} = \frac{\text{body weight}}{\text{body volume}}$$

$$\text{\% body fat} = (495 \div \text{body density}) - 450$$

For example, assume that the individual in the underwater weighing tank in Figure 7-7 has a body density of 1.06 grams per centimeter^3. We can use the second formula to calculate that he has 17% body fat ([495 ÷ 1.06] – 450 = 17).

Skinfold thickness is also a common anthropometric method to estimate total body fat content, although there are some limits to its accuracy. Clinicians use calipers to measure the fat layer directly under the skin at multiple sites and then plug these values into a mathematical formula (Fig. 7-9).

The technique of **bioelectrical impedance** is also used to estimate body fat content. The instrument sends a painless, low-energy electrical current to and from the

bioelectrical impedance The method to estimate total body fat that uses a low-energy electrical current. The more fat storage a person has, the more impedance (resistance) to electrical flow will be exhibited.

FIGURE 7-9 ▶ Skinfold measurements. Using proper technique and calibrated equipment, skinfold measurements around the body can be used to predict body fat content in about 10 minutes. Measurements are made at several locations including the suprailiac (photo) and triceps (drawing) skinfolds.

Muscle

Skin

Bone

Fat

Caliper

dual energy X-ray absorptiometry (DEXA) A highly accurate method of measuring body composition and bone mass and density using multiple low-energy X-rays.

upper-body obesity The type of obesity in which fat is stored primarily in the abdominal area; defined as a waist circumference more than 40 inches (102 centimeters) in men and more than 35 inches (89 centimeters) in women; closely associated with a high risk for cardiovascular disease, hypertension, and type 2 diabetes. Also known as android obesity.

lower-body obesity The type of obesity in which fat storage is primarily located in the buttocks and thigh area. Also known as gynoid or gynecoid obesity.

body via wires and electrode patches to estimate body fat. This estimation is based on the assumption that adipose tissue resists electrical flow more than lean tissue because it has a lower electrolyte and water content than lean tissue. More adipose tissue therefore means proportionately greater electrical resistance. Within a few seconds, bioelectrical impedance analyzers convert body electrical resistance into an approximate estimate of total body fat, as long as body hydration status is normal (Fig. 7-10).

A more advanced determination of body fat content can be made using **dual energy X-ray absorptiometry (DEXA)**. DEXA is considered the most accurate way to determine body fat, but the equipment is expensive and not widely available for this use. This X-ray system allows the clinician to separate body weight into three separate components—fat, fat-free soft tissue, and bone mineral. The usual whole-body scan requires about 5 to 20 minutes and the dose of radiation is less than a chest X ray. An assessment of bone mineral density and the risk of osteoporosis also can be made using this method (Fig. 7-11).

Another method to assess body fat is to measure total-body electrical conductance (TOBEC) when placed in an electromagnetic field. Still another method, convenient and inexpensive, but not very accurate is **near-infrared reactance**. This method exposes the bicep muscle to a beam of near-infrared light and assesses the interactions of the light beam with fat and lean tissues in the upper arm after only 2 seconds.

Using Body Fat Distribution to Further Evaluate Obesity

In addition to the amount of fat we store, the location of that body fat is an important predictor of health risks. Some people store fat in upper-body areas whereas others store fat lower on the body. Excess fat in either location generally spells trouble, but each storage space also has its unique risks. **Upper-body obesity**, characterized by a large abdomen, is more often related to cardiovascular disease, hypertension, and type 2 diabetes. Whereas other adipose cells empty fat into general blood circulation, the fat released from abdominal adipose cells goes directly to the liver, by way of the portal vein. This

FIGURE 7-10 ▶ Bioelectrical impedance. This method can estimate total body fat in less than 5 minutes and is based on the principle that fat in the body, because it is low in water and electrolytes, resists the flow of applied low-energy electricity. The degree of resistance to electrical flow is used to estimate body fatness.

FIGURE 7-11 ▶ Dual energy X-ray absorptiometry (DEXA). This method measures body fat by passing small doses of radiation through the body. The radiation reacts differently with fat, lean tissue, or bone allowing these components to be quantified. The scanner arm moves from head to toe and in doing so can determine body fat as well as bone density. DEXA is currently considered the most accurate method for determining body fat (as long as the person can fit under the arm of the instrument). The radiation dose is minimal.

process likely interferes with the liver's ability to use insulin and negatively affects lipoprotein metabolism by the liver. These abdominal adipose cells also make substances that increase insulin resistance, blood clotting, blood vessel constriction, and inflammation in the body. These changes can lead to long-term health problems.

High blood testosterone (primarily a male hormone) levels apparently encourage upper-body obesity, as does a diet with a high glycemic load, alcohol intake, and smoking. This characteristic male pattern of fat storage is also called android obesity and is commonly known as the apple shape (large abdomen [pot belly] and small buttocks and thighs). Upper-body obesity is assessed by measuring the waist at the widest point just above the hips when relaxed. A waist circumference more than 40 inches (102 centimeters) in men and more than 35 inches (88 centimeters) in women indicates upper-body obesity (Fig. 7-12). If BMI is also 25 or more, health risks are significantly increased.

Estrogen and progesterone (primarily female hormones) encourage lower-body fat storage and **lower-body (gynecoid** or **gynoid) obesity**—the typical female pattern. The small abdomen and much larger buttocks and thighs give a pear-like appearance. Fat deposited in the lower body often resists being shed. After menopause, blood estrogen falls, encouraging upper-body fat distribution.

FIGURE 7-12 ▶ Body fat distribution, showing upper-body and lower-body obesity. The upper-body (android) form brings higher risks for ill health associated with obesity. The woman has a waist circumference of 32 inches. The man has a waist circumference of 44 inches. Thus, the man has upper-body obesity, but the woman does not, based on the current cutoff of 40 inches for men and 35 inches for women.

CONCEPT CHECK

Overweight and obesity typically are associated with excessive body fat storage. The risk of health problems related to being overweight especially increases under the following conditions:

- A man's percentage of body fat exceeds 25%; a woman's exceeds about 35%.
- Excess fat is primarily stored in the upper-body region.
- Body mass index (BMI) is 30 or more (calculated as weight in kilograms divided by height squared in meters).

However, these are merely guidelines. A more individualized approach to assessment is warranted as long as a person is following a healthy lifestyle and has no existing health problems.

Body fat content can be estimated using a variety of methods such as underwater weighing, air displacement, skinfold thickness, bioelectrical impedance, and DEXA. Fat storage distribution further specifies an obese state as either upper-body or lower-body. Obesity leads to an increased risk for cardiovascular disease, some types of cancer, hypertension, type 2 diabetes, certain bone and joint disorders, and some digestive disorders. The risks for some of these diseases are greater with upper-body fat storage.

▲ Waist circumference is an important measure of weight-related health risk.

WHY SOME PEOPLE ARE OBESE— NATURE VERSUS NURTURE

Both genetic (nature) and environmental (nurture) factors can increase the risk for obesity (Table 7-2). The eventual location of fat storage is strongly influenced by genetics. Consider the possibility that obesity is nurture allowing nature to express itself. Some obese people begin life with a slower basal metabolism; maintain an inactive lifestyle; and consume highly-refined, calorie-dense diets. These people in turn are nurtured into gaining weight, promoting their natural tendency toward obesity.

Still, genes do not fully control destiny. With increased physical activity and decreased food consumption, even those with a genetic tendency toward obesity can attain a healthier body weight.

How Does Nature Contribute to Obesity?

Studies in pairs of **identical twins** give us some insight into the contribution of nature to obesity. Even when identical twins are raised apart, they tend to show similar weight gain patterns, both in overall weight and body fat distribution. It appears that nurture—eating habits and nutrition, which varies between twins raised apart—has

identical twins Two offspring that develop from a single ovum and sperm and, consequently, have the same genetic makeup.

less to do with obesity than nature does. In fact, research suggests that genes account for up to 70% of weight differences between people. A child with no obese parent has only a 10% chance of becoming obese. When a child has one obese parent (common in our society), that risk advances up to 40%, and with two obese parents, it soars to 80%. Our genes help determine metabolic rate, fuel use, and differences in brain chemistry—all of which affect body weight.

We also inherit specific body types. Tall, thin people appear to have an inherently easier time maintaining healthy body weight. This is probably because basal metabolism increases as body surface increases, and therefore taller people use more calories than shorter people, even at rest.

Many of us probably have inherited a thrifty metabolism that enables us to store fat more readily than the typical human, so that we require fewer calories to get through the day. In earlier times, when food supplies were scarce, a thrifty metabolism would have been a built-in safeguard against starvation. Now, with a general abundance of food, people operating in this low gear require much physical activity and wise food choices to prevent obesity. If you think you are prone to weight gain, you likely have inherited a thrifty metabolism.

TABLE 7-2 What Encourages Excess Body Fat Stores and Obesity?

Factor	How Fat Storage Is Affected
Age	Excess body fat is more common in adults and middle-age individuals.
Menopause	Increase in abdominal fat deposition is typical.
Gender	Females have more fat.
Positive energy balance	Over a long period promotes storage of fat.
Composition of diet	Excess calorie intake from fat, alcohol, and calorie dense (sugary, fat-rich) foods contributes to obesity.
Physical activity	Low physical activity ("couch potato") leads to positive energy balance and body fat storage.
Basal metabolism	A low BMR is linked to weight gain.
Thermic effect of food	Low for some obesity cases.
Increased hunger sensations	Some people have trouble resisting the abundant availability of food, which is likely linked to the activity of various brain chemicals.
Ratio of fat to lean tissue	A high ratio of fat mass to lean body mass is correlated with weight gain.
Fat uptake by adipose tissue	This is high in some obese individuals and remains high (perhaps even increases) with weight loss.
Variety of social and behavioral factors	Obesity is associated with socioeconomic status; familial conditions; network of friends; busy lifestyles that discourage balanced meals; binge eating; easy availability of inexpensive, "super-sized" high-fat food; pattern of leisure activities; television time; smoking cessation; excessive alcohol intake; and number of meals eaten away from home.
Undetermined genetic characteristics	These affect components of energy balance, particularly energy expenditure, the deposition of the energy surplus as adipose tissue or as lean tissue, and the relative proportion of fat and carbohydrate used by the body.
Race	In some ethnic groups, higher body weight may be more socially acceptable.
Certain medications	Food intake increases.
Childbearing	Women may not lose all weight gained in pregnancy.
National region	Regional differences, such as high-fat diets and sedentary lifestyles in the Midwest and areas of the South, lead to geographically different rates of obesity.

◄ Does the difference in body fat between the grandfathers and the grandsons arise from nature or nurture, or both?

Does the Body Have a Set Point for Weight?

The **set-point** theory of weight maintenance proposes that humans have a genetically predetermined body weight or body fat content, which the body closely regulates. Some research suggests that the hypothalamus monitors the amount of body fat in humans and tries to keep that amount constant over time. Recall from Chapter 1 that the hormone *leptin* forms a communication link between adipose cells and the brain, which allows for some weight regulation.

Several physiological changes that occur during calorie reduction and weight loss also endorse the set-point theory. For example, when calorie intake is reduced, the blood concentration of thyroid hormones falls, which slows basal metabolism. In addition, as weight is lost, the calorie cost of weight-bearing activity decreases, so that an activity that burned 100 kcal before weight loss may only burn 80 kcal after weight loss. Furthermore, with weight loss, the body becomes more efficient at storing fat by increasing the activity of the enzyme *lipoprotein lipase,* which takes fat into cells. All of these changes protect the body from losing weight.

If a person overeats, in the short run, basal metabolism tends to increase. This causes some resistance to weight gain. However, in the long run, resistance to weight gain is much less than resistance to weight loss. When a person gains weight and stays at that weight for a while, the body tends to establish a new set point.

Opponents of the set-point theory argue that weight does not remain constant throughout adulthood—the average person gains weight slowly, at least until old age. Also, if an individual is placed in a different social, emotional, or physical environment, weight can be altered and maintained markedly higher or lower. These arguments suggest that humans, rather than having a set point determined by genetics or the number of adipose cells, settle into a particular stable weight based on their circumstances, often regarded as a "settling point."

The size-acceptance nondiet movement, "Health at Every Size," indirectly refers to a set point for weight by defining healthy weight as the natural weight the body adopts, given a healthy diet and meaningful levels of physical activity. Overall, the set point is weaker in preventing weight gain than in preventing weight loss. Even with a set point helping us, the odds are in favor of eventual weight gain unless we devote effort to a healthy lifestyle.

Does Nurture Have a Role?

Some would argue that body weight similarities between family members stem more from learned behaviors rather than genetic similarities. Even couples, who have no genetic link, may behave similarly

set point Often refers to the close regulation of body weight. It is not known what cells control this set point or how it functions in weight regulation. There is evidence, however, that mechanisms exist that help regulate weight.

▲ Body weight is influenced by many factors related to both nature and nurture. We resemble our parents because of the genes we have inherited, as well as the lifestyle habits, including diet, that we have learned from them.

food insecurity A condition of anxiety regarding running out of either food or money to buy more food.

toward food and eventually assume similar degrees of leanness or fatness. Proponents of nurture pose that environmental factors, such as high-fat diets and inactivity, literally shape us. This seems likely when we consider that our gene pool has not changed much in the past 50 years, whereas according to the U.S. Centers for Disease Control and Prevention the ranks of obese people have grown in epidemic proportions over the last 10 years.

Is poverty associated with obesity? Ironically, the answer is often yes. North Americans of lower socioeconomic status, especially females, are more likely to be obese than those in upper socioeconomic groups. Are cultural expectations or socioeconomic stress (e.g., **food insecurity**) the cause of this?

Adult obesity in women is often rooted in childhood obesity. In addition, relative inactivity, periods of stress or boredom, as well as excess weight gain during pregnancy, contribute to female obesity. (Chapter 16 notes that breastfeeding one's infant contributes to loss of some of the excess fat associated with pregnancy.) These patterns suggest both social and genetic links. Male obesity, however, is not strongly linked to childhood obesity and, instead, tends to appear after age 30. This powerful and prevalent pattern suggests a primary role of nurture in obesity, with less genetic influence.

▲ Student life is often full of physical activity. This is not necessarily true for a person's later working life; hence, weight gain is a strong possibility.

FIGURE 7-13 ▶ Characteristics of a sound weight-loss diet. Use this checklist to evaluate any new diet plan before putting it into practice.

Rate of Loss

☐ Slow and steady weight loss, rather than rapid weight loss, is encouraged.

☐ Goal is 1 pound or so of fat loss per week.

☐ A period of weight maintenance for a few months following a loss of 10% of body weight.

☐ Evaluation of need for further dieting before more weight loss begins.

Flexibility

☐ Ability to participate in normal activities (e.g., parties, restaurants).

☐ Adaptations to individual habits and tastes.

Intake

☐ Nutritional needs are met (except for calories).

☐ Common foods are included, with no certain foods being promoted as magical.

☐ Use of a fortified ready-to-eat breakfast cereal or balanced multivitamin/mineral supplement is recommended, especially when consuming less than 1600 kcal per day.

☐ Use MyPyramid as a pattern for food choices.

Behavior Modification

☐ Maintenance of healthy lifestyle (and weight) is a key concern; there is a lifetime focus.

☐ Changes are reasonable and can be maintained.

☐ Social support is encouraged.

☐ Plans for relapse so one does not quit after a setback.

Overall Health

☐ Screening by a physician is required for persons with existing health problems, those over 40 (men) to 50 (women) years of age who plan to substantially increase physical activity, and those who plan to lose weight rapidly.

☐ Regular physical activity, proper rest, stress reduction, and other healthy changes in lifestyle are encouraged.

☐ Underlying psychological weight issues are addressed, such as depression or marital stress.

TREATMENT OF OVERWEIGHT AND OBESITY

Treatment of overweight and obesity should be long-term, similar to that for any chronic disease. Treatments require long-term lifestyle changes, rather than a quick fix promoted by many popular (also called fad) diet books. We often view a "diet" as something one goes on temporarily, only to resume prior (typically poor) habits once satisfactory results have been achieved. This is a big reason that so many people regain lost weight. Instead, an emphasis on healthy, active living with acceptable dietary modifications will promote weight loss and later weight maintenance.

What to Look for in a Sound Weight-Loss Plan

A dieter can develop a plan of action by seeking advice from a health professional, such as a registered dietitian, or by consulting current literature. Either way, a sound weight-loss program (Fig. 7-13) should especially include these components:

1. Control of calorie intake. One recommendation is to decrease calorie intake by 100 kcal per day (and increase physical activity by 100 kcal per day). This should allow for slow and steady weight loss.
2. Increased physical activity.
3. Acknowledgment that maintenance of a healthy weight requires lifelong changes in habits, not a short-term weight-loss period.

A one-sided approach that focuses only on restricting calories is a difficult plan of action. Instead, adding physical activity and an appropriate psychological component will contribute to success in weight loss and eventual weight maintenance (Fig. 7-14).

▶ The total cost attributable to weight-related disease is about $90 billion annually in the United States. Half of this cost is borne by the taxpayers through Medicare and Medicaid.

▶ **Weight-Control Objectives from *Healthy People 2010***

Increase by 40% the proportion of adults who are at a healthy weight (body mass index between 18.5 and 25).

Reduce by 50% the proportion of adults who are obese (body mass index of 30 or more).

Reduce by 50% the proportion of children and adolescents who are overweight or obese.

▲ Making a commitment to a healthier diet and lifestyle can be a challenge for many individuals. A sound weight-loss plan, however, does not require you to completely avoid certain favorite foods. Practical strategies include substituting lower-calorie choices, choosing high-calorie treats less often, and limiting portion sizes.

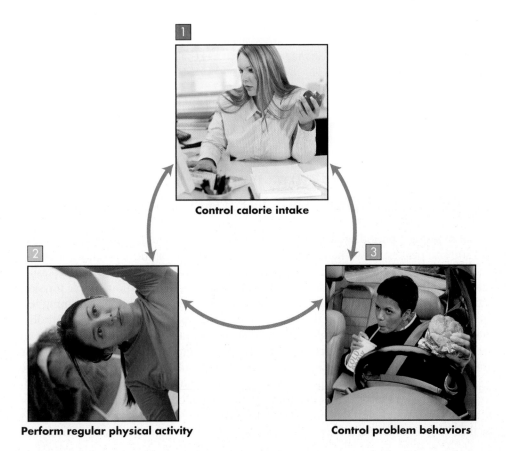

1 Control calorie intake

2 Perform regular physical activity

3 Control problem behaviors

FIGURE 7-14 ▶ Weight-loss triad. The key to weight loss and maintenance can be thought of as a triad which consists of three parts (1) controlling calorie intake, (2) performing regular physical activity, and (3) controlling problem behaviors. The three parts of the triad support each other in that without one part the triad, weight loss and later maintenance become unlikely.

▶ As you read brochures, articles, or research reports about specific diet plans, look beyond the weight loss promoted by the diet's advocate to see if the reported weight loss was maintained. If the weight maintenance aspect was missing, then the program was not successful.

▶ For more information on weight control, obesity, and nutrition, visit the Weight-Control Information Network (WIN) at www. niddk.nih.gov/index.htm or call 800-WIN-8098. Complete guidelines for weight management are available at www.nhlbi.nih. gov/guidelines/index.htm. Other websites include www.caloriecontrol.org, www. weight.com, www.obesity.org, and www. cyberdiet.com.

▲ Slow, steady weight loss is one of the characteristics of a sound weight-loss program.

Losing Body Fat

Rapid weight loss cannot consist primarily of fat loss because a high calorie deficit is needed to lose a large amount of adipose tissue. Adipose tissue, mostly fat, contains about 3500 kcal per pound. Weight loss, however, includes adipose tissue plus lean tissues that support it and represents approximately 3300 kcal per pound (about 7.2 kcal per gram). Therefore, to lose 1 pound of adipose tissue per week, calorie intake must be decreased by approximately 500 kcal per day, or physical activity must be increased by 500 kcal per day. Alternately, a combination of both strategies can be used. Diets that promise 10 to 15 pounds of weight loss per week cannot ensure that the weight loss is from adipose tissue stores alone. How many calories would need to be eliminated from the diet per day to lose 10 pounds per week? Is it possible to subtract enough calories from one's daily intake to lose that amount of adipose tissue? Lean tissue and water, rather than adipose tissue, account for the major part of the weight lost during these dramatic weight-loss programs.

Weight Loss in Perspective

These principles point to the importance of preventing obesity. This concept has wide support because conquering the disorder is so difficult. Public health strategies to address the current obesity problem must speak to all age groups. There is a particular need to focus on children and adolescents because patterns of excess weight and sedentary lifestyle developed during youth may form the basis for a lifetime of weight-related illness and increased mortality. In the adult population, attention should be directed toward weight maintenance and increased physical activity.

CONCEPT CHECK

Obesity is a chronic disease that necessitates lifelong treatment. Emphasis should be placed especially on preventing obesity, because overcoming this disorder is difficult. Appropriate weight-loss programs have the following characteristics in common: (1) They meet nutritional needs; (2) they can adjust to accommodate habits and tastes; (3) they emphasize readily obtainable foods; (4) they promote changing habits that discourage overeating; (5) they encourage regular physical activity; and (6) they help change obesity-promoting beliefs and rally healthy social support.

CONTROL OF CALORIE INTAKE—THE MAIN KEY TO WEIGHT LOSS AND WEIGHT MAINTENANCE

A goal of losing 1 pound or so of stored fat per week may require limiting calorie intake to 1200 kcal per day for women and 1500 kcal for men. The calorie allowance could also be higher for very active people. Keep in mind that, in our sedentary society, decreasing calorie intake is vital because it is difficult to burn much energy without ample physical activity. With regard to consuming fewer calories, some experts suggest consuming less fat (especially saturated fat and *trans* fat), while others suggest consuming less carbohydrate, especially refined (high glycemic load) carbohydrate sources. Protein intakes in excess of what is typically needed by adults are also receiving attention. Using all these approaches simultaneously is fine. At this time the low-fat, high-fiber approaches have been the most successful in long-term studies. There is no long-term evidence of the effectiveness of the other approaches. Finding what works for an individual is a process of trial and error. The notion that any type of diet promotes significantly greater calorie use by the body is unfounded, despite the marketing claims for low-carbohydrate diets.

FIGURE 7-15 ▶ Reading labels helps you choose foods with fewer calories. Which of these frozen desserts is the best choice, per ½ cup serving, for a person on a weight-loss diet? The % Daily Values are based on a 2000 kcal diet.

One way for a dieter to monitor calorie intake at the start of a weight-loss program is by reading labels. Label reading is important, because many foods are more energy dense than people suppose (Fig. 7-15). Another method is to write down food intake for 24 hours (Appendix E) and then calculate calorie intake from the food table in the text-book supplement or by using your diet analysis software. With knowledge of current calorie intake, future food choices can be adjusted as needed. People often underestimate portion size when recording food intake, so measuring cups and a food scale can help.

Table 7-3 shows how to start reducing calorie intake. As you should realize, it is best to consider eating healthy a lifestyle change, rather than a weight-loss plan. Also, liquids deserve attention, because liquid calories do not stimulate satiety mechanisms to the same extent as solid foods. The corresponding advice from experts is to use beverages that have few or no calories and limit sugar-sweetened beverages.

REGULAR PHYSICAL ACTIVITY—A SECOND KEY TO WEIGHT LOSS AND ESPECIALLY IMPORTANT FOR LATER WEIGHT MAINTENANCE

Regular physical activity is important for everyone, especially those trying to lose weight or maintain a lower body weight. Calorie burning is enhanced both during and after physical activity. Therefore, activity greatly complements a reduction in calorie intake for weight loss. Many of us rarely do more than sit, stand, and sleep. More calories are used during physical activity than at rest. Expending only 100 to 300 extra kcal per day above and beyond normal daily activity, while controlling calorie intake, can lead to a steady weight loss. Furthermore, physical activity has so many other benefits, including a boost for overall self-esteem. The latest advice for adults from the 2005 Dietary Guidelines is

▲ Physical activity complements any diet plan.

TABLE 7-3 Lowering Kcal: Point of Purchase and Consumption Decisions

Instead of	Try	Number of Kcal Saved
3 oz well-marbled meat (prime rib)	3 oz lean meat (eye of round)	140
½ chicken breast, batter-fried	½ chicken breast, broiled with lemon	175
½ cup beef stroganoff	3 oz lean roast beef (or use a fat-reduced recipe)	210
½ cup home-fried potatoes	1 medium baked potato	65
½ cup green bean-mushroom casserole	½ cup cooked green beans	50
½ cup potato salad	1 cup raw vegetable salad	140
½ cup pineapple chunks in heavy syrup	½ cup pineapple chunks canned in juice	25
2 tbsp bottled French dressing	2 tbsp low-calorie French dressing	150
⅛ 9-inch apple pie	1 baked apple, unsweetened	308
3 oatmeal-raisin cookies	1 oatmeal-raisin cookie	125
½ cup ice cream	½ cup ice milk	45
1 danish pastry	½ English muffin	150
1 cup sugar-coated corn flakes	1 cup plain corn flakes	60
1 cup whole milk	1 cup 1% low-fat milk	45
1-oz bag potato chips	1 cup plain popcorn	120
1/12 8-inch white layer cake with chocolate frosting	1/12 angel food cake, 10-inch tube	185
12 fluid ounce cola	12 fluid ounce diet cola	150

▶ The motivation to lose weight and keep it off generally comes with a proverbial "flip of the switch," in which the desire to lose weight finally becomes more important than the desire to overeat.

▲ Fruit is a great low-cal snack—high in nutrient density and low in calories.

60 minutes of physical activity per day to maintain body weight and prevent weight gain and 60 to 90 minutes per day for maintenance of weight loss.

Adding any of the activities in Table 7-4 to one's lifestyle can increase calorie use. Duration and regular performance, rather than intensity, are the keys to success with this approach to weight loss. One should search for activities that can be continued over time. In this regard, walking vigorously 3 miles per day can be as helpful as aerobic dancing or jogging, if it is maintained. Moreover, activities of lighter intensity are less likely to lead to injuries. Some resistance exercises (weight training) also should be added to increase lean body mass and, in turn, fat use (see Chapter 12). As lean muscle mass increases, so will one's overall metabolic rate. An added benefit of including exercise in a weight reduction program is maintenance of bone health.

Unfortunately, opportunities to expend calories in our daily lives are diminishing as technology systematically eliminates almost every reason to move our muscles. The easiest way to increase physical activity is to make it an enjoyable part of a daily routine. To start, one might pack a pair of sneakers and walk around the parking lot before coming home after school or work every day. Other ideas are avoiding elevators in favor of stairs and parking the car farther away from the shopping mall.

A pedometer is an inexpensive device that monitors activity as steps. A recommended goal for activity is to take at least 10,000 steps per day—typically we take half that many or less. A pedometer tracks this activity. Calorie counters, such as the Bodybugg, are new devices that track calorie expenditures throughout the day. The counters calculate calories by measuring heart rate, sweat rate, or heat loss and production. Like pedometers, calorie counters can motivate users to do more activity.

TABLE 7-4 Approximate Calorie Costs of Various Activities, and Specific Calorie Costs Projected for a 150-Pound (68 kilogram) Person

Activity	Kcal per kilogram per Hour	Total kcal per Hour	Activity	Kcal per kilogram per Hour	Total kcal per Hour
Aerobics—heavy	8.0	544	Horseback riding	5.1	346
Aerobics—medium	5.0	340	Ice skating (10 MPH)	5.8	394
Aerobics—light	3.0	204	Jogging—medium	9.0	612
Backpacking	9.0	612	Jogging—slow	7.0	476
Basketball—vigorous	10.0	680	Lying—at ease	1.3	89
Bowling	3.9	265	Racquetball—social	8.0	544
Calisthenics—heavy	8.0	544	Roller skating	5.1	346
Calisthenics—light	4.0	272	Running or jogging (10 MPH)	13.2	897
Canoeing (2.5 MPH)	3.3	224	Skiing downhill (10 MPH)	8.8	598
Cleaning (female)	3.7	253	Sleeping	1.2	80
Cleaning (male)	3.5	236	Swimming (.25 MPH)	4.4	299
Cooking	2.8	190	Tennis	6.1	414
Cycling (13 MPH)	9.7	659	Volleyball	5.1	346
Cycling (5.5 MPH)	3.0	204	Walking (3.75 MPH)	4.4	299
Dressing/showering	1.6	106	Walking (2.5 MPH)	3.0	204
Driving	1.7	117	Water skiing	7.0	476
Eating (sitting)	1.4	93	Weight lifting—heavy	9.0	612
Food shopping	3.6	245	Weight lifting—light	4.0	272
Football—touch	7.0	476	Window cleaning	3.5	240
Golf (using power cart)	3.6	244	Writing (sitting)	1.7	118

The values in Table 7-4 refer to total energy expenditure, including that needed to perform the physical activity, plus that needed for basal metabolism, the thermic effect of food, and thermogenesis. Use your diet analysis software for your personal estimate.

BEHAVIOR MODIFICATION—A THIRD STRATEGY FOR WEIGHT LOSS AND MANAGEMENT

Controlling calorie intake, so important to weight loss, also means modifying *problem* behaviors. Only the dieter can decide what behaviors keep him or her from reaching for the wrong foods at the wrong times for the wrong reasons.

What events cause us to start (or stop) eating? What factors influence food choices? Psychologists often use terms such as *chain-breaking, stimulus control, cognitive restructuring, contingency management,* and *self-monitoring* when discussing behavior modification (Table 7-5). These factors help place the problem in perspective and organize the intervention strategy into manageable steps.

Chain-breaking separates behaviors that tend to occur together—for example, snacking on chips while watching television. Although these activities do not have to

chain-breaking Breaking the link between two or more behaviors that encourage overeating, such as snacking while watching television.

▲ Large portions of food, such as this steak, provide us with many opportunities to overeat. It takes much perseverance to eat sensibly.

Successful weight losers and maintainers from the National Weight Control Registry:

• Eat a low-fat, high-carbohydrate diet (on average 25% of calorie intake as fat).
• Eat breakfast almost every day.
• Self-monitor by regularly weighing oneself and keeping a food journal.
• Exercise for about 1 hour per day.
• Eat at restaurants only once or twice per week.

Other recent studies support this approach, especially the last four characteristics.

TABLE 7-5 Behavior Modification Principles for Weight Loss

Shopping
1. Shop for food after eating—buy nutritious foods.
2. Shop from a list; limit purchases of irresistible "problem" foods. Shopping for fresh foods around the perimeter of the store first helps.
3. Avoid ready-to-eat foods.
4. Put off food shopping until absolutely necessary.

Plans
1. Plan to limit food intake as needed.
2. Substitute periods of physical activity for snacking.
3. Eat meals and snacks at scheduled times; don't skip meals.

Activities
1. Store food out of sight, preferably in the freezer, to discourage impulsive eating.
2. Eat all food in a "dining" area.
3. Keep serving dishes off the table, especially dishes of sauces and gravies.
4. Use smaller dishes and utensils.

Holidays and Parties
1. Drink fewer alcoholic beverages.
2. Plan eating behavior before parties.
3. Eat a low-calorie snack before parties.
4. Practice polite ways to decline food.
5. Don't get discouraged by an occasional setback.

Eating Behavior
1. Put fork down between mouthfuls.
2. Chew thoroughly before taking the next bite.
3. Leave some food on the plate.
4. Pause in the middle of the meal.
5. Do nothing else while eating (for example, reading, watching television).

Reward
1. Plan specific rewards for specific behavior (behavioral contracts).
2. Solicit help from family and friends and suggest how they can help you. Encourage family and friends to provide this help in the form of praise and material rewards.
3. Use self-monitoring records as basis for rewards.

Self-Monitoring
1. Note the time and place of eating.
2. List the type and amount of food eaten.
3. Record who is present and how you feel.
4. Use the diet diary to identify problem areas.

Cognitive Restructuring
1. Avoid setting unreasonable goals.
2. Think about progress, not shortcomings.
3. Avoid imperatives such as *always* and *never*.
4. Counter negative thoughts with positive restatements.

Portion Control
1. Make substitutions, such as a regular hamburger instead of a "quarter pounder" or cucumbers instead of croutons in salads.
2. Think small. Order the entrée and share it with another person. Order a cup of soup instead of a bowl or an appetizer in place of an entrée.
3. Use a doggie bag. Ask your server to put half the entrée in a doggie bag before bringing it to the table.

As we said at the start of this chapter, many of us need to become "defensive eaters." Know when to refuse food after satiety registers, and reduce portion sizes.

occur together, they often do. Dieters may need to break the chain reaction (see "Rate Your Plate" at the end of this chapter for more details).

Stimulus control puts us in charge of temptations. Options include pushing tempting food to the back of the refrigerator, removing fat-laden snacks from the kitchen counter, and avoiding the path by the vending machines. Provide a positive stimulus by keeping low-fat snacks available to satisfy hunger/appetite.

Cognitive restructuring changes our frame of mind. For example, after a hard day, avoid using alcohol or comfort foods as quick relief for stress. Instead, plan for healthful, relaxing activities for stress reduction. For example, take a walk around the neighborhood or have a satisfying talk with a friend.

Labeling some foods as "off limits" sets up an internal struggle to resist the urge to eat that food. This hopeless battle can keep us feeling deprived. We lose the fight. Managing food choices with the principle of moderation is best. If a favorite food becomes troublesome, place it off limits only temporarily, until it can be enjoyed in moderation.

Contingency management prepares us for potential pitfalls and high-risk situations. We might rehearse in advance some appropriate responses to pressures—such as food being passed around at a party.

A **self-monitoring** record can reveal patterns—such as unconscious overeating—that may explain problem eating habits. This record can encourage new habits that will counteract unwanted behaviors. Obesity experts note that this is the key behavioral tool to use in any weight-loss program.

Overall, it's important to address specific problems, such as snacking, compulsive eating, and mealtime overeating. Behavior modification principles (review Table 7-5) end up as critical components of weight reduction and maintenance. Without behavior modification, it is difficult to make lifelong lifestyle changes needed to meet weight-control goals.

Relapse Prevention Is Important

Preventing relapse is thought to be the hardest part of weight control—even harder than losing weight. A dieter can tolerate an occasional lapse but needs to plan for lapses. The key is not to overreact, but take charge immediately. Change responses such as "I ate that cookie; I'm a failure" to "I ate that cookie, but I did well to stop after only one!" When dieters lapse from their diet plan, newly learned food habits should steer them back toward the plan. This should enable dieters to avoid the lapse-relapse-collapse trap. Without a strong behavioral program for **relapse prevention** in place, a lapse frequently turns into a relapse. Once a pattern of poor food choices begins, dieters may feel that they have failed and stray farther from the plan. As the relapse lengthens, the diet plan collapses, and dieters fall short of their weight-loss goal. Even with a good behavioral plan, one may fail at a diet. Losing weight is difficult. Overall, maintenance of weight loss is fostered by the "3 Ms": motivation, movement, and monitoring.

Social Support Aids Behavioral Change

Healthy social support is helpful in weight control. Helping others understand how they can be supportive can make weight control easier. Family and friends can provide praise and encouragement. A registered dietitian or other weight-control professional can keep dieters accountable and help them learn from difficult situations. Long-term contact with a professional can be helpful for later weight maintenance. Groups of individuals attempting to lose weight or maintain losses can provide empathetic support.

Societal Efforts to Reduce Obesity

The incidence of obesity in the United States is now considered an epidemic. Public, private, and nonprofit organizations have begun to work together to address and reverse this public health crisis. For example, the U.S. Food and Drug Administration has brought

stimulus control Altering the environment to minimize the stimuli for eating—for example, removing foods from sight and storing them in kitchen cabinets.

cognitive restructuring Changing one's frame of mind regarding eating—for example, instead of using a difficult day as an excuse to overeat, substituting other pleasures for rewards, such as a relaxing walk with a friend.

contingency management Forming a plan of action to respond to a situation in which overeating is likely, such as when snacks are within arm's reach at a party.

self-monitoring Tracking foods eaten and conditions affecting eating; actions are usually recorded in a diary, along with location, time, and state of mind. This is a tool to help people understand more about their eating habits.

relapse prevention A series of strategies used to help prevent and cope with weight-control lapses, such as recognizing high-risk situations and deciding beforehand on appropriate responses.

CRITICAL THINKING

With regard to readiness to lose weight, what would you say to a young woman who has just had a baby, needs to find a new job, and recently has gone back to school part-time?

▲ Individuals who successfully maintain their weight loss employ a variety of strategies to cope with the stresses and challenges of changing problem behaviors.

together leaders from industry, government, academia, and the public health community to seek solutions to the obesity epidemic by making changes in foods eaten outside the home (restaurant and carry-out foods). These groups have collaborated and made recommendations to support the consumer's ability to manage calorie intake. Recommendations include "social marketing" programs that promote healthy eating and active living.

CONCEPT CHECK

Increasing physical activity in daily life should be part of any weight-loss plan. Daily activity, such as walking and stair climbing, is recommended. Behavior modification can improve conditions for losing weight. One key step is to break behavior chains that encourage overeating, such as snacking while watching television. Another tactic is to modify the environment to reduce temptation; for example, put foods into cupboards to keep them out of sight. In addition, rethinking attitudes about eating—for example, substituting pleasures other than food as a reward for coping with a stressful day—can be important for altering undesirable behavior. Advanced planning to prevent and deal with lapses is vital, as is rallying healthy social support. Finally, careful observation and recording of eating habits can reveal subtle cues that lead to overeating. Overall, weight loss and maintenance are fostered by controlling calorie intake, performing regular physical activity, and modifying "problem" behaviors.

PROFESSIONAL HELP FOR WEIGHT LOSS

The first professional to see for advice about a weight-loss program is one's family physician. Doctors are best equipped to assess overall health and the appropriateness of weight loss. The physician may then recommend a registered dietitian for a specific weight-loss plan and answers to diet-related questions. Registered dietitians are uniquely qualified to help design a weight-loss plan because they understand both food composition and the psychological importance of food. Exercise physiologists can provide advice about programs to increase physical activity. The expense for such professional interventions is tax deductible in the United States in some cases (see a tax advisor) and often covered by health insurance plans if prescribed by a physician.

Many communities have a variety of weight-loss organizations. These include self-help groups, such as Take Off Pounds Sensibly and Weight Watchers. Other programs, such as Jenny Craig and Physicians' Weight Loss Center, are less desirable for the average dieter. Often, the employees are not registered dietitians or other appropriately trained health professionals. These programs also tend to be expensive because of their requirements for intense counseling or mandatory diet foods and supplements. In addition, the Federal Trade Commission has charged these and other commercial diet-program companies with misleading consumers through unsubstantiated weight-loss claims and deceptive testimonials.

North Americans are willing to try almost anything to shed unwanted pounds. Operation Waistline is a program designed by the U.S. Federal Trade Commission to terminate fraudulent claims being made by weight-loss charlatans with regard to diet products. The program hopes to put an end to the $6 billion spent annually in the United States on counterfeit products. The Enforma Natural Products Corporation had to pay $10 million in response to false claims for its "Fat Trapper" product.

Medications for Weight Loss

Candidates for medications for obesity include those with a BMI of 30 or more, or a BMI of 27 to 29.9 with weight-related health conditions, such as type 2 diabetes, cardiovascular disease, hypertension, or excess waist circumference; those with no contraindications to use the medication; and those ready to undertake lifestyle change. Drug therapy alone has not been found to be successful. Success with medications has been shown only in those who also modify their behavior, decrease calorie intake, and increase physical activity. In addition, if a person has not lost at least 4.4 pounds (2 kilograms) after 4 weeks, it is not likely that the person will benefit from further use of the medication.

Three main classes of medications are used. An **amphetamine**-like medication (phenteramine [Fastin or Ionamin]) prolongs the activity of epinephrine and norepinephrine in the brain. This therapy is effective for some people in the short run but has not yet been proven effective in the long run. Most state medical boards limit use of this drug to 12 weeks unless the person is participating in a medical study using the product. The medication should not be used in pregnant or nursing women or those under 18 years of age.

Sibutramine (Meridia) is a second class of medication that has been approved by FDA for weight loss. It enhances both norepinephrine and serotonin activity in the brain by reducing reuptake of these neurotransmitters by nerve cells. The neurotransmitters then remain active in the brain for a longer time and so prolong a sense of reduced hunger. The most common side effects are constipation, dry mouth, insomnia, and a mild increase in blood pressure in some people. Thus, sibutramine should be used with caution in people with a history of hypertension (or cardiovascular disease). Studies have shown that it is effective in helping some people who already eat healthy diets, but just eat too much. The main effect is to moderately reduce appetite so that people eat less. Sibutramine is safe and effective only when combined with a comprehensive weight-control program and when supervised by a physician.

The third class of medication approved by FDA for weight loss is orlistat (Xenical). This medication reduces fat digestion by about 30% by inhibiting lipase enzyme action in the small intestine (Fig. 7-16). This cuts absorption of dietary fat by one-third for about 2 hours when taken along with a meal containing fat. This malabsorbed fat is deposited in the feces. *Fat intake has to be controlled,* however, because large amounts of fat in the feces cause numerous side effects, such as gas, bloating, and oily discharge. Interestingly, orlistat use can remind the person to follow a fat-controlled diet, as the symptoms resulting from consuming a high-fat meal are unpleasant and develop quickly. Orlistat is taken with each meal containing fat. The malabsorbed fat also carries fat-soluble vitamins into the feces, so the person taking orlistat must take a multivitamin and mineral supplement at bedtime. In this way, any micronutrients not absorbed during the day can be replaced; fat malabsorption from the dinner meal will not greatly influence micronutrient absorption in the late evening.

The only two weight-loss medications currently approved by FDA for long-term use are sibutramine (Meridia) and orlistat (Xenical). A low-dose form of orlistat (Alli™) is now available over-the-counter without a prescription. Drug companies are working on many other types of medications (e.g., rimonabant) and have high hopes that some of these will prove to be safe and effective for weight loss. In addition, physicians may prescribe medications not approved for weight loss *per se* but can have weight loss as a side effect. Certain antidepressants (e.g., bupropion [Wellbutrin]) are an example. Such an application is termed *off-label,* because the product label does not include weight loss as an FDA-approved use. Consumers need to educate themselves about weight-loss products before trying them. Over-the-counter medications and supplements are widely marketed as miracle cures for obesity, but in some cases, they do more harm than good. One woman developed liver failure after using a so-called weight-loss aid called usnic acid. Her purchase was via the Internet. Today more than ever, let the buyer beware concerning any purported weight-loss aid not prescribed by a physician.

▲ All weight loss programs should begin with a visit to your family physician.

amphetamine A group of medications that induce stimulation of the central nervous system and have other effects in the body. Abuse is linked to physical and psychological dependence.

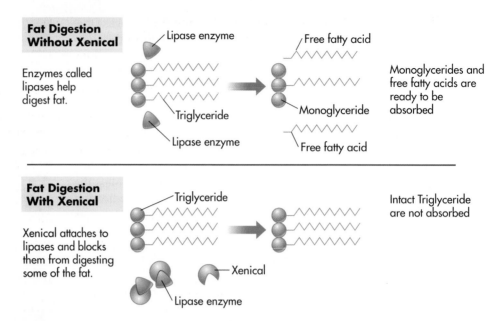

FIGURE 7-16 ▶ Xenical is a weight loss drug that works in the digestive system to block digestion of about one-third of the fat in the food we eat. A low-dose form of this drug (orlistat, Alli™) is now available without a prescription.

Overall, in skilled hands, prescription medications can aid weight loss in some instances. However, they do not replace the need for reducing calorie intake, modifying "problem" behaviors, and increasing physical activity, both during and after therapy. And, more often than not, any weight loss during drug treatment can be attributed mostly to the individual's hard work at balancing calorie intake with calorie output.

Treatment of Severe Obesity

Severe (morbid) obesity, having a BMI greater than or equal to 40 or weighing at least 100 pounds over healthy body weight (or twice one's healthy body weight), requires professional treatment. Because of the serious health implications of severe obesity, drastic measures may be necessary. Such treatments are recommended only when traditional diets and medications fail. Drastic weight-loss procedures are not without side effects, both physical and psychological, making careful monitoring by a physician a necessity.

very-low-calorie diet (VLCD) Known also as *protein-sparing modified fast (PSMF)*, this diet allows a person 400 to 800 kcal per day, often in liquid form. Of this, 120 to 480 kcal is carbohydrate, and the rest is mostly high-quality protein.

Very-Low-Calorie Diets. If more traditional diet changes have failed, treating severe obesity with a **very-low-calorie diet (VLCD)** is possible, especially if the person has obesity-related diseases that are not well controlled (e.g., hypertension, type 2 diabetes). Some researchers believe that people with body weight greater than 30% above their healthy weight are appropriate candidates. VLCD programs are offered almost exclusively by medical centers or clinics since careful monitoring by a physician is crucial throughout this very restrictive form of weight loss. Major health risks include heart problems and gallstones. Optifast is one such commercial program. In general, the diet allows a person to consume only 400 to 800 kcal per day, often in liquid form. (These diets were previously known as protein-sparing modified fasts.) Of this amount, about 30 to 120 grams (120 to 480 kcal) is carbohydrate. The rest is high-quality protein, in the amount of about 70 to 100 grams per day (280 to 400 kcal). This low carbohydrate intake often causes ketosis, which may decrease hunger. However, the main reasons for weight loss are the minimal energy consumption and the absence of food choice. About 3 to 4 pounds can be lost per week; men tend to lose at a faster rate than women. When physical activity and resistance training augment this diet, a greater loss of adipose tissue occurs.

Weight regain remains a nagging problem, especially without a behavioral and physical activity component. If behavioral therapy and physical activity supplement a long-term support program, maintenance of the weight loss is more likely but still difficult. Any program under consideration should include a maintenance plan. Today, antiobesity medications also may be included in this phase of the program.

Bariatric Surgery. Bariatrics is the medical specialty focusing on the treatment of obesity. Bariatric surgery is only considered for people with severe obesity and includes operations aimed at promoting weight loss. Two types of bariatric operations are now common and effective. Both procedures can be performed using an open incisions (8- to 10-inch) in the middle of the abdomen or a laparoscopic approach in which several smaller incisions (½- to 2-inch) are used that allow cameras and instruments to enter the abdomen. **Adjustable gastric banding** (also known as the lap-band procedure) is a restrictive procedure in which the opening from the esophagus to the stomach is reduced by a hollow gastric band. This creates a small pouch and a narrow passage into the rest of the stomach and thus decreases the amount of food that can be eaten comfortably. The band can be inflated or deflated via an access port placed just under the skin. Studies have demonstrated that adjustable gastric banding is more effective long term than a very low-calorie diet (500 kcal) for people who are about 50 pounds overweight.

Gastric bypass (also called **gastroplasty** or stomach stapling) is another bariatric surgical procedure used for treating severe obesity. The most common and effective approach (the Roux-en-Y gastric bypass procedure) works by reducing the stomach capacity to about 30 milliliters (the volume of one egg or shot glass) and bypassing a short segment of the upper small intestine (Fig. 7-17). Weight loss is promoted mainly because overeating of solid foods is now less likely due to rapid satiety and discomfort or vomiting after overeating. About 75% of people with severe obesity eventually lose 50% or more of excess body weight with this method. In addition, the surgery's success at long-term maintenance often leads to dramatic health improvements, such as reduced blood pressure and elimination of type 2 diabetes. Risks of the surgery include bleeding, blood clots, hernias, and severe infections. In the long run, nutrient deficiencies can develop if the person is not adequately treated in the years following the surgery. Anemia and bone loss might then be the result. Risk of death from this demanding surgery can be as high as 2% (less risk with experienced surgeons).

Patient selection criteria for bariatric surgery include:

- BMI should be greater than 40.
- BMI between 35 and 40 is considered when there are serious obesity-related health concerns.
- Obesity must be present for a minimum of 5 years, with several nonsurgical attempts to lose weight.
- There should be no history of alcoholism or major untreated psychiatric disorders.

The person also must consider that the surgery is costly ($12,000 to $40,000 or more) and may not be covered by medical insurance. In addition, follow-up surgery is often needed after weight loss to correct stretched skin, previously filled with fat. Furthermore, the surgery necessitates major lifestyle changes, such as the need to plan frequent, small meals. Therefore, the dieter who has chosen this drastic approach to weight loss faces months of difficult adjustments.

bariatrics The medical specialty focusing on the treatment of obesity.

adjustable gastric banding A restrictive procedure in which the opening from the esophagus to the stomach is reduced by a hollow gastric band.

gastroplasty Gastric bypass surgery performed on the stomach to limit its volume to approximately 30 milliliters. Also referred to as stomach stapling.

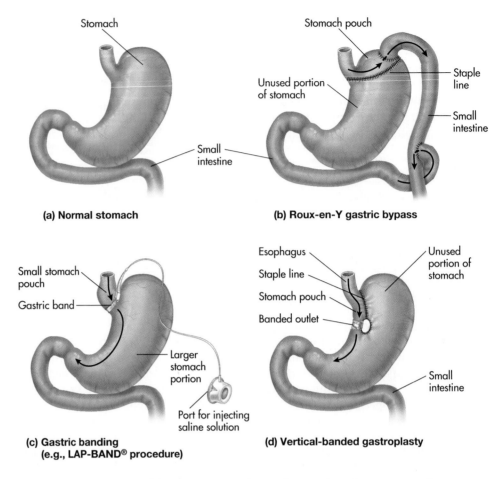

(a) Normal stomach

(b) Roux-en-Y gastric bypass

(c) Gastric banding (e.g., LAP-BAND® procedure)

(d) Vertical-banded gastroplasty

FIGURE 7-17 ▶ Three of the most common forms of gastroplasty for treatment of severe obesity. (b) The Roux-en-Y procedure is the most effective method but is more technically demanding for the surgeon than (c) gastric banding or (d) vertical-banded gastroplasty. In vertical-banded gastroplasty, the band prevents expansion of the outlet for the stomach pouch.

MAKING DECISIONS

Lipectomy

Spot-reducing by using diet and physical activity is not possible. "Problem" local fat deposits can be reduced in size, however, using suction lipectomy. Lipectomy means surgical removal of fat. A pencil-thin tube is inserted into an incision in the skin, and the fat tissue, such as that in the buttocks and thigh area, is suctioned. This procedure carries some risks, such as infection; lasting depressions in the skin; and blood clots, which can lead to kidney failure and sometimes death. The procedure is designed to help a person lose about 4 to 8 pounds per treatment. Cost is about $1600 per site; total costs range as high as $2600 to $9000.

CONCEPT CHECK

Severely obese people who have failed to lose weight with conservative weight-loss strategies may consider other options. Their doctors may recommend undergoing surgery such as reducing the volume of the stomach to approximately 30 milliliters or following a very-low-calorie diet plan containing 400 to 800 kcal per day. Careful monitoring by a physician is crucial in both cases.

TREATMENT OF UNDERWEIGHT

Underweight is defined by a BMI less than 18.5 and can be caused by a variety of factors, such as cancer, infectious disease (e.g., tuberculosis), digestive tract disorders (e.g., chronic inflammatory bowel disease), and excessive dieting or physical activity. Genetic background may also lead to a higher resting metabolic rate, a slight body frame, or both. Health problems associated with underweight include the loss of menstrual function, low bone mass, complications with pregnancy and surgery, and slow recovery after illness. Significant underweight is also associated with increased death rates, especially when combined with cigarette smoking. We frequently hear about the risks of obesity, but seldom of underweight. In our culture, being underweight is much more socially acceptable than being obese.

Sometimes being underweight requires medical intervention. A physician should be consulted first to rule out hormonal imbalances; depression; cancer; infectious disease; digestive tract disorders; excessive physical activity; and other hidden disease, such as a serious eating disorder (see Chapter 13 for a detailed discussion of eating disorders).

The causes of underweight are not altogether different from the causes of obesity. Internal and external satiety-signal irregularities, the rate of metabolism, hereditary tendencies, and psychological traits can all contribute to underweight.

In growing children, the high demand for calories to support physical activity and growth can cause underweight. During growth spurts in adolescence, active children may not take the time to consume enough calories to support their needs. Moreover, gaining weight can be a formidable task for an underweight person. An extra 500 kcal per day may be required to gain weight, even at a slow pace, in part because of the increased expenditure of energy in thermogenesis. In contrast to the weight loser, the weight gainer may need to increase portion sizes.

When underweight requires a specific intervention, one approach for treating adults is to gradually increase their consumption of calorie-dense foods, especially those high in vegetable fat. Italian cheeses, nuts, and granola can be good calorie sources with low saturated-fat content. Dried fruit and bananas are good fruit choices. If eaten at the end of a meal, they don't cause early satiety. The same advice applies to salads and soups. Underweight people should replace such foods as diet soft drinks with good calorie sources, such as fruit juices and smoothies.

Encouraging a regular meal and snack schedule also aids in weight gain and maintenance. Sometimes underweight people have experienced stress at work or have been too busy to eat. Making regular meals a priority may not only help them attain an appropriate weight but also help with digestive disorders, such as constipation, sometimes associated with irregular eating times.

Excessively physically active people can reduce activity. If their weight remains low, they can add muscle mass through a resistance training (weight-lifting) program, but they must also increase their calorie intake to support that physical activity. Otherwise, weight gain will be hindered.

If these efforts fail to help a person achieve a healthy weight, they should at least prevent the health problems associated with being underweight. After achieving that, they may have to accept their lean frames.

▲ Underweight is frequently the result of gastrointestinal disorders such as inflammatory bowel disease.

underweight   A body mass index below 18.5. The cutoff is less precise than for obesity because this condition has been less studied.

Many overweight people try to help themselves by using the latest popular (also called fad) diet book. But, as you will see, most of these diets do not help, and some can actually harm those who follow them (Table 7-6). Research has shown that early dieting and other unhealthful weight control practices in adolescents lead to an increased risk of weight gain, overweight, and eating disorders.

Recently, weight-loss experts came together at the request of the USDA to evaluate weight-loss diets. They came to this conclusion: Forget these fads when it comes to dieting. Most of the popular diets are nutritionally inadequate and include certain foods that people would not normally choose to consume in large amounts. The experts stated that eating less of one's favorite foods and becoming more physically active can be much more effective when trying to implement a weight-loss diet. People need a plan that they can live with in the long run so that weight control becomes permanent. The goal should be weight control over a lifetime, not immediate weight loss. Every popular diet leads to some immediate weight loss simply because daily intake is monitored and monotonous food choices are typically part of the plan. A well-known example of the effectiveness of monotony contributing to weight loss is the experience of Jared Fogle. He ate primarily Subway sandwiches for 11 months and lost 245 pounds. He notes however that this is not a miracle diet—it takes a lot of hard work to lead to the success he experienced. There are also many other examples where diet monotony has led to weight loss. Overall, a traditional moderate diet coupled with regular physical activity is adequate for weight loss.

People on diets often fall within a healthy BMI of 18.5 to 25. Rather than worrying about weight loss, these individuals should be focusing on a healthy lifestyle that allows for weight maintenance. Incorporating necessary lifestyle changes and learning to accept one's particular body characteristics should be the overriding goals.

The dieting mania can be viewed as mostly a social problem, stemming from unrealistic weight expectations (especially for women) and lack of appreciation for the natural variety in body shape and weight. Not every woman can look like a fashion model, nor can every man look like a Greek god, but all of us can strive for good health and, if physically possible, an active lifestyle.

The size-acceptance nondiet movement, "Health at Every Size," has attempted to shift the paradigm away from the use of "popular" weight loss diets. The goals of the movement are all independent of body weight and include improvement of self-image, normalization of eating behavior, and increase in physical activity.

HOW TO RECOGNIZE AN UNRELIABLE DIET

The criteria for evaluating weight-loss programs with regard to their safety and effectiveness were discussed previously (review Fig. 7-13). In contrast, unreliable diets typically share some common characteristics:

1. They promote quick weight loss. This is the primary temptation that the dieter falls for. As mentioned, this initial weight loss primarily results from water loss and lean muscle mass depletion.

2. They limit food selections and dictate specific rituals, such as eating only fruit for breakfast or cabbage soup every day.

3. They use testimonials from famous people and tie the diet to well-known cities, such as Beverly Hills and South Beach.

TABLE 7-6 Summary of Popular Diet Approaches to Weight Control

Approach	Examples*	Characteristics	Dietitian's Review
Moderate calorie restriction	• *Dieting for Dummies* (2003) • *Dieting with the Duchess* (2000) • *Dr. Phil's Ultimate Weight Solution* (2003, 2005) • Jenny Craig (1980s) • *Picture Perfect Weight Loss* (2003) • Slim-fast (1980s) • *Sonoma Diet* (2005) • *Volumetrics* (2000) • *Wedding Dress Diet* (2000) • Weight Watchers (1960s)	• Generally 1200 to 1800 kcal per day • Moderate fat intake • Reasonable balance of macronutrients • Encourage exercise • May use behavioral approach	These diets are acceptable if a multivitamin and mineral supplement is used and permission of family physician is granted.
Carbohydrate focused	• *Carbohydrate Addicts Diet* (1993, 2001) • *Dr. Atkin's Diet Revolution* (1973, 2002) • *Dr. Gott's No Flour, No Sugar Diet* (2006) • *Eat, Drink & Weigh Less* (2006) • *G.I. (Glycemic Index) Diet* (2003) • *Healthy for Life* (2005) • *New Glucose Revolution* (2002) • Nutrisystem (2003) • *South Beach Diet* (especially initial phases) (2003) • *Sugar Busters Diet* (1998, 2003) • *Zone Diet* (1995)	• Restricted carbohydrate diets generally advise consumption of less than 100 grams of carbohydrate per day • Some plans focus on carbohydrate choces (e.g., choosing low rather than high glycemic index foods)	Selecting high-fiber, whole-grain sources of carbohydrates is an advisable practice for weight control and prevention of several chronic diseases. However, severe carbohydrate restriction may lead to ketosis, reduced exercise capacity (due to poor glycogen stores in the muscles), excessive animal fat intake, constipation, headaches, halitosis (bad breath), and muscle cramps. Severe carbohydrate restriction is not a nutritionally sound, long-term, weight-loss solution.
Low fat	• 20/30 Fat and Fiber Diet Plan (2000) • *Complete Hip and Thigh Diet* (1989, 1999) • *Eat More, Weigh Less* (1993, 2001) • *Fit or Fat* (1977, 2005) • *Foods That Cause You to Lose Weight* (1992, 2003) • *McDougall Program* (1983, 1995) • Pritikin Diet (1984, 1995) • *Rice Diet Solution* (2005) • *T-Factor Diet* (1989, 2001) • *Okinawa Program* (2002)	• Generally less than 20% of calories from fat • Limited (or elimination of) animal protein sources; also limited plant oils, nuts, seeds	Low-fat diet plans are not necessarily to be avoided, but certain aspects may be unacceptable. Some potentially negative outcomes include flatulence, poor mineral absorption (from excess fiber intake), and a sense of deprivation (due to limited food choices).
Novelty diets	• *3-Hour Diet* (2005) • *Beverly Hills Diet* (1981, 1996) • Cabbage-Soup Diet (2004) • *Eat Right 4 Your Type* (1996) • *Fat Smash Diet* (2006) • *Fit for Life* (1987, 2001) • *Metabolic Typing Diet* (2002) • *New Hilton Head Metabolism Diet* (1983, 1996) • *Ultrametabolism* (2006) • *Weigh Down Diet* (2002)	• Promote certain nutrients, foods, or combinations of foods as having unique, magical, or previously undiscovered qualities	Novelty diets are usually not nutritionally balanced, thus malnutrition is a possible result. Also, failure to make long-term changes may lead to relapse, and unrealistic food choices lead to possible bingeing.

*Dates listed are original release date followed by most recent release date, if applicable.

4. They bill themselves as cure-alls. These diets claim to work for everyone, whatever the type of obesity or the person's specific strengths and weaknesses.

5. They often recommend expensive supplements.

6. No attempts are made to change eating habits permanently. Dieters follow the diet until the desired weight is reached and then revert to old eating habits—they are told, for example, to eat rice for a month, lose weight, and then return to old habits.

7. They are generally critical of and skeptical about the scientific community. The lack of a quick fix from medical and dietetic professionals has led some of the public to seek advice from those who appear to have the answer.

8. They claim that there is no need to exercise.

Probably the cruelest characteristic of these diets is that they essentially guarantee failure for the dieter. The diets are not designed for permanent weight loss. Habits are not changed, and the food selection is so limited that the person cannot follow the diet in the long run. Although dieters assume they have lost fat, they have lost mostly muscle and other lean tissue mass. As soon as they begin eating normally again, much of the lost tissue is replaced. In a matter of weeks, most of the lost weight is back. The dieter appears to have failed, when actually the diet has failed. The gain and loss cycle is called weight cycling or "yo-yo" dieting. This whole scenario can add more blame and guilt, challenging the self-worth of the dieter. It can also come with some health costs, such as increased upper-body fat deposition. If someone needs help losing weight, professional help is advised. It is unfortunate that current trends suggest that people are spending more time and money on "quick fixes" rather than on such professional help.

TYPES OF POPULAR DIETS

Low- or Restricted-Carbohydrate Approaches

Low-carbohydrate diets have recently been the most popular diets. The low-carbohydrate intake leads to less glycogen synthesis, and therefore less water in the body (about 3 grams of water are stored per gram of glycogen). As discussed in Chapter 4, a very-low-carbohydrate intake also forces the liver to produce needed glucose. The source of carbons for this glucose is mostly proteins from tissues such as muscle resulting in loss of protein tissue, about 72% water. Essential ions, such as potassium are also lost in the urine. With the loss of glycogen stores, lean tissue and water, the dieter loses weight very rapidly. When a normal diet is resumed, the protein tissue is rebuilt and the weight is regained.

Low-carbohydrate diets work in the short run primarily because they limit total food intake. In long-term studies these diets have not shown a distinct advantage compared to diets that limit calorie intake in general.

The most popular diet using a low-carbohydrate approach is the Dr. Atkins' New Diet Revolution. More moderate approaches are found in the various Zone diets (40% of calorie intake as carbohydrate), Sugar Busters diet, and the South Beach diet (especially initial phases).

Carbohydrate-Focused Diets

Several recent diets, including Sugar Busters the Glucose Revolution, and Eat, Drink and Weigh Less, do not restrict carbohydrates, but rather emphasize the "good" carbohydrates in place of the "bad" or "harmful" ones. These diets recommend eating plenty of fruits, vegetables, whole grains, and cutting out simple sugars and processed grains. The carbohydrate-focused diets rely largely on low glycemic index and low glycemic load foods. In theory, these foods will cause a slow, steady rise in blood sugar, which will help control hunger.

Low-Fat Approaches

The very-low-fat diets contain approximately 5% to 10% of calories as fat and are very high in carbohydrates. The most notable are the Pritikin Diet and the Dr. Dean Ornish "Eat More, Weigh Less" diet plans. This approach is not harmful for healthy adults, but it is difficult to follow.

People are quickly bored with this type of diet because they cannot eat many of their favorite foods. These dieters eat primarily grains, fruits, and vegetables, which most people cannot do for very long. Eventually, the person wants some foods higher in fat or protein. These diets are just too different from the typical North American diet for many adults to follow consistently, but may be acceptable for some people.

Novelty Diets

A variety of diets are built on gimmicks. Some novelty diets emphasize one food or food group and exclude almost all others. A rice diet was designed in the 1940s to lower blood pressure; now it has resurfaced as a weight-loss diet. The first phase consists of eating only rice and fruit. On the Beverly Hills Diet, you eat mostly fruit.

The rationale behind these diets is that you can eat only rice or fruit for just so long before becoming bored and, in theory, reducing your calorie intake. However, chances are that you will abandon the diet entirely before losing much weight.

The most questionable of the novelty diets propose that "food gets stuck in your body." Fit for Life, the Beverly Hills Diet, and Eat Great, Lose Weight are examples. The supposition is that food gets stuck in the intestine, putrefies, and creates toxins, which invade the blood and cause disease. In response, recommendations are to not consume meat with potatoes or to consume fruits only after noon. These recommendations make no physiological sense.

Meal Replacements

Meal replacements come in many forms, including beverages or formulas, frozen or shelf-stable entrees, and meal or snack bars. Most meal replacements are fortified with vitamins and minerals and are appropriate to replace one or two regular meals or snacks per day. Although they are not a "magic bullet" for weight loss, they have been shown to help some people lose weight. Advantages of these convenient products are that they provide portion- and calorie-controlled foods that can serve as a visual education on appropriate portion sizes.

Quackery Is Characteristic of Many Popular Diets

Many popular diets fall under the category of quackery—people taking advantage of others. They usually involve a product or service that costs a considerable amount of money. Often, those offering the product or service don't realize that they are promoting quackery, because they were victims themselves. For example, they tried the product and by pure coincidence it worked for them, so they wish to sell it to all their friends and relatives.

Numerous other gimmicks for weight loss have come and gone and are likely to resurface. If in the future an important aid for weight loss is discovered, you can feel confident that major journals, such as the *Journal of the American Dietetic Association,* the *Journal of the American Medical Association,* or *The New England Journal of Medicine,* will report it. You don't need to rely on paperback books, infomercials, billboards, or newspaper advertisements for information about weight loss.

◀ In time, the very-low-carbohydrate, high-protein diets typically leave a person wanting more variety in meals, and so the diets are abandoned. Dropout rates are high on these diets.

CASE STUDY

Choosing a Weight-Loss Program

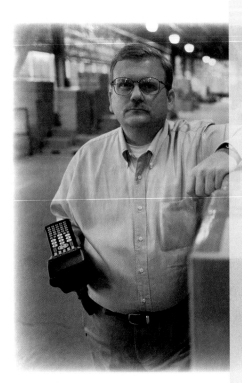

Joe has a hectic schedule. During the day he works full-time at a warehouse distribution center filling orders. At night, three times a week, he attends class at the local community college in pursuit of computer certification. On weekends he likes to watch sports on TV, spend time with family and friends, and study. Joe has little time to think about what he eats—convenience rules. He stops for coffee and a pastry on his way to work, has a burger or pizza for lunch at a quick service restaurant, and for dinner picks up fried chicken or fish at the drive-through on his way to class. Unfortunately, over the past few years Joe's weight has been climbing. Watching a game on television a few nights ago, he saw an infomercial for a product that promises he can eat large portions of tasty foods but not gain weight. A famous actor supports the claim that this product allows one to eat at will and not gain weight. This claim is tempting to Joe.

Answer the following questions, and check your response in Appendix A.

1. Has Joe been experiencing positive or negative energy balance over the past few years?
2. What aspects of Joe's lifestyle (other than diet) are causing this effect on his energy balance? What changes could Joe make in his habits to promote weight loss or maintenance?
3. What changes could Joe make in his diet that would promote weight loss or maintenance?
4. Why should Joe be skeptical of the claims he heard about the weight-loss product in the infomercial?
5. What advice can you offer Joe for evaluation of weight-loss programs?

▲ What changes can Joe make in his daily routine and diet to stop his weight gain?

SUMMARY

1. Energy balance considers energy intake and energy output. Negative energy balance occurs when energy output surpasses energy intake, resulting in weight loss. Positive energy balance occurs when calorie intake is greater than output, resulting in weight gain.

2. Basal metabolism, the thermic effect of food, physical activity, and thermogenesis account for total energy use by the body. Basal metabolism, which represents the minimum amount of calories required to keep the resting, awake body alive, is primarily affected by lean body mass, surface area, and thyroid hormone concentrations. Physical activity is energy use above that expended at rest. The thermic effect of food describes the increase in metabolism that facilitates digestion, absorption, and processing of the nutrients recently consumed. Thermogenesis is heat production caused by shivering when cold, fidgeting, and other stimuli. In a sedentary person, about 70%

to 80% of energy use is accounted for by basal metabolism and the thermic effect of food.

3. A person of healthy weight shows good health and performs daily activities without weight-related problems. A body mass index (weight in kilograms ÷ height^2 in meters) of 18.5 to 25 is one measure of healthy weight, although weight in excess of this value may not lead to ill health. A healthy weight is best determined in conjunction with a thorough health evaluation by a physician.

4. A body mass index of 25 to 29.9 represents overweight. Obesity is defined as a total body fat percentage over 25% (men) or 35% (women) or a body mass index of 30 or more.

5. Fat distribution greatly determines health risks from obesity. Upper-body fat storage, as measured by a waist circumference greater than 40 inches (102 centimeters) for men or 35 inches (88 centimeters) for women typically

results in higher risks of hypertension, cardiovascular disease, and type 2 diabetes than does lower-body fat storage.

6. A sound weight-loss program meets the dieter's nutritional needs by emphasizing a wide variety of low-calorie, bulky foods; adapts to the dieter's habits; consists of readily obtainable foods; strives to change poor eating habits; stresses regular physical activity; and stipulates the supervision by a physician if weight is to be lost rapidly or if the person is over the age of 40 (men) or 50 (women) and plans to perform substantially greater physical activity than usual.

7. A pound of adipose tissue contains about 3500 kcal. Loss or gain of a pound of adipose tissue—the fat itself plus lean support tissue—represents approximately 3300 kcal. Thus, if energy output exceeds calorie intake by about 500 kcal per day, a pound of adipose tissue can be lost per week.

8. Physical activity as part of a weight-loss program should be focused on duration rather than intensity. Ideally, vigorous activity for 60 minutes should be part of each day to prevent adult weight gain.

9. Behavior modification is a vital part of a weight-loss program because the dieter may have many habits that discourage weight maintenance. Specific behavior modification techniques, such as stimulus control and self-monitoring, can be used to help change problem behavior.

10. Medications to blunt appetite, such as phenteramine (Fastin) and sibutramine (Meridia), can aid weight-reduction strategies. Orlistat (Xenical) reduces fat absorption from a meal when taken with the meal. Weight-loss drugs are reserved for those who are obese or have weight-related problems, and they must be administered under close physician supervision.

11. The treatment of severe obesity may include surgery to reduce stomach volume to approximately 30 milliliters (1 ounce) or very-low-calorie diets containing 400 to 800 kcal per day. Both of these measures should be reserved for people who have failed at more conservative approaches to weight loss. They also require close medical supervision.

12. Underweight can be caused by a variety of factors, such as excessive physical activity and genetic background.

Sometimes being underweight requires medical attention. A physician should be consulted first to rule out underlying disease. The underweight person may need to increase portion sizes and learn to like calorie-dense foods. In addition, encouraging a regular meal and snack schedule aids in weight gain, as well as weight maintenance.

13. Many overweight people try popular diets that most often are not helpful and may actually be harmful. Unreliable diets typically share some common characteristics, including promoting quick weight loss, limiting food selections, using testimonials as proof, and requiring no exercise.

STUDY QUESTIONS

1. After re-examining the nature and nurture aspects of weight control, propose two hypotheses for the development of obesity.

2. Propose two hypotheses for the development of obesity, based on the four contributors to energy expenditure.

3. Define a healthy weight in a way that makes the most sense to you.

4. Describe a practical method to define obesity in a clinical setting.

5. What are the two most convincing pieces of evidence that both genetic and environmental factors play significant roles in the development of obesity?

6. List three health problems that obese people typically face. Describe a possible reason that each problem arises.

7. When searching for a sound weight-loss program, what three key characteristics would you look for?

8. Why is the claim for quick, effortless weight loss by any method always misleading?

9. Define the term *behavior modification*. Relate it to the terms *stimulus control, self-monitoring, chain-breaking, relapse prevention,* and *cognitive restructuring*. Give examples of each.

10. Why should the treatment of obesity be viewed as a lifelong commitment rather than just a short episode of weight loss?

CHECK YOUR KNOWLEDGE

Answers to the following multiple choice questions are in Appendix A.

1. Decreasing energy intake by about 400 to 500 kcal per day would mean a loss of about one pound of body fat stores in _____ days.
   a. 2
   b. 7
   c. 10
   d. 14

2. Thermic effect of food represents the energy cost of
   a. chewing food.
   b. peristalsis.
   c. basal metabolism.
   d. digesting, absorbing, and packaging nutrients.

3. A well-designed diet should
   a. increase physical activity.
   b. alter problem behaviors.
   c. reduce energy intake.
   d. All of the above.

4. Dr. Atkins' New Diet Revolution, The Zone, and the South Beach Diet are all examples of low- _____ diets.
   a. fat
   b. carbohydrate
   c. protein
   d. fiber

5. The intent of bariatric surgery is to
   a. limit stomach volume.
   b. speed transit time.
   c. surgically remove adipose tissue.
   d. prevent snacking.

6. Basal metabolism
   a. represents about 30% of total energy expenditure.
   b. is energy used to maintain heartbeat, respiration, and other basic functions and daily activities.
   c. represents about 60% to 70% of total calories used by the body during a day.
   d. includes the energy used to digest food.

7. All of the following factors are associated with a higher basal metabolic rate *except*
   a. stress.
   b. starvation.
   c. fever.
   d. pregnancy.

8. Probably the most important reason for obesity today in the United States is
   a. watching TV.
   b. snacking practices.
   c. inactivity.
   d. eating French fries.

9. The major goal for weight reduction in the treatment of obesity is the loss of
   a. weight.
   b. body fat.
   c. body water.
   d. body protein.

10. For most adults, the greatest portion of their energy expenditure is for
    a. physical activity.
    b. sleeping.
    c. basal metabolism.
    d. the thermic effect of food.

FURTHER READINGS (See also the May 2005 Supplement on Obesity in the Journal of the American Dietetic Association)

1. Adams KF and others: Overweight, obesity, and mortality in a large prospective cohort of persons 50 to 71 years old. *The New England Journal of Medicine* 355:763, 2006.

   Although obesity, defined by a body-mass index (BMI) of 30.0 or more, has been associated with an increased risk of death, the relationship between overweight (a BMI of 25.0 to 29.9) and the risk of death is not clear. BMI was prospectively examined in relation to the risk of death from any cause in 527,265 U.S. men and women 50 to 71 years old. Excess body weight during midlife was associated with an increased risk of death. Risk of death increased by 20 to 40 percent among overweight persons and by two to three times among obese persons.

2. Blackburn GL: Solutions in weight control: lessons from gastric surgery. *American Journal of Clinical Nutrition* 82:248S, 2005.

   Surgery is currently the only proven way to achieve significant long-term weight loss, improve obesity-related health problems, reduce the risk of premature death, and improve quality of life in a large proportion of obese individuals. Roux-en-Y gastric bypass, the most widely performed procedure in the United States, achieves permanent, significant weight loss in more than 90% of cases of severe obesity.

3. Booth KM and others: Obesity and the built environment. *Journal of the American Dietetic Association* 105:S110, 2005.

   Obesity is linked with many features of the "built environment": residence, neighborhood, resources, television, walkability, land use, and sprawl. Lower socioeconomic status neighborhoods are a primary concern, as residents in these areas may have less access to recreational facilities or food stores with healthful, affordable options. In the future, neighborhoods should be designed in ways that promote physical activity.

4. Dansinger ML and others: Comparison of the Atkins, Ornish, Weight Watchers, and Zone diets for weight loss and heart disease risk reduction: A randomized trial. *Journal of the American Medical Association* 293:43, 2005.

   All four popular diets (Atkins, Ornish, Weight Watchers, Zone) are equally effective for helping adults lose weight. Because success in this study directly correlated with adherence to the diet, it makes sense to help patients choose the diet that is easiest for them to follow, rather than preferentially encouraging one diet over any other.

5. Ello-Martin JA and others: The influence of food portion size and energy density on energy intake: Implications for weight management. *American Journal of Clinical Nutrition* 82:236S, 2005.

   Providing larger food portions can lead to significant increases in calorie intake. One strategy to address this effect of portion size is decreasing the energy density of foods. Eating satisfying portions of low-energy-dense foods maintains satiety while reducing calorie intake.

6. Foster GD and others: Behavioral treatment of obesity. *American Journal of Clinical Nutrition* 82:230S, 2005.

   The behavior change process is facilitated through the use of self-monitoring, goal-setting, and problem solving. Behavior therapy can help individuals develop a set of skills (such as eating a low-calorie, low-fat diet) to achieve a healthier weight.

7. Goldberg J and Bucciarelli A: A century of low-carbohydrate diets. *Nutrition Today.* 41(3):99, 2006.

   Low-carbohydrate diets have come and gone and been promising quick and easy weight loss for more than a century. This article is a review of the history of low-carbohydrate diets, their safety and effectiveness, and how they have performed in clinical trials.

8. Hu FB: Protein, body weight, and cardiovascular health. *American Journal of Clinical Nutrition* 82:242S, 2005.

   It may be beneficial to partially replace refined carbohydrates with protein sources low in saturated fat. Plant sources of protein and fat, such as nuts, legumes, soy, and vegetable oils, may provide even greater health benefits in place of refined carbohydrates and animal products.

9. Jakicic JM and Otto AD: Physical activity considerations for the treatment and prevention of obesity. *American Journal of Clinical Nutrition* 82:226S, 2005.

   Physical activity is an important component of long-term weight control, and therefore adequate levels of activity should be prescribed to combat the obesity epidemic. Although there is evidence that 30 minutes of moderate-intensity physical activity may improve health outcomes, a growing body of scientific literature suggests that at least 60 minutes of moderate-intensity physical activity may be necessary to maximize weight loss and prevent significant weight regain.

10. Kruger J and others: Dietary and physical activity behaviors among adults successful at weight loss maintenance. *International Journal of Behavioral Nutrition and Physical Activity* 3:17, 2006.

    Many individuals who lose weight do not keep the weight off and eventually regain most of the lost weight. In this study, weight-loss strategies among adults who reported successful weight-loss attempts (lost weight and were able to keep it off) were compared to persons whose previous attempts to lose weight were unsuccessful or who could not keep the lost weight off. Strategies practiced more frequently by successful weight losers included self-monitoring strategies such as weighing oneself, planning meals, tracking fat and calories, exercising 30 or more minutes daily, and adding physical activity to their daily routines.

11. Ledikwe JH and others: Low-energy density diets are associated with high diet quality in adults in the United States. *Journal of the American Dietetic Association* 106:1172, 2006.

    This study demonstrated the beneficial effects of a low-energy-density diet compared with a high-energy-density diet. Benefits included lower energy intakes, higher food intakes, and higher diet quality. A low-energy-density diet should include a variety of fruits and vegetables; low-fat/reduced-fat, nutrient dense, and/or water-rich grains; dairy products; and meats/meat alternatives.

12. Li Z and others: Meta-analysis: Pharmacologic treatment of obesity. *Annals of Internal Medicine* 142(7):532, 2005.

    Sibutramine, orlistat, and phentermine promote weight loss for at least 6 months when given along with recommendations for diet (and other behavioral and exercise interventions). The amount of extra weight loss attributable to these medications is modest, but still may be clinically significant. Use of each of these medications is reviewed in detail.

17. Spear BA: Does dieting increase the risk for obesity and eating disorders? *Journal of the American Dietetic Association* 106:523, 2006.

This editorial summarizes the results of recent studies on dieting and other unhealthful weight-control methods in adolescents that appear to predict and be associated with later weight gain, overweight, and eating disorders.

18. State-specific prevalence of obesity among adults—United States, 2005. *Morbidity and Mortality Weekly Report* 55(36):985, 2006.

This report indicates that the prevalence of obesity in adults at the state level, based on self-reported weight and height, increased significantly during 1995–2005. Age-adjusted obesity rates were 15.6%, 19.8%, and 23.7% for the 1995, 2000, and 2005 surveys, respectively. In 2005, 60.5% of the total U.S. adult population surveyed were overweight, 23.9% were obese and 3.0% were extremely obese. This increasing trend is moving states farther away from the Healthy People 2010 target of 15% prevalence of obesity.

19. Willett W, Katzen M: *Eat, Drink & Weigh Less,* Hyperion, 2006.

This diet book is written by top nutrition researcher, Willett and vegetarian cookbook author, Katzen. This diet recommends eating mostly fruits; vegetables; whole grains; nuts; legumes; olive oil; and proteins, such as beans, nuts, fish, and poultry. The diet limits red meat and processed foods.

20. Wing RR and Phelan S: Long-term weight loss maintenance. *American Journal of Clinical Nutrition* 82:222S, 2005.

National Weight Control Registry members provide evidence that long-term weight loss maintenance is possible and help identify the specific approaches associated with long-term success. The article reviews the habits of these participants, such as regularly eating breakfast, self-monitoring weight, and meeting the goal of 60 minutes of physical activity per day.

▶ **Check out the Contemporary Nutrition ARIS site**
www.mhhe.com/wardlawcontfa1 for quizzes, flash cards, other activities, and weblinks designed to further help you learn about what you eat and why.

I. A Close Look at Your Weight Status

Determine the following two indices of your body status: body mass index and waist circumference.

Body Mass Index (BMI)

Record your weight in pounds: _____ lb

Divide your weight in pounds by 2.2 to determine your weight in kilograms: _____ kilograms

Record your height in inches: _____ in

Divide your height in inches by 39.4 to determine your height in meters: _____ meters

Calculate your BMI using the following formula:

BMI = weight (kilograms)/height^2 (meters)

BMI = _____ kg/ _____ m^2 = _____

Waist Circumference

Use a tape measure to measure the circumference of your waist (at the umbilicus with stomach muscles relaxed). Circumference of waist (umbilicus) = _____ in

Interpretation

1. When BMI is greater than 25, health risks from obesity often begin. It is especially advisable to consider weight loss if your BMI exceeds 30. Does yours exceed 25 (or 30)?

   Yes _____   No _____

2. When a person has a BMI greater than 25 and a waist circumference of more than 40 inches (102 centimeters) in men or 35 inches (88 centimeters) in women, there is an increased risk of cardiovascular disease, hypertension, and type 2 diabetes. Does your waist circumference exceed the standard for your gender?

   Yes _____   No _____

3. Do you feel you need to pursue a program of weight loss?

   Yes _____   No _____

Application

From what you've learned in Chapter 7, what can you do to change your patterns of eating and physical activity to lose weight and help ensure maintenance of any loss?

_____

_____

_____

II. An Action Plan to Change or Maintain Weight Status

Now that you have assessed your current weight status, do you feel that you would like to make some changes? Following is a step-by-step guide to behavioral change. This process can be useful even for those satisfied with their current weight, as it can be applied to changing exercise habits, self-esteem, and a variety of other behaviors (Fig. 7-18).

NEW STATUS QUO

Changes become part of lifestyle

Develop a receptive framework for learning

Become aware of the problem

Gather baseline information

Set goals

Original status quo

Chart a plan of action

Success with changes

Unable or unwilling to commit to changes

Practice the plan

FIGURE 7-18 ▶ A model for behavior change. It starts with awareness of the problem and ends with the incorporation of new behaviors intended to address the problem.

Becoming Aware of the Problem

By calculating your current weight status, you have already become aware of the problem, if one exists. From here, it is important to find out more information about the cause of the problem and whether it is worth working toward a change.

1. What are the factors that most influence your eating habits? Do you eat due to stress, boredom, or depression? Is volume of food your problem, or do you eat mainly the wrong foods for you? Take some time to assess the root causes of your eating habits.

2. Once you have more information about your specific eating practices, you must decide if it is worth changing these practices. A benefits and costs analysis can be a useful tool in evaluating whether it is worth your effort to make life changes. Use the following example as a guide for listing benefits and costs pertinent to your situation (Fig. 7-19).

Setting Goals

What can we accomplish, and how long will it take? Setting a realistic, achievable goal and allowing a reasonable amount of time to pursue it increases the likelihood of success.

1. Begin by determining the outcome you would like to achieve. If you are trying to change your eating behaviors to be more healthy, list your reasons for doing so (e.g., overall health, weight loss, self-esteem).

Overall goal:

_____

_____

Reasons to pursue goal:

_____

_____

_____

FIGURE 7-19 ▶ Benefits and costs analysis applied to increasing physical activity. This process helps put behavior change into the context of total lifestyle.

Benefits and Costs Analysis

1 Benefits of changing eating habits?

What do you expect to get, now or later, that you want?
What may you avoid that would be unpleasant?

feel better physically and psychologically
look better

2 Benefits of not changing eating habits?

What do you get to do that you enjoy doing?
What do you avoid having to do?

no need for planning
can eat without feeling guilty

3 Costs involved in changing eating habits?

What do you have to do that you don't want to do?
What do you have to stop doing that you would rather continue doing?

take time to plan meals and shop
must give up some food volume

4 Costs of not changing eating habits?

What unpleasant or undesirable effects are you likely to experience now or in the future?
What are you likely to lose?

creeping weight gain
low self-esteem and poor health

2. Now list several steps that will be necessary to achieve your goal. Keep in mind, however, that it is generally best to change only a few specific behaviors at first—walking briskly for 60 minutes each day, reducing fat intake, using more whole-grain products, and not eating after 7 P.M. Attempting small and perhaps easier dietary changes first reduces the scope of the problem and increases the likelihood of success.

Steps toward achieving goal:

1. _____

2. _____

3. _____

If you are having trouble deciphering the steps needed to achieve your goal, health professionals are an excellent resource for aid in planning.

Measuring Commitment

Now that you have collected information and know what is required to reach your goal, you must ask yourself, "Can I do this?" Commitment is an essential component in the success of behavioral change. Be honest with yourself. Permanent change is not quick or easy. Once you have decided that you have the commitment required to see this through, continue on to the following sections.

Making It Official with a Contract

Drawing up a behavioral contract often adds incentive to follow through with a plan. The contract could list goal behaviors and objectives, milestones for measuring progress, and regular rewards for meeting the terms of the contract. After finishing a contract, you should sign it in the presence of some friends. This encourages commitment.

Initially, plans should reward positive behaviors, and then they should focus on positive results. Positive behaviors, such as regular physical activity, eventually lead to positive outcomes, such as increased stamina.

Figure 7-20 is a sample contract for increasing physical activity. Keep in mind that this sample contract is only a suggestion; you can add your ideas as well.

Psyching Yourself Up

Once your contract is in place, you need to psych yourself up. Discouragement from peers and your temptations to stray from your plan need to be anticipated. Psyching yourself up can enable you to progress toward your goals in spite of others' attitudes and opinions. Almost everyone benefits from some assertiveness training when it comes to changing behaviors. The following are a few suggestions. Can you think of any others?

- No one's feelings should be hurt if you say, "No, thank you," firmly and repeatedly when others try to dissuade you from a plan. Tell them you have new diet behavior and your needs are important.

- You don't have to eat a lot to accommodate anyone—your mother, business clients, or the chef. For example, at a party with friends, you may feel you have to eat a lot to participate, but you don't. Another trap is ordering a lot just because someone else is paying for the meal.

- Learn ways to handle put-downs—inadvertent or conscious. An effective response can be to communicate feelings honestly, without hostility. Tell criticizers that they have annoyed or offended you, that you are working to change your habits and would really like understanding and support from them.

Practicing the Plan

Once you've set up a plan, the next step is to implement it. Start with a trial of at least 6 to 8 weeks. Thinking of a lifetime commitment can be overwhelming. Aim for a total duration of 6 months of new activities before giving up. We may have to persuade ourselves more than once of the value of continuing the program. The following are some suggestions to help keep a plan on track:

- *Focus on reducing, but not necessarily extinguishing, undesirable behaviors.* For example, it's usually unrealistic to say, "I'll never eat a certain food again." It's better to say, "I won't eat that *problem* food as often as before."

- *Monitor progress.* Note your progress in a diary and reward yourself according to your contract. While conquering some habits and seeing improvement, you may find yourself quite encouraged, even enthusiastic, about your plan of action. That can give you the impetus to move ahead with the program.

- *Control environments.* In the early phases of behavioral change, try to avoid problem situations, such as parties, coffee breaks, and favorite restaurants. Once new habits are firmly established, you can probably more successfully resist the temptations of these environments.

Re-evaluating and Preventing Relapse

After practicing a program for several weeks to months, it is important to reassess the original plan. In addition, you may now be able to pinpoint other problem areas for which you need to plan appropriately.

1. Begin by taking a close and critical look at your original plan. Does it lead to the goals you set? Are there any new steps toward your goal that you feel capable of adding to your contract? Do you need new reinforcements? It may even be necessary to make a new contract. For permanent change, it is worth this time of reassessment.

2. In practicing your plan over the past weeks or months, you have likely experienced relapses. What triggered these relapses? To prevent a total retreat to your old habits, it is important to set up a plan for such relapses. You can do this by identifying high-risk situations, rehearsing a response, and remembering your goals.

You may have noticed a behavior chain in some of your relapses. That is, the relapse may stem from a series of interconnected habitual activities. The way to break the chain is to first identify the activities, pinpoint the weak links, break those links, and substitute other behaviors. Figure 7-21 illustrates a sample behavior chain and a substitute activities list. Consider compiling a list based on your behavior chains.

```
Name  Alan Young
_____

Goal
I agree to  ride my exercise bike
_____
                    (specify behavior)
_____

under the following circumstances  for 30 minutes, 4 times per week
in the evening       (specify where, when, how much, etc.)
_____

Substitute behavior and/or reinforcement schedule  I will reinforce myself
if I've achieved my goal after a month with a weekend off
campus with my roommate.

Environmental planning
In order to help me do this, I am going to (1) arrange my physical and social environment
by  buying a new portable CD player
_____

and (2) control my internal environment (thoughts, images) by  coordinating riding
the bike with the first T.V. watching I do in the evening

Reinforcements
Reinforcements provided by me daily or weekly (if contract is kept):
I will buy myself a new piece of clothing for off campus
trip

Reinforcements provided by others daily or weekly (if contract is kept):
at the end of a month if I've completed my goal my parents will
buy me a fitness club membership for winter.

Social support
Behavior change is more likely to take place when other people support you. During the
quarter/semester please meet with the other person at least three times to discuss your
progress.
The name of my "significant helper" is:  Mr. and Mrs. Young

This contract should include:
1. Baseline data (one week)
2. Well-defined goal
3. Simple method for charting progress (diary, counter, charts, etc.)
4. Reinforcements (immediate and long-term)
5. Evaluation method (summary of experiences, success, and/or new learnings about self).
```

FIGURE 7-20 ▶ Alan's behavior contract. Completing such a contract can help generate commitment to behavior change. What would your contract look like?

Epilogue

If you have used the activities in this section, you are well on your way to permanent behavioral change. Recall that this exercise can be used for a variety of desired changes, including quitting smoking, increasing physical activity, and improving study habits. It is by no means an easy process, but the results can be well worth the effort. Overall, the keys to success are motivation (keeping the problem in the forefront of your mind), having a plan of action, securing the resources and skills needed for success, and looking for help from family, friends, or a group.

ALTERNATIVE ACTIVITY SHEET

SUBSTITUTE ACTIVITIES

Pleasant activities
1. _Singing / washing hair_
2. _Reading comics / biking_
3. _Sewing / calling a friend_

Necessary activities
1. _Ironing_
2. _Vacuuming_
3. _Straightening apartment_

Situations when used
1. _Wanted ice cream – delayed with bath_
2. _Wanted wheat thins – cleaned up apt._
3. _Wanted snack – went for walk_
4. _Wanted cookies – did dishes first_
5. _Saw leftovers – went for bike ride_
6. _Tempted by cookies – set timer_
7. _Wanted snack – read comics_

BEHAVIOR CHAIN

Identify the links in your eating response chain on the following diagram. Draw a line through the chain where it was interrupted. Add the link you substituted and the new chain of behavior this substitution started.

FIGURE 7-21 ▶ Identifying behavior chains. This is a good tool for understanding more about your habits and pinpointing ways to change unwanted habits. The earlier in the chain you substitute a nonfood link, the easier it is to intervene. Four types of behaviors can be substituted in an ongoing behavior chain.

1. Fun activities (taking a walk, reading a book)
2. Necessary activities (cleaning a room, balancing your checkbook)
3. Incompatible activities (taking a shower)
4. Urge-delaying activities (setting a kitchen timer for 20 minutes before allowing yourself to eat)

Using activities to interrupt behavior patterns that lead to inappropriate eating (or inactivity) can be a powerful means of changing habits.

OVERVIEW OF THE MICRONUTRIENTS

Can food be medicine? Consider the following examples:

- Fatigue, bleeding gums, bruising, and scaly skin . . . these are the symptoms of **scurvy,** which plagued seamen during long ocean voyages until 1753, when James Lind, a physician in the British Navy, identified that consumption of citrus fruits could prevent this disease.
- Imagine the epidemic of **rickets** that occurred among children in post-Industrial Revolution Britain during the late eighteenth century. They suffered from bone pain; frequent fractures; weakness; and deformities, such as bowed legs. In 1922, cod liver oil was determined to be an effective treatment for rickets.
- First noted in medical literature in the mid-sixteenth century, **chlorosis** was a disorder characterized by a green skin color, extreme weakness, and poor appetite. Chlorosis was mainly described among adolescent women, so some physicians of the era declared it to be a hysterical condition. In the early 1700s, the British physician Thomas Sydenham prescribed that afflicted women should drink "mineral water impregnated with the Iron Mine."

How do citrus fruits, cod liver oil, and mineral water prevent or cure such serious ailments? As nutrition science has evolved, the discovery of essential compounds in the foods we eat has overturned old misconceptions about the origins of some diseases. These essential compounds are collectively known as **micronutrients.** Citrus fruits, sure cures for scurvy, contain vitamin C. Cod liver oil, a preventive treatment for rickets, is an excellent source of vitamin D. The mineral water prescribed by Sydenham supplied iron for his patients suffering from chlorosis, a form of iron-deficiency anemia.

Vitamin C, vitamin D, and iron are a few examples of micronutrients. In Chapters 4, 5, and 6, you learned about carbohydrates, lipids, and proteins. Along with water, these energy-yielding nutrients are known as macronutrients. These are essential components needed in relatively large amounts (grams) in the human diet. On the other hand, micronutrients yield no energy and are required in small amounts (milligrams or micrograms). However slight its requirement, each micronutrient is necessary for one or more functions in the body (Overview Figure 1). Too little or too much of any specific micronutrient leads to deterioration of physical health.

The micronutrients can be chemically grouped based upon the presence of carbon atoms bonded to hydrogen atoms in their chemical structures. Organic micronutrients are classified as **vitamins** and inorganic micronutrients are classified as **minerals.**

VITAMINS: VITAL DIETARY COMPONENTS

By definition, vitamins are essential organic (carbon-containing) substances needed in small amounts in the diet for normal function, growth, and maintenance of the body. In general, humans require a total of about 1 ounce (28 grams) of vitamins for every 150 pounds (70 kilograms) of food consumed. Vitamins can be divided into two broad classes based on solubility. Vitamins A, D, E, and

scurvy The vitamin C deficiency disease characterized by weakness, fatigue, slow wound healing, opening of previously healed wounds, bone pain, fractures, sore and bleeding gums, diarrhea, and pinpoint hemorrhages on the skin.

rickets A disease characterized by poor mineralization of newly synthesized bones because of low calcium content. Arising in infants and children, this deficiency is caused by insufficient amounts of the vitamin D hormone in the body.

chlorosis In traditional medical terminology, a form of iron-deficiency anemia characterized by pale or greenish skin, weakness, fatigue, and shortness of breath. In modern medical literature, chlorosis is termed hypochromic anemia.

micronutrient A nutrient needed in milligram or microgram quantities in a diet.

vitamin Compound needed in small amounts in the diet to help regulate and support chemical reactions and processes in the body.

mineral Element used in the body to promote chemical reactions and to form body structures.

OVERVIEW FIGURE 1 ▶ Micronutrients contribute to many functions in the body.

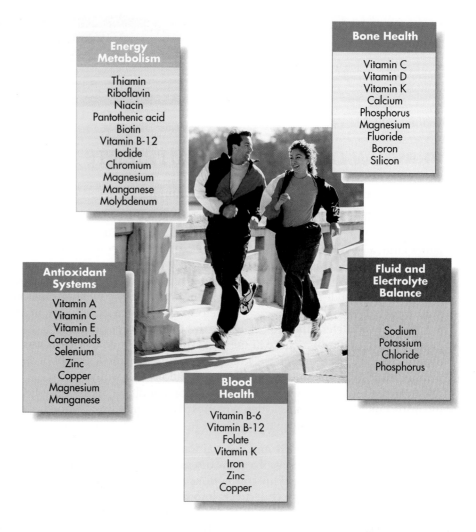

Energy Metabolism

Thiamin
Riboflavin
Niacin
Pantothenic acid
Biotin
Vitamin B-12
Iodide
Chromium
Magnesium
Manganese
Molybdenum

Bone Health

Vitamin C
Vitamin D
Vitamin K
Calcium
Phosphorus
Magnesium
Fluoride
Boron
Silicon

Antioxidant Systems

Vitamin A
Vitamin C
Vitamin E
Carotenoids
Selenium
Zinc
Copper
Magnesium
Manganese

Fluid and Electrolyte Balance

Sodium
Potassium
Chloride
Phosphorus

Blood Health

Vitamin B-6
Vitamin B-12
Folate
Vitamin K
Iron
Zinc
Copper

fat-soluble vitamins Vitamins that dissolve in fat and such substances as ether and benzene but not readily in water. These vitamins are A, D, E, and K.

water-soluble vitamins Vitamins that dissolve in water. These vitamins are the B vitamins and vitamin C.

K are **fat-soluble vitamin** (Overview Table 1), whereas the B vitamins and vitamin C are **water-soluble vitamin** (Overview Table 2). The B vitamins include thiamin, riboflavin, niacin, pantothenic acid, biotin, vitamin B-6, folate, and vitamin B-12. Choline is a related nutrient, but is not classified as a vitamin.

Vitamins are generally essential in human diets because they can't be synthesized in the human body or because their synthesis can be decreased by environmental factors. Notable exceptions to having a strict dietary need for a vitamin are vitamin A, which we can synthesize from certain pigments in plants; vitamin D, synthesized in the body if the skin is exposed to adequate sunlight; niacin, synthesized from the amino acid tryptophan; and vitamin K and biotin, synthesized to some extent by bacteria in the intestinal tract.

To be classified as a vitamin, a compound must meet the following criteria: (1) the body is unable to synthesize enough of the compound to maintain health; and (2) absence of the compound from the diet for a defined period produces deficiency symptoms that, if caught in time, are quickly cured when the substance is resupplied. A substance does not qualify as a vitamin merely because the body can't make it. Evidence must suggest that health declines when the substance is not consumed.

As scientists began to identify various vitamins, related deficiency diseases such as scurvy and rickets were dramatically cured. For the most part, as the vitamins were discovered, they were named alphabetically: A, B, C, D, E, and so on. Later, many substances originally classified as vitamins were found not to be essential for humans and were dropped from the list. Other vitamins, thought at first to be only one chemical turned out to be several chemicals, so the alphabetical names had to be broken down by numbers (B-6, B-12, and so on).

OVERVIEW TABLE 1 Summary of the Fat-Soluble Vitamins

Vitamin	Major Functions	RDA or Adequate Intake	Dietary Sources	Deficiency Symptoms	Toxicity Symptoms
Vitamin A (preformed vitamin A and provitamin A)	• Promote vision: night and color • Promote growth • Prevent drying of skin and eyes • Promote resistance to bacterial infection and overall immune system function	Females: 700 micrograms RAE Males: 900 micrograms RAE 2300–3000 IU if as preformed (vitamin A)	Preformed Vitamin A: • Liver • Fortified milk • Fortified breakfast cereals Provitamin A: • Sweet potatoes • Spinach • Greens • Carrots • Cantaloupe • Apricots • Broccoli	• Night blindness • Xerophthalmia • Poor growth • Dry skin	• Fetal malformations • Hair loss • Skin changes • Bone pain • Fractures Upper Level is 3000 micrograms of preformed vitamin A (10,000 IU) based on the risk birth defects and liver toxicity
Vitamin D	• Increase absorption of calcium and phosphorus • Maintain optimal blood calcium and calcification of bone	5–15 micrograms (200–600 IU)	• Vitamin D fortified milk • Fortified breakfast cereals • Fish oils • Sardines • Salmon	• Rickets in children • Osteomalacia in adults	• Growth retardation • Kidney damage • Calcium deposits in soft tissue Upper Level is 50 micrograms (2000 IU) based on the risk of elevated blood calcium
Vitamin E	• Antioxidant prevents breakdown of vitamin A and unsaturated fatty acids	15 milligrams alpha-tocopherol 22 IU natural form, 33 IU (synthetic form)	• Plant oils • Products made from plant oils • Some greens • Some fruits • Nuts and seeds • Fortified breakfast cereals	• Hemolysis of red blood cells • Nerve degeneration	• Muscle weakness • Headaches • Nausea • Inhibition of vitamin K metabolism Upper Level is 1000 milligrams (1100 IU synthetic form, 1500 IU natural form) based on the risk of hemorrhage
Vitamin K	• Activation of blood-clotting factors • Activation of proteins involved in bone metabolism	Females: 90 micrograms Males: 120 micrograms	• Green vegetables • Liver • Some plant oils • Some calcium supplements	• Hemorrhage • Fractures	No Upper Level has been set

Abbreviations: RAE = retinol activity equivalents; IU = international units

OVERVIEW TABLE 2 Summary of the Water-Soluble Vitamins and Choline

Vitamin	Major Functions	RDA or Adequate Intake	Dietary Sources*	Deficiency Symptoms	Toxicity Symptoms
Thiamin	• Coenzyme of carbohydrate metabolism • Nerve function	1.1–1.2 milligrams	• Sunflower seeds • Pork • Whole and enriched grains • Dried beans • Peas	*Beriberi* • Nervous tingling • Poor coordination • Edema • Heart changes • Weakness	None
Riboflavin†	• Coenzyme of carbohydrate metabolism	1.1–1.3 milligrams	• Milk • Mushrooms • Spinach • Liver • Enriched grains	• Inflammation of the mouth and tongue • Cracks at the corners of the mouth • Eye disorders	None
Niacin	• Coenzyme of energy metabolism • Coenzyme of fat synthesis • Coenzyme of fat breakdown	14–16 milligrams (niacin equivalents)	• Mushrooms • Bran • Tuna • Salmon • Chicken • Beef • Liver • Peanuts • Enriched grains	*Pellagra* • Diarrhea • Dermatitis • Dementia • Death	Upper Level is 35 milligrams from supplements, based on flushing of skin
Pantothenic acid	• Coenzyme of energy metabolism • Coenzyme of fat synthesis • Coenzyme of fat breakdown	5 milligrams	• Mushrooms • Liver • Broccoli • Eggs *Most foods have some*	• No natural deficiency disease or symptoms	None
Biotin	• Coenzyme of glucose production • Coenzyme of fat synthesis	30 micrograms	• Cheese • Egg yolks • Cauliflower • Peanut butter • Liver	• Dermatitis • Tongue soreness • Anemia • Depression	Unknown
Vitamin B-6†	• Coenzyme of protein metabolism • Neurotransmitter synthesis • Hemogloblin synthesis Many other functions	1.3–1.7 milligrams	• Animal protein foods • Spinach • Broccoli • Bananas • Salmon • Sunflower seeds	• Headache • Anemia • Convulsions • Nausea • Vomiting • Flaky skin • Sore tongue	Upper Level is 100 milligrams, based on nerve destruction
Folate (folic acid)†	• Coenzyme involved in DNA synthesis *Many other functions*	400 micrograms (dietary folate equivalents)	• Green leafy vegetables • Orange juice • Organ meats • Sprouts • Sunflower seeds	• Megaloblastic anemia • Inflammation of tongue • Diarrhea • Poor growth • Depression	None likely Upper Level for adults set at 1000 micrograms for synthetic folic acid (exclusive of food folate), based on masking of B-12 deficiency

Vitamin	Major Functions	RDA or Adequate Intake	Dietary Sources*	Deficiency Symptoms	Toxicity Symptoms
Vitamin B-12†	• Coenzyme of folate metabolism • Nerve function *Many other functions*	2.4 micrograms *Older adults and vegans should use fortified foods or supplements.*	• Animal foods (not natural in plants) • Organ meats • Oysters • Clams • Fortified, ready-to-eat breakfast cereals	• Macrocytic anemia • Poor nerve function	None
Vitamin C	• Connective tissue synthesis • Hormone synthesis • Neurotransmitter synthesis • Possible antioxidant activity	75–90 milligrams *Smokers should add 35 milligrams*	• Citrus fruits • Strawberries • Broccoli • Greens	• Scurvy • Poor wound healing • Pinpoint hemorrhages • Bleeding gums	Upper Level is 2 grams, based on development of diarrhea Can also alter some diagnostic tests
Choline†	• Neurotransmitter synthesis • Phospholipid synthesis	425–550 milligrams	Widely distributed in foods and synthesized by the body	No natural deficiency	Upper Level is 3.5 grams per day based on development of fishy body odor and reduced blood pressure

*Fortified ready-to-eat breakfast cereals are good sources for most of these vitamins and a common source of B vitamins for many of us.

†These nutrients also participate in homocysteine metabolism, which in turn may reduce the risk of developing cardiovascular disease.

In addition to their use in correcting deficiency diseases, a few vitamins have also proved useful in treating several nondeficiency diseases. These medical applications require administration of **megadoses,** well above typical human needs for the vitamins. For example, megadoses of a form of niacin can be used as part of blood cholesterol-lowering treatment for certain individuals. Still, any claimed benefits from use of vitamin supplements, especially intakes in excess of the Upper Level (if set), should be viewed critically because unproved claims are common.

Plant and animal foods supply vitamins in the human diet. Vitamins isolated from foods or synthesized in the laboratory are the same chemical compounds and work equally well in the body. Contrary to claims in the health-food literature, "natural" vitamins isolated from foods are, for the most part, no more healthful than those synthesized in a laboratory, but there are exceptions. Vitamin E is much more potent in its natural form. In contrast, synthetic folic acid, the form of the vitamin added to ready-to-eat breakfast cereals and flour, is 1.7 times more potent than the natural vitamin form.

megadose Intake of a nutrient beyond estimates of needs to prevent a deficiency or what would be found in a balanced diet; two to 10 times human needs is a starting point for such a dosage.

Absorption and Storage of Vitamins in the Body

The fat-soluble vitamins A, D, E, and K are absorbed along with dietary fat. These vitamins then travel with dietary fats as part of chylomicrons through the bloodstream to reach body cells. Special carriers in the bloodstream help distribute some of these vitamins. Fat-soluble vitamins are stored mostly in the liver and fatty tissues.

When fat absorption is efficient, about 40% to 90% of the fat-soluble vitamin is absorbed. Anything that interferes with normal digestion and absorption of fats, however, also interferes with fat-soluble vitamin absorption. For example, people with cystic fibrosis, a disease that often hampers fat absorption, may develop deficiencies of fat-soluble vitamins. Some medications, such as the weight-loss drug orlistat (Xenical), discussed in Chapter 7, also interfere with fat absorption. Unabsorbed fat carries these vitamins to the large intestine, where they are excreted in the feces. People with such conditions are especially susceptible to vitamin K deficiency because body stores of vitamin K are lower than those of the other fat-soluble vitamins. Vitamin supplements, taken under a physician's guidance, are part of the treatment for preventing a vitamin deficiency associated with fat malabsorption. Finally, people who use mineral oil as a laxative at mealtimes risk fat-soluble vitamin deficiencies. The intestine does not absorb mineral oil, so fat-soluble vitamins are eliminated with the mineral oil in the feces.

Water-soluble vitamins are handled much differently than fat-soluble vitamins. After being ingested, the B vitamins are first broken down from their active coenzyme forms into free vitamins in the stomach and small intestine. The vitamins are then absorbed, primarily in the small intestine. Typically, about 50% to 90% of the B vitamins in the diet are absorbed, which means they have relatively high **bioavailability.** Water-soluble vitamins are transported to the liver via the portal vein and are distributed to body tissues. Once inside cells, the active coenzyme forms are resynthesized. There is no need to consume the coenzyme forms. Some vitamins are sold in their coenzyme forms but these are broken down during digestion and we activate them when needed.

Except for vitamin K, the fat-soluble vitamins are not readily excreted from the body. In contrast, excesses of the water-soluble vitamins are rapidly lost from the body, partly because the water in cells dissolves these vitamins and excretes them out of the body via the kidneys. Water-soluble vitamins B-6 and B-12 are exceptions; these are stored much more readily than the other water-soluble vitamins.

The limited storage of many vitamins dictates that they should be consumed in the diet daily, although an occasional lapse in the intake of even water-soluble vitamins causes no harm. Symptoms of a vitamin deficiency occur only when that vitamin is lacking in the diet and the body stores are essentially exhausted. For example, an average person must consume no thiamin for 10 days or no vitamin C for 20 to 40 days before developing the first symptoms of deficiency of these vitamins.

Vitamin Toxicity

Intakes in excess of daily needs for the water-soluble vitamins are rapidly lost from the body because the kidneys efficiently filter the excess from the blood and excrete these compounds in urine. Notable exceptions are vitamin B-6 and vitamin B-12, stored in the liver. Although they are water-soluble, these two B vitamins may accumulate to toxic levels.

In contrast to the water-soluble vitamins, fat-soluble vitamins are not readily excreted, so some can easily accumulate in the body and cause toxic effects. Although a toxic effect from an excessive intake of any vitamin is theoretically possible, toxicity of the fat-soluble vitamin A is the most frequently observed. Vitamin A causes toxicity in as little as two times human need. Vitamin E and the water-soluble vitamins niacin, vitamin B-6, and vitamin C can also cause toxic effects, but only when consumed in large amounts (15 to 100 times human needs or more). Vitamins are unlikely to cause toxic effects unless taken in supplement (pill) form.

Some people believe that consuming vitamins far in excess of their needs provides them with extra energy, protection from disease, and prolonged youth. They seem to think that if a little is good, then more must be better. A "one-a-day" type of multivitamin and mineral supplement usually contains less than two times the Daily Values of the components, so daily use of these products is unlikely to cause toxic effects in men and nonpregnant women. But consuming many vitamin pills, especially potent sources of vitamin A, can cause problems. Today, concentrated vitamin A supplements are widely available in grocery, drug, and health-food stores and pose risks for toxicity when used inappropriately.

Preservation of Vitamins in Foods

Good sources of vitamins can be found in all food groups, especially fruits and vegetables (Overview Figure 2). Substantial amounts of vitamins can be lost from the time a fruit or vegetable is picked until it is eaten. The water-soluble vitamins, particularly

MyPyramid: Sources of Vitamins and Choline

Grains	Vegetables	Fruits	Oils	Milk	Meat & Beans
• Thiamin • Riboflavin • Niacin • Folate	• Vitamin A • Vitamin K • Folate • Vitamin C	• Vitamin A • Vitamin C	• Vitamin E	• Vitamin D • Riboflavin • Vitamin B-12 • Choline	• Thiamin • Riboflavin • Niacin • Biotin • Vitamin B-6 • Vitamin B-12 • Choline

OVERVIEW FIGURE 2 ▶ Certain groups of MyPyramid are especially rich sources of various vitamins and choline. This is true for those listed. Each may be also found in other groups in the pyramid but in lower amounts. Pantothenic acid is also present in moderate amounts in many groups.

thiamin, vitamin C, and folate, can be destroyed with improper storage and excessive cooking. Heat, light, exposure to the air, cooking in water, and alkalinity are factors that can destroy vitamins. The sooner a food is eaten after harvest, the less chance of nutrient loss.

Frozen vegetables and fruits are often as nutrient-rich as freshly picked ones because fruits and vegetables are often frozen immediately after harvesting. As part of the freezing process, vegetables are quickly blanched in boiling water. This destroys the enzymes that would otherwise degrade the vitamins. If a food is not eaten within a few days, freezing is the best preservation method to retain nutrients.

MINERALS: AN OVERVIEW

Whereas vitamins are compounds consisting of many elements (e.g., carbon, oxygen, and hydrogen), minerals are individual chemical elements. The mineral content of foods is sometimes called "ash" because it is all that remains after the whole food has been destroyed by high temperatures or chemical degradation. In humans, minerals make up about 4% of adult body weight (Overview Figure 3). A mineral is essential for humans if a dietary inadequacy results in a physiological or structural abnormality, and its addition to the diet prevents such illness or reinstates normal health. Sixteen minerals are known to be essential in the diet.

Minerals are categorized based on the amount we need per day. Recall from Chapter 1 that if we require greater than 100 milligrams (1/50 of a teaspoon) of a mineral per day, it is considered a **major mineral** (Overview Table 3). These include calcium, phosphorus, magnesium, sulfur, sodium, potassium, and chloride. **Trace minerals** are required at levels less than 100 milligrams per day (Overview Table 4). Nine essential trace minerals (iron, zinc, copper, iodine, selenium, molybdenum, fluoride, manganese, and chromium) have been identified for humans. There are several additional trace minerals (sometimes called **ultratrace minerals**) found in the human

major mineral Vital to health, a mineral required in the diet in amounts greater than 100 milligrams per day.

trace mineral Vital to health, a mineral required in the diet in amounts less than 100 milligrams per day.

ultratrace mineral A mineral present in the human diet in trace amounts but that has not been shown to be essential to human health.

OVERVIEW FIGURE 3 ▶ Approximate amounts of various minerals present in the average human body. Other trace minerals of nutritional importance not listed include chromium, fluoride, molybdenum, selenium, and zinc.

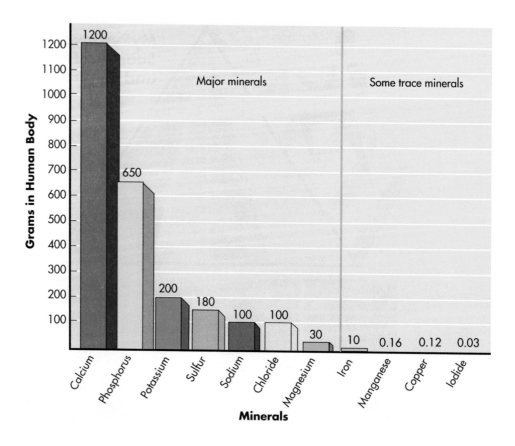

▶ If grains are leavened with yeast, as they are in bread making, enzymes produced by the yeast can break some of the bonds between phytic acid and minerals. This increases mineral absorption. The zinc deficiencies found among some Middle Eastern populations are attributed partly to their consumption of unleavened breads, resulting in low bioavailability of dietary zinc.

oxalic acid (oxalate) An organic acid found in spinach, rhubarb, and other leafy green vegetables that can depress the absorption of certain minerals present in the food, such as calcium.

phytic acid (phytate) A constituent of plant fibers that binds positive ions to its multiple phosphate groups.

body, but many of them have no known requirements. These include arsenic, boron, nickel, silicon, and vanadium.

Absorption and Storage of Minerals in the Body

Foods offer us a plentiful supply of many minerals, but the ability of our bodies to absorb and use them varies. The bioavailability of minerals depends on many factors, including many nonmineral components of foods. Age, gender, genetic variables, nutritional status, and diet will affect mineral absorption and bioavailability. Numerous prescription drugs also adversely affect mineral absorption. The mineral content listed in a food composition table for the amount of a mineral in a food is a starting point for estimating the contribution the food will make to our mineral needs.

Components of fiber, such as **phytic acid (phytate)** and **oxalic acid (oxalate),** can limit absorption of some minerals by binding to them. Spinach, for example, contains plenty of calcium, but only about 5% (compared to the typical 25% bioavailability of calcium from foods) of it can be absorbed because of the vegetable's high concentration of oxalic acid, which binds calcium. High-fiber diets—particularly those in excess of current recommendations of 25 (adult women) to 38 (adult men) grams of fiber per day—can decrease the absorption of iron, zinc, and possibly other minerals.

Many minerals, such as magnesium, calcium, iron, and copper, are of similar sizes and electrical charges. Having similar sizes and the same electrical charge causes these minerals to compete with each other for absorption, and therefore they affect each other's bioavailabilty. An excess of one mineral decreases the absorption and metabolism of other minerals. For example, a large intake of zinc decreases copper absorption. Therefore, people should avoid taking individual mineral supplements unless a dietary deficiency or medical condition specifically warrants it. Food sources, however, pose little risk for these mineral interactions, giving us another reason to emphasize foods in meeting nutrient needs.

OVERVIEW TABLE 3 Summary of the Major Minerals

Mineral	Major Functions	RDA, or Adequate Intake	Dietary Sources	Deficiency Symptoms	Toxicity Symptoms
Sodium	• Major positive ion of the extracellular fluid • Aids nerve impulse transmission • Water balance	*Age 19–50 years:* 1500 milligrams *Age 51–70 years:* 1300 milligrams *Age > 70 years* 1200 milligrams	• Table salt • Processed foods • Condiments • Sauces • Soups • Chips	• Muscle cramps	• Contributes to hypertension in susceptible individuals • Increases calcium loss in urine • Upper Level is 2300 milligrams
Potassium	• Major positive ion of intracellular fluid • Aids nerve impulse transmission • Water balance	4700 milligrams	• Spinach • Squash • Bananas • Orange juice • Milk • Meat • Legumes • Whole grains	• Irregular heart beat • Loss of appetite • Muscle cramps	• Slowing of the heartbeat, as seen in kidney failure
Chloride	• Major negative ion of extracellular fluid • Participates in acid production in stomach • Aids nerve impulse transmission • Water balance	2300 milligrams	• Table salt • Some vegetables • Processed foods	• Convulsions in infants	• Linked to hypertension in susceptible people when combined with sodium • Upper Level is 3600 milligrams
Calcium	• Bone and tooth structure • Blood clotting • Aids in nerve impulse transmission • Muscle contractions • Other cell functions	*Age 9–18 years:* 1300 milligrams *Age > 18 years:* 1000–1200 milligrams	• Dairy products • Canned fish • Leafy vegetables • Tofu • Fortified orange juice (and other fortified foods)	• Increased risk of osteoporosis	• May cause kidney stones and other problems in susceptible people • Upper Level is 2500 milligrams
Phosphorus	• Major negative ion of intracellular fluid • Bone and tooth strength • Part of various metabolic compounds • Acid/base balance	*Age 9–18 years:* 1250 milligrams *Age > 18 years:* 700 milligrams	• Dairy products • Processed foods • Fish • Soft drinks • Bakery products • Meats	• Possibility of poor bone maintenance	• Impairs bone health in people with kidney failure • Poor bone mineralization if calcium intakes are low • Upper Level is 3 to 4 grams
Magnesium	• Bone formation • Aids enzyme function • Aids nerve and heart function	*Men:* 400–420 milligrams *Women:* 310–320 milligrams	• Wheat bran • Green vegetables • Nuts • Chocolate • Legumes	• Weakness • Muscle pain • Poor heart function	• Causes diarrhea and weakness in people with kidney failure • Upper Level is 350 milligrams, but refers to nonfood sources (e.g., supplements) only
Sulfur	• Part of vitamins and amino acids • Aids in drug detoxification • Acid/base balance	None	• Protein foods	• None observed	• None likely

OVERVIEW TABLE 4 A Summary of Key Trace Minerals

Mineral	Major Functions	RDA, or Adequate Intake	Dietary Sources	Deficiency Symptoms	Toxicity Symptoms
Iron	• Components of hemoglobin and other key compounds used in respiration • Immune function • Cognitive development	*Men:* 8 milligrams *Premenopausal Women:* 18 milligrams	• Meats • Seafood • Broccoli • Peas • Bran • Enriched breads	• Fatigue • Anemia • Low blood hemoglobin values	• Liver and heart damage (extreme cases) • GI upset • Upper Level is 45 milligrams
Zinc	• Required for nearly 200 enzymes • Growth • Immunity • Alcohol metabolism • Sexual development • Reproduction • Antioxidant protection	*Men:* 11 milligrams *Women:* 8 milligrams	• Seafood • Meats • Greens • Whole grains	• Skin rash • Diarrhea • Decreased appetite and sense of taste • Hair loss • Poor growth and development • Poor wound healing	• Reduced copper absorption • Diarrhea • Cramps • Depressed immune function • Upper Level is 40 milligrams
Selenium	• Part of an antioxidant system	55 micrograms	• Meats • Eggs • Fish • Seafood • Whole grains	• Muscle pain • Weakness • Form of heart disease	• Nausea • Vomiting • Hair loss • Weakness • Liver disease • Upper Level is 400 micrograms
Iodide	• Component of thyroid hormones	150 micrograms	• Iodized salt • White bread • Saltwater fish • Dairy products	• Goiter • Mental retardation • Poor growth in infancy when mother is iodide deficient during pregnancy	• Inhibition of thyroid gland function • Upper Level is 1.1 milligrams
Copper	• Aids in iron metabolism • Works with many antioxidant enzymes • Involved with enzymes of protein metabolism and hormone synthesis	900 micrograms	• Liver • Cocoa • Beans • Nuts • Whole grains • Dried fruits	• Anemia • Low white blood cell count • Poor growth	• Vomiting • Nervous system disorders • Upper Level is 8–10 milligrams
Fluoride	• Increases resistance of tooth enamel to dental caries	*Men:* 3.8 milligrams *Women:* 3.1 milligrams	• Fluoridated water • Toothpaste • Tea • Seaweed • Dental treatments	• Increased risk of dental caries	• Stomach upset • Mottling (staining) of teeth during development • Bone pain • Upper Level is 10 milligrams for adults
Chromium	• Enhances insulin action	25–35 micrograms	• Egg yolks • Whole grains • Pork • Nuts • Mushrooms • Beer	• High blood glucose after eating	Caused by industrial contamination, not dietary excesses, so no Upper Level has been set
Manganese	• Cofactor of some enzymes, such as those involved in carbohydrate metabolism • Works with some antioxidant systems	1.8–2.3 milligrams	• Nuts • Oats • Beans • Tea	None observed in humans	• Nervous system disorders • Upper Level is 11 milligrams
Molybdenum	• Aids in action of some enzymes	45 micrograms	• Beans • Grains • Nuts	None observed in healthy humans	• Poor growth in laboratory animals • Upper Level is 2 milligrams

Several beneficial vitamin-mineral interactions occur during nutrient absorption and metabolism. When consumed in conjunction with vitamin C, absorption of certain forms of iron—such as that in plant products—improves. The active form of vitamin D hormone improves calcium absorption. Many vitamins require specific minerals to act as components in their structure and function. For example, the thiamin coenzyme requires magnesium or manganese to efficiently function.

The average North American diet derives minerals from both plant and animal sources. Overall, minerals from animal products are better absorbed than those from plants because binders such as fiber are not present to hinder absorption. The mineral content of plants greatly depends on mineral concentrations of the soil in which they are grown. Vegans must be aware of the potentially poor mineral content of some plant foods and choose some concentrated sources of minerals. Soil conditions have less of an influence on the mineral content of animal products because livestock usually consume a variety of plant products grown from soils of differing mineral contents.

Like vitamins, the majority of the minerals are absorbed in the small intestine. Minor amounts may be absorbed in the stomach, and some sodium and potassium is absorbed in the large intestine. After minerals are absorbed, some travel freely in the bloodstream, but many are carried by specific transport proteins to their site of action or storage. Calcium is one example of a mineral that can travel as an ion in the blood or bound to a blood protein called albumin. Iron, on the other hand, has damaging effects in its unbound form, so it is transported bound to proteins, such as transferrin. Minerals are stored in various tissues throughout the body. Some minerals must remain in the bloodstream to maintain fluid balance and supply body functions. Others, such as calcium, phosphorus, magnesium, and fluoride, are stored mainly in bones. Iron, copper, zinc, and many trace minerals are stored in the liver. Still others are stored in muscle tissue, organs, or glands.

Mineral Toxicities

An excessive mineral intake, especially of trace minerals such as iron and copper, can have toxic results. For many trace minerals, the gap between just enough and too much is small. Taking minerals as supplements poses the biggest threat for mineral toxicity, whereas food sources are unlikely culprits. Mineral supplements exceeding current standards for mineral needs—especially those that supply more than 100% of the Daily Values on supplement labels—should be taken only under a physician's supervision. The Daily Values are for the most part higher than our current standards (e.g., Recommended Dietary Allowances [RDA]) for mineral needs. Without close monitoring, doses of minerals should not exceed any Upper Level set on a long-term basis.

The potential for toxicity is not the only reason to carefully consider the use of mineral supplements. Harmful interactions with other nutrients are possible. Also, contamination of mineral supplements—with lead, for example—is a possibility. Use of brands approved by the United States Pharmacopeia (USP) lessens this risk. Even with the best intentions, people may harm themselves using mineral supplements.

Preservation of Minerals in Foods

Minerals are found in plant and animal foods (Overview Figure 4), but as you previously read, the bioavailability of minerals varies widely. Minerals are not typically lost from animal sources during processing, storage, or cooking, but for plant sources, significant amounts may be lost during food processing. When grains are refined, the final products have lost the majority of their vitamin E, many B vitamins, and trace minerals. The more refined a plant food, as in the case of white flour, the lower its mineral content. During the enrichment of refined grain products, iron is the only mineral added, whereas the selenium, zinc, copper, and other minerals lost during

MyPyramid: Sources of Minerals

Grains	Vegetables	Fruits	Oils	Milk	Meat & Beans
• Sodium chloride • Calcium (fortified products) • Phosphorus • Magnesium • Iron • Zinc • Copper • Selenium • Chromium	• Potassium • Magnesium	• Potassium • Boron	• None	• Calcium • Phosphorus • Zinc	• Sodium chloride (processed foods) • Potassium • Phosphorus • Magnesium • Selenium • Iron • Zinc • Copper

OVERVIEW FIGURE 4 ▶ Certain groups of MyPyramid are especially rich sources of various minerals. This is true for the minerals listed. Each mineral may also be found in other groups, but in lower amounts. Other trace minerals are also present in moderate amounts in many groups. With regard to the grains group, whole-grain varieties are the richest sources of most trace minerals listed.

refinement are not replaced. Following the recommendation of the 2005 Dietary Guidelines for Americans to "make half your grains whole" will effectively preserve the mineral content of foods.

THE FUNCTIONAL ROLES OF MICRONUTRIENTS

The next four chapters will explore the vitamins and minerals from a functional perspective. The micronutrients will be grouped and discussed as they apply to various metabolic roles in the body. Keep in mind that each vitamin and mineral has multiple roles in metabolism. For example, calcium, best known for its role in bone formation, is also crucial for the transmission of nerve impulses through the body and plays a role in blood clotting. Vitamin C contributes to cellular antioxidant function, bone health, and metabolism of proteins. At all levels—cellular, tissue, organ, and whole body—vitamins and minerals clearly play important and interrelated roles in maintaining healthy body functions.

Chapter 8 focuses on the roles of the micronutrients in fluid and electrolyte balance. Water balance requires sodium, potassium, chloride, and phosphorus. Levels of these minerals in the blood are tightly regulated by the body and imbalances can have dire consequences. In addition to maintaining the delicate balance between intracellular and extracellular water, these minerals participate in the transmission of nerve impulses and acid-base balance.

Chapter 9 will enhance your understanding of the body's antioxidant systems and how various vitamins and minerals take part in protecting tissues from oxidative damage. Vitamin E, vitamin C, vitamin A and its precursor carotenoids, as well as selenium are discussed in this chapter. In addition, the roles of beneficial plant chemicals in protection of human health will be explored.

Before moving ahead in your study of vitamins and minerals as they participate in antioxidant systems (and energy metabolism, discussed in Chapter 11), it is important to understand how enzymes work.

Enzymes are catalysts for biochemical reactions in living organisms. A catalyst is a compound that speeds the rate of a reaction but is not altered by the reaction. Most of the chemical reactions in the body would not occur, or would occur only at very slow rates, in the absence of catalysts. Enzymes allow for the breakdown of carbohydrates, lipids, and proteins to generate energy. They also catalyze synthetic reactions, such as the assembly of triglycerides for storage in adipose tissue. Enzymes are crucial players in antioxidant reactions, which neutralize damaging free radicals in the body. Beyond these few roles, thousands of other enzymes have been identified and studied.

Typically, enzymes are made of proteins, but many such proteins require the aid of another compound (a **cofactor**, such as a **coenzyme**) for biological activity (Overview Figure 5). Frequently, the assisting compound is a vitamin or mineral, such as copper or selenium. In some reactions, numerous vitamins and minerals are required as coenzymes. Requirements for an enzyme and its coenzymes are specific, with little or no enzymatic activity observed if another coenzyme is substituted for the required one. Minerals are required as coenzymes for activation of about 30% of all known enzymes. A cofactor is a general term referring to any organic or inorganic substance that binds to an enzyme to aid enzyme activity. A coenzyme is one type of cofactor that is organic. In our discussion of vitamins and minerals, vitamins (organic molecules) are called coenzymes and minerals (inorganic molecules) are called cofactors.

In Chapter 10, you will learn how micronutrients are vital to bone health. When we think of bone, we often imagine the hard, lifeless architecture of a skeleton hanging in the back of our high school science classroom. However, bone is a living and dynamic tissue that supports growth, houses nerves and blood vessels, produces blood cells, and helps regulate blood levels of certain minerals. This chapter explores the roles of calcium, phosphorus, vitamin D, vitamin K, magnesium, fluoride, and some other vitamins and ultratrace minerals in bone health.

Chapter 11 delves into the roles of vitamins and minerals in energy metabolism and blood health. Although vitamins and minerals yield no energy to the body, they often participate as coenzymes in energy-yielding reactions. All of the B vitamins are involved in metabolism of the macronutrients, as are many trace minerals. Blood health encompasses immune function; clotting ability; and transport of oxygen, nutrients, and waste products. Blood health is influenced by vitamin K, iron, zinc, copper, and various B vitamins.

Micronutrients are vital to every aspect of human health. Although requirements for vitamins and minerals are small, depriving the body of any one of these important dietary factors can be debilitating or deadly. For most healthy children and adults, foods are safe, effective, and enjoyable sources of vitamins and minerals, although dietary supplements may be useful under some circumstances. As you study the next four chapters, prepare to be amazed by the intricate interplay of micronutrients and human health.

Inactive enzyme

Vitamin coenzyme

Active enzyme

OVERVIEW FIGURE 5 ▶ Coenzymes, such as those formed from B vitamins, aid in the function of various enzymes. Without the coenzyme, the enzyme cannot function, and deficiency symptoms associated with the missing vitamin eventually appear. Health-food stores sell the coenzyme forms of some vitamins. These more expensive forms of vitamins are unnecessary. The body makes all the coenzymes it needs from vitamin precursors.

enzyme A compound that speeds the rate of a chemical reaction but is not altered by the reaction. Almost all enzymes are proteins (some are made of genetic material).

cofactor A substance that binds to a specific region on a protein, such as an enzyme, and is necessary for the protein's function.

coenzyme A compound (frequently a water-soluble vitamin or mineral) that combines with an inactive enzyme to form a catalytically active form. In this manner, coenzymes aid in enzyme function.

CHAPTER 8 Nutrients Involved in Fluid and Electrolyte Balance

CHAPTER OBJECTIVES Chapter 8 is designed to allow you to:

1. List and explain the functions of water in the body.

2. List the four minerals that function as electrolytes.

3. Describe how electrolytes control fluid balance.

4. Describe the control mechanisms that regulate water intake and output.

5. Identify sources of water.

6. Describe the health consequences of dehydration.

7. Describe factors that can contribute to the development of hypertension.

CHAPTER OUTLINE

NUTRIENT INTAKE, ENVIRONMENTAL CONDITIONS, AND THE LEVEL OF PHYSICAL ACTIVITY VARY TREMENDOUSLY THROUGHOUT THE DAY AND FROM DAY TO DAY. Despite these ever-changing conditions, the composition of the internal and external environment of the trillions of cells in the human body remains relatively constant. This relatively static environment is critical for cells to function properly. Three critical factors are under tight intracellular and extracellular control: water and electrolyte distribution and pH.

Water (H_2O) is the most abundant molecule found in the human body. Water is constantly lost from the body through respiration, perspiration, urine, and feces. Water is not stored in the human body, therefore death will occur in a few days without consuming water. The distribution of intracellular and extracellular water is controlled by the concentrations of dissolved minerals called **electrolytes.** The membrane surrounding all cells is freely permeable to water. Water moves into or out of cells depending upon the concentration of the electrolytes. The pH of cells and blood is also under tight control, and this is also principally regulated by electrolytes.

Refresh Your Memory

As you begin the study of water and other nutrients involved in fluid balance in Chapter 8, you may want to review:

- Cell structure and function, digestion and absorption of nutrients, cardiovascular function, immunity, and endocrine function in Chapter 3.
- The functions of phosphorus related to bone health in Chapter 10.

Electrolytes   Minerals that separate into positively or negatively charged ions in water. They are able to transmit an electrical current.

Intracellular fluid   Fluid contained within a cell; it represents about two-thirds of body fluid.

Ion   A positively or negatively charged atom.

Extracellular fluid   Fluid found outside the cells; it represents about one-third of all body fluid.

INTRACELLULAR AND EXTRACELLULAR FLUID DISTRIBUTION—A DELICATE BALANCE BETWEEN WATER AND ELECTROLYTES

The cells of the body are surrounded by a membrane. Water found inside the cell membrane is part of the **intracellular fluid.** Intracellular fluid accounts for 63% of fluid in the body. This should not be surprising when you consider the body contains trillions of cells. The remaining body fluid is found outside of cells in one of two extracellular spaces. The fluid portion of blood (plasma) and lymph account for 7% of body fluid and the fluid between cells (interstitial) makes up 30% of the body fluid (Fig. 8-1).

The distribution of water between the intracellular and extracellular compartments is tightly regulated. Water can freely travel into and out of cells across the cell membrane. The body controls the amount of water in the intracellular and extracellular compartments mainly by controlling ion concentrations. **Ions** are minerals that dissolve in water and are either positively or negatively charged. These charged ions allow the transfer of electrical current so they are called electrolytes. Four electrolytes predominate: sodium (Na^+) and chloride (Cl^-) are primarily found in the **extracellular fluid,** and potassium (K^+) and phosphate $PO4^-$) are the principle electrolytes in the intracellular fluid (Fig. 8-2). Water likes electrolytes and is attracted to electrolytes, so water is slightly charged.

FRANK & ERNEST by Bob Thaves

Replacing fluids—water as part of foods, beverages, and water itself—is an important daily task. Why is this so critical for maintaining health? And why are infants, athletes, and older adults particularly at risk for dehydration? In addition, how does water interact with some of the minerals used by the body? Chapter 8 provides some answers.

FRANK & ERNEST © Reprinted by permission of Newspaper Enterprise Association, Inc.

FIGURE 8-1 ▶ Fluid compartments in the body. Total fluid volume is about 40 liters (about 165 cups).

Fluid compartments

3 Liters
Blood plasma

14 Liters
Fluid between cells
Lymph
Gastrointestinal fluid
Spinal column fluid
Fluid in eyes
Tears
Synovial fluid (in joints)

25 Liters
Fluid found inside every type of cell, e.g., blood, bone, muscle, adipose

Extracellular fluid (37%)

Intracellular fluid (63%)

Total fluid (40 liters)

Liters

Intracellular Fluid

Mg⁺⁺
Na⁺
Ca⁺⁺
K⁺

Positively charged electrolytes

SO4⁼
HCO3⁻
Protein
HPO4⁼
Cl⁻
Organic acids

Negatively charged electrolytes

FIGURE 8-2 ▶ Intracellular and extracellular percent distribution of electrolytes. Each figure shows the percent distribution of electrolytes inside and outside cells. The total concentration of positively and negatively charged electrolytes is equal in the intracellular and extracellular fluid.

Extracellular Fluid

Mg⁺⁺   Ca⁺⁺   K⁺
Na⁺

Positively charged electrolytes

HPO4⁼
Organic acids
HCO3⁻
Protein
Cl⁻
SO4⁼

Negatively charged electrolytes

FIGURE 8-3 ▶ Effects of various ion concentrations in a fluid on red blood cells. This shows the process of osmosis. Fluid is shifting in and out of the red blood cells in response to changing ion concentrations in the flasks.

Red blood cell

H_2O

Dilute solution   Normal concentration   Concentrated solution

(a) A dilute solution with a low ion concentration results in swelling (black arrows) and subsequent rupture (puff of red in the lower left part of the cell) of a red blood cell placed into the solution.

(b) A normal concentration (a concentration of ions outside the cell equal to that inside the cell) results in a typically shaped red blood cell. Water moves into and out of the cell in equilibrium (black arrows), but there is no net water movement.

(c) A concentrated solution, with a high ion concentration, causes shrinkage of the red blood cell as water moves out of the cell and into the concentrated solution (black arrows).

Osmosis The passage of water through a membrane from a less concentrated compartment to a more concentrated compartment.

The term **osmosis** is used to describe the passage of water through a membrane from an area of lower electrolyte concentration to an area of higher electrolyte concentration. Cells regulate the balance of intra- and extracellular fluid through the use of pumps located in the cell membrane that, with the help of energy (ATP), actively pump electrolytes across the cell membrane (Fig. 8-3). If the intracellular concentration of electrolytes is greater than the extracellular concentration, water will freely flow into the cell. If too much water flows into the cells, the cell can burst—similar to filling a balloon with too much air. The opposite can also occur, where the intracellular concentration of electrolytes is relatively low compared to the extracellular environment and water will exit the cell leading to cell shrinkage. Under normal conditions, the flow of electrolytes is controlled in such a way that water movement into and out of the cell is in equilibrium.

The principle of osmosis is used by the digestive tract to absorb water from the colon. Consumed water from drink and food, in addition to intestinal tract secretions, makes the contents of the intestinal tract very high in water as it enters the colon from the small intestine. Cells that line the colon actively absorb sodium, and this in turn causes large amounts of water to be absorbed from the colon. As a result, daily water loss from feces is low—approximately 150 milliliters, or 5 ounces. Osmosis can lead to life-threatening medical conditions in response to long bouts of diarrhea and vomiting due to eating disorders or foodborne illnesses. The large loss of fluid from the intestinal tract causes a loss of water from the extracellular space, resulting in a high concentration of electrolytes in the extracellular space. Intracellular water exits the cells in an attempt to balance the water loss from the extracellular space. There is then an imbalance in fluid and electrolyte concentration across the cell membrane. This imbalance can lead to a decreased ability of cells to function normally. In the heart this imbalance can lead to a decreased ability of the heart to pump blood and, ultimately, to cardiac failure.

ELECTROLYTES—ESSENTIAL FOR NERVE FUNCTION

Sodium, potassium, chloride, and phosphate ions are found in very different concentrations on either side of the cell membrane. These ions are charged, so there is an electrochemical gradient across the cell membrane. Let's investigate this a little further.

(a) Resting state   (b) Depolarization   (c) Repolarization

FIGURE 8-4 ▶ Electrolytes control the conduction of a nerve impulse. (a) Under resting conditions the intracellular fluid has slightly more electrolytes with a negative charge. (b) Nervous stimulation cause the influx of sodium into the interior of the cell. The intracellular charge changes from slightly negative to slightly positive (depolarization). This results in an electrical signal (action potential) transmitted along the surface of the membrane. (c) The flow of potassium ions from the intracellular to the extracellular space allows the membrane to return to the resting state. This process is called repolarization.

All membranes contain an energy dependent pump that transfers sodium from inside to outside the cell. As Na^+ is actively pumped out of the cell, K^+ enters the cell to balance the loss of positively charged sodium ions. The sum of positive and negative charges are slightly different between the intracellular and extracellular fluid resulting in a slight charge separate at the cell membrane. The inside of the cell is slightly negatively charged relative to the outside. It is this difference in electrical charge that allows a transmission of nerve impulse (Fig. 8-4).

Nerve impulses are transmitted along a cell by the following process. In response to stimulation, positively charged sodium ions rush into the cell causing the cell to become less negatively charged. The change in electrical charge is transmitted from one cell to the next (like dominos falling), which leads to the electrical signal being transmitted from one nerve cell to the next. Immediately after the change in electrolyte balance, sodium is actively pumped out of the cell to reestablish the normal electrolyte balance.

Acid-Base Balance

The electrolytes provide another critical function by maintaining fluid **pH** in a very narrow range. Even small deviations from the normal range of pH will negatively impact the ability of hemoglobin to bind to oxygen and the rate at which chemical reactions take place within the body. The pH of blood, foods, and other common substances is shown in Figure 8-5. The pH scale is logarithmic. The pH of a fluid is determined by the concentration of hydrogen ion (H^+). A change of 1 pH unit (e.g., 8 to 7) is equivalent to a 10-fold increase in the hydrogen ion concentration.

As carbohydrates, lipids, and proteins are used by the body to provide energy to the cells, acids are continuously produced as a by-product of these reactions. These acids must be neutralized; otherwise the pH of the body would become acidic. Under normal conditions, the body is easily able to maintain a pH of 7.4 in the extracellular fluids. A large production of acids occurs in poorly controlled diabetes, starvation, and conditions where excessive production of carbon dioxide occurs for an extended time. Under these conditions, to maintain normal pH the control systems may be inadequate.

Regulation of pH is complex involving **buffer** systems, the respiratory system, and kidney secretion of excess acid or base. Proteins have a critical function in the buffer

pH   A measure of the concentration of hydrogen ions. A pH below 7.0 is acidic.

Buffer   Compounds that function to take up or release hydrogen ions thereby causing a fluid to resist changes in pH.

FIGURE 8-5 ▶ pH scale. The diagonal line indicates the proportionate number of hydrogen ions to hydroxide ions. Any pH value above 7 is basic, and any pH value below 7 is acidic.

system as they bind or release hydrogen ions to control pH. The respiratory system can increase or decrease the amount of carbon dioxide exhaled when breathing. Increased production and release of carbon dioxide can lower pH because CO_2 is an acidic compound. Electrolytes, especially sodium, function in the kidney to control the release of acid and base in the urine to maintain pH balance. Phosphate is also an important buffering agent in the body. Sodium and potassium salts of phosphoric acid are among the most widely used buffers in the scientific laboratory.

WATER

Solvent A liquid substance in which other substances dissolve.

Water provides a number of vital functions essential for life. Water is the perfect medium for body processes to occur in because it acts as a universal **solvent.** Carbohydrates, proteins, minerals, water-soluble vitamins, and many enzymes and hormones dissolve in water. The primary component of blood is water, making it an excellent transportation medium. Lipids do not mix or dissolve in water, so the ability to transport lipids in the blood could be a serious problem. To solve this problem, lipids are coated with a layer of water-soluble protein which allows them to be dispersed throughout the body via the blood. These lipid transport vehicles are called lipoproteins. In addition to its function as a solvent, water has a number of other critical functions in the body, including (Fig. 8-6):

- Providing a medium in which chemical reactions take place
- Active participant in many chemical reactions
- Distributing nutrients to cells in the body
- Removing waste products from cells for elimination
- Acting as a lubricant for joints
- Moistening the respiratory, gastrointestinal, urogenital tracts, as well as the eyes and skin
- Maintaining body temperature
- As the major component of blood, maintaining blood volume

FIGURE 8-6 ▶ Water has many essential functions in the body.

A Closer Look at the Functions of Water

Water Contributes to Body Temperature Regulation. Water temperature changes slowly because it has a great ability to hold heat. It takes much more energy to heat water than it does to heat air. Water molecules are polar (charged) so they are attracted to each other. This attractive force is strong and it requires energy to separate the water molecules. The human body is 50% to 70% water (Fig. 8-7); therefore, a lot of energy is required to change body temperature.

When overheated, the body secretes fluids in the form of perspiration, which evaporates through skin pores. As water evaporates from the skin, heat energy is required. So, as perspiration evaporates, heat energy is removed from the skin, cooling it in the process (Fig. 8-8). In response to an increased body temperature, blood vessels in the skin become larger allowing greater water loss through perspiration. Each quart (liter) of perspiration evaporated represents approximately 600 kilocalories of energy lost from the skin and surrounding tissues. For this reason, fever increases the need for calories.

When carbohydrate, lipid, and protein are used by cells in the body, energy is released in the form of heat. About 60% of the chemical energy in food is turned into body heat; the other 40% is converted to forms of energy that cells can use (principally ATP). Almost

Healthy Man

170-lb Man

105 lbs of water (62%)

27 lbs of protein (16%)

27 lbs of fat (16%)

10 lbs of minerals (6%)

1 lb of glycogen (<1%)

Healthy Woman

130-lb. woman

74 lbs. of water (57%)

17 lbs. of protein (13%)

32 lbs. of fat (25%)

7 lbs. of minerals (5%)

1 lb. of glycogen (<1%)

FIGURE 8-7 ▶ Although the percentages vary for men and women, the main constituent of the body is water.

FIGURE 8-8 ▶ Body temperature is reduced when heat is transported from the body through the bloodstream to the surface of the skin. The water evaporates from the surface of the skin and heat is removed with it. This cools the blood, which circulates back to the body reducing body temperature.

Heat released from skin

Hair shaft

Sweat evaporates and cools skin and blood at skin surface

Blood vessels

Blood travels to capillary beds under the surface of skin

Cooled blood flows back to body

Body temperature decreases

Sweat gland

all of that energy eventually leaves the body in the form of heat. If this heat could not be dissipated, the body temperature would rise enough to prevent enzyme systems from functioning efficiently, ultimately leading to death. Perspiration is the primary way to prevent this rise in body temperature.

Water Dissolves and Transports Substances Throughout the Body. Water is an important vehicle to transport nutrients to the cells and remove waste products. The majority of the nutrients consumed are water soluble and therefore are dissolved in blood and therefore can move into the water-based environment within and around cells and tissues. Most unusable substances or waste products in the body can dissolve in water and exit the body through the urine.

When carbohydrate and lipids are used as an energy source, water and carbon dioxide are produced. Protein breakdown also results in the production of water and carbon dioxide; however, the body cannot use the nitrogen portion of amino acids in energy production. The nitrogen by-product is converted into urea by the liver. The more protein consumed in excess of needs, the more nitrogen must be excreted in the form of urea in the urine. Likewise, the more sodium we consume, the more sodium we excrete in the urine. Overall, the amount of urine a person needs to produce is determined primarily by excess protein and salt intake. By limiting excess protein and salt intakes, it is possible to limit urine output—a useful practice in space flights. This type of diet is also used to treat some kidney diseases wherein the ability to produce urine is hampered.

Typical urine volume is about 1 liter, depending mostly on the intake of fluid, protein, and sodium. A somewhat greater urine output than that is fine, but less—especially less than 500 milliliters (2 cups)—forces the kidneys to form concentrated urine. The simplest way to determine if water intake is adequate is to observe the urine color. Urine should be clear or pale yellow with adequate hydration, concentrated urine is dark yellow. The heavy ion concentration, in turn, increases the risk of kidney stone formation in susceptible people (generally men). Kidney stones form from minerals and other substances that have precipitated out of the urine and accumulate in the kidney.

Water Functions as an Important Lubricant. The body secretes many fluids that are primarily water. Water-based solutions are produced by the digestion tract, respiratory tract, urogenital tract, eyes, and skin. Saliva acts as a lubricant allowing food to pass through the esophagus to the stomach. Mucus provides a protective fluid coating throughout the digestive tract. The lungs are coated with a layer of mucus that provides an important immunologic function. Water helps form the lubricant found in knees and other joints of the body. Water is also the basis of amniotic fluid, which functions as a shock absorber surrounding the growing fetus in the mother's womb. Without adequate availability of water, the ability of the body to produce these critical secretions will be limited.

▲ Regular intake of water and water-rich fluids are essential to replace daily fluid losses. One trend in North America is to carry bottles of water.

Water Balance

Every cell, tissue, and organ contains water, although the percentage of water varies tremendously between tissues. For example, muscle is 73% water, adipose tissue is 10 to 20% water, and bone contains approximately 20% water. The human body contains 50% to 70% water. As the fat content of the body increases, the percentage of lean decreases and subsequently the total body water content decreases. When body composition measurements are performed on extremely lean athletes, the percentage body water will be around 70%.

If you don't drink enough water, your body eventually lets you know by signaling thirst. Your brain is communicating the need to drink. This thirst mechanism can lag behind actual water loss during prolonged exercise and illness, as well as in the elderly. For this reason, athletes should monitor fluid status. They should weigh themselves before and after training sessions to determine their rate of water loss and, thus, their water needs. The goal for athletes is to consume at least 2 cups of fluid for every pound lost. Sick children, especially those with fever, vomiting, diarrhea, and increased perspiration, and older persons often need to be reminded to drink plenty of fluids.

Once the body registers a shortage of available water, it increases fluid conservation. Two hormones that participate in this process are **antidiuretic hormone (ADH)** and **aldosterone.** The pituitary gland, located in the brain, releases ADH to force the kidneys to conserve water. The kidneys respond by reducing urine production and output. As fluid volume decreases in the bloodstream, blood pressure decreases. ADH also causes blood vessel constriction, which acts to raise blood pressure. Low blood pressure triggers the release of the hormone aldosterone, which signals the kidneys to retain more sodium and, in turn, more water via osmosis.

However, despite mechanisms that work to conserve water, fluid continues to be lost via the feces, skin, and lungs. Those losses must be replaced. In addition, there is a limit to how concentrated urine can become. Eventually, if fluid is not consumed, the body becomes dehydrated and suffers ill effects.

By the time a person loses 1% to 2% of body weight in fluids, he or she will be thirsty. Even this small water deficit can cause one to feel tired and uncomfortable. At a 4% loss of body weight, muscles lose significant strength and endurance, central nervous system function is negatively impacted (e.g., memory and reaction time are compromised). By the time the body weight is reduced by 10% to 12%, heat tolerance is decreased and weakness results. Ultimately **dehydration**

Antidiuretic hormone A hormone secreted by the pituitary gland when blood volume is low. It causes the kidneys to decrease water excretion, which increases blood volume.

Aldosterone A hormone, produced by the adrenal glands, that acts on the kidneys to conserve sodium (and therefore water).

Dehydration Inadequate intake of water to replace losses.

TABLE 8-1 Water Content
(by Weight) of Various Foods

Food	Water %
Lettuce	95
Tomato	95
Beer	90
Milk	89
Orange	87
Apple	86
Banana	75
Potato	75
Chicken	64
Steak	50
Bread, whole wheat	38
Jam	28
Honey	20
Butter	16
Crackers, saltine	4
Shortening	0

Metabolic water When carbohydrates, lipids, and proteins are used as an energy source, carbon dioxide and water are formed as a by-product.

Hyponatremia Dangerously low blood sodium level.

Water intoxication Potentially fatal condition that occurs with a high intake of water which results in a severe dilution of the blood and other fluid compartments.

will lead to kidney failure, coma, and death. Dehydration is a contributing factor to the development of the very serious condition, heat stroke. Performing strenuous physical activity in hot, humid conditions can lead to dehydration and the inability to control body temperature. In addition to an elevated body temperature and dehydration, heart rate is increased and the skin becomes dry. Unabated the individual will become unconscious and die. Adequate fluid intake and cessation of physical activity in hot, humid conditions are the best recommendations to prevent heat illness.

Water Intake and Output

The Adequate Intake (AI) for total water intake is 2.7 liters (11 cups) for adult women and 3.7 liters (15 cups) for adult men. This is based primarily on average water intake from fluids and foods. For fluid alone this corresponds to about 2.2 liters (9 cups) for women and about 3 liters (13 cups) for men.

Drinking water is not the only way we consume water. We also consume water in fruit juice, coffee, tea, soft drinks, and water. Nearly all foods contain water. Many fruits and vegetables are more than 80% water and many meats contain at least 50% water (Table 8-1). The body produces 250 to 350 milliliters (1–1 1/2 cups) of water each day as a result of the chemical reactions used to metabolize energy. The amount of **metabolic water** produced can double in physically active people.

Urinary excretion of water accounts for the greatest source of output. Average urinary water loss per day is approximately 1650 milliliters. The daily amount of urine produced is variable depending upon water intake. To remove the waste products generated each day, the minimum daily water excretion is about 500 milliliters.

Water is also lost through the skin in the form of perspiration and from the lungs. On days of low physical activity these losses amount to about 1 liter. Under hot, humid conditions or with strenuous physical activity loss can be much greater than 1 liter per day. A relatively small amount of water is lost daily in the feces. When we consider the large amount of water used to lubricate the digestive tract, the loss of only 100 milliliters (5 ounces) of water each day through the feces is remarkable. About 8000 milliliters of water enter the digestive tract daily through secretions from the mouth, stomach, intestine, pancreas, and other organs, while the diet supplies an additional 30% to 50% or more. The small intestine reabsorbs most of this water, while the colon takes up a lesser, but still important, amount. The kidneys also greatly conserve water. They can reabsorb as much as 97% of the water filtered each day.

The volume of water intake and output shown in Figure 8-9 are estimates. Altitude, caffeine intake, alcohol intake, ambient temperature, humidity, and physical activity will influence water loss.

MAKING DECISIONS

Can a Person Consume Too Much Water?

It is possible to consume too much water, however it is rare. As water intake increases above what is needed, the kidneys process the excess fluid and excrete dilute urine. If intake of water exceeds the kidneys' ability to excrete the excess, overhydration and a severe dilution of sodium in the blood occurs. This condition is called **hyponatremia.** Symptoms of **water intoxication** include blurred vision, headaches, confusion, seizures, coma, and death.

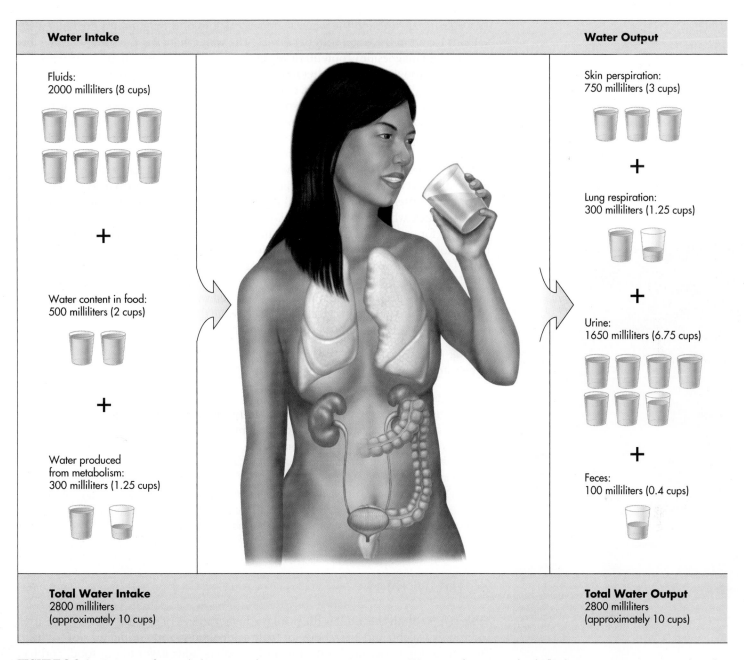

Water Intake

Fluids:
2000 milliliters (8 cups)

+

Water content in food:
500 milliliters (2 cups)

+

Water produced
from metabolism:
300 milliliters (1.25 cups)

Total Water Intake
2800 milliliters
(approximately 10 cups)

Water Output

Skin perspiration:
750 milliliters (3 cups)

+

Lung respiration:
300 milliliters (1.25 cups)

+

Urine:
1650 milliliters (6.75 cups)

+

Feces:
100 milliliters (0.4 cups)

Total Water Output
2800 milliliters
(approximately 10 cups)

FIGURE 8-9 ▶ Estimate of water balance—intake versus output—in a woman. We primarily maintain body fluids at an optimum amount by adjusting water output to intake. As you can see for this woman, most water comes from the liquids we consume. Some comes from the moisture in more solid foods, and the remainder is manufactured during metabolism. Water output includes that lost via lungs, urine, skin, and feces.

Water Sources

Water consumed each day comes from one of the following sources: well, spring, public water supply, or bottled water. The water source and how it is processed will influence the composition of the water. Water can be classified as either hard or soft. **Hard water** contains relatively large levels of the minerals calcium and magnesium. It is easy to determine if the water is hard or soft. When washing with hard water it is difficult to work up lather, and hard water will leave a pronounced ring around the bathtub or sink. **Soft water** does a better job of cleaning clothes and feels much better when bathing. Naturally occurring soft water is usually high in sodium. Hard water can be converted into soft water through the use of a commercial water softener.

Hard water   Water that contains high levels of calcium and magnesium.

Soft water   Water that contains a high level of sodium.

As water travels through the water softener, calcium and magnesium exchange with sodium found in the water softener device. The water that exits the softener has a low calcium and magnesium content; however the sodium content is high. Water can also be passed through a charcoal filter to remove off-flavors. Home-installed filtration systems designed to remove chlorine may also remove the tooth decay fighting mineral, fluoride. The additional intake of sodium from soft water is undesirable for people restricting sodium intake due to **hypertension.** The additional intake of calcium and magnesium afforded by consumption of hard water would be more beneficial than increasing sodium intake through the use of soft water.

Bottled water is a popular alternative to consuming tap water. Rather than using chlorine to disinfect water, most bottled water is treated with ozone, which does not impart a flavor in the water. The Environmental Protection Agency regulates and monitors public water supplies, whereas the Food and Drug Administration regulates bottled water. The standards for quality and contaminants are identical for both regulatory agencies so the perception that bottled water is safer is unfounded. Much of the bottled water produced in the United States is processed municipal tap water. Very few bottled water manufacturers add the cavity preventative mineral fluoride to the water. The large amount of plastic used to package the over 6 billion gallons of bottled water consumed by Americans each year creates a huge energy, recycling, and solid waste disposal concern. There is also concern about the safety of beverages stored in plastic containers.

Hypertension High blood pressure. The pressure inside the blood vessels exceeds 140/90 millimeters of mercury.

▲ Bottled water pouring into glass

CONCEPT CHECK

Water dissolves substances, serves as a medium for chemical reactions and as a lubricant, and aids in temperature regulation. Water is the most abundant molecule in the body, however we cannot store water. Daily water intake is balanced with output. Water accounts for 50% to 70% of body weight and distributes itself throughout the body in intracellular and extracellular fluids. The distribution of water between cellular compartments is tightly regulated. The AI for total water intake is 2.7 liters (11 cups) for women and 3.7 liters (15 cups) for men. Thirst is the body's first sign of dehydration. If the thirst mechanism is faulty, as it may be during vigorous exercise, illness, or as a natural part of aging, hormonal mechanisms also help to conserve water by reducing urine output. Excess fluid intake can be dangerous, even fatal.

SODIUM (Na)

Table salt (sodium chloride) is the primary dietary source of sodium. Table salt is 40% sodium by weight, and 1 teaspoon of table salt contains 2400 milligrams of sodium. This mineral is an essential constituent of our diets, adds flavor to our food, and has been used as a preservative for many generations. There is concern that high intakes of sodium may have harmful health effects.

Functions of Sodium

The digestive tract absorbs nearly all consumed sodium. When sodium chloride (NaCl) is dissolved in water the chemical bond holding the two atoms together breaks and the charged ions Na^+ and Cl^- are released. These electrolytes, as well as others, attract water. The concentration of intracellular and extracellular water is controlled by the concentration of the electrolytes. Fluid balance is maintained by moving or actively pumping sodium ions where more water is needed. Sodium ions also function in nerve impulse conduction and absorption of some nutrients (e.g., glucose).

Sodium consumption varies tremendously from day to day. The kidneys function to tightly regulate the amount of sodium found in the blood. In most instances consumption of sodium is well in excess of that required each day. As blood flows through the functional unit of the kidney, sodium is filtered out of the blood. To maintain the appropriate concentration of sodium in the blood, the appropriate amount of sodium is then added back to the blood by this same apparatus in the kidney. The excess sodium is then excreted by the kidney into urine so it can be eliminated from the body. A diet low in sodium, coupled with excessive perspiration and persistent vomiting or diarrhea, has the ability to deplete the body of sodium. This state can lead to muscle cramps, nausea, vomiting, dizziness, and later shock and coma. The likelihood of this occurring is low because the kidney is efficient at conserving sodium under conditions of low sodium status.

Only when weight loss from perspiration exceeds 2% to 3% of total body weight (or about 5 to 6 pounds) should sodium losses raise concern. Even then, merely salting food is sufficient to restore body sodium for most people. Athletes that perspire for hours during endurance activities may need to consume electrolyte replacement drinks during competition to avoid depletion of sodium, which can lead to hyponatremia. Perspiration contains about two-thirds the sodium concentration found in blood or about 1 gram of sodium per liter.

▲ Deli meats, such as ham, are high in sodium (salt).

Sodium Sources and Needs

About 80% of the sodium we consume is added during food manufacturing and food preparation at restaurants. Sodium added while cooking at home provides about 10% of our intake, and naturally occurring sodium in foods provides the remaining 10%. Most unprocessed foods are relatively low in sodium; milk is one exception (about 120 milligrams per cup).

The more processed and restaurant food consumed, the higher one's sodium intake. Conversely, the more home cooked meals prepared, the more control a person has over the sodium content of the food. Major contributors of sodium in the adult diet are white bread and rolls; hot dogs and lunch meat; cheese; soups; and foods with tomato sauce, partly because these foods are consumed so often. Other foods that can be major contributors to sodium intake include salted snack foods, French fries, potato chips, sauces, and gravies.

If we ate only unprocessed foods and added no salt, we would consume about 500 milligrams of sodium per day. The Dietary Reference Intakes recommended for sodium is 1500 milligrams for adults less than age 51, 1300 milligrams for people ages 51 through 70, and 1200 milligrams for those over 70. If we compare 500 milligrams of sodium from a diet consisting of unprocessed foods with the 2300 to 4700 milligrams or more typically consumed by adults, it is clear that food processing and salt added while cooking are the major contributors to sodium intake. When dietary sodium must be restricted, attention to food labels is valuable to monitor sodium intake. The Daily Value (DV) on food labels is 2400 milligrams.

Most people can adapt to wide variations in dietary sodium intakes—today's sodium intake is in tomorrow's urine. However, approximately 10% to 15% of adults are sodium sensitive. For these people, sodium intake has a direct relationship on blood pressure. As sodium intake increases, blood pressure increases. Lower sodium diets (about 2000 milligrams daily) often lower blood pressure. Groups that appear to be especially affected are African-Americans and people who have diabetes and/or are overweight. Lifestyle factors such as being overweight and inactive are the major contributors to the development of hypertension.

The medical community suggests that adults should reduce sodium consumption to limit the risk of developing hypertension later in life. It is also a good idea to have your blood pressure checked regularly. If you are diagnosed with hypertension, you should reduce sodium intake as you follow a comprehensive plan to treat this disease. Reducing sodium intake also helps to maintain a healthy calcium status, as sodium intake greater than about 2000 milligrams per day may increase urinary calcium loss as the sodium is excreted. The effect of this increased urinary calcium loss on bone health is controversial.

It is not hard to follow a low-sodium diet, but many typical food choices will have to be limited (Fig. 8-10). At first, foods may taste bland, but eventually you will perceive more

FIGURE 8-10 ▶ Food sources of sodium compared to the Adequate Intake.

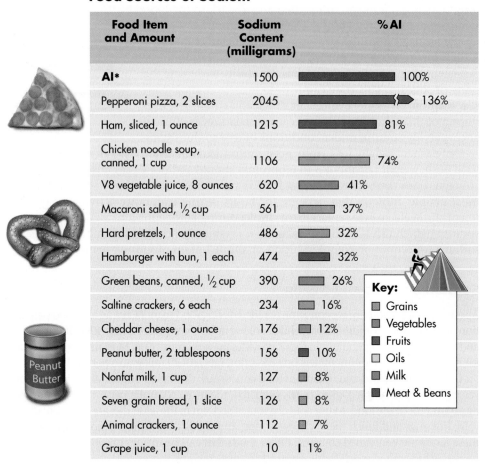

Food Sources of Sodium

Food Item and Amount	Sodium Content (milligrams)	% AI
AI*	1500	100%
Pepperoni pizza, 2 slices	2045	136%
Ham, sliced, 1 ounce	1215	81%
Chicken noodle soup, canned, 1 cup	1106	74%
V8 vegetable juice, 8 ounces	620	41%
Macaroni salad, ½ cup	561	37%
Hard pretzels, 1 ounce	486	32%
Hamburger with bun, 1 each	474	32%
Green beans, canned, ½ cup	390	26%
Saltine crackers, 6 each	234	16%
Cheddar cheese, 1 ounce	176	12%
Peanut butter, 2 tablespoons	156	10%
Nonfat milk, 1 cup	127	8%
Seven grain bread, 1 slice	126	8%
Animal crackers, 1 ounce	112	7%
Grape juice, 1 cup	10	1%

Key:
- ■ Grains
- ■ Vegetables
- ■ Fruits
- □ Oils
- ■ Milk
- ■ Meat & Beans

* For adults; See the DRI table in the back of this book for age-specific recommendations.

flavor as the taste receptors in the tongue become more sensitive to the salt content of foods. By slowly reducing dietary sodium and substituting lemon juice, herbs, and spices, you can eventually become accustomed to a diet that contains minimal amounts of salt. Many cookbooks offer excellent recipes for flavorful low-sodium foods.

Upper Level for Sodium

The Upper Level (UL) for sodium for adults is 2300 milligrams (2.3 grams), approximately 1 teaspoon. Intakes exceeding this amount typically increase blood pressure. About 95% of North American adults have sodium intakes that exceed that UL.

CONCEPT CHECK

Sodium is the major positive ion in the extracellular fluid. It is important for maintaining fluid balance and conducting nerve impulses. Sodium depletion is unlikely, because the typical diet has abundant sources of sodium. Compared to dining out or buying commercially prepared foods, preparation of foods in the home allows greater control over sodium intake. The AI for sodium for adults is 1500 milligrams per day. The average adult consumes 2300 to 4700 milligrams or more daily. Some adults are sensitive to sodium intake, and blood pressure will increase as sodium intake increases. Sodium in the North American diet is provided predominantly through processed and restaurant foods.

POTASSIUM (K)

Potassium performs many of the same functions as sodium, such as water balance and nerve impulse transmission. It is the principal positively charged ion inside cells. Intracellular fluids contain 95% of the potassium in the body. Higher potassium intake is associated with lower rather than higher blood pressure values. Approximately 90% of the potassium consumed is absorbed.

Low blood potassium is a life-threatening problem. Symptoms often include a loss of appetite, muscle cramps, confusion, and constipation. Eventually the heart beats irregularly, decreasing its capacity to pump blood.

Potassium Sources and Needs

Unprocessed foods are rich sources of potassium. This includes fruits, vegetables, milk, whole grains, dried beans, and meats (Fig. 8-11). Major contributors of potassium to the adult diet include milk, potatoes, beef, coffee, tomatoes, and orange juice (Fig. 8-12).

The Adequate Intake for potassium for adults is 4700 milligrams (4.7 grams) per day. The DV used on food and supplement labels is 3500 milligrams. Typically, North Americans consume on average 2000 to 3000 milligrams per day. Thus, many of us need to increase potassium intake, preferably by increasing fruit and vegetable intake.

Diets are more likely to be lower in potassium than sodium because we generally do not add potassium to foods. Some **diuretics** used to treat high blood pressure also deplete the body's potassium. Thus, people who take potassium-wasting diuretics need to monitor their

▲ Vegetables in general are a rich source of potassium, as are fruits.

Diuretic A substance that increases urinary fluid excretion.

FIGURE 8-11 ▶ Food sources of potassium compared to the Adequate Intake.

Food Sources of Potassium

Food Item and Amount	Potassium (milligrams)	% AI
AI*	4700	100%
Kidney beans, 1 cup	715	15%
Winter squash, ¾ cup	670	14%
Plain yogurt, 1 cup	570	12%
Orange juice, 1 cup	495	11%
Cantaloupe, 1 cup	495	11%
Lima beans, ½ cup	480	10%
Banana, 1 medium	470	10%
Zucchini, 1 cup	450	10%
Soybeans, ½ cup	440	9%
Artichoke, 1 medium	425	9%
Tomato juice, ¾ cup	400	9%
Pinto beans, ½ cup	400	9%
Baked potato, 1 small	385	8%
Buttermilk, 1 cup	370	8%
Sirloin steak, 3 ounces	345	7%

Key:
- Grains
- Vegetables
- Fruits
- Oils
- Milk
- Meat & Beans

* For adults; See the DRI table in the back of this book for age-specific recommendations.

FIGURE 8-12 ▶ Sources of potassium from MyPyramid. The height of the background color (none, 1/3, 2/3, or completely covered) within each group in the pyramid indicates the average nutrient density for potassium in that group. Overall, the vegetables group and the fruits group contain many foods that are nutrient-dense sources of potassium, with the milk group and meat & beans group following close behind. With regard to physical activity, potassium is especially needed for cardiovascular function.

MyPyramid: Sources of Potassium

Grains	Vegetables	Fruits	Oils	Milk	Meat & Beans
• Whole-wheat bread • Whole-grain products	• Spinach • Squash • Potatoes • Tomatoes • Lettuce • Lima beans	• Pears • Prunes • Peaches • Avocados • Cantaloupes • Bananas	• None	• Milk • Yogurt • Cottage cheese • Ricotta cheese	• Meat • Chicken • Fish • Shrimp • Beans

potassium intake carefully. For these people, high-potassium foods are good additions to the diet, as are potassium chloride supplements prescribed by a physician.

A continually deficient food intake, as may be the case in alcoholism, can result in a potassium deficiency and low blood potassium levels called hypokalemia. People with certain eating disorders whose diets are poor and whose bodies can be depleted of nutrients because of vomiting and diarrhea are also at risk for potassium deficiency. Other populations especially at risk for potassium deficiency include people on low-calorie diets and athletes who exercise heavily. These people should compensate for potentially low body potassium by consuming potassium-rich foods.

Upper Level of Potassium

If the kidneys function normally, typical food intakes will not lead to potassium toxicity. Thus no Upper Level for potassium has been set. When the kidneys function poorly, potassium builds in the blood. This inhibits heart function, causing slowed heartbeat. If untreated, this can be fatal, as the heart eventually stops beating. Consequently, in cases of reduced kidney function, close monitoring of blood levels of potassium and potassium intake becomes critical.

CHLORIDE (Cl)

Chloride is a negative ion found primarily in the extracellular fluid. Chlorine (Cl_2) is a poisonous gas used to disinfect municipal water supplies. Chloride ions are a component of the acid produced in the stomach (hydrochloric acid) and are also used during immune responses as white blood cells attack foreign cells. In addition, nerve function relies on the presence of chloride. As is the case with sodium, nearly all the consumed chloride is efficiently absorbed and the principle route of excretion is by the kidneys; some is lost in perspiration. It has also been linked to the blood pressure-raising ability of sodium chloride. Vomiting that takes place for an extended period can lead to a disturbance of the body's acid-base balance due to the large loss of stomach acid.

A chloride deficiency is unlikely because our dietary sodium intake is so high. Frequent and lengthy bouts of vomiting, if coupled with a nutrient-poor diet, can contribute to a deficiency because stomach secretions contain a lot of chloride.

Chloride Sources and Needs

A few fruits and some vegetables are naturally good sources of chloride. Chlorinated water is also a source. Most chloride is consumed as salt added to foods. Knowing a food's salt content allows for a close prediction of its chloride content. Salt is 60% chloride.

The Adequate Intake for chloride for adults is 2300 milligrams per day. This is based on the 40:60 ratio of sodium to chloride in salt (1500 milligrams of sodium in a diet is accompanied by 2300 milligrams of chloride). The DV used on food and supplement labels is 3400 milligrams. If the average adult consumes about 9 grams of salt daily, that yields 5.4 grams (5400 milligrams) of chloride.

Upper Level of Chloride

The UL of chloride is 3600 milligrams. Thus, the average adult typically consumes an excess of this ion.

CONCEPT CHECK

Potassium performs functions similar to those of sodium, except that it is the main positive ion found inside cells. Potassium is vital to fluid balance and nerve transmission. A potassium deficiency—caused by an inadequate intake of potassium, persistent vomiting, or use of some diuretics—can lead to loss of appetite, muscle cramps, confusion, and heartbeat irregularities. Fruits and vegetables are good sources of potassium. Potassium intake can be toxic if a person's kidneys do not function properly. Chloride is the major negative ion found in the extracellular fluid. Chloride also functions in digestion as part of hydrochloric acid and in immune and nervous system responses. Deficiencies of chloride are highly unlikely because we eat so much salt.

▲ Chloride is likely part of the blood pressure-raising property of sodium chloride (salt).

PHOSPHORUS (P)

Phosphorus is a negatively charged ion found mainly in the intracellular fluid and in the body fluids primarily bound to hydrogen and oxygen ($H_2PO_4^-$ and HPO_4^{2-}).

Functions of Phosphorus

As the principle negatively charged electrolyte found inside cells, phosphorus functions to maintain fluid balance. Phosphorus has many other critical functions in the body. The majority of phosphorus in the body is found chemically combined with calcium to form the structural component of the bone. Phosphorus also has an important structural function as a component of phospholipids. Phospholipids are the principle component of cell membranes. Phosphorus is an important structural component of the chemicals that make the genetic material in the human body (deoxyribonucleic acid-DNA and ribonucleic acid-RNA). The activity of many enzymes is controlled by the addition and removal of phosphorus. The primary chemicals used by cells as an energy source contain phosphorus (adenosine triphosphate [ATP] and creatine phosphate). Phosphorus also has an important function in the maintenance of acid-base balance. For a complete review of how phosphorus functions in the maintenance of bone refer to Chapter 10.

Phosphorus Sources and Needs

Phosphorus is found in many commonly consumed foods. Protein-rich foods and many animal products (milk and other dairy products, unprocessed and processed meats) are good sources of phosphorus. Phosphorus deficiency is rare because of the diversity of foods that are rich sources. Phosphorus is commonly added to foods because of its water-binding capacity and antimicrobial function as a component of phosphoric acid. Figure 8-13 lists the phosphorus content of a variety of foods. Low phosphorus status can be observed in premature infants, alcoholics, and the elderly. There are a couple of conditions that can induce phosphorus deficiency: vitamin D deficiency and excessive secretion of parathyroid hormone by the parathyroid gland.

Upper Level of Phosphorus

Compromised kidney function can prevent an appropriate amount of phosphorus excretion leading to elevated blood levels (hyperphosphatemia). Excessive vitamin D supplementation or high consumption of phosphorus-containing antacids can also lead to hyperphosphatemia.

▲ Meats are rich in phosphorus.

CONCEPT CHECK

Phosphorus is the major negatively charged ion in the intracellular fluid. Phosphorus deficiency is unlikely because the typical diet has abundant food sources of phosphorus. Phosphorus is an important component of bone, cell membranes, DNA, and enzymes.

FIGURE 8-13 ▶ Food sources of phosphorus compared to the RDA.

Food Sources of Phosphorus

Food Item and Amount	Phosphorus (milligrams)	% RDA
RDA*	700	100%
Plain yogurt, 1 cup	350	50%
Swiss cheese, 2 ounces	345	49%
Almonds, ½ cup	340	49%
Sunflower seeds, 1 ounce	330	47%
1% milk, 1 cup	235	34%
Cheddar cheese, 1.5 ounces	220	31%
Salmon, 3 ounces	220	31%
Raisin Bran cereal, 1 cup	215	31%
Sirloin steak, 3 ounces	210	30%
Egg, 2 hard boiled	200	29%
Chicken breast, 3 ounces	180	26%
Roasted turkey, 3 ounces	180	26%
Pot roast, 3 ounces	170	24%
Lean ham, 3 ounces	165	24%
American cheese, 1 slice	155	22%

Key:
- ■ Grains
- ■ Vegetables
- ■ Fruits
- □ Oils
- ■ Milk
- ■ Meat & Beans

*For adults; See the DRI table in the back of this book for age-specific recommendations.

Among North Americans, an estimated 1 in 5 adults has hypertension. Over the age of 65, the number rises to 1 in every 2 adults. Only about half of cases are being treated. Blood pressure is expressed by two numbers. The higher number represents systolic blood pressure, the pressure in the arteries when the heart muscle is contracting and pumping blood into the arteries. Optimal systolic blood pressure is 120 millimeters of mercury (mm Hg) or less. The second value is diastolic blood pressure, the artery pressure when the heart is relaxed. Optimal diastolic blood pressure is 80 mm Hg or less. Elevations in both systolic and diastolic blood pressure are strong predictors of disease (Fig. 8-14).

Hypertension is defined as sustained systolic pressure exceeding 139 mm Hg or diastolic blood pressure exceeding 89 mm Hg. Most cases of hypertension (about 95%) have no clear-cut cause. It is described as primary, or essential (i.e., essential hypertension). Kidney disease, sleep-disordered breathing (sleep apnea), and other causes often lead to the other 5% of cases, known as secondary hypertension. African-Americans are more likely than Caucasians to develop hypertension and to do so earlier in life.

Unless blood pressure is periodically measured, the development of hypertension is easily overlooked. Thus, it's described as a silent disorder, because it usually does not cause symptoms.

WHY CONTROL BLOOD PRESSURE?

Blood pressure needs to be controlled mainly to prevent cardiovascular disease, kidney disease, strokes and related declines in brain function, poor blood circulation in the legs, problems with vision, and sudden death. These conditions are much more likely to be found in individuals with hypertension than in people with normal blood pressure. Smoking and elevated blood lipoproteins make these diseases even more likely. Individuals with hypertension need to be diagnosed and treated as soon as pos-

sible, as the condition generally progresses to a more serious stage over time and even resists therapy if it persists for years.

CAUSES OF HYPERTENSION

A family history of hypertension is a risk factor, especially if both parents have (or had) the problem. In addition, blood pressure usually increases as a person ages. Some increase is caused by atherosclerosis. As plaque builds up in the arteries, the arteries become less flexible and cannot expand. When vessels remain rigid, blood pressure remains high. Eventually, the plaque begins to decrease the blood supply to the kidneys, decreasing their ability to control blood volume and, in turn, blood pressure.

An enzyme secreted by the kidneys and some hormonelike compounds are designed to maintain a healthy blood pressure. When blood pressure is elevated, the effect of these compounds can be reduced by antihypertension medications.

Overweight people have six times greater risk of having hypertension than lean people. Overall, obesity is considered the number one lifestyle factor related to hypertension. This is especially the case in minority populations.

How High is High?

If your systolic and diastolic pressures fall into different categories, your risk depends on the higher category.

	SYSTOLIC	DIASTOLIC
Hypertension (High)		
	140	90
Pre-hypertension		
	120	80
Normal		

Numbers (in millimeters of mercury) apply to adults who aren't taking drugs to lower their blood pressure.

FIGURE 8-14 ▲ The cut-off for hypertension is 140/90 mm Hg but the risk of heart attacks and stroke precedes the rise in blood pressure.

▲ Older adults are particularly at risk of hypertension.

Additional blood vessels develop to support excess tissue in overweight and obese individuals, and these extra miles of associated blood vessels increase work by the heart and also blood pressure. Hypertension is linked to obesity if elevated blood insulin levels result from insulin-resistant adipose cells. This increased insulin level increases sodium retention in the body and accelerates atherosclerosis. A weight loss of as little as 10 to 15 pounds often can help treat hypertension.

Inactivity is considered the number two lifestyle factor related to hypertension. If an obese person can engage in regular physical activity (at least 5 days per week for 30 to 60 minutes) and lose weight, blood pressure often returns to normal.

Third, excess alcohol intake is responsible for about 10% of all cases of hypertension, especially in middle-aged males and among African-Americans in general. When hypertension is caused by excessive alcohol intake, it is usually reversible. A sensible alcohol intake for people with hypertension is two or fewer drinks per day for men and one or no drinks per day for women and all older adults. Did you recognize that this is the same recommendation given in the 2005 Dietary Guidelines for Americans? Some studies suggest that such a minimal alcohol intake may reduce the risk of ischemic stroke. These data, however, should not be used to encourage alcohol use.

In some people, particularly African-Americans and older overweight persons, blood pressure is especially sensitive to sodium. In these people, excess salt leads to fluid retention by the kidney and a corresponding increase in blood volume, which therefore increases blood pressure. It is not clear whether the sodium ion or the chloride ion is most responsible for the effect. Still, as reviewed in this chapter, if one reduces sodium intake, chloride intake naturally falls; the opposite is also true. For the most part, a recommendation to consume less sodium is equivalent to a call for less salt in the diet. Only some North Americans are susceptible to increases in blood pressure from salt intake, so it is only the number four lifestyle factor related to hypertension. It is unfortunate that salt intake receives the major portion of public attention with regard to hypertension. Efforts to prevent hypertension should also focus on obesity, inactivity, and alcohol abuse.

OTHER MINERALS AND BLOOD PRESSURE

Minerals such as calcium, potassium, and magnesium also deserve attention when it comes to prevention and treatment of hypertension. Studies show that a diet rich in these minerals and low in salt can decrease blood pressure within days of beginning this type of diet, especially among African-Americans. The response is even similar to that seen with commonly used medications. The diet is called the Dietary Approaches to Stop Hypertension (DASH) diet (Table 8-2). The diet, rich in calcium, phosphorus, and

▲ Opting for the fruits, vegetables, foods recommended by the DASH diet is good nutrition advice regardless of hypertension.

magnesium and low in salt, takes a standard MyPyramid food plan and adds 1 to 2 extra vegetables and fruits servings and a serving of nuts, seeds, or legumes (beans) 4 to 5 days of the week. In DASH studies, participants also consumed no more than 3 grams of sodium and no more than one to two alcoholic drinks per week. A DASH 2 diet trial tested three daily sodium intakes (3300 milligrams, 2400 milligrams, and 1500 milligrams). People showed a steady decline in blood pressure on the DASH diet as sodium intake declined. Over all, the DASH diet is seen as a total dietary approach to treating hypertension. It is not clear which

TABLE 8-2 What Is the DASH Diet?
The DASH diet is characterized as low in fat and sodium and rich in fruits, vegetable fat dairy products. Here is the breakdown:

Per Day	Per Week
6–8 servings of grains and grain products	4–5 servings of nuts, seeds, or legumes
4–5 servings of fruit	5 servings of sweets and added sugars
4–5 servings of vegetables	
2–3 servings of low-fat or fat-free dairy products	
2 or less servings of meats, poultry, and fish	
2–3 servings of fats/oils	

of the many healthful practices of this diet are responsible for the fall in blood pressure.

Other studies also show a reduction in stroke risk among people who consume a diet rich in fruits, vegetables, and vitamin C (recall that fruits and vegetables are rich in vitamin C). Overall, a diet low in salt and rich in low-fat and fat-free dairy products, fruits, vegetables, whole grains, and some nuts can substantially reduce hypertension and stroke risk in many people, especially those with hypertension.

MEDICATIONS TO TREAT HYPERTENSION

Diuretic medications are one class of drugs used to treat hypertension. These "water pills" work to reduce blood volume (and therefore blood pressure) by increasing fluid output in the urine. Other medications act by slowing heart rate or by causing relaxation of blood vessels. A combination of two or more medications is commonly required to treat hypertension that does not respond to diet and lifestyle therapy.

PREVENTION OF HYPERTENSION

Many of the risk factors for hypertension and stroke are controllable, and appropriate lifestyle changes can reduce a person's risk (Fig. 8-15). Experts also recommend that those with hypertension lower blood pressure through diet and lifestyle changes before resorting to blood pressure medications.

▲ Regular, moderate physical activity contributes to better blood pressure control.

FIGURE 8-15 ▶ What works? If your blood pressure is high, here's how much lifestyle changes should lower it.

Advice	Details	Drop in Systolic Blood Pressure
Lose excess weight	For every 20 pounds you lose	5 to 20 points
Follow a DASH diet	Eat a lower-fat diet rich in vegetables, fruits, and low-fat dairy foods	8 to 14 points
Exercise daily	Get 30 minutes a day of aerobic activity (such as brisk walking)	4 to 9 points
Limit sodium	Eat no more than 2400 mg per day (1500 mg per day is better)	2 to 8 points
Limit alcohol	Have no more than 2 drinks per day for men, 1 drink per day for women (1 drink = 12 oz. beer, 5 oz. wine, or 1.5 oz. 80-proof whiskey)	2 to 4 points

Source: *The Seventh Report of the Joint National Committee on Prevention, Detection, Evaluation, and Treatment of High Blood Pressure* (www.nhibl.hih.gov/guidelines/hypertension).

CASE STUDY

Under Pressure

Last spring, Greg graduated from college with a degree in computer science and started a full-time job as a programmer. Over the past few months, his life has been consumed by his new job, which requires long hours of intense concentration at his desk. He loves the work, but his supervisor's many demands sometimes leave him feeling stressed. Although he used to participate in intramural sports in college, life as a working adult has not afforded him much time to exercise, and he has put on about 15 pounds over the past few months. Greg usually skips breakfast, microwaves a frozen entrée for lunch, and buys snacks like pretzels and potato chips from the vending machine if he gets hungry later in the day. By the time he fights traffic to get home in the evening, he doesn't feel much like cooking or doing anything else, so Greg usually orders take-out pizza or Chinese food and eats his dinner in front of the television, where he remains for the rest of the evening.

At a recent health fair, Greg had his blood pressure checked and the nurse informed him it was 135/88. She told Greg that he should make some changes to his lifestyle to get his blood pressure under control, warning him that if his blood pressure gets much higher, he may have to start taking medications.

Answer the following questions about Greg's health and check your responses in Appendix A.

1. How does Greg's blood pressure compare to current recommendations from the American Heart Association? What should be his blood pressure goal?
2. Identify some lifestyle factors that may contribute to Greg's elevated blood pressure. Provide some suggestions for lifestyle changes Greg could make to lower his blood pressure.
3. What is the AI for sodium for an adult? How do you think Greg's sodium intake compares to the AI?
4. How does sodium influence blood pressure? Would you guarantee that following a low-sodium diet will decrease Greg's blood pressure? Besides sodium, what other micronutrients affect blood pressure?
5. Point out three important health reasons for Greg to lower his blood pressure.

SUMMARY

1. Water constitutes 50% to 70% of the human body. Its unique chemical properties enable it to dissolve substances as well as serve as a medium for chemical reactions, temperature regulation, and lubrication. Water also helps regulate the acid-base balance in the body. For adults, daily water needs from the combination of food and drink are estimated at 9 cups (women) and 13 cups (men) per day.

2. Many minerals are vital for sustaining life. For humans, animal products are the most bioavailable sources of most minerals. Supplements of minerals exceeding 100% of the Daily Values listed on the label should be taken only under a physician's supervision. Toxicity and nutrient interactions are especially likely if the UL (when set) is exceeded on a long-term basis.

3. Sodium, the major positive ion found outside cells, is vital in fluid balance and nerve impulse transmission. The North American diet provides abundant sodium through processed foods and table salt. About 10% to 15% of the adult population are sensitive to sodium intake. Overweight people are especially at risk for developing hypertension from consuming excessive sodium.

4. Potassium, the major positive ion found inside cells, has a similar function to sodium. Milk, fruits, and vegetables are good sources.

5. Chloride is the major negative ion found outside cells. It is important in digestion as part of stomach acid and in immune and nerve functions. Table salt supplies most of the chloride in our diets.

6. Controlling weight and alcohol intake; exercising regularly; decreasing salt intake; and ensuring adequate potassium, magnesium, and calcium in the diet all can play a part in controlling high blood pressure.

STUDY QUESTIONS

1. Approximately how much water do you need each day to stay healthy? Identify at least two situations that increase the need for water. Then list three sources of water in the average person's diet.

2. List five functions of water in the body.

3. What is the relationship between sodium and water balance, and how is that relationship monitored as well as maintained in the body?

4. Describe the effects of antidiuretic hormone (ADH) and aldosterone on body water.

5. What are two similarities and differences between sodium and potassium? Sodium and chloride?

6. How do sodium and potassium participate in nerve impulse transmission?

7. What metabolic processes affect the pH of body fluids? Why is it important for pH to be maintained within a narrow range?

8. What are some possible health effects of excess sodium in the body? What are the effects of sodium depletion? How might sodium depletion occur?

9. What foods are good sources of phosphorus? Describe three functions of phosphorus in the body.

10. Of the micronutrients discussed in this chapter, which are typically consumed in excess? Which of the micronutrients in this chapter are typically lacking in North American diets?

CHECK YOUR KNOWLEDGE

Answers to the following multiple choice questions are in Appendix A.

1. Which compartment contains the greatest amount of body fluid?
   a. intracellular
   b. extracellular
   c. They contain the same amount.

2. Minerals involved in fluid balance are
   a. calcium and magnesium.
   b. copper and iron.
   c. calcium and phosphorus.
   d. sodium and potassium.

3. The primary function of sodium is to maintain
   a. bone mineral content.
   b. hemoglobin concentration.
   c. immune function.
   d. fluid distribution.

4. Chloride is
   a. a component of hydrochloric acid.
   b. an intracellular fluid ion.
   c. a positively charged ion.
   d. converted to chlorine in the intestinal tract.

5. Hypertension is defined as a blood pressure greater than
   a. 110/60.
   b. 120/65.
   c. 140/90.
   d. 190/80.

6. A compound that separates into positive or negative ions when dissolved in water and conducts electricity is known as a(n)
   a. atom.
   b. electrolyte.
   c. solvent.
   d. solution.

7. A hormone that causes the kidneys to conserve sodium is called
   a. glucagon.
   b. parathyroid hormone.
   c. antidiuretic hormone.
   d. aldosterone.

8. Total water needs are about _____ cups per day for women and about _____ cups per day for men.
   a. 8, 10
   b. 9, 13
   c. 11, 15
   d. 15, 18

9. The major intracellular positive ion is
   a. sodium.
   b. potassium.
   c. chloride.
   d. calcium.

10. Food sources of potassium include
    a. milk.
    b. kidney beans.
    c. orange juice.
    d. All of the above.

FURTHER READINGS

1. America's pressure cooker. *Nutrition Action HealthLetter* July/August:3, 2005.

   This article summarizes three recent trials (TOHP II, TONE, and DASH) on diet and hypertension and provides lists of the sodium content of several common foods and of many restaurant foods. Healthy lifestyle changes are outlined, including losing excess weight, following a DASH diet, and limiting sodium and alcohol. Finally, foods rich in potassium are suggested as a "sodium antidote."

2. Appel LJ and others: Dietary approaches to prevent and treat hypertension: A scientific statement from the American Heart Association. *Hypertension* 47:296, 2006.

   The authors provide the latest advice from the American Heart Association on diet and hypertension. Key preventive factors are to avoid overweight and inactivity and to moderate alcohol and salt intake.

3. Food and Nutrition Board, Institute of Medicine: *Dietary Reference Intakes for water, potassium, sodium, chloride, and sulfate.* Washington, DC: National Academies Press, 2004.

   Dietary standards for water, potassium, sodium, and chloride are discussed. The rationale used to derive the Adequate Intakes, as well as the Upper Levels, is presented along with information on function, intake, and deficiency.

4. Hollenberg NK: The influence of dietary sodium on blood pressure. *Journal of the American College of Nutrition* 25:240S, 2006.

   Evidence relating salt intake to blood pressure is reviewed. The merit of maintaining a reduction in salt intake is discussed. The author indicates that the evidence supporting such a policy is inconsistent and small. The importance of antihypertensive drugs is emphasized.

5. Popkin BM and others: A new proposed guidance system for beverage consumption in the United States. *American Journal of Clinical Nutrition* 83:529, 2006.

   Drinking water is recommended as the preferred beverage to fulfill water needs, with tea, coffee, and low-fat and skim milk also ranked high. The Beverage Guidance Panel suggests that beverages with no or few calories should be consumed more often than calorie-containing beverages. An intake of 98 fluid ounces is rec-ommended daily for a person consuming 2200 calories.

6. Adrogue HJ and Madias NE: Sodium and potassium in the pathogenesis of hypertension. *New England Journal of Medicine* 356:1966, 2007.

   The roles of sodium and potassium in hypertension are explored in great detail with an interesting evolutionary perspective. The article provides several illustrations of pathways involved in mediation of hypertension. The authors advocate a return to the high-potassium, low-sodium dietary patterns of our ancestors and call upon not only consumers, but also food manufacturers, to put this dietary goal into action.

7. Haddy FJ and others: Role of potassium in regulating blood flow and blood pressure. *American Journal of Physiology—Regulatory, Integrative, and Comparative Physiology* 290: R546, 2006.

   There may be multiple mechanisms by which potassium decreases hypertension. High potassium intake increases urinary excretion of sodium. Potassium also causes vasodilation through its action on the smooth muscle of arterial walls. The effects of potassium on blood pressure take about four weeks to appear, but taking advantage of the beneficial effects of dietary changes may lessen the need for prescription medications.

8. Havas S and others: The urgent need to reduce sodium consumption. *Journal of the American Medical Association* 298(12): 1439, 2007.

   In this commentary, the authors call for drastic public policy changes to decrease sodium consumption in the United States. They emphasize the high burden of hypertension in terms of mortality, morbidity, and health care costs, and review the overwhelming evidence linking overconsumption of sodium with hypertension. Several other countries have already adopted public health policies to decrease sodium content of processed and restaurant foods. The authors report that a 50% reduction in sodium intake would translate into 150,000 fewer deaths per year in the United States.

9. Heird WC and others: Current electrolyte intakes of infants and toddlers. *Journal of the American Dietetic Association* 106:S43, 2006.

   Results of the Feeding Infants and Toddlers Study revealed that the sodium and chloride intakes of more than half of infants and toddlers exceed the Upper Limit for these micronutrients. Potassium intakes are much lower. It is becoming increasingly evident that many chronic diseases originate during childhood and that health habits established early in life persist throughout adulthood. Parents and other caregivers need to focus on better nutrition for infants and toddlers.

10. LaRowe TL and others: Beverage patterns, diet quality, and body mass index of US preschool and school-age children. *Journal of the American Dietetic Association* 107:1124, 2007.

    Previous studies have shown an increase in calories consumed as beverages to be related to the rise in childhood overweight and obesity. In this study, diet quality, as measured by the Healthy Eating Index, suffered with the inclusion of calorically sweetened beverages. High-calorie beverages such as fruit drinks and soft drinks crowd out water and dairy products as sources of hydration. The authors recommend that preschool and school-age children reduce their intakes of calorically-sweetened beverages and increase their consumption of micronutrient-dense foods.

11. Sawka MN and others: Exercise and fluid replacement. *Medicine and Science in Sports and Exercise* 39(2):377, 2007.

    Dehydration affects physical performance and can lead to serious illness. Factors that affect hydration during exercise include gender, age, and food intake. This position statement of the American Society of Sports Medicine outlines updated recommendations for fluid replacement before, during, and after exercise.

12. Sharp RL: Role of sodium in fluid homeostasis with exercise. *Journal of the American College of Nutrition* 25(3):231S, 2006.

    In this article, the importance of sodium replacement along with fluid replacement after sporting events is described. Hyponatremia, or sodium depletion, is defined and discussed. Due to its role in fluid retention, sodium can help to rapidly normalize fluid status after a sporting event.

▶ Check out the **Contemporary Nutrition ARIS site**
www.mhhe.com/wardlawcontfa1 for quizzes, flash cards, other activities, and weblinks designed to further help you learn about what you eat and why.

I. How High Is Your Sodium Intake?

Complete this questionnaire to evaluate your sodium habits with respect to typically rich sources.

How Often Do You . . .	Rarely	Occasionally	Often	Regularly (Daily)
1. Eat cured or processed meats, such as ham, bacon, sausage, frankfurters, and other luncheon meats?				
2. Choose canned or frozen vegetables with sauce?				
3. Use commercially-prepared meals, main dishes, or canned or dehydrated soups?				
4. Eat cheese, especially processed cheese?				
5. Eat salted nuts, popcorn, pretzels, corn chips, or potato chips?				
6. Add salt to cooking water for vegetables, rice, or pasta?				
7. Add salt, seasoning mixes, salad dressings, or condiments—such as soy sauce, steak sauce, catsup, and mustard—to foods during preparation or at the table?				
8. Salt your food before tasting it?				
9. Ignore labels for sodium content when buying foods?				
10. When dining out, choose obviously salty sauces or foods?				

The more checks you put in the "often" or "regularly" columns, the higher your dietary sodium intake. However, not all the habits in the table contribute the same amount of sodium. For example, many natural cheeses such as cheddar are relatively moderate in sodium, whereas processed cheeses and cottage cheese are much higher. To moderate sodium intake, choose lower-sodium foods from each food group more often and balance high-sodium food choices with low-sodium ones.

Adapted from *USDA Home and Garden Bulletin* No. 232-6, April 1986.

II. Rate Your Beverage Choices

Water is the key component in the beverage consumption guidelines that have been recently developed (Table 8-3). These recommendations give guidance on the health and nutritional benefits as well as the risks of various beverage categories. The basis of the Beverage Guidance System is that fluids should not provide a significant amount of the energy nutrients in a healthy diet. More specifically, the system recommends that beverages provide less than 10% of total calories consumed for a 2200 kcal diet.

TABLE 8-3 The Beverage Guidance System

Level	Category*	Recommended Servings per day
1	Water	50 fluid ounces (1.7 liters)
2	Tea or coffee, unsweetened	0 to 40 fluid ounces (0 to 1.4 liters)
3	Low-fat and skim milk and soy beverages	0 to 16 fluid ounces (0 to 0.5 liter)
4	Non-calorically sweetened beverages (diet drinks)	0 to 32 fluid ounces (0 to 1 liter)
5	Calorie beverages with some nutrients (100% fruit juices, alcoholic beverages, whole milk, sports drinks)	0 to 8 fluid ounces 100% fruit juices (0 to 0.25 liter) 0 to 1 alcoholic drinks for women 0 to 2 alcoholic drinks for men
6	Calorically-sweetened beverages (regular soft drinks)	0 to 8 fluid ounces (0 to 0.25 liter)

*Categories established based on their possible health benefits or risks.
Adapted from Popkin and others: *Am J Clin Nutr* 83:529, 2006.

1. Think of all the beverages you drank yesterday, from the time you woke up to the time you went to bed. Do your best to recall the types and amounts of your fluid intake in the space below.

   _____

   _____

   _____

   _____

2. Next to each beverage choice you listed for question 1, indicate its category from the Beverage Guidance System.

3. Did you come close to the recommendation to consume 50 fluid ounces (1.7 liters) of fluid in the form of water yesterday?

   _____

   _____

4. How many fluid ounces of your beverages fit into categories 2, 3, 4, or 5? Did you exceed the recommended servings per day for these categories?

   _____

   _____

5. What changes could you make in your beverage choices to follow the Beverage Guidance System more closely? How does following the Beverage Guidance System contribute to good health?

   _____

   _____

Metabolic water   When carbohydrates, lipids, and proteins are used as an energy source, carbon dioxide and water are formed as a by-product.

CHAPTER 9 Nutrients That Function as Antioxidants

CHAPTER OBJECTIVES Chapter 9 is designed to allow you to:

1. Define the term free radical and understand how they can alter normal cell function.

2. Describe how antioxidants function to neutralize free radicals.

3. List the important micronutrients shown to have antioxidant properties.

4. List major food sources of the antioxidants.

5. List the human diseases that have been linked to oxidative damage.

6. Define functional foods and phytochemicals.

7. Describe the relationship between consumption of nutrients that are rich sources of antioxidants and a decreased risk for disease.

CHAPTER OUTLINE

OXIDATION AND REDUCTION

To have an understanding of how antioxidants function, a brief review of the anatomy of an atom is necessary. Atoms contain protons and neutrons found in the nucleus. Electrons circle the nucleus. The electrons are found in pairs. The nucleus is positively charged and the electrons are negatively charged, and the positive and negative charges are balanced so there is no overall charge.

Atoms are joined together to form molecules. For example, hydrogen (H) and oxygen (O) are atoms, and they combine to form a molecule of water (H_2O). Carbohydrates, lipids, and proteins are examples of molecules. Approximately half of all enzymatic chemical reactions in the body involve the exchange of electrons between atoms and molecules. The gain of a negatively charged electron is called reduction, and the loss of an electron is termed oxidation (Fig. 9-1).

Oxidation frequently involves reactions with oxygen, hence the name. As food is oxidized by the trillions of cells in the body, an even number of electrons are transferred between atoms and molecules. The key to human life is respiration, where breathed oxygen reacts with the atoms and molecules in food to produce carbon dioxide, water and the energy found in the chemical bonds of food is converted into ATP and other high-energy containing compounds that can be used by the body to perform work (Fig. 9-2).

There are instances when an atom loses a single electron during an oxidation reaction. This results in a situation where the number of positive charges contributed by the nucleus of the atom is no longer equal to the number of negative charges

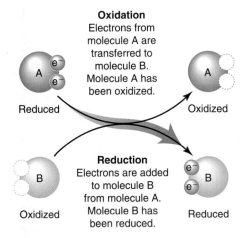

Oxidation
Electrons from molecule A are transferred to molecule B. Molecule A has been oxidized.

Reduced — Oxidized

Reduction
Electrons are added to molecule B from molecule A. Molecule B has been reduced.

Oxidized — Reduced

FIGURE 9-1 ▶ Electrons are transfered between molecules in oxidation reduction reactions.

in the electrons surrounding the nucleus. These chemically unstable atoms are classified as **free radicals.** Free radicals are chemically reactive and sometimes aggressive. To reestablish a balance between positive and negative charges, the free radical pilfers an electron from an adjacent atom or molecule. With the loss of an electron, the nearby molecule becomes a free radical and it looks to acquire an electron from another adjacent molecule. This leads to a chain reaction. The body's natural defenses and repair systems try to control the destruction caused by free radicals, but these systems are not 100% effective.

The production of free radicals is a normal consequence of cellular respiration. In some instances free radical production is important for human health. The aggressive oxidizing capacity and potentially damaging effects of free radicals is used by the immune system in the destruction of disease-causing microorganisms. White blood cells produce highly reactive free radicals that assist in the destruction of bacteria, viruses, and fungi. The production of free radicals has also been shown to be an important component of the mechanism by which the body destroys altered cells, which could potentially proceed to cancerous growth. On the other hand, free radicals can also be deleterious to healthy cells. They can aggressively remove electrons from cellular constituents including: nucleic acid in DNA, proteins, and polyunsaturated fatty acids found in membranes surrounding the cell or organelles. Once formed, free radicals give rise to the production of more free radicals and thus more damage. The chemical damage produced by free radicals has been linked to numerous diseases including:

cancer	kidney disease
atherosclerosis	Alzheimer's disease
arthritis	Parkinson's disease
diabetes	cataracts
emphysema	

Environmental substances have been shown to accelerate the formation of free radicals. Examples are excessive sunlight, water and air pollution, radiation, asbestos, ozone, and toxic chemicals.

DEFENSE AGAINST FREE RADICALS

The body has two principle defense mechanisms to limit or defend against the adverse effects of free radicals: enzyme systems and antioxidant chemicals. The enzyme systems have a close relationship with nutrition in that their activity requires the presence of minerals such as selenium, manganese, zinc, iron, and copper. These enzyme systems detoxify specific free radicals or related compounds at specific locations within cells.

Chemicals that function as antioxidants include **vitamins,** a vitamin precursor, and **phytochemicals.** These antioxidants principally function by donating an electron or hydrogen atom to reactive molecules to stabilize their structure (Fig. 9-3). The antioxidants

Antioxidant A substance that has the ability to prevent or repair the damage caused by oxidation.

Free radical An unstable atom with an unpaired electron in its outermost shell.

Vitamin Compound needed in small amounts to help regulate and support chemical reactions and processes in the body.

Phytochemicals Chemicals found in plants that have health protective actions.

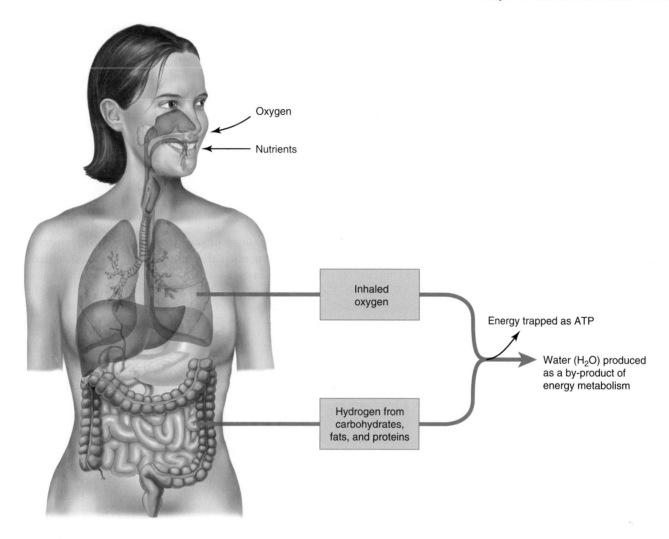

FIGURE 9-2 ▶ The process of consuming oxygen in air (breathing) and consuming food (eating) allowing the body to convert the energy found in food into a form the body can use (ATP). Atoms of oxygen and hydrogen are combined during this process to make water as a by-product.

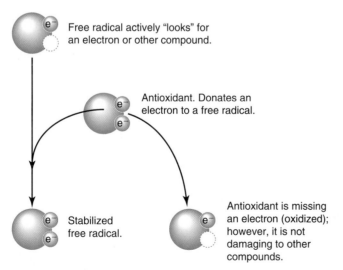

Free radical actively "looks" for an electron or other compound.

Antioxidant. Donates an electron to a free radical.

Stabilized free radical.

Antioxidant is missing an electron (oxidized); however, it is not damaging to other compounds.

FIGURE 9-3 ▶ Antioxidants stabilize free radicals by donating electrons to them. Free radicals are dangerous to cells, because they seek to fill their outer shells by removing electrons from other substances such as DNA, proteins, and lipids.

then become chemically unstable but because of their unique structure they are not reactive molecules prone to induce cellular damage. The enzyme systems and dietary antioxidants work in concert to limit free radical formation, destroy free radicals, and assist in repairing oxidative damage induced by reactive molecules. Dietary recommendations, including those found in MyPyramid and the Five-A-Day program, are based on the premise that increased consumption of fruits and vegetables will increase intake of fiber; antioxidant vitamins and minerals; and phytochemicals, which have important functions in the detoxification of reactive molecules, including free radicals.

NUTRIENTS THAT PROVIDE AN ANTIOXIDANT ROLE

Carotenoids Pigment materials that range in color from yellow to orange to red; three of the carotenoids are converted into Vitamin A. Many are antioxidants.

The antioxidant minerals and vitamins, along with phytochemicals, may help prevent or postpone diseases that have oxidation as a component to their development. These nutrients must be consumed in the diet as the body cannot synthesize them. The principle antioxidant vitamins are E and C. Vitamin A and its precursor, the **carotenoids,** are also discussed in this chapter as they have antioxidant properties. The antioxidant function of phytochemicals, selenium, and, to a lesser extent, other minerals is also examined in this chapter.

CONCEPT CHECK

As cells in the body use the molecules found in foods in metabolism, atoms gain pairs of electrons (reduction) and lose pairs of electrons (oxidation). Free radicals are formed when atoms contain an unpaired electron and form naturally in metabolic reactions, and a number of environmental factors (pollution, radiation) increase their formation. Free radicals are chemically destructive, aggressive, and play a role in the development of numerous diseases. Numerous vitamins and minerals function as antioxidants to stabilize or detoxify free radicals, thereby reducing the cellular damage they can induce.

VITAMIN E

Functions of Vitamin E

Vitamin E is a family of four tocopherols and four tocotrienols called alpha, beta, gamma, and delta. The tocopherols have a saturated side chain whereas the tocotrienols have an unsaturated side chain. Alpha-tocopherol is the main form in the human body, and alpha- and gamma-tocopherol are the principle forms in food. In the 1920s a fat-soluble compound was found to be essential for fertility in rats. This compound was named tocopherol from the Greek words *tokos*, meaning birth, and *phero*, meaning to bring forth. Later this essential nutrient was named vitamin E. Vitamin E is unique in that in many animal species it has an essential function in fertility, whereas it does not appear to have this same function in humans. It is, however, important for the development of muscles and the central nervous system in early human development.

The principle function of vitamin E in humans is as an antioxidant. Vitamin E resides primarily in cell membranes. Membranes surrounding cells and organelles are made up of two layers of lipid (phospholipids bilayer). Vitamin E is a fat-soluble vitamin found primarily in adipose tissue and cell membranes. Many of the lipids within these membranes are polyunsaturated fatty acids particularly susceptible to oxidative attack by free radicals. The formation of free radicals may destabilize the cell membrane, which may ultimately alter the ability of the cell to function properly. Vitamin E can donate electrons or hydrogen to free radicals found in membranes thereby making them more stable (Fig. 9-4). The antioxidant function of vitamin E appears to be critical in cells continually exposed to high levels of oxygen, particularly red blood cells and the lungs.

The ability of vitamin E to lower the risk of developing coronary heart disease and cataracts has been studied. Oxidative damage is largely responsible for the

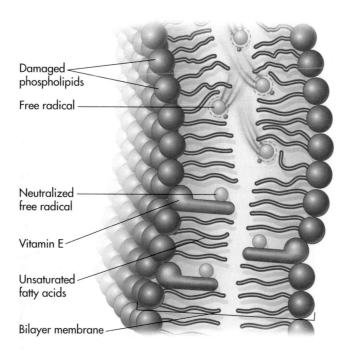

Damaged phospholipids

Free radical

Neutralized free radical

Vitamin E

Unsaturated fatty acids

Bilayer membrane

FIGURE 9-4 ▶ Fat-soluble vitamin E can insert itself into cell membranes, where it helps stop free-radical chain reactions. If not interrupted, these reactions cause extensive oxidative damage to cells and ultimately cell death.

development of these diseases. Oxidized cholesterol is a major component of the plaque that develops in arteries, which leads to atherosclerosis. Vitamin E is thought to have a beneficial effect on the development of atherogenic plaque due to its ability to prevent or reduce the formation of oxidized cholesterol. Oxidative damage to proteins in the eye leads to the development of cataracts. Oxidized proteins combine and precipitate in the lens, causing cloudiness and decreasing visual acuity. Low intakes of foods that are good sources of antioxidants have been shown to be related to an increased incidence of these diseases.

Experts do not know whether supplementation with **megadoses** of vitamin E can confer any additional protection against diseases linked to oxidative damage. The consensus among the scientific community is that the proven benefits of lifestyle choices have a far greater effect than any postulated benefits of antioxidant supplementation. The position of scientific research groups (American Heart Association, U.S. Preventative Services Task Force) conclude that it is premature to recommend vitamin E supplements to the general population, based on current knowledge and the failure of large clinical trials to show any consistent benefit. This conclusion is an agreement with the latest report on vitamin E by the Food and Nutrition Board of the National Academy of Sciences. In addition, the Food and Drug Administration has denied the request of the dietary supplement industry to make a health claim that vitamin E supplements reduce the risk of cardiovascular disease and cancer.

Vitamin E has been shown to improve vitamin A absorption if the dietary intake of vitamin A is low. Vitamin E also functions in the metabolism of iron within cells, and it helps maintain nervous tissue and immune function.

Megadose Intake of a nutrient beyond estimates of needs to prevent a deficiency or what would be found in a balanced diet; two to 10 times human needs is a starting point for such a dosage.

Vitamin E Sources and Needs

Major sources of vitamin E include plant oils (e.g., salad dressings and mayonnaise), ready-to-eat breakfast cereals, some fruits and vegetables, eggs, and margarine (Fig. 9-5). Other good sources of Vitamin E include whole grains, nuts (e.g., almonds), and seeds (e.g., sunflower seeds).

Plant oils are made up of mainly unsaturated fatty acids, and the relatively high amount of vitamin E in plant oils provides a natural function of protecting these unsaturated lipids from oxidation. Animal products (meat, dairy, eggs) and fish oils, on the other hand, have almost

▲ Plant oils are good sources of vitamin E.

no vitamin E (Fig. 9-6). Vitamin E is susceptible to destruction by oxygen, metals, light, and especially repeated use in deep-fat frying, so the vitamin E content of a food depends on how it is harvested, processed, stored, and cooked. Approximately two-thirds of the vitamin found in cooking oils is lost during processing. The majority of vitamin E is lost during the processing of wheat to produce flour through the removal of the germ and bleaching process.

The Recommended Dietary Allowances (RDA) of vitamin E for adults is 15 milligrams per day of alpha-tocopherol, the most active form of vitamin E (d isomer) or 22.5 milligrams of the synthetic source (dl isomer). Typically, North American adults consume about two-thirds of the RDA for vitamin E from food sources. The Daily Value used on food and supplement labels is 20 milligrams.

Several population groups are especially susceptible to developing marginal Vitamin E status. Preterm infants tend to have low vitamin E stores because this vitamin is transferred from mother to baby during the late stages of pregnancy. The potential for oxidative damage, which could cause the cell membranes of red blood cells to break (hemolysis), is of particular concern for preterm infants. The rapid growth of preterm infants, coupled with the high oxygen needs of their immature lungs, greatly increases the stress on red blood cells. Special formulas and supplements designed for preterm infants compensate for lack of vitamin E through fortification. Smokers are another group at high risk for vitamin E deficiency, as smoking readily destroys vitamin E in the lungs. Others at risk of vitamin E deficiency include adults on very low-fat diets or those with fat malabsorption.

Upper Level for Vitamin E

The Upper Level for vitamin E is 1000 milligrams per day of supplemental alpha-tocopherol. Excessive intake of vitamin E can interfere with vitamin K's role in the

Food Sources of Vitamin E

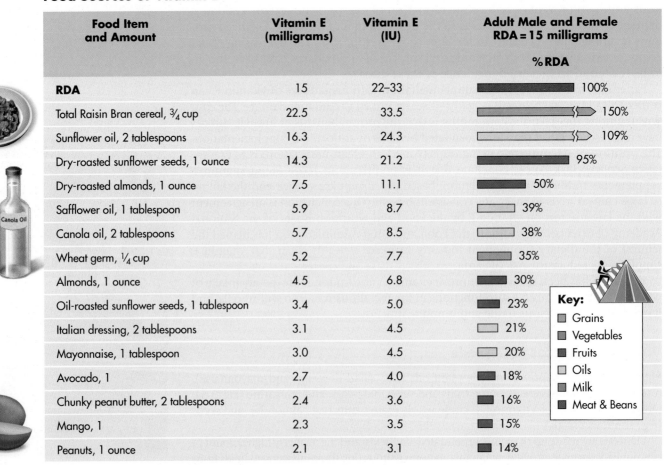

Food Item and Amount	Vitamin E (milligrams)	Vitamin E (IU)	Adult Male and Female RDA = 15 milligrams %RDA
RDA	15	22–33	100%
Total Raisin Bran cereal, ¾ cup	22.5	33.5	150%
Sunflower oil, 2 tablespoons	16.3	24.3	109%
Dry-roasted sunflower seeds, 1 ounce	14.3	21.2	95%
Dry-roasted almonds, 1 ounce	7.5	11.1	50%
Safflower oil, 1 tablespoon	5.9	8.7	39%
Canola oil, 2 tablespoons	5.7	8.5	38%
Wheat germ, ¼ cup	5.2	7.7	35%
Almonds, 1 ounce	4.5	6.8	30%
Oil-roasted sunflower seeds, 1 tablespoon	3.4	5.0	23%
Italian dressing, 2 tablespoons	3.1	4.5	21%
Mayonnaise, 1 tablespoon	3.0	4.5	20%
Avocado, 1	2.7	4.0	18%
Chunky peanut butter, 2 tablespoons	2.4	3.6	16%
Mango, 1	2.3	3.5	15%
Peanuts, 1 ounce	2.1	3.1	14%

Key:
- Grains
- Vegetables
- Fruits
- Oils
- Milk
- Meat & Beans

FIGURE 9-5 ▶ Food sources of vitamin E compared to the RDA for adults.

**MyPyramid:
Sources of Vitamin E**

Grains	Vegetables	Fruits	Oils	Milk	Meat & Beans
• Wheat germ (whole grains) • Some fortified breakfast cereals	• Cabbage • Asparagus • Sweet potatoes • Tomatoes	• Apples • Avocados • Mango	• Plant oils • Margarines • Salad dressings	• None	• Nuts • Seeds • Shrimp • Peanut butter

FIGURE 9-6 ▶ Sources of Vitamin E from MyPyramid. The height of the background color (none, 1/3, 2/3, or completely covered) within each group in the pyramid indicates the average nutrient density for Vitamin E in that group. Overall, plant oils are the richest source, followed by nuts and seeds in the meat & beans group. With regard to physical activity, Vitamin E has no primary role in the related energy metabolism per se but likely limits some oxidant damage during such endeavors.

clotting mechanism, leading to hemorrhage. The risk of insufficient blood clotting is especially high if vitamin E is taken in conjunction with anticoagulant medications (e.g., Coumadin or heavy aspirin use).

There is additional concern that consumption of large amounts of alpha-tocopherol supplements might decrease the **bioavailability** and activity of the other forms of vitamin E in the body. Some experts recommend that vitamin E supplements should contain a mixture of the naturally occurring forms of vitamin E found in food (i.e., mixed tocopherols). This form is more expensive, however, than natural or synthetic alpha-tocopherol alone.

Bioavailability The degree to which an ingested nutriat is absorbed and thus is available to the body.

CONCEPT CHECK

Enzymes and other body mechanisms scavenge and minimize the formation of free radicals and other oxidative compounds, but they are not 100% effective. Hence, diet-derived antioxidants may be critical in diminishing oxidative damage and helping us to stay healthy. Vitamin E functions primarily as an antioxidant. By providing electrons to free radicals, vitamin E helps prevent oxidative damage, especially of cell membranes. When more plant oils are consumed, more vitamin E is needed to protect the double bonds found in plant oils from oxidation. The vitamin E content in plant oils is high. Preterm infants are particularly susceptible to oxidative breakdown of their red blood cell membranes (hemolysis) because of their poor Vitamin E status. Among adults deficiency is rare. People who smoke or experience long-term fat malabsorption run the biggest risk of vitamin E deficiency. There is a controversy about whether taking large amounts of vitamin E in supplement form over a long period provides any special health benefits; research is ongoing. Megadose use of vitamin E reduces blood clotting, possibly leading to a hemorrhage.

FIGURE 9-7 ▶ Pinpoint hemorrhages of the skin—an early symptom of vitamin C deficiency and scurvy. The spots on the skin are caused by slight bleeding into hair follicles. Vitamin C deficiency also slows wound healing.

VITAMIN C

On long sea voyages, half or more of sailing crews died due to scurvy, the Vitamin C deficiency disease. In 1740, the Englishman Dr. James Lind first showed that citrus fruits—two oranges and one lemon a day—could prevent the development of scurvy. Fifty years after Lind's discovery, daily rations for British sailors included limes (thus their nickname, limeys). Even after this discovery, scurvy continued to affect many people as thousands died during the American Civil War due to inadequate intake of vitamin C. Intestinal absorption of vitamin C is dependant on intake. When a person consumes between 15 and 200 milligrams per day, the absorption percentage is high whereas ingestion of greater levels will decrease absorption efficiency.

Functions of Vitamin C

Vitamin C has a specific function in the synthesis of numerous compounds in the body, including collagen; carnitine; and two neurotransmitters, serotonin and norepinephrine. Vitamin C also has a more general function by acting as an antioxidant because it can readily accept and donate electrons. The best understood function of vitamin C is its role in the synthesis of collagen. This protein is highly concentrated in connective tissue, bone, teeth, tendons, and blood vessels. The important function of vitamin C in the formation of connective tissue is exemplified in the early symptoms of a deficiency: pinpoint hemorrhages under the skin (Fig. 9-7), bleeding gums, and joint pain. Vitamin C is also important for wound healing and increases the cross-connections between amino acids found in collagen, greatly strengthening the structural tissues it helps form. Vitamin C is required for the synthesis of carnitine, a compound required for the transport of fatty acids into the mitochondria.

Vitamin C has antioxidant properties. These antioxidant properties have been postulated to reduce the formation of cancer-causing nitrosamines in the stomach. Vitamin C also aids in the reactivation of vitamin E after it has donated an electron to a free radical. Population studies suggest that the antioxidant properties of vitamin C may be effective in the prevention of certain cancers (esophagus, mouth, and stomach) and cataracts. The extent to which vitamin C functions in the reduction of diseases is debatable based on the scientific studies to this point.

Vitamin C (ascorbic acid) enhances iron absorption by keeping iron in its most absorbable form, especially as the mineral travels through the alkaline environment of the small intestine. A vitamin C intake of 75 milligrams or more at a meal significantly increases iron absorption. Increasing intake of vitamin C-rich foods is beneficial for those with poor iron status. Iron deficiency anemia is common in the United States and is the number one worldwide nutritional deficiency.

Vitamin C is vital for the function of the immune system, especially for the activity of certain cells in the immune system. Thus, disease states that increase the need for immune function can increase the need for vitamin C. It is unknown if this increased need is greater than the RDA. Partly on the basis of this observation, Nobel laureate Dr. Linus Pauling, claimed that supplementation with large doses of vitamin C could combat the common cold. In the 1970s he advocated the consumption of at least 1000 milligrams of vitamin C daily. As a result of the popularity of his books and the respectability of his scientific credentials, millions of North Americans supplement their diets with vitamin C.

Does vitamin C reliably and effectively function against the likelihood of developing an upper respiratory infection? Numerous well-designed, double-blind studies have failed to show that vitamin C prevents colds, though it does appear to reduce the duration of symptoms by a day or so. The effect of vitamin C on cold symptoms may be due to a general role in stimulating immune function and its ability to increase the breakdown of histamine. The reaction of vitamin C with the oxidized products formed in upper respiratory infection minimizes the inflammatory effects of these oxidized products and therefore may reduce the severity of these infections.

Food Sources of Vitamin C

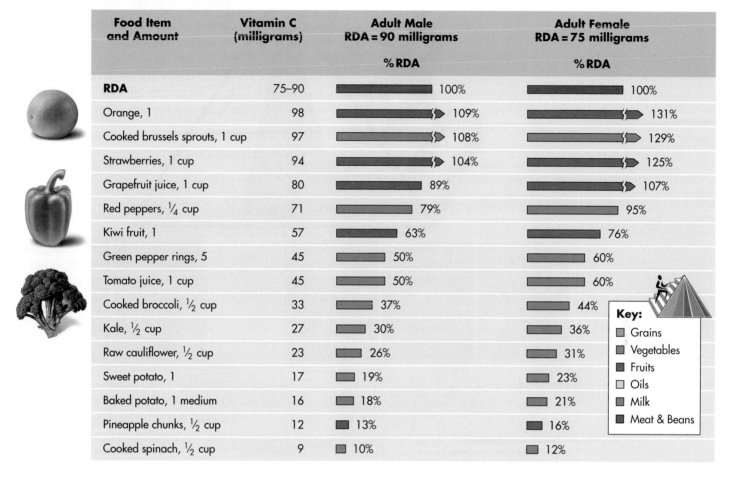

Food Item and Amount	Vitamin C (milligrams)	Adult Male RDA = 90 milligrams %RDA	Adult Female RDA = 75 milligrams %RDA
RDA	75–90	100%	100%
Orange, 1	98	109%	131%
Cooked brussels sprouts, 1 cup	97	108%	129%
Strawberries, 1 cup	94	104%	125%
Grapefruit juice, 1 cup	80	89%	107%
Red peppers, ¼ cup	71	79%	95%
Kiwi fruit, 1	57	63%	76%
Green pepper rings, 5	45	50%	60%
Tomato juice, 1 cup	45	50%	60%
Cooked broccoli, ½ cup	33	37%	44%
Kale, ½ cup	27	30%	36%
Raw cauliflower, ½ cup	23	26%	31%
Sweet potato, 1	17	19%	23%
Baked potato, 1 medium	16	18%	21%
Pineapple chunks, ½ cup	12	13%	16%
Cooked spinach, ½ cup	9	10%	12%

Key:
- Grains
- Vegetables
- Fruits
- Oils
- Milk
- Meat & Beans

FIGURE 9-8 ▶ Food sources of Vitamin C compared to the RDA for adult males and females.

The percent of vitamin C absorbed from usual dietary intakes (60 to 100 milligrams/day) is 80% to 90%. Most vitamin C consumed in large doses in supplements ends up in the feces or the urine. Only a small fraction of such large doses can be used. The kidneys start rapidly excreting vitamin C when intakes exceed 100 milligrams per day. As the amount ingested increases, the percent absorbed decreases precipitously. Absorption efficiency decreases to approximately 50% when 1000 milligrams per day are ingested and 20% when 6000 milligrams are ingested daily.

Vitamin C Sources and Needs

Major sources of vitamin C are citrus fruits, strawberries, green peppers, cauliflower, broccoli, cabbage, papayas, and romaine lettuce (Fig. 9-8). Ready-to-eat breakfast cereals, potatoes, and fortified fruit drinks are also good sources of vitamin C (Fig. 9-9). The five to nine servings of fruit and vegetables from the Food Guide Pyramid can easily provide enough vitamin C. Vitamin C is rapidly lost in processing and cooking as it is unstable in the presence of heat, iron, copper, or oxygen, and is water soluble. When fruits and vegetables are boiled for an extended time, much of the vitamin C is destroyed or leached out of the food and found in the often discarded water.

The adult RDA of vitamin C is 75 to 90 milligrams per day. The Daily Value used on food and supplement labels is 60 milligrams. Tobacco users need to add an extra 35 milligrams per day to the RDA. The toxic by-products of cigarette smoke and the oxidizing agents found in tobacco products increase the need for the antioxidant effects of vitamin C. Average daily

Grains	Vegetables	Fruits	Oils	Milk	Meat & Beans
• Fortified break- fast cereals	• Tomatoes • Potatoes • Cauliflower • Green vegetables	• Citrus fruits • Pineapple • Strawberries	• None	• None	• None

FIGURE 9-9 ▶ Sources of Vitamin C from MyPyramid. The height of the background color (none, 1/3, 2/3, or completely covered) within each group in the pyramid indicates the average nutrient density for Vitamin C in the group. Overall, the vegetables group and the fruits group contain many foods that are nutrient-dense sources of Vitamin C. With regard to physical activity, Vitamin C has no primary role in the related energy metabolism per se, but likely limits some oxidant damage during such endeavors.

consumption of vitamin C in the United States is 70 to 100 milligrams. Nutrition experts who advocate increased consumption of vitamin C recommend intakes of about 200 milligrams per day. This amount can be obtained through consumption of additional amounts of vegetables and fruit. People at risk for vitamin C deficiency are alcoholics who consume nutrient-poor diets and some older persons with inadequate food intakes.

Upper Level for Vitamin C

The Upper Level (UL) of vitamin C is 2000 milligrams. Regular consumption of more than 2000 milligrams per day may cause stomach inflammation and diarrhea. Ingestion of large amounts of vitamin C supplements is discouraged in people predisposed to kidney stones and people who absorb too much iron or have excessive iron stores. High doses of vitamin C may interfere with medical tests for diabetes or blood in the feces. Physicians may misdiagnose conditions when large doses of vitamin C are consumed without their knowledge.

CONCEPT CHECK

Vitamin C functions as an antioxidant by donating electrons that chemically stabilize free radicals. Vitamin C also regenerates vitamin E after vitamin E has stabilized free radicals. Vitamin C is also required for the synthesis of collagen, and neurotransmitters. A vitamin C deficiency causes scurvy, marked by many changes in the skin and gums, because of reduced collagen synthesis. Vitamin C also modestly improves iron absorption and is involved in the synthesis of certain hormones. Many fruits and vegetables are good sources of vitamin C. Fresh or lightly cooked foods are the best sources because loss of vitamin C in cooking can be high.

VITAMIN A

Vitamin A was the first fat-soluble vitamin to be recognized as an important constituent of food essential for human health. A deficiency and toxicity of this vitamin can cause severe problems. In addition, there is a narrow range of optimal intakes between these two states. Vitamin A has many important functions in the body. The best known and most clearly understood is its role in vision. Vitamin A may have antioxidant functions in the body; however the precursors of vitamin A have profound antioxidant properties, therefore both of these nutrients are discussed in this chapter.

Functions of Vitamin A

Vision. The link between Vitamin A and night vision has been known since ancient Egyptian times when juice extracted from liver was used as a cure for **night blindness.** Vitamin A performs important functions in light-dark vision and, to a lesser extent, color vision. Light entering the back of the eye reaches a lining called the **retina.** The retina consists of rods, cones, and nerve cells. Rods detect black and white and are responsible for night vision. Cones are responsible for color vision. Rods and cones require vitamin A for normal function. One form of vitamin A (retinal) allows certain cells in the eye to adjust from dim light (such as after seeing the headlines of an oncoming car) (Fig. 9-10). Without sufficient dietary vitamin A, the cells in the eye cannot quickly readjust to dim light. This condition is known as night blindness.

Night blindness A vitamin A-deficiency disorder that results in loss of the ability to see under low-light conditions.

Retina A light-sensitive lining in the back of the eye. It contains retinal.

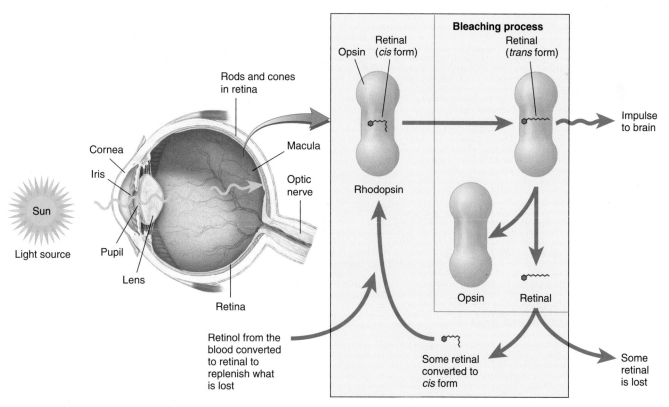

FIGURE 9-10 ▶ Vitamin A functions to maintain vision. Light enters the eye through the cornea, and lens, and hits the retina. The light reacts with vitamin A containing rhodopsin stored in the rod cells of the retina, which allows us to see black-and-white images. The retinal is cleaned from the rhodopsin (bleaching) which stimulates an electrical impulse to the brain, a new molecule of vitamin A combines with opsin to regenerate rhodopsin.

FIGURE 9-11 ▶ Vitamin A deficiency that eventually led to blindness. Note the severe effects on this eye. This problem is commonly seen today in southeast Asia.

Xerophthalmia Hardening of the cornea and drying of the surface of the eye, which can result in blindness.

If vitamin A deficiency progresses, the cells that line the cornea of the eye (the clear window of the eye) lose the ability to produce mucus. The eye then becomes dry. Eventually, dirt particles scratch the dry surface of the eye, leading to blindness. This disease is called **xerophthalmia,** which means dry eye. Xerophthalmia can progress to the stage where there is an accumulation of dead cells and secretions on the surface of the eye. This condition is called Bitot's spots (Fig. 9-11).

Vitamin A deficiency is the leading cause of blindness worldwide (Fig. 9-12). North Americans are at little risk because of good diets. However, poor vitamin A intakes, low-fat intakes that do not allow for sufficient vitamin A absorption, and low stores of vitamin A lessen the ability of children to meet high needs during rapid childhood growth. Hundreds of thousands of children in developing nations, especially Asia, become blind each year because of vitamin A deficiency. Some of these children ultimately die from infections. Worldwide attempts to reduce this problem have included giving large doses of vitamin A twice yearly and fortifying sugar, margarine, and monosodium glutamate with vitamin A. These food vehicles are used because they are commonly consumed by the populations of less-developed nations. This effort has proven effective in some countries.

Health of Other Cells. Vitamin A maintains the health of cells that line internal and external surfaces of the lungs, intestines, stomach, vagina, urinary tract, and bladder, as well as those of the eyes and skin. These cells (called epithelial cells) serve as important barriers to bacterial infection. One form of vitamin A (retinoic acid) is required for immature epithelial cells to develop into mature fully functional epithelial cells. As just noted for the eye, some epithelial cells secrete mucus, a needed lubricant. Without vitamin A, mucus-forming cells deteriorate and no longer synthesize mucus.

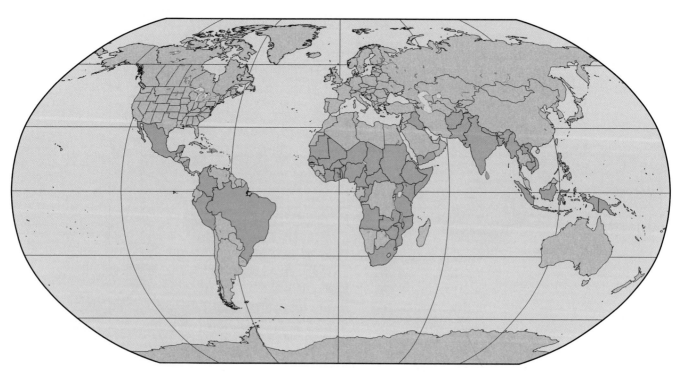

FIGURE 9-12 ▶ Areas of the world where vitamin A represents a major malnutrition problem. Every year 250,000 to 500,000 children become blind due to vitamin A deficiency.

Source: WHO

Vitamin A deficiency also causes insufficient mucus production in the intestines and lung cells and poor health of cells in general. Hyperkeratosis, a condition in which skin cells produce too much keratin occurs as a result of vitamin A deficiency. The excessive keratin in these skin cells causes the skin to be hard and dry. Vitamin A deficiency also reduces the activity of certain immune system cells. Together, these effects leave the vitamin A-deficient person at great risk for infections. For many years, vitamin A has been dubbed the "anti-infection" vitamin.

Growth, Development, and Reproduction. Vitamin A participates in the processes of growth, development, and reproduction in several ways. This role has been best illustrated in children experiencing growth retardation as a result of deficiencies of this vitamin and in whom supplementation with vitamin A has been shown to increase their growth. At the genetic level, vitamin A binds to receptors on DNA to increase synthesis of a variety of proteins. Some of these proteins are required for growth, such as bone growth. During early fetal growth, vitamin A functions in the differentiation and maturation of cells, which ultimately form tissues and organs. In laboratory animals, another consequence of vitamin A deficiency is an inability to reproduce.

Cancer Prevention. Vitamin A has been shown to play an important role in immune function. Vitamin A-deficient animals and humans have an increased infection rate and when they are supplemented with vitamin A the immune response improves. Vitamin A plays a role in cellular differentiation and embryonic development. Numerous studies have found that diets rich in vitamin A or **provitamin A** carotinoids are associated with a lower risk of skin, lung, bladder, and breast cancers. Still, because of the potential for toxicity, unsupervised use of megadose vitamin A supplementation to reduce cancer risk is not advised. More about the effects of carotenoids on the incidence of cancer is covered later in this chapter.

Provitamin A A substance that can be converted into vitamin A.

Vitamin A Analogs for Acne. The acne medication tretinoin (Retin-A) is made of one analog form of vitamin A. It is used as a topical treatment (applied to the skin) for acne. It appears to work by altering cell activity in the skin (gene expression role discussed earlier). Another derivative of vitamin A, 13-*cis* retinoic acid (Accutane), is an oral drug used to treat serious acne. Taking high doses of vitamin A would not be safe. Even Accutane, a less potentially toxic form, can induce toxic symptoms, as well as birth defects in the offspring of women using during pregnancy. A pregnancy test is required before Accutane is prescribed to women.

Vitamin A Sources and Needs

Preformed vitamin A is found in liver, fish, fish oils, fortified milk and yogurt, and eggs (Fig. 9-14). Margarine is also fortified with Vitamin A. About 65% of the vitamin A in the typical North American diet comes from preformed vitamin A sources, whereas provitamin A dominates in the diet among poor people in other parts of the world.

The RDA for vitamin A is 700 to 900 micrograms of retinol activity equivalents (RAEs). These RAE units take into account the activity of both preformed vitamin A and the three carotenoids that also yield vitamin A in humans. The total RAE value for a food is calculated by adding the concentration of preformed vitamin A to the amount of provitamin A carotenoids in the food that will be converted to vitamin A. The Daily Value used on food and supplement labels is 1000 micrograms (5000 IU).

▲ Vegetables are rich sources of provitamin A carotenoids.

Food Sources of Vitamin A

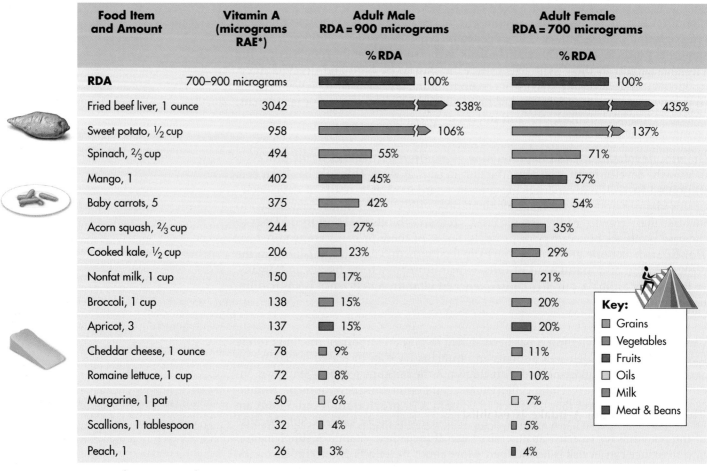

Food Item and Amount	Vitamin A (micrograms RAE*)	Adult Male RDA = 900 micrograms %RDA		Adult Female RDA = 700 micrograms %RDA	
RDA	700–900 micrograms		100%		100%
Fried beef liver, 1 ounce	3042		338%		435%
Sweet potato, ½ cup	958		106%		137%
Spinach, ⅔ cup	494		55%		71%
Mango, 1	402		45%		57%
Baby carrots, 5	375		42%		54%
Acorn squash, ⅔ cup	244		27%		35%
Cooked kale, ½ cup	206		23%		29%
Nonfat milk, 1 cup	150		17%		21%
Broccoli, 1 cup	138		15%		20%
Apricot, 3	137		15%		20%
Cheddar cheese, 1 ounce	78		9%		11%
Romaine lettuce, 1 cup	72		8%		10%
Margarine, 1 pat	50		6%		7%
Scallions, 1 tablespoon	32		4%		5%
Peach, 1	26		3%		4%

Key:
- ▢ Grains
- ▢ Vegetables
- ▢ Fruits
- ▢ Oils
- ▢ Milk
- ▢ Meat & Beans

* Retinol activity equivalents

FIGURE 9-13 ▶ Food sources of vitamin A compared to the RDA for adult males and females.

FIGURE 9-14 ▶ Sources of vitamin A from MyPyramid. The height of the background color (none, 1/3, 2/3, or completely covered) within each group in the pyramid indicates the average nutrient density for Vitamin A in that group. Overall, the vegetables group, fruits group and certain choices in the meat & beans group provide the richest sources. The grains group contains some foods that are nutrient-dense sources of vitamin A because they are fortified with the vitamin. With regard to physical activity, vitamin A plays no specific role per se in such endeavors.

MyPyramid: Sources of Vitamin A

Grains	Vegetables	Fruits	Oils	Milk	Meat & Beans
• Fortified breakfast cereals • Fortified meal replacement bars	• Carrots • Broccoli • Spinach • Squash • Sweet potatoes	• Peaches • Apricots • Cantaloupes • Mangoes • Papayas	• Some forms of palm oil • Fish oil	• Fortified milk • Fortified yogurt • Cheese	• Liver • Eggs • Fish

MAKING DECISIONS

Most nutrient amounts in foods, including vitamin A, were formerly expressed in less accurate international units (IUs). Some food and supplement labels still show the IU for vitamin A. To compare the older IU standards to current RAE recommendations, assume that for any preformed vitamin A in a food or added to food, 3.3 IU = 1RAE. The same is true for any beta-carotene added to foods.

There is no easy way to convert IU units to RAE units for foods that naturally contain provitamin A carotenoids, such as carrots, spinach, and apricots. A general rule is to divide the IU units for foods containing carotenoids by 2, then divide the result by 3.3 as just described.

Average intakes of vitamin A for North American adult women meet the RDA. Most adults in North America have liver reserves of vitamin A three to five times higher than needed to provide good health. Thus, the use of vitamin A supplements by most people is unnecessary. Deficient vitamin A status in North America may be seen in preschool children who do not eat enough vegetables. The urban poor, older adults, and people with alcoholism or liver disease (which limits vitamin A storage) can also show diminished vitamin A status, especially with respect to stores. Finally, children and adults with severe fat malabsorption may also experience vitamin A deficiency.

Upper Level for Vitamin A

The UL for vitamin A intake is established at 3000 micrograms of preformed vitamin A (3000 RAE or 10,000 IU) per day for adult men and women. This is based on the increases in birth defects and liver toxicity that accompany intakes in excess of 3000 micrograms of vitamin A per day. Above the Upper Level, other possible side effects include an increased risk of hip fracture and poor pregnancy outcomes.

During the early months of pregnancy, a high intake of preformed vitamin A is especially dangerous because it may cause fetal malformations and spontaneous abortions. This is because vitamin A binds to DNA and thus influences cell development. Food and Drug Administration (FDA) recommends that women of childbearing age limit their overall intake of preformed vitamin A to a total of about 100% of the Daily Value (1000 micrograms REA or 5000 IU). In addition, it is also important to limit consumption of rich food sources, such as liver. These precautions also apply to women who may possibly become pregnant. Because vitamin A is stored in the body for long periods, women who ingest large amounts during the months before pregnancy place their fetus at risk.

CONCEPT CHECK

Vitamin A has diverse functions. The binding of a form of vitamin A to DNA can influence cell growth and differentiation. Vitamin A is important for maintaining vision and epithelial tissues, reproduction, growth, and ensuring proper function of the immune system. The role of vitamin A as an antioxidant is questionable. Vitamin A in the diet comes in two forms: **retinoids** (preformed vitamin A) and certain carotenoids (provitamin A). Major food sources of vitamin A include liver, carrots, eggs, tomatoes, milk, and many vegetables. North Americans most at risk for poor vitamin A status are preschool children and alcoholics. Large doses of retinoids can be toxic, even at chronic dosages only about two to four times the RDA, especially during early pregnancy. Symptoms of toxicity include birth defects, poor vision, and liver damage. Deficiency symptoms include poor growth, increased infection rates, and night blindness.

Retinoids Chemical forms of preformed vitamin A; one source is animal foods.

CAROTENOIDS

Plants contain pigments called carotenoids, which can be turned into vitamin A as needed. Thus, they can be termed provitamin A. Only three of the more than 600 carotenoids found in nature are known to serve as provitamin A in humans, but there may be more. Beta-carotene, the orange-yellow pigment in carrots, is the most potent form of provitamin A. The other two carotenoids that can be converted into vitamin A are alpha-carotene and beta-cryptoxanthin. Other carotenoids that may play a role in human health but are not vitamin A precursors include lycopene, zeaxanthin, and lutein. These carotenoids are called phytochemicals. Beta-carotene is split in half by cells in the body to form two molecules of retinal. The conversion of the provitamin A carotenoids into vitamin A is not an efficient process. In addition, the absorption of these carotenoids is not as efficient as the absorption of vitamin A. Therefore, 12 milligrams of provitamin A is equivalent to 1 milligram of vitamin A. Together, preformed vitamin A from animal sources and provitamin A carotenoids make up what is called vitamin A.

▲ Provitamin A carotenoids are the safest way to meet vitamin A needs. Brightly colored fruits and vegetables are typically good food sources of carotenoids.

Functions of the Carotenoids

Vision. Age-related macular degeneration is a leading cause of legal blindness among North American adults over the age of 65 (Fig. 9-15). The disease is associated with changes in the macular area of the eye, which provides the most detailed vision. Age, smoking, and genetics are risk factors. The macula contains the carotenoids lutein and zeaxanthin in high enough concentrations to impart a yellow color. In one study, the higher the total number of carotenoids (beta-carotene, lutein, and zeaxanthin) consumed in the diet, the lower was the risk for age-related macular degeneration.

These carotenoids may also decrease the risk of cataracts in the eyes. Although these are interesting hypotheses, consumption of fruits and vegetables high in carotenoids may reduce the risk for these eye disorders rather than the intake of these specific carotenoids. Multivitamin and mineral supplements formulated for older adults (e.g., Centrum Silver™) are being marketed as a source of lutein.

(a)   (b)

FIGURE 9-15 ▶ (a) Age related degeneration of the macular region. (b) The blurry center of the image simulates the vision of a person with macular degeneration

◀ Microscopic image of cancerous lung more research is needed to understand the relationship of carotenoids and cancer prevention.

Cardiovascular Disease Prevention. Carotenoids may play a role in preventing cardiovascular disease in persons at high risk. This may be linked to carotenoids ability to inhibit the oxidation of low-density lipoproteins. Until definitive studies are complete, many scientists recommend that we consume a total of at least five servings of a combination of fruits and vegetables per day as part of an overall effort to reduce the risk of cardiovascular disease.

Cancer Prevention. Carotenoids by themselves also may prevent cancer, acting again as antioxidants. Population studies show that regular consumption of foods rich in carotenoids decreases the risk of lung and oral cancers. The carotenoid lycopene may decrease skin cancer risk. In contrast, recall from Chapter 1 that studies from the United States and Finland failed to show a reduction in lung cancer in male smokers and nonsmokers given supplements of the carotenoid beta-carotene for five or more years. In fact, beta-carotene use in male smokers increased the number of lung cancer cases compared with control groups. No comparable studies have been done with women. Although further research continues, most researchers are convinced that beta-carotene supplementation offers no protection against cancer. Again, the best advice is to rely on food sources for this or any other carotenoids.

Cancer of the **prostate gland** is one of the most common cancers among North American men. The dietary carotenoid lycopene (the red pigment found in tomatoes, watermelon, and several other fruits) seems to protect against this type of cancer. The proposed biological role of lycopene again appears to be that of an antioxidant. Some food companies (e.g., Campbell Soup Company), are even marketing their products as important sources of lycopene.

Prostate gland A solid, chestnut-shaped organ surrounding the first part of the urinary tract in the male. The prostate gland secretes substances into the semen.

Carotenoid Sources and Needs

The provitamin A carotenoids are mainly found in dark green and yellow-orange vegetables and some fruits. Carrots, spinach and other greens, winter squash, sweet potatoes, broccoli, mangoes, cantaloupe, peaches, and apricots are examples of such sources. Many vegetables are good sources of beta-carotene and the other two provitamin A carotenoids. Beta-carotene accounts for some of the orange color of carrots. In vegetables such as broccoli, this yellow-orange color is masked by dark-green chlorophyll pigments. Still, green vegetables contain provitamin A. Green, leafy vegetables, such as spinach and kale, have high concentrations of lutein and zeaxanthin. Tomato juice and other tomato products, such as pizza sauce, contain significant amounts of lycopene. In contrast to many other nutrients, cooking food improves the digestion and subsequent absorption of the carotenoids because they are tightly bound to constituents within the plant cell. Cooking helps to release them and make them more bioavailable. There is no separate RDA for beta-carotene or any of the other provitamin A carotenoids.

Upper Level for Carotenoids

The ingestion of large amounts of vitamin A-yielding carotenoids does not cause toxic effects. A high carotenoid concentration in the blood can occur if someone consumes large amounts of carrots, takes pills containing beta-carotene (more than 30 milligrams daily), or if infants eat a great deal of squash. This can turn the skin yellow-orange. The palms of the hands and soles of the feet, in particular, become colored. This condition does not appear to cause harm and disappears when carotenoid intake decreases. Dietary carotenoids do not produce toxic effects because (1) their rate of conversion into vitamin A is relatively slow and regulated; and (2) the efficiency of carotenoid absorption from the small intestine decreases markedly as oral intake increases.

CONCEPT CHECK

The carotenoids are a chemically similar group of over 600 compounds found in plants. Three carotenoids can be converted into vitamin A by the body (provitamin A). Carotenoids act as antioxidants and have been shown to have beneficial effects in the prevention of oxidative damage and subsequent development of macular degeneration, cardiovascular disease, and cancer. Many fruits and vegetables are good sources of the carotenoids. No toxicity of deficiency symptoms has been reported.

PHYTOCHEMICALS

In addition to the approximately 45 essential nutrients, there are thousands of other substances in food. For many years, much of the nutrition research concentrated on gaining knowledge about carbohydrates, lipids, proteins, vitamins, and minerals. There is interest in gaining knowledge about the potential health benefits of other substances found in food. Foods that are sources of the chemicals that provide health benefits beyond being dietary essential nutrients are termed **functional foods.** These chemicals are placed into one of two categories: **zoochemicals,** health-promoting compounds found in animal food, and phytochemicals, health-promoting compounds found in plant food. Phytochemicals are responsible for the colors observed in plants and their unique flavors. Improved health has been shown by consuming diets high in plant foods, so most of the nutrition research on functional foods has focused on phytochemicals. Some of the phytochemicals being studied include allicin, carotenoids, dithiolthione, ellagic acid, flavonoids, glucarates, indoles, isothiocynates, lignans, phthalides, phytoestrogens, polyacetylenes, saponins, stanols, and terpenes. Examples of foods that contain rich sources of phytochemicals include apples, celery, citrus fruit, cruciferous vegetables, garlic, green tea, soybeans, tomatoes, whole grains, and a number of herbs and spices. Many individual foods contain hundreds of different phytochemicals.

Functional foods Foods that have health benefits beyond basic nutrition.

Zoochemicals Chemicals found in animal products that have health protective actions.

Functions of Phytochemicals

Phytochemicals are not essential nutrients because a deficiency disease is not observed when they are removed from the diet. The phytochemicals cannot be synthesized in the body, therefore we must ingest them from food. Although the study of the metabolic actions of phytochemicals is relatively new, numerous functions of phytochemicals have been elucidated. Phytochemicals have the following functions:

- Act as antioxidants
- Inhibit the initiation and proliferation of cancer and stimulate spontaneous cell death
- Alter the absorption, production, and metabolism of cholesterol
- Mimic or inhibit hormones and enzymes
- Decrease the formation of blood clots

A number of phytochemicals are strong antioxidants. As mentioned in the previous section, beta-carotene has been shown to have powerful antioxidant properties. Other carotenoids prevalent in foods that have antioxidant properties include alpha-carotene, beta-cryptoxanthin, lycopene, lutein, and zeaxanthin. Over 600 carotenoids are found in plants, and their potential health benefits have yet to be determined. Lycopene, a red carotenoid found in tomatoes and strawberries, appears to have stronger antioxidant properties than beta-carotene. Rich sources of flavonoids are blueberries, chocolate, citrus fruit, and raspberries. Flavonoids function as antioxidants by inhibiting the oxidation of cholesterol, an initial step in the development of athlerogenic plaque. Not all of the naturally occurring phytochemicals in foods are beneficial to health. Plants produce chemicals that act as toxins that have important insecticide properties.

There are no specific dietary recommendations for the amount of phytochemicals that should be consumed. Following the recommendations in MyPyramid will provide a diet rich in phytochemicals (at least five servings of fruits and vegetables). In the United States, average consumption of fruits and vegetables falls far short of these recommendations. Media reports of the potential benefits of phytochemicals have stimulated a plethora of dietary supplements containing them. The evidence that these phytochemicals extracted from foods has health benefits is minimal. The digestion, absorption, and use of phytochemicals depends on the presence of other nutrients and phytochemicals consumed. Many of the phytochemicals interact with other phytochemicals and nutrients, which ultimately influence their ability to function. Therefore it is recommended that foods rather than supplements be consumed to ingest these powerful substances.

SELENIUM (Se)

Selenium is a trace mineral that exists in many readily absorbed chemical forms. Trace minerals are required by the body in an amount of 100 milligrams or less per day or present in the body in an amount of 0.01% or less of body weight. Selenium's best understood role is aiding the activity of the enzyme (glutathione peroxidase) that participates in reducing the damage that electron-seeking, free-radicals can do.

Glutathione peroxidase chemically converts potentially damaging peroxides (hydrogen peroxide, for example) into water. Selenium also functions by activating thyroid hormone and immune function.

Low blood levels of selenium have been linked with an increased incidence of some forms of cancer, specifically prostate cancer. Although selenium could prove to have a role in prevention of cancers, it is premature to recommend megadose selenium supplementation for this purpose. Animal studies in this area are conflicting; studies with humans using supplemental intakes of 200 micrograms per day are under way to help clarify what role, if any, selenium plays in cancer prevention.

Selenium deficiency symptoms in humans include muscle pain and wasting and a certain form of heart damage. In some areas of China, people develop characteristic muscle and heart disorders associated with inadequate selenium intake. Other factors probably also contribute.

Selenium Sources and Needs

Fish, meat (especially organ meats), shellfish, and eggs are good animal sources of selenium (Fig. 9-16). Grains and seeds grown in soils containing selenium are good plant sources. Major selenium contributors to the adult diet are animal and grain products. We eat a varied diet of foods supplied from many geographic areas, so it is unlikely that low soil selenium in a few locations will mean inadequate selenium in our diets.

The RDA for selenium is 55 micrograms per day for adults. This intake maximizes the activity of selenium-dependent enzymes. The Daily Value used on food and supplement labels is 70 micrograms. Adults meet the RDA, consuming on average 105 micrograms each day.

Upper Level Selenium

Selenium toxicity has not been reported from eating food. Supplementation for an extended period has been shown to be toxic. The UL for selenium is 400 micrograms per day for adults. This is based on overt signs of selenium toxicity, such as hair loss, weakness, and cirrhosis.

FIGURE 9-16 ▶ Food sources of selenium compared to the RDA.

Food Sources of Selenium

Food Item and Amount	Selenium (micrograms)	%RDA
RDA*	55	100%
Tuna, 3 ounces	68	124%
Sirloin steak, 5 ounces	47	85%
Lean ham, 3 ounces	42	76%
Clams, 3 ounces	41	75%
Salmon, 3 ounces	40	73%
Egg noodles, 1 cup	35	64%
Chicken breast, 3 ounces	20	36%
Special K cereal, 1 cup	17	31%
Oat bran cereal, 1 cup	14	25%
Whole-wheat bread, 1 slice	10	18%
Cooked oatmeal, 1 cup	10	18%
White bread, 1 slice	9	16%
Raisin bran cereal, 1 cup	4	7%

Key:
- Grains
- Vegetables
- Fruits
- Oils
- Milk
- Meat & Beans

*For adults; See DRI table in the back of this book for gender-and age- specifc recommendations.

CONCEPT CHECK

Selenium activates an enzyme (glutathione peroxidase) that helps change electron-seeking free-radical (oxidizing) compounds into less toxic compounds so these do not attack and break down cell membranes. Selenium also has an antioxidant function in the maintenance of the immune system and production of thyroid hormones. A selenium deficiency results in muscle and heart disorders. Animal products and grains are good selenium sources; however, the selenium content in plants depends on the selenium concentration in the soil. The misuse of selenium supplements can readily lead to toxicity. Toxic symptoms include brittle hair and nails, vomiting, and liver damage.

CASE STUDY

Choosing a Dietary Supplement

Amy works the predawn shift as a baker at a popular bistro. Amy is also a full-time student, and the combination of taking a full course load at college and working early hours while her friends are sleeping has created a lot of stress for her. Amy's many commitments also make it important that she not become ill. Recently, one of her co-workers suggested that she take Nutramega supplements to help prevent colds, flu, and other illnesses. The product's label suggests that Nutramega helps prevent such problems, especially those associated with the changing of seasons. The label recommends taking two to three tablets daily for health maintenance and two to three tablets every 3 hours at the first sign of feeling ill. Amy looks at the Supplement Facts label on the bottle and finds that each tablet contains (as percent of the DV): 33% for vitamin A (three-quarters is preformed vitamin A), 700% for vitamin C, 50% for zinc, and 10% for selenium. A month's supply costs about $50.

Answer the following questions and check your responses in Appendix A.

1. Are there any health risks associated with taking the "maintenance" dose of two to three tablets per day? How does this dose compare with the Upper Tolerable Intake Levels for the four nutrients?

2. How many tablets would be taken per day if Amy was feeling ill?

   a. For Vitamin A, use the % Daily Value to calculate the micrograms RAE that would be in this larger dose. How does this compare to the UL for vitamin A?

   b. Use the % Daily Value to calculate the milligrams of vitamin C in this larger dose. How does this compare to the UL for vitamin C?

   c. Use the % Daily Value to calculate the milligrams of zinc in this larger dose. How does this compare to the UL for zinc?

   d. Use the % Daily Value to calculate the micrograms of selenium in this larger dose. How does this compare to the UL for selenium?

   e. Does the recommended dosage of any of these nutrients pose any health risks?

3. Does the cost of this supplement seem reasonable? How does it compare to the cost of a typical multivitamin/mineral supplement available at your local drug store?

4. Should Amy be concerned about meeting her nutrient needs? Does the type of stress she is under increase her nutrient needs?

5. After studying Chapter 9, what diet and supplement advice would you offer to Amy?

▲ Is a dietary supplement a safe way for Amy to prevent colds and the flu?

SUMMARY

1. Vitamins are carbon-containing compounds we need daily in small amounts from foods. They yield no energy directly, but many contribute to energy-yielding chemical reactions in the body and promote growth and development. Many vitamins act as coenzymes, which help enzymes function. Vitamins A, D, E, and K are fat soluble, whereas the B vitamins and vitamin C are water soluble.

2. Vitamin A is a family of compounds that includes several forms of preformed vitamin A. Three forms of carotenoids can also yield vitamin A; some also function as antioxidants. Vitamin A contributes to vision, immune function, and cell development. Vitamin A is found in liver and fish oils; carotenoids are especially plentiful in dark green and orange vegetables. Vitamin A can be toxic, even when taken at just three times the RDA for preformed vitamin A (the upper level). High vitamin A intakes are especially dangerous during pregnancy.

3. Vitamin E functions primarily as an antioxidant and is found in plant oils. By donating electrons to electron-seeking free radical (oxidizing) compounds, it neutralizes them. This effect shields cell membranes and red blood cells from breakdown. Claims are made about the curative powers of vitamin E but more information is needed before megadose vitamin E recommendations for healthy adults can be made with certainty. The Upper Level is set at about 50 times adult needs.

4. Vitamin C is a potent antioxidant and also functions to synthesize collagen, some hormones, and neurotransmitters. A vitamin C deficiency results in scurvy, evidenced by pinpoint hemorrhages in the skin, bleeding gums, and joint pain. Vitamin C also modestly enhances iron absorption. Fresh fruits and vegetables, especially citrus fruits, are good sources. A great amount of vitamin C is lost in cooking, therefore the diet should emphasize fresh or minimally cooked vegetables. Deficiencies can occur in people with alcoholism and those whose diets lack sufficient fruits and vegetable intakes. Smoking increases the possibility of vitamin C deficiency. The Upper Level is set at about 20 times adult needs.

5. Taking a multivitamin and mineral supplement to help meet nutrient needs is recommended by some experts, while other experts suggest that only some in the population need such supplementation. Taking many nutrient supplements can lead to nutrient-related toxicity, so any such use should be carefully considered. The clearest evidence is for a diet rich in fruits and vegetables and whole-grain breads and cereals, not reliance on supplements.

STUDY QUESTIONS

1. What is the difference between reduction and oxidation? How do free radicals arise?

2. Identify two beneficial roles of free radicals in the body.

3. Name three micronutrients involved in enzyme systems that quench free radicals. Identify at least one good food source of each of these micronutrients.

4. Name three micronutrients that act as antioxidants by donating electrons or hydrogen atoms to unstable free radicals. Identify at least one good food source of each of these micronutrients.

5. What is the role of vitamin E in the prevention of cardiovascular disease? Should people at risk for cardiovascular disease take vitamin E supplements?

6. How would you determine which fruits and vegetables displayed in the produce section of your supermarket are likely to provide plenty of carotenoids?

7. Describe how vitamin A functions as an antioxidant.

8. Other than its role as an antioxidant, describe three functions of vitamin C.

9. Identify one similarity in the antioxidant roles of vitamin E and vitamin C. Describe one way in which these two vitamins are different in their antioxidant activities. How do vitamin E and vitamin C work together?

10. Is it necessary for North Americans to consume a great excess of vitamin C to avoid the possibility of a deficiency? Do vitamin C intakes well above the RDA have any negative consequences?

CHECK YOUR KNOWLEDGE

Answers to the following multiple choice questions are in Appendix A.

1. Vitamin E functions as a(n)
   a. coenzyme.
   b. antioxidant.
   c. hormone.
   d. peroxide.

2. A deficiency of vitamin A can lead to the disease called
   a. xerophthalmia.
   b. osteomalacia.
   c. scurvy.
   d. pellagra.

3. A high intake of vitamin E can
   a. inhibit vitamin K metabolism.
   b. result in lead poisoning.
   c. inhibit copper absorption.
   d. cause baldness.

4. Vitamin C is necessary for the production of
   a. stomach acid.
   b. collagen.
   c. hormones.
   d. clotting factors.

5. Damage caused by free radicals is thought to contribute to
   a. atherosclerosis.
   b. diabetes.
   c. Alzheimer's disease.
   d. All of the above.

6. Good food sources of vitamin E include
   a. meats.
   b. white bread.
   c. nuts.
   d. All of the above.

7. Which of the following micronutrients is NOT involved in immune function?
   a. Vitamin A
   b. Vitamin C
   c. Vitamin E
   d. None of the above.

8. Excessive intake of preformed vitamin A can lead to
   a. birth defects.
   b. night blindness.
   c. xerophthalmia.
   d. decreased blood clotting.

9. Phytochemicals are
   a. a new type of vitamin.
   b. plant chemicals that protect health.
   c. plant pigments that may be converted into vitamin A.
   d. animal chemicals that protect health.

10. Selenium is an antioxidant micronutrient because it
    a. donates electrons to free radicals.
    b. accepts electrons from free radicals.
    c. aids glutathione peroxidase activity.
    d. enhances the absorption of vitamin E.

FURTHER READINGS

1. Food and Nutrition Board, Institute of Medicine: *Dietary Reference Intakes for vitamin C, vitamin E, selenium, and carotenoids.* Washington, DC: The National Academy Press, 2000.

   The functions of antioxidant nutrients, how the RDA and related standards were determined, and deficiency and toxicity symptoms are explained. This is the definitive report by the panel of experts on nutrient needs for dietary antioxidants.

2. Lee I and others: Vitamin E in the primary prevention of cardiovascular disease and cancer: The women's health study: A randomized controlled trial. *Journal of the American Medical Association* 294:56, 2005.

   The data from this large trial indicated that 600 IU of natural-source vitamin E taken every other day provided no overall benefit for major cardiovascular events or cancer. These data do not support recommending vitamin E supplementation for cardiovascular disease or cancer prevention among healthy women, but more research is warranted, because a decrease in sudden cardiac death was seen in a subset of older women in this study.

3. Lichtenstein AH and Russell RM: Essential nutrients: Food or supplement? Where should the emphasis be? *Journal of the American Medical Association* 294:351, 2005.

   There is insufficient evidence to justify a shift in public health policy from one that emphasizes a food-based diet to fulfill nutrient requirements and promote optimal health to one that emphasizes dietary supplementation. Targeted nutrient supplementation is appropriate in some cases, however, as reviewed by these authors.

4. NIH State-of-the-Science Panel: National Institutes of Health state-of-the-science conference statement: Multivitamin/mineral supplements and chronic disease prevention. *Annals of Internal Medicine* 145(5):364, 2006.

   This report is the result of a thorough assessment of current medical knowledge of multivitamin/mineral supplements (MVMs). The effectiveness and safety of MVMs in relation to chronic disease prevention was systemically evaluated. The panel found few rigorous studies on which to base conclusions and recommendations. Only a few trials of vitamins and minerals demonstrate beneficial effects for the prevention of chronic disease, including increased bone mineral density and decreased fractures in postmenopausal women who use calcium and vitamin D supplements. In contrast, several other studies provide disturbing evidence of risk, such as increased lung cancer with beta-carotene use among smokers. The report concludes that the present evidence is

   insufficient to recommend either for or against the use of MVMs by the American public to prevent chronic disease. This conclusion is important to remember because manufacturers of these products are not required to report adverse events, and the FDA has no regulatory authority to require labeling or to help inform the public of these issues and concerns.

5. Voutilainen S and others: Carotenoids and cardiovascular health. *American Journal of Clinical Nutrition* 83:1265, 2006.

   This report reviews the role of carotenoids in the prevention of heart disease. Although fruits and vegetables are recognized as having protective effects against cardiovascular disease, the role of a single group of compounds such as carotenoids cannot be ascertained. Therefore, the consumption of carotenoids in supplemental forms cannot be recommended.

6. Flores-Mateo G and others: Selenium and coronary heart disease: A meta-analysis. *American Journal of Clinical Nutrition* 84(4):762, 2006.

   The meta-analysis of studies of selenium and coronary heart disease show an inverse association between selenium concentrations and coronary heart disease risk in observational studies. The validity of this association is uncertain because the results of observational studies have been misleading for other antioxidants. Only a few randomized trials have addressed the efficacy of selenium supplementation on cardiovascular health and their findings are inconclusive. Large ongoing trials are needed to establish if low selenium concentrations are a cardiovascular disease risk factor. Therefore, selenium supplements are not recommended for cardiovascular disease prevention.

7. Bleys J and others: Vitamin-mineral supplementation and the progression of atherosclerosis: A meta-analysis of randomized controlled trials. *American Journal of Clinical Nutrition* 84(4):880, 2006.

   The results of previous studies suggest that antioxidant and B vitamin supplementation may prevent atherosclerosis. This meta-analysis showed no evidence of a protective effect of antioxidant or B vitamin supplements on the progression of atherosclerosis as measured by imaging techniques. These results provide an explanation for the lack of effect of these supplements on clinical cardiovascular health.

8. Johnson IT: Phytochemicals and cancer. *Proceedings of the Nutrition Society* 66:207, 2007.

   The author reviews current evidence on the roles of phytochemicals in the prevention of cancer, including a discussion of possible mechanisms of action. An important research need is to conduct in vivo studies, as in vitro studies may overestimate the bioavailability and overlook metabolism of phytochemicals.

9. Kaliora AC and others: Dietary antioxidants in preventing atherogenesis. *Atherosclerosis* 187:1, 2006.

   The role of oxidation in the development of cardiovascular disease is well accepted. This article reviews the evidence for antioxidant nutrients, including vitamin C, vitamin E, phytochemicals, and coenzyme Q10, in prevention of LDL oxidation and plaque formation. The authors highlight the anticipated importance of nutrigenomics in the prevention of cardiovascular disease.

10. Rayman MP. Selenium in cancer prevention: A review of the evidence and mechanism of action. *Proceedings of the Nutrition Society* 64:527, 2005.

    Adequate selenium intake has been implicated in prevention of many types of cancer, including prostate, esophageal, colorectal, and lung. This article provides a review of studies that lay the groundwork for the link between selenium and cancer, providing insight into potential mechanisms by which selenium exerts its protective effects.

11. Ryan-Harshman M and Aldoori W. The relevance of selenium to immunity, cancer, and infectious/inflammatory diseases. *Canadian Journal of Dietetic Practice and Research* 66:98, 2005.

    This review article examines the potential roles of selenium in the prevention of cancer, promotion of immune function, and treatment of infectious diseases. Particular attention is given to the individualized nutrient needs of at-risk populations, such as patients with HIV/AIDS.

12. Sebastian RS and others: Older adults who use vitamin/mineral supplements differ from nonusers in nutrient intake adequacy and dietary attitudes. *Journal of the American Dietetic Association* 107:1322, 2007.

    As reported in previous studies, those who use supplements typically have more nutritious diets than those who do not use supplements. In this study of older adults, dietary vitamin and mineral supplements were found to be useful in meeting requirements of nutrients such as vitamin E, folate, and magnesium. However, use of dietary supplements may increase risk for toxicity of some nutrients, particularly iron and preformed vitamin A. The authors concluded that dietary vitamin and mineral supplements are a useful addition to the diets of older adults, but that oversupplementation with iron and vitamin A should be avoided.

13. Singh U and others: Vitamin E, oxidative stress, and inflammation. *Annual Review of Nutrition* 25:151, 2005.

    Vitamin E has been promoted for the prevention of cardiovascular disease based on its antioxidant and anti-inflammatory functions. However, results of clinical studies of the effectiveness of vitamin E supplementation have been equivocal. The authors review the mechanisms by which vitamin E may promote cardiovascular health and suggest explanations for the contradictory results of previous studies. They suggest that alpha-tocopherol is the form of vitamin E that will prove most beneficial for at-risk populations.

14. Stimpson JP and others: Acculturation in the United States is associated with lower serum carotenoid levels: Third National Health and Nutrition Examination Survey. *Journal of the American Dietetic Association* 107:1218, 2007.

    Despite public health campaigns promoting fruit and vegetable consumption, intakes of fruits and vegetables remain below recommendations for the majority of Americans. This study showed that for Mexican-Americans, acculturation is associated with declines in fruit and vegetable intake, as reflected by declines in serum carotenoid levels. Among immigrant populations, targeted public health messages should focus on maintenance of existing positive dietary habits.

15. Timbo BB and others: Dietary supplements in a national survey: Prevalence of use and reports of adverse events. *Journal of the American Dietetic Association* 106:1966, 2006.

    Data from the U.S. Food and Drug Administration's Health and Diet Survey was used to examine dietary supplement use. As other authors have reported, dietary supplement use is on the rise, with 74% of noninstitutionalized adults using at least one dietary supplement during the last 12 months. The most popular supplements were multivitamin/mineral supplements. Users of dietary supplements tend to be white, women, and have higher income and education than nonusers. Many adults take supplements with prescription medications, which could lead to harmful interactions. Supplement users may not report their supplement use to their health care providers or may choose to use herbs or botanicals in place of prescribed medications. These findings highlight the importance of probing to learn about dietary supplement use in the health care setting.

16. Valko M and others: Free radicals and antioxidants in normal physiological functions and human disease. *International Journal of Biochemistry and Cell Biology* 39:44, 2007.

    Clearly, overproduction of free radicals has deleterious effects. However, free radicals do play important roles in normal human physiology. For example, free radicals are involved in cellular signaling pathways that protect the body against pathogens or identify and destroy tumors. This article reviews the roles of free radicals—good and bad—in human health.

▶ Check out the **Contemporary Nutrition ARIS site**

www.mhhe.com/wardlawcontfa1 for quizzes, flash cards, other activities, and weblinks designed to further help you learn about what you eat and why.

RATE YOUR PLATE

I. Spotting Fraudulent Claims on the Internet

Search for vitamins and vitaminlike substances sold over the Internet. Then write a report concerning any claims, that you consider fraudulent or misleading, made on behalf of these products. Are the websites selling vitamins, or are they a cover for selling something else? Compare the price of the vitamins from these sites with the price you would pay at the local supermarket or drugstore. Do any of these sites display any disclaimers or warnings about the products?

II. A Closer Look at Supplement Use

With the popularity of vitamin and mineral supplements, it is important to understand how to evaluate a supplement. Study the label of a supplement you use or one readily available from a friend or the supermarket. Then answer the following questions.

1. What is the recommended dosage of this supplement?

   _____

   _____

2. Based on the recommended dosage, are there any individual vitamins for which the intake would be greater than 100% of the DV? List these vitamins.

   _____

   _____

3. Are any suggested intakes above the UL for the nutrient?

   _____

   _____

4. Are there any superfluous ingredients, such as herbs or flavors, in the supplement? You can often determine these by looking for ingredients that do not have a percent of DV.

   _____

   _____

5. Does at least 50% of the vitamin A in the product come from beta-carotene or other provitamin A carotenoids (to reduce risk of preformed vitamin A toxicity)?

   _____

   _____

6. Are there any warnings on the label as to populations who should not consume the product?

   _____

   _____

7. Are there any other signs that tip you off that this product may not be safe?

   _____

   _____

CHAPTER 10 Nutrients Involved in Bone Health

THE HUMAN SKELETAL SYSTEM CAN BE THOUGHT OF AS THE BRICKS AND MORTAR THAT PROVIDE THE STRUCTURAL SUPPORT FOR THE BODY. One major difference however, is that bone is a vibrant, living tissue that flexes and undergoes constant breakdown and resynthesis. It is estimated that in the middle-aged adult, every year 9% of bone is removed and replaced by new bone. In addition to providing architectural framework, bone contains nerves and cartilage and is the site of red and white blood cell synthesis, as well as the production of platelets required for blood clotting. Numerous minerals and vitamins are essential to synthesize and maintain bone. This chapter will explore how these nutrients function to achieve optimal bone health.

Maintenance of healthy bone is critical for an active, productive life. The human body contains 206 bones, infiltrated by blood vessels that supply nutrients and hormones to the cells found in bone. To achieve and maintain healthy bone, an appropriate balance between nutrients, hormones, and lifestyle choices is necessary. Genetics also plays a role, as heredity will determine frame size and a genetic predisposition for bone disease.

Refresh Your Memory

As you begin the study of nutritional factors which influence bone health in Chapter 10, you may want to review:

- Implications of the Dietary Supplement Health and Education Act (DSHEA) in Chapter 1.
- Cell structure, function, digestion and absorption of nutrients in Chapter 3.
- The role of vitamin C in collagen synthesis in Chapter 9.

BONE STRUCTURE

To understand how bone health is achieved, it is important to study the anatomy of bone. The solid portions of bone consist of networks of strong protein fibers (called the "protein matrix") embedded with mineral crystals. The surface of bone is called **periosteum.** This thin layer consists of connective tissue, nerves, and blood vessels.

Beneath the surface, two types of bone are found: **cortical bone** and **trabecular bone.** Cortical bone is sometimes referred to as "compact bone" and trabecular bone is called "spongy bone." The outer layer of all bones is composed of dense, strong cortical bone. The principle function of cortical bone is to provide strength. Cortical bone contains microscopic openings through which blood vessels and nerves pass allowing nutrient delivery to the bone cells. Cortical bone comprises the outer portion of all bones and nearly all of the bones in the hands, wrist, and feet. The interior of most bones is a mixture of cortical and trabecular bone.

Trabecular bone is less dense than cortical bone and has a much more open or porous structure (Fig. 10-1). This more open lattice of the trabecular bone is the location of blood vessels, lymphatic vessels, and nerves, important for the transport of nutrients and hormones to the cells found in bone. Trabecular bone is also the location of bone marrow, where cells are located to synthesize red blood cells, white blood cells, and platelets. The proportion of cortical and trabecular bone varies depending upon the anatomical location of the bone. Trabecular bone is predominant in the ends of the long bones, vertebrae, ribcage, and the flat bones of the pelvis. The human skeleton contains approximately 80% cortical bone and 20% trabecular bone. Teeth have the same properties as bone plus a hard, protective outer covering called enamel, not infiltrated by blood vessels or nerves.

Periosteum A specialized connective tissue covering all bones and having bone-forming potentialities.

Cortical bone The compact or dense bone found on the outer surfaces of bone.

Trabecular bone The less dense, more open structure bone found in the inner layer of bones.

FIGURE 10-1 ▶ Bone consists of two types of bone: cortical and trabecular bone. Cortical bone forms the shafts of bones and the outer mineral covering. Trabecular bone supports the outer shell of cortical bone in various bones of the body.

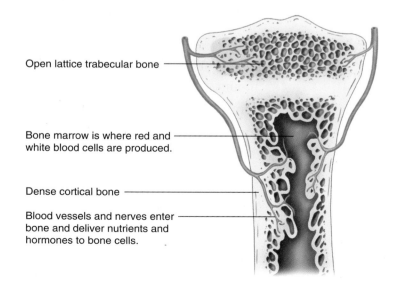

Open lattice trabecular bone

Bone marrow is where red and white blood cells are produced.

Dense cortical bone

Blood vessels and nerves enter bone and deliver nutrients and hormones to bone cells.

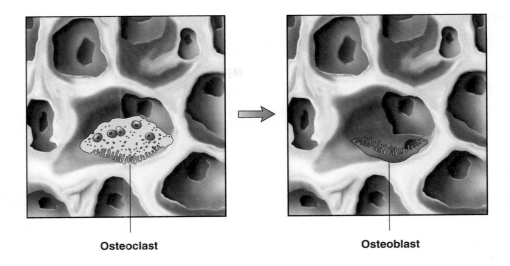

FIGURE 10-2 ▶ Bone turnover involves two cell types with opposing actions. Osteoclast's dissolve bone through secretion of enzymes and acids. Osteoblasts form a collagen matrix infiltrated by minerals to form new bone.

Osteoclast   Osteoblast

BONE CELLS

Bone is composed of approximately 65% minerals and 35% connective tissue. Minerals provide the strength and rigidity, whereas the connective tissue provides flexibility. There are two principle types of bone cells responsible for growth, maintenance, and repair of bone. These are the **osteoblast** and **osteoclast.** Bone synthesis is the function of the osteoblast. These cells form a collagen matrix infiltrated with a complex mixture of calcium and phosphorus called hydroxyapatite. Osteoblasts embedded within the bone matrix are called **osteocytes.** In contrast to the osteoblast, osteoclasts dissolve the mineralized bone through the secretion of enzymes and acids. Osteoblasts and osteoclasts work in concert to maintain bone health (Fig. 10-2).

BONE GROWTH AND REMODELING

Bone growth occurs in length and width during the first two decades of life. The rate of bone formation exceeds the rate of bone breakdown during infancy, childhood, and young adulthood. The majority of bone growth occurs before adulthood, although in both males and females peak bone mass is usually achieved a few years before age 30. Genetics as well as nutrient intake, drugs, hormones, physical activity, and lifestyle choices will influence the age at which peak bone mass occurs. People with a larger frame size and body weight will have a greater bone mass due to the additional stress on the bone associated with the additional weight.

The growth, maintenance, and repair of bone involve a complex relationship between the synthesis of new bone by the osteoblasts and the breakdown of bone by osteoclasts. The degradation and resynthesis of bone is termed **bone remodeling.** The optimal situation throughout adulthood would be to maintain peak bone mass through an equal amount of bone degradation (resorption) and resynthesis. However, after 30 years of age, bone resorption occurs at a faster rate than synthesis, resulting in a loss of bone mass and a decrease in bone mineral density. Bone mineral density is the concentration of mineral found in the bone and is used as an indicator of bone health.

FACTORS THAT INFLUENCE BONE HEALTH

The rate of bone remodeling is different between trabecular and cortical bone. The breakdown and resynthesis of trabecular bone occurs at a faster rate when compared to cortical bone. This subsequently makes the trabecular bone more responsive to factors that

Osteoblast Bone cells that initiate the synthesis of new bone.

Osteoclast Bone cells that breakdown bone and subsequently release bone minerals into the blood.

Osteocyte Osteoblast embedded into the bone matrix.

Bone remodeling The chemical process by which bone is broken down and replaced by new bone.

▲ Ninety-nine percent of calcium in the body is in bones.

TABLE 10-1 Biological Factors Associated with Bone Status

Biological Factors	Effect on Bone Status
Sex	Women have lower bone mass and density than men
Age	Bone loss occurs after age 40
Ethnicity	Caucasian or Asian heritage are at greater risk for poor bone health than individuals of African decent
Frame size	People with "small bones" have a lower bone mass

influence bone remodeling. Biological and lifestyle factors have a large role in the growth, maintenance, and overall health of bone.

Biological factors (Table 10-1) are predetermined by genetics; subsequently an individual has little or no ability to change these factors. Contrast this to lifestyle factors (Table 10-2) that can be modified. People with larger frames tend to have higher peak bone mass than do people with smaller frames, and women have lower peak bone mass than men. The greater the bone mineral density, the stronger the bone. Individuals need to focus on meeting calcium, vitamin D, protein, and other nutrient needs to provide the building blocks to synthesize bone.

The hormone estrogen is a major contributor to bone maintenance because estrogen has been shown to stimulate osteoblast activity. Therefore any sign of menstrual irregularities is reason to see a physician. Some nonmenstruating female athletes and other women with irregular menstrual cycles (e.g., women with eating disorders) typically exhibit low bone mineral density. Physical activity alone cannot prevent bone

TABLE 10-2 Modifiable Lifestyle Factors Associated with Bone Status

Lifestyle Factors	Call To Action
Adequate diet containing an appropriate amount of nutrients	• Follow MyPyramid with special emphasis on adequate amounts of fruits, vegetables, and low-fat and fat-free dairy products • Consider use of fortified foods (or supplements) to make up for specific nutrient shortfalls, such as vitamin D and calcium
Healthy body weight	• Low body weight concomitant with small frame size increases the risk for low bone mass
Normal menses	• During childbearing years, seek medical advice if menses cease (such as in cases of anorexia nervosa or extreme athletic training) • Women at menopause and beyond should consider use of current medical therapies to reduce bone loss linked to the fall in estrogen output
Weight-bearing physical activity	• Perform weight-bearing activity as this contributes to bone maintenance, where as bed rest and a sedentary lifestyle lead to bone loss. Strength training is especially helpful to bone maintenance.
Smoking	• Smoking lowers estrogen synthesis in women. Cessation is advised.
Medications	• Some medications (thyroid hormone, cortisol, diuretics) stimulate urinary calcium secretion.
Excessive intake of protein, phosphorus, sodium, caffeine, wheat bran, alcohol	• Moderate intake of these dietary constituents is recommended. Problems primarily arise if adequate calcium is not consumed. • Excessive soft drink consumption is especially discouraged.

Biceps brachii muscle

Weights used as resistance

Skeletal muscle pulls against the bone, causing it to rebuild and become denser

FIGURE 10-3 ▶ The stress of muscles pulling on bone during exercise increases bone mineral density.

loss associated with irregular menstruation. Even though female athletes may perform an extensive amount of weight-bearing physical activity, high levels of physical activity not balanced with energy intake results in "low energy availability" to support reproductive function. The hormone estrogen also plays an important role in the decline of bone mass and bone mineral density in later life. Estrogen is a female reproductive hormone produced in the ovaries. When a woman reaches menopause and the ovaries stop producing estrogen, bone loss accelerates.

An active lifestyle that includes weight-bearing physical activity is also an important factor in bone health. The increased muscle mass that stems from weight bearing physical activity is associated with greater bone mineral density, as muscle keeps tension on bone and the hormonal changes that occur with the stress associated with exercise cause bones to retain and possibly gain density (Fig. 10-3).

Older adults especially need to stay physically active—including some weight-bearing and resistance activities. At any age, smoking and excessive alcohol intake decrease bone mass. Smoking lowers the estrogen concentration in the blood in women, increasing bone loss. Alcohol is toxic to bone cells for both men and women, and alcoholism is probably a major undiagnosed and unrecognized cause of low bone mineral density. Excessive intakes of phosphorus, caffeine, and sodium adversely affect bone health.

Osteoporosis The presence of a stress-induced fracture or a T-score of −2.5 or lower. The bones are porous and fragile due to low mineral density.

OSTEOPOROSIS

Healthy People 2010 identified the prevention of bone disease, or osteoporosis, as one of its major focus areas. It is estimated that 8 million women and 2 million men have osteoporosis and another 34 million Americans have low bone mass, placing them at risk for osteoporosis. Osteoporosis leads to approximately 1.5 million bone fractures per year in the United States, including 300,000 broken hips (Fig. 10-4). The health care costs associated with these fractures is about $17 billion per year. The National Osteoporosis Foundation estimates these costs to reach more than $60 billion by the year 2020. Women tend to lose 1% to 3% of their bone mass each year after menopause. Men also lose bone mass as they age, but the loss is more gradual. When the bone breakdown activities of osteoclasts exceed the bone-building activities of osteoblasts, bone mass declines. This

▲ Women with osteoporosis typically develop abnormal curvature of the upper spine. This results from fractures of the weakened vertebrae. This can lead to both physical and emotional pain.

FIGURE 10-4 ▶ Osteoporosis leads to 300,000 hip fractures per year in the United States.

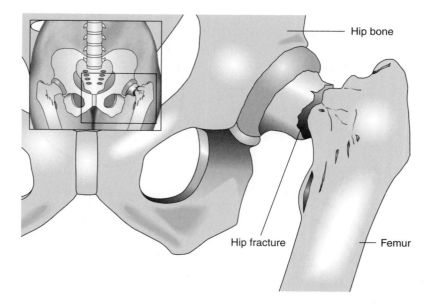

Hip bone

Hip fracture

Femur

FIGURE 10-5 ▶ Corotical and trabecular bone. Cortical bone forms the shafts of bones and their outer mineral covering. Trabecular bone supports the outer shell of cortical bone in various bones of the body, as in the illustration, Note how the osteoporotic bone has much less trabecular bone. This leads to a more fragile bone and is not reversible to any major extent with current therapies.

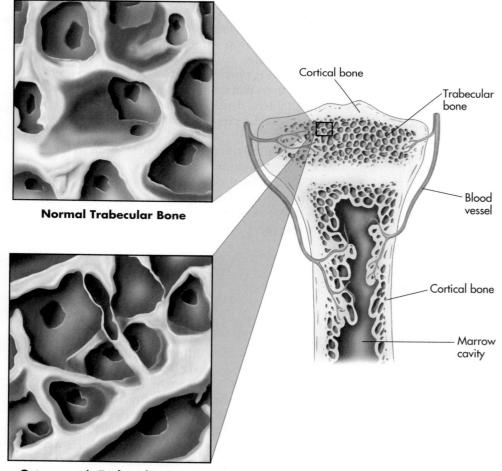

Normal Trabecular Bone

Osteoporotic Trabecular Bone

Cortical bone

Trabecular bone

Blood vessel

Cortical bone

Marrow cavity

is a normal part of aging and does not always lead to unhealthy bones. However, if bone mass is low when this process begins, even moderate bone demineralization can lead to a condition called **osteopenia.** As more bone is lost, the entire matrix of the bone tissue also begins to break down. When this occurs, osteoporosis is likely to result. About 25% of women older than age 50 develop or have osteoporosis. Among people older than age 80, osteoporosis becomes the rule, not the exception.

Osteopenia A bone disease defined by low mineral density.

Type I Osteoporosis Porous trabecular bone characterized by rapid bone demineralization following menopause.

Type 1 and Type 2 Osteoporosis

There are two types of osteoporosis. **Type 1 osteoporosis,** also called postmenopausal osteoporosis, typically occurs in women between 50 and 60 years of age. This type of osteoporosis is directly linked to decreased estrogen concentrations that occur at menopause. Type 1 osteoporosis most dramatically affects trabecular bone as this type of bone undergoes faster remodeling than cortical bone (Fig. 10-5). A women can lose 20% to 30% of trabecular bone and 5% to 10% of cortical bone between age 50 and 60 (Fig. 10-6).

Trabecular bone has a much higher density of osteoblast and osteoclast cells than cortical bone. The osteoblast cells require estrogen for maximal activity. After menopause osteoblast activity decreases; however, osteoclast activity remains high. The result is that bone is broken down at a faster rate than it is synthesized (Fig. 10-7). The trabecular-rich bones of the pelvis, vertebrae, and portions of long bones are at greatest risk for fracture in people with osteoporosis (Fig. 10-8).

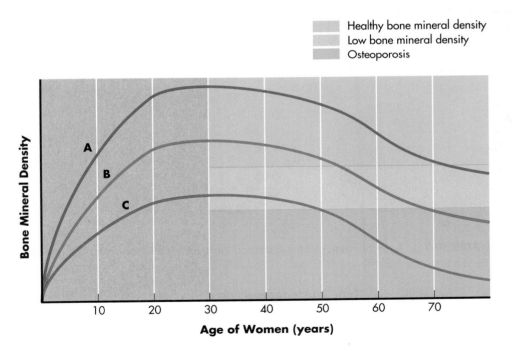

Healthy bone mineral density
Low bone mineral density
Osteoporosis

FIGURE 10-6 ▶ The relationship between peak bone mass and the ultimate risk of developing osteoporosis and related bone fractures. Women A developed a high peak bone mass by age 30, bone loss was slow and steady age 30 and age 50, and sped up somewhat after age 50 due to the effects of menopause. Still, by age 75, the woman had a healthy bone mineral density value and did not show evidence of osteoporosis. Woman B developed an average peak bone mass and experienced the same rate of bone loss as woman A. By age 65, woman B had low bone mineral density and evidence of osteoporosis. She was not at risk of related fractures. Woman C achieved a low peak bone mass, and by following the typical pattern for bone loss, at age 50, she already showed evidence of low bone mineral density and osteoporosis. Given the low calcium intakes common among young women, line C is a sobering reality. Ideally, by following a diet and lifestyle pattern that contributes to maximal bone mineral density, more women will follow line A, in turn significantly reducing their risk of developing osteoporosis in their lifetimes.

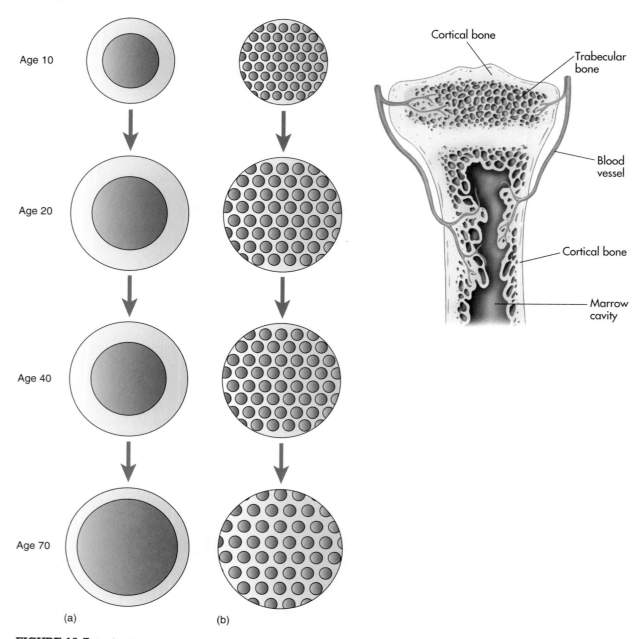

FIGURE 10-7 ▶ A representation of the width and density changes that occur in (a) cortical and (b) trabecular bone as a person ages.

Type II Osteoporosis Porous trabecular and cortical bone observed in men and women after the age of 60.

Kyphosis Abnormally increased bending of the spine.

Type 2 osteoporosis occurs in both men and women and tends to be diagnosed later in life (70 to 75 years of age). Type 2 osteoporosis is a result of breakdown of both cortical and trabecular bone and is due to a combination of dietary and age-related factors. People with either form of osteoporosis can lose significant height and experience severe pain, especially in the vertebrae. A woman may lose an inch or more in height as the bone is demineralized and develop a curvature in the upper spine called **kyphosis** or dowager's hump (Fig. 10-9). Kyphosis is a major concern because the bending of the spine may decrease the volume of the chest cavity, resulting in difficulty breathing, abdominal pain, decreased appetite, and premature satiety. Osteoporotic bone is also more susceptible to fracture following a fall. Approximately one in four people who fracture a hip die within a year. Bone fractures often result in hospitalization and loss of the ability to live independently, so preventing osteoporosis means enhanced health and well being as we age.

The most effective way to treat osteoporosis in women is the use of hormone replacement therapy (HRT), a combination of the hormones estrogen and progesterone or estrogen alone. However, HRT may increase the risk of other health problems, such as vaginal bleeding, increased risk for some cancers (breast, cervical, ovarian, uterine), and increased risk for cardiovascular disease. Women considering HRT should consult a doctor to evaluate whether HRT is the appropriate therapy. Some studies suggest that consuming phytoestrogens, estrogenlike phytochemicals found primarily in soy products, may help maintain bone health after menopause. Other medications, such as selective estrogen receptor modulators (SERM) and bisphosphonates may also help reduce bone loss. SERMs mimic the beneficial effects of estrogen on bone density without some of the risks associated with HRT. **Bisphosphonates** work by inhibiting bone breakdown, specifically by inhibiting osteoclast activity. An example of a bisphosphonate is Fosamax, commonly prescribed to people with reduced bone mass or osteoporosis.

The incidence of osteoporosis increases as a person ages. Its importance as a personal and public health problem is intensifying as the U.S. population ages. It appears, however, that a large percentage of the cases of osteoporosis can be prevented. The key to prevention is to build dense bones during the first 30 years of life and then limit the amount of bone loss in adulthood. People with higher peak bone mass have more calcium to lose before bones become weak and fracture easily. A higher peak bone mass is also the reason males experience osteoporosis less often than females do; they have more bone mass to lose.

Bisphosphonates Drugs that bind minerals and prevent osteoclast breakdown of bone. Examples are alendronate (Fosamax) and risedronate (Actonel).

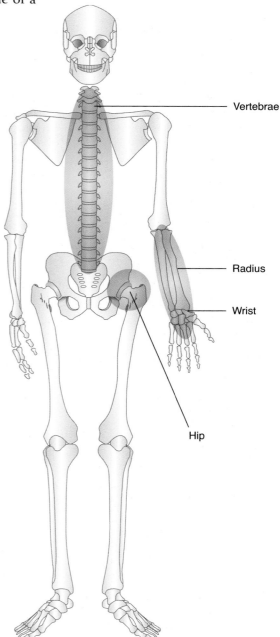

FIGURE 10-8 ▶ Regions of skeleton most susceptible to low bone density and osteoporosis.

FIGURE 10-9 ▶ Normal and Osteoporotic woman. Osteoporotic bones have less substance, so osteoporosis generally leads to loss of height, distorted body shape, fractures, and loss of teeth. Monitoring changes in adult height is one way to detect early evidence of osteoporosis.

BONE HEALTH ASSESSMENT

Until recently there were no convenient clinical measurement devices health care professionals could use to assess bone health. The presence of a hairline fracture of the vertebrae was used as the diagnosis of the presence of osteoporosis. This was a diagnosis of the presence of osteoporosis; however, it was not a predictive diagnostic tool. In the past few decades scientific instruments have been developed that can quantitate bone mass and bone density and subsequently the likelihood of a person developing bone disease.

Duel energy X-ray absorptiometry (DEXA) A scientific tool used to measure bone mineral density.

Techniques available to obtain information on bone mass and quality include: single or **dual energy X-ray absorptiometry (DEXA)**, quantitative computer tomography, and quantitative ultrasound. Single energy X-ray absorptiometry is a less accurate measurement tool than the DEXA. The single energy X-ray absorptiometry involves measurement of bone density at a single site, usually the wrist or heel. The quantitative ultrasound technique uses sound waves to measure the density of bone in the heel, shin, and kneecap. These technologies are frequently used at health fairs because the machines are portable and provide results faster than the traditional DEXA.

The most accurate screening involves a DEXA bone scan of the whole body. The DEXA procedure is simple, painless, safe, and noninvasive. The DEXA test requires a person lie on their back while a movable imaging arm moves over the length of the body. The procedure usually takes 20 to 30 minutes. The ability of a bone to block the path of the low-level X-ray is used as a measure of bone mineral density. A very low dose of radiation is used for the DEXA—about one-tenth of the exposure from a chest X-ray.

From the DEXA measurement of bone density, a T score is generated, which compares the observed bone density to that of a person at peak bone mass (e.g., age 30). The T score is interpreted as follows:

0 to –1	Normal
–1 to –2.4	Low bone mineral density
–2.5 or lower	Osteoporosis

The National Osteoporosis Foundation recommends DEXA testing for the following people.

- All women aged 65 and older.
- Younger postmenopausal women with one or more risk factors (other than being white, postmenopausal, and female) including estrogen deficiency, steroid therapy, or thyroid dysfunction.
- Postmenopausal women who have already had a fracture.

The incidence of osteoporosis is far less in many other countries than the United States. Although genetic and other factors play a role, the causes of osteoporosis are mainly related to diet and other lifestyle behaviors. That means that osteoporosis can largely be prevented.

To synthesize, maintain, and repair bone requires several vitamins, minerals, and hormones. The key nutrients include vitamins D and K, and the minerals calcium, phosphorus, magnesium, and fluoride. Other nutrients required by bone but of lesser importance include vitamin C, boron, and silicon. In addition, adequate protein must be consumed, especially in the elderly, to reduce bone loss.

CRITICAL NUTRIENTS REQUIRED FOR BONE GROWTH, MAINTENANCE, AND REPAIR

Calcium (Ca)

All cells require calcium to function, however more than 99% of the calcium in the body is used to strengthen bones and teeth. Calcium represents 40% of all the minerals present in the body and equals about 2.5 pounds (1200 grams) in the average person. Less than 1% of calcium is found in blood but this circulating calcium is critical to supply the needs of cells other than bone cells (e.g. muscle, nerve).

Bone growth, development, and maintenance require an adequate calcium intake. Calcium requires an acidic environment in the gastrointestinal tract to be absorbed efficiently. Absorption occurs primarily in the upper part of the small intestine. This area tends to remain acidic because it receives the acidic stomach contents. After the first loop of the small intestine, secretions from the pancreas enter the small intestine and the pH becomes neutral to slightly basic, which decreases calcium absorption. Efficient calcium absorption in the upper small intestine depends on the presence of the active form of vitamin D.

Adults absorb about 25% of the calcium in the foods eaten, but during times when the body needs extra calcium, such as in infancy and pregnancy, absorption increases to as high as 60%. Young people tend to absorb calcium better than do older people, especially those older than 70.

Many factors enhance calcium absorption, including:

- Blood levels of **parathyroid hormone** and vitamin D
- The presence of glucose and lactose in the diet
- The flow rate (motility) of digestive contents through the intestine
- Acidic environment of the stomach

Many factors limit calcium absorption, including:

- Large amounts of **phytic acid** and fiber from grains
- **Oxalates** found in vegetables
- Great excess of phosphorus, magnesium, sodium, and zinc in the diet
- Tannins (polyphenols) in tea and some legumes
- A vitamin D deficiency
- Diarrhea
- Old age
- Some medications (anticonvulsants, cortisone, antacids)

Tight regulation of a constant blood calcium concentration is maintained regardless of dietary intake. If dietary calcium intake is inadequate and blood calcium concentration begins to decrease, three hormonally controlled actions are stimulated to reestablish calcium blood levels. Bones release calcium, intestines absorb more calcium, and the kidneys retain more calcium. The skeleton provides the framework of the body and it functions as a bank from which calcium can be added or withdrawn. Bone loss caused by inadequate calcium intake and/or absorption can proceed slowly over many years. Only after many years are clinical symptoms apparent. By not meeting calcium needs, some people, especially women, are most likely setting the stage for osteoporosis and future bone fractures.

Additional Functions of Calcium Forming and maintaining bones are calcium's major roles in the body. However, calcium is critical for many other processes. Calcium is essential for formation of a blood clot. Muscle contraction is activated by calcium release and the flow of calcium along the surface of the muscle cell. If blood calcium falls below a critical point, muscles cannot relax after contraction; the body stiffens and shows involuntary twitching, called tetany. In nerve transmission, calcium assists in the release of neurotransmitters and permits the flow of ions in and out of nerve cells. Without sufficient calcium, nerve function fails, opening another path to tetany. Calcium helps regulate cellular metabolism by influencing the activities of various enzymes and hormonal responses. Calcium also functions in the maintenance of cell membrane integrity, normal blood pressure, regulation of glucose concentration and cellular differentiation. It is the tight regulation of the concentration of calcium in the blood that keeps these processes going, even if a person fails to consume enough dietary calcium.

Other Possible Health Benefits of Calcium Researchers have been examining links between calcium intake and risks for a wide array of diseases. An adequate calcium intake can reduce the risk of colon cancer, especially in people who consume a high-fat

Parathyroid hormone (PTH) A hormone made by the parathyroid gland that increases synthesis of the active form of vitamin D. This hormone works with vitamin D to increase blood levels of calcium.

Phytic acid (phytate) A constituent of plant fiber that chemically binds minerals and prevents their absorption.

Oxalic acid (Oxalate) An organic acid, found in spinach, kale, and other leafy green vegetables, that can depress the absorption of certain minerals, such as calcium.

diet. A decreased risk of some forms of kidney stones and reduced lead absorption are other possible benefits when calcium is part of a meal. Calcium intakes of 800 to 1200 milligrams per day can also decrease blood pressure, compared with intakes of 400 milligrams per day or less. Calcium intakes of 1200 milligrams per day in combination with a low-fat, low-cholesterol diet can help people with elevated LDL improve their blood lipid profiles. For women, an adequate calcium intake might also reduce the risk of premenstrual syndrome and high blood pressure that can develop during pregnancy. Overall, the benefits of a diet providing adequate calcium extend beyond bone health.

Calcium Sources and Needs Calcium is found in both plant and animal foods, although the best sources are dairy products. Milk is also a source of vitamin D and lactose, two nutrients that enhance calcium absorption. Dairy products, such as milk and cheese, provide about 75% of the calcium in North American diets. An exception is cottage cheese, because most calcium is lost during production.

Bread, rolls, crackers, and foods made with milk products are secondary contributors. Other calcium sources are leafy greens (such as spinach), broccoli, some legumes, sardines, and canned salmon. Overall, fat-free milk is the most nutrient-dense (milligrams per kcal) source of calcium because of its relatively high **bioavailability** and low calorie content, with some of the vegetables noted following close behind (Fig. 10-10). Calcium-fortified foods such as orange juice, breakfast cereals, breakfast bars, waffles, and soy products provide considerable amounts of calcium. Through the production of more products fortified with calcium, food and beverage companies are responding to consumers' desire to increase consumption of calcium (Fig. 10-11).

Bioavailability The degree to which a consumed nutrient is adsorbed and used by the body.

▼ Milk is a rich as well as convenient source of calcium.

Food Sources of Calcium

Food Item and Amount	Calcium (milligrams)	%AI
AI*	1000	100%
Plain yogurt, 1 cup	450	45%
Parmesan cheese, 1 ounce	390	39%
Fortified orange juice, 1 cup	350	35%
Romano cheese, 1 ounce	300	30%
1% milk, 1 cup	300	30%
Buttermilk, 1 cup	285	29%
Swiss cheese, 1 ounce	275	28%
Spinach, 1 cup	250	25%
Salmon (with bones), 3 ounces	210	21%
Cheddar cheese, 1 ounce	200	20%
Total Raisin Bran cereal, ¾ cup	180	18%
Sardines (with bones), 2 ounces	170	17%
Chocolate pudding, ½ cup	160	16%
Tofu, ½ cup	140	14%

Key:
- Grains
- Vegetables
- Fruits
- Oils
- Milk
- Meat & Beans

*For adults; See the DRI table in the back of this book for age-specific recommendations.

FIGURE 10-10 ▶ Food sources of calcium compared to the Adequate Intake.

MyPyramid: Sources of Calcium

Grains	Vegetables	Fruits	Oils	Milk	Meat & Beans
• Calcium-fortified snack foods • Calcium-fortified flour tortillas • Calcium-fortified breakfast cereals	• Greens • Spinach • Broccoli • Green beans	• Calcium-fortified orange juice	• None	• Milk • Yogurt • Cheese	• Tofu • Almonds • Shrimp • Sardines • Canned salmon

FIGURE 10-11 ▶ Sources of calcium form MyPyramid. The height of the background color (none, 1/3, 2/3, or completely covered) within each group in the pyramid indicates the average nutrient density in the pyramid indicates the average nutrient density for calcium in that group. Overall, foods from the milk group and many fortified foods are nutrient-dense and bioavailable sources of calcium. Addition calcium-fortified foods appear in stores each year and thus will add to the food sources listed for various groups. With regard to physical activity, calcium is especially important for related muscle contraction and as well to maintain a strong skeleton to support the body.

A serving of some calcium-fortified foods may exceed the amount of calcium contained in a cup of milk. An 8-ounce glass of calcium-fortified orange juice provides approximately 350 milligrams of calcium. Another source of calcium is soybean curd (tofu) if it is made with calcium carbonate (check the label). It is easy to assess the calcium content of foods because the Nutrition Facts panel on food labels must list the amount of 2 minerals in the product (calcium and iron). The Daily Value (DV) for calcium used for food and supplement labels is 1000 milligrams. To determine the amount of calcium in a food, use this trick. If a food label states a serving supplies 30% of the DV for calcium, convert this to milligrams by adding a 0, so 30% is the same as 300 milligrams.

Many factors can influence the ability of the calcium to be absorbed and efficiently used by the body. Calcium absorption can be reduced by the presence of oxalates, tannins, and phytic acid. These compounds chelate (chemically bind) calcium in the digestive tract. Oxalates are found in cocoa, tea, collard greens, spinach, and numerous other vegetables. Tea and some legumes are rich sources of tannins. Phytates are found in whole grains, raw beans, and nuts. Although some foods, such as spinach, contain high amounts of calcium, much of it cannot be absorbed because of the high concentration of oxalates, tannins, or phytic acid. It is estimated that a person would have to consume over eight servings (8 cups) of spinach to absorb the same amount of calcium present in one serving (1 cup) of milk. Diets high in dietary fiber reduce mineral absorption. Other factors such as age also influence the bioavailabilty of calcium. Calcium absorption decreases in the fifth decade of life making it more difficult for older people to meet their need for calcium.

There are insufficient data to generate Recommended Dietary Allowances (RDA) for calcium. An Adequate Intake (AI) of 1000 milligrams/day has been established for adults up to 50 years of age. The AI is 1200 milligrams/day for older adults. The AI is based on the amount of calcium needed each day to offset calcium losses in urine, feces, and other routes. The AI for young people includes an additional amount to allow for increases in bone mass during growth and development. Most

▲ Spinach is often touted as a rich source of calcium, but little of the calcium present is bioavailable—that which is available to the body.

FIGURE 10-12 ▶ The gap between recommended daily intake of calcium and daily consumption of calcium in males and females in the United States.

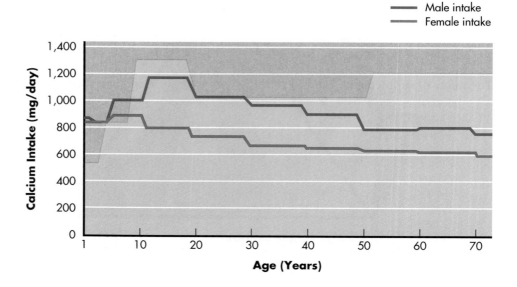

older children and adolescents in the United States do not consume the recommended amount of calcium. In the United States, average daily calcium intakes are approximately 800 milligrams for women and 1000 milligrams for men. Approximately half of adult women in the United States consume less than 60% of the recommended intake of calcium (Fig. 10-12). Many women have low calcium intake for several reasons. Dairy products are perceived to be high in calories. The food industry has responded to this concern through the introduction of many reduced-fat dairy products. Many adults report losing a taste for milk as they age. In addition, lactose intolerance becomes more prevalent as people age.

Thus, dietary intakes of calcium by many women, especially young women, are below the AI, whereas intakes by most men are roughly equivalent to the AI. It is also important for vegans to focus on eating good plant sources of calcium, as well as on the total amount of calcium ingested.

MAKING DECISIONS

To estimate your calcium intake, use the rule of 300's. Count 300 milligrams for the calcium provided by foods scattered throughout the diet. Add to that another 300 milligrams for every cup of milk or yogurt or 1.5 ounces of cheese. If you eat a lot of tofu, almonds, or sardines, or drink calcium-fortified beverages use Figure 10-10 or diet analysis software to get a more accurate calculation of calcium intake.

Calcium Supplements. People who do not like milk or who cannot incorporate enough calcium-containing foods into their diets can increase calcium intake through the use of calcium supplements. Calcium carbonate, the form found in calcium-based antacid tablets, is the most common supplement used. People should take this supplement with or just after meals in doses not to exceed 500 milligrams so that stomach acid produced during digestion can aid with absorption of this mineral. On the other hand, a supplement containing calcium citrate, which is acidic, can be consumed between or with meals or at bedtime. Intake of calcium from supplements and/or food above 500 milligrams at any time significantly reduces the percent absorbed. High intake of calcium at one time may also inhibit absorption of other minerals.

With calcium supplements, interactions with other minerals are a concern. There is evidence that calcium supplements may decrease zinc, iron, and other mineral absorption. An effect of calcium supplementation on iron absorption is possible; however, this appears to be small over the long term. To be safe, people using a calcium supplement on a regular basis should notify their physician of the practice.

The safety of supplements is not determined only by the amount consumed. Potential contamination with lead and/or aluminum is a problem recognized over 50 years ago. Supplements derived from bone meal, dolomite, and oyster shells have been found to contain unhealthy levels of contaminants. The FDA has issued warnings and is in the process of enacting measures toward reducing permissible levels of lead and aluminum exposure. Tablet or liquid calcium supplements with the United States Pharmacopeia (USP) seal of approval are less likely than others to contain high concentrations of contaminants.

Upper Level for Calcium The Upper Level (UL) for calcium intake is 2500 milligrams per day, based on the observation that greater intakes increase the risk for some forms of kidney stones. Excessive calcium intakes by some people can also cause high blood and urinary calcium concentrations, irritability, headache, kidney failure, soft tissue calcification, and decreased absorption of other minerals, as noted previously.

So which is better: calcium from food or supplements? Taking 1000 milligrams of calcium carbonate or calcium citrate daily in divided doses (about 500 milligrams per tablet) is probably safe in many instances. However, people often have difficulty adhering to a supplement regimen. Modification of eating habits to include foods that are good sources of calcium is a better plan of action. In addition to this important mineral, foods that contain calcium also supply other vitamins, minerals, phytochemicals, and fats needed to support health. Problems associated with excessive consumption of calcium are not likely when foods are the primary sources of calcium.

CONCEPT CHECK

About 99% of calcium in the body is found in the bones and teeth. Aside from its critical role in bone, calcium also functions in blood clotting, muscle contraction, nerve-impulse transmission, and cell metabolism. Calcium requires the vitamin D hormone for efficient absorption. Factors that reduce calcium absorption include a vitamin D deficiency, ingestion of large amounts of fiber, oxalate, phytate, and old age. Blood calcium is regulated primarily by hormones and does not closely reflect daily intake.

Dairy products are rich food sources of calcium. Other foods, such as calcium-fortified beverages, are rich sources as well. Supplemental forms, such as calcium carbonate, are well absorbed by most people. However, overzealous supplementation can also result in the development of kidney stones and other health problems.

Phosphorus (P)

Functions of Phosphorus. Phosphorus is the second most abundant mineral in the body. Approximately 85% of phosphorus is found as a component of hydroxyapatite crystals that make up the functional component of bone and teeth providing strength. The remaining 15% of phosphorus has numerous other critical functions within the body. Phosphorus is part of DNA and RNA, the genetic code material present in every cell. Therefore, phosphorus is critical for cellular replication and growth because DNA and RNA are responsible for mitosis and protein synthesis.

▲ Meats are rich in phosphorus.

Phosphorus is also a primary component of adenosine triphosphate (ATP), the energy molecule that fuels body functions. Phosphorus is essential for the activation and deactivation of many enzymes. Many enzymes and the B vitamins are functional only when a phosphate group is attached. A major class of lipids contains phosphorus (phospholipids). Phospholipids are the principle structural component of cell membranes, making up approximately 60% of membranes. These phospholipid membranes regulate the transport of nutrients and waste products into and out of cells. Phosphorus also functions to maintain blood pH and fluid balance because phosphates can accept and donate charged hydrogen atoms.

Phosphorus Sources and Needs. In contrast to calcium, phosphorus is naturally abundant in many foods. Milk, cheese, meat, and bread provide most of the phosphorus in the adult diet. Nuts, fish, Breakfast cereals, bran, and eggs are also good sources (Fig. 10-13). About 20% to 30% of dietary phosphorus comes from food additives, especially in baked goods, cheeses, processed meats, and many soft drinks (about 75 milligrams per 12 ounces). Phosphorus is considered a GRAS (generally recognized as safe) substance, and its function as a food additive is to increase water binding and taste. Phosphoric acid will also significantly lower the pH of a food or beverage (pH of a soft drink is less than 3). Absorption of phosphorus is high; however phosphorus absorption in grains is reduced because of the high phytic

FIGURE 10-13 ▶ Food sources of phosphorous compared to the RDA.

Food Sources of Phosphorus

Food Item and Amount	Phosphorus (milligrams)	%RDA
RDA*	700	100%
Plain yogurt, 1 cup	350	50%
Swiss cheese, 2 ounces	345	49%
Almonds, ½ cup	340	49%
Sunflower seeds, 1 ounce	330	47%
1% milk, 1 cup	235	34%
Cheddar cheese, 1.5 ounces	220	31%
Salmon, 3 ounces	220	31%
Raisin Bran cereal, 1 cup	215	31%
Sirloin steak, 3 ounces	210	30%
Egg, 2 hard boiled	200	29%
Chicken breast, 3 ounces	180	26%
Roasted turkey, 3 ounces	180	26%
Pot roast, 3 ounces	170	24%
Lean ham, 3 ounces	165	24%
American cheese, 1 slice	155	22%

Key:
■ Grains
■ Vegetables
■ Fruits
□ Oils
■ Milk
■ Meat & Beans

*For adults; See the DRI table in the back of this book for age-specific recommendations.

acid content. Average daily adult consumption is about 1000 to 1600 milligrams. Thus, deficiencies of phosphorus are unlikely in healthy adults, especially because it is so efficiently absorbed.

Marginal phosphorus status can be found in preterm infants, vegans, people with alcoholism, older people on nutrient-poor diets, and people with long-term bouts of diarrhea.

Upper Level for Phosphorus. The UL for phosphorus intake is 3 to 4 grams per day. Intakes greater than this can result in mineralization of soft tissues. The kidney appears to be the most sensitive organ. High intakes can lead to serious problems in people with certain kidney diseases. In addition, chronic imbalance in the calcium-to-phosphorus ratio in the diet, resulting from a high phosphorus intake coupled with a low calcium intake, also can contribute to bone loss. This situation most likely arises when the AI for calcium is not met, as can occur in adolescents and adults who regularly substitute soft drinks for milk or otherwise underconsume calcium.

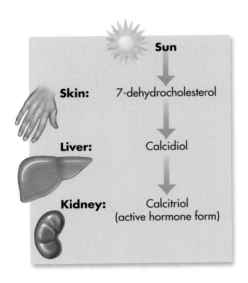

▲ Solar radiation on the skin provides about 80% to 100% of the vitamin D humans use. This is also the most reliable way to maintain vitamin D status. Dietary vitamin D is also effective, but less so.

CONCEPT CHECK

Phosphorus absorption is efficient and is enhanced by the active vitamin D hormone. Urinary excretion mainly controls body content. Phosphorus aids enzyme function and is part of key metabolic compounds and cell membranes. No distinct deficiency symptoms caused by an inadequate phosphorus intake have been reported. Food sources for phosphorus include dairy products, baked goods, and meat. The RDA is met by most North Americans. An excess intake of phosphorus can compromise bone health, if sufficient calcium is not otherwise consumed, and can impair kidney function.

Vitamin D

Vitamin D is a unique nutrient in that it can be efficiently produced in the skin when the skin is exposed to ultraviolet light. Cholesterol is the building block or precursor of vitamin D found in the skin. Regardless of whether the body manufactures vitamin D or obtains it from food, chemical modifications of the vitamin D precursor must occur before the vitamin D becomes active. One chemical reaction occurs in the liver followed by another in the kidney. The cells that participate in the synthesis of vitamin D are different from the cells that respond to vitamin D, namely bone and intestinal cells; therefore, vitamin D is considered a hormone. The definition of a hormone is a compound manufactured by one organ of the body that then enters the bloodstream and has a physiological effect on another organ or tissue. A precursor to vitamin D (7-dehydrocholesterol) is synthesized by cells in the skin. This precursor then travels via the blood to the liver and kidney where it is chemically converted into the active form of vitamin D (calcitriol) (Fig. 10-14). The active form of vitamin D then enters the blood and has a physiologic effect on cells throughout the body. Overall, sun exposure provides about 80% to 100% of vitamin D requirements.

The amount of sun exposure needed by individuals to produce vitamin D depends on skin color, age, time of day, season, and location. Exposure of hands, face, and arms for about 15 minutes at least two to three times a week will provide the required amount of ultraviolet light to synthesize an adequate amount of the vitamin D precursor to meet weekly requirements for children and adults. However, seniors and persons with dark skin would need about three to five times the amount of sun exposure to synthesize an equivalent amount of vitamin D. The pigment that imparts color to skin, melanin, is a potent natural sunscreen.

FIGURE 10-14 ▶ A precursor to vitamin D is synthesized when skin is exposed to sunlight. Previtamin D must be further modified by the liver and kidney for maximal activity.

FIGURE 10-15 ▶ Seasonal variations to sunlight intensity. If you live north of the 37th parallel, the angle of the winter sun is such that the sun's rays must pass through more of the atmosphere than at other times of the year. As a result, skin forms less prohormone vitamin D in the winter.

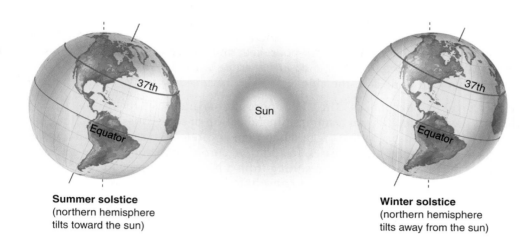

Summer solstice
(northern hemisphere
tilts toward the sun)

Winter solstice
(northern hemisphere
tilts away from the sun)

Sun exposure is only effective for vitamin D synthesis if sunscreen over SPF 8 is not used while the skin is exposed to the sun. In addition, the amount of vitamin D produced is reduced with smog or overcast weather, as these conditions reduce the amount of ultraviolet light reaching the skin. Skin synthesis of vitamin D is negligible in the winter months in northern climates (Fig. 10-15). Vitamin D synthesized in the warm summer months is stored in the liver and adipose cells; however it is advised that people residing in northern climates should find alternative (dietary) sources in the winter months. Overall, anyone who does not receive enough direct exposure to sunshine to synthesize an adequate amount of vitamin D must have a dietary source of the vitamin. Many tanning machines produce ultraviolet light of the appropriate wavelength to cause vitamin D synthesis in the skin. Relying on tanning machines is not recommended by the Food and Drug Administration and American Academy of Dermatology because of the potential health hazards (burns, damage to eyes, and skin cancer) associated with this practice.

Functions of Vitamin D. The main function of vitamin D (calcitriol) is to maintain the normal range of calcium and phosphorus in the blood. In concert with the hormones parathyroid hormone (PTH) and calcitonin, vitamin D closely maintains blood calcium in a narrow range. This tight regulation of blood calcium level assures that an appropriate amount of calcium is available to all cells. Vitamin D functions to regulate calcium by three methods: (1) regulates absorption of calcium and phosphorus from the small intestine; (2) in combination with PTH and calcitonin it regulates calcium excretion via the kidney; and (3) through bone remodeling.

When blood levels of calcium begin to drop from the normal range, PTH stimulates the synthesis of the most active form of vitamin D (calcitriol) by the kidney. The calcitriol increases the production of proteins in the small intestine required for calcium absorption from the gut. The subsequent effect is to increase the amount of calcium absorbed from the intestinal tract. Vitamin D also functions in concert with PTH to (1) cause the kidneys to reduce calcium excretion in the urine and (2) release calcium from bone by stimulating osteoclast activity. When calcium levels reach the normal range, PTH release is inhibited and calcitonin is released, which has the opposite effects of PTH. One way to think about PTH and calcitonin is that they have opposing effects similar to insulin and glucagon in the regulation of blood glucose levels in the normal range.

It has been discovered that vitamin D has other critical functions in many cells throughout the body. Vitamin D binds to and subsequently affects cells of the immune system, brain and nervous system, pancreas, skin, muscles, and reproductive organs. Of particular interest is that vitamin D is also capable of influencing normal development of some cells, such as skin, colon, prostate, ovary, and breast cells, in turn reducing cancer risk in these sites. Vitamin D also controls the growth of the parathyroid gland, aids in the function of the immune system, and contributes to skin cell development. Studies have shown that vitamin D deficiency can be a problem in individuals with dark skin, the elderly, babies breastfeeding without supplementation, insufficient exposure to sunlight, and with the use of nonfortified food (e.g., cereal and dairy products).

Without adequate levels of vitamin D in the blood, calcium absorption from the small intestine decreases. Subsequently, calcium and phosphorus deposition during bone synthesis is reduced resulting in weak bones especially in the legs where a characteristic bowed leg appearance is observed. Symptoms also include an enlarged head, joints, and rib cage and a deformed pelvis. A child with these symptoms has the disease **rickets** (Fig. 10-16). For the prevention of rickets, infants should be provided supplemental vitamin D (under a physician's guidance). Keep in mind, however, that supplements need to be used carefully to avoid vitamin D toxicity in the infant. Rickets in children is also associated with fat malabsorption, which can occur in children with cystic fibrosis.

Osteomalacia, which means soft bone, is an adult disease comparable to rickets. It results from inadequate calcium intake, inefficient calcium absorption in the intestine, or poor conservation of calcium by the kidneys. This condition leads to a decrease in bone mineral density and subsequently bones become porous and weak and break easily. One study showed that treatment with 10 to 20 micrograms (400 to 800 IU) per day of vitamin D, in conjunction with adequate dietary calcium, greatly decreased fracture risk in older people in nursing homes. Follow-up studies support this role of vitamin D in reducing hip fracture risk. AI or synthesis of vitamin D is no less important than calcium for bone health. An analysis of many human studies concluded that vitamin D decreases the incidence of vertebral fractures and may decrease nonvertebral fractures, as well. Vitamin D supplementation was also found to reduce the risk of fracture from falls among institutionalized elderly by more than 20%. Aging decreases production of vitamin D in the skin by about 70% by age 70.

Osteomalacia in adults occurs most commonly in people with kidney, stomach, gallbladder, or intestinal disease (especially when most of the intestine has been removed) and in people with cirrhosis of the liver. These diseases affect both vitamin D activation and calcium absorption. Adults with limited sun exposure and/or dark skin are more prone to develop this disease. The combination of sun exposure and adequate dietary intake can prevent this problem.

Vitamin D Sources and Needs. Dietary sources of vitamin D are limited. Rich sources are fatty fish (e.g., salmon and sardines), fortified dairy products, and many breakfast cereals (Fig. 10-17). In the United States and Canada, milk is usually fortified with 10 micrograms (400 IU) per quart. Consumption of at least 2 cups of vitamin D-fortified milk a day is advisable for people at risk for vitamin D deficiency. Although eggs, butter, liver, and a few brands of margarine contain some vitamin D, large servings must be eaten to obtain an appreciable amount of the vitamin; therefore, these foods are not considered significant sources. Without adequate exposure to direct sunlight, consumption of fortified foods, or supplementation, a vegan diet cannot meet vitamin D requirements. It is advisable for vegans to consume vitamin D fortified soy milk.

Rickets The vitamin D deficiency disease observed in infants and children. Mineral content of the bones is markedly reduced.

Osteomalacia Adult form of rickets. The bones have low mineral density and subsequently are at risk for fracture.

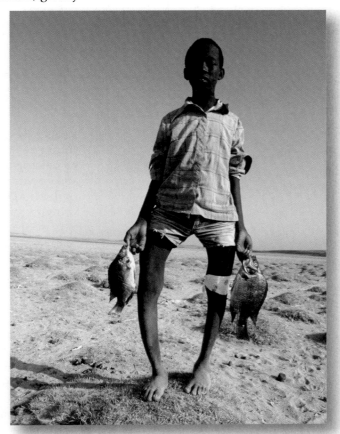

FIGURE 10-16 ▶ Vitamin D deficiency causes rickets, in which the bones and teeth do not develop normally.

Food Sources of Vitamin D

Food Item and Amount	Vitamin D (micrograms)	Vitamin D (IU)	Adult Male and Female AI = 5 micrograms %AI
AI	5	200	100%
Baked herring, 3 ounces	44.4	1775	888%
Smoked eel, 1 ounce	25.5	1020	510%
Baked salmon, 3 ounces	6.0	238	119%
Sardines, 1 ounce	3.4	136	68%
Canned tuna, 3 ounces	3.4	136	68%
1% milk, 1 cup	2.5	99	50%
Nonfat milk, 1 cup	2.5	98	49%
Soft margarine, 1 teaspoon	1.5	60	30%
Italian pork sausage, 3 ounces	1.1	44	22%
Soy milk, 1 cup	1.0	40	20%
Raisin Bran cereal, ¾ cup	1.0	38	19%
Baked bluefish, 3 ounces	0.9	34	17%
Special K cereal, ¾ cup	0.8	30	15%
Cooked egg yolk, 1	0.6	25	13%

Key: Grains, Vegetables, Fruits, Oils, Milk, Meat & Beans

FIGURE 10-17 Food sources of vitamin D Compared to the Adequate Intake for adults.

The AI set for vitamin D is 5 micrograms (200 IU) per day for people 50 and younger. The AI increases to 10 micrograms per day for those aged 51 to 70 and 15 micrograms per day for those over age 70, because of the reduced ability to absorb vitamin D from the intestine and decreased ability to synthesize it in the skin. An RDA has not been set because the amount produced by sunlight exposure is highly variable between individuals. The DV used on food and supplement labels is 10 micrograms (400 IU). As mentioned, young, light-skinned people can synthesize all the vitamin D needed from casual sun exposure. A number of experts suggest older adults, especially those over age 70 who have limited sun exposure or dark skin, receive about 25 micrograms (1000 IU) from a combination of vitamin D-fortified foods and a multivitamin and mineral supplement, with an individual supplement of vitamin D added if needed.

Upper Level for Vitamin D. The UL for vitamin D is 50 micrograms (2000 IU) per day. Too much vitamin D taken regularly can create serious health consequences in infants and children. Due to the role of vitamin D in calcium absorption, excretion, and release of calcium from bone, supplementation with high doses of vitamin D can cause calcium levels in the blood to increase above the normal range. The UL is based on the risk of overabsorption of calcium and eventual calcium deposits in the kidneys and other organs. Toxicity symptoms also include weakness, loss of appetite, diarrhea, vomiting, mental confusion, and increased urine output. Calcium deposits in organs cause metabolic disturbances and cell death. Vitamin D toxicity does not result from excessive exposure to the sun because the

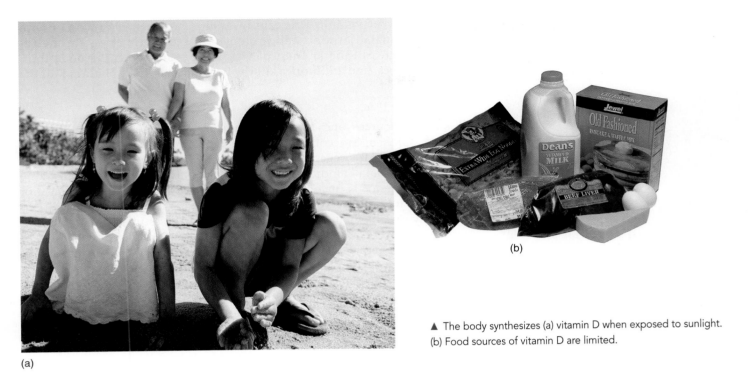

(a)

▲ The body synthesizes (a) vitamin D when exposed to sunlight. (b) Food sources of vitamin D are limited.

body regulates the amount made in the skin (i.e., as exposure to sunlight increases, vitamin D synthesis decreases).

CONCEPT CHECK

Vitamin D is a true vitamin only for people who fail to produce enough from sunlight, such as some older people or institutionalized people. Humans synthesize vitamin D from a cholesterol-like substance by the action of sunlight on their skin. The vitamin D is later acted on by the liver and kidneys to form the hormone calcitriol. This hormone increases calcium absorption in the intestines and works with another hormone PTH to maintain calcium in bones. Rich food sources of vitamin D are fish oils and fortified milk. Megadose vitamin D intake can be toxic, especially in infancy and early childhood.

Vitamin K

Vitamin K is similar to vitamin D in that it can be synthesized in the body. Bacteria that normally reside in the colon can make vitamin K, which is subsequently absorbed and used by the body. Vitamin K can be found in two different forms, both of which have a similar structure and function. Phylloquinone is the form found in the food we consume. Menaquinone is the form of vitamin K synthesized by the gut microflora.

Functions of Vitamin K. Vitamin K is vital for blood clotting, working along with various proteins and calcium. Vitamin K contributes to the activation of several blood-clotting factors. Vitamin K also activates proteins present in bone, muscle, and kidneys, thereby imparting calcium-binding potential to these organs. Vitamin K chemically modifies the protein, osteocalcin, required for calcium to be added and removed from bone. A poor vitamin K intake has been linked to an increase in hip fractures in women because of its effect on various proteins in bone. An active area of scientific research is to identify other proteins that require vitamin K for their normal function.

Inactive blood-clotting factors
↓ **Action of vitamin K**
Active blood-clotting factors

Deficiency of vitamin K is rare in adults, however, it can occur with chronic fat malabsorption and prolonged use of antibiotics. Fat malabsorption decreases the amount of vitamin K available to the body from dietary sources, and antibiotics kill the bacteria that make vitamin K in the intestinal tract.

Vitamin K Sources and Needs. Green leafy vegetables such as Brussels sprouts, spinach, broccoli, lettuce, and cabbage are good sources of vitamin K (Fig. 10-18). Vegetable oils, liver, milk, meat, eggs, and many other foods provide small amounts of vitamin K. Vitamin K is resistant to cooking losses. Deficiency is uncommon because of the widespread abundance of vitamin K in a balanced diet. Intestinal synthesis of vitamin K appears to be highly variable between individuals. It has been estimated that bacterial synthesis provides 10% to 30% of the required vitamin K. There is no RDA for vitamin K because of the variability in bacterial synthesis and the subsequent problems with determining the dietary requirement. AI for adult men is 120 micrograms and 90 micrograms for adult women. The DV used on food and supplement labels is 80 micrograms. Older adults may be at risk of deficiency because of low consumption of green vegetables. Oral vitamin K poses no risk of toxicity, so no UL has been set.

▲ A salad containing dark greens (or other green vegetables) each day provides abundant vitamin K for a diet.

Food Sources of Vitamin K

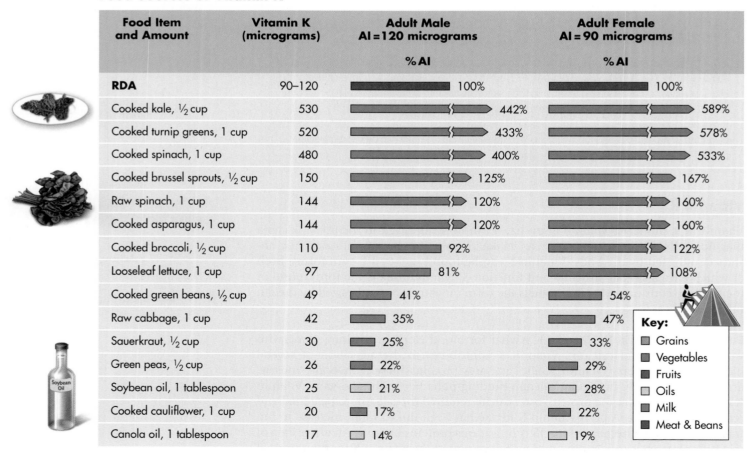

Food Item and Amount	Vitamin K (micrograms)	Adult Male AI=120 micrograms %AI	Adult Female AI=90 micrograms %AI
RDA	90–120	100%	100%
Cooked kale, ½ cup	530	442%	589%
Cooked turnip greens, 1 cup	520	433%	578%
Cooked spinach, 1 cup	480	400%	533%
Cooked brussel sprouts, ½ cup	150	125%	167%
Raw spinach, 1 cup	144	120%	160%
Cooked asparagus, 1 cup	144	120%	160%
Cooked broccoli, ½ cup	110	92%	122%
Looseleaf lettuce, 1 cup	97	81%	108%
Cooked green beans, ½ cup	49	41%	54%
Raw cabbage, 1 cup	42	35%	47%
Sauerkraut, ½ cup	30	25%	33%
Green peas, ½ cup	26	22%	29%
Soybean oil, 1 tablespoon	25	21%	28%
Cooked cauliflower, 1 cup	20	17%	22%
Canola oil, 1 tablespoon	17	14%	19%

Key: Grains, Vegetables, Fruits, Oils, Milk, Meat & Beans

FIGURE 10-18 ▶ Food sources of vitamin K compared to the Adequate Intake for adult males and females.

CONCEPT CHECK

Vitamin K plays a key role in efficient blood clotting; it contributes to the synthesis of calcium-binding proteins in some organs, such as bones. Between 10% to 30% of the vitamin K we absorb every day is synthesized by our intestinal bacteria; the rest comes from food. The amount in the diet alone meets our daily needs. Thus, except for newborns and possibly older adults, a deficiency of vitamin K is unlikely. Green vegetables and certain plant oils are good sources of vitamin K.

Magnesium (Mg)

Magnesium is important for nerve and heart function and aids in many enzyme reactions. Magnesium is similar to calcium and phosphorus in that most of the magnesium in the body is found in bones. Bone contains 60% of the body's magnesium. Magnesium serves a structural role in bones to help provide rigidity, and it also functions as a storage site drawn upon by other tissues when dietary intake is inadequate to meet the body's needs. Magnesium deficiency in animals has been shown to result in decreased bone strength and volume, poor bone development, reduced bone formation, and increased bone resorption. Magnesium also functions to relax muscles after contraction and promotes resistance to tooth decay by stabilizing calcium in tooth enamel. Over 300 enzymes use magnesium, and many energy-yielding compounds in cells require magnesium to function properly (e.g., ATP). Magnesium also plays a critical role in the synthesis of DNA and protein. Another notable function of magnesium as it relates to bone health is that magnesium is required for the synthesis of vitamin D in the liver.

In humans, a magnesium deficiency causes an irregular heartbeat, sometimes accompanied by weakness, muscle pain, disorientation, and seizures. Other possible benefits of magnesium in relation to cardiovascular disease include decreasing blood pressure by dilating arteries and preventing heart abnormalities. People with cardiovascular disease should closely monitor magnesium intake, especially because they are often on medications such as diuretics that reduce magnesium status. Keep in mind that a magnesium deficiency develops slowly because our bodies store it readily.

Magnesium Sources and Needs. Magnesium is found in the plant pigment chlorophyll, so rich sources for magnesium are plant products, such as squash, whole grains (like wheat bran), beans, nuts, seeds, and broccoli (Fig. 10-19). Animal products, such as milk and meats, and chocolate supply some magnesium, although less than the foods in the magnesium pyramid (Fig. 10-20). Two other sources of magnesium are hard tap water, which contains a high mineral content, and coffee.

The adult RDA for magnesium is about 400 milligrams per day for men and about 310 milligrams per day for women. This is based on the amount needed to offset daily losses. The DV used on food and supplement labels is 400 milligrams. Adult men consume an average of 320 milligrams daily, whereas women consume closer to 220 milligrams daily. This suggests that many of us should improve our intakes of magnesium-rich foods, such as whole-grain breads and cereals. The refined grain products that dominate the diets of many North Americans are poor sources of this mineral as refining reduces the magnesium content by as much as 80%. If dietary intake of magnesium is inadequate, a balanced multivitamin and mineral supplement containing approximately 100 milligrams of magnesium can help close the gap between intake and needs.

Poor magnesium status is especially found among users of certain diuretics. In addition, heavy perspiration for weeks in hot climates and bouts of long-standing diarrhea or vomiting cause significant magnesium loss. Alcoholism also increases the

Food Sources of Magnesium

Food Item and Amount	Magnesium (milligrams)	Adult Male RDA = 400 milligrams %RDA	Adult Female RDA = 310 milligrams %RDA
RDA	310–400	100%	100%
Spinach, 1 cup	157	39%	51%
Squash, 1 cup	105	26%	34%
Wheat germ, ¼ cup	90	23%	29%
Raisin Bran cereal, 1 cup	90	23%	29%
Navy beans, ½ cup	54	14%	17%
Peanut butter, 2 tablespoons	51	13%	16%
Black-eyed peas, ½ cup	46	12%	15%
Plain yogurt, 1 cup	43	11%	14%
Kidney beans, ½ cup	43	11%	14%
Sunflower seeds, ¼ cup	41	10%	13%
Broccoli, 1 cup	37	9%	12%
Banana, 1 medium	34	9%	11%
1% milk, 1 cup	34	9%	11%
Watermelon, 1 slice	32	8%	10%
Oatmeal, ½ cup	28	7%	9%
Whole-wheat bread, 1 slice	25	6%	8%

Key:
- Grains
- Vegetables
- Fruits
- Oils
- Milk
- Meat & Beans

FIGURE 10-19 ▶ Food sources of magnesium compared to the RDA for adult males and females.

risk of a deficiency because dietary intake may be poor and because alcohol increases magnesium excretion in the urine. The disorientation and weakness associated with alcoholism closely resembles the behavior of people with low blood magnesium.

Upper Level for Magnesium. The UL for magnesium intake is 350 milligrams per day, based on the risk of developing diarrhea. This guideline refers only to non-food sources such as antacids, laxatives, or supplements. Magnesium toxicity especially occurs in people who have kidney failure or who overuse over-the-counter medications that contain magnesium, such as certain antacids and laxatives (e.g., milk of magnesia). Older people are at particular risk, as kidney function may be compromised.

CONCEPT CHECK

Magnesium is required for nerve and heart function; it also aids activity for many enzymes. Food sources of magnesium are whole grains (wheat bran), vegetables, beef, coffee, beans, nuts, and seeds. People taking certain diuretics and people with alcoholism are at greatest risk of developing a deficiency. Magnesium toxicity is most likely in people with kidney failure or people using certain forms of laxatives and antacids.

MyPyramid:
Sources of Magnesium

Grains	Vegetables	Fruits	Oils	Milk	Meat & Beans
• Wheat bran • Wheat germ • Whole-grain products	• Spinach • Greens • Broccoli • Lima beans • Potatoes • Squash	• Figs • Peaches • Avocados • Bananas • Berries	• None	• Milk • Yogurt	• Tofu • Nuts • Shrimp • Kidney beans • Sunflower seeds

FIGURE 10-20 ▶ Sources of magnesium from MyPyramid. The height of the background color (non, 1/3, 2/3, or completely covered) within each group in the pyramid indicates the average nutrient density for magnesium in that group. Overall, the vegetables group provides the richest sources. Whole grain choices in the grains group are also rich sources. With regard to physical activity, magnesium is especially needed for the carbohydrate metabolism that takes place in such endeavors.

Fluoride (F)

The fluoride ion (F-) is the form of this trace mineral essential for human health. Nearly all (about 99%) of the fluoride in the body is associated with the teeth and skeleton. Dentists in the early 1900s noticed a lower rate of dental caries (cavities) in the southwestern United States. These areas contained high amounts of fluoride in the water. The amounts of fluoride were sometimes so high that small spots developed on the teeth (mottling). Even though mottled teeth were discolored, they contained few dental caries. Experiments in the early 1940s showed that fluoride in the water decreased the incidence of dental caries by 20% to 80% in children. Fluoridation of public water supplies in many parts of the United States has since been instituted.

Dentists can provide topical fluoride treatments and schools can provide fluoride tablets, but the most economical distribution method is to add fluoride to a community's drinking water. Numerous products are available to topically apply fluoride to teeth. These include gels applied at a dentists office, toothpaste, and mouth rinses. These products have a similar effect in reducing the incidence of dental caries. When water fluoridation and fluoridated topical products are used in combination, the reduction in dental caries are additive.

Functions of Fluoride. Fluoride functions in the following ways to prevent dental caries: (1) fluoride is incorporated into the tooth structure causing it to be stronger and more resistant to acid degradation from bacteria found in plaque; (2) stimulation of remineralization of enamel and inhibition of tooth demineralization; and (3) antibacterial effect on acid producing microorganisms found in plaque.

Fluoride has been shown to increase protein synthesis in the osteoblast and subsequently have an effect on the production of new bone. The combination of calcium and fluoride supplementation has been investigated to increase bone mass, however, to date the studies have been inconclusive.

▲ Example of mottling in a tooth caused by overexposure to fluoride.

▲ Fluoridated water is responsible for much of the decrease in dental caries throughout North America.

Fluorosis Discoloration of tooth enamel sometimes accompanied with pitting due to consuming a large amount of fluoride for an excessive period.

Fluoride Sources and Needs. Tea, seaweed, and some natural water sources are the only good food sources of fluoride. Most fluoride intake comes from fluoride added to drinking water and topical treatments. Fluoride is generally not added to bottled water. The trend to consume bottled water may result in an increase in the incidence of dental caries, especially in children.

The AI for fluoride for adults is 3.1 to 3.8 milligrams per day. This range of intake provides the benefits of resistance to dental caries without causing ill effects. Typical fluoridated water contains about 1 milligram per liter, which works out to about 0.25 milligrams per cup.

Upper Level for Fluoride. The UL for fluoride is set at 1.3 to 2.2 milligrams per day for young children and 10 milligrams per day for children over 9 years of age and adults, based on skeletal and tooth damage seen with higher doses. Children may swallow large amounts of fluoride toothpaste as part of daily tooth care and as result develop **fluorosis**. During tooth development (first decade of life), fluorosis permanently damages teeth. Fluorosis leads to stained and pitted teeth. Not swallowing toothpaste and limiting the amount used to "pea" size are the best ways to prevent this problem. In addition, children under 6 years should have tooth brushing supervised by an adult. In adults, fluorosis is associated with hip fractures, weak/stiff joints, and chronic stomach inflammation. There have been opponents to the fluoridation of public water supplies. These individuals claim that high fluoride intake can lead to a host of medical problems including cancer, bone disease, and Alzheimer's disease. These claims have been thoroughly investigated by independent researchers and government health organizations and none of the claims can be substantiated.

CONCEPT CHECK

Fluoride becomes incorporated into teeth during development and is present in salivary secretions. The presence of this trace mineral makes teeth resistant to acid and bacterial growth, in turn reducing development of dental caries. Fluoride also aids in the remineralization of teeth once decay begins. Most of us receive adequate amounts of fluoride from that added to drinking water and toothpaste. An excessive fluoride intake during tooth development can lead to spotted (i.e., mottled) teeth and possibly bone damage.

OTHER NUTRIENTS INVOLVED IN BONE HEALTH

In addition to these vitamins and minerals that play major roles in bone health (see Table 10-3), there are also a number of other nutrients that contribute to bone health.

Boron has been shown to have a role in the structure and strength of bone by influencing the transport of calcium across membranes and the synthesis of vitamin D. Elderly women fed a low-boron diet had low blood levels of calcium and magnesium. The estimated daily requirement is 1 milligram per day. The UL for boron is 20 milligrams per day. Silicon is required for normal growth and development of bone and connective tissue. Silicon is essential for synthesis of the collagen matrix upon which new bone is made. No UL for silicon has been established. Toxicity of silicon has been observed in people taking large amounts of silicon-containing antacids long term (for years). The consequences are an increased incidence of kidney stones and the level of some antioxidant enzymes is decreased. A serious respiratory condition called silicosis occurs with the inhalation of dust. Vitamin C is also critically important for the synthesis of the connective tissue upon which osteoblast cells build bone.

TABLE 10-3 Nutrients That Function In Bone Health

Nutrient	Primary Function in Bone	Common Food Sources
Calcium	Provides rigidity to bone. Ninety-nine percent of calcium in the human body is found in bones and teeth.	Milk, yogurt, fortified orange juice, sardines, canned salmon, fortified cereals
Phosphorus	Critical component of hydroxyapatite crystals in bone	Yogurt, almonds, milk, cheese, salmon, meats, eggs
Vitamin D	Regulates calcium and phosphorus levels for bone integrity and maintenance	Fish, milk, fortified cereals. Best source is sunlight.
Vitamin K	Activates proteins present in bone, muscle and kidney causing calcium-binding activity; blood clotting and activates several blood clotting factors. Increases bone density. Necessary for osteocalcin synthesis.	Brussels sprouts, dark green leafy vegetables, raw cabbage, green beans, asparagus, soybean oil, canola oil
Magnesium	Promotes resistance to tooth decay by holding calcium in tooth enamel. Stored in bone like calcium, works like calcium in blood-clot formation, necessary for hundreds of enzymatic reactions within the body	Dark green leafy vegetables, peanut butter, beans and peas, bananas, almonds
Fluoride	Strengthens bones and teeth. Stimulate osteoblasts.	Potatoes, legumes, canned salmon. Community water supplies have added fluoride. May not be present in bottled drinking water.

CASE STUDY

Giving Up Milk

Ashley, a 19-year-old sophomore in college, recently gave up drinking milk. She thought this would help her stay slim by avoiding the calories in milk. Ashley's mother is concerned about her diet change. One of her primary concerns is the future risk of osteoporosis. Ashley also started smoking, and her only physical activity is practice for the women's choir.

Ashley's typical diet consists of oatmeal made with water, a banana, and a cup of fruit juice for breakfast. At midmorning, she buys a snack cake or candy bar from the vending machine. At lunch, she has pasta with vegetables, bread with olive oil, a side salad, 1 ounce of mixed nuts, and a soft drink. For dinner, she has a chicken or hamburger sandwich along with mixed vegetables and another soft drink. As an evening snack, she has some cookies and hot tea.

Answer the following questions about Ashley's situation and check your responses in Appendix A.

1. What nutrients are low in Ashley's typical diet that put her at risk of osteoporosis in the future?
2. Which of Ashley's lifestyle factors contribute to this increased risk of osteoporosis?
3. Is there any evidence that consumption of milk or other dairy products leads to weight gain?
4. What changes to her current diet could reduce the risk of osteoporosis and also help Ashley maintain her weight?
5. What lifestyle changes (other than dietary changes) could Ashley make to decrease her risk of osteoporosis and maintain a healthy weight?

▲ Does giving up milk put Ashley at risk for osteoporosis?

SUMMARY

1. Calcium forms a part of bone structure and plays a role in blood clotting, muscle contractions, nerve transmission, and cell metabolism. Calcium absorption is enhanced by stomach acid and the active vitamin D hormone. Dairy products are important calcium sources. Women are particularly at risk for not meeting calcium needs.

2. Phosphorus aids enzyme function and forms part of the key metabolic compounds, cell membranes, and bone. It is efficiently absorbed, and deficiencies are rare, although there is some concern about possible poor intake by some older women. Good sources are daily products, bakery products, and meats.

3. Magnesium is a mineral found mostly in plant sources. It is important for nerve and heart function and as an activator for many enzymes. Whole-grain breads and cereals (bran portion), vegetables, nuts, seeds, milk, and meats are good food sources. Sulfur is incorporated into certain vitamins and amino acids.

4. Many minerals are vital for sustaining life. For humans, animal products are the most bioavailable sources of most minerals. Supplements of minerals exceeding 100% of the DV listed on the label should be taken only under a physician's supervision. Toxicity and nutrient interactions are especially likely if the UL (when set) is exceeded on a long-term basis.

5. Vitamin D is both a hormone and a vitamin. Human skin synthesizes it using sunshine and a cholesterol-like substance. If we don't spend enough time in the sun, such foods as fish and fortified milk can supply the vitamin. The active hormone form of vitamin D helps regulate blood calcium in part by increasing calcium absorption for the intestine. Infants and children who don't get enough vitamin D may develop rickets, and adults with inadequate amounts in the body develop osteomalacia. Older people and breastfed infants often need a supplemental source. Vitamin D is potentially a toxic substance in infancy and early childhood.

STUDY QUESTIONS

1. What are the differences between cortical and trabecular bone?

2. Describe the functions of two hormones that affect bone metabolism.

3. List three sources of dietary calcium. Identify two factors that negatively influence the absorption of calcium. Identify two factors that positively influence the absorption of calcium.

4. Other than its role in bone structure, what are three functions of phosphorus? List three food sources of this mineral.

5. What is the primary function of the vitamin D hormone? Which groups of people likely need to supplement their diets with vitamin D, and on what do you base your answer?

6. How does vitamin K contribute to bone health? Identify one other function of vitamin K.

7. List three roles of magnesium in the body. Identify two chronic diseases that may be affected by magnesium status.

8. What is peak bone mass? At what age is peak bone mass achieved? List three lifestyle factors that affect peak bone mass.

9. Describe the functions of fluoride in the body. List three sources of fluoride.

10. Describe two methods that can be used to assess bone density. What demographic groups should have bone density measured?

CHECK YOUR KNOWLEDGE

Answers to the following multiple choice questions are in Appendix A.

1. Vitamin D is called the sunshine vitamin because
   a. it is available in orange juice.
   b. exposure to sunlight converts a precursor to vitamin D.
   c. it can be destroyed by exposure to sunlight.
   d. All of the above.

2. Bowed legs, an enlarged and misshapen head, and enlarged knee joints in children are all symptoms of
   a. rickets.
   b. xerophthalmia.
   c. osteoporosis.
   d. vitamin D toxicity.

3. Ninety-nine percent of the calcium in the body is found in
   a. intracellular fluid.
   b. bones and teeth.
   c. nerve cells.
   d. the liver.

4. At the end of long bones, inside the spinal vertebrae, and inside the flat bones of the pelvis, is a spongy type of bone known as _____ bone.
   a. osteoclastic
   b. osteoblastic
   c. trabecular
   d. compact

5. Individuals in which of the following groups are most likely to develop osteoporosis?
   a. premenopausal women athletes
   b. women taking estrogen replacement therapy
   c. slender, inactive women who smoke
   d. women who eat a lot of high-fat dairy products

6. Vitamin D enhances absorption of
   a. calcium.
   b. phosphorus.
   c. both calcium and phosphorus.
   d. neither calcium nor phosphorus.

7. Fatty fish is a source of
   a. calcium.
   b. vitamin D.
   c. vitamin K.
   d. magnesium.

8. Food sources of vitamin K include all of the following except
   a. plant oils.
   b. green, leafy vegetables.
   c. oranges.
   d. liver.

9. Synthesis of the collagen matrix of bone requires all of the following except
   a. silicon.
   b. boron.
   c. vitamin C.
   d. protein.

10. Which of the following hormones acts to decrease calcium absorption?
    a. parathyroid hormone
    b. calcitriol
    c. estrogen
    d. calcitonin

FURTHER READINGS

1. Bischoff-Ferrari HA and others: Fracture prevention with vitamin D supplementation. *Journal of the American Medical Association* 293:2257, 2005.
   Providing about 800 IU/day of vitamin D to older adults reduced the risk of hip fracture in this study. It appears that 400 IU/day is not sufficient to provide the same benefit.

2. Food and Nutrition Board, Institute of Medicine: *Dietary Reference Intakes for calcium, phosphorus, magnesium, vitamin D, and fluoride.* Washington, DC: The National Academy Press, 1997.
   The RDAs and related standards for vitamin D and some minerals are discussed in detail. A major change in setting these new (and all other) estimates of human needs is the use of a specific biological marker or estimate of current intakes that shows adequacy.

3. Neld LS and others: Rickets: Not a disease of the past. *American Family Physician* 74(4),200:619, 2006.
   This review article emphasizes the need to screen for rickets even in developed countries. Background and support is given for the recent recommendation by the American Academy of Pediatrics (AAP) to provide a daily vitamin D supplement for all solely breastfed babies beginning in the first two months of life. Until recently, vitamin D supplementation was not advised for breastfed infants. Multiple case reports of nutritional rickets in the United States have prompted the AAP recommendation.

4. Tangpricha V and others: Tanning is associated with optimal vitamin D status (serum 25-hydroxyvitamin D concentration) and higher bone mineral density. *American Journal of Clinical Nutrition* 80:1645, 2004.
   A higher vitamin D status was correlated with higher bone mineral density in subjects exposed to UVB radiation by using a tanning bed at least once a week. Thus, tanning may have beneficial effects on the skeleton.

5. ADA Reports: Position of the American Dietetic Association: The impact of fluoride on health. *Journal of the American Dietetic Association* 105:1620, 2005.
   The American Dietetic Association reaffirms that fluoride is an important element for all mineralized tissues in the body. Appropriate fluoride intake is beneficial to bone and tooth health.

6. Heaney RP: Absorbability and utility of calcium in mineral waters. *American Journal of Clinical Nutrition* 84(2):371, 2006.
   Published absorbability and utility of high-calcium mineral waters are summarized in this article. The absorbability of all the high-calcium mineral waters was equal to or slightly better than milk calcium. The utility of calcium as measured by increased urinary calcium, decreased serum parathyroid hormone, decreased bone resorption biomarkers, and protection of bone mass indicated that a significant quantity of calcium was absorbed. High-calcium mineral waters, therefore, appear to provide useful quantities of bioavailable calcium.

7. Jackson RD and others: Calcium plus vitamin D supplementation and the risk of fractures. *New England Journal of Medicine* 354(7):669, 2006.
   Postmenopausal women, 50 to 79 years of age, enrolled in a Women's Health Initiative (WHI) clinical trial were assigned to receive daily doses of 1000 mg of elemental calcium as calcium carbonate (with 400 IU of vitamin D) or a placebo. Fracture occurrence and bone density were determined over 7 years. Calcium with vitamin D supplementation resulted in a small but significant increase in hip bone density, but did not significantly reduce hip fracture and increased the risk of kidney stones.

8. Keuhn BM: Better osteoporosis management a priority: Impact predicted to soar with aging population. *Journal of the American Medical Association* 293(20):2453, 2005.
   More than 2 million individuals in the United States will experience osteoporosis-related fractures this year, resulting in medical costs estimated to exceed $16.9 billion. By 2025, the number of fractures and the associated costs are expected to rise by 48%. Proper diet and exercise throughout life are now recognized as the most effective measures to maintain bone health.

9. Liebman B: Breaking up: Strong bones need more than calcium. *Nutrition Action Health Letter* 32(3):3, 2005.
   This article presents a good, basic overview of the latest research for preventing bone loss and maintaining bone health. The article includes specific recommendations for daily exercise and for intakes of calcium, vitamin A, vitamin D, vitamin K, protein, and potassium and for fruits and vegetables.

10. Nieves JW: Osteoporosis: The role of micronutrients. *American Journal of Clinical Nutrition* 81:1232S, 2005.
    The effects of calcium and vitamin D on bone cannot be considered in isolation from the other components of the diet. The other micronutrients needed for optimizing bone health include magnesium, potassium, vitamin C, and vitamin K. These needs can be met with a healthy diet high in fruits and vegetables (≥ 5 servings per day).

11. Raisz LG: Screening for osteoporosis. *The New England Journal of Medicine* 353:164, 2005.

    Measurement of bone mineral density at the lumbar spine and proximal femur by DEXA bone scans is a reliable and safe way to assess the risk of fracture in postmenopausal women. However, many other factors influence fracture risk, such as genetic background and race, and should be considered in making recommendations regarding bone densitometry and therapy.

12. Reid IR and others: Randomized controlled trial of calcium in healthy older women. *American Journal of Medicine* 119(9):777, 2006.

    In this study of postmenopausal women receiving 1 g/day as calcium citrate over 5 years, height loss was reduced by calcium but constipation was more common. The authors conclude that calcium results in a sustained reduction in bone loss and turnover, but its effect on fracture is uncertain.

13. Rosen CJ: Postmenopausal osteoporosis. *New England Journal of Medicine* 353:595, 2005.

    The diagnosis and treatment of osteoporosis, including use of current medications, is reviewed. The author recommends bisphosphonates as the most appropriate medication, as well as meeting calcium and vitamin D needs.

14. U.S. Preventive Services Task Force Recommendation Statement: Hormone therapy for the prevention of chronic conditions in postmenopausal women. *American Family Physician* 72(2):311, 2005.

    The U.S. Preventive Services Task Force (USPSF) recommends against routine use of combined estrogen and progestin for the prevention of chronic conditions in postmenopausal women. Any such use should be short term, such as for treating the initial symptoms of menopause. The American College of Obstetrics and Gynecology, the American Heart Association, the North American Menopause Society, and the Canadian Task Force on Preventive Health Care make similar recommendations.

15. Van Dam RM and others: Dietary calcium and magnesium, major food sources, and risk of type 2 diabetes in U.S. black women. *Diabetes Care* 29:2238, 2006.

    Magnesium and calcium intakes have been inversely associated with risk of type 2 diabetes in predominantly white populations. The results of this study of 41,186 participants of the Black Women's Health Study indicated that a diet high in magnesium-rich foods, particularly whole grains, is associated with a significantly lower risk of type 2 diabetes in U.S. black women.

16. Gonzalez AJ and others: Calcium intake and 10-year weight change in middle-aged adults. *Journal of the American Dietetic Association* 106:1066, 2006.

    Research into the relationship between dietary calcium from food and/or supplement sources and weight management has been inconsistent. This 10-year study of 10,591 middle-aged men and women who took dietary supplements showed that use of dietary calcium supplements was associated with lower weight gain over 10 years among women. Calcium from food sources was not associated with weight changes in this study. The authors do not recommend calcium supplementation for weight management, but suggest that weight control may be an added benefit of calcium supplementation to prevent osteoporosis.

17. Mark BL and Carson JS: Vitamin D and Autoimmune Disease—Implications for Practice from the Multiple Sclerosis Literature. *Journal of the American Dietetic Association* 106:418, 2006.

    Vitamin D is under study for its anti-inflammatory properties in many diseases, including arthritis, cancer, and some autoimmune diseases. Some evidence from studies conducted with multiple sclerosis (MS) patients suggests that vitamin D may be therapeutic, possibly lessening nerve damage and decreasing symptoms of MS. However, vitamin D is not currently a prescribed therapy because the high doses of vitamin D required to produce such effects may induce hypercalcemia. More research will be required before vitamin D may be prescribed for the treatment of autoimmune or other inflammatory disorders, but in the mean time, assessing dietary and supplemental vitamin D intake and promoting adequate consumption of this fat-soluble vitamin will aid in bone health with the possible benefit of reducing inflammation.

18. Pizzo G and others: Community water fluoridation and caries prevention: A critical review. *Clinical Oral Investigation* 11:189, 2007.

    Over the past 50 years, community water fluoridation has been a successful public health measure to reduce dental caries. However, now that oral hygiene has improved, access to regular dental care is widespread and other sources of fluoride are widely available, fluorosis is the emerging problem. The authors suggest that community water fluoridation may only now be necessary in disadvantaged communities.

19. Song WO and others: Ready-to-eat breakfast cereal consumption enhances milk and calcium intake in the U.S. population. *Journal of the American Dietetic Association* 106:1783, 2006.

    Milk consumption and total dietary calcium intake have declined over time. Possible reasons for these declines include concerns over heart health and weight control, as well as the availability of sweetened beverages. This study demonstrated that inclusion of ready-to-eat breakfast cereal improves calcium intake. Encouraging consumption of breakfast, particularly fortified, ready-to-eat breakfast cereal with fat-free or low-fat milk, is a simple way to promote bone health.

▶ **Check out the Contemporary Nutrition ARIS site**
www.mhhe.com/wardlawcontfa1 for quizzes, flash cards, other activities, and weblinks designed to further help you learn about what you eat and why.

I. Working for Denser Bones

Osteoporosis and related low bone mass affect many adults in North America, especially older women. One-third of all women experience fractures because of this disease, amounting to about 2 million bone fractures per year.

Osteoporosis is a disease you can do something about. Some risk factors can't be changed, but others, such as poor calcium intake, can. Is this true for you? To find out, complete this tool for estimating your current calcium intake. For all the following foods, write the number of servings you eat in a day. Total the number of servings in each category and then multiply the total number of servings by the amount of calcium for each category. Finally, add the total amount for each category to estimate your calcium intake for that day.

Does your intake meet your AI set for calcium?

Food	Serving Size	Number of Servings	Calcium (mg)	Total Calcium (mg)
Plain low-fat yogurt	1 cup	_____		
Fat-free dry milk powder	½ cup	_____		
	Total servings	_____	X 400	= _____ mg
Canned sardines (with bones)	3 ounces	_____		
Fruit-flavored yogurt	1 cup	_____		
Milk: fat-free, reduced-fat, whole, chocolate, buttermilk	1 cup	_____		
Calcium-fortified soy milk (e.g., Silk)	1 cup	_____		
Parmesan cheese (grated)	¼ cup	_____		
Swiss cheese	1 ounce	_____		
	Total servings	_____	X 300	= _____ mg
Cheese (all other hard cheese)	1 ounce	_____		
Pancakes	3	_____		
	Total servings	_____	X 200	= _____ mg
Canned pink salmon	3 ounces	_____		
Tofu (processed with calcium)	4 ounces	_____		
	Total servings	_____	X 150	= _____ mg
Collards or turnip greens, cooked	½ cup	_____		
Ice cream or ice milk	1 ounce	_____		
Almonds		_____		
	Total servings	_____	X 75	= _____ mg
Chard, cooked	½ cup	_____		
Cottage cheese	½ cup	_____		
Corn tortilla	1 medium	_____		
Orange	1 medium	_____		
	Total servings	_____	X 50	= _____ mg
Kidney, lima, or navy beans, cooked	½ cup	_____		
Broccoli	½ cup	_____		
Carrot, raw	1 medium	_____		
Dates or raisins	¼ cup	_____		
Egg	1 large	_____		
Whole-wheat bread	1 slice	_____		
Peanut butter	2 tablespoons	_____		
	Total servings	_____	X 25	= _____ mg
Calcium-fortified orange juice	6 ounces	_____		
Calcium-fortified snack bars	1 each	_____		
Calcium-fortified breakfast bars	½ bar	_____		
	Total servings	_____	X 200	= _____ mg
Calcium-fortified chocolate candies	1 each	_____	X 500	
Calcium supplements*	1 each	_____		
	Total servings	_____	Total calcium intake	= _____ mg = _____ mg

Other calcium sources to consider include many breakfast cereals (100–250 mg per cup) and some vitamin/mineral supplements (200–500 mg or more per tablet).
*Amount varies, so check the label for the amount in a specific product and then adjust the calculation as needed.
Reprinted with permission from *Topics in Clinical Nutrition*, "Putting Calcium into Perspective for Your Clients," G. Wardlaw and N. Weese, 11:1, © 1995 Aspen Publishers, Inc.

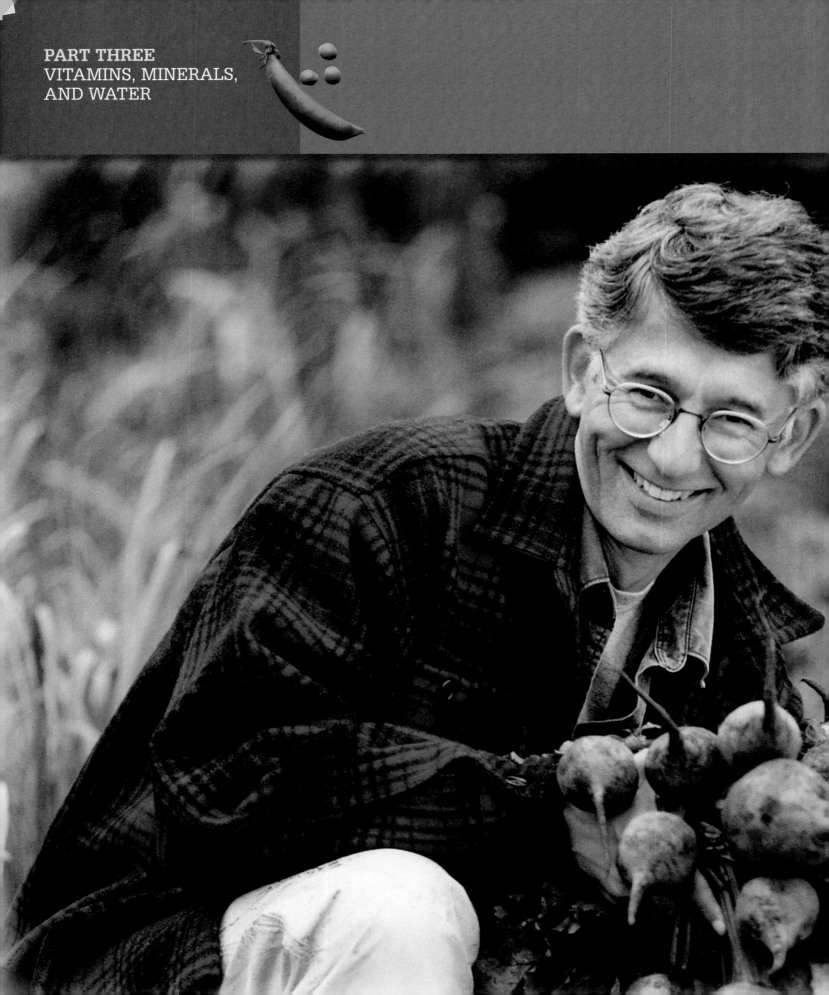

CHAPTER 11 Micronutrient Function in Energy Metabolism and Blood Health

CHAPTER OBJECTIVES   Chapter 11 is designed to allow you to:

1. Describe how vitamins and minerals function as coenzymes that allow chemical reactions in metabolism to occur.

2. List and describe how the eight B vitamins function to enhance energy metabolism.

3. Describe food sources, deficiency, and toxicity symptoms associated with the B vitamins.

4. List and describe the minerals involved in energy metabolism.

5. Describe the composition of blood.

6. List and describe the function of a vitamin and trace minerals in the maintenance of blood health.

7. Describe how nutrients influence the many forms of anemia observed.

CHAPTER OUTLINE

HOW DOES THE BODY CONVERT THE ENERGY FOUND IN FOOD INTO A FORM THAT THE CELLS CAN USE? The cells obtain energy from the chemical bonds found in the macronutrients (carbohydrates, lipids, and proteins). You learned previously that during the process of digestion, the macronutrients are chemically broken down into smaller substances (monosaccharides, fatty acids, monoglycerides, glycerol, and amino acids) that can be absorbed into the body via the small intestine. The circulatory system then transports these nutrients to the trillions of cells in the body. The cells use chemical reactions to further breakdown these substances into carbon dioxide and water. In the process, large amounts of energy are converted into a form that the cells can use to perform work. The chemical processes used by cells to extract energy from these nutrients is termed metabolism. A major function of the micronutrients (**vitamins** and

Vitamin Compound needed in very small amounts in the diet to help regulate and support chemical reactions and processes in the body

Coenzyme A compound that combines with an inactive enzyme to form a catalytically active form. In this manner, coenzymes aid in enzyme function.

Bioavailability The degree to which an ingested nutrient is absorbed and thus is available to the body.

Inactive enzyme

$+$

Vitamin coenzyme

Active enzyme

FIGURE 11-1 ▶ Coenzymes, such as those formed from B vitamins, aid in the function of various enzymes. Without the coenzyme, the enzyme cannot function, and deficiency symptoms associated with the missing vitamin eventually appear. Health-food stores sell the coenzyme forms of some vitamins. These more expensive forms of vitamins are unnecessary. The body makes all the coenzymes it needs from vitamin precursors.

minerals) is to assist enzymes in the chemical reactions in energy metabolism. These micronutrients are called **coenzymes** because they activate the enzymes and allow them to become chemically functional.

This chapter is divided into four sections. The first section will discuss the vitamins that function in energy metabolism. The second section will discuss the role that minerals function in energy metabolism. The third and fourth sections discuss the role in which vitamins and minerals function in the maintenance of blood health.

 Refresh Your Memory

As you begin study of nutrients that function in energy metabolism and blood health in Chapter 11, you might want to review:

- Implications of the Dietary Supplement Health and Education Act (DSHEA) in Chapter 1
- The gastrointestinal system for the digestion and absorption of nutrients in Chapter 3
- Carbohydrate metabolism in Chapter 4
- Lipid metabolism in Chapter 5
- Amino acid metabolism and protein synthesis in Chapter 6

THE ROLE OF WATER-SOLUBLE VITAMINS AND CHOLINE IN ENERGY METABOLISM

As coenzymes, the B vitamins and some minerals play many key roles in metabolism (Fig. 11-1). The metabolic pathways used to convert the energy found in carbohydrates, lipids, and amino acids into a form the cells can use require input from micronutrients. Many B vitamins are interdependent because they participate in the same processes (Fig. 11-2). Early symptoms of micronutrient deficiency typically occur in the brain and nervous system, skin, and gastrointestinal (GI) tract. Cells in these tissues are metabolically active, and those in the skin and GI tract are also constantly being replaced.

After being ingested, the B vitamins are first broken down from their coenzyme forms into free vitamins in the stomach and small intestine. The vitamins are then absorbed, primarily in the small intestine. Typically, about 50% to 90% of the B vitamins in the diet are absorbed, demonstrating their relatively high **bioavailability**. Once inside cells, the coenzyme forms are resynthesized. Although some vitamins are sold in their coenzyme forms in health-food stores, there is no need to consume the coenzyme forms. These are broken down during digestion and we make them when needed.

B Vitamin Intakes of North Americans

The nutritional health of most North Americans with regard to the B vitamins is good. Typical diets contain plentiful and varied natural sources of these vitamins. In addition, many common foods, such as ready-to-eat breakfast cereals, are fortified with one or more of the water-soluble vitamins. In some developing countries, however, deficiencies of the water-soluble vitamins are more common, and the resulting deficiency disease poses significant health problems. (A discussion of nutritional deficiencies worldwide is presented in the Overview of Micronutrients.)

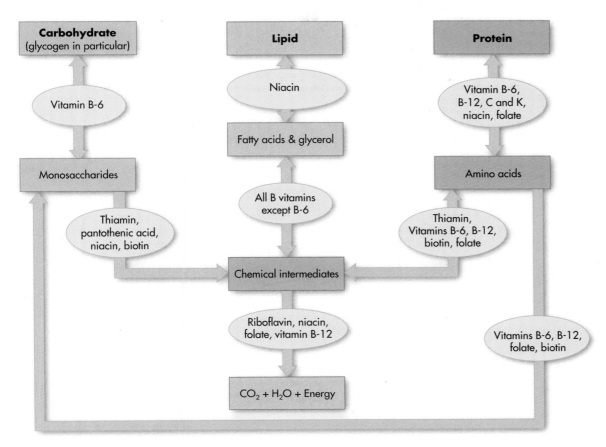

FIGURE 11-2 ▶ Examples of metabolic pathways for which water soluble vitamins are essential. The metabolism of energy-yielding nutrients requires vitamin input.

Most water-soluble vitamins are more readily excreted from the body than are fat-soluble vitamins. Any excess ends up in the urine or stool and little is stored, so it is important to regularly consume good sources of the water-soluble vitamins. Large amounts of these vitamins can be lost during food processing and preparation because they dissolve in water. Light cooking methods, such as stir-frying, steaming, and microwaving best preserve vitamin content (Table 11-1).

Despite good B vitamin status of North Americans, marginal deficiencies of the water-soluble vitamins may occur in some cases, especially in older people who eat little food, and in people who follow poor dietary patterns. The long-term effects of such marginal deficiencies are yet unknown, but increased risk of cardiovascular disease, cancer, and cataracts of the eye is suspected. However, in the short run, such a marginal deficiency in most people likely leads only to fatigue or other bothersome and unspecified physical effects. With rare exceptions, healthy adults do not develop the more serious B vitamin deficiency diseases from dietary inadequacy alone. The main exceptions are people with alcoholism. The combination of extremely unbalanced diets and alcohol-induced alterations of vitamin absorption and metabolism creates significant risks for serious nutrient deficiencies among people with alcoholism.

The milling of grains leads to losses of vitamins and minerals. In the milling process, seeds are crushed and the germ, bran, and husk layers are discarded, leaving just the starch-containing endosperm in the refined grains. The starch is used to make flour, bread, and cereal products. Unfortunately, many nutrients are lost along with the discarded germ, bran, and husk materials. To counteract these losses, in the United

▲ Rapid cooking of vegetables in minimal fluids aids in preserving vitamin content. Steaming is one effective method.

TABLE 11-1 Tips for Preserving the Vitamin Content of Foods

What to Do	Why
Keep fruits and vegetables cool.	Enzymes in food begin to degrade vitamins once the fruit or vegetable is picked. Chilling reduces this process. Refrigerate fresh produce (except for potatoes, tomatoes, onions, and bananas) until they are consumed.
Refrigerate foods in moisture-proof, air-tight containers.	Nutrients keep best at temperatures near freezing, at high humidity, and away from air.
Trim, peel, and cut fruits and vegetables minimally—just enough to remove rotten or inedible parts.	Oxygen breaks down vitamins faster when more surface is exposed. Outer leaves of lettuce and other greens have higher values of vitamins and minerals than the inner, tender leaves or stems. Potato skins and apple skins are higher in vitamins and minerals than the inner parts.
Microwave, steam, or use a pan or wok with small amounts of fat and a tight-fitting lid to cook vegetables.	More nutrients are retained when there is less contact with water and shorter cooking time. Whenever possible, cook fruits or vegetables in their skins.
Minimize reheating food.	Prolonged reheating reduces vitamin content.
Do not add fats to vegetables during cooking if you plan to discard the liquid.	Fat-soluble vitamins will be lost in discarded fat. Add fats to vegetables after they are fully cooked and drained.
Do not add baking soda to vegetables to enhance the green color.	Alkalinity destroys much vitamin D, thiamin, and other vitamins.
Store canned foods in a cool place.	Canned foods vary in the amount of nutrients lost, largely because of differences in storage time and temperatures. To get maximal nutritive value from canned goods, serve any liquid packed with the food whenever possible.

Anemia A decreased oxygen-carrying capacity of the blood. This can be caused by many factors, such as iron deficiency or blood loss.

Beriberi The thiamin deficiency disorder characterized by muscle weakness, loss of appetite, nerve degeneration, and sometimes edema.

▶ **The Whole-Grain Advantage**

Bread (whole-wheat vs. white)

vitamin E	↑	17%
vitamin B-6	↑	60%
potassium	↑	92%
magnesium	↑	70%
fiber	↑	66%

Rice (brown vs. white)

vitamin E	↑	800%
vitamin B-6	↑	93%
potassium	↑	280%
magnesium	↑	450%
fiber	↑	550%

States, bread and cereal products made from milled grains are enriched with four B vitamins (thiamin, riboflavin, niacin, and folic acid) and with the mineral iron.

Food enrichment was initiated by a legislative act in the 1930s to help combat nutrient deficiencies like pellagra (niacin deficiency) and iron-deficiency **anemia.** Federal regulations added folate to the list of nutrients required to be added to refined grain products in 1998. Unfortunately, these products remain lower in vitamin E, vitamin B-6, potassium, magnesium, fiber, and other nutrients than the whole grains. This is one reason why nutrient experts advocate regular consumption of whole-grain products, such as whole-wheat bread and brown rice, rather than refined grain products.

The B vitamins are thiamin, riboflavin, niacin, pantothenic acid, biotin, vitamin B-6, folate, and vitamin B-12. Choline is a related nutrient, but is not classified as a vitamin. The coenzyme function, recommended intake, and deficiency and toxicity symptoms of the B-complex vitamins follow.

VITAMINS AND MINERALS INVOLVED IN ENERGY METABOLISM

Thiamin (Vitamin B-1)

Thiamin was the first water-soluble vitamin to be discovered. A primary function is to help release energy from carbohydrate. Its coenzyme form participates in reactions in which a carbon dioxide (CO_2) is lost from a substrate. This reaction is particularly important in the body's ATP-producing energy pathways, which involve the breakdown of carbohydrates and certain amino acids (Fig. 11-2). Thiamin also functions in chemical reactions that make RNA, DNA, and neurotransmitters.

Thousands of years ago, the life-threatening condition of thiamin deficiency was described. The thiamin deficiency disease is called **beriberi,** a word that means "I can't, I can't" in the Sri Lanka language of Sinhalese. The symptoms include weakness, loss of appetite, irritability, nervous tingling throughout the body, poor arm and leg coordination, and deep muscle pain in the calves. A person with beriberi often develops an enlarged heart and sometimes severe edema.

Beriberi is seen in areas where rice is a staple and polished (white) rice is consumed rather than brown rice (whole-grain) rice. In most parts of the world, brown rice has had its bran and germ layer removed to make white rice, a poor source of thiamin, unless it is enriched.

Beriberi results when glucose, the primary fuel for brain and nerve cells, cannot be metabolized to release energy. The thiamin coenzyme participates in glucose metabolism, so problems with body functions associated with brain and nerve action are the first signs of a thiamin deficiency, some after only 10 days on a thiamin-free diet.

▲ Pork is a good source of thiamin.

Thiamin Sources and Needs. Major sources of thiamin include pork products, whole grains (wheat germ), ready-to-eat breakfast cereals, enriched grains, green beans, milk, orange juice, organ meats, peanuts, dried beans, and seeds (Fig. 11-3).

The adult RDA for thiamin is 1.1 to 1.2 milligrams per day. The Daily Value (DV) used on food and supplement labels is 1.5 milligrams. Average daily intakes for men exceed this by 50% or more, and women generally meet the RDA. Some groups, such as low-income and older people, may barely meet their needs for thiamin. A diet dominated by highly processed and unenriched foods, sugar, fat, and heavy alcohol intake and a poor diet also creates a potential for thiamin deficiency (Fig. 11-4). Oral

Food Sources of Thiamin

Food Item and Amount	Thiamin (milligrams)	Adult Male RDA = 1.2 milligrams %RDA	Adult Female RDA = 1.1 milligrams %RDA
RDA	1.1–1.2	100%	100%
Canned lean ham, 3 ounces	0.9	75%	82%
Pork chops, 4 ounces	0.6	50%	55%
Wheat germ, 1/4 cup	0.5	42%	45%
Canadian bacon, 2 ounces	0.5	42%	45%
Acorn squash, 1 cup	0.4	33%	36%
Soy milk, 1 cup	0.4	33%	36%
Flour tortilla, 1	0.4	33%	36%
Ham lunch meat, 2 pieces	0.3	25%	27%
Watermelon, 1 slice	0.2	17%	18%
Fresh orange juice, 1 cup	0.2	17%	18%
Cooked green peas, 1/2 cup	0.2	17%	18%
Baked beans, 1/2 cup	0.2	17%	18%
Navy beans, 1/2 cup	0.2	17%	18%
Corn, 1/2 cup	0.2	17%	18%

Key: Grains, Vegetables, Fruits, Oils, Milk, Meat & Beans

FIGURE 11-3 ▶ Food sources of thiamin compared to the RDA for adult males and females.

| Grains | Vegetables | Fruits | Oils | Milk | Meat & Beans |

MyPyramid: Sources of Thiamin, Riboflavin, and Niacin

FIGURE 11-4 ▶ Sources of thiamin, riboflavin, and niacin from MyPyramid. The height of the background color (none, 1/3, 2/3, or completely covered) within each group in the pyramid indicates the average nutrient density for these vitamins in that group. Overall, the meat & beans group and the grains group contain many foods that are nutrient-dense sources of thiamin, riboflavin, and niacin. As well, foods from the milk group are especially rich sources of riboflavin. With regard to physical activity, these vitamins play key roles in the increased energy metabolism that takes place during such endeavors.

thiamin supplements are typically nontoxic because thiamin is rapidly lost in the urine. Thus, no Upper Level (UL) has been set for thiamin.

MAKING DECISIONS

Alcohol Reduces Thiamin Status

People with alcoholism are at greater risk for thiamin deficiency because absorption and use of thiamin are profoundly diminished and excretion is increased by consumption of alcohol. Furthermore, the low-quality diet that often accompanies severe alcoholism makes matters worse. There is limited storage in the body, therefore an alcoholic binge lasting 1 to 2 weeks may quickly deplete already diminished amounts of the vitamin and result in deficiency symptoms. The beriberi associated with alcoholism is also called Wernicke-Korsakoff syndrome.

FIGURE 11-5 ▶ A painful, inflamed tongue (glossitis) can signal a deficiency of niacin, vitamin B-6, riboflavin, folate, or vitamin B-12. Often more than one deficiency is the cause.

Riboflavin (Vitamin B-2)

Riboflavin derives its name from its yellow color (*flavus* means yellow in Latin). The coenzyme forms of riboflavin participate in many energy-yielding metabolic pathways. For example, when fatty acids are broken down and used for energy, the coenzymes of riboflavin are used (Fig. 11-2). Some vitamin and mineral metabolism also requires riboflavin. In addition, because of its activation of certain enzymes, riboflavin has an antioxidant role in the body through its support of the enzyme glutathione peroxidase.

The symptoms associated with riboflavin deficiency (ariboflavinosis) include inflammation of the mouth and tongue, dermatitis, cracking of tissue around the corners of the mouth (called cheilosis), various eye disorders, sensitivity to the sun, and confusion (Fig. 11-5). Such symptoms develop after approximately 2 months on a riboflavin-poor diet. In addition, riboflavin deficiencies probably do not exist by themselves. Instead, a riboflavin deficiency would occur with deficiencies of niacin, thiamin, and vitamin B-6 because these nutrients often occur in the same foods.

Food Sources of Riboflavin

Food Item and Amount	Riboflavin (milligrams)	Adult Male RDA = 1.3 milligrams %RDA	Adult Female RDA = 1.1 milligrams %RDA
RDA	1.1–1.3	100%	100%
Multigrain Cheerios, ¾ cup	1.3	100%	110%
Fried beef liver, 1 ounce	1.2	92%	109%
Steamed oysters, 10	1.1	85%	100%
Plain yogurt, 1 cup	0.5	38%	45%
Raw mushrooms, 5	0.5	38%	45%
Braunschweiger sausage, 1	0.4	31%	36%
Cooked spinach, 1 cup	0.4	31%	36%
1% milk, 1 cup	0.4	31%	36%
Buttermilk, 1 cup	0.4	31%	36%
Boiled egg, 1	0.3	23%	27%
Sirloin steak, 3 ounces	0.3	23%	27%
Feta cheese, 1 ounce	0.2	15%	18%
Tortilla, 1	0.2	15%	18%
Lean ham, 3 ounces	0.2	15%	18%

Key:
- ▢ Grains
- ▢ Vegetables
- ▢ Fruits
- ▢ Oils
- ▢ Milk
- ▢ Meat & Beans

FIGURE 11-6 ▶ Food sources of riboflavin compared to the RDA for adult males and females.

Riboflavin Sources and Needs. Major sources of riboflavin are ready-to-eat breakfast cereals, milk and milk products, enriched grains, meat, and eggs (Fig. 11-6). Vegetables such as asparagus, broccoli, and various greens (e.g., spinach) are also good sources. Riboflavin is a relatively stable water-soluble vitamin; however, it is destroyed by light. Milk is sold in paper or plastic containers rather than clear glass to protect the riboflavin.

The adult RDA of riboflavin is 1.1 to 1.3 milligrams per day. The DV used on food and supplement labels is 1.7 milligrams. On average, daily intakes of riboflavin are slightly above the RDA. As with thiamin, people with alcoholism risk riboflavin deficiency because they eat nutrient-poor diets. No specific symptoms indicate that riboflavin taken in **megadoses** is toxic, so no UL has been set. Riboflavin supplementation can cause the urine to become bright yellow.

Niacin (vitamin B-3)

Niacin functions in the body as one of two related compounds: nicotinic acid and nicotinamide. The coenzyme forms of niacin function in many cellular metabolic pathways. When energy is being used, a niacin coenzyme is used. Synthetic pathways in the cell—those that make new compounds—also often use a niacin coenzyme. This is especially true for fatty acid synthesis (Fig. 11-2).

A coenzyme in over 200 enzymatic reactions, a niacin deficiency causes widespread changes in the body. The group of niacin deficiency symptoms is known as pellagra, which means rough or painful skin. The symptoms of the disease are **dementia,** diarrhea, and

Megadose Intake of a nutrient beyond estimates of needs to prevent a deficiency or what would be found in a balanced diet; two to 10 times human needs is a starting point for such a dose.

Dementia A general loss or decrease in mental function.

dermatitis (especially on areas of skin exposed to the sun) (Fig. 11-7). Later, death often results. Early symptoms include poor appetite, weight loss, and weakness.

Pellagra is the only dietary deficiency disease ever to reach epidemic proportions in the United States. It became a major problem in the southeastern United States in the late 1800s and persisted until the 1930s, when standards of living and diets improved. Today, pellagra is rare in Western societies, but can be seen in the developing world.

MAKING DECISIONS

Making Niacin Available

Niacin in corn is bound by a protein that hampers its absorption. Soaking corn in an alkaline solution, such as lime water (water with calcium hydroxide), releases bound niacin and renders it more usable. Hispanic people in North America traditionally soak corn in lime water before making tortillas. This treatment is one reason this Hispanic population never experienced much pellagra.

FIGURE 11-7 ▶ The dermatitis of a niacin deficiency called pellagra. Dermatitis on both sides of the body (bilateral) is a typical symptom. Sun exposure worsens the condition.

Niacin Sources and Needs. Major sources of niacin are tuna, poultry, peanuts, fish, ready-to-eat cereals, beef, and asparagus (Fig. 11-8). Coffee and tea also contribute some niacin to the diet. Niacin is heat stable; little is lost in cooking.

Food Sources of Niacin

Food Item and Amount	Niacin (milligrams)	Adult Male RDA = 16 milligrams %RDA	Adult Female RDA = 14 milligrams %RDA
RDA	14–16	100%	100%
Tuna, 3 ounces	11.3	71%	81%
Roasted chicken, 3 ounces	10.1	63%	72%
Peanuts, ½ cup	9.9	62%	71%
Baked salmon, 3 ounces	8.6	54%	61%
Turkey lunch meat, 3 ounces	5.4	34%	39%
Ground beef, 3 ounces	5.0	31%	36%
Raw mushrooms, 5	4.7	29%	34%
Lean steak, 4 ounces	4.5	28%	32%
Chunky peanut butter, 2 tablespoons	4.4	28%	31%
Fried beef liver, 1 ounce	4.1	26%	29%
Raisin Nut Bran cereal, ¾ cup	3.8	24%	27%
Tortilla, 1	2.6	16%	19%
Baked cod, 3 ounces	2.1	13%	15%
Potato, 1	2.1	13%	15%
Broiled halibut, 3 ounces	1.6	10%	11%

Key:
- ▢ Grains
- ▢ Vegetables
- ▢ Fruits
- ▢ Oils
- ▢ Milk
- ▢ Meat & Beans

FIGURE 11-8 ▶ Food sources of niacin compared to the RDA for adult males and females.

Besides the preformed niacin found in protein foods, we can synthesize niacin from the amino acid tryptophan: 60 milligrams of tryptophan in a diet yield about 1 milligram of niacin. In this manner, we synthesize about 50% of the niacin required each day. This reaction requires two other vitamins (riboflavin and vitamin B-6) to function as coenzymes in this chemical conversion.

The adult RDA of niacin is 14 to 16 milligrams per day. The RDA is expressed as niacin equivalents (NE) to account for niacin received intact from the diet, as well as that made from tryptophan. The DV used on food and supplement labels is 20 milligrams. Intakes of niacin by adults are about double the RDA, without considering the contribution from tryptophan. (Tables of food composition values also ignore this contribution.) Although pellagra was once common, today it is typically only seen associated with chronic alcoholism in conjunction with poverty and malnutrition and in those with rare disorders of tryptophan metabolism.

▲ Chicken is a good source of niacin. The tryptophan present can also be metabolized to niacin.

Upper Level for Niacin. The UL for niacin is 35 milligrams per day of the nicotinic acid form. Effects include headache; itching; and increased blood flow to the skin, causing blood vessel dilation or flushing in various parts of the body, especially when intakes are above 100 milligrams per day. In the long run, GI tract and liver damage are possible, so any use of megadoses, including large doses recommended for treatment for cardiovascular disease, requires close physician scrutiny. Nicotinic acid has been promoted as a natural method to lower blood lipids, however due to potential adverse side effects, its use is discouraged.

CONCEPT CHECK

The B vitamins thiamin, riboflavin, and niacin are important in the metabolism of carbohydrates, proteins, and fats. Energy metabolism in particular requires adequate amounts of the coenzyme forms of these three vitamins. Deficiency symptoms typically occur in the brain and nervous system, skin, and GI tract. Cells in these tissues are metabolically active, and those in the skin and GI tract are also constantly being replaced. Enriched grains are adequate sources of all three vitamins, as are ready-to-eat breakfast cereals. Otherwise, pork is an excellent source of thiamin; milk is an excellent source of riboflavin; and protein foods in general, such as chicken, are excellent sources of niacin. Deficiencies of all three vitamins can occur with alcoholism; a thiamin deficiency is the most likely of the three.

Pantothenic Acid

Pantothenic acid functions as a coenzyme in chemical reactions, which allow the release of energy from carbohydrates, lipids, and protein. This water-soluble vitamin also activates fatty acids so they can yield energy (Fig. 11-2). It is also used in the initial steps of fatty acid synthesis. Pantothenic acid is so widespread in foods that a nutritional deficiency among healthy people who eat varied diets is unlikely. *Pantothen* means "from every side" in Greek.

Pantothenic Acid Sources and Needs. Rich sources of pantothenic acid are sunflower seeds, mushrooms, peanuts, and eggs (Fig. 11-9). Other rich sources are meat, milk, and many vegetables.

The Adequate Intake (AI) set for pantothenic acid is 5 milligrams per day for adults. Average consumption is well in excess of this amount. The DV on food and supplement

FIGURE 11-9 ▶ Food sources of pantothenic acid compared to the Adequate Intake for adults.

Food Sources of Pantothenic Acid

Food Item and Amount	Panthothenic Acid (milligrams)	Adult Male and Female AI = 5 milligrams %AI
AI	5	100%
Total corn flakes cereal, ¾ cup	11.8	236%
Power bar, 1	10.0	200%
Luna bar, 1	9.9	198%
Sunflower seeds, ¼ cup	2.3	46%
Fried beef liver, 1 ounce	1.7	34%
Raw mushrooms, 5	1.7	34%
Plain yogurt, 1 cup	1.5	30%
Acorn squash, 1 cup	1.2	24%
Peanuts, ½ cup	1.0	20%
1% milk, 1 cup	0.9	18%
Roasted chicken breast, 3 ounces	0.8	16%
Broccoli, 1 cup	0.8	16%
Baked potato, 1	0.7	14%
Legumes, ½ cup	0.7	14%
Cooked egg yolk, 1	0.6	12%

Key:
- Grains
- Vegetables
- Fruits
- Oils
- Milk
- Meat & Beans

labels is 10 milligrams. A deficiency of pantothenic acid might occur in alcoholism along with a nutrient-deficient diet. However, the symptoms would probably be hidden among deficiencies of thiamin, riboflavin, vitamin B-6, and folate, so the pantothenic acid deficiency might be unrecognizable. No toxicity is known for pantothenic acid, so no UL has been set.

Biotin

In its coenzyme form, biotin aids in dozens of chemical reactions. Biotin assists in the addition of carbon dioxide to other compounds. These reactions are critical for the synthesis of glucose and fatty acids, while also helping to breakdown certain amino acids. Symptoms of biotin deficiency include a scaly inflammation of the skin, changes in the tongue and lips, decreased appetite, nausea, vomiting, a form of anemia, depression, muscle pain and weakness, and poor growth.

Biotin Sources and Needs. Egg yolks, peanuts, and cheese are good sources of biotin (Fig. 11-10). Intestinal bacteria synthesize and supply some biotin, making a biotin deficiency unlikely. However, scientists are not sure how much of the bacteria-synthesized biotin in our intestines is absorbed. If intestinal bacteria synthesis is not sufficient, as in people who are missing a large part of the colon or who take antibiotics for many months, special attention should be paid to meeting biotin needs. A protein called avidin in raw egg whites binds biotin and inhibits its ab-

Food Sources of Biotin

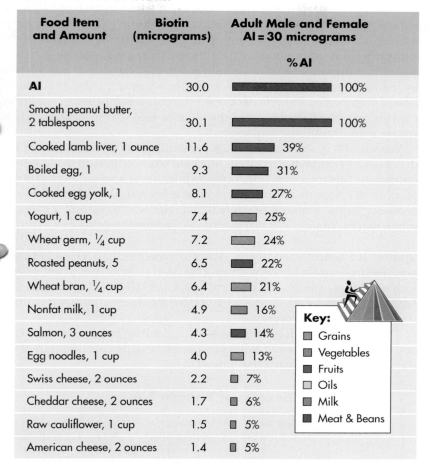

Food Item and Amount	Biotin (micrograms)	Adult Male and Female AI = 30 micrograms %AI	
AI	30.0	▬▬▬▬▬▬	100%
Smooth peanut butter, 2 tablespoons	30.1	▬▬▬▬▬▬	100%
Cooked lamb liver, 1 ounce	11.6	▬▬▬	39%
Boiled egg, 1	9.3	▬▬	31%
Cooked egg yolk, 1	8.1	▬▬	27%
Yogurt, 1 cup	7.4	▬▬	25%
Wheat germ, ¼ cup	7.2	▬	24%
Roasted peanuts, 5	6.5	▬▬	22%
Wheat bran, ¼ cup	6.4	▬	21%
Nonfat milk, 1 cup	4.9	▬	16%
Salmon, 3 ounces	4.3	▬	14%
Egg noodles, 1 cup	4.0	▬	13%
Swiss cheese, 2 ounces	2.2	▪	7%
Cheddar cheese, 2 ounces	1.7	▪	6%
Raw cauliflower, 1 cup	1.5	▪	5%
American cheese, 2 ounces	1.4	▪	5%

Key:
- ▪ Grains
- ▪ Vegetables
- ▪ Fruits
- ▪ Oils
- ▪ Milk
- ▪ Meat & Beans

FIGURE 11-10 ▶ Food sources of biotin compared to the Adequate Intake for adults.

sorption. Consuming many raw egg whites eventually leads to biotin deficiency disease. Cooking denatures the protein avidin in eggs such that it cannot bind biotin.

The AI set for biotin is 30 micrograms per day for adults. Our food supply is thought to provide 40 to 60 micrograms per person per day. The DV used on food and supplement labels is 300 micrograms, 10 times the estimate of needs. Biotin is relatively nontoxic. Large doses have been given over an extended period without harmful side effects to children who exhibit defects in biotin metabolism. Thus, no UL for biotin has been set.

Vitamin B-6

Vitamin B-6 is a family of three structurally similar compounds. All can be converted into the active vitamin B-6 coenzyme. The general name and form added to foods is called pyridoxine.

Functions of Vitamin B-6. The coenzymes of vitamin B-6 are needed for the activity of numerous enzymes involved in carbohydrate, protein, and fat metabolism. Vitamin B-6 is required in so many areas of metabolism, so a deficiency results in widespread symptoms, such as depression, vomiting, skin disorders, irritation of the nerves, and impaired immune response.

▲ Bananas are a plant source of vitamin B-6.

A key function of vitamin B-6 concerns protein because it functions as a coenzyme in over 100 chemical reactions that involve the metabolism of amino acids and proteins (Fig. 11-2). By helping split the nitrogen group ($-NH_2$) from an amino acid and making it available to another amino acid, the coenzyme participates in reactions that allow the synthesis of nonessential (dispensable) amino acids.

Another important role of vitamin B-6 is the synthesis of many neurotransmitters including serotonin and gamma aminobutyric acid. In the 1950s, infants fed overheated commercial formula developed vitamin B-6 deficiency symptoms, particularly convulsions. The heat destroyed the vitamin B-6, which subsequently leads to inadequate neurotransmitter synthesis.

Vitamin B-6 is also important for the synthesis of heme portion of **hemoglobin.** A deficiency of vitamin B-6 results in small red blood cells, with reduced hemoglobin concentration. This condition (microcytic hypochromic anemia) decreases a cell's ability to produce ATP because aerobic metabolism is limited. The vitamin B-6 coenzyme is also necessary for the synthesis of white blood cells, which perform a major role in the immune system. Vitamin B-6 also plays a role in **homocysteine** metabolism.

Vitamin B-6 Sources and Needs. Major sources of vitamin B-6 are potatoes, animal products, and ready-to-eat breakfast cereals (Fig. 11-11). Other sources are vegetables and fruits such as potatoes, spinach, bananas, and cantaloupes (Fig. 11-12). Overall animal sources and fortified products are the most reliable because the vitamin B-6 they contain is more absorbable than that in plant foods.

The adult RDA of vitamin B-6 is 1.3 to 1.7 milligrams per day. The DV used on food and supplement labels is 2 milligrams. Average daily consumption of vitamin B-6 for men and women is greater than the RDA.

Hemoglobin The iron-containing part of the red blood cell that carries oxygen to the cells and carbon dioxide away from the cells. The heme iron portion is also responsible for the red color of blood.

Homocysteine An amino acid that arises from the metabolism of methionine. Adequate levels of vitamin B-6, folate, and vitamin B-12 are required for its metabolism. Elevated levels are associated with an increased risk of cardiovascular disease.

FIGURE 11-11 ▶ Food sources of vitamin B-6 compared to the RDA for adults.

Food Sources of Vitamin B-6

Food Item and Amount	Vitamin B-6 (milligrams)	Adult Male and Female RDA = 1.3 milligrams %RDA
RDA	1.3	100%
Baked salmon, 3 ounces	0.8	62%
Baked potato, 1 medium	0.7	54%
Banana, 1	0.7	54%
Avocado, 1	0.6	46%
Roasted chicken breast, 3 ounces	0.5	38%
Acorn squash, 1 cup	0.5	38%
Special K cereal, 3/4 cup	0.5	38%
Fried beef liver, 1 ounce	0.4	31%
Roasted turkey lunch meat, 3 ounces	0.4	31%
Sirloin steak, 3 ounces	0.4	31%
Lean ham, 3 ounces	0.4	31%
Watermelon, 1 slice	0.3	23%
Sunflower seeds, 1/4 cup	0.3	23%
Cooked spinach, 1/2 cup	0.2	15%

Key:
- Grains
- Vegetables
- Fruits
- Oils
- Milk
- Meat & Beans

MyPyramid: Sources of Vitamin B-6

Grains	Vegetables	Fruits	Oils	Milk	Meat & Beans
• Fortified breakfast cereals • Wheat germ (whole-wheat products)	• Potatoes • Spinach • Cauliflower	• Avocados • Bananas • Dates • Cantaloupe • Watermelon	• None	• Milk • Yogurt • Cottage cheese	• Meat • Poultry • Fish • Beans • Nuts • Seeds

FIGURE 11-12 ▶ Sources of vitamin B-6 from MyPyramid. The height of the background color (none, 1/3, 2/3, or completely covered) within each group in the pyramid indicates the average nutrient density for vitamin B-6 in that group. Overall, the meat group especially contains many foods that are nutrient-dense sources of vitamin B-6. With regard to physical activity, vitamin B-6 participates in the related energy metabolism during such endeavors.

Athletes may need slightly more vitamin B-6 than sedentary adults. The athlete's body processes large quantities of glycogen and protein, and the metabolism of these compounds requires vitamin B-6. However, athletes are likely to consume plenty of protein—enough to supply needed amounts of vitamin B-6.

People with alcoholism are susceptible to a vitamin B-6 deficiency because a metabolite formed in alcohol metabolism can displace the coenzyme form from enzymes, increasing its tendency to be destroyed. In addition, alcohol decreases the absorption of vitamin B-6 and decreases the synthesis of its coenzyme form. Cirrhosis and hepatitis (both of which accompany alcoholism) also disable liver tissue from actively metabolizing vitamin B-6, which in turn decreases synthesis of its coenzyme form. Vitamin B-6 is relatively unstable. Heating and freezing can destroy it.

Carpal tunnel syndrome, a nerve disorder in the wrist, has been treated successfully with large daily doses of vitamin B-6 in some people. However, because of defects in the design of trials and conflicting data on its effectiveness, vitamin B-6 is not routinely recommended for this condition. The inconsistent results of studies of vitamin B-6 and **premenstrual syndrome (PMS)** also make a definitive recommendation for taking vitamin B-6 controversial. Some physicians, however, advise doses of 50 to 100 milligrams per day as a possible part of therapy. Such large doses may also help treat "morning sickness" that develops during pregnancy.

Upper Level for Vitamin B-6. The UL for vitamin B-6 is 100 milligrams per day, based on the risk of developing nerve damage. Studies have shown that intakes of 2 to 6 grams of vitamin B-6 per day for 2 or more months can lead to irreversible nerve damage. Symptoms of vitamin B-6 toxicity include walking difficulties and hand and foot numbness. Some nerve damage in individual sensory neurons is probably reversible, but damage to the ganglia (where many nerve fibers converge) appears to be permanent. With 500 milligram tablets of vitamin B-6 available in health-food stores, taking a toxic dose is easy.

Premenstrual syndrome (PMS) A disorder found in some women a few days before a menstrual period begins. It is characterized by depression, anxiety, headache, bloating, and mood swings. Severe cases are termed premenstrual dysphoric disorder (PDD).

CONCEPT CHECK

Pantothenic acid and biotin both participate in the metabolism of carbohydrate and fat. A deficiency of either vitamin is unlikely, pantothenic acid is found widely in foods, and our need for biotin is partially met by intestinal synthesis from bacteria. Vitamin B-6 is important for protein metabolism, neurotransmitter synthesis, homocysteine metabolism, and other key metabolic functions. Headache, a form of anemia, nausea, and vomiting can result from a vitamin B-6 deficiency. Increased risk of cardiovascular disease is also likely. Animal foods, ready-to-eat breakfast cereals, broccoli, spinach, and bananas are some food sources of vitamin B-6. Megadose supplements of vitamin B-6 can lead to nerve damage.

Folate

The term folate encompasses a variety of food forms of the vitamin. Folic acid is the chemical form added to foods and present in supplements.

Functions of Folate. A key role of the folate coenzyme is to supply or accept single carbon compounds. In this role, the coenzymes help form DNA and also metabolize amino acids and their derivatives, such as homocysteine.

One major result of a folate deficiency is that in the early phases of red blood cell synthesis, the immature cells cannot divide because they cannot form new DNA. The cells grow progressively larger because they can still synthesize enough protein and other cell parts to make new cells. When the time comes for the cells to divide, however, the amount of DNA is insufficient to form two nuclei. The cells then remain in a large immature form, known as a **megaloblast** (Fig. 11-13).

Few mature red blood cells (**erythrocytes**) arrive in the bloodstream because the bone marrow of a folate-deficient person produces mostly immature megaloblast cells. When fewer mature red blood cells are present, the blood's capacity to carry oxygen decreases, causing a form of anemia. In short, a folate deficiency causes megaloblastic anemia (also called macrocytic or large cell anemia).

The changes in red blood cell formation occur after 7 to 16 weeks on a folate-free diet, depending on the person's folate stores. White blood cell formation is also affected, but to a lesser degree. In addition, cell division throughout the entire body is disrupted. Clinicians focus primarily on red blood cells because they are easy to collect and examine. Other symptoms of folate deficiency are inflammation of the tongue, diarrhea, poor growth, mental confusion, depression, and problems in nerve function.

Megaloblast A large, immature red blood cell that results from the inability of the cell to divide normally.

Erythrocyte Mature red blood cell. They have no nucleus and a life span of about 120 days; they contain hemoglobin, which transports oxygen and carbon dioxide.

MAKING DECISIONS

Some forms of cancer therapy provide a vivid example of the effects of a folate deficiency on DNA metabolism. A cancer drug, methotrexate, closely resembles a form of folate but cannot act in its place. When methotrexate is taken in high doses, because of this resemblance, it hampers folate metabolism. Methotrexate crowds out folate in the metabolic pathways. As a consequence DNA synthesis is retarded and cell division decreases. Cancer cells are among the most rapidly dividing cells in the body, so they are among those first affected. However, other rapidly dividing cells, such as intestinal cells and skin cells, are also affected. Not surprisingly, typical side effects of methotrexate therapy are diarrhea, vomiting, and hair loss. These are also typical symptoms of folate deficiency. Today when patients are given methotrexate, they need to consume a folate-rich diet or take folic acid supplements because this reduces the toxic side effects of the drug. High supplemental doses have little or no influence on methotrexate's effectiveness as a cancer therapy.

Normal blood cells in the bloodstream. The size, shape, and color of the red blood cells show that they are normal. Mature red blood cells have lost their nuclei.

Red blood cell precursor (stem cell)

Folate and vitamin B-12 adequate

Cells divide normally

Folate or vitamin B-12 deficient

Cells are unable to divide

Megaloblastic blood cells seen here in the bone marrow are arrested at an immature stage of development. They still have their nuclei and are slightly larger than normal red blood cells.

FIGURE 11-13 ▶ Megaloblastic anemia occurs when blood cells are unable to divide, leaving large, immature red blood cells. Either a folate or vitamin B-12 deficiency may cause this condition. Measurements of blood concentrations of both vitamins are taken to help determine the cause of the anemia.

Maternal deficiencies of folate along with a genetic abnormality related to folate metabolism have been linked to development of **neural tube defects** in the fetus (Fig. 11-14). These defects include spina bifida (spinal cord or spinal fluid bulge through the back) and anencephaly (absence of a brain). Annually, about 2000 infants are affected with neural tube defects in the United States. Victims of spina bifida exhibit paralysis, incontinence, learning disabilities, and other health problems. Children born with anencephaly die shortly after birth. Adequate folate nurture is crucial for all women of childbearing age because the neural tube closes within the first 28 days of pregnancy, a time when many women are not even aware that they are pregnant. Hence a recommendation is made that ample folate, specifically 400 micrograms of synthetic folic acid per day, be consumed at least 6 weeks before conception.

Almost all related research has been done with synthetic folic acid supplementation, and it appears that even women with varied diets may not consume adequate synthetic folic acid to prevent neural tube defects unless specific attention to rich sources is given. As many as 70% of these defects could be avoided by adequate folate status before conception. (Women who have had a child with a neural tube defect are advised to consume 4000 micrograms per day of folic acid, beginning at least one month before any future pregnancy. This must be done under strict physician supervision.)

Consuming ready-to-eat breakfast cereals that contain 100% of the DV for folate (this is the same as the RDA) is a good practice for meeting the goal for synthetic folic acid intake. A multivitamin and mineral supplement can also be used to supply adequate synthetic folic acid, but women should be careful to monitor the amount of any accompanying preformed vitamin A content (don't exceed 100% the DV).

Neural tube defects A defect in the formation of the neural tube occurring during early fetal development. This type of defect results in various nervous system disorders, such as spina bifida. Folate deficiency in the pregnant woman increases the risk that the fetus will develop this disorder.

FIGURE 11-14 ▶ Neural tube defects result from a developmental failure affecting the spinal cord or brain in the embryo. Very early in fetal development, a ridge of neural-like tissue forms along the back of the embryo. As the fetus develops, this material develops into both the spinal cord and nerves at the lower end and into the brain at the upper end. At the same time, the bones that make up the back gradually surround the spinal cord on all sides. If any part of this sequence goes awry, many defects can appear. The worst case is total lack of a brain (anencephaly). Spina bifida, in which the back bones do not form a complete ring to protect the spinal cord, is much more common. Deficient folate status in the mother during the beginning of pregnancy, especially in combination with a genetic abnormality in folate metabolism, greatly increases the risk of neural tube defects.

Research is underway on the link between folate and cancer protection. Folate aids in DNA synthesis, so it is hypothesized that even mild folate deficiency contributes to abnormal DNA integrity, which in turn affects certain cancer-producing genes. Meeting the RDA for folate is thought to be one way to reduce cancer risk.

A final function of folate is the formation of neurotransmitters in the brain. Meeting folate needs can improve the depressed state in some cases of mental illness.

Folate Sources and Needs. Green, leafy vegetables (folate is derived from the Latin word *folium*, which means foliage or leaves), other vegetables; orange juice; dried beans; and organ meats are the richest sources of folate (Fig. 11-15). The vitamin C in orange juice also reduces folate destruction. Ready-to-eat breakfast cereals, bread, and milk also are important sources of folate for many adults (Fig. 11-16).

Folate is susceptible to destruction by heat. Food processing and preparation destroy 50% to 90% of the folate in food. This underscores the importance of regularly eating fresh fruits and raw or lightly cooked vegetables.

The RDA of folate for adults is 400 micrograms per day, as is the DV used on food and supplement labels. Folate recommendations for all but women of childbearing age are based on dietary folate equivalents (DFE). To compute folate intake in DFE units, one has to determine how much of a day's folate intake comes from food folate and how much comes from synthetic folic acid added to foods. When in doubt, assume all folate in a diet is in the food form, except that coming from ready-to-eat breakfast cereals and refined grain products. Also included in this second category is any folic acid consumed as part of supplements. To calculate the DFE, multiply total synthetic folic acid intake by 1.7, and add that value to the food folate consumed. For example, if a person consumed 300 micrograms as food folate and 200 micrograms from a ready-to-eat breakfast cereal, total folate DFE would be 640 micrograms (300 + (200 × 1.7) = 640). Compared to the RDA of 400 micrograms, this intake would be sufficient.

Prior to 1998, average daily folate intakes in the United States were approximately 320 micrograms for men and 220 micrograms for women. In 1998, the Food and Drug Administration (FDA) mandated the fortification of grain products with folate with the aim of

Food Sources of Folate

Food Item and Amount	Folate (micrograms)	Adult Male and Female RDA = 400 micrograms %RDA
RDA	400	100%
Asparagus, 1 cup	263	66%
Cooked spinach, 1 cup	262	66%
Cooked lentils, ½ cup	179	45%
Black-eyed peas, ½ cup	179	45%
Romaine lettuce, 1½ cups	114	29%
Great Grains cereal, ¾ cup	114	29%
Tortilla, 1	89	22%
Cooked turnips, ½ cup	85	21%
Cooked broccoli, 1 cup	78	20%
Sunflower seeds, ¼ cup	76	19%
Fresh orange juice, 1 cup	75	19%
Cooked beets, ½ cup	68	17%
Kidney beans, ½ cup	65	16%
Fried beef liver, 1 ounce	62	16%

Key:
- ☐ Grains
- ☐ Vegetables
- ☐ Fruits
- ☐ Oils
- ☐ Milk
- ☐ Meat & Beans

FIGURE 11-15 ▶ Food sources of folate compared to the RDA for adults.

MyPyramid: Sources of Folate

Grains	Vegetables	Fruits	Oils	Milk	Meat & Beans
• Fortified breakfast cereals • Wheat germ (whole-wheat products) • Enriched grains	• Asparagus • Leafy green vegetables	• Oranges • Strawberries • Cantaloupes and other melons	• None	• Cottage cheese • Yogurt	• Liver • Eggs • Beans • Sunflower seeds

FIGURE 11-16 ▶ Sources of folate from MyPyramid. The height of the background color (none, 1/3, 2/3, or completely covered) within each group in the pyramid indicates the average nutrient density for folate in that group. Overall, the vegetables group provides the richest sources, but the fruits group and the grains group contain some foods that are nutrient-dense sources of folate.

reducing birth defects of the spine. With this mandate, average intakes have increased by about 200 micrograms per day. Studies have shown this practice has decreased rates of neural tube defects in infants as well as decreased blood homocysteine levels in adults in the United States. The decline in neural tube defects is estimated to be 15% to 30% in the United States since folate enrichment in refined grains was mandated. Other factors (genetics, environment) play a role in the development of neural tube defects.

Pregnant women need extra folate (a total of 600 micrograms DFE) to accommodate the increased rates of cell division and DNA synthesis in their bodies and in the developing fetus. A healthy diet easily supplies this much. Still, prenatal care often includes a specially formulated multivitamin and mineral supplement enriched with synthetic folic acid to help compensate for the extra needs associated with pregnancy.

Older people are also at risk for folate deficiency, possibly due to a combination of inadequate folate intake and decreased absorption. Perhaps these people fail to consume sufficient amounts of fruits and vegetables because of poverty or physical problems, such as poor dental health. In addition, folate deficiencies often occur with alcoholism, due mostly to poor intake and absorption. Symptoms of a folate-related anemia can alert a physician to the possibility of alcoholism.

MAKING DECISIONS

Food Folate Content

The use of dietary folate equivalents (DFEs) instead of the actual amount of folate in a food has some important implications. Typically, many foods will be richer in folate than the Nutrition Facts label suggests because folate content is due primarily to synthetic folic acid added to the foods, such as in enriched grains and ready-to-eat breakfast cereals. This contributes substantially to the DFE calculation. Another implication is that food composition tables and diet analysis software programs also underestimate the true folate contribution of a diet compared to folate needs because these have not been updated to DFE units.

Upper Level for Folate. The UL for folate is 1 milligram (1000 micrograms), but only refers to the synthetic source. This is because folate naturally present in foods has limited absorption. Large doses of folate can hide the signs of vitamin B-12 deficiency and therefore complicate its diagnosis. Specifically, regular consumption of large amounts of folate can prevent the appearance of an early warning sign of vitamin B-12 deficiency—enlarged red blood cell size. To prevent such masking of vitamin B-12 deficiency, it is the goal of FDA, through its enactment of folate fortification grains, to increase the folate status of women of childbearing age without causing excessive intake (over 1 milligram of synthetic folic acid per day) by other groups. Also, because of risk of masking a vitamin B-12 deficiency, FDA limits supplements for nonpregnant adults and food fortification to 400 microgram amounts.

Vitamin B-12

Vitamin B-12 represents a family of compounds that contain the mineral cobalt. Vitamin B-12 compounds are synthesized by bacteria, fungi, and other lower organisms.

The body's complex means of absorbing vitamin B-12 is unique to this vitamin. Vitamin B-12 in food is chemically bound to other substances like protein. Stomach acid liberates bound vitamin B-12. The free vitamin B-12 in the stomach binds with a substance originally produced by the salivary glands in the mouth, and then later is again freed during digestion. The vitamin then binds in the small intestine with a compound made in the stomach called **intrinsic factor.** The resulting intrinsic factor/vitamin B-12

Intrinsic factor A protein-like compound produced by the stomach that enhances vitamin B-12 absorption in the ileum.

complex travels to the last portion of the small intestine (ileum) for absorption. After these digestion steps, approximately 50% of dietary vitamin B-12 is absorbed, depending on the body's need for it. Any failure in this system results in only 1% to 2% absorption of the dietary vitamin.

If a defect in the digestion and absorption of vitamin B-12 develops, the person usually takes monthly injections of vitamin B-12, uses nasal gels of the vitamin to bypass the need for absorption, or takes megadoses of a supplemental form (300 times the RDA). In this latter case, the vitamin B-12 absorption defect is overcome by providing enough of the vitamin via simple diffusion across the intestinal tract.

About 95% of cases of vitamin B-12 deficiencies in healthy people result from defective absorption, rather than from inadequate intakes. This is especially true for older people. As we age, our stomachs have a decreased ability to synthesize the intrinsic factor needed for vitamin B-12 absorption.

Functions of Vitamin B-12. Vitamin B-12 participates in a variety of cellular processes. The most important function is in folate metabolism. It is required to convert folate coenzymes to the active forms needed for metabolic reaction, such as DNA synthesis. Without vitamin B-12, reactions that require certain active forms of folate do not take place in the cell. Thus, a deficiency can result in symptoms of a folate deficiency. Another vital function of vitamin B-12 is maintaining the myelin sheaths that insulate neurons from each other. People with vitamin B-12 deficiencies have destruction of segments of the myelin sheaths. This destruction eventually causes paralysis and, perhaps, death. Vitamin B-12, folate, and vitamin B-6 are necessary to metabolize homocysteine. Homocysteine is produced during the breakdown of the amino acid, methionine. When vitamin B-12, folate, or vitamin B-6 intake is inadequate, homocysteine concentration in the blood becomes elevated. High blood level of homocysteine is linked to an increased risk of heart disease.

In the past, the inability to absorb enough vitamin B-12 eventually led to death, mainly because it destroyed nerves. This phenomenon was called **pernicious anemia** (pernicious literally means "leading to death"). Clinically, the anemia looks much like a folate-deficient anemia, characterized by the appearance of many large red blood cells in the bloodstream. However, the true cause of pernicious anemia is poor vitamin B-12 absorption rather than inadequate folate intakes.

Pernicious anemia The anemia that results from a lack of vitamin B-12 absorption; it is pernicious because of associated nerve degeneration that can result in eventual paralysis and death.

Some symptoms of pernicious anemia include weakness, sore tongue, back pain, apathy, and tingling in the extremities. We are able to store significant amounts of vitamin B-12, therefore symptoms of nerve destruction do not develop until after about 3 years from the onset of the disease. Unfortunately, significant nerve destruction often occurs before the anemia is detected, and this destruction is irreversible. Pernicious anemia and its accompanying nerve destruction start after middle age, affecting up to 20% of older adults. The explanation for this age-associated pernicious anemia is twofold. First, aging is often associated with reduced production of stomach acid. Thus vitamin B-12 is not cleaved from substances to which it is bound. Second, aging may be accompanied by reduced output of intrinsic factor, resulting in decreased absorption of the vitamin.

Infants breastfed by vegetarian mothers are at risk for vitamin B-12 deficiency accompanied by anemia and long-term nervous system problems, such as diminished brain growth, degeneration of the spinal cord, and poor intellectual development. The problems may have their origins during pregnancy, when the mother is deficient in vitamin B-12. Vegan diets supply little vitamin B-12 unless they include vitamin B-12-enriched food or supplements, so achieving an adequate vitamin B-12 intake is a key diet planning goal for vegans.

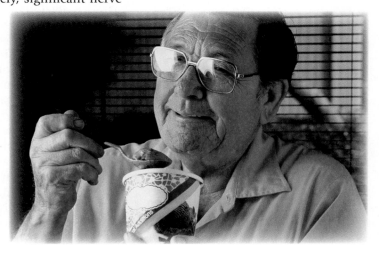

▲ As we age our digestive system absorbs vitamin B-12 from food less efficiently.

FIGURE 11-17 ▶ Food sources of vitamin B-12 compared to the RDA for adults.

Food Sources of Vitamin B-12

Food Item and Amount	Vitamin B-12 (micrograms)	Adult Male and Female RDA = 2.4 micrograms %RDA
RDA	2.4	100%
Fried beef liver, 1 ounce	31.7	1321%
Baked clams, 1 ounce	15.7	654%
Boiled oysters, 2	14.4	600%
Lobster, 3 ounces	2.7	113%
Pot roast, 3 ounces	2.5	104%
Plain yogurt, 1 cup	1.4	58%
Corn Flakes cereal, ¾ cup	1.1	46%
Shrimp, 3 ounces	1.0	42%
1% milk, 1 cup	0.9	38%
Soy milk, 1 cup	0.8	33%
Boiled egg, 1	0.6	25%
Lean ham, 3 ounces	0.6	25%
Beef hot dog, 1	0.5	21%
Ham lunch meat, 2 ounces	0.4	17%

Key:
- Grains
- Vegetables
- Fruits
- Oils
- Milk
- Meat & Beans

▲ Seafood, especially clams and lobster, are good sources of vitamin B-12.

Vitamin B-12 Sources and Needs. Organ meats (especially liver, kidneys, and heart) are especially rich sources of vitamin B-12. Other major sources of vitamin B-12 include meat, seafood, ready-to-eat breakfast cereals, milk, and eggs (Fig. 11-17). Adults over age 50 are encouraged to seek a synthetic vitamin B-12 source to aid absorption, which can be limited due to reduced intrinsic factor and stomach acid output. Synthetic vitamin B-12 is not food bound, so it doesn't need stomach acid to release it from foods. Thus, it will be more readily absorbed than the form found in food. Ready-to-eat breakfast cereals and a multivitamin and mineral supplement are two possible synthetic sources.

The RDA of vitamin B-12 for adults is 2.4 micrograms per day. The DV used on food and supplement labels is 6 micrograms. On average, adults consume two times the RDA or more. This high intake provides the average meat-eating person with 2 to 3 years' storage of vitamin B-12 in the liver.

It takes approximately 20 years of consuming a diet essentially free of vitamin B-12 to exhibit nerve destruction caused by a diet deficiency. (Still, vegans, who eat no animal products, should find a reliable source of vitamin B-12, such as fortified soybean milk, ready-to-eat breakfast cereals, and a form of yeast grown on media rich in vitamin B-12. Use of a multivitamin and mineral supplement containing vitamin B-12 is another option). Pernicious anemia most frequently develops after a few years of the loss of vitamin B-12 absorption capacity. The quicker appearance is because of the reduced ability to reabsorb vitamin B-12 excreted into the GI tract during digestion, coupled with reduced absorption of dietary sources. Vitamin B-12 supplements are essentially nontoxic, so no UL has been set.

CONCEPT CHECK

Folate is needed for cell division because it is required for DNA synthesis. A folate deficiency results in megaloblastic (macrocytic) anemia, as well as elevated homocysteine, inflammation of the tongue, diarrhea, and poor growth. Excess folate intake can mask a vitamin B-12 deficiency because these vitamins work together in metabolism. Folate is found in fruits and vegetables, beans, and organ meats. Emphasizing fresh and lightly cooked vegetables in the diet is important because much folate is lost during cooking. Women of childbearing age should meet needs by consuming a source of synthetic folic acid. Folate needs during pregnancy are especially high; a deficiency around time of conception and in the first month of pregnancy may lead to neural tube defects in the fetus.

Vitamin B-12 is necessary for folate metabolism. Without dietary vitamin B-12, folate deficiency symptoms, such as **macrocytic anemia** develop. In addition, vitamin B-12 is necessary for maintaining the nervous system. Paralysis can develop from a vitamin B-12 deficiency. The vitamin also participates in homocyteine metabolism. The absorption of vitamin B-12 requires a number of specific factors. If absorption is inhibited, the resulting deficiency can lead to pernicious anemia and nerve destruction. Concentrated amounts of vitamin B-12 are found only in animal foods; meat-eaters generally have a 2- to 3-year supply stored in the liver. Vegans need to find an alternate source. Vitamin B-12 absorption may decline as we age. Monthly injections, nasal gels, or megadoses can make up for this.

Macrocytic anemia Anemia characterized by the presence of abnormally large red blood cells.

Choline

The dietary component choline is the latest addition to the list of essential nutrients. Choline is part of acetylcholine, a neurotransmitter associated with attention, learning and memory, muscle control, and many other functions. It is also part of phospholipids, such as lecithin, the major component of the cell membrane. Finally, choline participates in some aspects of homocysteine metabolism.

There has been only one published study examining the effect of inadequate dietary intake of choline in healthy humans. The study of male volunteers showed decreased choline stores and liver damage when humans were fed choline-deficient total parenteral (intravenous) nutrition solutions. Based on this one study, plus laboratory animal studies, choline has been deemed essential, but is not yet classified as a vitamin.

Choline Sources and Needs. Choline is widely distributed in foods (Fig. 11-18). Milk, beef, and peanut butter are sources. Lecithin is often added to food during processing, so this is yet another source. There is so much choline available in ordinary foods that it is unlikely that a dietary deficiency exists naturally. Choline also can be synthesized from the nonessential (dispensable) amino acid serine.

The AI for choline for adults is 425 to 550 milligrams per day. We don't know if a dietary supply is needed at all life stages. Although AI are set for choline, it may be that the choline requirements can be met by body synthesis at some or all stages of life. We consume ample choline from food, at least 700 to 1000 milligrams per day.

▲ Nuts, such as peanuts, are a good source of choline. Body cells also produce choline.

Food Sources of Choline

Food Item and Amount	Choline (milligrams)	Adult Male AI = 550 milligrams %AI	Adult Female AI = 425 milligrams %AI
AI	425–550	100%	100%
Egg, 1 each	126	23%	30%
Cod, 3 ounces	70	13%	16%
Chicken, 3 ounces	56	10%	13%
Fat-free milk, 1 cup	37	7%	9%
Beef, 3 ounces	36	7%	8%
Yogurt, 1 cup	31	6%	7%
Wheat germ, 2 tablespoons	21	4%	5%
Peanut butter, 2 tablespoons	20	4%	5%
Cottage cheese, ½ cup	20	4%	5%
Orange, 1 each	12	2%	3%
Broccoli, ½ cup	7	1%	2%
Squash, ½ cup	7	1%	2%
Whole-wheat bread, 1 slice	7	1%	2%
Apple, 1 each	7	1%	2%
Romaine lettuce, 4 leaves	6	1%	1%
White bread, 1 slice	3	1%	1%

Key: Grains, Vegetables, Fruits, Oils, Milk, Meat & Beans

FIGURE 11-18 ▶ Food sources of choline compared to the Adequate Intake for adult males and females.

Upper Level of Choline. The UL for adults is 3.5 grams per day. This is based on development of a fishy body odor and low blood pressure at excessive intakes.

Table 11-2 summarizes much of what we know about the water-soluble B-complex vitamins and choline. Figure 11-19 provides an overview of rich sources of the vitamins and choline in the six food groups of MyPyramid. Figure 11-20 shows how the vitamins and related nutrients work together to maintain health.

Sulfur (S)

Major mineral A mineral vital to health; required in amounts greater than 100 milligrams per day.

Sulfur is a **major mineral** found in many important compounds in the body including the vitamins biotin and thiamin. The amino acids methionine and cysteine contain sulfur, which functions to stabilize the three-dimensional structure of proteins. Sulfur helps in the balance of acids and bases in the body and is an important part of the liver's drug-detoxifying pathways. Proteins supply the sulfur we need, so it is not an essential nutrient. Sulfur containing compounds have been used for centuries to preserve foods. There are no known deficiency or toxicity symptoms associated with sulfur.

TABLE 11-2 Summary of the Water-Soluble Vitamins and Choline

Vitamin	Major Functions	RDA or Adequate Intake	Dietary Sources*	Deficiency Symptoms	Toxicity Symptoms
Thiamin	• Coenzyme of carbohydrate metabolism • Nerve function	1.1–1.2 milligrams	• Sunflower seeds • Pork • Whole and enriched grains • Dried beans • Peas	*Beriberi* • Nervous tingling • Poor coordination • Edema • Heart changes • Weakness	None
Riboflavin	• Coenzyme of carbohyrate metabolism	1.1–1.3 milligrams	• Milk • Mushrooms • Spinach • Liver • Enriched grains	• Inflammation of the mouth and tongue • Cracks at the corners of the mouth • Eye disorders	None
Niacin	• Coenzyme of energy metabolism • Coenzyme of fat synthesis • Coenzyme of fat breakdown	14–16 milligrams (niacin equivalents)	• Mushrooms • Bran • Tuna • Salmon • Chicken • Beef • Liver • Peanuts • Enriched grains	*Pellagra* • Diarrhea • Dermatitis • Dementia • Death	Upper level is 35 milligrams from supplements, based on flushing of skin
Panthothenic acid	• Coenzyme of energy metabolism • Coenzyme of fat synthesis • Coenzyme of fat breakdown	5 milligrams	• Mushrooms • Liver • Broccoli • Eggs *Most foods have some*	• No natural deficiency disease or symptoms	None

*Fortified ready-to-eat breakfast cereals are good sources for most of these vitamins and a common source of B vitamins for many of us.

MyPyramid: Sources of Vitamins and Choline

FIGURE 11-19 ▶ Certain groups of MyPyramid are especially rich sources of various vitamins and choline. This is true for those listed. Each may be also found in other groups in the pyramid but in lower amounts. Pantothenic acid is also present in moderate amounts in many groups.

Grains	Vegetables	Fruits	Oils	Milk	Meat & Beans
• Thiamin • Riboflavin • Niacin • Folate	• Vitamin A • Vitamin K • Folate • Vitamin C	• Vitamin A • Vitamin C	• Vitamin E	• Vitamin D • Riboflavin • Vitamin B-12 • Choline	• Thiamin • Riboflavin • Niacin • Biotin • Vitamin B-6 • Vitamin B-12 • Choline

FIGURE 11-20 ▶ Vitamins and related nutrients work together to maintain health.

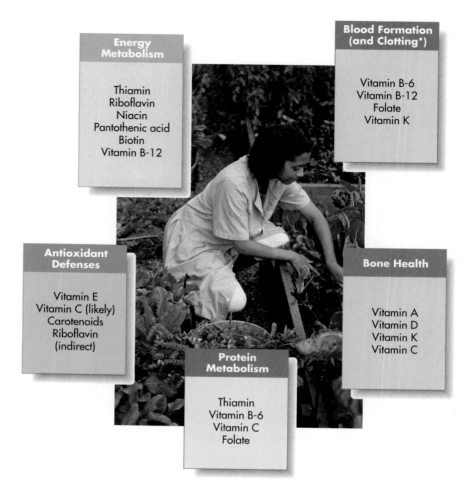

Energy Metabolism

Thiamin
Riboflavin
Niacin
Pantothenic acid
Biotin
Vitamin B-12

Blood Formation (and Clotting*)

Vitamin B-6
Vitamin B-12
Folate
Vitamin K

Antioxidant Defenses

Vitamin E
Vitamin C (likely)
Carotenoids
Riboflavin
(indirect)

Bone Health

Vitamin A
Vitamin D
Vitamin K
Vitamin C

Protein Metabolism

Thiamin
Vitamin B-6
Vitamin C
Folate

Trace mineral A mineral vital to health; required in the diet in amounts less than 100 milligrams per day.

Goiter An enlargement of the thyroid gland; this is often caused by insufficient iodide in the diet.

TRACE MINERALS—AN OVERVIEW

Information about **trace minerals** is perhaps the most rapidly expanding area of knowledge in nutrition. With the exceptions of iron and iodide, the importance of trace minerals to humans has been recognized only within the last 40 years. Although we need 100 milligrams or less of each trace mineral daily, they are as essential to good health as are major minerals.

In some cases, discovering the importance of a trace mineral reads like a detective story, and the evidence is still unfolding. In 1961, researchers linked dwarfism in Middle Eastern villagers to a zinc deficiency. Other scientists recognized that a rare form of heart disease in an isolated area of China was linked to a selenium deficiency. In North America, some trace mineral deficiencies were first observed in the late 1960s and early 1970s when the minerals were not added to synthetic formulas used for intravenous feeding.

It is difficult to define precisely our trace mineral needs because we need only minute amounts. Highly sophisticated technology is required to measure such small amounts in both food and body tissues.

Iodide (I)

Iodine, a trace mineral, is found in an ion form in foods called iodide. During World War I, a link was discovered between a deficiency of iodide and the production of a

goiter, an enlarged thyroid gland. Men drafted from areas such as the Great Lakes Region of the United States had a much higher rate of goiter than did men from other areas of the country. The soils in these areas have low iodide contents. In the 1920s, a researcher in Ohio found that low doses of iodide given to children over a 4-year period could prevent goiter. That finding led to the addition of iodide to salt beginning in the 1920s.

Today, many nations, such as Canada, require iodide fortification of salt. In the United States, salt can be purchased either iodized or plain. Check for this on the label of a package of salt next time you are in a grocery store. Some areas of Europe, such as northern Italy, have very low soil levels of iodide, but have yet to adopt an iodide fortification program. People in these areas, especially women, still suffer from goiter, as do people in areas of Latin America, the Indian subcontinent, Southeast Asia, and Africa. About 2 billion people worldwide are at risk of iodide deficiency, and approximately 800 million of these people have suffered the widespread effects of such a deficiency. Eradication of iodide deficiency is a goal of many health-related organizations worldwide.

Functions of Iodide. The thyroid gland actively accumulates and traps iodide from the bloodstream to support thyroid hormone synthesis. Thyroid hormones are synthesized using iodide and the amino acid, tyrosine. These hormones help regulate metabolic rate and promote growth and development throughout the body, including the brain.

If a person's iodide intake is insufficient, the thyroid gland enlarges as it attempts to take up more iodide from the bloodstream. This eventually leads to goiter. Simple goiter is a painless condition, but if uncorrected can lead to pressure on the trachea (windpipe), which may cause difficulty in breathing. Although iodide can prevent goiter formation, it does not significantly shrink a goiter once it has formed. Surgical removal may be required in severe cases.

If a woman has an iodide-deficient diet during the early months of her pregnancy, the fetus suffers iodide deficiency because the mother's body uses up the available iodide. The infant then may be born with short length and develop mental retardation. The stunted growth and mental retardation that results is known as **cretinism.** Cretinism appeared in North America before iodide fortification of table salt began. Today, cretinism still appears in Europe, Africa, Latin America, and Asia.

Iodide Sources and Needs. Iodized salt, dairy products, and grain products contain various forms of iodide (Fig. 11-21). Sea salt found in health-food stores, however, is not a good source because the iodide is lost during processing.

The RDA for iodide for adults is 150 micrograms to support thyroid gland function. This is the same as the DV used on food and supplement labels. A half teaspoon of iodide-fortified salt (about 2 grams) supplies that amount. Most adults consume more iodide than the RDA—an estimated 190 to 300 micrograms daily, not including that from use of iodized salt at the table. This extra amount adds up because dairies use it as a sterilizing agent, bakeries use it as a dough conditioner, food producers use it as part of food colorants, and it is added to salt. There is concern, however, that vegans may not consume enough unless iodized salt is used.

Upper Level for Iodide. The UL for iodide is 1.1 milligrams per day. When high amounts of iodide are consumed, thyroid hormone synthesis is inhibited, as in a deficiency. This can appear in people who eat a lot of seaweed, because some seaweeds contain as much as 1% iodide by weight. Total iodide intake then can add up to 60 to 130 times the RDA.

▲ Iodide deficiency leads to a goiter. The mother on the left has a goiter, but is otherwise normal. Her daughter on the right has a goiter and is mentally retarded, deaf, and mute.

Cretinism The stunting of body growth and poor development in the offspring that result from inadequate maternal intake of iodide during pregnancy.

FIGURE 11-21 ▶ Food sources of iodide Compared to the RDA.

Food Sources of Iodide

Food Item and Amount	Iodide (micrograms)	%RDA
RDA*	150	100%
Iodized table salt, ½ cup	195	130%
Plain yogurt, ½ cup	87	56%
Buttermilk, 1 cup	60	40%
1% milk, 1 cup	59	39%
Luna bar, 1	38	25%
Soy protein bar, 1	38	25%
Egg, 1 large	35	23%
1% cottage cheese, ½ cup	28	19%
Mozzarella cheese, 1 ounce	10	7%

Key:
- Grains
- Vegetables
- Fruits
- Oils
- Milk
- Meat & Beans

*For adults; See the DRI table in the back of this book for gender- and age-specific recommendations.

Chromium (Cr)

Chromium is required for glucose uptake into cells by aiding insulin function. Marginal-to-low chromium intakes may contribute to an increased risk for developing type 2 diabetes, but opinions are mixed on the true degree of this effect.

A chromium deficiency is characterized by impaired blood glucose control and elevated blood cholesterol and triglycerides. The mechanism by which chromium influences cholesterol metabolism is not known but involves enzymes that control cholesterol synthesis. Chromium deficiency appears in people maintained on intravenous total parenteral nutrition solutions not supplemented with chromium and in children with malnutrition. Marginal deficiencies may go undetected, because sensitive measures of chromium status are not available.

Chromium Sources and Needs. Specific data regarding the chromium content of various foods are scant, and most food composition tables do not include values for this trace mineral. Egg yolks, whole grain (bran), organ meats, other meats, mushrooms, nuts, and beer are good sources. Yeast is also a source. The amount of chromium in foods is related to the soil content in which the food was grown.

The AI for chromium is 25 to 35 micrograms per day, based on the amount present in a balanced diet. The DV used on food and supplement labels is 120 micrograms. Average adult intakes in North America are estimated at about 30 micrograms per day, but could be somewhat higher.

No UL for chromium has been set because toxicity for that present in foods has not been observed. Chromium toxicity, however, has been reported in people exposed to industrial waste and in painters who use art supplies with high chromium content. Liver damage and lung cancer can result. Use of any supplement should normally not exceed the DV set unless supervised by a physician, because of the risk of toxicity.

▲ Mushrooms are a good source of chromium.

Manganese (Mn)

The mineral manganese is easily confused with magnesium. Not only are their names similar, but they also often substitute for each other in metabolic processes. Manganese is needed by some enzymes, such as those used in carbohydrate and free-radical metabolism (via superoxide dismutase). Manganese is also important in bone formation.

No human deficiency symptom is associated with a low manganese intake. Animals on manganese-deficient diets suffer alterations in brain function, bone formation, and reproduction. If human diets were low in manganese, these symptoms would probably appear as well. As it happens, our need for manganese is very low, and our diets tend to be adequate in this trace mineral.

Good food sources of manganese are nuts, rice, oats, and other whole grains, beans, and leafy vegetables. The AI for manganese is 1.8 to 2.3 milligrams to offset daily losses. Average intakes fall within this range. The DV used on food and supplement labels is 2 milligrams. Manganese is toxic at high doses.

▲ Nuts are rich in manganese.

Upper Level for Manganese. The UL is 11 milligrams per day. This is based on the development of nerve damage.

Molybdenum (Mo)

Several human enzymes use molybdenum. No molybdenum deficiency has been reported in people who consume diets orally. Deficiency symptoms have appeared in people maintained on intravenous total nutrition devoid of this trace mineral. Symptoms include increased heart and respiratory rates, night blindness, mental confusion, edema, and weakness.

Good food sources of molybdenum include milk and dairy products, beans, whole grains, and nuts. The RDA for molybdenum is 45 micrograms to offset daily losses. The DV used on food and supplement labels is 75 micrograms. Our daily intakes average 75 to 110 micrograms.

Upper Level for Molybdenum. The Upper Level for molybdenum is 2 milligrams per day. When consumed in high doses, molybdenum causes toxicity in laboratory animals, resulting in weight loss and decreased growth.

CONCEPT CHECK

Chromium contributes to insulin function. The amount of chromium found in food depends on chromium content of the soil in which it was grown. Meats, whole grains, and egg yolks are good sources. Manganese is a component of bone and is used by many enzymes, including those involved in glucose production. Our need for manganese is low, so deficiencies are rare. Nuts, rice, oats, and beans are good food sources. Molybdenum is another trace mineral required by a few enzymes. Good sources include milk, beans, whole grains, and nuts. Deficiencies have appeared only in people nourished by unsupplemented total parenteral nutrition. The needs for some other trace minerals, such as boron, nickel, arsenic, and vanadium, have not been fully established in humans. If required, these minerals are needed in such small amounts that current diets are probably adequate sources.

FIGURE 11-22 ▶ When placed in a centrifuge, whole blood separates into its four components: red blood cells, white blood cells, platelets, and plasma.

(a) Centrifuged Blood Sample

Plasma

White blood cells and platelets

Red blood cells

White blood cells

Platelets

Red blood cell

Plasma

(b) Blood Components

VITAMINS AND MINERALS INVOLVED IN BLOOD HEALTH

The human body has a number of elaborate systems to keep the roughly 100 trillion cells alive and properly functioning. The digestive tract allows the extraction of nutrients consumed in food so that they can be used by cells. The circulatory system is another elaborate system that delivers oxygen and nutrients to the cells so they can be used by the cells. Blood is the conduit through which nutrients are disseminated throughout the body. Blood consists of four distinct elements (Fig. 11-22). The most prevalent component of blood is the red blood cells or erythrocytes. They transport oxygen to the cells and remove carbon dioxide from the cells. Leukocytes (white blood cells) are critical for immune function. **Platelets** function in the blood-clotting process. They clump together at the site of injury and form a plug that slows the rate of bleeding until a permanent clot can form. **Plasma** is the largest portion of blood (approximately 55% of the total volume). Substrates (proteins, carbohydrates, and lipids), enzymes, hormones, and electrolytes are critical components of plasma. Vitamins and minerals function as coenzymes, which provide a critical function in the maintenance of blood health.

Platelets A protoplasmic disc smaller than a red blood cell that promotes coagulation.

Plasma The fluid, extracellular portion of blood.

The Role of Vitamins in Blood Health

Vitamin K, vitamin B-6, folate, and vitamin B-12 all function to maintain blood health. Vitamin B-6, folate, and vitamin B-12 have been covered adequately in previous sections of this chapter.

Vitamin K

A family of compounds known collectively as vitamin K is found in plants, plant oils, fish oils, and animal products. Vitamin K is also synthesized by bacteria in the human colon. It is estimated that colonic synthesis accounts for approximately 10% of requirements.

Functions of Vitamin K. Vitamin K in combination with a number of proteins and calcium is vital for the life-and-death process of blood clotting (Fig. 11-23). The K stands for koagulation in the Danish language. Danish researchers first noted the relationship between vitamin K and blood clotting. As described in the chapter on bone health, vitamin K also activates proteins present in bone, muscle, and kidneys, and doing so it allows calcium-binding in these organs.

At birth a newborn's intestinal tract lacks a sufficient amount of bacteria to produce enough vitamin K to allow for effective blood clotting if the infant is injured or needs surgery. Therefore, vitamin K is routinely administered by injection shortly after birth. In adults, deficiencies of vitamin K have occurred when

FIGURE 11-23 ▶ Vitamin K works to activate clotting factors, then able to bind calcium. This calcium binding to clotting factors is necessary for clot formation.

a person takes antibiotics for an extended time (this destroys the bacteria that normally produce some of the vitamin K subsequently absorbed) and when fat absorption is limited.

Vitamin K Sources and Needs. Major food sources of vitamin K are liver, green leafy vegetables, broccoli, peas, and green beans (Fig. 10-17). Vitamin K is widespread in foods, therefore a deficiency is rare. Vitamin K is resistant to cooking losses.

The AI for vitamin K is 90 to 120 micrograms per day for adults. The DV used on food labels is 80 micrograms. Intake of an adequate amount of vitamin K can be a problem in the elderly due to low consumption of vegetables.

A UL has not been established for vitamin K because no reports of toxicity have been published. Megadoses or inconsistent dietary intake of vitamin K have been reported to reduce the effectiveness of medications used to reduce clotting (e.g., Coumadin). These medications are frequently used in patients prone to blood-clotting disorders or those who have recently undergone cardiovascular surgery.

THE ROLE OF MINERALS IN BLOOD HEALTH

Iron (Fe)

Although the importance of dietary iron has been recognized for many years, iron deficiency is the most common nutrient deficiency worldwide. Iron is the only nutrient for which young women have a greater RDA than do adult men.

Absorption and Distribution of Iron. Iron absorption is tightly regulated. Controlling absorption is important because the human body cannot easily eliminate excess iron once it is absorbed. Overall, iron absorption depends on its form in food, the person's iron status, and other dietary components found in food. Relative to most other nutrients, iron absorption is low. If iron status is adequate, absorption can be as low as 1%; however, if iron status is depressed, absorption can be as high as 40%. Healthy people with adequate iron stores absorb between 5% to 15% of dietary iron.

The form of iron in foods influences how much is absorbed. About 40% of the total iron in animal flesh is found as hemoglobin and **myoglobin** (found primarily in muscle). Iron found as a component of hemoglobin and myoglobin is called **heme iron.** Heme iron is absorbed two to three times more efficiently than **nonheme iron.** Nonheme iron makes up 60% of the iron found in meat, as well as eggs, milk, vegetables, grains, and other plant foods.

Meats, fish, and poultry contain a special meat factor that aids non-heme absorption. Overall, eating meat with vegetables and grain products enhances the absorption of all nonheme iron present.

Production of adequate hydrochloric acid by the stomach is important for iron absorption. The acidic environment helps solubilize the iron and keeps the iron in a form more readily absorbed. Iron absorption is less efficient in people as they age because less gastric acid tends to be produced. Long-term consumption of antacids raises the pH in the stomach and subsequently has a negative impact on iron absorption. Vitamin C (ascorbic acid) in amounts of about 75 milligrams can increase nonheme iron absorption. Consuming a glass of orange juice with an iron containing supplement will increase the iron absorbed from that supplement. Consuming foods that are rich sources of vitamin C is advisable if blood indicators of low blood iron status are low.

Myoglobin Iron-containing protein that binds oxygen in muscle tissue.

Heme iron Iron provided from animal tissues in the form of hemoglobin and myoglobin. Approximately 40% of the iron in meat is heme iron; it is readily absorbed.

Nonheme iron Iron provided from plant sources and animal tissues other than in the forms of hemoglobin and myoglobin. Nonheme iron is less efficiently absorbed than heme iron; absorption is closely dependent on body needs.

▲ Red meat is a major source of iron in the North American diet. The heme iron present is better absorbed than the nonheme iron found in meats and plants.

Numerous substances reduce the ability to absorb iron. **Phytic acid** and other grain fibers and **oxalic acid** in vegetables can bind iron and reduce its absorption. Polyphenols (tannins) found in tea and beans also reduce nonheme iron absorption. Moderation of fiber and tannin intake is ideal if iron deficiency anemia has been diagnosed. High zinc and calcium supplementation also interfere with nonheme iron absorption.

The most important factor influencing nonheme iron absorption is body need. Iron needs are increased during pregnancy and growth. At high altitudes, the lower oxygen concentration of the air causes an increase in the hemoglobin concentration of blood and thus an increase in iron needs. When iron stores are inadequate, the main protein that carries iron (transferrin) readily binds more iron, shifting it from intestinal cells into the bloodstream. If iron stores are adequate and the iron-binding protein in the blood is fully saturated with iron, absorption from the intestinal cells is minimal. The iron remains in the intestinal cells. This mechanism allows iron to be absorbed as needed. When intestinal cells shed at the end of their 2- to 5-day life span, unabsorbed iron returns to the lumen of the intestinal tract and is subsequently excreted. High doses of iron can still be toxic, but absorption is carefully regulated under most dietary conditions. Except for bleeding associated with menstruation, injury, or childbirth, body loss of iron is minimal. The principle mechanism to regulate iron content in the body is by tight control of absorption.

Function of Iron. Iron is part of the hemoglobin in red blood cells and myoglobin in muscle cells. Hemoglobin molecules in red blood cells transport oxygen (O_2) from the lungs to cells and transport carbon dioxide (CO_2) from cells to the lungs for excretion. In addition, iron is used as part of many enzymes, some proteins, and compounds that cells use in energy production. Iron is also needed for brain and immune function and contributes to drug detoxification in the liver and to bone health.

If neither the diet nor body stores can supply the iron needed for hemoglobin synthesis, the concentration of hemoglobin and red blood cells decreases. Medical professionals use both the percentage of red blood cells (**hematocrit**) and the hemoglobin concentration to assess iron status. Other measures indicative of poor iron status include the concentration of iron and iron-containing proteins in blood. When hematocrit and hemoglobin fall, an iron deficiency is suspected. In severe deficiency, hemoglobin and hematocrit fall so low that the amount of oxygen carried in the bloodstream is decreased. This condition is called anemia.

Iron deficiency can be categorized into three stages. The body depletes iron stores, however no physiological impairment is observed in the first stage. The second stage involves depletion of circulating iron in transferrin and some physiological impairment occurs. Heme production is decreased and enzymes that require iron as a cofactor are impaired. The last stage is iron-deficiency anemia where the red blood cells are small, pale, and their number is reduced.

There are many conditions that lead to an anemic state; iron-deficiency anemia is the most prevalent worldwide. About 30% of the world's population is anemic, and about half of those cases are caused by an iron deficiency. Probably about 10% of North Americans in high-risk categories have iron-deficiency anemia. This appears most often in infancy, the preschool years, and at puberty for both males and females. Growth, with accompanying expansion of blood volume and muscle mass, increases iron needs, making it difficult to consume enough iron. Women are also vulnerable during childbearing years from blood loss during menstruation. In addition, anemia is often found in pregnant women. Iron-deficiency anemia in adult men is usually caused by blood loss from ulcers, colon cancer, or hemorrhoids. Athletes can have increased iron requirements due to increased blood loss in feces and urine and chronic lysis of red blood cells in the feet due to the trauma of running.

Phytic acid A constituent of plants that binds positive ions to its multiple phosphate groups.

Oxalic acid An organic acid found in spinach, rhubarb, and other leafy green vegetables that can depress the absorption of certain minerals present in the food, such as calcium.

Hematocrit The percentage of blood made up of red blood cells.

▲ Pregnancy greatly increases iron needs, as does growth in childhood.

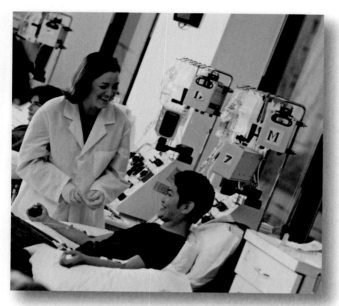

▲ Young adult women should avoid frequent blood donations because a significant amount of iron is lost in each donation.

Clinical symptoms of iron-deficiency anemia include pale skin, fatigue upon exertion, poor temperature regulation, loss of appetite, and apathy. Poor iron stores may decrease learning ability, attention span, work performance, and immune status even before a person is anemic. More North Americans have an iron deficiency without anemia than have iron-deficiency anemia. Their blood hemoglobin values are still normal, but they have no stores to draw from in times of pregnancy or illness, and basic functioning may be at decreased levels. That could mean anything from too little energy to perform everyday tasks in an efficient manner to difficulties staying mentally alert.

To cure iron-deficiency anemia, a person needs to take iron supplements. A physician should also find the cause so that the anemia does not reoccur. Changes in diet may prevent iron-deficiency anemia, but supplemental iron is the only reliable cure once it has developed.

Iron Sources and Needs. Animal sources contain approximately 40% heme iron, the most bioavailable form. The major iron sources in the adult diet are ready-to-eat breakfast cereals, beans, and animal products (Fig. 11-24). Iron is added to flour during the enrichment process. Other iron sources are spinach, peas, and legumes, but the absorption of nonheme iron found in these products is relatively low (Fig. 11-25).

Milk is a poor source of iron. A common cause of iron-deficiency anemia in children is due to high consumption of milk, coupled with insufficient meat intake. Vegan

Food Sources of Iron

Food Item and Amount	Iron (milligrams)	Adult Male RDA = 8 milligrams %RDA	Adult Female RDA =18 milligrams %RDA
RDA		100%	100%
Oat bran cereal, 1 cup	15	188%	83%
Baked clams, 3 ounces	14	175%	78%
Spinach, 1 cup	6.4	80%	36%
Kidney beans, 1 cup	5.3	66%	29%
Pot roast, 4 ounces	3.9	49%	22%
Sirloin steak, 4 ounces	3.8	48%	21%
Parsley, 1 cup	3.7	46%	21%
Fried beef liver, 2 ounces	3.6	45%	20%
Shrimp, 3 ounces	2.7	34%	15%
Braunschweiger sausage, 1 piece	2.7	34%	15%
Flour tortilla, 1	2.4	30%	13%
Garbanzo beans, ½ cup	2.4	30%	13%
Navy beans, ½ cup	2.3	29%	13%
Baked potato, 1	1.7	21%	9%
Artichoke, 1	1.6	20%	9%

Key: Grains, Vegetables, Fruits, Oils, Milk, Meat & Beans

FIGURE 11-24 ▶ Food sources of iron compared to the RDA for adult males and females.

FIGURE 11-25 ▸ Sources of iron from My-Pyramid. The height of the background color (none, 1/3, 2/3, or completely covered) within each group in the pyramid indicates the average nutrient density for iron in the group. Overall, the meat & beans group and the grains group contain many foods that are nutrient-dense sources of iron. Still, the iron content of a food containing mostly nonheme iron is only an approximate measure of the amount delivered to body cells, as body need greatly influences the absorption of nonheme iron. With regard to physical activity, iron is especially needed as part of the hemoglobin that carries oxygen in the red blood cells to muscle (and other) cells.

Grains	Vegetables	Fruits	Oils	Milk	Meat & Beans
• Whole grains • Enriched grains • Wheat germ • Oatmeal	• Spinach • Peas • Potatoes • Green beans • Broccoli	• Peaches • Prune juice • Dried apricots	• None	• None	• Beef • Tofu • Beans • Seafood • Organ meats

vegetarians are particularly susceptible to iron-deficiency anemia because of their lack of dietary heme iron.

The daily adult RDA for iron is 8 milligrams for men, as well as for women over 50 years, and 18 milligrams for women ages 19 to 50 years. The higher RDA in younger women is based on the amount needed to counter iron losses due to menstruation. Menstrual blood loss is highly variable, making it difficult to set an RDA for women. Women who menstruate more heavily and longer may need even more iron than those who have lighter and shorter flows. The DV used on food and supplement labels is 18 milligrams.

Most women do not consume 18 milligrams of iron daily. The average daily amount consumed by women is closer to 13 milligrams, while in men it is about 18 milligrams per day. Women can close this gap between average daily intakes and needs by seeking out iron-fortified foods, such as ready-to-eat breakfast cereals that contain at least 50% of the DV. Use of a balanced multivitamin and mineral supplement containing up to 100% of the DV for iron is another option. Consuming more than that much iron is not advised unless recommended by a physician.

MAKING DECISIONS

Blood Donation

The adult human body contains about 21 cups (5 liters) of blood. Blood donations are 2 cups (500 milliliters). Thus, a blood donor gives about 10% of the total blood found in the body. Healthy people can generally donate blood two to four times a year without harmful consequences. As a precaution, blood banks first screen potential donors' blood for the presence of anemia. Red blood cells contain about two-thirds of total body iron and have a life span of about 120 days. At the end of the life span of a red blood cell the iron is efficiently recycled or stored for later use.

Hemochromatosis A disorder of iron metabolism characterized by increased iron absorption and deposition in the liver and heart. This eventually poisons the cells in those organs.

▲ Minimal intakes of protein and zinc limit growth in people worldwide, such as seen in these Bolivian children and adults.

Upper Level for Iron. The UL for iron is 45 milligrams per day. Higher amounts can lead to stomach irritation. Although iron overload is not as common as iron deficiency, it can be a serious result of misuse because it can easily build up in the body and lead to toxic symptoms. Even a large single dose of 60 milligrams of iron can be life threatening to a 1-year-old. Children are frequently victims of iron poisoning because iron pills and supplements containing iron are tempting and available when accessible on kitchen tables and even from cabinets. FDA requires that all iron supplements must carry a warning about toxicity, and those with 30 milligrams of iron or more per tablet must be individually wrapped.

Smaller doses of iron (but still greater than what is needed) over a long period can also cause problems. A form of iron toxicity, for example has been observed in an African tribe that brews beer in iron pots. Repeated blood transfusions can also lead to iron toxicity.

Iron toxicity accompanies the genetic disease called hereditary **hemochromatosis.** The disease is associated with a substantial increase in iron absorption. Iron in the body builds up to dangerous levels, especially in the blood and liver. Some iron is deposited in the muscles, pancreas, and heart. If not treated, the excess iron deposits contribute to severe organ damage, especially in the liver and heart.

Development of hereditary hemochromatosis requires that a person carry two defective copies of a particular gene. People with one defective gene and one normal gene, called carriers, may also absorb too much dietary iron but not to the same extent as those with two defective genes. About 5% to 10% of North Americans of Northern European descent are carriers of hemochromatosis. Approximately 1 in 250 North Americans has both hemochromatosis genes. These numbers are high considering that many physicians regard hemochromatosis as a rare disease and therefore do not routinely test for it.

A reasonable approach is for you to ask to be screened for iron overload. At your next visit to a physician ask for a transferrin saturation test to assess iron stores. A ferritin test may also be added to assess iron stores. Hemochromatosis can go undetected until a person is in their 50s or 60s, so some experts recommend screening for anyone over the age of 20. If the disease goes untreated, many organs will have become irreversibly damaged by midlife. Treatment of hemochromatosis is relatively easy. Regular blood donations and avoiding iron-rich foods and iron containing supplements are effective mechanisms to reduce iron content of the body.

CONCEPT CHECK

Iron absorption depends on its form and the body's need for it. Absorption is affected by iron needs but excess iron intake can override the body's ability to effectively control absorption, leading to toxicity. Nonheme iron absorption increases in the presence of vitamin C and meat protein and decreases in the presence of large amounts of some components of grain, such as fiber and phytic acid. Iron is used in synthesizing hemoglobin and myoglobin, supporting immune function, and metabolizing energy. An iron deficiency can cause decreased red blood cell synthesis, which can lead to anemia. It is particularly important for women of childbearing age to consume adequate iron, primarily to replace that lost in menstrual blood. Sources include red meat, pork, liver, enriched grains and cereals, and oysters. Iron toxicity causes overabsorption and accumulation of iron, which can result in severe liver and heart damage. Any use of iron supplements should be supervised by a physician, because of the risk of toxicity.

Zinc (Zn)

Zinc deficiency was first recognized in the early 1960s in Egypt and Iran. Zinc deficiencies were determined to cause growth retardation and poor sexual development in some groups of people, even though zinc content of their diets was fairly high. However, the customary diet contained unleavened bread almost exclusively and little animal protein. Unleavened bread is high in phytic acid and other factors that decrease zinc bioavailability. Parasite infestation and the practice of eating clay and other parts of soil also contributed to the severe zinc deficiency.

In North America, zinc deficiencies were first observed in the early 1970s in hospitalized patients fed only intravenously via total parenteral nutrition. The protein source in earlier intravenous solutions was based on milk protein or a blood protein, both naturally rich in zinc. When the solutions were changed to include mostly individual amino acids as the protein source, deficiency symptoms quickly developed because of their low zinc content.

Like iron, zinc absorption is influenced by the foods a person ingests. About 40% of dietary zinc is absorbed, especially when animal protein sources are used and when the body needs more zinc. Most people worldwide rely on cereal grains (low in zinc) for their source of protein, calories, and zinc. This makes consuming adequate zinc a problem. In addition, high-dose calcium supplementation with meals decreases zinc absorption. Finally, zinc competes with copper and iron for absorption, and vice versa, when supplemental sources are consumed.

Functions of Zinc. Approximately 200 enzymes require zinc as a cofactor for activity. Adequate zinc intake is necessary to support many bodily functions, such as:

- DNA synthesis and function
- Protein metabolism, wound healing, and growth
- Immune function (intakes in excess of the RDA do not provide any extra benefit to immune function)
- Development of sexual organs and bones
- Storage, release, and function of insulin
- Cell membrane structure and function
- Component of superoxide dismutase, an enzyme that aids in the prevention of oxidative damage to cells. Zinc, therefore, has an indirect antioxidant function.

Other possible functions of zinc are slowing the progression of macular degeneration of the eye and reducing the risk for developing certain forms of cancer.

Symptoms of adult zinc deficiency include an acnelike rash, diarrhea, lack of appetite, reduced sense of taste and smell, and hair loss. In children and adolescents with zinc deficiency, growth, sexual development, and learning ability may also be hampered.

Zinc Sources and Needs. Protein-rich diets are rich in zinc. Animal foods supply almost half of zinc intake. Major sources of zinc are beef, fortified breakfast cereals, wheat germ, and some cheese (Fig. 11-26). The food source influences bioavailability of zinc. Zinc found in animal foods is better absorbed than that found in plants due to phytic acid binding. Plant sources of zinc do contribute to zinc intake (Fig. 11-27). The form generally used in multivitamin and mineral supplements (zinc oxide) is not as well-absorbed as zinc found naturally in foods, but still contributes to meeting zinc needs.

The adult RDA for zinc is 11 milligrams for men and 8 milligrams for women, based on the amount to cover daily losses of zinc. The DV used on food and supplement labels is 15 milligrams. The average North American consumes 10 to 14 milligrams of zinc a day, with men consuming the higher values. There are no indications of moderate or severe zinc deficiencies in an otherwise healthy adult population. It is likely, however, that some North Americans—especially some women, poor children, vegans, and older people with alcoholism—have a marginal zinc status. These and other people who show deterioration in taste sensation, recurring infections, poor growth, or depressed wound healing should have their zinc status checked.

Upper Level for Zinc. The UL for zinc is 40 milligrams per day. Excessive zinc intake over time can lead to problems by interfering with copper metabolism. The interference

▲ Chocolate is a good source of zinc and magnesium. Eaten in moderation, chocolate like other foods, can be part of a healthy diet.

Food Sources of Zinc

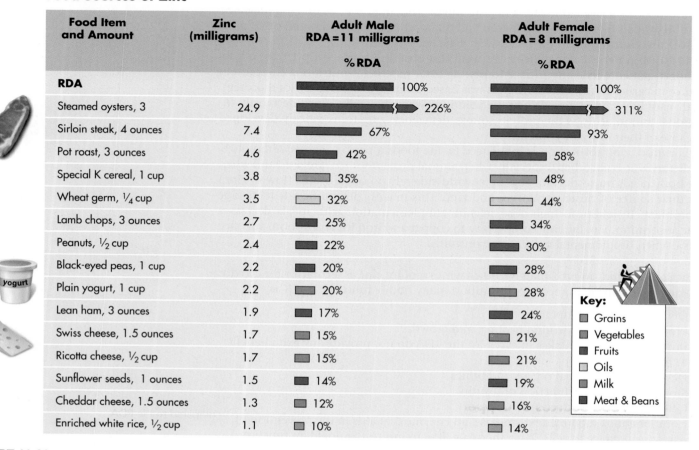

Food Item and Amount	Zinc (milligrams)	Adult Male RDA =11 milligrams %RDA	Adult Female RDA = 8 milligrams %RDA
RDA		100%	100%
Steamed oysters, 3	24.9	226%	311%
Sirloin steak, 4 ounces	7.4	67%	93%
Pot roast, 3 ounces	4.6	42%	58%
Special K cereal, 1 cup	3.8	35%	48%
Wheat germ, 1/4 cup	3.5	32%	44%
Lamb chops, 3 ounces	2.7	25%	34%
Peanuts, 1/2 cup	2.4	22%	30%
Black-eyed peas, 1 cup	2.2	20%	28%
Plain yogurt, 1 cup	2.2	20%	28%
Lean ham, 3 ounces	1.9	17%	24%
Swiss cheese, 1.5 ounces	1.7	15%	21%
Ricotta cheese, 1/2 cup	1.7	15%	21%
Sunflower seeds, 1 ounces	1.5	14%	19%
Cheddar cheese, 1.5 ounces	1.3	12%	16%
Enriched white rice, 1/2 cup	1.1	10%	14%

Key:
- Grains
- Vegetables
- Fruits
- Oils
- Milk
- Meat & Beans

FIGURE 11-26 ▶ Food sources of zinc compared to the RDA for adult males and females.

FIGURE 11-27 ▶ Sources of zinc from MyPyramid. The height of the background color (none, 1/3, 2/3, or completely covered) within each group in the pyramid indicates the average nutrient density for zinc in that group. Overall, the meat & beans group and the grains group contain many foods that are nutrient-dense sources of zinc. With regard to physical activity, zinc is especially needed to support muscle growth and muscle healing.

MyPyramid: Sources of Zinc

Grains	Vegetables	Fruits	Oils	Milk	Meat & Beans
• Whole-grain breads and cereals • Fortified breakfast cereals	• Spinach • Peas • Asparagus	• Avocados • Dried fruit	• None	• Milk • Yogurt • Cheese	• Beef • Eggs • Beans • Nuts • Shellfish • Poultry

with copper metabolism is the basis for setting the UL. If a person uses megadose supplementation, they should be under close medical supervision and also take a supplement containing copper (2 milligrams per day). Zinc intakes over 100 milligrams per day also result in diarrhea, cramps, nausea, vomiting, and depressed immune system function, especially if intake exceeds 2000 milligrams per day.

Copper (Cu)

Copper and iron are similar in terms of food sources, absorption, and functions. Copper functions in the synthesis of hemoglobin. A copper-containing enzyme aids in the release of iron from storage. Copper is needed by enzymes that create cross-links in connective tissue proteins. Copper is also needed by other enzymes, such as those that defend the body against free-radical damage (e.g., superoxide dismutase) and those that act in the brain and nervous system. Finally, copper performs in immune system function, blood clotting, and blood lipoprotein metabolism. Copper absorption is highly variable with higher intakes associated with lower absorption. Absorption takes place in the stomach and upper small intestine. Excess copper is not stored to a great extent, so when intake exceeds needs, the liver incorporates it into bile, excreted by the feces. Phytates, fiber, as well as zinc and iron supplements, may all interfere with copper absorption. Symptoms of copper deficiency include a form of anemia, low white blood cell count, bone loss, poor growth, and some forms of cardiovascular disease.

Copper Sources and Needs. Rich sources of copper include liver, legumes, seeds, whole-grain breads and cereals, and cocoa (Fig. 11-28).

Food Sources of Copper

FIGURE 11-28 ► Food sources of copper compared to the RDA.

Food Item and Amount	Copper (micrograms)	% RDA
RDA*	900	100%
Fried beef liver, 3 ounces	3800	422%
Power bar, 1	700	78%
Walnuts, ½ cup	600	67%
Kidney beans, ½ cup	500	56%
Lobster, 3 ounces	400	44%
Molasses, 3 tablespoons	300	33%
Sunflower seeds, 2 tablespoons	300	33%
Shrimp, 3 ounces	300	33%
Raisin Bran cereal, 1 cup	300	33%
Great Grains cereal, 1 cup	300	33%
Black-eyed peas, ½ cup cooked	200	22%
Wheat germ, ¼ cup	200	22%
Milk chocolate, 1 ounce	110	12%
Whole-wheat bread, 1 slice	80	9%

Key:
- Grains
- Vegetables
- Fruits
- Oils
- Milk
- Meat & Beans

*For adults; See the DRI table in the back of this book for gender- and age-specific recommendations.

▲ Seafood is one source of copper in the diet.

The RDA for copper is 900 micrograms daily for adults, based on the amount needed for activity of copper-containing proteins and enzymes. The DV used on food and supplement labels is 2 milligrams. The average adult intake is about 1 to 1.6 milligrams per day. Women consume the smaller amount. The form of copper typically found in multivitamin and mineral supplements (copper oxide) is not readily absorbed. It is best to rely on food sources to meet copper needs. The copper status of adults appears to be good, although sensitive laboratory tests to determine copper status is lacking.

The groups most likely to develop copper deficiencies are preterm infants recovering from semistarvation on a milk-dominated diet (a poor source of copper) and people recovering from intestinal surgery. A copper deficiency can result from over-zealous supplementation of zinc, because zinc and copper compete with each other for absorption.

Upper Level for Copper. The UL for copper is 10 milligrams per day. High doses of copper can cause toxicity with a single dose of greater than 10 milligrams. Other forms of toxicity (e.g., liver damage) are also observed with consumption of megadoses.

CASE STUDY

Anemia

Anita is a 60-year-old woman who prides herself on taking charge of her health. She exercises daily, whether it's walking her dog, playing golf, or a tai chi class at the senior center. She follows the 2005 Dietary Guidelines for Americans, choosing a variety of whole grains; at least five servings per day of fruits and vegetables; and keeping her saturated fat, *trans* fat, cholesterol, and sodium intakes to a minimum. She eats lean sources of protein, choosing poultry, fish, or vegetable sources of protein instead of red meat. She maintains a healthy body weight, has never had high blood pressure or high blood sugar, and doesn't take any medications or supplements.

Last week, she went to a blood drive at her church with the intent of donating blood, but she was turned away because her hematocrit (a measure of the percentage of red blood cells in the blood) was slightly below the requirements for donation. Anita was surprised because she'd never had a problem donating blood before. The nurse told Anita that her low hematocrit level was indicative of anemia, which has many possible causes. As Anita thought about it, she realized that she had been feeling more tired than usual.

Answer the following questions and check your responses in Appendix A.

1. Iron deficiency is the most common form of anemia. What role does iron play in the health of red blood cells? From the description, is it possible that Anita has low iron stores? What dietary changes could Anita make to improve her iron status?

2. A deficiency of vitamin B-6 is another possible cause of anemia. What role does vitamin B-6 play in the health of red blood cells? From the description, is it likely that Anita is deficient in vitamin B-6?

3. Folate deficiency may lead to anemia. What role does folate play in the health of red blood cells? From the description, is it likely that Anita is deficient in folate?

4. Low vitamin B-12 may result in anemia. What role does vitamin B-12 play in the health of red blood cells? Suggest an explanation for why Anita may have low vitamin B-12 status even with adequate dietary intake of vitamin B-12. What dietary changes could Anita make to improve her vitamin B-12 status?

5. What should Anita do now that she knows she is anemic? Will changes to her food choices suffice to resolve the problem?

SUMMARY

1. Vitamins are carbon-containing compounds we need daily in small amounts from foods. They yield no energy directly, but many contribute to energy-yielding chemical reactions in the body and promote growth and development. Many vitamins act as coenzymes, which help enzymes function.

2. Thiamin, riboflavin, and niacin play key roles as coenzymes in energy-yielding reactions. They help metabolize carbohydrates, fats, and proteins. Alcoholism and a poor diet can create deficiencies of these three nutrients, which often show up as symptoms in the brain and nervous system, skin, and GI tract. Enriched grain products are common sources of these vitamins. Only niacin has an UL (2.5 times adult needs).

3. Pantothenic acid, which participates in many aspects of cell metabolism, is widely distributed among foods. Biotin, which participates in glucose productions, fatty acid synthesis, and DNA synthesis, can be synthesized by bacteria in the intestine. Biotin comes from foods such as eggs, peanuts, and cheese. No ULs have been set for either vitamin.

4. Vitamin B-6 performs a vital role in protein metabolism, especially in synthesizing nonessential amino acids. It also helps synthesize neurotransmitters and performs other metabolic roles, such as metabolism of homocysteine. Headaches, a form of anemia, nausea, and vomiting result from a B-6 deficiency. Regular consumption of animal protein foods and rich plant sources, such as broccoli, provide needed vi-

tamin B-6. Taking high doses causes damage to the nervous system. The UL is about 60 times adult needs.

5. Folate plays an important role in DNA synthesis and homocysteine metabolism. Symptoms of a deficiency include poor cell division in various areas of the body, megaloblastic anemia, tongue inflammation, diarrhea, and poor growth. Pregnancy puts high demands for folate in the body; deficiency during the first month of pregnancy can result in neural tube defects in offspring. A deficiency can also occur in people with alcoholism. Food sources are leafy vegetables, organ meats, and orange juice. Women of childbearing age need to meet the Daily Recommended Allowances (DRA) with synthetic folic acid. Excess folate in the diet can mask a vitamin B-12 deficiency, as an UL has been set at 2 ½ times adult needs (refers to synthetic folic acid only).

6. Vitamin B-12 is needed to metabolize folate and homocysteine and maintain the insulation surrounding nerves. A deficiency results in anemia (because of its relationship to folate) and nerve degeneration. Older people often suffer from inefficient absorption of vitamin B-12, in which case they can benefit from monthly injections or megadoses of the vitamin. A dietary deficiency is unlikely because vitamin B-12 is highly concentrated in animal products, which constitute a major part of the North American diet. Vitamin B-12 does not occur naturally in plant foods. Vegans need a supplemental source, as found

in ready-to-eat breakfast cereals. No UL has been set.

7. Choline is a dietary component available from a wide variety of foods and is synthesized in the body. It is used to form a neurotransmitter, among other functions, such as homocysteine metabolism. Nutritional needs have been set. No natural deficiency of choline has been reported. The UL is set at about eight times adult needs.

8. The vitaminlike compounds carnitine, inositol, taurine, and lipoic acid, while participating in many important chemical reactions in the body, are not true vitamins because they can be synthesized in the body from readily available building blocks; they are also obtained from the diet.

9. Taking a multivitamin and mineral supplement to help meet nutrient needs is recommended by some experts, while other experts suggest that only some in the population need such supplementation. Taking many nutrient supplements can lead to nutrient-related toxicity, so any such use should be carefully considered. The clearest evidence is for a diet rich in fruits and vegetables and whole-grain breads and cereals, not reliance on supplements.

10. Magnesium is a mineral found mostly in plant sources. It is important for nerve and heart function and as an activator for many enzymes. Whole-grain breads and cereals (bran portion), vegetables, nuts, seeds, milk, and meats are good food sources. Sulfur is incorporated into certain vitamins and amino acids.

STUDY QUESTIONS

1. Describe how the RDA, DV, and UL for vitamin B-6 should be used in everyday life. How do the RDA and DV for vitamin B-6 differ?

2. Athletes have increased needs for certain micronutrients. Name two such

micronutrients and explain why this is the case.

3. Take one of the B vitamins that might be low in the North American diet and explain why a deficiency might occur.

4. Milling (refining) grains removes which vitamins and minerals? Which of these are replaced during processing?

5. Why does the FDA limit the amount of folate that may be included in supplements and fortified foods?

6. What are the best food sources for zinc and copper?

7. Describe the symptoms of iron-deficiency anemia and explain possible reasons they occur.

8. What are the practical consequences of the DV on food and supplement labels

exceeding the RDA or AI for many trace minerals?

9. Name two vitamins and two minerals that function as coenzymes. How do the deficiency diseases (if any) associated with inadequate supply of these

micronutrients relate to their coenzyme functions?

10. Explain the difference between heme and nonheme iron. Name one food source of each. How does the body's need for iron influence the absorption of heme and nonheme iron?

CHECK YOUR KNOWLEDGE

Answers to the following multiple choice questions are in Appendix A.

1. A vitamin synthesized by bacteria in the intestine is
   a. A.
   b. D.
   c. E.
   d. K.

2. Thiamin, riboflavin, and niacin are called the "energy" vitamins because they
   a. can be broken down to provide energy.
   b. are coenzymes needed for release of energy from carbohydrates, fats, and proteins.
   c. are ingredients in energy drinks such as Powerade.
   d. are needed in large amounts by competitive athletes.

3. A deficient intake of _____ has been shown to increase the risk of having a baby with a neural tube defect such as spina bifida.
   a. thiamin
   b. biotin
   c. iron
   d. folic acid

4. Dietary heme iron is derived from
   a. elemental iron in food.
   b. animal flesh.
   c. breakfast cereal.
   d. vegetables.

5. In a situation where there is an insufficient intake of dietary iodide, the thyroid-stimulating hormone promotes the enlargement of the thyroid gland. This condition is called
   a. Grave's disease.
   b. goiter.
   c. hyperparathyroidism.
   d. cretinism.

6. Strict vegetarians (vegans) are at risk for deficiency of which of the following micronutrients?
   a. Vitamin B-6
   b. Vitamin B-12
   c. folate
   d. magnesium

7. Avidin, a component in raw egg whites, may decrease the absorption of
   a. biotin.
   b. iron.
   c. zinc.
   d. riboflavin.

8. Which of the following micronutrients participates in DNA synthesis?
   a. folate
   b. zinc
   c. biotin
   d. All of the above

9. Anemia may result from deficiency of all of the following micronutrients except
   a. copper.
   b. zinc.
   c. vitamin B-6.
   d. vitamin B-12.

10. Impaired glucose tolerance may result from a deficiency of
    a. chromium.
    b. iodide.
    c. iron.
    d. zinc.

FURTHER READINGS

1. ADA Reports: Position of the American Dietetic Association: Fortification and nutritional supplements. *Journal of the American Dietetic Association* 105:1300, 2005.

   The best nutritional strategy for promoting optimal health and reducing the risk of chronic disease is to wisely choose a wide variety of foods. Additional vitamins and minerals from fortified foods and/or supplements can help some people meet their nutritional needs as set by science-

based nutrition standards (e.g., the Dietary Reference Intakes).

2. Andres E and others: Food-cobalamin malabsorption in elderly patients: Clinical manifestations and treatments. *American Journal of Medicine* 118:1154, 2005.

   About 15% of older adults show defective vitamin B-12 absorption. This condition especially affects absorption of the vitamin B-12 found naturally in foods. Consumption of crystalline

vitamin B-12 in contrast is not so affected and was found to be a useful form of therapy for the older adults in this study.

3. Are you getting enough of this vitamin? *Harvard Health Letter* 30(10):1, 2005.

   Those at risk for B-12 deficits include older adults and strict vegans. Although a severe deficiency is fairly unlikely in older adults, mild shortfalls may affect balance, memory, and perhaps mood.

4. Aufiero E and others: Pyridoxine hydrochloride treatment of carpal tunnel syndrome: A review. *Nutrition Reviews* 62(3):96, 2004.

Some, but not all, studies have found megadose vitamin B-6 therapy effective in helping treat carpal tunnel syndrome. This article discusses the latest findings on this topic.

5. Baily LB and others: Folic acid supplementation and fortification affect the risk for neural tube defects, vascular disease and cancer: Evolving science. *Journal of Nutrition* 133:1961S, 2003.

Adequate folic acid status before and during pregnancy reduces the risk of neural tube defects by about 70%. The ability of folic acid to reduce the risk of cancer and cardiovascular disease are interesting scientific theories that need more research before clear recommendations can be made.

6. Bentley TGK and others: Population-level changes in folate intake by age, gender, and race/ethnicity after folic acid fortification. *American Journal of Public Health* 96:2040, 2006.

The impact of the 1998 U.S. FDA folic acid fortification policy was quantified by estimating folate intake at the population level. After fortification, mean food and total folate intake increased by about 100 µg/day. The number of women of childbearing age who consume more than 400 µg/day of folate increased after fortification, but has not yet reached the FDA's target of 50%. Although folic acid intake has increased among the U.S. population since fortification, there are substantial variations by age, gender, and race/ethnicity.

7. Food and Nutrition Board, Institute of Medicine: Dietary Reference Intakes for thiamin, riboflavin, niacin, vitamin B-6, folate, vitamin B-12, pantothenic acid, biotin, and choline. Washington, DC: *The National Academy Press*, 1998.

This work outlines how nutrient recommendations were established for the B vitamins and choline, with specific reference to establishing the RDA and related standards. The functions of each of the B vitamins and choline are explained.

8. Food and Nutrition Board, Institute of Medicine: Dietary Reference Intakes for vitamin A, vitamin K, arsenic, boron, chromium, copper, iodine, iron, manganese, molybdenum, nickel, silicon, vanadium, and zinc. Washington, DC: *The National Academy Press*, 2001.

Recommendations for vitamin A and vitamin K intake are listed. The rationale used to set the RDA or AI and UL for these nutrients is discussed in detail.

9. McCormick DB: The dubious use of vitamin-mineral supplements in relation to cardiovascular disease. *American Journal of Clinical Nutrition* 84(4):680; 2006.

This editorial supports the findings of studies, including the meta-analysis by Bleys and others, that antioxidants and B vitamins should not be used to prevent cardiovascular disease. The author hopes that these recent findings, "which carefully separate fact from faith," will decrease the extensive use of vitamin-mineral supplements.

10. Franchini M and Veneri D: Hereditary hemochromatosis. *Hematology* 10(2):145, 2005.

Hereditary hemochromatosis is a disorder of iron metabolism characterized by progressive tissue iron overload, which leads to irreversible organ damage if not treated in time. Transferrin saturation and serum ferritin are the most reliable tests for the detection of subjects with hereditary hemochromatosis. Therapeutic phlebotomy is the mainstay of treatment. If phlebotomy is started before the onset of irreversible organ damage, the life expectancy of these patients is similar to that of the normal population.

11. Hubbs-Tait L and others. Zinc, iron, and lead: Relations to Head Start children's cognitive scores and teachers' ratings of behavior. *Journal of the American Dietetic Association* 107:128, 2007.

Research points to interactions between essential micronutrients (e.g., iron and zinc) and toxic elements (e.g., lead) and their effects on cognition and behavior. In this small study, higher levels of lead were associated with lower levels of iron and zinc. Low zinc levels were associated with higher anxiety in boys. High lead levels were associated with lower social skills in girls. This study emphasizes the importance of

micronutrient status for learning and behavior among young children and also highlights the detrimental effect of lead exposure.

12. Lichtenstein AH and others: Diet and lifestyle recommendations revision 2006: A scientific statement from the American Heart Association Nutrition Committee. *Circulation* 114:82, 2006.

Supplementation with several B vitamins (folate, vitamin B-6, and vitamin B-12) has been proposed as a preventive measure to protect against cardiovascular disease due to the involvement of these micronutrients in homocysteine metabolism. However, despite effectiveness in lowering serum homocysteine levels, clinical studies have failed to show an effect of these dietary supplements on cardiovascular events. Thus, there is insufficient evidence to recommend dietary supplementation to prevent cardiovascular disease. A diet rich in whole grains, fruits, and vegetables, coupled with regular physical activity, remain the best strategies for prevention of cardiovascular disease.

13. Pitkin RM. Folate and neural tube defects. *American Journal of Clinical Nutrition* 85:285S, 2007.

The ability of adequate folic acid during the periconceptional period to prevent neural tube defects is well-established. This article reviews important research that has led to advancements in the prevention of neural tube defects, discusses recommendations for intake (0.4 mg/d for all women of childbearing age or 4 mg/d for high-risk women), and examines the success of the folic acid fortification program instituted in 1998 in the United States.

14. Zeisel SH. Choline: Critical role during fetal development and dietary requirements in adults. *Annual Review of Nutrition* 26:229, 2006.

The author reviews recommendations for intake of choline and calls for updates to the AIs based on evidence from animal and human studies. Choline requirements are influenced by age, gender, and genetic conditions. The importance of choline during pregnancy, particularly in fetal brain development, is emphasized. In addition, the role of choline in cardiovascular health is discussed.

► Check out the **Contemporary Nutrition ARIS site**
www.mhhe.com/wardlawcontfa1 for quizzes, flash cards, other activities, and weblinks designed to further help you learn about what you eat and why.

RATE YOUR PLATE

I. Boosting Your Micronutrient Intake

For each of the following meal options, choose the one that would supply the most of the given micronutrient.

1. Which meal supplies the most iron?

A	B
• Roast beef sandwich on whole-grain bread with lettuce, tomato, and mustard	• Roast beef sandwich on whole-grain bread with lettuce, tomato, and mustard
• Grapes	• Grapes
• Skim milk	• Orange juice

2. Which meal supplies the most vitamin K?

A	B
• Pasta with shrimp, tomatoes, and spinach	• Pasta with shrimp, tomatoes, and feta cheese
• Italian bread with olive oil	• Italian bread with butter
• White wine	• White wine

3. Which meal supplies the most zinc?

A	B
• Cheerios	• Blueberry bagel with cream cheese
• Banana	• Banana
• Orange juice	• Orange juice

4. Which meal supplies the most vitamin B-12?

A	B
• Cheeseburger	• Veggie burger
• Baked potato with sour cream	• Baked potato with sour cream
• Diet cola	• Iced tea

CHAPTER 12 Nutrition: Fitness and Sports

ATHLETES INVEST A LOT OF TIME AND EFFORT IN TRAINING. Most athletes don't want to miss out on any advantage, whether real or perceived, that might give them the winning edge. Athletes often seek ways to enhance their diets to improve performance, so they make easy targets for purveyors of nutrition misinformation.

Although good eating habits can't substitute for physical training and genetic endowment, proper food and beverage choices are crucial for top-notch performance, contributing to endurance and helping to speed the repair of injured tissues.

Although experts might disagree on how much carbohydrate, protein, and fat we should consume, there is no argument over the health benefits of regular physical activity. It is even beneficial for overweight people who remain at that excess weight. As the comic in this chapter suggests, it takes a strong commitment to reap the benefits.

In Chapter 12, you will discover how physical fitness benefits the entire body and how nutrition relates to fitness and sports performance.

Refresh Your Memory

As you begin your study of nutrition for fitness and sports in Chapter 12, you may want to review:

- The current trend of consuming "energy bars" in Chapter 1
- Components of the cell in Chapter 3
- Concept of glycemic load in Chapter 4
- Various food sources of carbohydrates, proteins, and lipids in Chapters 4–7
- Food sources of calcium and iron in Chapters 10 and 11

THE CLOSE RELATIONSHIP BETWEEN NUTRITION AND FITNESS

The ability to engage routinely in vigorous physical activity requires good health. Peak performance also depends on a diet that supplies all the needed nutrients.

The type of fuel used by muscles depends on how physically fit the athletes are and how hard each one performs. This **physical fitness**—defined as the ability to perform moderate to vigorous activity without undue fatigue—especially affects fat use by the body. As one's level of physical fitness improves, so does one's ability to mobilize fat stores for energy needs—especially during activities that last for 20 minutes or more.

Beyond affecting fuel use, the benefits of regular physical activity include enhancement of several aspects of heart function, less injury, better sleep habits, and improvement in body composition (less body fat, more muscle mass). Physical activity also can reduce stress and positively affect blood pressure, blood cholesterol, blood glucose regulation, and immune function. In addition, physical activity aids in weight control, both by raising resting energy expenditure for a short time after exercise and by increasing overall energy expenditure. See Figure 12-1 for a further look at those and other benefits of a physically active lifestyle.

Unfortunately, as noted in Chapter 7, many North American adults lead sedentary lives. Most adults do not practice moderate to vigorous physical activity on a regular basis, and about half of all adults quit an exercise program within 3 months of onset.

physical fitness The ability to perform moderate to vigorous activity without undue fatigue.

Sherman's Lagoon by J.P. Toomey

Why is regular physical activity—including some strength-building activities— generally advocated for all of us? What benefits accrue from this practice? How do strength-training and endurance athletes need to tailor their diets to support their vigorous physical activities? Chapter 12 provides some answers.

Strengthens bones and joints

Reduces blood pressure

Improves blood glucose regulation

Increases cardiovascular function and improves blood lipid profile

Reduces stress and improves self-image

Aids in weight loss/weight control

Increases flexibility and balance

Increases muscle mass and strength

Improves immune function

Improves GI tract peristalsis

Reduces risk of colon cancer, prostate cancer, and likely breast cancer

Improves sleep (if activity is done in the morning or afternoon)

FIGURE 12-1 ▶ Exercise is medicine—the benefits of regular, moderate physical activity. There is also evidence that regular physical activity slows the aging process.

Healthy People 2010 has set a number of specific objectives, for U.S. adults, related to physical activity and exercise:

- Reduce by 50% the proportion of adults engaging in no leisuretime physical activity (currently 27% of adults).
- Double the proportion of adults engaging regularly, preferably daily, in moderate exercise for at least 30 minutes per day (currently 45% of adults).
- Increase by 50% the proportion of adults who perform physical activities that enhance and maintain muscular strength and endurance (currently 19% of adults).

To help yourself stay with an exercise program, experts recommend the following:

- Start slowly.
- Vary your activities; make it fun.
- Include friends and others.
- Set specific attainable goals and monitor progress.
- Set aside a specific time each day for exercise; build it into your routine, but make it convenient.
- Reward yourself for being successful in keeping up with your goals.
- Don't worry about occasional setbacks; focus on the long-term benefits to your health.

The *2005 Dietary Guidelines for Americans* recommends three different time goals for physical activity (review Chapter 2).

- 30 minutes/day of moderate-intensity physical activity, in addition to usual activity, for individuals trying to reduce their risk of chronic disease in adulthood. Doing more than 30 minutes or increasing the intensity of the workout could lead to even greater benefits.

▲ What is the best exercise? One you want to continue to do.

▶ One day in December 2000, Joe Decker:

bicycled 100 miles,

ran 10 miles, hiked 10 miles,

power-walked 5 miles,

kayaked 6 miles,

skied on a NordicTrack 10 miles,

rowed 10 miles, swam 2 miles,

did 3000 abdominal crunches,

did 1100 jumping jacks,

did 1000 leg lifts, did 1100 push-ups.

And he lifted weights for a cumulative total of 278,540 lb.

For his efforts (and pains), he earned a place in the *Guinness Book of World Records* as the fittest man alive.

- 60 minutes/day of moderate- to vigorous-intensity physical activity to help adults manage body weight and prevent gradual weight gain
- 90 minutes/day of moderate-intensity physical activity may be needed for some adults to sustain weight loss; at the same time, these individuals also need to monitor their calorie intakes.

MAKING DECISIONS

Planning Your Exercise

Consider applying the dietary principles of variety, balance, and moderation to your exercise plan:

- Variety: Enjoy many different activities to exercise different muscles.
- Balance: Different activities have different benefits, so balance your exercise pattern. For overall fitness, you need exercises that build cardiovascular endurance, muscular strength, and flexibility.
- Moderation: Exercise to keep fit without overdoing it. You don't need a heavy workout every day to achieve fitness.

CONCEPT CHECK

Regular physical activity is a vital part of a healthy lifestyle, ideally consisting of a total of at least 30 minutes (and preferably 60, especially if weight loss/weight control is an issue) of aerobic activity on most (or all) days. Physically active people benefit from lower risks of cardiovascular disease, type 2 diabetes, obesity, and other common chronic diseases.

GUIDELINES FOR ACHIEVING AND MAINTAINING PHYSICAL FITNESS

For healthy people, a gradual increase to a goal of regular physical activity is recommended. Men 40 years of age or older and women 50 years of age or older who have been inactive for many years, or who have an existing health problem, should discuss their fitness goals with their physician before increasing activity. Health problems that require medical evaluation before beginning an exercise program are obesity, cardiovascular disease (or family history of it), hypertension, diabetes (or family history), shortness of breath after mild exertion, and arthritis.

During the first phase of a fitness program to promote health, you should begin to incorporate short periods of physical activity into the daily routine. This includes walking, taking the stairs instead of the elevator, house cleaning, gardening, and other activities that cause you to "huff and puff" a bit. The goal is a total of 30 minutes of this moderate type of physical activity on most (and preferably all) days. If necessary, this can be broken up into increments lasting at least 10 minutes. Experts suggest starting with short intervals, building up to a total of 30 minutes of activity incorporated into each day's tasks. If there is not much time for activity, you can even go for more intensity in the activities over shorter periods to get the same benefits. Clearly, many of the activities just recommended are not very vigorous.

Once you can perform physical activity for 30 minutes per day, turn your attention to more specific goals, such as increasing muscle mass and strength, to reap even more benefits. Guidelines for designing a fitness program are listed in Table 12-1. Aerobic, strength, and stretching activities are included, as well as considerations for duration, frequency, intensity, and progression.

Begin by warming up with 5 to 10 more minutes of low-intensity exercises, such as walking, slow jogging, or any slow version of the anticipated activity. This warms up

TABLE 12-1 Designing a Fitness Program

Type of Activity	Aerobic (uses large muscle groups in rhythmic fashion)	Strength (resistance activity)	Stretching (uses major muscle groups; important during warm-up and cooldown)
Examples	Brisk walking, running, cycling, swimming, basketball, tennis, soccer	Weight-lifting, pilates, push-ups, pull-ups	Yoga
Duration (time spent in exercise session)	20 to 60 minutes	8 to 12 repetitions of 8 to 10 different exercises	4 repetitions of 10 to 30 seconds per muscle group
Frequency (times activity is performed)	5 days per week	2 to 3 days per week	2 to 3 days per week and during warm-up and cooldown
Intensity (level of exertion)	55% to 90% maximum heart rate or RPE of 4 or above (see Figure 12-2)	Enough to condition major muscle groups of the upper and lower body	5 to 10 minutes during warm-up and cooldown
Progression (increase in frequency, intensity, and duration over time)	**Initiation phase:** 3 to 6 weeks **Improvement phase:** 5 to 6 months **Maintenance phase:** plateau in gains in fitness		Start with smaller muscle groups (e.g., arms) and work toward large muscle groups (e.g., legs and abdomen)

your muscles so that muscle filaments more easily slide over one another to increase range of motion and decrease the risk of injury.

Aerobic Workout

Daily aerobic activity is recommended. Health benefits from regular physical activity are especially seen when you can achieve a moderate level of intensity of exercise.

There are a few ways to determine the intensity of exercise. A popular and simple method is to use a percentage of your age-predicted maximum heart rate. To find maximum heart rate, subtract your age from 220. Multiplying maximum heart rate by 0.60 and 0.90 will result in a range of heart rates, sometimes called the *target zone*. For a 20-year-old person beginning an exercise program, maximum heart rate equals 200 beats per minute (220 – 20 = 200). Then, (200 × 0.6) and (200 × 0.9) yields a target zone of 120 to 180 beats per minute. Measuring heart rate (pulse) is easy: Stop and count your pulse for 10 seconds and then multiply that number by 6 to determine your heart rate for one minute. There are also watches available that contain heart rate monitors.

At the initiation of an exercise program, aim for the lower end of the target zone. As you progress and become more physically fit, you can work up to a higher heart rate. As with many of the prediction formulas, calculation of maximum heart rate is just an estimate. Medications, such as those for hypertension and other health conditions, may impact heart rate. If you have health concerns, a physician can help to personalize your target zone.

▲ Taking one's pulse determines if exercise output is in the target zone.

RPE Scale*

Nothing at all   Very weak   Weak   Moderate   Somewhat strong   Strong   Very strong   Very, very strong

0   1   2   3   4   5   6   7   8   9   10

* Rating of Perceived Exertion (RPE) beyond 10 is considered maximal

FIGURE 12-2 ▶ Rating of Perceived Exertion scale. When exercising, a rating of 4 or above is advocated for building/maintaining physical fitness.

Another way of determining the intensity of exercise is the Rating of Perceived Exertion scale (RPE). One version includes a range of 1 to 10, with each number corresponding to a subjective feeling of exertion. For example, the number 0 is "nothing at all" (sitting at a table) and the number 10 is considered close to maximal effort or "very, very strong" (all-out sprint) (Figure 12-2).

When using the RPE scale, the goal is to aim for the number 4, which corresponds to the beginning of "somewhat strong." This is the point at which you begin to see significant fitness results. You should be working hard, but still be able to talk to an exercise partner (sometimes called the "talk test").

During cooldown, follow a reverse pattern of the warm-up: 5 to 10 minutes of low-intensity activity and add 5 to 10 minutes of stretching. The same exercises performed during warm-up are appropriate. The cooldown is essential to the prevention of injury and soreness.

ENERGY SOURCES FOR EXERCISING MUSCLES

Like other cells, muscle cells cannot directly use the energy released from breaking down glucose or triglycerides. Muscle cells need a specific form of energy for contraction. Body cells must first convert food energy (i.e., calories) to **adenosine triphosphate (ATP).**

The chemical bonds between phosphates in ATP and related molecules are high-energy bonds. Using the energy obtained from foodstuffs, cells make ATP from its breakdown product **adenosine diphosphate (ADP)** and a phosphate group (abbreviated Pi).

$$ADP + Energy\ from\ food + Pi \rightarrow ATP$$

Conversely, to release energy from ATP, cells partially break the compound down into ADP and Pi. The released energy is used for many cell functions.

$$ATP \rightarrow Energy\ to\ do\ work + ADP + Pi$$

Essentially, ATP is the immediate source of energy for body functions (Table 12-2). The primary goal in the use of any fuel, whether carbohydrate, fat, or protein, is to make ATP. A resting muscle cell contains only a small amount of ATP that can be used immediately. This amount of ATP could keep the muscle working maximally for only about 2 to 4 seconds if no resupply of ATP were possible. Fortunately, another type of high-energy compound—**phosphocreatine (PCr)**—is also present in muscle cells and can be quickly broken down to release enough energy to make more ATP. This helps resupply ATP until use of carbohydrate and fat fuels begins in earnest. Overall, cells must constantly and repeatedly use and then re-form ATP, using a variety of energy sources.

Adenosine — Pi ⁓ Pi ⁓ Pi

High-energy bonds

Structure of ATP

adenosine triphosphate (ATP) The main energy currency for cells. ATP energy is used to promote ion pumping, enzyme activity, and muscular contraction.

adenosine diphosphate (ADP) A breakdown product of ATP. ADP is synthesized into ATP using energy from foodstuffs and a phosphate group (abbreviated Pi).

phosphocreatine (PCr) A high-energy compound that can be used to re-form ATP. It is used primarily during bursts of activity, such as lifting and jumping.

TABLE 12-2 Energy Sources Used by Resting and Working Muscle Cells

Energy Source*	When in Use	Activity
ATP	At all times	All types
Phosphocreatine (PCr)	All exercise initially; short bursts of exercise thereafter	Shotput, high jump, bench press
Carbohydrate (anaerobic)	High-intensity exercise, especially lasting 30 seconds to 2 minutes	200-yard (about 200 meters) sprint
Carbohydrate (aerobic)	Exercise lasting 2 minutes to 3 hours or more; the higher the intensity (for example, running a 6-minute mile), the greater the use	Basketball, swimming, jogging, power walking, soccer, tennis
Fat (aerobic)	Exercise lasting more than a few minutes; greater amounts are used at lower exercise intensities	Long-distance running, long-distance cycling; much of the fuel used in a 30-minute brisk walk is fat
Protein (aerobic)	Low amount during all exercise; slightly more in endurance exercise, especially when carbohydrate fuel is lacking	Long-distance running

*At any given time, more than one source is used. The relative amount of use differs during various activities.

▲ Bursts of muscle activity use a variety of energy sources, including PCr and ATP.

creatine An organic (i.e., carbon-containing) molecule in muscle cells that serves as a part of a high-energy compound (termed creatine phosphate or phosphocreatine) capable of synthesizing ATP from ADP.

Phosphocreatine Is the First Line of Defense for Resupplying ATP in Muscles

As soon as ATP stored in muscle cells begins to be used, another source of energy just mentioned, PCr, is used to produce ATP. An enzyme in the muscle cell is activated to split PCr into phosphate and **creatine.** This releases energy that can be used to re-form ATP from its breakdown products. If no other source of energy for ATP resupply were available, PCr could probably maintain maximal muscle contractions for about 10 seconds. Other sources of ATP resupply kick in, however, so PCr ends up as a source of energy for events lasting about 1 minute or less.

$$PCr + ADP \rightarrow ATP + Cr$$

The main advantage of PCr is that it can be activated instantly and can replenish ATP at rates fast enough to meet the energy demands of the fastest and most powerful actions, including jumping, lifting, throwing, and sprinting. The disadvantage of PCr is that not much of it is made and stored in the muscles. Strength-training athletes have begun to use creatine supplements in an effort to increase PCr in muscles.

 See the *Nutrition and Your Health Section: Ergogenic Aids and Athletic Performance* at the end of Chapter 12.

Carbohydrate Fuel for Muscles

Carbohydrates are an important fuel for muscles. The most useful form of carbohydrate fuel is the simple sugar glucose, available to all cells from the bloodstream. As you will recall from Chapter 4, glucose is stored as glycogen in the liver and muscle cells. Blood glucose is maintained by the breakdown of liver glycogen. Breakdown of glycogen stored in a specific muscle also helps meet the carbohydrate demand of that muscle, but the actual amount of glycogen stored in muscle is limited (about 350 grams, which would yield about 1400 kcal).

Depending on whether oxygen is available to exercising muscles, use of glucose to make ATP can be either anaerobic or aerobic.

pyruvic acid A three-carbon compound formed during glucose metabolism; also called *pyruvate*.

lactic acid A three-carbon acid formed during anaerobic cell metabolism; a partial breakdown product of glucose; also called *lactate*.

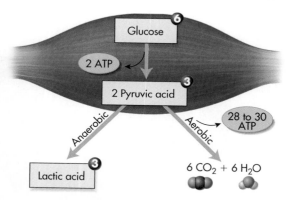

FIGURE 12-3 ▶ ATP yield from aerobic versus anaerobic glucose use.

Anaerobic Glucose Breakdown Yields Energy Fast. When oxygen supply in the muscle is limited (anaerobic conditions), glucose is broken down into a three-carbon compound called **pyruvic acid.** The pyruvic acid accumulates in the muscle and is then converted to **lactic acid.** Only about 5% of the total amount of ATP that could be formed from complete breakdown of glucose, is released through this anaerobic process (glucose →→ lactic acid).

The advantage of anaerobic glucose breakdown is that it is the fastest way to resupply ATP, other than PCr breakdown. It therefore provides most of the energy needed for events that require a quick burst of energy, ranging from about 30 seconds to 2 minutes. Examples of activities that primarily rely on anaerobic glucose breakdown include sprinting 400 meters or swimming 100 meters.

The two major disadvantages of the anaerobic process are that (1) the high rate of ATP production cannot be sustained for long periods, and (2) the rapid accumulation of lactic acid greatly increases the acidity of the muscle. Acidity inhibits the activities of key enzymes in the muscle cells, slowing anaerobic ATP production and causing short-term fatigue. The acidity also leads to a net potassium loss from muscle cells, providing another cause of fatigue. We learn by trial-and-error a pace that will control muscle lactic acid concentrations during these anaerobic events.

For the most part, lactic acid builds up in active muscle cells until it is released into the bloodstream. The liver (and the kidneys, to some extent) takes up the lactic acid and resynthesizes it into glucose. Glucose can then reenter the bloodstream, where it is available for cell uptake and breakdown.

Aerobic Glucose Breakdown Is a Sustained Energy Source. If plenty of oxygen is available in the muscle (aerobic conditions), such as when the exercise is of low to moderate intensity, the bulk of the three-carbon pyruvic acid is shuttled to the mitochondria of the cell, where it is further and fully metabolized into carbon dioxide (CO_2) and water (H_2O) (Fig. 12-4). This aerobic breakdown of glucose yields approximately 95% of the ATP made from complete glucose metabolism (glucose →→ CO_2 + H_2O).

Aerobic glucose breakdown supplies more ATP than does the anaerobic process, but it releases the energy more slowly. This slower rate of aerobic energy supply can be sustained for hours. One reason is that the products are carbon dioxide and water, not lactic acid. Aerobic glucose breakdown makes a major energy contribution to activi-

▶ Sprinting relies primarily on anaerobic glucose breakdown.

FIGURE 12-4 ▶ Simplified view of ATP formation from carbohydrate, fat, and protein. Along with phosphocreatine (PCr), all three nutrients may be used for ATP synthesis, but glucose and fatty acids are primary sources. Glucose may be broken down anaerobically or may undergo complete aerobic metabolism. The products of fatty acid breakdown are channeled into aerobic metabolism. Although limited, products of amino acid breakdown are channeled into the aerobic pathway as well. Recall also from Chapters 8 and 9 that many vitamins and minerals participate in these metabolic pathways.

ties that last anywhere from 2 minutes to 3 hours or more. Examples of such activities include jogging or distance swimming (review Table 12-2).

Many researchers have studied the ability of various types of carbohydrate feedings to maximize glucose supply to muscles during prolonged exercise. Overall, the techniques have succeeded. Consuming about 30 to 60 grams of carbohydrate per hour during strenuous endurance exercise that lasts 1 hour or more, such as cycling, can aid in maintaining adequate blood glucose, resulting in a delay of fatigue by 30 to 60 minutes. This attention to carbohydrate intake also helps one tolerate vigorous training on a daily basis.

As blood glucose declines during exercise, so does mental function. Cyclists refer to this diminished mental ability as "bonking." The fall in blood glucose is related to depletion of liver glycogen, not muscle glycogen, because liver glycogen is used to maintain blood glucose. See the later section, "Sports Drinks," to learn more about carbohydrate replacement during exercise (see Figure 12-6 on page 445).

CRITICAL THINKING

Marty started going to the gym about 8 weeks ago. At first, he noticed that he began "huffing and puffing" about 7 minutes into his aerobic workout. Now, however, he can work out for about 25 minutes without tiring. What is a possible explanation for this ability to work out longer?

16-carbon
fatty acid

about 108 ATP
for cell use

$CO_2 + H_2O$

ATP yield from aerobic fatty acid utilization.

 See the *Nutrition and Your Health Section: Ergogenic Aids and Athletic Performance* at the end of Chapter 12.

▲ Fatty acids can come from all over the body, not necessarily from fat stored near the active muscles. *This is why spot reducing does not work.* Exercise can tone the muscles near adipose tissue but does not preferentially use those stores.

Carbohydrate intake during exercise is not as important in shorter events (e.g., 30 minutes or so) because the muscles do not take up much blood glucose during short-term exercise, relying instead primarily on their glycogen stores for fuel.

Fat: The Main Fuel for Prolonged Low-Intensity Activity

When fat stores in body tissues begin to be broken down for energy, each triglyceride first yields three fatty acids and a glycerol. The majority of the stored energy is found in the fatty acids. During physical activity, the fatty acids are released from various adipose tissue depots into the bloodstream and travel to the muscles, where they are taken into each cell and broken down aerobically to carbon dioxide and water. Some of the fat stored in muscles also is used, especially as activity increases from a low to a moderate pace.

The rate at which muscles use fatty acids partly depends on the concentration of fatty acids in the bloodstream. In other words, the more fatty acids released from adipose tissue stores into the bloodstream, the more fat will be used by the muscles. Some cyclists and other endurance athletes have attempted to raise their blood concentrations of fatty acids by consuming caffeinated beverages. This practice can actually increase fatty acid release from the adipose tissue depots and is therefore helpful to certain athletes, but it is illegal under NCAA rules if the amount of caffeine in the body exceeds the equivalent of 6 to 8 cups of coffee (see the "Nutrition and Your Health" section at the end of this Chapter).

Fat is not a very useful muscle fuel for intense, brief exercise, but it becomes a progressively more important energy source as duration increases, especially when exercise remains at a low or moderate (aerobic) rate for more than 20 minutes (Fig. 12-5). The reason for this is that some of the steps involved in fat breakdown cannot occur fast enough to meet the ATP demands of short-duration, high-intensity exercise. If fat were the only available fuel, we would be unable to exercise beyond a fast walk or jog.

The advantage of fat fuel is that it provides stores of energy in a relatively concentrated form, and we generally have a lot of it stored. For a given weight of fuel, fat supplies more than twice as much energy as carbohydrate does. For lengthy activities at a moderate pace (for example, hiking) or even sitting at a desk for 8 hours a day, fat supplies about 70% to 90% of the energy required. Carbohydrate use is much less. As intensity increases, such as in a 3-hour marathon run at a competitive pace, muscles use about a 50:50 ratio of fat to carbohydrate. In comparison, for short events, such as a 100-meter sprint or even a 1500-meter race, the contribution of fat to resupply ATP is minimal. To summarize, remember that the only fast-paced (anaerobic) fuel we eat is carbohydrate; slow and steady (aerobic) activity uses much fat in addition to carbohydrate.

MAKING DECISIONS

Training Effect

As people start exercising regularly four or five times per week, they experience a "training effect." Initially, these individuals might be able to exercise for 20 minutes before tiring. Months later, exercise can be extended to an hour before they feel tired. During the months of training, muscle cells have produced more mitochondria and thus can burn more fat. Training also increases the number of capillaries in muscles, which increases oxygen supply to the muscles. As a result, lactic acid production from anaerobic glucose metabolism decreases. Lactic acid contributes to short-term muscle fatigue, so the less lactic acid produced, the longer the exercise can be sustained. Other contributors to the training effect include increased aerobic efficiency of the heart and muscles and elevations in muscle triglyceride content, with an enhanced ability of muscles to use triglycerides for energy needs.

FIGURE 12-5 ► Rough estimates of fuel use during various forms of physical activity. With regard to the weightlifting session, carbohydrate use could be somewhat greater and fat use somewhat less if the session is intense and fast-paced (e.g., circuit training). Fat use generally is higher because much of the time spent weight lifting is for rest periods and equipment-related activities.

Protein: A Minor Fuel Source, Primarily for Endurance Exercise

Although amino acids derived from protein can be used to fuel muscles, their contribution is relatively small, compared with that of carbohydrate and fat. As a rough guide, only about 5% of the body's general energy needs, as well as the typical energy needs of exercising muscles, is supplied by the metabolism of amino acids.

During endurance exercise, proteins can contribute importantly to energy needs, perhaps as much as 10% to 15%, especially as glycogen stores in the muscle are exhausted. Most of the energy supplied from protein comes from metabolism of the branched-chain amino acids—leucine, isoleucine, and valine. A normal diet provides ample branched chain amino acids to supply this amount of fuel, so protein or amino acid supplements are not needed. Contrary to what many athletes believe, protein is used for fuel less in resistance types of exercise (e.g., weightlifting) than in endurance exercise (e.g., running) (review Fig. 12-5). The primary muscle fuels for weightlifting are phosphocreatine (PCr) and carbohydrate for the brief bursts of activity, with fat providing energy during the resting stages, and with little use of protein overall. Despite this, high-protein products such as Pro-Complex, Amino Fuel 2000, High Voltage Protein Drink, and Instant Egg Protein are marketed specifically to weightlifters and bodybuilders in nearly every health-food and fitness store. Consuming high-carbohydrate, moderate-protein foods immediately after a weight-training workout enhances the muscle-building effect of the activity, most likely by increasing the concentrations of insulin and growth hormone released into the blood and contributing

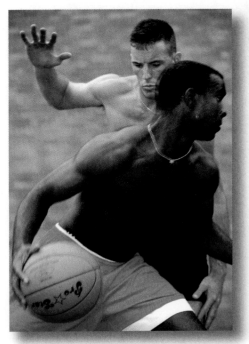

▲ The calories needed to perform come from carbohydrate, fat, and protein. The relative mix depends on the pace.

to protein synthesis. Still, it is impossible to increase muscle mass simply by eating protein. Putting physical strain on muscle through strength training or other physical activity is needed.

CONCEPT CHECK

Adenosine triphosphate (ATP) is the main form of energy used by cells. Cells use food energy to form ATP. Phosphocreatine (PCr) can rapidly re-form ATP from its breakdown product adenosine diphosphate (ADP), but PCr supplies are limited. Carbohydrate metabolism to form ATP begins as glucose becomes available from the absorption of carbohydrates from the diet or glycogen breakdown. In a muscle cell, each glucose molecule is broken down through a series of steps to yield either lactic acid or carbon dioxide (CO_2) plus water (H_2O). The process that occurs when glucose is broken down into carbon dioxide and water is called *aerobic* because oxygen is used. The conversion of glucose to lactic acid is called *anaerobic* because no oxygen is used. The anaerobic process allows the cell to quickly re-form ATP and supports the demand for energy during intense exercise. Fat is a key aerobic fuel for muscle cells, especially at low exercise outputs. At rest and during light activity, muscles burn primarily fat for energy needs. In comparison, little protein generally is used to fuel muscles. At most, protein supplies 10% to 15% of energy needs during endurance activities, especially when glycogen stores are depleted.

▲ Athletes often expend much energy. In such cases, their increased food intake should easily provide ample protein and other nutrients to support activity.

▶ Review Table 7-5 in Chapter 7, which listed the energy costs of typical forms of physical activity.

POWER FOOD: DIETARY ADVICE FOR ATHLETES

Athletic training and genetic makeup are two important determinants of athletic performance. A good diet won't substitute for either factor, but diet can help to enhance and maximize an athlete's potential. On the other hand, a poor diet can seriously reduce performance.

Calorie Needs

Athletes need varying amounts of calories, depending on each athlete's body size, body composition, and the type of training or competition being considered. A small person may need only 1700 kcal daily to sustain normal daily activities without losing body weight; a large, muscular man may need 4000 kcal. These rough estimates can be viewed as starting points that need to be individualized by trial and error for each athlete.

An estimate of the calories required to sustain moderate activity is 5 to 8 kcal per minute. The calories required for sports training or competition then have to be added to those used to carry on normal activities. For example, an hour of bowling requires few calories in addition to that required to sustain normal daily living. At the other extreme, a 12-hour endurance bicycle race over mountains can require an additional 4000 kcal per day. Therefore, some athletes may need as much as 7000 kcal or more daily to maintain body weight while training, whereas others may need 1700 kcal or less. If an athlete experiences daily fatigue, the first consideration should be whether he or she is consuming enough food. Up to six meals per day may be needed, including one before each workout.

How can we know if an athlete is getting enough calories? Estimating daily intake from a food diary kept by the athlete is one way. Another step is to estimate the athlete's body fat percentage via skinfold measurements, bioelectrical impedance, or underwater weighing (review Chapter 7). Body fat should be the typical amount found for athletes in the specific sport practiced. This corresponds to 5% to 18% for most male athletes and 17% to 28% for most female athletes. The next step is to monitor body weight changes on a daily or weekly basis. If body weight starts to fall, calories should be increased; if weight rises and it is because of increases in body fat, the athlete should eat less.

MAKING DECISIONS

Making Weight

Wrestlers, boxers, judoists, jockeys, and oarsmen often try to lose weight before a competition, so that they can be certified to compete in a lower weight class. This helps them gain a mechanical advantage over an opponent of smaller stature. They usually lose this weight before stepping on the scale for weight certification. Athletes can lose up to 22 pounds (10 kilograms) of body weight as water in 1 day by sitting in a sauna, exercising in a plastic sweat suit, or taking diuretic drugs, which speed water loss from the kidneys. Losing as little as 2% of body weight by dehydration, however, can adversely affect endurance and performance, especially in hot weather. A pattern of repeated weight loss or gain of more than 5% of body weight by dehydration carries risk of kidney malfunction and heat-related illness. Death is also a possibility.

To prevent future deaths from such weight loss in athletes, the National Collegiate Athletic Association and many states have authorized physicians or athletic trainers to set safe weight and body fat content minimums (e.g., 7% or more of total body weight for male athletes and 12% or more for females) in weight-class sports. Under new guidelines, athletes are assigned to weight classes at the beginning of the season and are not allowed to "cut weight" to gain a competitive advantage. Weight gain in the days after a competition (reflecting regain of body water) can now be no greater than 2 pounds. If athletes, such as wrestlers, wish to compete in a lower-bodyweight class and have enough extra fat stores, they should begin a gradual, sustained reduction in calorie intake long before the competitive season starts.

If the body composition test shows that an athlete has too much body fat, the athlete should lower food intake by about 200 to 500 kcal per day, while maintaining a regular exercise program, until the desirable fat percentage is achieved. Reducing fat intake is the best nutrient-related approach. On the other hand, if an athlete needs to gain weight, increasing food intake by 500 to 700 kcal per day will eventually lead to the needed weight gain. A mix of carbohydrate, fat, and protein is advised, coupled with exercise to make sure this gain is mostly in the form of lean tissue and not fat stores.

Carbohydrate Needs

Anyone who exercises vigorously, especially for more than 1 hour per day on a regular basis, needs to consume a diet that includes moderate to high amounts of carbohydrates. The diet should provide a variety of foods, such as those recommended by MyPyramid. Numerous servings of grains, starchy vegetables, and fruits provide enough carbohydrate to maintain adequate liver and muscle glycogen stores, especially for replacing glycogen losses from workouts on the previous day. Relatively low-carbohydrate/high-protein diets, such as *The Zone Diet*, are not recommended. Recall that Chapter 7 discussed the Zone Diet. The carbohydrate content of this diet is only 40% of calories, rather than the 60% or more typically recommended for athletes.

Carbohydrate intake should be at least 5 grams per kilogram body weight. People engaged in aerobic training and endurance activities (duration 60 minutes or more per day) may need as much as 7 grams per kilogram body weight. When exercise duration approaches several hours per day, the carbohydrate recommendation increases to up to 10 grams per kilogram of body weight. In other words, triathletes and marathoners should consider eating close to 500 to 600 grams of

▲ High-carbohydrate foods should form the basis of the diet for athletes.

carbohydrates daily, and even more if necessary, to (1) prevent chronic fatigue and (2) load the muscles and liver with glycogen. Attention to carbohydrate intake is especially important when performing multiple training bouts in a day, such as swim practices, or heavy training on successive days, as in cross-country running. Depletion of carbohydrate ranks just behind depletion of fluid and electrolytes as a major cause of fatigue. Table 12-3 shows sample menus, based on MyPyramid, for diets providing food energy ranging from 1500 to 5000 kcal per day. In addition, the Exchange System described in Appendix D is a very useful tool for planning all types of diets, including high-carbohydrate diets for athletes.

TABLE 12-3 Sample Daily Menus Based on MyPyramid That Provide Various Total Calorie Intakes

1500 kcal Diet	2000 kcal Diet	3000 kcal Diet	4000 kcal Diet	5000 kcal Diet
Breakfast Fat-free milk, 1 cup Cheerios, 1/2 cup Bagel, 1/2 Cherry jam, 2 tsp Margarine, 1 tsp	**Breakfast** Fat-free milk, 1 cup Cheerios, 1 cup Bagel, 1/2 Cherry jam, 1 tbsp Margarine, 1tsp	**Breakfast** Fat-free milk, 1 cup Cheerios, 2 cups Bagel, 1 Cherry jam, 2 tsp Margarine, 1 tsp Oat bran muffins, 2	**Breakfast** Fat-free milk, 1 cup Cheerios, 2 cups Orange, 1 Bran muffins, 2	**Breakfast** Fat-reduced milk, 1 cup Cheerios, 2 cups Bran muffins, 2 Orange, 1
			Snack Chopped dates, 3/4 cup	**Snack** Low-fat yogurt, 1 cup Chopped dates, 1 cup

Lunch
Chicken breast (roasted),
  2 oz
Figs, 1
Fat-free milk, 1/2 cup
Banana, 1
	Lunch
	Chicken breast (roasted),
	  2 oz
	Wheat bread, 2 slices
	Mayonnaise, 1 tsp
	Raisins, 1/4 cup
	Cranberry juice,
	  1 1/2 cups
	Banana, 1
		Lunch
		Chicken breast (roasted),
		  2 oz
		Wheat bread, 2 slices
		Provolone cheese, 1 oz
		Mayonnaise, 1 tsp
		Raisins, 1/3 cup
		Cranberry juice,
		  1 1/2 cups
		Low-fat fruit yogurt, 1 cup
			Lunch
			Romaine lettuce, 1 cup
			Garbanzo beans, 1 cup
			Grated carrots, 1/2 cup
			French dressing, 2 tbsp
			Macaroni and cheese,
			  3 cups
			Apple juice, 1 cup
				Lunch
				Apple juice, 1 cup
				Chicken enchilada, 1
				Romaine lettuce, 1 cup
				Garbanzo beans, 1 cup
				Shredded carrots, 3/4 cup
				Chopped celery, 1/2 cup
				Seasoned croutons, 1 oz
				French dressing, 2 tbsp
				Wheat bread, 2 slices
				Margarine, 1 tbsp

Snack Oatmeal-raisin cookie, 1 Low-fat fruit yogurt, 1 cup	**Snack** Oatmeal-raisin cookies, 3 Low-fat fruit yogurt, 1 cup	**Snack** Banana, 1 Oatmeal-raisin cookies, 3	**Snack** Wheat bread, 2 slices Margarine, 1 tsp Jam, 2 tbsp	**Snack** Banana, 1 Bagel, 1 Cream cheese, 1 tbsp

Dinner
Spaghetti w/meatballs,
  1 cup
Romaine lettuce, 1 cup
Italian dressing, 2 tsp
Green beans, 1/2 cup
Cranberry juice, 1 1/2 cups
	Dinner
	Broiled beef sirloin, 3 oz
	Romaine lettuce, 1 cup
	Italian dressing, 2 tsp
	Green beans, 1 cup
	Fat-free milk, 1/2 cup
		Dinner
		Broiled beef sirloin, 3 oz
		Romaine lettuce, 1 cup
		Garbanzo beans, 1 cup
		Italian dressing, 2 tsp
		Spinach pasta noodles,
		  1 1/2 cups
		Margarine, 1 tsp
		Green beans, 1 cup
		Fat-free milk, 1/2 cup
			Dinner
			Skinless turkey breast, 2 oz
			Mashed potatoes, 2 cups
			Peas and onions, 1 cup
			Banana, 1
			Fat-free milk, 1 cup
				Dinner
				Fat-reduced milk, 1 cup
				Beef sirloin, 5 oz
				Mashed potatoes, 2 cups
				Spinach pasta noodles,
				  1 1/2 cups
				Grated parmesan cheese,
				  2 tbsp
				Green beans, 1 cup
				Oatmeal-raisin cookies, 3

			Snack Pasta, 1 cup cooked Margarine, 2 tsp Parmesan cheese, 2 tbsp Cranberry juice, 1 cup	**Snack** Cranberry juice, 2 cups Air-popped popcorn, 4 cups Raisins, 1/3 cup
18% protein (68 grams) 64% carbohydrate (240 grams) 19% fat (32 grams)	17% protein (85 grams) 63% carbohydrate (315 grams) 20% fat (44 grams)	17% protein (128 grams) 62% carbohydrate (465 grams) 21% fat (70 grams)	14% protein (140 grams) 61% carbohydrate (610 grams) 26% fat (116 grams)	14% protein (175 grams) 63% carbohydrate (813 grams) 24% fat (136 grams)

As noted, athletes should obtain at least 60% of their total energy needs from carbo-hydrate (rather than the 50% typical of most North American diets), especially if exercise duration is expected to exceed 2 hours and total caloric intake is about 3000 kcal per day or less. Diets providing 4000 to 5000 kcal per day can be as low as 50% carbohydrate, as these will still provide sufficient carbohydrate (e.g., 500 to 600 grams or so per day).

One does not have to give up any specific food when planning a high-carbohydrate diet. The focus is to include more high-carbohydrate foods while moderating con-centrated fat sources. Sports nutritionists emphasize the difference between a high-carbohydrate meal and a high-carbohydrate/high-fat meal. Before endurance events, such as marathons or triathlons, some athletes seek to increase their carbohydrate reserves by eating foods such as potato chips, French fries, banana cream pie, and pastries. Although such foods provide carbohydrate, they also contain a lot of fat. Better high-carbohydrate food choices include pasta, rice, potatoes, bread, fruit and fruit juices, and many breakfast cereals (check the label for carbohydrate content)

CRITICAL THINKING

Joe is a wrestler who qualified for the 125-pound weight classification in the an-nual state high school competition. After a few matches, Joe began to feel dizzy and faint. He was disqualified because he was unable to continue the match. Later, the coach found out that Joe had spent 2 hours in the sauna before weighing in, which had made him dehydrated. What are the consequences of dehydration? What can you suggest as a safer alterna-tive for weight loss?

TABLE 12-4 Grams of Carbohydrate Based on Serving Size of Typical Carbohydrate-Rich Foods

Starches—15 grams Carbohydrate per Serving (80 kcal)

One Serving

dry breakfast cereal*, 1/2–3/4 cup	baked potato, 1/4 large
cooked breakfast cereal, 1/2 cup	bagel, 1/4 (4 oz)
cooked grits, 1/2 cup	English muffin, 1/2
cooked rice, 1/3 cup	bread, 1 slice
cooked pasta, 1/3 cup	pretzels, 3/4 oz
baked beans, 1/3 cup	saltine crackers, 6
cooked corn, 1/2 cup	pancake, 4 inches in diameter, 1
cooked dry beans, 1/2 cup	taco shells, 2 (add 45 kcal)

Vegetables—5 grams Carbohydrate per Serving (25 kcal)

One Serving
cooked vegetables, 1/2 cup
raw vegetables, 1 cup
vegetable juice, 1/2 cup
Examples: carrots, green beans, broccoli, cauliflower, onions, spinach, tomatoes, vegetable juice

Fruits—15 grams Carbohydrate per Serving (60 kcal)

One Serving

canned fruit or berries, 1/2 cup	grapes (small), 17
fruit juice, 1/2 cup	grapefruit, 1/2
figs (dried), 1 1/2	dates, 3
apple or orange, 1 small	peach, 1
apricots (dried), 8	watermelon cubes, 1 1/4 cups
banana, 1 small	

Milk—12 grams Carbohydrate per Serving

One Serving   soymilk, 1 cup
milk, 1 cup
plain low-fat yogurt, 2/3 cup

Sweets—15 grams Carbohydrate per Serving (variable calories)

One Serving

cake, 2-inch square	ice cream, 1/2 cup
cookies, 2 small	sherbet, 1/2 cup

*The carbohydrate content of dry cereal varies widely. Check the labels of the ones you choose and adjust the serving size accordingly.

Modified from *Exchange Lists for Meal Planning* by the American Diabetes Association and American Dietetic Association, 2003, Chicago, American Dietetic Association.

carbohydrate loading A process in which a high carbohydrate intake is consumed for 6 days before an athletic event while tapering exercise duration in an attempt to increase muscle glycogen stores.

Carbohydrate Loading May Be Beneficial for These Activities

Marathons

Long-distance swimming

Cross-country skiing

30-kilometer runs

Triathlons

Tournament-play basketball

Soccer

Cycling time trials

Long-distance canoe racing

Carbohydrate Loading Is Not Beneficial for These Activities

American football games

10-kilometer or shorter runs

Walking and hiking

Most swimming events

Single basketball games

Weightlifting

Most track and field events

▲ Carbohydrate loading is appropriate only for endurance activities such as a long-distance race.

(Table 12-4). Sports drinks appropriate for carbohydrate loading, such as GatorLode and UltraFuel, can also help. Consuming a moderate rather than a high amount of fiber during the final day of training is a good precaution to reduce the chances of bloating and intestinal gas during the next day's event.

Carbohydrate Loading

For athletes who compete in continuous, intense aerobic events lasting more than 60 to 90 minutes (or in shorter events taking place more than once within a 24-hour period), a **carbohydrate-loading** regimen can help to maximize the amount of energy stored in the form of muscle glycogen for the event. (However, this amount of activity applies to few athletes.) In one possible regimen, during the week prior to the event, the athlete gradually reduces the intensity and duration of exercise ("tapering") while simultaneously increasing the percentage of total calories supplied by carbohydrate.

For example, consider the carbohydrate-loading schedule of a 25-year-old man preparing for a marathon. His typical calorie needs are about 3500 kcal per day. Six days before competition, he completes a final hard workout of 60 minutes. On that day, carbohydrates contribute 45% to 50% of his total calorie intake. As he goes through the rest of the week, the duration of his workouts decreases to 40 minutes, and then to about 20 minutes by the end of the week. Meanwhile, he increases the amount of carbohydrate in his diet to reach 70% to 80% of total calorie intake as the week continues. Total calorie intake should decrease as exercise time decreases throughout the week. On the final day before competition, he rests while maintaining the high-carbohydrate intake.

Carbohydrate Loading Regimen

Days Before Competition	6	5	4	3	2	1
Exercise time (minutes)	60	40	40	20	20	Rest
Carbohydrate (grams)	450	450	450	600	600	600

This carbohydrate-loading technique usually increases muscle glycogen stores by 50% to 85% over typical conditions (that is, when dietary carbohydrate constitutes only about 50% of total calorie intake).

A potential disadvantage of carbohydrate loading is that additional water (about 3 grams) is incorporated into the muscles along with each gram of glycogen. Although the additional water aids in maintaining hydration, for some individuals this additional water weight and related muscle stiffness detract from their sports performance, making carbohydrate loading inappropriate. Athletes considering a carbohydrate-loading regimen should try it during training (and well before an important competition) to experience its effects on performance. They can then determine whether it is worth the effort. Also, consuming carbohydrates during a competition provides about the same advantage as carbohydrate loading prior to the event. Expert advice is shifting away from carbohydrate loading and more toward this second method, coupled with a daily diet high in carbohydrate. In addition, remember the importance of the "training effect" discussed in "Making Decisions: Training Effect" on page 434.

Fat Needs

A diet containing up to 35% of calories from fat is generally recommended for athletes. Rich sources of monounsaturated fat, such as canola oil, should be emphasized, and saturated fat and *trans* fat intake should be limited.

Protein Needs

For most athletes, typical recommendations for protein intake range from 1.0 to 1.6 grams of protein per kilogram of body weight. This is considerably higher than the RDA of 0.8 grams per kilogram body weight for nonathletes recommended by the Food and Nutrition Board for all adults, including athletes (Table 12-5).

For athletes beginning a strength-training program, some experts recommend up to 1.7 grams of protein per kilogram of body weight. That is more than twice the RDA for protein. To date, the value of such an excessive protein intake during the initial phases of strength training has not been supported by sufficient research. In addition, protein intakes above this amount result in an increased use of amino acids for energy needs; no further increase in muscle protein synthesis is seen. Recall from earlier in this chapter that phosphocreatine and carbohydrate (not extra protein) primarily fuel the body during strength-training activities. The extra protein, theoretically, is required for the synthesis of new muscle tissue brought on by the loading effect of strength training. Once the desired muscle mass is achieved, protein intake need not exceed 1.2 grams per kilogram of body weight.

▲ High-protein products, often marketed to athletes, are unnecessary. The same holds true for high-protein bars, a trend in marketing products to athletes.

Table 12-5 summarizes recommended ranges of protein intakes for various types of activity. Any athlete not specifically on a low-calorie regimen can easily meet these protein recommendations by eating a variety of foods (review Table 12-3). To illustrate, a 123-pound (53-kilogram) woman performing endurance activity can consume 64 grams of protein (53 × 1.2) during a single day by including 3 ounces of chicken (one chicken breast), 3 ounces of beef (a small, lean hamburger), and two glasses of milk in her diet. Similarly, a 180-pound (77-kilogram) man who aims to gain muscle mass through strength training needs to consume only 6 ounces of chicken (a large chicken breast), ½ cup of cooked beans, a 6-ounce can of tuna, and three glasses of milk to achieve an intake of 130 grams of protein (77 × 1.7) in a day. And, for both athletes, these calculations do not even include the protein present in grains or vegetables they will also eat. As you can see, by meeting their calorie needs, many athletes consume much more protein than is required. Despite marketing claims, protein supplements are an expensive and unnecessary part of a fitness plan.

Consuming excessive amounts of protein has drawbacks. As noted in Chapter 6, it increases calcium loss somewhat in the urine. It also leads to increased urine production, possibly compromising body hydration. It also may lead to kidney stones in people with a history of this or other kidney problems. Finally, enough carbohydrate

TABLE 12-5 Recommendations for Protein Intake Based on Kilograms Body Weight*

Activity Group	grams/kilograms	Amount for a 70-kilogram (154 lb) Person (grams)
Sedentary	0.8	56
Strength trained, maintenance	1.0–1.2	70–84
Strength trained, gain muscle mass	1.5–1.7	105–119
Moderate intensity endurance activities	1.2	84
High-intensity endurance training	1.6	112

*Calculate kilograms by dividing pounds by 2.2.

Source: Burke L, Deakin V: Clinical Sports Nutrition, McGraw-Hill, Roseville NSW2069, Australia, 2000.

▲ Weight-restricted athletes especially should make sure they are consuming enough protein as well as other essential nutrients.

► Recall from Chapter 9 that nutrients in dietary supplement should not exceed any Upper Levels set over the long term. As well, men should be cautious about any use of supplements containing iron.

► Blood doping is the injection of red blood cells, naturally containing iron, to enhance aerobic capacity. This is an illegal practice under Olympic guidelines.

 See the *Nutrition and Your Health Section: Ergogenic Aids and Athletic Performance* at the end of Chapter 12.

fuel may not be consumed on such a diet, leading to fatigue. Athletes who either feel they must significantly limit their calorie intake or are vegetarians should specifically determine how much protein they eat. They should make sure to follow a diet that provides at least 1.2 grams of protein per kilogram of body weight per day, the upper recommendation for most athletes.

Vitamin and Mineral Needs

Vitamin and mineral needs are the same or slightly higher for athletes, compared with those of sedentary adults. Athletes usually have high calorie intakes, so they tend to consume plenty of vitamins and minerals. An exception is athletes consuming low-calorie diets (about 1200 kcal or less), such as seen with some female athletes participating in events in which maintaining a low body weight is crucial. These diets may not meet B-vitamin and other micronutrient needs. Vegetarian athletes are also a concern. In these cases, consuming fortified foods, such as ready-to-eat breakfast cereals or a balanced multivitamin and mineral supplement is recommended.

Athletes' needs for antioxidants such as vitamin E and vitamin C may be somewhat greater because of the potential protection these nutrients provide; this effect could be especially important in the face of high oxygen use by muscles. The use of large doses of vitamin E and vitamin C, however, requires more study and is not currently an accepted part of the dietary guidance for athletes. Experts suggest consuming a diet containing foods rich in antioxidants, such as fruits, vegetables, whole-grain breads and cereals, and vegetable oils. In addition, there is evidence that antioxidant systems in the body increase in activity as exercise training progresses. There is also speculation that the "oxidative stress" produced during exercise might have benefits, such as for muscle adaptation to exercise, and so trying to block this process may not be advantageous.

Iron Deficiency Impairs Performance. Iron is involved in red blood cell production, oxygen transport, and energy production, so a deficiency of this mineral can noticeably detract from optimal athletic performance. The potential causes for iron deficiency in athletes vary. As in the general population, female athletes are most susceptible to low iron status due to monthly menstrual losses. Special diets followed by athletes, such as low-calorie and vegetarian (especially vegan) diets are likely to be low in iron. Distance runners should pay special attention to iron intake, because their intense workouts may lead to gastrointestinal bleeding. Another concern is *sports anemia*—which occurs because exercise causes blood plasma volume to expand, particularly at the start of a training regimen before the synthesis of red blood cells increases. This results in dilution of the blood. In this case, even if iron stores are adequate, blood iron tests may appear low.

Sports anemia is not detrimental to performance, but it is hard to differentiate between sports anemia and true anemia. If iron status is low and not replenished, iron-deficiency anemia and markedly impaired endurance performance can eventually result. Although true anemia (a depressed blood hemoglobin level) is not that common among athletes, it is a good idea, especially for adult women athletes, to have their iron status checked at the beginning of a training season and at least once during midseason and to monitor dietary iron intake.

Any blood test indicating low iron status—sports anemia or not—is cause for follow-up. For some, the use of iron supplements may be advisable. However, indiscriminate use of iron supplements is not advised because toxic effects are possible. It is important that physicians investigate the cause of the deficiency because iron deficiency can be caused by blood loss. If caught early, some serious medical conditions such as this can be treated or prevented.

Some studies have suggested that iron deficiency without anemia may also have a negative effect on physical activity and performance. Also, once depleted, iron stores can take months to replenish. For this reason, athletes must be especially careful to meet iron needs.

Calcium Intake Is Important, Especially in Women. Athletes, especially women trying to lose weight by restricting their intake of dairy products, can have marginal or low dietary intakes of calcium. This practice compromises optimal bone health. Of still greater concern are women athletes who have stopped menstruating because their arduous exercise training and low body fat content interferes with the normal secretion of reproductive hormones. Disturbing reports show that female athletes who do not menstruate regularly have spinal bones far less dense than those of both non-athletes and female athletes who menstruate regularly. This places them at increased risk for bone fractures during training and competition and osteoporosis in later life. The negative impacts of low dietary calcium intake and irregular menses in female athletes outweigh the benefits of weight-bearing exercise on bone density. This topic is discussed further in Chapter 13, with respect to the female athlete triad, and in Chapter 10, where osteoporosis was reviewed in detail.

Research has clearly documented the importance of regular menstruation to maintain bone mineral density. Studies show that a woman runner who does not menstruate regularly may also have a higher risk for the development of a **stress fracture.** Thus, female athletes whose menstrual cycles become irregular should consult a physician to determine the cause. Decreasing the amount of training or increasing energy intake and body weight often restores regular menstrual cycles. If irregular menstrual cycles persist, severe bone loss (much of which is not reversible) and osteoporosis can result. Extra calcium in the diet does not necessarily compensate for the effects of menstrual irregularities, but inadequate dietary calcium can make matters worse.

stress fracture A fracture that occurs from repeated jarring of a bone. Common sites include bones of the foot.

A FOCUS ON FLUID NEEDS

Fluid needs for an average adult are about 9 cups per day for women and 13 cups per day for men. Athletes generally need even more water to maintain the body's ability to regulate internal temperature and to keep cool. Most energy released during metabolism appears immediately as heat. Furthermore, heat production in contracting muscles can rise 15 to 20 times above that of resting muscles. Unless this heat is quickly dissipated, heat exhaustion, heat cramps, and deadly heat-stroke may ensue.

Athletes must avoid becoming dehydrated not only for the sake of athletic performance, but to prevent heat exhaustion, heat cramps, and potentially fatal heatstroke. Fluid intake during exercise, when possible, should be adequate to minimize body-weight loss; following this practice is a good idea even when sweating can go unnoticed, such as when swimming or during the winter. To replace fluids lost in sweat, regulate body temperature, and prevent dehydration and low blood sodium levels, the American College of Sports Medicine recommends appropriate fluid intake before, during, and after physical activity. Fluid and electrolyte needs vary widely, so an athlete should aim to replace the total amount of fluid lost during exercise. This can be accomplished by knowing their body's hourly sweat rate, which can be calculated from the weight lost during exercise per hour plus the fluid consumed during exercise per hour.

The recommended fluid status goal is a loss of no more than 2% of body weight during exercise, especially in hot weather. Athletes should first calculate 2% of their body weight and then by trial and error determine how much fluid they must take in to avoid losing more than this amount of weight during exercise. This determination will be most accurate if an athlete is weighed before and after a typical workout. For every 1 pound (½ kilogram) lost, 2½ to 3 cups (about 0.75 liters) of water should be consumed during exercise or immediately afterward. The fluid recommendations replace the previous recommendation of 2 cups per pound, as some of the fluid replacement will quickly be lost via increased sweating after exercise and increased urine output. Much of this fluid replacement will have to take place after exercise because it is difficult to consume enough fluid during exercise to prevent weight loss. If weight change can't be monitored, urine color is another measure of hydration status. Urine color should be no more yellow than lemonade.

▲ Dehydration, which can lead to illness and death, is a problem that must be avoided during physical activity in hot, humid environments.

▲ Fluid intake before, during, and after physical activity is important.

Thirst is a late sign of dehydration and so is not a reliable indicator of an athlete's need to replace fluid during exercise. An athlete who drinks only when thirsty is likely to take 48 hours to replenish fluid losses. After several days of training, an athlete relying on thirst as an indicator can build up a fluid debt that will impair performance. The following fluid replacement approach can meet athletes' fluid needs in most cases:

- Freely drink beverages (e.g., water, diluted fruit juice, sports drinks) during the 24-hour period before an event, even if not particularly thirsty.
- Drink 1½ to 2½ cups of fluid (400 to 600 milliliters) 2 to 3 hours before exercise. This allows time for both adequate hydration and excretion of excess fluid.
- During events lasting more than 30 minutes, consume about ½ to 1½ cups (150 to 350 milliliters) of fluid every 15 to 20 minutes throughout the exercise. Consuming more than 1 quart (1 liter) per hour can cause discomfort. On hot days, cold drinks are preferable to help cool the body. Again, the athlete should not wait until he or she feels thirsty. In many cases, athletes, especially children and teenagers, need to be reminded to do this.
- Within 4 to 6 hours after exercise, about 2½ to 3 cups of fluid should be consumed for every pound lost, as mentioned. It is also important that weight be restored before the next exercise period. Skipping fluids before or during events will almost certainly impair performance. Also, because caffeine has a dehydrating effect on the body, fluids containing it should not be part of any hydration plan before, during, or after exercise. Alcoholic beverages also have a diuretic effect.

Heat exhaustion occurs when heat stress causes loss of body fluid and then depletion of blood volume. Maintaining adequate body fluid is important. As environmental temperature rises above 95°F (35°C), virtually all body heat is lost through the evaporation of sweat from the skin. Sweat rates during prolonged exercise range from 3 to 8 cups (750 to 2000 milliliters) per hour. However, as the humidity rises, especially above 75%, evaporation slows and sweating becomes an inefficient way to cool the body. The result is rapid fatigue, increased work for the heart, and difficulty with prolonged exertion. Clearly, the combination of high heat and humidity (e.g., 95°F and 90% humidity) can be as dangerous as extreme cold.

Increased body temperature associated with dehydration is evident when the amount of water loss exceeds only 2% of body weight, especially in hot weather. This dehydration then leads to a decline in endurance, strength, and overall performance. Wearing football equipment in hot weather can lead to a loss of 2% of body weight in 30 minutes. Marathon runners have been shown to lose 6% to 10% of body weight during a race.

Common symptoms of heat exhaustion include profuse sweating, headache, dizziness, nausea, vomiting, muscle weakness, visual disturbances, and flushing of the skin. A person with heat exhaustion should be taken to a cool environment immediately, and excess clothing should be removed. The body should be sponged with tap water. Fluid replacement, as tolerated, then should suffice to correct the condition.

Heat cramps are a frequent complication of heat exhaustion, but they may appear without other symptoms of dehydration. Cramps usually occur in individuals who have exercised for several hours in a hot climate, experienced significant sweating, and have consumed a large volume of water without replacing sodium losses. It is important not to confuse heat cramps with other forms of muscle cramps, such as those caused by GI tract upset. Heat cramps occur in skeletal muscles, including those of the abdomen and extremities. They consist of a contraction lasting 1 to 3 minutes at a time. The cramp moves down the muscle and is associated with excruciating pain. The best way to prevent heat cramps is to exercise moderately at first and to have adequate salt intake before engaging in long, strenuous activity in the heat, and not become dehydrated.

Heatstroke can occur when the internal body temperature reaches 104°F or more. Related symptoms include nausea, confusion, irritability, poor coordination, seizures, and coma. Exertional heatstroke results from high blood flow to exercising muscles, which overloads the body's cooling capacity. Sweating generally ceases, and the body temperature may become dangerously high. If left untreated, circulatory collapse, ner-

heat exhaustion The first stage of heat-related illness that occurs because of depletion of blood volume from fluid loss by the body. This increases body temperature and can lead to headache, dizziness, muscle weakness, and visual disturbances, among other effects.

heat cramps A frequent complication of heat exhaustion. They usually occur in people who have experienced large sweat losses from exercising for several hours in a hot climate and have consumed a large volume of water. The cramps occur in skeletal muscles and consist of contractions for 1 to 3 minutes at a time.

heatstroke Heatstroke can occur when internal body temperature reaches 104°F. Sweating generally ceases if left untreated, and blood circulation is greatly reduced. Nervous system damage may ensue, and death is likely. Often the skin of individuals who suffer heatstroke is hot and dry.

vous system damage, and death are likely. The death rate from heatstroke is high, approximately 10%. Typically three to five athletes die each year of heatstroke. In 2001, both college and professional football players died this way.

Many individuals faint during heatstroke, and their skin becomes hot and dry. Cooling the skin with ice packs or cold water is the usual recommended immediate treatment until medical help can be summoned. To decrease the risk of developing heatstroke, athletes should watch for rapid body-weight changes (2% or more of body weight), replace lost fluids, and avoid exercising under extremely hot, humid conditions.

Sports Drinks

A question that often arises is whether to drink water or a sports-type carbohydrate-electrolyte drink (e.g., All Sport, Exceed Energy Drink, Gatorade, PowerAde, and Amino Force) during competition (Fig. 12-6). For sports that require less than 60 minutes of exertion or when total weight loss is less than 5 to 6 pounds, the primary concern is replacing the water lost in sweat, because losses of carbohydrate stores and electrolytes (sodium, chloride, potassium, and other minerals) are not usually very great. Although electrolytes are lost in sweat, the quantities lost in exercise of brief to moderate duration can be easily replaced later by consuming normal foods, such as orange juice, potatoes, and tomato juice. Keep in mind that sweat is about 99% water and only 1% electrolytes and other substances.

When exercise extends beyond 60 minutes, electrolyte (especially sodium) and carbohydrate replacement becomes increasingly important. Use of sports drinks during these longer bouts of exercise—even more so in hot weather—offers several distinct advantages over water alone.

Water by itself, as you have learned, increases blood volume to allow for efficient cooling and transport of fuels and waste products to and from cells. The addition of carbohydrate to a sports drink supplies glucose to muscles as they become depleted of glycogen, and thus can enhance performance when administered during endurance activities (see the later section on carbohydrate replacement). Carbohydrate also adds flavor, which encourages athletes to drink. Finally, the electrolytes in sports drinks help to maintain blood volume, enhance the absorption of water and carbohydrate from the intestine, and stimulate thirst. For these reasons, some experts prefer sports drinks over water for all athletes.

Overall, the decision to use a sports drink hinges primarily on the duration of the activity. As the projected duration of continuous activity approaches 60 minutes or longer, the advantages of the use of a sports drink over plain water clearly emerge. However, athletes should first experiment with sports drinks during practice, instead of trying them for the first time during competition.

It is also possible for some athletes to drink too much water. Endurance athletes (especially poorly trained individuals) may compete at relatively low exercise intensities for prolonged periods and therefore may not sweat as much as one might predict. Thus, water losses are not high. Drinking less fluid, choosing a sports drink containing sodium (usually in the form of sodium chloride), and not gaining weight during the activity can help prevent this problem. (A drop in blood sodium can occur in both hot and cold weather.)

FIGURE 12-6 ▶ Sports drinks for fluid and electrolyte replacement typically contain a form of simple carbohydrate plus sodium and potassium. The various sugars in this product total 14 grams per 1 cup (240 milliliters) serving. In percentage terms based on weight, the sugar content is about 6% ([14 grams sugar per serving ÷ 240 grams per serving] × 100 = 5.8%). Sports drinks typically contain about 6% to 8% sugar. This provides ample glucose and other monosaccharides to aid in fueling working muscles, and it is well tolerated. Drinks with a sugar content above 10%, such as soft drinks or fruit juices, may cause stomach distress and so are not recommended.

SPECIALIZED DIETARY ADVICE FOR BEFORE, DURING, AND AFTER ENDURANCE EXERCISE

A light meal supplying up to 1000 kcal should be eaten about 2 to 4 hours before an endurance event to top off muscle and liver glycogen stores, prevent hunger during the event, and provide extra fluid. The longer the period before an event, the larger the meal can be, because there will be more time available for digestion. A pre-event meal should consist primarily of carbohydrate (about 200 grams), have little fat or

General Guide for Approximate Pre-event Carbohydrate Intake

Hours Before	Grams per kilogram Body Weight	For a 70-kilogram Person
1	1	70
2	2	140
3	3	210
4	4	280

fiber, and include a moderate amount of protein (Table 12-6). A meal eaten 1 hour or so before an event should be blended or liquid to promote rapid stomach emptying. Examples are low-fat smoothies, juices, and sports drinks.

Good food choices for a pre-event meal include spaghetti, muffins, bagels, pancakes with fresh fruit topping, oatmeal with fruit, baked potato topped with yogurt or a small amount of sour cream, toasted bread with jam, bananas, apples, oranges, pears, plums, nuts, and low-sugar breakfast cereals with reduced-fat or fat-free milk. Liquid meal-replacement formulas, such as Carnation Instant Breakfast, also can be used. Foods especially rich in fiber should be eaten the previous day to help empty the colon before an event, but they should not be eaten the night before or in the morning before the event. Avoid fatty or fried foods, such as sausage, bacon, sauces, and gravies.

Replenishing Fuel During Endurance Exercise

We've already established the importance of consuming adequate fluids during endurance exercise. For sporting events longer than 60 minutes, consumption of carbohydrate during activity can also improve athletic performance. This is

TABLE 12-6 Convenient Pre-event Meals

Breakfast

Cheerios, ¾ cup Reduced-fat milk, 1 cup Blueberry muffin, 1 Orange juice, 4 oz	450 kcal 92 grams (82%) carbohydrate
or	
Low-fat fruit yogurt, 1 cup Plain bagel, ½ Apple juice, 4 oz Peanut butter (for bagel), 1 tbsp	482 kcal 84 grams (68%) carbohydrate
or	
Whole-wheat toast, 1 slice Jam, 1 tsp Apple, 1 large Reduced-fat milk, 1 cup Oatmeal, ½ cup (with reduced-fat milk, ½ cup)	507 kcal 98 grams (73%) carbohydrate

Lunch or Dinner

Chili; with beans, 8 oz Baked potato with sour cream and chives Chocolate milk shake	900 kcal 150 grams (65%) carbohydrate
or	
Spaghetti noodles, 2 cups Spaghetti sauce, 1 cup Reduced-fat milk, 1½ cups Green beans, 1 cup	761 kcal 129 grams (66%) carbohydrate
or	
Orange, 1 large Reduced-fat milk, 1½ cups Chicken noodle soup, 1 cup Saltine crackers, 12 Buttered beans, 1 cup Corn, 1 cup Angel food cake, 1 slice	829 kcal 160 grams (70%) carbohydrate

With regard to the timing of pre-activity meals, a general guide is to allow 4 hours for a big meal (about 1200 kcal), 3 hours for a moderate meal (about 800 to 900 kcal), 2 hours for a light meal (about 400 to 600 kcal), and an hour or less for a snack (about 300 kcal).

because prolonged exercise depletes muscle glycogen stores and low levels of blood glucose lead to fatigue, both physical and mental. When the supply of carbohydrate calories runs low, athletes often complain of "hitting the wall," the point at which maintaining a competitive pace seems impossible. One way to overcome this obstacle is to maintain normal blood glucose concentrations by carbohydrate feedings. As mentioned, a general guideline for endurance events is to consume 30 to 60 grams of carbohydrate per hour; however, an athlete should experiment during training sessions to establish the level that leads to optimal performance.

In the previous section on fluid needs, you learned that sports drinks are a good source of carbohydrate calories during endurance events. They supply the necessary fluid, electrolytes, and carbohydrate to keep an athlete performing at his or her best. As an alternative to sports drinks, some athletes have begun to use carbohydrate gels (e.g., PowerGel and Clif Shot) and energy bars (e.g., PowerBar). Check the label on these products to gauge the amount of gel or bar that provides 30 to 60 grams of carbohydrate per hour. Gels contain about 25 grams of carbohydrate per serving, and depending on the type, popular energy bars range from 2 to 45 grams of carbohydrate per serving (Table 12-7). Sports drinks, by comparison, contain about 14 grams

▲ Carbohydrate intake during endurance exercise helps maintain this source of energy for the body.

TABLE 12-7 Calorie and Macronutrient Contents of Popular Energy Bars and Gels

Product	Energy (kcal)	Carbohydrates (g)	Fiber (g)	Protein (g)	Fat (g)
Balance Bar (chocolate)	200	22	<1	14	6
Balance CarbWell (chocolate fudge)	190	23	2	14	6
Balance Gold (rocky road)	210	22	1	15	7
Clif Bar (chocolate chip)	250	45	5	10	5
Clif Shot (vanilla)	100	25	0	0	0
Genisoy Bar (cookies & cream)	240	35	1	14	4.5
Kashi GoLean Bar (malted chocolate crisp)	290	49	6	13	6
Luna Bar (cherry-covered chocolate)	180	28	3	9	5
PowerBar Gel (strawberry banana)	110	27	0	0	0
PowerBar Performance (chocolate)	230	45	3	10	2
PowerBar Pria (French vanilla crisp)	110	17	5	5	3
PowerBar ProteinPlus (cookies & cream)	300	38	1	23	6
PowerBar Triple Threat (s'mores)	230	30	4	10	8
Snickers Marathon (multigrain crunch)	220	32	2	10	7
Zone Perfect (apple cinnamon)	210	21	1	15	7

Overall, choosing energy bars is preferable to choosing candy bars and packaged cakes. When used in sports situations, energy bars can be handy. Better yet, however, is to eat a variety of wholesome foods; these offer more health-protective compounds. This is also a less expensive choice, especially for day-to-day snacking. An additional concern is that micronutrient toxicity might occur if numerous bars are eaten in a day, as many are highly fortified. Vitamin A and iron are two nutrients of special concern in this regard.

▶ It cannot be emphasized enough that any nutrition strategies should be tested during practice and trial runs before being used in a meet or key event. An athlete should never try a new food or beverage on the day of competition. Some food items and beverages may not be well tolerated, and the day of competition is not the time to find out.

of carbohydrate per 8-oz serving. The wide range of carbohydrate content in energy bars is due to a variety of marketing trends in the sports supplement industry. Overall, choosing a bar with about 40 grams of carbohydrate and no more than 10 grams of protein, 4 grams of fat, and 5 grams of fiber is recommended. The bars are also typically fortified with vitamins and minerals, often up to 100% of the Daily Values. As such, these bars can be seen as a convenient, although somewhat expensive, source of nutrients. Caution should be exercised, however, because the highly fortified nature of these bars may also lead to nutrient toxicities such as with vitamin A, if overused.

MAKING DECISIONS

Fat for Endurance?

Why hasn't fat been mentioned as a way to improve athletic performance during an endurance event? While fat is used along with carbohydrate as fuel during prolonged aerobic activity, the processes of digestion, absorption, and metabolism of fat are relatively slow. Therefore, consumption of fat during activity is not likely to translate into better athletic performance.

If solid sources of carbohydrate are one's preference, fig cookies, Gummy Bears, and jellybeans can also yield a quick source of glucose and with a much lower cost. However, any carbohydrate-containing food, including energy bars and gels, must be accompanied by fluid to ensure adequate hydration.

MAKING DECISIONS

Energy Bars

As discussed, food manufacturers have begun to promote meal replacement bars (also called "energy" bars) to all kind of athletes. These bars typically contain about 180 to 250 kcal, with a macronutrient distribution typical of common diets. However, some bars replace much of the carbohydrate with protein. The bars are fortified with vitamins and minerals in amounts ranging from about 25% to 100% of typical human needs. Some people find these bars provide a convenient way to consume a meal (or snack) on the run, while also focusing on certain nutrients they may underconsume, such as the B vitamin folate or the mineral calcium. These bars generally cost $1 to $2. The energy and nutrient content of popular energy bars are shown in Table 12-7. Critics suggest these products are essentially the nutritional equivalent of a cup of low-fat yogurt and piece of fruit.

▲ Elite athletes such as Olympic beach volleyball gold medal winner Kerri Walsh are well aware that modifying their diet and training regimen to match the specific needs of their sport is key to optimum performance. Replenishing carbohydrate and fluids is especially important when training.

Carbohydrate Intake During Recovery from Prolonged Exercise

Carbohydrate-rich foods providing 1 to 2 grams of carbohydrate per kilogram body weight should be consumed within 2 hours after extended (endurance) exercise, and the sooner the better (Table 12-8). Immediately after exercise is when glycogen synthesis is greatest, because the muscles are insulin-sensitive at this point. This process should then be repeated over the next 2-hour interval. Athletes training hard can consume a sugar candy, sugared soft drink, fruit or fruit juice, or a sports-type carbohydrate supplement right after training as they attempt to reload their muscles with glycogen.

TABLE 12-8 Sample Postexercise Meals for Rapid Muscle Glycogen Replacement

Option 1
1 regular bagel
2 tbsp peanut butter, smooth
8 fl oz fat-free milk
1 medium banana
562 kcal, 77 grams carbohydrate, 23 grams protein, 18 grams fat

Option 2
1 packet Carnation Instant Breakfast
8 oz fat-free milk
1 medium banana
1 tbsp peanut butter
Blend until smooth
438 kcal, 70 grams carbohydrate, 17 grams protein, 10 grams fat

Option 3
1.5 cans GatorPro (11 fl oz per can)
559 kcal, 89 grams carbohydrate, 26 grams protein, 11 grams fat

▶ For more information on sports nutrition, visit the Gatorade Sport Science Institute webpage (www.gssiweb.com). For more information on sports medicine, visit www.physsportsmed.com. This homepage of *The Physician and Sportsmedicine* journal details current issues in sports medicine, including injury prevention, nutrition, and exercise. Also helpful are the webpages of the American College of Sports Medicine (www.acsm.org), Centers for Disease Control and Prevention Division of Nutrition and Physical Activity (www.cdc.gov/nccdphp/dnpa), and the American Council on Exercise (www.acefitness.org).

Later, enriched bread, mashed potatoes, and short-grain white rice can contribute to additional carbohydrate consumption. These high-glycemic-load carbohydrates especially contribute to glycogen synthesis. Recall that Table 4-4 shows the glycemic load for various foods. Adding an appropriate amount of protein (3 grams of carbohydrate: 1 gram of protein) during recovery can be especially helpful for meeting overall calorie and nutrient needs. For a 154-pound (70-kilogram) athlete, this corresponds to about 70 grams of carbohydrate and 25 grams of protein in each 2-hour interval (Table 12-8 contains sample meals of this composition). In summary, the following are key factors for achieving the most rapid replenishment of muscle glycogen after exercise: (1) availability of adequate carbohydrate, (2) ingestion of carbohydrate as soon as possible after completion of exercise, and (3) selection of high-glycemic-load carbohydrates.

Fluid and electrolyte (i.e., sodium and potassium) intake is also an essential component of an athlete's recovery diet. This helps replenish body fluids as quickly as possible. This is especially important if two workouts a day are performed or if the environment is hot and humid. If food and fluid intake is sufficient to restore weight loss, it generally will also supply enough electrolytes to meet needs during recovery from endurance activities.

CONCEPT CHECK

All athletes would do well to plan a diet following MyPyramid. High-carbohydrate foods should be emphasized, and these should dominate in pre-event meals. Protein intake above 1.7 grams per kilogram of body weight is not supported by scientific evidence. Most athletes easily consume enough protein from typical food choices. If nutrient supplements are used, dosages generally should not exceed the Upper Level set for each nutrient. Fluid should be consumed as liberally as possible before, during, and after an event. Carbohydrate and electrolytes in the fluid are especially helpful to help delay fatigue and maintain electrolyte balance when exercise duration exceeds 60 minutes.

NUTRITION AND YOUR HEALTH
Ergogenic Aids and Athletic Performance

ERGOGENIC AIDS TO ENHANCE ATHLETIC PERFORMANCE

Extreme diet manipulation to improve athletic performance is not a recent innovation. As long as 30 years ago, American football players were encouraged on hot practice days to "toughen up" for competition by liberally consuming salt tablets before and during practice and by not drinking water. Now it is widely recognized that this practice can be fatal. Today's athletes are as likely as their predecessors to experiment with artichoke hearts, bee pollen, dried adrenal glands from cattle, seaweed, freeze-dried liver flakes, gelatin, and ginseng. These are just some of the ineffective substances used by athletes in hopes of gaining an **ergogenic** (work-producing) edge.

Based on what is known at this time, today's athletes can benefit from scientific evidence documenting the ergogenic properties of a few dietary substances. These ergogenic aids include sufficient water and electrolytes, lots of carbohydrates, and a balanced and varied diet consistent with MyPyramid. Protein and amino acid supplements are not among those aids because athletes can easily meet protein needs from foods, as Table 12-3 demonstrated.

The use of nutrient supplements should be designed to meet a specific dietary shortcoming, such as an inadequate iron intake. These and other aids, which often have dubious benefits and may pose health risks, must be given close scrutiny before use. The risk-benefit ratio of any ergogenic aid merits careful evaluation.

As summarized in Table 12-9, no scientific evidence supports the effectiveness of many substances touted as performance-enhancing aids. Many are useless; some are dangerous. Athletes should be skeptical of any substance until its ergogenic effect is scientifically verified. FDA has a limited ability to regulate these dietary supplements (review Chapter 1), and the manufacturing processes for dietary supplements are not as tightly regulated by FDA as they are for prescription drugs. Some supplements may contain substances that will cause athletes to "test positive" for various banned substances. This was demonstrated in the 2002 Winter Olympics. Studies also have called into question the quality control associated with the manufacturing of dietary supplements. Many do not contain the substance and/or the amount listed on the label.

These results add yet another worry for the athlete. Not only must he or she determine whether there is evidence that a dietary supplement is safe and effective

---

MAKING DECISIONS

NCAA and Supplements

The NCAA's Committee on Competitive Safeguards and Medical Aspects of Sports has developed lists of permissible and nonpermissible supplements for athletic departments to dispense. Following are key examples:

Permissible	**Nonpermissible**
Vitamins and minerals	Amino acids
"Energy" bars (if no more than 30% protein)	Creatine
Sports drinks	Glycerol
Meal replacement drinks such as Ensure Plus or Boost	HMB
	L-carnitine
	Protein powders

---

ergogenic Work-producing. An ergogenic aid is a mechanical, nutritional, psychological, pharmacological, or physiological substance or treatment intended to directly improve exercise performance.

TABLE 12-9 An Evaluation of Current Ergogenic Aids

Substance/Practice	Rationale	Reality
Useful in Some Circumstances		
Creatine	Increase phosphocreatine (PCr) in muscles to keep ATP concentration high	Use of 20 grams per day for 5 to 6 days and then a maintenance dose of 2 grams per day may improve performance in those who undertake repeated bursts of activity, such as in sprinting and weightlifting. Vegetarian athletes benefit the most because their diets are low in or void of creatine. Some of the muscle weight gain noted with use results from water contained in muscles. Endurance athletes do not benefit from use. Little is known about the safety of long-term creatine use. Continual use of high doses has led to kidney damage in a few cases. Cost: $25 to $65 per month.
Sodium Bicarbonate (baking soda)	Counter lactic acid buildup	Partially effective in some circumstances (when lactic acid is rapidly produced), such as wrestling, but induces nausea and diarrhea. The dose used is 300 milligrams/kilogram, given 1 to 3 hours before exercise. Cost: nil.
Caffeine	Increase use of fatty acids to fuel muscles, promote mental alertness	Drinking two to three 5-ounce cups of coffee (equivalent to 3 to 9 milligrams of caffeine per kilogram of body weight) about 1 hour before events lasting about 5 minutes or longer is useful for some athletes; benefits are less apparent in those who have ample stores of glycogen, are highly trained, or habitually consume caffeine; intake of more than about 600 milligrams (six to eight cups of coffee) elicits a urine concentration illegal under NCAA rules (greater than 15 micrograms per milliliter). A possible side effect is reduced body hydration and shakiness. Cost: $0.08 per 300 milligrams.
Possibly Useful, Still Under Study		
Beta-hydroxy-beta methylbutyric acid (HMB)	Decrease protein catabolism, causing a net growth-promoting effect	Research in livestock and humans suggests that supplementation with this substance may increase muscle mass. Still, safety and effectiveness of long-term HMB use in humans is unknown. Cost: $100 per month.
Glutamine (an amino acid)	Enhance immune function, preserve lean body mass	Some preliminary studies show decreased occurrence of upper respiratory tract infections in athletes with use. It also may promote muscle growth, but long-term studies are lacking. Protein foods are a rich source of glutamine. Cost: $10 to $20 per month for 1 to 2 grams per day.
Branched-chain amino acids (BCAA) (leucine, isoleucine, valine)	Important energy source, especially when carbohydrate stores are depleted	Supplementation of BCAA (10 to 30 grams per day) during exercise can increase BCAA in the blood when it has been lowered due to exercise, but there is no consistent evidence of improved performance. Carbohydrate feeding, by delaying use of BCAA as fuel, may negate the need for BCAA supplementation. Preliminary studies show that BCAA use increases muscle mass more than does carbohydrate supplementation alone in swimmers, but there are no studies regarding resistance training. Protein-rich foods (especially dairy proteins) are also rich in BCAA. Cost: $20 per month.

TABLE 12-9 *(continued)*

Substance/Practice	Rationale	Reality
Dangerous or Illegal Substances/Practices		
Anabolic steroids (and related substances, such as androstenedione and tetrahydrogestrinone)	Increase muscle mass and strength	Although effective for increasing protein synthesis, anabolic steroids are illegal in the United States unless prescribed by a physician. They have numerous potential side effects, such as premature closure of growth plates in bones (thus possibly limiting the adult height of a teenage athlete), bloody cysts in the liver, increased risk of cardiovascular disease, increased blood pressure, and reproductive dysfunction. Possible psychological consequences include increased aggressiveness, drug dependence (addiction), withdrawal symptoms (such as depression), sleep disturbances, and mood swings (known as "roid rage"). Use of needles for injectable forms adds further health risk. Banned by the International Olympic Committee.
Growth hormone	Increase muscle mass	At critical ages, may increase height; may also cause uncontrolled growth of the heart and other internal organs and even death; potentially dangerous; requires careful monitoring by a physician. Use of needles for injections adds further health risk. Banned by the International Olympic Committee.
Blood doping	To enhance aerobic capacity by injecting red blood cells harvested previously from the athlete, or alternately the athlete may use the hormone erythropoietin (Epogen) to increase red blood cell number	May offer aerobic benefit; very serious health consequences are possible, including thickening of the blood, which puts extra strain on the heart; is an illegal practice under Olympic guidelines.
Gamma hydroxybutyric acid (GHB)	Promoted as a steroid alternative for bodybuilding	FDA has never approved it for sale as a medical product; is illegal to produce or sell GHB in the United States. GHB-related symptoms include vomiting, dizziness, tremors, and seizures. Many victims have required hospitalization, and some have died. Clandestine laboratories produced virtually all of the chemical accounting for GHB abuse. FDA is working with the U.S. Attorney's office to arrest, indict, and convict individuals responsible for the illegal operations.

Substances promoted to athletes but that have yet to show any clear ergogenic effects include pyruvic acid (pyruvate), glycerol, chromium, coenzymeQ10, ribose, medium chain triglycerides, L-carnitine, conjugated linoleic acid (CLA), bovine colostrum, insulin, and amino acids not already mentioned in this section. Any use of these products is not recommended at this time. These substances are defined in the glossary.

(FDA does not closely regulate dietary supplements), but must also question if the dietary supplement contains what it is supposed to contain.

Even substances whose ergogenic effects have been supported by systematic scientific studies should be used with caution, as the testing conditions may not match those of the intended use.

Finally, rather than waiting for a magic bullet to enhance performance, athletes are advised to concentrate their efforts on improving their training routines and sport techniques, while consuming well-balanced diets as described in this chapter.

▲ Attention to carbohydrate and fluid needs—along with meeting overall nutrient needs—is the most important ergogenic aid.

CASE STUDY

Planning a Training Diet

Michael is training for a 10K run coming up in 3 weeks. He has read a lot about sports nutrition and especially about the importance of eating a high-carbohydrate diet while in training. He also has been struggling to keep his weight in a range that he feels contributes to better speed and endurance. Consequently he is also trying to eat as little fat as possible. Unfortunately, over the past week his workouts in the afternoon have not met his expectations. His run times are slower, and he shows signs of fatigue after just 20 minutes into his training program.

His breakfast yesterday was a large bagel, a small amount of cream cheese, and orange juice. For lunch, he had a small salad with fat-free dressing, a large plate of pasta with marinara sauce and broccoli, and a diet soft drink.

For dinner, he had a small broiled chicken breast, a cup of rice, some carrots, and iced tea. Later, he snacked on fat-free pretzels.

Answer the following questions, and check your responses in Appendix A.

1. Is the high-carbohydrate diet a good idea during Michael's training?
2. Are there any important components missing in Michael's diet? Are missing components contributing to his fatigue?
3. Describe some changes that should be made in Michael's diet including some specific foods that should be included.
4. How should fluid needs be met during workouts?
5. Should Michael focus on fueling his body before, during, or after workouts?

SUMMARY

1. A gradual increase in regular physical activity is recommended for all healthy persons. A minimum plan includes 30 minutes of physical activity on most (or all) days; 60 minutes per day provides even more benefit, especially if weight control is an issue. An intense program lasting about 60 to 90 minutes should begin with warm-up exercises to increase blood flow and warm the muscles and end with cooldown exercises. Regular resistance activities and stretching add further benefits.

2. Human metabolic pathways extract chemical energy from food and transform it into ATP, the compound that provides energy for body functions.

3. In carbohydrate fuel use, glucose is broken down into the three-carbon compound pyruvic acid, yielding some ATP. This is metabolized further via the aerobic pathway to form carbon dioxide (CO_2) and water (H_2O) or via the anaerobic pathway to form lactic acid.

4. At rest, muscle cells mainly use fat for fuel. For intense exercise of short duration, muscles mostly use phosphocreatine (PCr) for energy. During more sustained intense activity, muscle glycogen breaks down to lactic acid, providing a small amount of ATP. For endurance exercise, both fat and carbohydrate are used as fuels; carbohydrate is used increasingly as activity intensifies. Little protein is used to fuel muscles.

5. Anyone who exercises regularly should consume a diet that meets calorie needs and is moderate to high in carbohydrates and fluid and adequate in other nutrients such as iron and calcium.

6. Athletes should consume enough fluid to both minimize loss of body weight and ultimately restore pre-exercise weight. Sports-drinks help replace fluid, electrolytes, and carbohydrates lost during workouts. Their use is especially appropriate when continuous activity lasts beyond 60 minutes.

7. Plenty of carbohydrates should be in the pre-event meal, especially for endurance athletes. High-glycemic-load carbohydrates should be consumed by an athlete within 2 hours after a workout to begin restoration of muscle glycogen stores. Some protein in the meal is also helpful.

STUDY QUESTIONS

1. How does greater physical fitness contribute to better overall health? Explain the process.

2. The store of ATP in muscle is rapidly depleted once muscle contraction begins. For physical activity to continue, ATP must be resupplied immediately. Describe how this occurs after initiation of exercise and at various times thereafter.

3. What is the difference between anaerobic and aerobic exercise? Explain why aerobic metabolism is increased by a regular exercise routine.

4. What is glycogen? How is it used during exercise?

5. Is fat from adipose tissue used as an energy source during exercise? If so, when?

6. What are some typical measures used to assess whether an athlete's calorie intake is adequate?

7. List five specific nutrients that athletes need and the appropriate food sources from which these nutrients can be obtained.

8. What conditions might contribute to the inability to get all required nutrients from food, thus requiring use of a multivitamin and mineral supplement?

9. What advice would you give your neighbor, planning to run a 5-kilometer (km) race, concerning fluid intake before and during the event?

10. One of your friends, a competitive athlete, asks your opinion about an amino acid supplement sold in a local sporting-goods store. She has read that such supplements can help improve athletic performance. What would you tell her about the general effectiveness of such products?

CHECK YOUR KNOWLEDGE

Answers to the following questions are in Appendix A.

1. An energy-rich compound, phosphocreatine (PCr), is found in _____ tissue.
   a. adipose
   b. muscle
   c. liver
   d. kidney

2. Carbohydrate loading is a process designed to increase
   a. fat stores.
   b. blood glucose concentrations.
   c. liver glucose levels.
   d. muscle glycogen stores.

3. During muscle-building regimes, athletes should consume _____ grams of protein per kilogram body weight.
   a. 0.5 to 0.7
   b. 0.8
   c. 1.5 to 1.7
   d. 2 to 2.5

4. Which of these foods is the best choice for carbohydrate loading before endurance events?
   a. potato chips
   b. French fries
   c. All-Bran (high-fiber) cereal
   d. rice

5. It is a good idea, especially for adult women athletes, to have blood hemoglobin checked regularly to detect for a possible deficiency of what mineral?
   a. calcium
   b. potassium
   c. copper
   d. iron

6. Additional fluid should be consumed _____ an athletic event.
   a. before
   b. during
   c. after
   d. a, b, and c.

7. How many cups of fluid are required to replace each pound of weight loss during an athletic event or workout?
   a. 0.5 to 0.75
   b. 1 to 1.5
   c. 2.5 to 3
   d. 4 to 5

8. The benefit of a "sports" drink is to provide
   a. water to hydrate.
   b. electrolytes to enhance water absorption in the intestine and maintain blood volume.
   c. carbohydrate for energy.
   d. All of the above.

9. A light meal is best eaten before participating in a sporting event.
   a. immediately
   b. 2 to 4 hours
   c. 4 to 6 hours
   d. 8 to 10 hours

10. Caffeine is used as an ergogenic aid by some athletes because it is thought to
    a. increase use of fatty acids.
    b. decrease the buildup of lactic acid.
    c. serve as an energy source.
    d. increase muscle mass and strength.

FURTHER READINGS

1. Adamidou J, Bell-Wilson J: Iron deficiency anemia and exercise. *IDEA Fitness Journal* May:82, 2006.
   This article reviews why athletes may have increased iron requirements. The best food sources to prevent iron depletion and sports anemia are also suggested.

2. Almond CSD and others: Hyponatremia among runners in the Boston Marathon. *The New England Journal of Medicine* 352:1550, 2005.
   Low blood sodium (technically called hyponatremia) is a potential problem if runners drink too much water during a prolonged race. This is especially seen in poorly trained runners in comparison to elite athletes. Any fluid replacement

needs to be carefully monitored to avoid weight gain during prolonged physical activity.

3. Bell-Wilson J, Nisevich P: Eating for endurance: Nutrition needs of power players. *Today's Dietitian* 8(3): 2006.
   Endurance athletes need fuel for their rigorous workouts. Guidelines for proper carbohydrate and fluid intake at all stages of activity—before, during, and after—are offered.

4. Casa DJ and others: American College of Sports Medicine Roundtable on Hydration and Physical Activity: Consensus Statements. *Current Sports Medicine Reports* 4:115, 2005.
   This report by an international panel of experts concludes that appropriate fluid intake before,

during, and after physical activity is important to replace fluids lost in sweat and to regulate body temperature. An athlete should aim to replace the total amount of fluid lost during exercise. This can be accomplished by knowing their body's hourly sweat rate, which can be calculated from the weight lost during exercise per hour + fluid consumed during exercise per hour.

5. Denny S: What are the guidelines for prevention of hyponatremia in individuals training for endurance sports, as well as other physically active adults? *Journal of the American Dietetic Association* 105:1323, 2005.
   To decrease the risk of hyponatremia (low blood sodium levels), experts agree that endurance athletes should replace body fluids by drinking

beverages, such as sports drinks, that contain carbohydrate and electrolytes in addition to water.

6. Dunford M: Supplements for athletes. Safe? Effective? *Today's Dietitian* p. 4, March 2005.

   The supplements that have the most support in the sports nutrition literature are creatine for weight lifters and caffeine for some aerobic sports. A number of other supplements reviewed in this article have little or no support for use, including chromium and ribose. The author recommends visiting the website www.ais.org.au/ nutrition/supplements.asp to learn more about the various supplements marketed to athletes.

7. Glazer JL: Management of heat stroke and heat exhaustion. *American Family Physician* 71:2133, 2005.

   Heat exhaustion and heat stroke are common and preventable conditions that affect athletes (and other individuals such as older adults). Treatment of heat exhaustion involves putting the person in a cool shady environment and ensuring adequate hydration. Treating heat stroke is much more complicated, as outlined in the article.

8. Harber VJ: Energy balance and reproductive function in active women. *Canadian Journal of Applied Physiology* 29:48, 2004.

   It is important for female athletes engaged in rigorous training programs to meet their calorie needs. If not, the resulting negative calorie balance will likely lead to a variety of menstrual cycle disturbances that can lead to other health problems. The article discusses this problem in detail and provides treatment strategies for problems that may develop.

9. Hew-Butler T and others: Updated fluid recommendation: Position statement from the International Marathon Medical Directors Association (IMMDA). *Clinical Journal of Sport Medicine* 16:283, 2006.

   This position statement is the result of an extensive review by the IMMDA of current scientific evidence regarding the physiological processes that regulate fluid balance in marathon runners. Studies have shown that thirst is a more dynamic cue to maintaining fluid balance than are static approaches such as estimating fluid or weight loss. To prevent dehydration due to fluid loss while exercising, the key recommendation is to drink when thirsty. Avoiding drinking when not thirsty is recommended to avoid the risk of dangerously low sodium levels caused by excessive fluids. Runners are also advised to follow their body's cues as to whether to drink plain water or sports drinks, which provide sodium and other minerals.

10. Kunstel K: Calcium requirements for the athlete. *Current Sports Medicine Reports* 4:203, 2005.

    Adequate calcium intake is needed to maintain bone health and prevent osteoporosis in all individuals.

This article points out that the increased physical activity of athletes does not necessarily require an increased intake of dietary calcium or other micronutrients. Calcium may be lost in sweat, however, so athletes are advised to replenish it by consuming a diet including calcium-rich foods or by taking a calcium supplement.

11. Laaksonen DE and others: Physical activity in the prevention of Type 2 diabetes: The Finnish Diabetes Prevention Study. *Diabetes* 54:158, 2005.

    Regular physical activity can substantially reduce the risk of developing type 2 diabetes in high risk individuals. People who increased their activity from moderate to vigorous amounts reduce their risk of developing type 2 diabetes by 65% compared to people who remained inactive. Even typical low intensity activities, such as walking, conferred similar benefits in this study.

12. Lukaski HC: Vitamin and mineral status: Affects on physical performance. *Nutrition* 20:632, 2004.

    Physically active people generally consume sufficient vitamins and minerals to support such activity. The clearest indication for use of vitamin and mineral supplements by athletes is to treat existing nutrition deficiencies or bridge gaps in nutrient intake versus nutrient needs. Use of vitamin and mineral supplements does not improve measures of performance in people consuming adequate diets.

13. McCaffree J: Managing the diabetic athlete. *Journal of the American Dietetic Association* 106(8): 2006.

    Compared to other athletes and other diabetics, the athlete with diabetes faces challenges in terms of balancing their insulin/medications, food, and exercise. This article offers advice for diabetic athletes and their health care providers on when and what to eat. In addition, the difference between type 1 and type 2 diabetes is addressed. Guidelines are also provided for specific nutrients and for hydration.

14. Powers SK and others: Dietary antioxidants and exercise. *Journal of Sports Sciences* 22:81, 2004.

    After careful review of the scientific literature, the authors could find little evidence for the effectiveness of antioxidant supplements in preventing exercise-related muscle damage. Therefore, they recommend that antioxidant supplements cannot be recommended at this time.

15. Sawka MN and others: Human water needs. *Nutrition Reviews* 63:S30, 2005.

    This review summarizes the water intake recommendations for healthy humans emphasizing that hydration is well maintained as long as food and fluid are readily available. The effect of strenuous physical exercise and heat stress on water needs is also reviewed. The review

concludes that exercise and heat can greatly increase water needs, and that the individual variability between athletes can be significant.

16. Shirreffs SM: The importance of good hydration for work and exercise performance. *Nutrition Reviews* 63:S14, 2005.

    This review summarizes the published literature on the influence of hydration status on exercise performance, especially endurance exercise performance. The review concludes that exercising in a hot environment (30°C or more) can cause dehydration by 2% of body mass or more, which impairs exercise performance and increases the possibility of suffering a heat injury. It is emphasized that heat is a significant factor. Studies have shown that some individuals can tolerate body water losses up to 2% of body mass without risk to physical well-being or endurance exercise performance when the environment is cold (for example 5°C-10°C) or temperate (for example 20°C-22°C).

17. Sinclair LM, Hinton PS: Prevalence of iron deficiency with and without anemia in recreationally active men and women. *Journal of the American Dietetic Association* 105:975, 2005.

    Both male and female athletes are at risk of exhibiting poor iron stores and even iron deficiency anemia, with females being at much higher risk. The authors recommend that athletes be screened for iron deficiency anemia, and as well have their current state of iron storage tested. Poor iron status can lead to poor work performance, and therefore should be avoided.

18. Spano M: Ergogenic aids: Fueling the sports nutrition industry. *Today's Dietitian* 8(3): 2006.

    This article reviews the trends in sports nutrition and the influence of research, consumer demand, and legislation. The industry is improving with the top companies basing new products on scientific research and with more qualified sports nutritionists positioning themselves as professionals.

19. Suedekum NA, Dimeff RJ: Iron and the athlete. *Current Sports Medicine Reports* 4:1999, 2005.

    Iron deficiency can occur in the athlete at different levels with a higher incidence in female athletes compared with males. Symptoms can range from none to severe fatigue. Iron deficiency can occur without anemia and may decrease athletic performance. This article discusses various causes of iron deficiency including poor intake, menstrual losses, gastrointestinal and genitourinary losses due to exercise-induced ischemia or organ movement, foot strike hemolysis, thermohemolysis, and sweat losses.

20. Williams MH: *Nutrition for health, fitness & sport.* 7th ed. Boston: McGraw-Hill, 2005.

    Excellent textbook for reviewing nutrient needs of athletes, as well as learning more about ergogenic aids; also provides a detailed look at metabolism in exercise.

▶ ## Check out the **Contemporary Nutrition ARIS site**

   www.mhhe.com/wardlawcontfa1 for quizzes, flash cards, other activities, and weblinks designed to further help you learn about what you eat and why.

RATE YOUR PLATE

I. Evaluating Protein Intake—A Case Study

Mark is a college student who has been lifting weights at the student recreation center. The trainer at the center recommended a protein drink to help Mark build muscle mass. Answer the following questions about Mark's current food intake and determine whether a protein drink is needed to supplement Mark's diet.

1. The following is a tally of yesterday's intake.

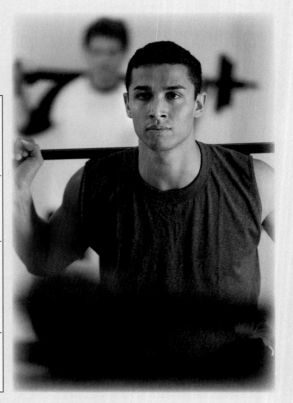

Breakfast	Frosted Mini-Wheats cereal, 2 oz 1% milk, 1½ cups Orange juice, chilled, 6 oz Glazed yeast doughnut, 1 Brewed coffee, 1 cup
Lunch	Double hamburger with condiments, 1 French fries, 30 Cola, 12 oz Medium apple, 1
Dinner	Frozen lasagna w/meat, 2 pieces 1% milk, 1 cup Looseleaf lettuce, chopped, 1 cup Creamy Italian salad dressing, 2 tsp Medium tomato, ½ Whole carrot, raw, 1
Evening snack	Vanilla ice milk, 1 cup Hot fudge chocolate topping, 2 tsp Soft chocolate chip cookies, 2

Evaluate Mark's diet using NutritionCalc Plus—is he meeting the minimum recommendations of MyPyramid?

_____

2. Mark's weight has been stable at 70 kilograms (154 pounds). Determine his protein needs based on the RDA (0.8 grams per kilogram).
   a. Mark's estimated protein RDA: _____
   b. What are the maximum recommendations for protein intake for strength-training athletes (see p. 441)? _____
   c. Calculate the maximum protein recommendation for Mark. _____

   _____

3. An analysis of the total calorie and protein content of Mark's current diet is 3470 kcal, 125 grams of protein (14% of total calories supplied by protein). This diet is representative of the food choices and amounts of food that Mark chooses on a regular basis.
   a. What is the difference between Mark's estimated protein needs as an athlete (from number 2) and the amount of protein that his current diet provides? _____
   b. Is his current protein intake inadequate, adequate, or excessive? _____

4. Mark takes his trainer's advice and goes to the supermarket to purchase a protein drink to add to his diet. Four products are available; they contain the following label information.

	Amino Fuel	Joe Weider's Sugar-Free 90% Plus Protein	Joe Weider's Dynamic Muscle Builder	Victory Super Mega Mass 2000
Serving size	3 tbsp	3 tbsp	3 tbsp	¼ scoop
Kcal	104	110	103	104
Protein (grams)	15	24	10	5

The trainer recommends adding the supplement to Mark's diet two times a day. Mark chooses the Muscle Builder protein drink.

a. How much protein would be added to Mark's diet daily from two servings of the supplement alone (prior to mixing it with a beverage)?

b. Mark mixes the powder with the milk he already consumes at breakfast and dinner. How much protein total would Mark now consume in 1 day? (Add the protein amount from the nutrition analysis to the value from question 4a.)

c. What is the difference between Mark's estimated protein needs as an athlete and this total value?

5. What is your conclusion—does Mark need the protein supplement?

Answers to Calculations

2a. Mark's estimated protein RDA: 70 kilograms × 0.8 grams per kilogram = 56 grams.
2b. Maximum recommendation for protein intake for athletes = 1.8 grams per kilogram.
2c. Applied to Mark: 1.8 × 70 = 126 grams.
3a. Difference between Mark's estimated maximum protein needs if an athlete and the amount of protein provided by his current diet: 126 − 125 = 1 gram protein.
3b. Mark's current diet is adequate.
4a. Two servings of protein supplement alone = 20 grams of protein.
4b. Mark's total protein consumption: 125 grams + 20 grams = 145 grams protein.
4c. Difference between Mark's estimated maximum protein needs as an athlete and total value (from above): 145 grams − 126 grams = 19 grams protein.

457

II. How Physically Fit Are You?

The fitness assessments presented here are easy to do and require little equipment. Also included are charts to compare your results to those typical of your peers.

Cardiovascular Fitness: One-Mile Walk

Measure a mile on a running track (usually four laps) or on a little-trafficked neighborhood street (use a car's odometer to get the right distance). With a stopwatch or watch with a second hand, walk the mile as fast as you can. Note the time it took.

Strength: Push-Ups

Men: Get up on your toes and hands. Keep your back straight, with hands flat on the floor directly below your shoulders.
Women: Same position, but you can support your body on your knees if necessary.
   Lower your body, bending your elbows, until your chin grazes the floor. Push back up until your arms are straight. Continue until you can't do any more push-ups (you can rest when in the up position).

Strength: Curl-Ups

Lie on the floor on your back with your knees bent, feet flat. Your hands should rest on your thighs. Now squeeze your stomach muscles, push your back flat, and raise your upper body high enough for your hands to touch the tops of your knees. Don't pull with your neck or head, and keep your lower back on the floor. Count how many curl-ups you can do in one minute.

Flexibility: Sit-and-Reach

Place a yardstick on the floor and apply a two-foot piece of tape on the floor perpendicular to the yardstick, crossing at the 15-inch mark. Sit on the floor with your legs extended and the soles of your feet touching the tape at the 15-inch mark, the zero-inch facing you. Your feet should be about 12 inches apart. Put one hand on the other, exhale, and very slowly reach forward as far as you can along the yardstick, lowering your head between your arms. Don't bounce! Note the farthest inch mark you reach. Don't hurt yourself by reaching farther than your body wants to. Relax, and then repeat two more times.
   Now check your results. Want to improve? You know the answer:

- Do aerobic exercise that makes you breathe hard for at least half an hour on almost or all days of the week.
- Lift weights that challenge you two to three times per week.
- Stretch after activity at least a couple of times per week.
- Walk more.

Cardiovascular: One-Mile Walk (time, in minutes)

| | Under 40 | | Over 40 | |
	Men	Women	Men	Women
Excellent	13:00 or less	13:30 or less	14:00 or less	14:30 or less
Good	13:01–15:30	13:31–16:00	14:01–16:30	14:31–17:00
Average	15:31–18:00	16:01–18:30	16:31–19:00	17:01–19:30
Below average	18:01–19:30	18:31–20:00	19:01–21:30	19:31–22:00
Poor	19:31 or more	20:01 or more	21:31 or more	22:01 or more

Source: Copper Institute

Strength: Push-Ups (number completed without rest)

	Age	17–19	20–29	30–39	40–49	50–59	60–65
Men							
Excellent		>56	>47	>41	>34	>31	>30
Good		47–56	39–47	34–41	28–34	25–31	24–30
Above average		35–46	30–39	25–33	21–28	18–24	17–23
Average		19–34	17–29	13–24	11–20	9–17	6–16
Below average		11–18	10–16	8–12	6–10	5–8	3–5
Poor		4–10	4–9	2–7	1–5	1–4	1–2
Very poor		<4	<4	<2	0	0	0

	Age	17–19	20–29	30–39	40–49	50–59	60–65
Women							
Excellent		>35	>36	>37	>31	>25	>23
Good		27–35	30–36	30–37	25–31	21–25	19–23
Above average		21–27	23–29	22–30	18–24	15–20	13–18
Average		11–20	12–22	10–21	8–17	7–14	5–12
Below average		6–10	7–11	5–9	4–7	3–6	2–4
Poor		2–5	2–6	1–4	1–3	1–2	1
Very poor		0–1	0–1	0	0	0	0

Source: Golding LA: *YMCA Fitness Testing and Assessment Manual.* YMCA of the USA, 4th ed, 2000. topendsports.com

Strength: Curl-Ups (number completed in 60 seconds)

	Men					
Age	**18–25**	**26–35**	**36–45**	**46–55**	**56–65**	**65+**
Excellent	>49	>45	>41	>35	>31	>28
Good	44–49	40–45	35–41	29–35	25–31	22–28
Above average	39–43	35–39	30–34	25–28	21–24	19–21
Average	35–38	31–34	27–29	22–24	17–20	15–18
Below average	31–34	29–30	23–26	18–21	13–16	11–14
Poor	25–30	22–28	17–22	13–17	9–12	7–10
Very poor	<25	<22	<17	<13	<9	<7

	Women					
Age	**18–25**	**26–35**	**36–45**	**46–55**	**56–65**	**65+**
Excellent	>43	>39	>33	>27	>24	>23
Good	37–43	33–39	27–33	22–27	18–24	17–23
Above average	33–36	29–32	23–26	18–21	13–17	14–16
Average	29–32	25–28	19–22	14–17	10–12	11–13
Below average	25–28	21–24	15–18	10–13	7–9	5–10
Poor	18–24	13–20	7–14	5–9	3–6	2–4
Very poor	<18	<13	<7	<5	<3	<2

Source: Golding LA: *YMCA Fitness Testing and Assessment Manual*. YMCA of the USA, 4th ed, 2000.

Flexibility: Sit-and-Reach (in inches)

	Men	Women	
Super	>+27	>+30	
Excellent	+17–+27	+21–+30	
Good	+6–+16	+11–+20	
Average	0–+5	+1–+10	
Fair	−8−−1	−7–0	
Poor	−19−−9	−14−−8	
Very poor	<−20	<−15	

Source: Golding LA: *YMCA Fitness Testing and Assessment Manual*. YMCA of the USA, 4th ed, 2000.

These charts are typical charts used by health and fitness experts. For a more thorough assessment of fitness or for development of an exercise plan appropriate for your fitness level, consult a certified personal trainer or other fitness professional.

CHAPTER 13 Eating Disorders:
Anorexia Nervosa, Bulimia Nervosa, and Other Conditions

CHAPTER OBJECTIVES Chapter 13 is designed to allow you to:

1. Contrast healthy attitudes toward uses of food with behavior patterns that could lead to unhealthy uses of food.

2. Outline the causes of, effects of, typical persons affected by, and treatment for anorexia nervosa.

3. Outline the causes of, effects of, typical persons affected by, and treatment for bulimia nervosa.

4. Describe still other forms of eating disorders: binge-eating disorder, night eating syndrome, and the female athlete triad.

5. Relate the presence of eating disorders to current social trends.

6. Describe methods to reduce the development of eating disorders, including the use of warning signs to identify early cases.

CHAPTER OUTLINE

MANY OF US OCCASIONALLY EAT UNTIL WE'RE STUFFED AND UNCOMFORTABLE, SUCH AS AT THANKSGIVING DINNER. Faced with savory and tempting foods, we find that we can't easily stop eating. Usually we forgive ourselves, vowing not to overeat the next time. Nevertheless, many of us have problems controlling our food intake and body weight. Although progressive weight gain can eventually lead to medical problems, it is usually associated with simple overeating, coupled with too little physical activity.

Actually, obesity, now considered a chronic disease, is the most common eating disorder in our society; however, the eating disorders explored in Chapter 13 involve much more severe distortions of the eating process. The eating disorders discussed here are just as serious, if not more, than obesity, and can develop into life-threatening conditions if left untreated. What's most alarming about these disorders—anorexia nervosa, bulimia nervosa, binge-eating disorder, and the female athlete triad—is the increasing number of cases reported each year.

Some people are more susceptible to these eating disorders than other people are—for genetic, psychological, and physical reasons. Successful treatment of eating disorders, therefore, is complex and must go beyond nutritional therapy. And keep in mind that eating disorders are not restricted to any socio-economic class or ethnicity. They can also strike, as suggested in the comic in this chapter, at any age in both females and males. Let's examine the causes and treatments of these conditions in detail, because these eating disorders touch many of our lives.

 Refresh Your Memory

As you begin your study of eating disorders, such as anorexia nervosa and bulimia nervosa, in Chapter 13, you may want to review:

- The effects of neurotransmitters on food intake in Chapter 1
- The role of genetic risk in disease susceptibility in Chapter 3
- Calculation of BMI in Chapter 7
- The effects and treatment of osteoporosis in Chapter 10
- The effects and treatment of iron-deficiency anemia in Chapter 11

FROM ORDERED TO DISORDERED EATING HABITS

Eating—a completely instinctive behavior for animals—serves an extraordinary number of psychological, social, and cultural purposes for humans. Eating practices may take on religious meanings; signify bonds within families and ethnic groups; and provide a means to express hostility, affection, prestige, or class values. Within the family, supplying, preparing, and distributing food may be a means of expressing love, hatred, or even power.

We are bombarded daily with images of our society's portrayal of the "ideal" body. Dieting is promoted to achieve this ideal body—eternally young and admired. Television programs, billboard advertisements, magazine pictures, movies, and newspapers suggest that an ultraslim body will bring happiness, love, and ultimately, success. This fantasy notion is contradictory to the fact that much of society is becoming fatter, even

FOR BETTER OR FOR WORSE

Concern with body image often starts early in life. Why do you think this is so? What societal trends have fostered this concern? Are some people more vulnerable, based on genetics and environment? Chapter 13 provides some answers.

obese. In response to this social pressure, some of us take an extreme approach—the pathological pursuit of weight control or weight loss.

Early in life, we develop images of "acceptable" and "unacceptable" body types. Of the attributes that constitute attractiveness, many people view body weight as the most important, partly because we can control our weight somewhat. Fatness is the most dreaded deviation from our cultural ideals of body image, the one most derided and shunned, even among schoolchildren.

It is difficult to resist comparing ourselves to the "ideal" body. Not everyone can look like a fashion model. People who are overly impressed by these messages, especially those with genetic, psychological, and physical influences, may be more likely than others to develop eating disorders in an effort to close the gap between reality and the perceived ideal.

Given the multiple functions associated with normal eating and the media bombardment with the ideal body image, it is not surprising that some people progress from typical responses to hunger and satiety cues to obsessive weight-loss behaviors, and then to a full-blown eating disorder.

Food: More than Just a Source of Nutrients

From birth, we link food with personal and emotional experiences. As infants, we associate milk with security and warmth so the breast or bottle becomes a source of comfort as well as food. As noted in Chapter 1, even when older, most people continue to derive comfort and great pleasure from food. This is both a biological and a psychological phenomenon. Food can be a symbol of comfort, but eating can also stimulate the release of certain neurotransmitters (e.g., serotonin) and *natural opioids* (including **endorphins**), which produce a sense of calm and euphoria in the human body. Thus, in times of great stress, some people turn to food for a druglike, calming effect.

Food is also used as a reward or a bribe. Haven't you heard or spoken something similar to the following comments?

You can have your dessert if you eat five more bites of your vegetables.
You can't play until you clean your plate.
I'll eat the broccoli if you let me watch TV.
If you love me, you'll eat your dinner.

On the surface, using food as a reward or bribe seems harmless enough. Eventually, however, this practice encourages both caregivers and children to use food to achieve goals other than satisfying hunger and nutrient needs. Food may then become much more than a source of nutrients. Regularly using food as a bargaining chip can contribute to abnormal eating patterns. Carried to the extreme, these patterns can lead to **disordered eating.**

Disordered eating can be defined as mild and short-term changes in eating patterns that occur in response to a stressful event, an illness, or even a desire to modify the diet for a variety of health and personal appearance reasons. The problem may be no more than a bad habit, a style of eating adapted from friends or family members, or an aspect of preparing for athletic competition. While disordered eating can lead to weight loss or weight gain, as well as certain nutritional problems, it rarely requires in-depth professional attention. If, however, disordered eating becomes sustained, distressing, or starts to interfere with everyday activities and linked to physiological changes, it may require professional intervention.

Overview of Anorexia Nervosa and Bulimia Nervosa

Given the common practice of dieting in North America, it can sometimes be difficult to tell where disordered eating stops and an **eating disorder** begins. Indeed, many eating disorders start with a simple diet. Eating disorders then go on to involve physiological changes associated with food restriction, binge eating, purging, and fluctuations in

▲ Maintaining an anorexic body type is an all too common goal in today's culture. The media and the fashion world bombard us with body images that are unrealistic for most people.

endorphins Natural body tranquilizers that may be involved in the feeding response and function in pain reduction.

disordered eating Mild and short-term changes in eating patterns that occur in relation to a stressful event, an illness, or a desire to modify one's diet for a variety of health and personal appearance reasons.

eating disorder Severe alterations in eating patterns linked to physiological changes. The alterations are associated with food restriction, binge eating, purging, and fluctuations in weight. They also involve a number of emotional and cognitive changes that affect the way a person perceives and experiences his or her body.

anorexia nervosa An eating disorder involving a psychological loss or denial of appetite, followed by self-starvation; related in part to a distorted body image and to various social pressures commonly associated with puberty.

bulimia nervosa An eating disorder in which large quantities of food are eaten at one time (binge eating) and then purged from the body by vomiting, or misuse of laxatives, diuretics, or enemas. Alternate means to counteract the binge behavior are fasting and excessive exercise.

binge-eating disorder An eating disorder characterized by recurrent binge eating and feelings of loss of control over eating that have lasted at least 6 months. Binge episodes can be triggered by frustration, anger, depression, anxiety, permission to eat forbidden foods, and excessive hunger.

weight. They also involve a number of emotional and cognitive changes that affect the way a person perceives and experiences his or her body, such as feelings of distress or extreme concern about body shape or weight. Eating disorders are not due to a failure of will or behavior; rather, they are real, treatable medical illnesses in which certain maladaptive patterns of eating take on a life of their own.

The main types of eating disorders are **anorexia nervosa** and **bulimia nervosa.** Other types, including **binge-eating disorder** and night eating syndrome, have been suggested but have not yet been approved as formal psychiatric diagnoses. More than 5 million people in North America have one of these disorders; females outnumber males 5 to 1. Eating disorders frequently (85% of the time) develop during adolescence or early adulthood but some reports indicate their onset can occur during childhood or later in adulthood. Eating disorders frequently co-occur with other psychological disorders such as depression, substance abuse, and anxiety disorders. *People who suffer from eating disorders, especially anorexia nervosa and bulimia nervosa, can experience a wide range of physical health complications, including serious heart conditions and kidney failure, which may even lead to death.* Recognition of eating disorders as important and treatable diseases, therefore, is critical.

Currently, up to 5% of women in North America develop some form of anorexia nervosa or bulimia nervosa in their lifetimes. This section provides a brief description of the characteristics and diagnoses of the two primary eating disorders that primarily afflict those of college age and younger. A detailed discussion of these and related disorders, including treatment, then follows.

Anorexia nervosa is characterized by extreme weight loss, a distorted body image, and an irrational, almost morbid, fear of obesity and weight gain. Anorexic patients irrationally believe they are fat, even though others constantly comment on their thin physique. Some anorexics realize they are thin but continue to be haunted by certain areas of their bodies that they believe to be fat (such as thighs, buttocks, and stomach).

Common to both eating disorders, *nervosa* refers to an attitude of disgust with one's body. The term *anorexia* implies a loss of appetite; however, a denial of one's appetite more accurately describes the behavior of people with anorexia nervosa. By rough estimate, approximately 1 in 200 (0.5%) adolescent girls in North America eventually develops anorexia nervosa. This high number may be due to the tendency for females to blame themselves for weight gain typical of their age group. Men only account for approximately 10% of the cases of anorexia nervosa, partly because the ideal image conveyed for men is big and muscular. Among men, athletes are most prone to develop this and other eating disorders, especially those who participate in sports that require weight classes, such as boxers, wrestlers, and jockeys. Other activities that may foster eating disorders in men include swimming, dancing, and modeling.

Bulimia nervosa (*bulimia* means "great [ox] hunger") is characterized by episodes of binge eating followed by attempts to purge the calories consumed by vomiting or misusing laxatives, diuretics, or enemas. People with this disorder may be difficult to identify because they keep their binge-purge behaviors secret, and their symptoms are not obvious. Four percent or more of adolescent and college-age women suffer from bulimia nervosa. And, as with anorexia nervosa, about 10% of the cases occur in men.

Specific criteria are used by clinicians to diagnose eating disorders (e.g., *Diagnostic and Statistical Manual of Mental Disorders* of the American Psychiatric Association). Some characteristics are listed in Table 13-1. It is possible that people exhibit some symptoms of eating disorders, but not enough to enable a medical worker to diagnose one of the two diseases. Also, as suggested in the diagnostic criteria, some people show characteristics of both anorexia nervosa and bulimia nervosa because the dis-

▲ Self-image is an important part of adolescence. For people with eating disorders, the difference between the real and desired body images may be too difficult to accept. See the website www.4women.gov/bodyimage.

Progression from Ordered to Disordered Eating

Attention to hunger and satiety signals; limitation of calorie intake to restore weight to a healthful level

↓

Some disordered eating habits begin as weight loss is attempted, such as very restricted eating

↓

Clinically evident eating disorder recognized

TABLE 13-1 Typical Characteristics of Anorexic and Bulimic Persons

Anorexia Nervosa	Bulimia Nervosa
• Rigid dieting causing dramatic weight loss, generally to less than 85% of what would be expected for one's age (or BMI of 17.5 or less) • False body perception—thinking "I'm too fat," even when extremely underweight; relentless pursuit of control • Rituals involving food, excessive exercise, and other aspects of life • Maintenance of rigid control in lifestyle; security found in control and order • Feeling of panic after a small weight gain; intense fear of gaining weight • Feelings of purity, power, and superiority through maintenance of strict discipline and self-denial • Preoccupation with food, its preparation, and observing another person eat • Helplessness in the presence of food • Lack of menstrual periods (after what should be the age of puberty) for at least 3 months • Possible presence of bingeing and purging practices	• Secretive binge eating; generally not overeating in front of others • Eating when depressed or under stress • Bingeing on a large amount of food, followed by fasting, laxative or diuretic abuse, self-induced vomiting, or excessive exercise (at least twice a week for 3 months) • Shame, embarrassment, deceit, and depression; low self-esteem and guilt (especially after a binge) • Fluctuating weight (±10 pounds or 5 kilograms) resulting from alternate bingeing and fasting • Loss of control; fear of not being able to stop eating • Perfectionism, "people pleaser"; food as the only comfort/escape in an otherwise carefully controlled and regulated life • Erosion of teeth, swollen glands • Purchase of syrup of ipecac, a compound sold in pharmacies that induces vomiting

Those who exhibit only one or a few of these characteristics may be at risk but probably do not have either disorder. They should, however, reflect on their eating habits and related concerns and take appropriate action, such as seeking a careful evaluation by a physician.

▲ Anorexia nervosa is characterized by a feeling of panic after only a small weight gain; bulimia nervosa is characterized by frequent weight fluctuations from alternate bingeing and fasting.

eases overlap considerably. About half of the women diagnosed as having anorexia nervosa eventually develop bulimic symptoms. As shown in Table 13-1, bulimic characteristics also can be seen in anorexia nervosa, which blurs the distinction. Still, appreciating the differences between the disorders helps us to understand the various approaches to prevention and treatment.

Until recently, most researchers have reported that eating disorders primarily affect middle- and upper-class Caucasian women. Now, studies show greater similarities in the rates of body dissatisfaction and disordered eating behaviors across ethnic and cultural groups. Perhaps minorities with eating disorders have been less likely to seek help in the past due to fear of shame or stigma, lack of resources, or language barriers. It seems more likely, however, that health care workers are less likely to diagnose non-Caucasians as having eating disorders. Previously, it seemed that non-Caucasian cultures were more accepting of larger body shapes, but mainstream pressures for thinness now seem to cut across racial differences. Our overall cultural change may be associated with increased vulnerability to eating disorders.

Do you know someone who is at risk of these eating disorders? If so, suggest that the person seek a professional evaluation because, the sooner treatment begins, the better the chances for recovery. However, do not try to diagnose eating disorders in your friends or family members. Only a professional can exclude other possible diseases and correctly evaluate the diagnostic criteria required to make a diagnosis of anorexia nervosa or bulimia nervosa. Once an eating disorder is diagnosed, immediate treatment is advisable. As a friend, the best you can do is to encourage an affected

▶ Our passion for thinness may have its roots in the Victorian era of the nineteenth century, which specialized in denying "unpleasant" physical realities, such as appetite and sexual desire. Flappers of the 1920s cemented the twentieth century trend for thinness. Since 1922, the BMI values of Miss America winners have steadily decreased; during the last three decades, most winners had a BMI in the "underweight" range (less than 18.5).

▲ Eating disorders are commonly seen in people who must maintain low body weight, such as ballet dancers.

▶ A person with anorexia nervosa may use the disorder to gain attention from the family, sometimes in hopes of holding the family together.

person to seek professional help. Such help is commonly available at student health centers and student guidance/counseling facilities on college campuses.

There are no simple causes of eating disorders, and there are no simple treatments. Stress may have an especially strong role in the development of eating disorders. An underlying commonality seems to be the lack of appropriate coping mechanisms as individuals begin to reach adolescence and young adulthood, coupled with dysfunctional family relationships.

A few research studies have investigated the possible link between genetic factors and the development of eating disorders. These studies have involved a comparison of identical twins with fraternal twins and the incidence of eating disorders. In general, these studies have shown that identical twins have a higher likelihood of sharing eating disorders than do fraternal twins. This indicates that genetics is a strong risk factor in development of such disorders, because identical twins share the same DNA. One study found genetic background to describe 50% of the overall risk of developing anorexia nervosa. Identifying genes that cause eating disorders eventually could help in tailoring prevention efforts to those who are at risk, but affected individuals would still need the same counseling that is part of therapy today.

A CLOSER LOOK AT ANOREXIA NERVOSA

Anorexia nervosa evolves from a dangerous mental state to an often life-threatening physical condition. As first described in the early medical literature in 1689, people suffering from this disorder think they are fat and intensely fear obesity and weight gain. They lose much more weight than is healthful. Although food is entwined in this disease, it stems more from psychological conflict.

About 10% of people with anorexia nervosa eventually die from the disease—from suicide, heart ailments, and infections. About one quarter of those with anorexia nervosa recover within 6 years, whereas the rest simply exist with the disease or go on to develop another form of eating disorder. The longer someone suffers from this eating disorder, the poorer the chances for complete recovery. A young patient with a brief episode and a cooperative family has a better outlook than those without these factors. Overall, prompt and vigorous treatment with close follow-up improves the chances for success.

Anorexia nervosa may begin as a simple attempt to lose weight. A comment from a well-meaning friend, relative, or coach suggesting that the person seems to be gaining weight or is too fat may be all that is needed. The stress of having to maintain a certain weight to look attractive or competent on a job can also lead to disordered eating. Physical changes associated with puberty, the stress of leaving childhood, or the loss of a friend may serve as another trigger for extreme dieting. Leaving home for boarding school or college or starting a job can reinforce the desire to appear more "socially acceptable." Still, looking "good" does not necessarily help people deal with anger, depression, low self-esteem, or past experiences with sexual abuse. If these issues are behind the disorder and are not resolved as weight is lost, the individual may intensify efforts to lose weight "to look even better," rather than work through unresolved psychological concerns.

During adolescence, a period of turbulent sexual and social tensions, teenagers seek—and are often expected—to establish separate and independent lives. While declaring independence, they seek acceptance and support from peers and parents and react intensely to how they think others perceive them. At the same time, their bodies are changing, and much of the change is beyond their control. In response to the adolescent's or teenager's lack of control and coping mechanisms, dieting may start and then lead to a failure to gain appropriate weight-for-height. This may not be readily identified as a problem because the child has not actually lost any weight. Stunting (failure to grow in height) may also occur if inadequate calories are ingested during a period of growth. If anorexia develops before puberty, sexual maturation and menstruation also may be delayed.

Teens with chronic illnesses, such as type 1 diabetes or asthma, are at even greater risk for disordered eating. Any evidence of poor weight gain/maintenance or excessive exercise among these individuals needs to be investigated as a possible sign of disordered eating.

Extreme dieting is the most important predictor of an eating disorder. (Adolescents expressing concern about their weight should be advised to focus on exercise, which does not appear to impart a risk for subsequent problems.) Once dieting begins, a person developing anorexia nervosa does not stop. The result is a long period of rigidly self-enforced semistarvation, practiced almost with a vengeance, in a relentless pursuit of control. Anorexia nervosa may eventually lead to bingeing on large amounts of food in a short time, then purging. Purging occurs primarily through vomiting, but laxatives, diuretics, and enemas are also used. Thus, a person with anorexia nervosa may exist in a state of semistarvation or may alternate periods of starvation with periods of bingeing and purging.

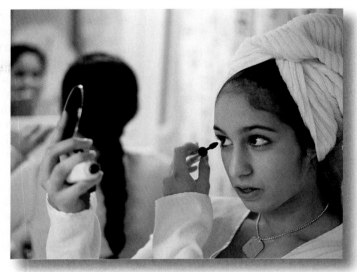

▲ Concern over appearance begins early in life; a focus on a healthful outlook with regard to body weight should also begin at this time.

Profile of the Typical Person with Anorexia Nervosa

A person with anorexia nervosa refuses to eat enough food to maintain an acceptable weight. This refusal is a hallmark of the disease, whether or not other practices, such as binge-purge cycles, appear. The most typical anorexic person is a Caucasian female from the middle or upper socioeconomic class. Perhaps her mother also has distorted views of desirable body shape and acceptable food habits. The girl is often described by parents and teachers as responsible, meticulous, and obedient.

She is competitive and often obsessive. Her parents set high standards for her. At home, she may not allow clutter in her bedroom. Physicians note that, after a physical examination, she may fold her examination gown very carefully and clean up the examination room before leaving. Even though such behavior may seem odd, only a skilled professional can tell the difference between anorexia nervosa and other adolescent complaints, such as delayed puberty, fatigue, and depression.

A common thread underlying many—but not all—cases of anorexia nervosa is conflict within the family structure, typically with an overbearing mother and an emotionally absent father. When family expectations are always too high—including those regarding body weight—frustration results and leads to fighting. Overinvolvement, rigidity, overprotection, and denial are typical daily transactions of such families.

Issues of control are central to the development of anorexia nervosa. Often, the eating disorder allows an anorexic person to exercise control over an otherwise powerless existence. Losing weight may be the first independent success the person has had. People with anorexia evaluate their self-worth almost entirely in terms of self-control. Some sexually abused children develop anorexia nervosa, believing that if they control their appetite for food, sexual relations, and human contact, they will feel in control and competent and will eliminate shameful feelings. Moreover, food restriction, which arrests development and shuts down sexual impulses, may be a strategy to prevent future victimization and guilt feelings. Often anorexic persons feel hopeless about human relationships and socially isolated because of their dysfunctional families. They focus on food, eating, and weight instead of human relationships.

▶ By severely limiting calorie intake for long periods, adolescent girls and young adult women greatly compromise their nutritional status, impair their reproductive systems, and restrict growth. The harm produced by milder, shorter periods of diet restriction is not clear. Evidence, however, suggests that even moderate diet restriction, if continued, contributes to the risks for various forms of anemia, future pregnancy complications and delivery of low-birth-weight infants, and permanently reduced bone mass.

Early Warning Signs

A person developing anorexia nervosa exhibits important warning signs. At first, dieting becomes the life focus. The person may think, "The only thing I am good at is dieting. I can't do anything else." This innocent beginning often leads to very abnormal self-perceptions and eating habits, such as cutting a pea in half before eating it. Other habits

▲ Anorexia nervosa occurs much more frequently in young women than in young men.

▶ Parents may not consider a teenager mature enough to make decisions. If the teen disagrees and the situation is very tense, she may turn to purging or starving as a way to show her power: "You may try to control my life, but I can do anything I want with my body."

In the words of one young woman, "I couldn't get angry, because it would be like destroying someone else, like my mother. It felt like she would hate me forever. I got angry through anorexia nervosa. It was my last hope. It's my own body and this was my last-ditch effort."

CRITICAL THINKING

Jennifer is an attractive 13-year-old. However, she's very compulsive. Everything has to be perfect—her hair, her clothes, even her room. Her body is beginning to mature, so she's obsessed with having perfect physical features as well. Her parents are worried about her behavior. The school counselor told them to look for certain signs that could indicate an eating disorder. What might those signs be?

include hiding and storing food and or spreading food around a plate to make it look as if much has been eaten. An anorexic person may cook a large meal and watch others eat it while refusing to eat anything. Anorexic persons may also exercise compulsively to the point that it is obsessive and driven. Exercise can interfere with life activities or occur at unusual times or settings—for example, doing squats while brushing teeth.

As the disorder progresses, the range of foods may narrow and be rigidly divided into safe and unsafe ones, with the list of safe foods becoming progressively shorter. For people developing anorexia nervosa, these practices say "I am in control." These people may be hungry, but they deny it, driven by the belief that good things will happen by just becoming thin enough. It becomes a question of willpower.

People with anorexia become irritable and hostile and begin to withdraw from family and friends. School performance generally crumbles. They refuse to eat out with family and friends, thinking, "I won't be able to have the foods I want to eat," or "I won't be able to throw up afterward."

Anorexic persons see themselves as rational and others as irrational. They also tend to be excessively critical of themselves and others. Nothing is good enough. Because it cannot be perfect, life appears meaningless and hopeless. A sense of joylessness pervades everything.

As stress increases in the person's life, sleep disturbances and depression are common. Many of the psychological and physical problems associated with anorexia nervosa arise from insufficient calorie intake, as well as deficiencies of nutrients, such as thiamin and vitamin B-6. For a female, the combination of problems—coupled with lower and lower body weight and fat stores—causes menstrual periods to cease. This may be the first sign of the disease that a parent notices and represents an additional hallmark of the disease.

Ultimately, an anorexic person eats very little food; 300 to 600 kcal daily is not unusual. In place of food, the person may consume up to 20 cans of diet soft drinks and chew many pieces of sugarless gum each day.

Physical Effects of Anorexia Nervosa

Rooted in the emotional state of the victim, anorexia nervosa produces profound physical effects. The anorexic person often appears to be skin and bones. Body weight less than 85% of that expected is one clinical indicator of anorexia nervosa. This percentage can be calculated using the Metropolitan Life Insurance Company tables (see Appendix G), but body build and weight history should also be used when estimating an appropriate weight. BMI is a more reliable indicator of the degree of malnourishment; generally, a BMI of 17.5 or less indicates a severe case (review Chapter 7 for more on BMI). For children under age 18, growth charts should be used to assess weight status (see Chapter 17).

The state of semistarvation disturbs many body systems as it forces the body to conserve energy stores as much as possible (Fig. 13-1). This attempt to conserve energy stores is the cause of most of the physical effects. Thus, many complications can be reversed by returning to a healthy weight, provided the duration of the insult has not been too long. The following are predictable effects caused by hormonal responses to and deficient nutrient intakes from semistarvation:

- Lowered body temperature and cold intolerance from loss of insulating fat layer
- Slowed metabolic rate from decreased synthesis of thyroid hormones
- Decreased heart rate as metabolism slows, leading to premature fatigue, fainting, and an overwhelming need for sleep. Other changes in heart function may occur as well, including loss of heart tissue and irregular heart rhythm.
- Iron-deficiency anemia, which leads to further weakness
- Rough, dry, scaly, and cold skin, which may show multiple bruises because of the loss of the protective fat layer normally present under the skin
- Low white blood cell count, which increases the risk of infection—one cause of death in people with anorexia nervosa

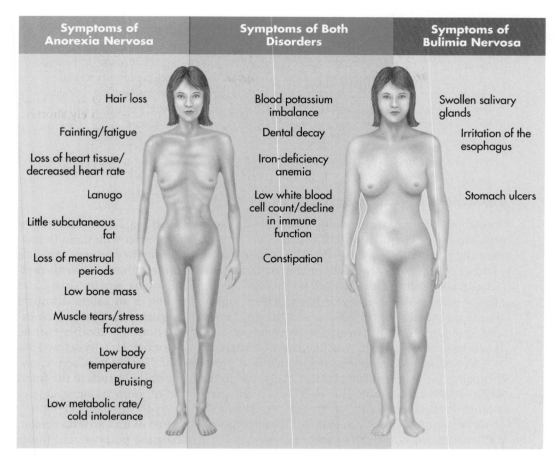

Symptoms of Anorexia Nervosa	Symptoms of Both Disorders	Symptoms of Bulimia Nervosa
Hair loss	Blood potassium imbalance	Swollen salivary glands
Fainting/fatigue	Dental decay	Irritation of the esophagus
Loss of heart tissue/ decreased heart rate	Iron-deficiency anemia	
Lanugo	Low white blood cell count/decline in immune function	Stomach ulcers
Little subcutaneous fat		
Loss of menstrual periods	Constipation	
Low bone mass		
Muscle tears/stress fractures		
Low body temperature		
Bruising		
Low metabolic rate/ cold intolerance		

FIGURE 13-1 ▶ Signs and symptoms of eating disorders. A vast array of physical effects are associated with anorexia nervosa and bulimia nervosa. This figure contains many, but is not an exhaustive list of all, potential consequences. These physical effects can also serve as warning signs that a problem exists. Professional evaluation is then indicated.

- Abnormal feeling of fullness or bloating, which can last for several hours after eating
- Loss of hair
- Appearance of **lanugo**—downy hairs on the body that trap air to partially counteract heat loss that occurs with loss of fat tissue
- Constipation due to deterioration of the gastrointestinal tract and abuse of laxatives
- Low blood potassium, worsened by potassium losses during vomiting and use of some types of diuretics. This increases the risk of heart rhythm disturbances, another leading cause of death in anorexic people.
- Loss of menstrual periods because of low body weight, low body fat content, and the stress of the disease. Accompanying hormonal changes cause a loss of bone mass and increase the risk of osteoporosis later in life.
- Changes in neurotransmitter function in the brain, which lead to depression
- Eventual loss of teeth caused by acid erosion of tooth enamel if frequent vomiting occurs. Until vomiting ceases, one way to reduce this effect on teeth is to rinse the mouth with water right away and brush the teeth as soon as possible. Loss of teeth (along with low bone mass) can be lasting signs of the disease, even if the other physical and mental problems are resolved.
- Muscle tears and stress fractures in athletes because of decreased bone and muscle mass

A person with this disorder is psychologically and physically ill and needs help.

lanugo Down-like hair that appears after a person has lost much body fat through semi-starvation. The hair stands erect and traps air, acting as insulation for the body to compensate for the relative lack of body fat, which usually functions as insulation.

▶ Erika Goodman, former dancer with the Joffrey Ballet, is now in her fifties and is crippled from osteoporosis resulting from years of restricting food intake to maintain a low body weight. Her food restriction led to irregular or absent menstrual periods for many years.

CONCEPT CHECK

Anorexia nervosa is an eating disorder characterized by semistarvation. It is found primarily—but not exclusively—in adolescent girls, starting at or around puberty. People with anorexia dwindle essentially to skin and bones yet still believe they are fat. Semistarvation produces hormonal changes and nutrient deficiencies, which lower body temperature; slow the heart rate; decrease immune response; stop menstrual periods; and contribute to hair, muscle, and bone loss. It is a serious disease, which often produces lifelong consequences and may be fatal.

Treatment of Anorexia Nervosa

▶ Singer Karen Carpenter's death from complications of anorexia nervosa in 1983 increased awareness of the serious nature of this disease. Currently, the average time for recovery from anorexia nervosa is 7 years; many insurance companies cover only a fraction of the estimated $150,000 cost of treatment.

People with anorexia often sink into shells of isolation and fear. They deny that a problem exists. Frequently, their friends and family members meet with them to confront the problem in a loving way. This is called an *intervention*. They present evidence of the problem and encourage immediate treatment. Treatment then requires a multidisciplinary team of experienced physicians, registered dietitians, psychologists, and other health professionals working together. An ideal setting is an eating disorders clinic in a medical center. Outpatient therapy generally begins first. This may be extended to 3 to 5 days per week. Day hospitalization (6 to 12 hours) is another option, as is total hospitalization. Hospitalization is necessary once a person falls below 75% of expected weight, experiences acute medical problems, and/or exhibits severe psychological problems or suicidal risk. Still, even in the most skilled hands at the finest facilities, efforts may fail. This tells us that the prevention of anorexia nervosa is of utmost importance.

Once a medical team has gained the cooperation and trust of an anorexic person, the team attempts to work together to restore a sense of balance, purpose, and future possibilities. As previously stated, anorexia nervosa is usually rooted in psychological conflict. However, the anorexic person who has been barely existing in a state of semistarvation cannot focus on much besides food. Dreams and even morbid thoughts about food will interfere with therapy until sufficient weight is regained.

▶ A young woman in a self-help group for those with anorexia nervosa explained her feelings to the other group members: "I have lost a specialness that I thought it gave me. I was different from everyone else. Now I know that I'm somebody who's overcome it, which not everybody does."

Nutrition Therapy. The first goal of nutrition therapy is to gain the person's cooperation and trust, with the ultimate objective of increasing oral food intake. Ideally, weight gain must be enough to raise the metabolic rate to normal and reverse as many physical signs of the disease as possible. Food intake is designed first to minimize or stop any further weight loss. Then, the focus shifts to restoring appropriate food habits. After this, the expectation can be switched to slowly gaining weight. A gain of 2 to 3 pounds per week is appropriate. Tube and/or intravenous (IV) feeding is used only if immediate renourishment is required, as this can frighten the person and cause him or her to distrust medical staff.

Persons with anorexia nervosa need considerable reassurance during the refeeding process because of uncomfortable and unfamiliar effects—such as bloating, increase in body heat, and increase in body fat. This is a frightening process because these changes can symbolize a loss of control. Rapid changes in electrolytes and minerals in the blood associated with refeeding, especially potassium, phosphorus, and magnesium, can be dangerous. Therefore, monitoring blood levels of these minerals is of critical importance during the process of incorporating more food into the diet.

In addition to helping persons with anorexia nervosa reach and maintain adequate nutritional status, the registered dietitian on the medical team provides accurate nutrition information throughout the treatment, promotes a healthy attitude toward food, and helps the person learn to eat in response to natural hunger and satiety cues. The focus then turns to identifying healthy and adequate food choices that promote weight gain to achieve and maintain a clinically estimated goal weight (e.g., BMI of

20 or more). As noted, nutrient deficiencies are commonly seen in anorexic persons. A multivitamin and mineral supplement will be added, as well as enough calcium to raise intake to about 1500 milligrams per day.

Excessive physical activity prevents weight gain, so professionals must help anorexic persons moderate their activity. At many treatment centers, moderate bed rest is used in the early stages of treatment to help promote weight gain.

Experienced professional help is the key. An anorexic person may be on the verge of suicide and starvation. In addition, anorexic people are often very clever and resistant to therapy. They may try to hide weight loss by wearing many layers of clothes, putting coins in their pockets or underwear, and drinking numerous glasses of water.

Psychological and Related Therapy. Once the physical problems of anorexia nervosa are addressed, the treatment focus shifts to the underlying emotional problems that led to excessive dieting and other symptoms of the disorder. To heal, these anorexic persons must reject the sense of accomplishment they have associated with an emaciated body and begin to accept themselves at a healthy body weight. If therapists can discover reasons for the disorder, they can develop strategies for restoring normal weight and eating habits that involve resolving psychological conflicts. Education about the medical consequences of semistarvation is also helpful. A key aspect of psychological treatment is showing affected individuals how to regain control of other facets of their lives and cope with difficult situations. As eating evolves into a normal routine, they can turn to previously neglected activities.

Therapists may use **cognitive behavior therapy,** which involves helping the person confront and change irrational beliefs about body image, eating, relationships, and weight. Underlying issues that may be the cause for the disease, such as sexual abuse, also must be identified and addressed by the therapist.

Family therapy often is important in treating anorexia nervosa, especially for younger persons who still live with their families. It focuses on the role of the illness among family members, the reactions of individual family members and ways in which their subconscious behavior might contribute to the abnormal eating patterns. Frequently, a therapist finds family struggles at the heart of the problem. As the disorder resolves, patients must relate to family members in new ways to gain the attention that was needed and previously tied to the disease. For example, the family may need to help the young person ease into adulthood and accept its responsibilities as well as its advantages. Self-help groups for anorexic (and bulimic) people, as well as their families and friends, represent nonthreatening first steps into treatment.

Food is the drug of choice in the treatment of anorexic patients. Generally, medications are not effective in management of the primary symptoms of anorexia nervosa. Fluoxetine (Prozac®) and related medications may stabilize recovery once 85% of expected body weight has been attained. These medications work by prolonging serotonin activity in the brain, which in turn regulates mood and feelings of satiety. A variety of other pharmacologic agents, such as olanzapine (Zyprexa®), may have some role in treating mood changes, anxiety, or psychotic symptoms associated with anorexia nervosa, but they have limited value unless weight gain is also achieved.

With professional help, many people with anorexia nervosa can lead normal lives. Although they may not be totally cured, anorexic individuals do not have to depend on unusual eating habits to cope with daily problems. They recover a sense of normalcy in their lives. No universal approach exists, because each case is unique. Establishing a strong relationship with either a therapist or another supportive person is an especially important key to recovery. Once anorexic persons feel understood and accepted by another person, they can begin to build a sense of self and exercise some autonomy. As they learn alternative coping mechanisms, they can relinquish their dysfunctional relationships with food and instead develop healthy personal relationships.

▶ A disturbing trend is the attempt to promote eating disorders as a way of life. Some anorexic individuals have personified their illness into a role model named "Ana," who tells them what to eat and mocks them when they don't lose weight. Ana websites reject the serious health risks of anorexia behaviors and instead dispense unsafe "thinspiration" to vulnerable individuals.

cognitive behavior therapy Psychological therapy in which the person's assumptions about dieting, body weight, and related issues are confronted. New ways of thinking are explored and then practiced by the person. In this way, an individual can learn new ways to control disordered eating behaviors and related life stress.

▲ Early treatment for an eating disorder, such as anorexia nervosa, improves chances of success.

A CLOSER LOOK AT BULIMIA NERVOSA

▶ Bingeing and purging (via vomiting) was evident in pre-Christian Roman times, but was practiced in a group setting. The eating disorder bulimia nervosa is generally practiced in private. It was first described in the medical literature in 1979.

Bulimia nervosa involves episodes of binge eating followed by various means to purge the food. It is most common among young adults of college age, although some high school students are also at risk. Susceptible people often have genetic factors and lifestyle patterns that predispose them to becoming overweight, and many try frequent weight-reduction diets as teenagers. Like people with anorexia nervosa, those with bulimia nervosa are usually female and successful. Unlike anorexic individuals, however, they are usually at or slightly above a normal weight. Females with bulimia nervosa are also more likely to be sexually active than those with anorexia nervosa.

The person with bulimia nervosa may think of food constantly. But unlike the anorexic person, who turns away from food when faced with problems, the bulimic person turns toward food in critical situations. Also, unlike those with anorexia nervosa, people with bulimia nervosa recognize their behavior as abnormal. These people often have low self-esteem and are depressed. Approximately half of the people with bulimia nervosa have major depression. Lingering effects of child abuse may be one reason for these feelings. Many bulimic persons report that they have been sexually abused. They appear competent to outsiders, while they actually feel out of control, ashamed, and frustrated.

Bulimic people tend to be impulsive, which may be expressed in behaviors such as stealing, increased sexual activity, drug and alcohol abuse, self-mutilation, or attempted suicide. Some experts have suggested that part of the problem may actually arise from an inability to control responses to impulse and desire. Some studies have demonstrated that bulimic people tend to come from disengaged families—ones that are loosely organized. In these families, roles for family members are not clearly defined, rules are disregarded, and a great deal of conflict exists. (In contrast, anorexic people tend to have families so actively engaged that roles may be too well defined.)

Typical Behavior in Bulimia Nervosa

It is likely that many people with bulimic behavior are never diagnosed; the diagnostic criteria specify that a person must binge and purge at least twice a week for 3 months. People with bulimia nervosa lead secret lives, hiding their abnormal eating habits. Moreover, it is impossible to recognize the disorder simply by appearance. Most diagnoses of bulimia nervosa rely on self-reports, so estimates of the number of cases are probably low. The disorder, especially in its milder forms, may be much more widespread than commonly thought.

For intake to qualify as a binge, an atypically large amount of food must be consumed in a short time and the person must exhibit a lack of control over his or her behavior. Among sufferers of bulimia nervosa, bingeing often alternates with attempts to rigidly restrict food intake. Elaborate food rules are common, such as avoiding all sweets. Thus, eating just one cookie or donut may cause individuals with this disorder to feel as though they have broken a rule. At that point, in the mind of a bulimic person, the objectionable food must be eliminated. Usually this leads to further overeating, partly because it is easier to regurgitate a large amount of food than a small amount.

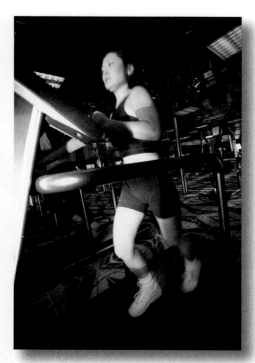

▲ Excessive exercising can be one component of bulimia if it is used as a way to offset the calorie intake from a binge. Exercise is considered excessive when it is done at inappropriate times or settings or when a person does it despite injury or other medical complications.

Binge-purge cycles may be practiced daily, weekly, or across longer intervals. A specific time often is set aside. Most binge eating occurs at night, when other people are less likely to interrupt, and usually lasts from ½ to 2 hours. A binge can be triggered by a combination of stress, boredom, loneliness, and depression. It often follows a period of strict dieting and thus can be linked to intense hunger. The binge is not at all like normal eating; once begun, it seems to propel itself. The person not only loses control, but generally doesn't even taste or enjoy food during a binge. This separates the practice from overeating.

Most commonly, bulimic people consume cakes, cookies, ice cream, and other high-carbohydrate convenience foods during binges because these foods can be purged relatively easily and comfortably by vomiting. In a single binge, foods supplying 3000 kcal or more may be eaten. Purging follows in hopes that no weight will be gained. However, even when vomiting follows the binge, 33% to 75% of the calories taken in is still absorbed, inevitably causing some weight gain. When laxatives or enemas are used, about 90% of the calories are absorbed, as laxatives act in the large intestine, beyond the point of most nutrient absorption. The belief that purging soon after bingeing will prevent excessive calorie absorption and weight gain is a misconception.

At the onset of bulimia nervosa, sufferers often induce vomiting by placing their fingers deep into the mouth. They may bite down on these fingers inadvertently, resulting in bite marks and scars around the knuckles, a characteristic sign of this disorder. Once the disease is established, however, a person may be able to vomit simply by contracting the abdominal muscles. Vomiting may also occur spontaneously.

Another way bulimic persons attempt to compensate for a binge and control their weight is by engaging in excessive exercise to expend a large amount of calories. In this practice, referred to as "debting," bulimic individuals try to estimate the amount of calories eaten during a binge, and then exercise to counteract the excess.

People with bulimia nervosa are not proud of their behavior. After a binge, they usually feel guilty and depressed. Over time, they experience low self-esteem, feel hopeless about their situation, and are caught in a vicious cycle of obsession (Fig. 13-2). Compulsive lying, shoplifting to obtain food, and drug abuse can further intensify these feelings. Bulimic people discovered in the act of bingeing by a friend or family member may order the intruder to "get out" and "go away." Sufferers gradually distance themselves from others, spending more time preoccupied by and engaging in bingeing and purging.

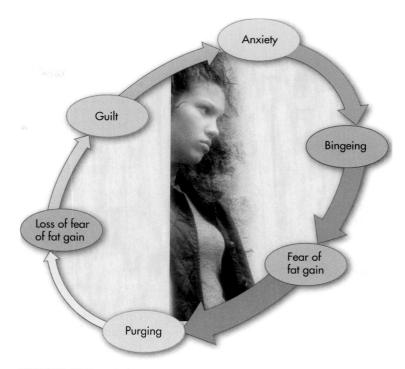

FIGURE 13-2 ▶ Bulimia nervosa's vicious cycle of obsession.

Health Problems Stemming from Bulimia Nervosa

The vomiting that many bulimic sufferers induce is a physically destructive method of purging. Indeed, the majority of health problems associated with bulimia nervosa, as noted here, arise from vomiting:

- Repeated exposure of teeth to the acid in vomit causes demineralization, making the teeth painful and sensitive to heat, cold, and acids. Eventually, the teeth may decay severely, erode away from fillings, and finally fall out (Fig. 13-3). Dental professionals are sometimes the first health professionals to notice signs of bulimia nervosa. As noted, it is important to rinse the mouth with water after any vomiting episode, especially before brushing the teeth.
- Blood potassium can drop significantly with regular vomiting or the use of certain diuretics. This can disturb the heart's rhythm and even produce sudden death.

FIGURE 13-3 ▶ Excessive tooth decay is common in bulimic patients.

- Salivary glands may swell as a result of infection and irritation from persistent vomiting.
- Stomach ulcers and bleeding and tears in the esophagus develop in some cases.
- Constipation may result from frequent laxative use.
- Ipecac syrup, sometimes used to induce vomiting, is toxic to the heart, liver, and kidneys. It has caused accidental poisoning when taken repeatedly.

Overall, bulimia nervosa is a potentially debilitating disorder that can lead to death, usually from suicide, low blood potassium, or overwhelming infections.

Treatment of Bulimia Nervosa

Therapy for bulimia nervosa, as for anorexia nervosa, requires a team of experienced clinicians. Bulimic individuals are less likely than those with anorexia to enter treatment in a state of semistarvation. However, if a bulimic person has lost significant weight, this must be treated before psychological treatment begins. Although clinicians have yet to agree on the best therapy for bulimia nervosa, they generally agree that treatment should last at least 16 weeks. Hospitalization may be indicated in cases of extreme laxative abuse, regular vomiting, substance abuse, and depression, especially if physical harm is evident.

▶ The binge-purge cycle can create an initial state of euphoria in the person. Giving up this euphoria has been equated to giving up an addiction. Still, it is important to do so.

The first goal of treatment for bulimia nervosa is to decrease the amount of food consumed in a binge session to decrease the risk of esophageal tears from related purging by vomiting. A decrease in the frequency of this type of purging will also decrease damage to the teeth.

The primary aim of psychotherapy is to improve a persons' self-acceptance and help one to be less concerned about body weight. Cognitive behavior therapy is generally used. Psychotherapy helps correct the all-or-none thinking typical of bulimic persons: "If I eat one cookie, I'm a failure and might as well binge." The premise of this psychotherapy is that, if abnormal attitudes and beliefs can be altered, normal eating will follow. In addition, the therapist guides the person in establishing food habits that will minimize bingeing: avoiding fasting, eating regular meals, and using alternative methods—other than eating—to cope with stressful situations. Group therapy is often useful to foster strong social support. One goal of therapy is to help bulimic persons accept some depression and self-doubt as normal.

Although pharmacological agents should not be used as the sole treatment for bulimia nervosa, studies indicate that some medications may be beneficial in conjunction with other therapies. Fluoxetine (Prozac®) is the only antidepressant that has been approved by FDA for use in the treatment of bulimia nervosa, but physicians also may prescribe other similar forms of antidepressants, other classes of psychiatric medications, or certain antiseizure medications, (e.g., topiramate [Topamax®]).

Nutritional counseling has two main goals: correcting misconceptions about food and re-establishing regular eating habits. Bulimic persons are given information about bulimia nervosa and its consequences. Avoiding binge foods and not constantly stepping on a scale may be recommended early in treatment. The primary goal, however, is to develop a normal eating pattern. To achieve this goal, some specialists encourage these individuals to develop daily meal plans and keep a food diary in which they record food intake, internal sensations of hunger, environmental factors that precipitate binges, and thoughts and feelings that accompany binge-purge cycles. Keeping a food diary not only is an accurate way to monitor food intake but also may help identify situations that seem to trigger binge episodes. With the help of a therapist, bulimic persons can develop alternative coping strategies.

In general, the focus is not on stopping bingeing and purging *per se* but on developing regular eating habits. Once this is achieved, the binge-purge cycle should start to break down. Individuals are discouraged from following strict rules about healthy food choices, because this mimics the typical obsessive attitudes associated with bulimia nervosa. Rather, encouraging a mature perspective on nutrient intake—that is, regular consumption of moderate amounts of a variety of foods balanced among the food groups—helps one overcome this disorder.

Setting time limits for the completion of meals and snacks is important for people with eating disorders. Many bulimic persons eat quickly, reflecting their difficulties with satiety. Suggesting that the person put his or her utensil down after each bite is a behavioral technique that a therapist might try during recovery for bulimia. (In comparison, many anorexic persons eat in an excessively slow manner—for example, taking 1 hour to eat a muffin cut into tiny, bite-size pieces.)

People with bulimia nervosa must recognize that they have a serious disorder that can have grave medical complications if not treated. Relapse is likely, so therapy should be long term. Those with bulimia nervosa need professional help because they can be very depressed and are at a high risk for suicide. About 50% of people with bulimia nervosa recover completely from the disorder. Others continue to struggle with it to varying degrees for the rest of their lives. This underscores the need for prevention because treatment is difficult.

CONCEPT CHECK

Bulimia nervosa is characterized by episodes of binge eating followed by purging, usually by vomiting. Vomiting is very destructive to the body, often causing severe dental decay, stomach ulcers, irritation of the esophagus, and blood potassium imbalances. Treatment using nutrition counseling and psychotherapy attempts to restore normal eating habits, to help the person correct distorted beliefs about diet and lifestyle, and to find tools to cope with the stresses of life. Medications, such as fluoxetine (Prozac®), can aid recovery when added to this regimen.

OTHER DISORDERED EATING PATTERNS

In recent years, other patterns of disordered eating have been recognized. Several of these patterns fall under the diagnosic category, *eating disorder not otherwise specified* (EDNOS). EDNOS is described in the American Psychiatric Association diagnostic manual as a "category [of] disorders of eating that do not meet the criteria for any specific eating disorder."

The EDNOS category is frequently used for people who have some, but not all, of the characteristics of anorexia nervosa or bulimia nervosa. Each EDNOS has distinctive qualities. For example, a person may experience episodes of bingeing and purging, but not frequently enough to meet the diagnosis of bulimia nervosa. A person may also engage in bingeing episodes without the use of inappropriate compensatory behaviors; this is referred to as binge-eating disorder. Another disordered eating pattern under study is night eating syndrome. **Night eating syndrome** is characterized by eating a lot of food in the late evening and nocturnal awakening with ingestion of food. Finally, the **female athlete triad** is a condition characterized by disordered eating, lack of menstrual periods, and osteoporosis. These conditions have been recognized as requiring professional treatment and are discussed in the following sections.

Binge-Eating Disorder

The typical characteristics for binge-eating disorder are listed in Table 13-2. Generally, it can be defined as binge-eating episodes not accompanied by purging (as typifies bulimia nervosa) at least two times per week for at least 6 months. First officially described in 1994, today health care professionals recognize binge-eating disorder as a growing, complex, and potentially serious problem.

Approximately 30% of subjects in organized weight-control programs have binge-eating disorder, whereas among the general U.S. population, about 4 million have this disorder. However, many more people in the general population are likely to have less severe forms of the disorder that do not meet all the criteria that describe the problem. The number of cases of binge-eating disorder is far greater than that of either

▲ Eventually stopping the binge-purge cycle is central to the treatment of bulimia nervosa.

night eating syndrome Eating a lot of food in the late evening and nocturnal awakenings with ingestion of food.

female athlete triad A condition characterized by disordered eating, lack of menstrual periods (amenorrhea), and osteoporosis.

TABLE 13-2 Some Characteristics of Binge-Eating Disorder

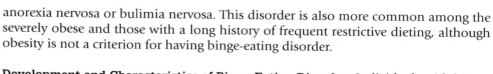

A. Recurrent episodes of binge eating, an episode characterized by:
   (1) Eating, in a discrete period (e.g., within any 2-hour period), an amount of food definitely larger than most people would eat during a similar period in similar circumstances
   (2) A sense of lack of control during the episodes (e.g., a feeling that one can't stop eating or control what or how much one is eating)

B. During most binge episodes, at least three of the following occur:
   (1) Eating much more rapidly than usual
   (2) Eating until feeling uncomfortably full
   (3) Eating large amounts of food when not feeling physically hungry
   (4) Eating alone because of being embarrassed by how much one is eating
   (5) Feeling disgusted with oneself, depressed, or guilty after overeating

C. Marked distress regarding binge eating

D. The binge eating occurs, on average, at least 2 days a week for 6 months.

E. The behavior does not occur only during the course of bulimia nervosa or anorexia nervosa.

Based on information from the *Diagnostic and Statistical Manual of Mental Disorders*, Fourth Edition (DSM-IV-TR). Washington DC: American Psychiatric Association, 2000.

▲ Binge-eating disorder is seen in both men and women.

▶ As noted in Chapter 2, spreading one's dietary intake into numerous, small meals (grazing) over a day provides some health advantages if overall calorie intake remains appropriate.

anorexia nervosa or bulimia nervosa. This disorder is also more common among the severely obese and those with a long history of frequent restrictive dieting, although obesity is not a criterion for having binge-eating disorder.

Development and Characteristics of Binge-Eating Disorder. Individuals with binge-eating disorder (about 40% of whom are males) often perceive themselves as hungry more often than normal. They usually started dieting at a young age, began bingeing during adolescence or in their early twenties, and did not succeed in commercial weight-control programs. Almost half of those with severe binge-eating disorder exhibit clinical depression. Some people also may have a genetic predisposition for this disorder.

Typical binge eaters isolate themselves and eat large quantities of a favorite food. Stressful events and feelings of depression or anxiety can trigger this behavior. Giving themselves permission to eat a forbidden food can also precipitate a binge. Other triggers include loneliness, anxiety, self-pity, depression, anger, rage, alienation, and frustration. They sometimes binge on whatever is easy to eat in large amounts—noodles, rice, bread, leftovers. Characteristically, however, binge eaters consume foods that carry the social stigma of "junk" or "bad" foods—ice cream, cookies, sweets, potato chips, and similar snack foods.

In general, people engage in binge eating to induce a sense of well-being and perhaps even numbness, usually in an attempt to avoid feeling and dealing with emotional pain and anxiety. They eat without regard to biological need and often in a recurrent, ritualized fashion. Some people with this disorder eat food continually over an extended period, called *grazing;* others cycle episodes of bingeing with normal eating. For example, someone with a stressful or frustrating job might come home every night and graze until bedtime. Another person might eat normally most of the time but find comfort in consuming large quantities of food when an emotional setback occurs.

Although people with anorexia nervosa and bulimia nervosa exhibit persistent preoccupation with body shape, weight, and thinness, binge eaters do not necessarily share these concerns. Thus, neither purging nor prolonged food restriction is characteristic of binge-eating disorder. Some physicians classify binge-eating disorder as an addiction to food, involving psychological dependence. The person becomes attached to the behavior and has a drive to continue it, senses only limited control over it, and needs to persist at it despite negative consequences. Food is used to reduce stress, produce feelings of power and well-being, avoid feelings of intimacy with others, and avoid life problems. Obesity and binge eating are not necessarily linked. Not all obese people are binge eaters, and, although obesity may result from trying to numb emotional pain with food, it is not necessarily an outcome of binge eating.

Binge-eating disorder is most likely to develop in people who never learned to express and deal appropriately with their feelings. Rather than face their frustration, anger, and pain, they turn to food. The frustration will continue because they never confront the basic problem. Binge eating makes them feel they cannot control the behavior pattern and therefore cannot control their lives. Worse, the binge eating usually increases feelings of guilt, embarrassment, and shame.

Often, people who practice binge eating have been shaped by families who do not address and express feelings in healthful ways. The parents nurture and comfort their children with food rather than engage in healthy exchanges of self-disclosure of feelings and potential solutions. Members of such families learn to eat in response to emotional needs and pain instead of hunger. Those who regularly practice binge eating may grow up nurturing others instead of themselves, avoiding their own feelings and taking little time for themselves. Not knowing how to satisfy their personal and emotional needs in more healthful ways, people in these families turn to food.

For some people, frequent dieting beginning in childhood or adolescence is a precursor to binge-eating disorder. During periods when little food is eaten, they get very hungry and obsessive about food. When allowed to eat more food, they feel driven to eat in a compulsive, uncontrolled way. The pattern of strict dieting alternating with binge eating may continue over time.

▶ People with binge-eating disorder may come from families with alcoholism or may have suffered sexual abuse. Members of such dysfunctional families often do not know how to deal effectively with emotions. They cope by turning to substances. Family members learn to cover up dysfunctional patterns for the alcoholic person and to nurture him or her at the expense of each other and their own needs.

Help for the Person with Binge-Eating Disorder. Those with binge-eating disorder must learn to eat in response to hunger—a biological signal—rather than in response to emotional needs or external factors (such as the time of day or the simple presence of food). Counselors often direct binge eaters to record their perceptions of physical hunger throughout the day and at the beginning and end of every meal. These people must learn to respond to a prescribed amount of fullness at each meal. They should initially avoid weight-loss diets because feelings of food deprivation can lead to more disruptive emotions and a greater sense of unmet needs. Diets are likely to encourage more intense problems, such as extreme hunger. Many people with binge-eating disorder may experience difficulty in identifying personal emotional needs and expressing emotions. This problem is a common predisposing factor in binge eating, so communication issues should be addressed during treatment. Binge eaters often must be helped to recognize their buried emotions in anxiety-producing situations, and then encouraged to share them with their therapist or therapy group. Learning simple but appropriate phrases to say to oneself can help stop bingeing when the desire is strong.

Self-help groups, such as Overeaters Anonymous, aim to help recovery from binge-eating disorder. Their treatment philosophy, which parallels that of Alcoholics Anonymous, attempts to create an environment of encouragement and accountability to overcome this eating disorder. Dietary advice typically ranges from avoiding restraint in eating in general to limiting binge foods. Some experts feel that learning to eat all foods—but in moderation—is an effective goal for binge eaters. This practice can prevent the feelings of desperation and deprivation that come from limiting particular foods. Antidepressants, such as fluoxetine (Prozac®), and other types of medications (e.g., topiramate [Topamax®]) also have been found to help reduce binge eating in these individuals by decreasing depression. Overall, people who have this disorder are usually unsuccessful in controlling it on their own. Professional help is advised.

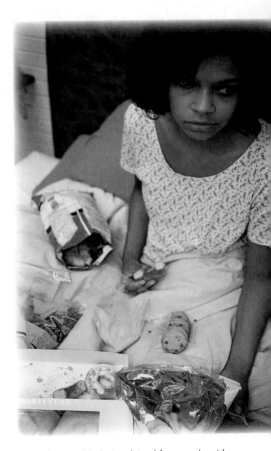

▲ Professional help is advised for people with a binge-eating disorder.

▲ Night eating syndrome is characterized by waking at least once during the night and needing to eat to be able to fall asleep again.

Night Eating Syndrome

Night eating syndrome is characterized by evening hyperphagia (eating more than one-third of total daily calories after the evening meal) and nighttime awakening accompanied by the ingestion of food. Although night eating syndrome was first observed among obese patients, it also occurs among nonobese persons. It has been estimated to occur in 1.5% of the general population and in 8.9% of persons treated in obesity clinics.

Signs and Symptoms of Night Eating Syndrome
- Not feeling hungry in the morning and delaying the first meal until several hours after waking
- Overeating in the evening with more than one-third of daily food intake after dinner
- Difficulty falling asleep and a need to eat something to help fall asleep faster
- Waking at least once during the night and a need to eat to be able to fall asleep again
- Eating produces feelings of guilt and shame
- Feeling depressed, especially at night

Research shows that the cause of night eating syndrome may be an abnormal food cycle in the body, resulting in a delayed intake of food during the day. The circadian rhythm (your body's 24-hour clock) of food intake appears to be disturbed in night eating syndrome. Studies have also shown that night eating syndrome is prevalent among outpatients with psychiatric conditions and that the symptoms, including nocturnal ingestion and evening hyperphagia, are significantly improved with use of the antidepressant setraline (Zoloft®).

Female Athlete Triad

▶ A female high school athlete recently admitted her 3-year struggle with anorexia nervosa and bulimia nervosa. Even after her athletic performance declined and she suffered a sports-related injury, which sidelined her for a year and required surgery, she continued to think that controlling her weight and eating behaviors would make her the best—academically and physically. This example demonstrates several important points about eating disorders: certain groups of people are at greater risk for developing eating disorders; these people are often high achievers and are careful about concealing their eating disorder; and eating disorders such as the female athlete triad, bulimia nervosa, and anorexia nervosa frequently overlap.

▶ It is often difficult to get female athletes to accept necessary treatment plans. They frequently have a single-minded approach to their sport, while ignoring future health consequences.

Women participating in appearance-based and endurance sports are at risk of developing an eating disorder. One study of college-age female athletes found that 15% of swimmers, 62% of gymnasts, and 32% of varsity athletes exhibited disordered eating patterns. Estimates of eating disorders for college women not involved in competitive sports are much lower.

In addition to disordered eating, college women athletes tend to experience irregular menstruation more frequently than other college women. Disordered eating, particularly food restriction, and stress can precipitate this, causing women to have less dense and weaker bones than normal because of lower estrogen concentrations in the blood. Some of these young women have bone mass values equivalent to those of 50- to 60-year-olds, increasing their risk for bone and stress fractures during sports as well as general activities. Much of the bone loss is irreversible.

The American College of Sports Medicine (ACSM) has named this syndrome "female athlete triad" because it consists of three parts: disordered eating, lack of menstrual periods, and osteoporosis (Fig. 13-4). The ACSM has issued a plea to teachers, coaches, health professionals, and parents to educate female athletes about the triad and its health consequences.

Many coaches/trainers and even some health professionals wrongly believe that loss of menstrual periods is a normal consequence of a high level of physical activity. However, loss of menstrual periods in female athletes stems from a dramatic decrease in female reproductive hormones, particularly estrogen. Loss of estrogen has other negative consequences on the body, such as fragile bones, as mentioned. Correcting the hormonal imbalance and menstrual irregularities by increasing caloric intake should stabilize bone mass. During therapy, a physician may prescribe a multivitamin and mineral supplement as well as calcium supplements as needed to maintain an intake of 1200 to 1500 milligrams.

Those exhibiting symptoms of the female athlete triad should seek treatment from a multidisciplinary team of health professionals. Involving the coach or trainer in therapy is usually a key factor in the success of the treatment plan. Suggestions for treatment are as follows:

- Reduce preoccupation with food, weight, and body fat.
- Gradually increase meals and snacks to an appropriate amount.
- Achieve an appropriate weight-for-height.
- Establish regular menstrual periods.
- Decrease training time and/or intensity by 10% to 20%.

The tragic case of Christy Henrich illustrates why anyone at risk for the female athlete triad should seek professional help. As a young teenager, Christy weighed 95 pounds and was 4 feet 11 inches tall. She showed promise as a gymnast but was told that she was too fat to excel in gymnastics. Christy continued her training but often starved herself, some days consuming just an apple and frequently purging by vomiting. Her success in gymnastics continued, but at age 22 her weight had fallen to 52 pounds, and she died from the effects of long-term semistarvation.

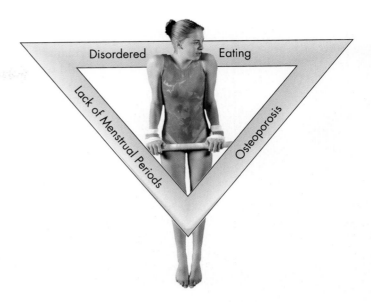

FIGURE 13-4 ▶ The female athlete triad occurs when the athlete has disordered eating, lack of menstrual periods, and osteoporosis. Stress fractures and chronic fatigue also occur. This triad often is seen in appearance-related sports, such as gymnastics. Long-term health is at risk; thus, prevention and early treatment is most beneficial.

PREVENTION OF EATING DISORDERS

A key to developing and maintaining healthful eating behavior is to realize that some concern about diet, health, and weight is normal. It is also normal to experience variation in what we eat, how we feel, and even how much we weigh. For example, it is normal to experience some minimal weight change (up to 2 to 3 pounds) throughout the day and even more over the course of a week. A large weight fluctuation or ongoing weight gain or weight loss is more likely to indicate that a problem is present. If you notice a large change in your eating habits, how you feel, or your body weight, it is a good idea to consult your personal physician. Treating physical and emotional problems early helps lead you to peace of mind and good health.

With a view on society as a whole, many people begin to form opinions about food, nutrition, health, weight, and body image prior to or during puberty. Parents, friends, and professionals working with young adults should consider the following advice for preventing eating disorders:

- Discourage restrictive dieting and meal skipping. Fasting is also discouraged (except for religious occasions).
- Provide information about normal changes that occur during puberty.
- Correct misconceptions about nutrition, healthy body weight, and approaches to weight loss.
- Carefully phrase any weight-related recommendations and comments.
- Don't overemphasize numbers on a scale. Instead, primarily promote healthful eating.
- Encourage normal expression of disruptive emotions.
- Encourage children to eat only when they're hungry.
- Teach the basics of proper nutrition and regular physical activity in school and at home.
- Provide adolescents with an appropriate, but not unlimited, degree of independence, choice, responsibility, and self-accountability for their actions.

CRITICAL THINKING

Tom, a high school teacher, is concerned about eating disorders. He wants to try to prevent young adults from falling into the discouraging traps of anorexia nervosa and bulimia nervosa. What are some of the topics and issues he should discuss with students in his health classes?

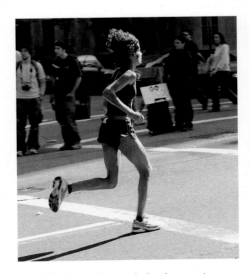

▲ Low body weight coupled with excessive exercise can lead to amenorrhea and ultimately the female athlete triad.

▲ Bulimia nervosa affects many college students. Counselors are aware of this and are available to help.

- Increase self-acceptance and appreciation of the power and pleasure emerging from one's body.
- Enhance tolerance for diversity in body weight and shape.
- Build respectful environments and supportive relationships.
- Encourage coaches to be sensitive to weight and body-image issues among athletes.
- Emphasize that thinness is not necessarily associated with better athletic performance.

Our society as a whole can benefit from a fresh focus on nutritious food practices and a healthful outlook toward food and body weight. Not only is treatment of eating disorders far more difficult than prevention, these disorders also have devastating effects on the entire family. For this reason, caregivers and health care professionals must emphasize the importance of an overall healthful diet that focuses on moderation, as opposed to restriction and perfection. Restricted diets are especially detrimental to children because they do not supply enough calories to sustain growth. In response, nutritional counseling can assure caregivers that including some sweets and fast-food in a child's diet is appropriate (see Chapter 17 for more details).

Overall, the challenge facing many North Americans is achieving a healthy body weight without excessive dieting. This means adopting and maintaining sensible eating habits, a physically active lifestyle, and realistic and positive attitudes and emotions while practicing creative ways to handle stress. Eating disorders develop in part from certain cultural values; changing these values might reduce the pressures predisposing some people to various types of disordered eating behavior. Some feminists, for example, assert that true liberation means being free to find one's natural weight. Women who combine careers and motherhood are saying that they have more important things to worry about; some fashion leaders are tolerating more curves; exercise programs are encouraging regular brisk walking, rather than high-intensity activities such as jogging. Finally, writers, therapists, and registered dietitians are working to help women accept their bodies, as noted in the "size acceptance" approach discussed in Chapter 7.

MAKING DECISIONS

Polycystic Ovary Syndrome and Eating Disorders

Polycystic ovary syndrome (PCOS) is a complex hormonal disorder and is the leading cause of infertility. PCOS is characterized by hormonal imbalances in women with high levels of male hormones such as testosterone secreted by the ovaries. The hormonal imbalance causes tiny cysts to surround the ovaries like a strand of pearls. The signs and symptoms of PCOS include difficulty losing weight, intense cravings for carbohydrates, and irregular or absent periods. Most of these have a direct effect on body image and self-esteem, so a relationship between PCOS and eating disorders is suspected. The overlap in symptoms means it is important that persons with these characteristics be screened for both PCOS and eating disorders before recommendations for treatment are made.

CONCEPT CHECK

Food bingeing (without purging) and grazing are two characteristic behaviors of binge-eating disorder. Treatment addresses the deeper emotional issues that undermine healthy eating practices, while shifting the person's focus away from food deprivation and restrictive diets and toward more normal eating behaviors. Night eating syndrome involves overeating in the evening and a need to eat to be able to fall asleep. The female athlete triad consists of disordered eating, amenorrhea, and osteoporosis, and most commonly affects those in appearance-related and endurance sports. Parents, coaches, teachers, and health professionals need to initiate efforts to prevent and treat this problem.

For further information on eating disorders, contact:

Academy for Eating Disorders, 60 Revere Drive, Suite 500, Northbrook, IL 60062, 847-498-4274; **www.aedweb.org**

The National Eating Disorders Association, 603 Stewart St., Suite 803, Seattle, WA 98101; 206-382-3587 or 800-931-EDAP; **www. nationaleatingdisorders.org**

The National Institute of Mental Health has published a concise review of eating disorders (**www.nimh.nih.gov/publicat/ eatingdisorders.cfm**).

THOUGHTS OF AN ANOREXIC WOMAN

It was the spring of my freshman year of high school, and I had just turned 15. I wanted to get a leading role in the upcoming high school musical *West Side Story*. I thought I should lose some weight to look more attractive to the student director Shawn, so I decided to give up "junk" food. The next day my friend Sandra looked at my lunch, spread out neatly on a napkin before me, and squawked, "Dill pickles?! Who brings dill pickles for lunch in a zip-lock baggie?" The other girls at the table fell into a fit of hysterics. "Casting for *West Side Story* is coming up," I said, "and I gave up 'junk' food to try to lose a few pounds." One of my friends thought it would be funny to give me an M&M—just to smell. Ha, ha. I put it in a little Tupperware container and kept it for days in my backpack as a reminder. Every once in a while, I did smell it.

For the next few weeks there were times when I would find myself cracking open the refrigerator door and just staring down what I knew to be a deliciously crunchy, crisp, and cold Kit Kat bar in the dairy bin. I didn't eat it though. At the mall with my friends (since

▲ A history of anorexia nervosa can harm physical as well as mental health.

at 15, that's about all my parents allowed me to do), Bridgette and Nora wanted to stop and get a cinnamon bun. They chided me, but I didn't budge. The cinnamon bun smelled so good. But as I sat opposite them in the food court and watched them overdramatize its ooey-gooey goodness, I felt a sense of pride that I could make a decision and stick with it. I could see that they were jealous of my willpower.

When Easter came around, I took a look at the contents of the Easter basket my mom insisted on preparing and turned up my nose at it. I had proven to myself that I could resist temptation . . . why stop now?

I was eventually offered only a minor part in the musical, but I wasn't that disappointed. I was looking so much better as the pounds kept coming off. Every morning, just after going to the bathroom and before getting any breakfast, I would pop onto the scale in my mom's bathroom. One hundred and fifteen pounds and still going. At 5 feet 7 inches, that wasn't too bad.

Also at this time, I started running, and my friend Laura became my running partner. She was getting in shape for the next season of field hockey. After school, we met in the locker room, changed out of our school clothes, and out we went. I had never been much of an athlete—I thought that being part of a team, whether in sports or academics, diluted the excellence I could achieve on my own. Running, however, could just be me and the road—no mediocrity there.

Cheese and butter had made it to the "no" list by the time I was 16 and down to 105 pounds. Fat-free was my mantra. For my 16th birthday, my friends threw a little surprise party for me. Nora, knowing I would put up a fight, made me a cake. "It's your birthday! You can have a piece of cake!" I politely said no, that I would cut it for everyone else, but I really didn't want any. They pestered me and Nora started to feel offended, so finally I took a few bites so she wouldn't burst into tears. It had been so long since I'd had so much sugar. I felt bloated and sick. I ate nothing for the rest of the day, and only 6 saltines, 1 apple, and 2 stalks of celery the next day. Those foods were on the "yes" list. Salads also were okay, but only lettuce with salt and vinegar. I told my parents that the dissections in biology class had given me a distaste for meat, but really, I just didn't want all those calories. For a while, I craved food day and night, but I was getting better and better at holding my ground.

By my senior year, I was skipping lunches altogether, opting instead to hang out in the library and read over my AP Bio text. "Where were you at lunch today?" Bridgette would ask later. "Oh, I had some reading to do. The AP exam is going to be tough." At 100 pounds, I was getting closer to finding out what "tough" really meant.

Even though Laura moved out of state, I didn't give up on exercising. Now, the stair stepper in the gym was my favorite. I'd take my microbiology notes, prop them up in front of me, and step-step-step until I had burned 400 kcal. I felt so efficient being that I could multi-task. Sometimes I'd go twice a day. As senior year wore on, though, it got harder and harder to get up in the morning and put on my tennis shoes. And then one morning, in the shower, I just collapsed under the stream of hot water.

I ended up in this hospital bed with an IV tube in my arm. At 92 pounds, my body was starving. As it turns out, if you don't give your body any fuel, you start to cannibalize yourself, in a sense. My body had been so hungry, my muscles had been wasting away, and the episode in the shower was due to a problem with my heart. It's a problem I have created . . . not my parents or my distant group of friends . . . just me. My mom was there, next to me, caressing the arm with the IV tube, putting her whole life on hold because of me. Isn't this what I'd wanted—to be in control of my own destiny?

Where do I go from here?

THOUGHTS OF A BULIMIC WOMAN

From Hall L, Cohn L: *Bulimia—A Guide to Recovery.* Gurze Books: Carlsbad, CA, 1992.

I am wide awake and immediately out of bed. I think back to the night before, when I made a new list of what I wanted to get done and how I wanted to be. My husband is not far behind me on his way into the bathroom to get ready for work. Maybe I can sneak onto the scale to see what I weigh this morning before he notices me. I am already in my private world. I feel overjoyed when the scale says that I stayed the same weight as I was the night before, and I can feel that slightly hungry feeling. Maybe it will stop today; maybe today everything will change. What were the projects I was going to get done?

We eat the same breakfast, except that I take no butter on my toast, no cream in my coffee, and never take seconds (until Doug gets out the door). Today I am going to be really good, and that means eating certain predetermined portions of food and not taking one more bite than I think I am allowed. I am very careful to see that I don't take more than Doug. I judge myself by his body. I can feel the tension building. I wish Doug would hurry up and leave so I can get going!

As soon as he shuts the door, I try to get involved with one of the myriad responsibilities on my list. I hate them all! I just want to crawl into a hole. I don't want to do anything. I'd rather eat. I am alone; I am nervous; I am no good; I always do everything wrong anyway; I am not in control; I can't make it through the day, I know it. It has been the same for so long. I remember the starchy cereal I ate for breakfast. I am into the bathroom and onto the scale. It measures the same, but I don't want to stay the same! I want to be thinner! I look into the mirror. I think my thighs are ugly and deformed looking. I see a lumpy, clumsy, pear-shaped wimp. There is always something wrong with what I see. I feel frustrated, trapped in this body, and I don't know what to do about it.

I float to the refrigerator knowing exactly what is there. I begin with last night's brownies. I always begin with the sweets. At first I try to make it look like nothing is missing, but my appetite is huge and I resolve to make another batch of brownies. I know there is half of a bag of cookies in the bathroom, thrown out the night before, and I polish them off imme-diately. I take some milk so my vomiting will be smoother. I like the full feeling I get after downing a big glass. I get out six pieces of bread and toast one side of each in the broiler, turn them over and load them with pats of butter, and put them under the broiler again until they are bubbling. I take all six pieces on a plate to the television and go back for a bowl of cereal and a banana to have along with them. Before the last piece of toast is finished, I am already preparing the next batch of six more pieces. Maybe another brownie or five, and a couple of large bowls full of ice cream, yogurt, or cottage cheese.

My stomach is stretched into a huge ball below my rib cage. I know I'll have to go into the bathroom soon, but I want to postpone it. I am in never-never land. I am waiting, feeling the pressure, pacing the floor in and out of the rooms. Time is passing. Time is passing. It is getting to be time. I wander aimlessly through each of the rooms again, tidying, making the whole house neat and put back together. I finally make the turn into the bathroom. I brace my feet, pull my hair back and stick my finger down my throat, stroking twice, and get up a huge pile of food. Three times, four times, and another pile of food. I can see everything come back. I am so glad to see those brownies because they are so fattening. The rhythm of the emptying is broken and my head is beginning to hurt. I stand up feeling dizzy, empty, and weak. The whole episode has taken about an hour.

▲ Bulimic episodes add to the despair felt in this disorder.

CASE STUDY

Eating Disorders—Steps to Recovery

At age 16, Sarah suddenly became self-conscious about her body when her peers teased her about being overweight. She began exercising to an aerobics video for an hour each day and found that she had success in losing weight; this was the beginning of her obsession to be thin. Next, Sarah turned to eating less food to lose even more weight and began eliminating certain foods from her diet, such as candy and meat. She increased her water and vegetable intake and chewed sugarless gum to curb her appetite. Once she began dieting, it was impossible for her to stop. She enjoyed having a high degree of self-control over her body. Still, she was literally obsessed with food, even staring at others while they were eating a meal. She occasionally cooked large meals and then refused to eat all but a few bites. By the time Sarah was 19 years old and 5 feet 6 inches tall, her weight had dropped from 150 pounds to 85 pounds in 20 months. Her family was concerned about her weight status, demanding that she go to a physician for an evaluation. Sarah was not happy about this idea but believed that her family would stop pestering her if she went. Sarah did not think she had a problem; she thought she was still grotesquely overweight.

She did notice, however, that she was intolerant of cold temperatures and was concerned that she had not menstruated in a year.

Answer the following questions, and check your responses in Appendix A.

1. Sarah appears to have an eating disorder. Which eating disorder best describes her behavior?
2. List the behaviors that Sarah developed between age 16 and 19 years that are signs of the development of this eating disorder.
3. What physical symptoms of this disorder does Sarah have (review Fig. 13-1)?
4. What types of therapy do you think the physician will suggest for Sarah?
5. Do you think Sarah has developed any vitamin or mineral deficiencies? Which ones would be most likely? How could these deficiencies be best treated?
6. Where could she go for the therapy she needs?
7. What type of professionals would most likely provide therapy for Sarah's condition?
8. What is the likelihood that she will fully recover from her condition?

SUMMARY

1. Anorexia nervosa is most common among high-achieving, perfectionist girls from families marked by conflict, high expectations, rigidity, and denial. The disorder usually starts with dieting in early puberty and proceeds to the near-total refusal to eat. Early warning signs include intense concern about weight gain and dieting, as well as abnormal food habits, such as cooking food that they won't allow themselves to eat.

2. Anorexic persons become irritable, hostile, overly critical, and joyless; they tend to withdraw from family and friends. Eventually, anorexia nervosa can lead to numerous physical effects, including a profound decrease in body weight and body fat, a fall in body temperature and

heart rate, iron-deficiency anemia, a low white blood cell count, hair loss, constipation, low blood potassium, and the loss of menstrual periods. Those with anorexia nervosa are in a state of physical illness.

3. Treatment of anorexia nervosa includes increasing food intake to support gradual weight gain. Psychological counseling attempts to help establish regular food habits and to find means of coping with the life stresses that led to the disorder. Hospitalization may be necessary, as well as use of certain medications.

4. Bulimia nervosa is characterized by secretive bingeing on large amounts of food within a short time span, and then purging by vomiting or misusing

laxatives, diuretics, or enemas. Alternately, fasting and excessive exercise may be used. Both men and women are at risk. Vomiting as a means of purging is especially destructive to the body; it can cause severe tooth decay, stomach ulcers, irritation of the esophagus, low blood potassium, and other problems. Bulimia nervosa poses a serious health problem and is associated with significant risk of suicide.

5. Treatment of bulimia nervosa includes psychological as well as nutritional counseling. During treatment, bulimic persons learn to accept themselves and to cope with problems in ways that do not involve food. Regular eating patterns are developed as these bulimic

persons begin to plan meals in an informed, healthful manner. Certain medications can be a helpful addition to the regimen.

6. Binge-eating disorder, more widespread than either anorexia nervosa or bulimia nervosa, is most common among people with a history of frequent, unsuccessful dieting. Binge eaters typically either practice bingeing (without purging) or grazing (i.e., eating continually over extended periods).

Emotional disturbances are often at the root of this disordered form of eating. Treatment addresses deeper emotional issues, discourages food deprivation and restrictive diets, and helps restore normal eating behaviors. Certain medications may be a useful addition to this therapy.

7. Night eating syndrome is overeating in the evening with more than one-third of daily food intake after dinner, difficulty falling asleep and a need to eat

something to help fall asleep faster, and waking at least once during the night and a need to eat to be able to fall asleep again.

8. The female athlete triad consists of disordered eating, loss of menstrual periods, and osteoporosis. It is particularly common in appearance-related and endurance sports. If not corrected, this disorder eventually leads to decreased athletic performance and general health problems.

STUDY QUESTIONS

1. What are the typical characteristics of a person with anorexia nervosa? What may influence a person to begin rigid, self-imposed dietary patterns?

2. List the detrimental physical and psychological side effects of bulimia nervosa. Describe important goals of the psychological and nutrition therapy used to treat bulimic patients.

3. What is the current thinking concerning medication use for anorexia nervosa and bulimia nervosa?

4. Explain the role of excessive exercise in eating disorders.

5. How might parents significantly contribute to the development of an eating disorder? Suggest an attitude that a

parent or an adult friend of yours displayed that may not have been conducive to developing a normal relationship to food.

6. Based on your knowledge of good nutrition and sound dietary habits, answer the following questions:
   a. How can repeated bingeing and purging lead to significant nutrient deficiencies?
   b. How can significant nutrient deficiencies contribute to major health problems in later life?
   c. A friend asks you, the nutrition expert, if it is okay to "cleanse" the body by eating only grapefruit for a week. What is your response?

7. How, in your opinion, has society contributed to the development of various forms of disordered eating? Provide an example.

8. List the three symptoms that constitute the female athlete triad. What is the major health risk associated with loss of menstrual periods in the female athlete?

9. How does binge-eating disorder differ from bulimia nervosa? Describe the factors that contribute to the development and treatment of binge-eating disorder.

10. Provide two recommendations to reduce the problem of eating disorders in our society.

CHECK YOUR KNOWLEDGE

Answers to the following multiple choice questions are in Appendix A.

1. Anorexia nervosa generally is a disease of
   a. children.
   b. middle-aged women.
   c. young boys.
   d. teenage women.

2. Anorexia nervosa can be defined as
   a. compulsive eating.
   b. hyperactivity.
   c. psychological denial of appetite.
   d. purging.

3. A long-term health consequence of anorexia nervosa could be
   a. fractures resulting from bone loss.
   b. atherosclerotic heart disease.
   c. esophageal ulcers.
   d. cancer.

4. Bulimia is most frequently diagnosed by a
   a. dietitian.
   b. physician.
   c. dentist.
   d. physical therapist.

5. The *major* health risk from frequent vomiting due to bulimia nervosa is
   a. a drop in blood potassium.
   b. constipation.
   c. weight gain.
   d. a swelling of salivary glands.

6. Initial treatment of bulimia nervosa includes all of the following *except*
   a. psychotherapy to improve body image.
   b. emphasis on regular eating habits.
   c. nutritional counseling.
   d. refeeding via tube feedings.
   e. Both a and c.

7. Binge-eating disorder can be characterized as
   a. bingeing accompanied by purging.
   b. secretive eating.
   c. eating to avoid feeling and dealing with emotional pain.
   d. the early phase of bulimia nervosa.

8. Binge-eating disorder is different from anorexia nervosa, and particularly bulimia nervosa, because it doesn't necessarily involve
   a. females.
   b. a persistent concern with body shape, weight, and thinness.

c. purging, such as regular vomiting.
d. health risks.
e. Both b and c.

9. Night eating syndrome is characterized by
   a. eating dinner but no breakfast or lunch.
   b. the need to eat to fall asleep.
   c. waking at night to purge by vomiting.
   d. consuming all of the daily calories at night.

10. Female athlete triad consists of
    a. anorexia nervosa, lack of family support, and overtraining.
    b. disordered eating, overtraining, and lack of menstrual periods.
    c. osteoporosis, lack of menstrual periods, and disordered eating.
    d. osteoporosis, lack of sleep, and disordered eating.

FURTHER READINGS

1. ADA Reports: Position of the American Dietetic Association: Nutrition intervention in the treatment of anorexia nervosa, bulimia nervosa, and eating disorders not otherwise specified (EDNOS). *Journal of the American Dietetic Association* 101:810, 2001.

   Eating disorders are complex and serious illnesses, as described in detail in this article. To be effective in treating individuals who suffer from these illnesses, the expert interaction between professionals in many disciplines is required.

2. American Academy of Pediatrics: Identifying and treating eating disorders. *Pediatrics* 111:204, 2003.

   Eating disorders are becoming more common in our society. This article reviews the current diagnostic and treatment options for such disorders.

3. American Psychiatric Association: Practice guidelines for the treatment of patients with eating disorders (revision). *American Journal of Psychiatry* 157(suppl):4, 2000.

   People with eating disorders display a broad range of symptoms that occur along a continuum between those of anorexia nervosa and those of bulimia nervosa. The care of these people requires a comprehensive array of approaches to provide the best chance of treatment success.

4. Couturier J, Lock J: What is recovery in adolescent anorexia nervosa? *International Journal of Eating Disorders* 39:550, 2006.

   A range of definitions are used to define recovery from anorexia nervosa including percent ideal body weight, psychological recovery, and combinations of these variables. In this study of adolescents treated for anorexia nervosa, the recovery rates ranged from 57% to 94% depending on the definition used. Mean time to remission for weight ranged from 11 to 22 months. A consistent definition of recovery is needed that includes both weight and psychological symptoms.

5. Grassi A: Are polycystic ovary syndrome & eating disorders related? *Today's Dietitian* p. 32, October 2006.

   Polycystic ovary syndrome (PCOS) is a complex hormonal disorder and is the leading cause of infertility. The symptoms of polycystic ovary syndrome and certain eating disorders are similar. In addition, the symptoms of PCOS have a direct effect on body image and self-esteem and may lead to the development of eating disorders. This article discusses these relationships.

6. Jackson K: Eating disorders revealed. *Today's Dietitian* p. 37, March 2004.

   Eating disorders are often hard to recognize as individuals may hide the various practices. This article discusses the many characteristics of eating disorders that can be used in the diagnosis.

7. Jackson K: Exercise abuse: Too much of a good thing. *Today's Dietitian* p. 51, March 2005.

   Regularly performing an excessive amount of exercise has deleterious effects on the body, including the skeleton. This author discusses the problem of exercise abuse and reviews treatment options.

8. Kouba S and others: Pregnancy and neonatal outcomes in women with eating disorders. *Obstetrics and Gynecology* 105: 255, 2005.

   Pregnant women with past or ongoing eating disorders such as anorexia nervosa and bulimia nervosa have a greater risk for delivering infants with low birth weight. The authors suggest that these women receive careful medical follow up during pregnancy.

9. Lamberg L: Advances in eating disorders offer food for thought. *Journal of the American Medical Association* 290:1437, 2003.

   The latest research shows that genetic background provides a major risk factor for the development of eating disorders and is possibly implicated in 50% to 80% of cases. The current thinking is that today's societal emphasis on thinness brings out the genetic propensity in certain individuals to develop an eating disorder.

10. Lundgren JD and others: Prevalence of the night eating syndrome in a psychiatric population. *American Journal of Psychiatry* 163 (1):156, 2006.

    The night eating syndrome is a pattern of disordered eating characterized by evening hyperphagia (eating more than one-third of total daily calories after the evening meal) and nocturnal awakening with ingestion of food. The results of this study show that night eating syndrome is a common disorder among psychiatric outpatients and is associated with substance use and obesity.

11. Mehler PS: Bulimia nervosa. *The New England Journal of Medicine* 349:875, 2003.

    The combination of cognitive behavior therapy and antidepressant medications provides the best hope for treatment of bulimia nervosa. Nutritional counseling also has a role, such as addressing concerns about specific "forbidden" foods.

12. Miller KK and others: Medical findings in out-patients with anorexia nervosa. *Archives of Internal Medicine* 165: 561, 2005.

    Medical problems are typically seen in people with anorexia nervosa. Examples are lowered immune system status and bone loss with related history of bone fractures.

13. Mond JM and others: An update on the definition of "excessive exercise" in eating disorders research. *International Journal of Eating Disorders* 39:147, 2006.

    The relationship between exercise behavior and eating-disordered behavior was studied in 3,472 women aged 18–42 years who exercised regularly. The results of the study indicated that exercise was excessive when its postponement was followed by intense guilt and when it was undertaken solely to influence weight or shape.

Women who reported these exercise characteristics had significantly greater levels of eating disorder psychopathology. Therefore these variables could be a useful indicator of eating disorders.

14. Norris ML and others: Ana and the Internet: A review of pro-anorexia websites. *International Journal of Eating Disorders* 39:443, 2006.

    Searching for "anorexia" using common search engines results in hundreds of links, many of which are "pro-anorexia." These websites provide information that is supportive of anorexia nervosa but is largely controversial and dangerous. This study was conducted to identify key characteristics of pro-anorexia websites. Themes that were most common were control, success, and perfection. Photo galleries are prevalent that serve as motivators for weight loss. It is important that health care providers and caregivers be aware of these websites and their content.

15. Pritts SD, Susman J: Diagnosis of eating disorders in primary care. *American Family Physician* 67:297, 2003.

    Eating disorders can lead to devastating medical and psychological consequences. Treatment, as outlined in this article, needs to be instituted as soon as possible to improve chances of a successful outcome.

16. Ringham R and others: Eating disorder symptomatology among ballet dancers. *International Journal of Eating Disorders* 39:503, 2006.

    Ballet dancers are at high risk of developing eating disorders. In this study, 29 female ballet dancers were compared to women with anorexia nervosa, bulimia nervosa, and not eating pathology. The results showed that the eating patterns of dancers were more similar to eating-disordered individuals than to control individuals. The majority of the dancers (83%) met lifetime criteria for eating disorders.

17. Shanta-Retelny V: Binge eating into obesity. *Today's Dietitian* p. 34, May 2004.

    Binge-eating disorder is a common problem in people seeking therapy for obesity. The combination of cognitive behavior therapy and certain psychiatric and antiseizure medications currently provides the greatest likelihood for successful therapy. Not skipping meals is a key part of the nutrition therapy.

18. Spear BA: Does dieting increase the risk for obesity and eating disorders? *Journal of the American Dietetic Association* 106:523, 2006.

    This editorial summarizes the results of recent studies on dieting and other unhealthful weight control methods in adolescents that appear to predict and be associated with later weight gain, overweight, and eating disorders.

19. Wolfe BE: Reproductive health in women with eating disorders. *Journal of Obstetric, Gynecologic, and Neonatal Nursing* 34:255, 2005.

    Medical complications from eating disorders include symptoms associated with reproductive health. This review discusses the reproductive health issues that may occur in women with anorexia nervosa and bulimia nervosa as well as the clinical implications.

20. Yager J, Andersen AA: Anorexia nervosa. *The New England Journal of Medicine* 353:1481, 2005.

    Excellent review of eating disorders by noted experts. Both diagnosis and treatment are highlighted.

▶ Check out the **Contemporary Nutrition ARIS site**

www.mhhe.com/wardlawcontfa1 for quizzes, flash cards, other activities, and weblinks designed to further help you learn about what you eat and why.

RATE YOUR PLATE

I. Assessing Risk of Developing an Eating Disorder

British investigators have developed a five-question screening tool called the **SCOFF** Questionnaire for recognizing eating disorders:[†]

1. Do you make yourself **S**ick because you feel full?
2. Do you lose **C**ontrol over how much you eat?
3. Have you lost more than **O**ne stone (about 13 pounds) recently?
4. Do you believe yourself to be **F**at when others say you are thin?
5. Does **F**ood dominate your life?

Two or more positive responses suggest an eating disorder.

1. After completing this questionnaire, do you feel that you might have an eating disorder or the potential to develop one?

   _____

   _____

2. Do you think any of your friends might have an eating disorder?

   _____

   _____

3. What counseling and education resources exist in your area or on your campus to help with a potential eating disorder?

   _____

   _____

4. If a friend has an eating disorder, what do you think is the best way to assist him or her in getting help?

   _____

   _____

[†]Morgan JF and others: The SCOFF Questionnaire, *British Medical Journal* 319:1467, 1999.

II. Helping Prevent Eating Disorders

You have been asked to speak to a junior high school class about eating disorders. What are four major points that you would make to help prevent disordered eating in this population?

1. _____
2. _____
3. _____
4. _____

Here are points you may consider:

1. Extreme thinness is oversold in the media. Extremely low weight (i.e., BMI of less than 17.5) is generally not healthy.
2. Self-induced vomiting is dangerous. Damage to the teeth, stomach, and esophagus often results.
3. Loss of menstrual periods is a sign of illness. It is important to see a physician about this. Bone deterioration is a common result.
4. The treatment of eating disorders in early phases aids success. These diseases are difficult to treat once firmly established.

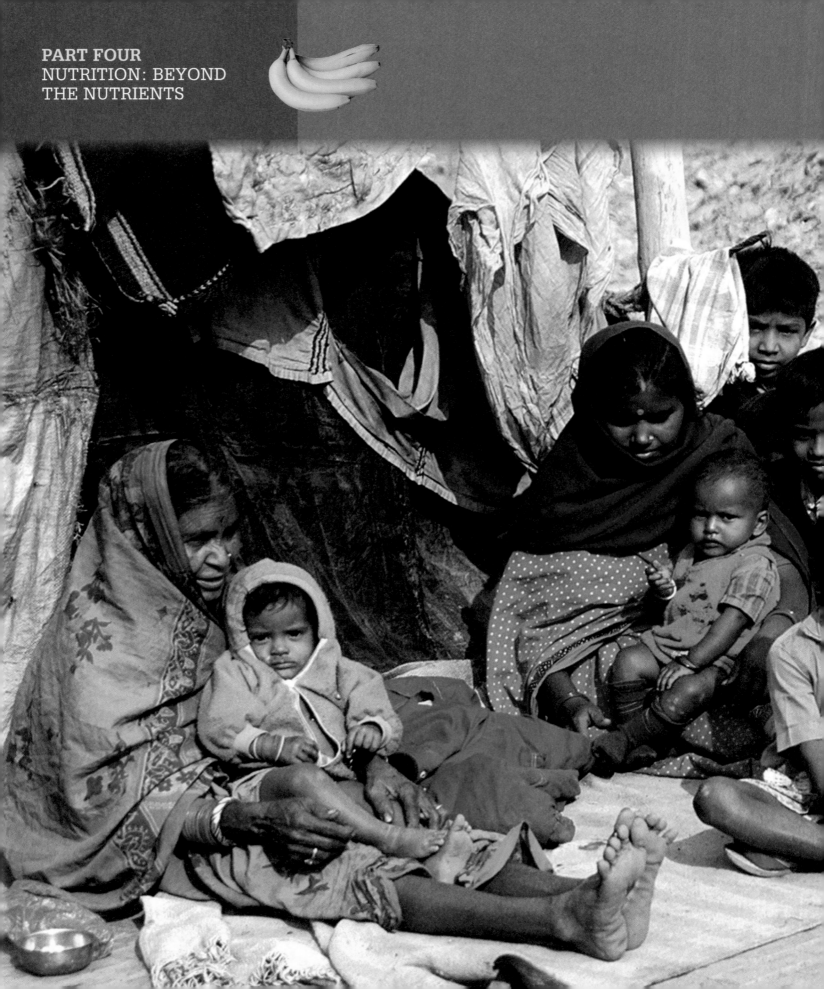

CHAPTER 14 Undernutrition Throughout the World

CHAPTER OBJECTIVES Chapter 14 is designed to allow you to:

1. Define and characterize the terms *hunger, malnutrition,* and *undernutrition.*
2. Evaluate the consequences of undernutrition during critical periods in a person's life.
3. Examine undernutrition in the United States and highlight several programs established to combat this problem.
4. Examine undernutrition in the developing world and evaluate the major obstacles that hinder a solution.
5. Outline some possible solutions to undernutrition in the developing world.
6. List the worldwide effects of AIDS.
7. Consider how biotechnology may help solve the food shortage/distribution problem in the developing world.

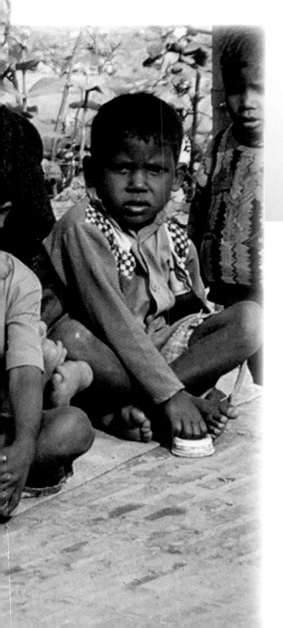

CHAPTER OUTLINE

Chapter Objectives

Refresh Your Memory

World Hunger: A Continuing Plague

World Hunger Today

Undernutrition in the United States

Undernutrition in the Developing World

The Role of Biotechnology in Expanding Worldwide Food Availability

The New Biotechnology

Role of the New Biotechnology in the Developing World

Some Concluding Thoughts

Nutrition and Your Health: Undernutrition at Critical Life Stages

Case Study: Undernutrition During Childhood

Summary/Study Questions/Check Your Knowledge/Further Readings

Rate Your Plate

THE IMAGES ARE VIVID AND APPALLING. Emaciated children with haunting eyes and distended stomachs who are too weak to cry, stare at us from news photos and television screens. Nearly 12 million children under age 5 die each year in developing countries; 55% of the deaths are attributable to undernutrition.

Today, nearly one in six people worldwide is chronically undernourished—too hungry to lead a productive, active life. Over the past 10 years, this problem has worsened. Throughout the world, the problems of poverty and undernutrition are widespread and growing—even though there is enough food available to sufficiently feed all of us.

The majority (two-thirds) of undernourished people live in Asia. However, the largest increase in numbers of chronically hungry people have recently occurred in eastern Africa, particularly in Ethiopia, Sudan, Rwanda, Burundi, Sierra Leone, Kenya, Somalia, Eritrea, and Tanzania.

Chapter 14 examines the problem of undernutrition, the conditions that create it, and some possible solutions. If we are to eradicate undernutrition, we all have to understand the problem and, as the comic in the chapter suggests, assume responsibility for supplying solutions. It is important to recognize that many political, economic, and social factors worldwide contribute directly and indirectly to the hunger problem.

 Refresh Your Memory

As you begin your study of world hunger in Chapter 14, you may want to review:

- The health effects of protein-calorie malnutrition in Chapter 6
- The role of vitamin A and rich food sources in Chapter 9
- The roles and rich food sources of iron, zinc, and iodide in Chapter 11

▲ Every year, crises that develop worldwide put many people at risk of undernutrition.

WORLD HUNGER: A CONTINUING PLAGUE

In November 1974, the United Nations World Food Conference proclaimed its bold objective "that within a decade no child will go to bed hungry, that no family will fear for its next day's bread, and that no human being's future and capacities will be stunted by malnutrition." Today, this promise remains unfulfilled: Uncertainty regarding the source of one's next meal remains a daily experience for one in six people in the developing world (800 million to 1.1 billion) and one in ten households in North America.

We must face the reality that the United Nations' members have yet to meet their current pledge to elevate 3 billion people (half of the world's population) out of poverty (living on less than $2 per day). We also have to consider that 45% of the world's income currently goes to the 12% of the world's people who live in rich industrial nations such as the United States and Canada.

Millions of people worldwide die each year from health problems related to undernutrition. War and environmental catastrophe combine with the global threat of AIDS as important causes. Why must we act today to stem this tide of undernutrition? Why is Ziggy's concern an important one? Chapter 14 provides some answers.

WORLD HUNGER TODAY

Let's begin our look at the problem of world hunger and malnutrition today by defining some key terms.

Hunger is the physiological state that results when not enough food is eaten to meet energy needs. It also describes an uneasiness, a discomfort, a weakness, or a pain caused by lack of food. The medical and social costs of the undernutrition that can result from hunger are high—preterm births, mental disabilities, inadequate growth and development in childhood, poor school performance, decreased work output in adulthood, and chronic disease (Table 14-1). Although malnutrition does occur in North America, it is not due to extreme poverty over a large section of the population. Instead, there are usually specific causes such as an eating disorder, alcoholism, problems in nursing home settings, or homelessness. There is also some degree of moderate malnutrition in some of the poorer segments of North American society (i.e., those earning less than the current poverty level). Fortunately, there are resources

hunger The primarily physiological (internal) drive to find and eat food.

acquired immune deficiency syndrome (AIDS) A disorder in which a virus (human immunodeficiency virus [HIV]) infects specific types of immune system cells. This leaves the person with reduced immune function and, in turn, defenseless against numerous infectious agents; typically contributes to the person's death.

TABLE 14-1 The Realities of Worldwide Undernutrition

- Nearly one in six people worldwide is chronically undernourished—too hungry to lead a productive, active life. This includes one-third of the world's children.

- About 55,000 people die of hunger each day—two-thirds of them are children.

- About 2 billion people in the world suffer from a micronutrient deficiency.

- About 1 billion people in the world have iron deficiency. The same is true for zinc deficiencies.

- Up to 500,000 children are permanently blinded each year simply from lack of vitamin A. About 100 million to 140 million children are deficient in vitamin A.

- About 50 million people worldwide have developed brain damage from maternal iodide deficiency; currently, 2 billion people are at risk for iodide deficiency.

- Residents in developed countries spend more money on pet food, perfumes, and cosmetics than it would take to provide basic education, water, sanitation, health care, and nutrition for all those now deprived of it.

- Every day the world produces enough food to provide about 2400 kcal for each person, generally meeting average calorie needs. A daily intake less than 2100 kcal would not likely sustain an older child or adult, depending on workload.

- Poor women in developing countries face a 50- to 200-fold increased risk of death in pregnancy, compared with women in North America.

- In many developing countries, life expectancy of the population is one-half to two-thirds that of North Americans.

- Almost half of the world's people earn less than $200 a year—many use 80% to 90% of that income to obtain food. About $2000 to $3000 of income each year is needed for a person to reach the life expectancy seen in North America.

- Of the 6.2 billion people in the world, about 1.1 billion drink contaminated water. In India alone, 300,000 children die each year from drinking polluted water.

- About 2 billion people in the world live without proper sanitation, such as reliable toilet facilities.

- Developing countries have 95% of the **acquired immune deficiency syndrome (AIDS)** cases worldwide.

- Developing countries bear 93% of the world's disease burden but use only 11% of the world's health care resources.

food insecurity A condition of anxiety regarding running out of either food or money to buy more food.

malnutrition Failing health that results from longstanding dietary practices that do not coincide with nutritional needs.

undernutrition Failing health that results from a longstanding dietary intake that is not enough to meet nutritional needs.

famine An extreme shortage of food, which leads to massive starvation in a population; often associated with crop failures, war, and political unrest.

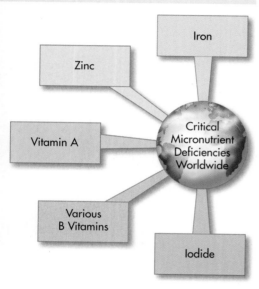

FIGURE 14-1 ▶ Critical micronutrient deficiencies worldwide.

▶ Blood loss caused by intestinal and blood-borne parasite infections is another common cause of anemia among poor populations, especially when people do not wear shoes. Parasites, such as hookworms, can easily penetrate the soles of the feet and legs and enter the bloodstream. Although hookworm disease has been largely eradicated through improved sanitation in the United States and other industrialized nations, it continues to plague more than one-eighth of the world's population, mostly in tropical regions.

▶ The Irish potato famine of 1840 to 1850 caused an estimated 2 million deaths and resulted in nearly as many people emigrating to other countries, such as the United States and Canada. More than 3 million people may have perished in the great famine of 1943 in Bengal, India. In 1974, another 1.5 million starved in the country of Bangladesh. China suffered a famine from 1959 to 1961—estimates of mortality range from 16 million to 64 million.

such as food banks and food stamps, though sometimes there are bureaucratic obstacles to getting these resources to the people who need them. In addition, there is also a problem known as **food insecurity** which describes a state of anxiety about running out of food or running out of money to buy more food. In 2002, over 11% of households in the United States reported that they experienced food insecurity. Of these, 3% reported that they experienced hunger at least one time during that year. Food insecurity is also a problem in Canada.

According to UNICEF (United Nations Children's Fund), the United States ranks eleventh out of sixteen industrialized countries for child poverty. Fortunately, the United States does have food assistance programs for low-income families, and therefore most children in the United States are shielded from hunger.

Malnutrition is a condition of impaired development or function caused by either a long-term deficiency or excess in calorie and/or nutrient intake. When food supplies are low and the population is large, **undernutrition** is common, leading to nutritional deficiency diseases, such as goiter (from an iodide deficiency) and xerophthalmia (eye problems caused by poor vitamin A intake). However, when the food supply is ample or overabundant, incorrect food choices coupled with an excessive intake can lead to overnutrition-related chronic diseases, such as type 2 diabetes.

Undernutrition is the most common form of malnutrition among the poor in both developing and developed countries. About half of the 4 million African children under 5 years of age who die annually are undernourished. Undernutrition is also the primary cause of specific nutrient deficiencies that can result in muscle wasting, blindness, scurvy, pellagra, beriberi, anemia, rickets, goiter, and a host of other problems (Table 14-2).

The most critical micronutrients missing from diets worldwide (see Fig. 14-1) are iron, vitamin A, iodide, zinc, and various B vitamins (e.g., folate), as well as selenium and vitamin C. About 1 billion people, mostly in the developing world, are affected by iron deficiency. The same is true for zinc deficiencies. With poor iron status, cognitive development will likely be impaired, particularly if prolonged deficiency occurs during early infancy. An estimated 50 million people worldwide also suffer brain damage from preventable maternal iodide deficiency. Although severe vitamin A deficiency, which causes blindness, is on the decline, up to 500,000 preschool-age children are still blinded by it each year. UNICEF reports that the lives of 1 million to 3 million children could be saved annually in the developing world if vitamin A supplements were provided a few times each year. The annual cost per child would be about 6 cents.

Of the 6.2 billion people in the world, about 2 billion may experience episodes of food shortages and be affected by some form of micronutrient malnutrition. Death and disease from infections, particularly those causing acute and prolonged diarrhea or respiratory disease, increase dramatically when the infections occur during a state of chronic undernutrition. Chronic undernutrition leaves many people in the developing world in a continual state of depressed immune function, in turn greatly increasing the risk of death, especially in childhood.

Protein-calorie malnutrition (PCM) is a form of undernutrition caused by an extremely deficient intake of calories or protein generally accompanied by an illness. The dramatic results of PCM—kwashiorkor and marasmus—were described in Chapter 6. This chapter focuses on the more subtle effects of a chronic lack of food.

Famine is the extreme form of chronic hunger. Periods of famine are characterized by large-scale loss of life, social disruption, and economic chaos that slows food production. As a result of these extreme events, the affected community experiences a downward spiral characterized by human distress; sales of land, livestock, and other farm assets; migration; division and impoverishment of the poorest families; crime; and the weakening of customary moral codes, as seen in Sudan and Rwanda. In the midst of all this, undernutrition rates soar; infectious diseases, such as cholera, spread; and many people die.

Special efforts are needed to eradicate the fundamental causes of famine. Causes vary by region and decade, but the most common is crop failure. The most obvious reasons for crop failure are bad weather, war, and civil strife. War deserves a special focus and will be specifically addressed in a separate section on war and political/civil unrest.

TABLE 14-2 Nutrient-Deficiency Diseases That Commonly Accompany Undernutrition

Disease and Key Nutrient Involved	Typical Effects	Foods Rich in Deficient Nutrient	Target Populations for Intervention
Xerophthalmia Vitamin A	Blindness from chronic eye infections, restricted growth, dryness and keratinization of epithelial tissues	Liver, fortified milk, sweet potatoes, spinach, greens, carrots, cantaloupe, apricots	Asia, Africa
Rickets Vitamin D	Poorly calcified bones, bowed legs, other bone deformities	Fortified milk, fish oils, sun exposure	Asia, Africa, and parts of the world where religious dress codes prevent women and children from receiving adequate sun exposure; older adults in developed nations
Beriberi Thiamin	Nerve degeneration, altered muscle coordination, cardiovascular problems	Sunflower seeds, pork, whole and enriched grains, dried beans	Victims of famine in Africa
Ariboflavinosis Riboflavin	Inflammation of tongue, mouth, face and oral cavity, nervous system disorders	Milk, mushrooms, spinach, liver, enriched grains	Victims of famine in Africa
Pellagra Niacin	Diarrhea, dermatitis, dementia	Mushrooms, bran, tuna, chicken, beef, peanuts, whole and enriched grains	Victims of famine in Africa, survivors of war-torn Eastern Europe
Megaloblastic anemia Folate	Enlarged red blood cells, fatigue, weakness	Green leafy vegetables, legumes, oranges, liver	Asia, Africa
Scurvy Vitamin C	Delayed wound healing, internal bleeding, abnormal formation of bones and teeth	Citrus fruits, strawberries, broccoli	Victims of famine in Africa
Iron-deficiency anemia Iron	Reduced work output, retarded growth, increased health risk in pregnancy	Meats, seafood, broccoli, peas, bran, whole-grain and enriched breads	Worldwide
Goiter Iodide	Enlarged thyroid gland in teenagers and adults, possible mental retardation, cretinism	Iodized salt, saltwater fish	South America, Eastern Europe, Africa

Although the nutrients are listed separately to illustrate the important role of each one, often two or more nutrition-deficiency diseases are found in an undernourished person in the developing world.

General Effects of Semistarvation

In the initial stages, the results of undernutrition from semistarvation are often so mild that physical symptoms are absent and blood tests do not usually detect the slight metabolic changes. Even in the absence of clinical symptoms, however, undernourishment may affect reproductive capacity, resistance to and recovery from disease, physical activity and work output, and lead to fatigue and behavior problems. Recall from Chapter 2 that, as tissues continue to be depleted of nutrients, blood tests eventually detect biochemical changes, such as a drop in blood hemoglobin concentration. Physical symptoms, such

▶ The effects of hunger are widespread:
- Reduced energy and strength
- Diminished concentration
- Impaired ability to learn
- Lowered productivity
- Worsening of chronic health conditions
- Increased susceptibility to infectious diseases
- Deterioration of mood
- Slowed recovery from illness and injury

FIGURE 14-2 ▶ The downward spiral of poverty and illness can ultimately end in death (based on World Food Program graphic).

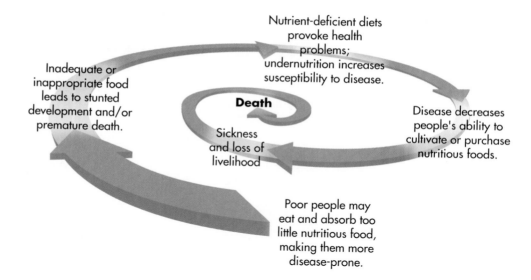

Nutrient-deficient diets provoke health problems; undernutrition increases susceptibility to disease.

Inadequate or inappropriate food leads to stunted development and/or premature death.

Death

Sickness and loss of livelihood

Disease decreases people's ability to cultivate or purchase nutritious foods.

Poor people may eat and absorb too little nutritious food, making them more disease-prone.

▶ In the 1940s a group of researchers led by Dr. Ansel Keys examined the general effects of undernutrition on adults. The researchers maintained 32 previously healthy men on a diet averaging about 1800 kcal daily for 6 months. During this time, the men lost an average of 24% of their body weight. After about 3 months, the participants complained of fatigue, muscle soreness, irritability, intolerance to cold, and hunger pains. They exhibited a lack of ambition, self-discipline, and concentration, and were often moody, apathetic, and depressed. Their heart rate and muscle tone decreased and they developed edema. When the men were permitted to eat normally again, feelings of recurrent hunger and fatigue persisted even after 12 weeks of rehabilitation. Full recovery required about 8 months. This study tells us a lot about the general state of undernourished adults worldwide.

as body weakness, appear with further depletion. Finally, the full-blown symptoms of the predominating deficiency are recognizable, such as when blindness accompanies a vitamin A deficiency.

When a few people in a population develop a severe deficiency, this may represent only the "tip of the iceberg." Typically, a much greater number have milder degrees of undernutrition. These deficiencies should not, therefore, be dismissed as trivial, especially in the developing world. It is becoming clear that combined deficiencies of specific vitamins and the minerals iron and zinc can seriously reduce work performance, even when they do not cause obvious physical symptoms. This resulting state of ill health, in turn, diminishes the ability of individuals, communities, and even whole countries to perform at peak levels of physical and mental capacity (Fig. 14-2).

Added to their lack of nourishment, the inhabitants of poorer countries must also contend with recurrent infections, poor sanitation, extreme weather conditions, and regular exposure to infectious diseases. They require greater amounts of certain nutrients—especially iron—to combat rampant parasite and other infections. Deficiencies of both iron and zinc can lead to reduced immune function and thereby increase the risk of diseases, such as diarrhea and pneumonia.

CONCEPT CHECK

Hunger provokes uneasiness and pain when insufficient food is eaten to meet calorie needs. Food insecurity is anxiety about running out of food or money to buy more food. Chronic hunger leads to undernutrition, which can cause growth failure in children and physical weakness in adults. Risk of infection increases, and nutrient-deficiency diseases result. The primary cause of undernutrition is poverty. The critical periods for undernutrition occur during pregnancy, infancy, childhood, and old age. Chronic undernutrition decreases work performance, motivation, and immune function. The adverse effects in pregnancy and infancy are dramatic, as evidenced by mortality rates much higher than those of healthy populations. Irreversible developmental damage in surviving children is also common.

UNDERNUTRITION IN THE UNITED STATES

About 33 million (12%) people in the United States live at or below the poverty level, estimated at about $18,400 annually for a family of four (Table 14-3). Of those 33 million, 12 million (37%) are children.

TABLE 14-3 The Realities of Poverty and Undernutrition in the United States

- About 7% of infants born in the United States are low birth weight. This accounts for more than half of all infant deaths and for 75% of deaths of babies under 1 month of age.

- The infant mortality rate in the United States is higher than that of 26 other industrialized countries. Teenage pregnancy contributes to infant mortality in part because young mothers frequently don't meet their nutrient needs.

- Single-parent families constitute about 25% of all families with children. The poverty rate (40%) for the approximately 19 million children in such families is five times higher than that for children in two-parent families.

- About 33 million people in the United States live at or below the poverty level. These poor include about 16% of all children; children, in fact, comprise 37% of the poor. Hunger frequently accompanies poverty.

- A family of four in the United States at the bottom 20% of household income has an average income one-fifth of that of the average income of the top 20% of households.

- In the United States, an estimated 12 million people, or 6.5% of all adults, have experienced homelessness sometime during their lives. An episode of homelessness nearly always lasts for at least 1 week and often for a month or more.

- The Food Stamp Program for low-income people provides each household with $190 per month. About 1 person in 16 participates in this program.

- Second Harvest, the largest U.S. food bank, estimates that more than 23 million people, or more than 1 person in 10, rely on food depositories and soup kitchens to feed themselves and their families. Most of these people, the organization reports, are workers who have lost their jobs.

- Food thrown out in U.S. cafeterias, supermarkets, and restaurants could feed 49 million people per year.

Eight percent of Caucasians, 24% of African-Americans, and 23% of Hispanics live in poverty. Many Native Americans are also poor, as are 11% of Asian Americans. (Many Native Americans in Canada also live in poverty.)

The poor often face difficult choices: whether to buy groceries for the family or pay this month's rent; whether to have dental work done or pay the current utility bill; whether to replace clothes the children have outgrown or pay for transportation to apply for a job. Food is one of the few flexible items in a poor person's budget. Whereas housing and utility costs, medical care, and transportation fares are non-negotiable, a person can always eat less. The short-term consequences of eating less may be less dramatic than getting evicted, but the long-term cumulative effects are significant.

Helping the Hungry in the United States

Until the twentieth century, individuals and a wide variety of charitable, often church-related organizations, provided most of the help to poor, undernourished people in the United States. Early programs rarely distributed direct cash payments to poor people because these were thought to reduce recipients' motivation to improve their circumstances or change behaviors, such as excessive drinking, that contributed to their poverty. Beginning in the early 1900s, the involvement of local, county, and state governments in providing assistance to the poor has steadily increased.

After observing extensive hunger and poverty during his presidential campaign in the 1960s, John F. Kennedy revitalized the Food Stamp Program, which had begun two decades earlier, and expanded commodity distribution programs. Today the Food Stamp Program for low-income people allows recipients to use an Electronic Benefit Transfer (EBT) card to purchase food and garden seeds—but not tobacco, cleaning

▲ Food insecurity is part of the North American landscape. A "safety net" of programs exists, but it is "porous."

items, alcoholic beverages, and nonedible products—at stores authorized to accept them. Each participating household receives about $190 per month, on average. About 21 million people in the United States participate in this program (Table 14-4).

The U.S. Congress established the School Breakfast Program in 1965 as politicians became aware of the number of hungry children coming to school. School breakfast and lunch programs still enable low-income students—8.4 million for breakfast and 27 million for lunch—to receive meals free or at reduced cost if certain income guidelines are met (under $23,920 to $34,040, respectively, for annual income of a family of four). In the same year, the U.S. Congress funded group noontime (called *congregate*) meals and home-delivered meals for all citizens over 60 years of age, regardless of income (donations

TABLE 14-4 Some Current Federally Subsidized Programs That Supply Food for People in the United States

Program	Eligibility	Description
Food Stamp Program	Low-income families	Electronic Benefit Transfer (debit) cards are given to purchase food at grocery stores; the amount is based on size of household and income.
The Emergency Food Assistance Program (TEFAP)	Low-income families	Provides nutrition assistance to needy Americans through distribution of USDA food commodities.
Commodity Supplemental Food Program	Certain low-income populations, such as pregnant women, children until the age of 6 years, and seniors	USDA surplus foods are distributed by county agencies; not found in all states; may be based on nutritional risk.
Special Supplemental Nutrition Program for Women, Infants, and Children (WIC)	Low-income pregnant/lactating women, infants, and children less than 5 years old at nutritional risk	Coupons are given to purchase milk, cheese, fruit juice, cereal, infant formula, and other specific food items at grocery stores; includes nutrition education component.
National School Lunch Program	Low-income children of school age	Free or reduced-price lunch is distributed by the school; meal follows USDA pattern based on MyPyramid; cost for the child depends on family income. For students who do not participate in the lunch program, special milk program may be available.
School Breakfast Program	Low-income children of school age	Free or reduced-price breakfast is distributed by the school; meal follows USDA pattern; cost for the child depends on family income.
Child and Adult Care Food Program	Child enrolled in organized child-care program and seniors in adult-care programs; income guidelines are the same as those for the School Lunch Program	Reimbursement is given for meals supplied to children at the site; meals must follow USDA guidelines based on MyPyramid.
Congregate Meals for the Elderly	Age 60 or over (no income guidelines)	Free noon meal is furnished at a site; meal follows specific pattern based on one-third of nutrient needs.
Home-Delivered Meals	Age 60 or over, homebound	Noon meal is delivered at no cost or for a donation at least 5 days a week. Sometimes additional meals for later consumption are delivered at the same time; often referred to as "Meals on Wheels."
Summer Food Service Program	Residence in a low-income neighborhood or participation in a program	Free, nutritious meals and snacks are given to children in a low-income area at a central site, such as a school or a community center during long school vacations.
Food Distribution Program on Indian Reservations	Low-income American Indian and non-Indian households on reservations; members of federally recognized tribes	Alternative to Food Stamp Program, distribution of monthly food packages; includes nutrition education component.

are requested, however). Both remain active programs, serving about 1 million meals each day, but they still do not reach all who need help. In addition, in 1972, the Special Supplemental Nutrition Program for Women, Infants, and Children (WIC) was authorized. This program provides food vouchers and nutrition education to low-income pregnant and lactating women and their young children. It serves about 7.6 million people.

Between 1969 and 1971, some already large federal food programs were expanded and others were created. For example, the Food Stamp Program served only 2 million people in 1968, but by 1971 it was serving 11 million. The National School Lunch Program, which served only 2 million poor children before 1970, was serving 8 million children by 1971. Soon after, the School Breakfast Program, a pilot program for children living in impoverished areas, became available nationally.

Sometimes, severe undernutrition due to involuntary hunger does occur in the United States. More often, though, Americans experience periodic episodes of hunger and food insecurity. Unemployment, medical and housing expenses, and even occasional holiday shopping can cause a household to be hungry or food insecure.

Government food assistance programs are like a "safety net"—they are strong, yet porous. Privately funded programs have stepped in to add to state and federal efforts to combat hunger and related food insecurity in the United States. There are more than 150,000 charitable food providers (such as food banks and food pantries) helping to cope with this problem. They serve about 23 million Americans. Many low-income U.S. households rely on food pantries, and one survey found that slightly more than two of every three people requesting such emergency food assistance are members of families—children and their parents.

MAKING DECISIONS

Food Insecurity and Overweight?

Undernutrition in North America is a much more subtle problem than in developing countries. To the untrained eye, undernourished children may just seem skinny, when, in fact, their growth is being stunted by insufficient nutrients. More likely, though, children from food-insecure households are prone to be overweight. This may be the result of considerable reliance on convenience foods that provide mostly fat and sugar. Also, food-insecure families may buy candies and snack foods as treats when expensive toys and clothing aren't affordable.

The availability of cooking facilities affects nutrient intake among the poor. Without cooking facilities, people may buy expensive convenience foods that require no preparation. These are typically highly processed snack foods, which provide calories but are often lacking in nutrients.

Socioeconomic Factors Related to Undernutrition

In the United States, persistent hunger and food insecurity are largely associated with two interrelated conditions: poverty and homelessness. Thus, the economic, social, and political changes that lead to an increase in the number of poor or homeless people also tend to intensify the problem of undernutrition.

Poverty. Underemployment leads to poverty. An overabundance of unskilled manual laborers exists throughout North America. Many such people (and their families) suffer hardships when layoffs occur seasonally or because of changes in the economy. Contrary to common perceptions, the parents in most poor families are working—nearly two in three families contain at least one worker. Often, the jobs available to untrained adults are in the service sector, such as the food service and retail industries, which pay minimum wage and may not offer health and other benefits to employees. Even when one or

▲ Food pantries and soup kitchens are important sources of nutrients for a growing number of people in the United States. Consider volunteering some of your time to a local program.

both parents work at these low-paying jobs, their families may still be left with the choice of either paying rent or buying groceries.

Another primary factor contributing to poverty has been the dramatic increase in the number of single-parent families in the United States, the result of high rates of divorce and out-of-wedlock births. There are about 4 million single-parent families. The poverty rate (40%) for the approximately 19 million children in single-parent families is five times higher than the rate for children in two-parent families.

Homelessness. Homelessness is much more evident now than in 1980 as the economics of poverty and undernutrition has changed in an important way. The economic status of the working poor has declined because affordable housing is harder for them to find. Due to the nation's rising affluence, higher-income tenants have bid up the prices of the apartments in some cities beyond the financial resources of poorer tenants. The U.S. government considers housing costs, which include rent and utilities, to be affordable if they make up no more than 30% of a family's income. One U.S. government report stated that 1 in 8 low-income families pay more than half their incomes for housing or live in dilapidated units. These families, although not homeless, are likely to experience undernutrition without direct food assistance. Families with children account for about 43% of the homeless. An estimated 12 million people in the United States, or 1 in 15 of all adults, have experienced homelessness sometime during their lives. This statistic rises to about 1 in 7 when it includes people who have moved into someone else's residence during periods when they had nowhere else to live. Moreover, the continuing changes in the economic circumstances they face could force such low-income families into homelessness, at least temporarily.

Other important causes of homelessness include unemployment, personal crises, and widespread release of mentally ill patients from mental institutions in the 1980s. The abuse of alcohol and crack cocaine is another notable cause. Up to 85% of homeless people in large cities in the United States abuse alcohol or drugs or have a mental illness. Most people with such problems are unable to find and hold employment; without support from family or friends, they and their dependents will probably become homeless.

Possible Solutions to Poverty and Hunger in the United States

Few would dispute the importance of supporting physically and mentally challenged adults and the multitude of poor children in the United States. The debate begins when able-bodied adults are receiving public aid. Many of these people have extenuating circumstances or have dug such a deep financial hole for themselves that it is difficult to get out. The United States has enough resources to feed every citizen; government-funded food assistance programs have helped to alleviate some problems of undernutrition in the United States. The question is, *Can government programs provide a permanent solution to poverty and undernutrition . . . and should they?*

Private emergency food network systems are also important to consider, but are not sufficient to meet all food needs in the United States. Furthermore, most of the donated items are limited in nutritional value. By necessity, processed and canned grocery items predominate, rather than fresh or frozen fruits and vegetables, or protein-rich foods such as milk.

Some observers believe that publicly–funded assistance programs have self-propagated—that they provide an incentive for poor, single women to have more children, because more children entitle a family to more benefits. New welfare reform laws have addressed this issue by requiring able-bodied adults to get jobs and by limiting future direct support to 5 years in a lifetime. It is up to each state to determine how to implement this work requirement and establish exceptions for certain situations, as in the case of disability, short-term downturns in the economy, or other overwhelming hardships.

▲ Homelessness can be the result of many problems, including poverty.

Many states are improving child care, teaching parenting skills, and expanding job opportunities as they help people end their dependence on welfare payments. Nation-wide, the number of people on welfare has fallen 60% since 1992, but the number has stabilized, and in some states has increased slightly.

Despite even the highest motivation, the outlook is bleak for many people who attempt to gain independence from assistance programs. Teen pregnancy may have cut short the education or vocational training of one or both parents, thwarting efforts to earn adequate income. Often, the expense of reliable and safe child care far exceeds the meager income from a minimum-wage job. Illness of either the parents or children may prevent the adults from holding steady employment. Poor communication skills, inability to relocate, and a lack of economic reserves also complicate financial independence. Regardless of how wasteful government assistance appears to some people, it will probably always be necessary to some extent.

Many in the United States consider an increase in individual responsibility as a critical goal. Government programs cannot easily fix poverty and the resulting hunger that stem from irresponsible individual behavior. Government programs can, however, help reduce or prevent the poverty that results largely from lack of education or opportunity.

Long-term undernutrition—especially among children—has both individual and societal consequences, so everyone in the United States is affected by this problem, either directly or indirectly. The next few years are likely to bring further changes in both government and private assistance programs, demanding new initiatives. As the welfare system is further reformed and government programs are redesigned, it is likely that some will suffer. The hope is that these new approaches will lead to long-term progress and the eventual relief of poverty and hunger.

▶ One goal of *Healthy People 2010* is to increase food security among U.S. households from the current 88% to 94%. Another is to reduce growth retardation to 5% among low-income children under age 5.

CONCEPT CHECK

In response to reports of widespread poverty and hunger during the 1960s, the U.S. Congress established several food assistance programs and substantially increased funding for already existing programs. Largely as a result of these federal programs, undernutrition had decreased substantially by the mid-1970s. The presence of poverty, homelessness, and undernutrition is influenced by economic, cultural, and individual factors, as well as government policies. The serious questions about the long-term effectiveness of many government assistance programs are causing major changes in their program design. All citizens can help reduce the problem of undernutrition.

UNDERNUTRITION IN THE DEVELOPING WORLD

Undernutrition in the developing world is also tied to poverty, and any true solution must address this problem. However, these countries have a multitude of problems so complex and interrelated that they cannot be treated separately. Programs that have proved immensely helpful in the United States (and throughout the rest of North America) are only a starting point in this context. The following major obstacles challenge those seeking a solution:

- Extreme imbalances in the food/population ratio in different regions of a country
- War and political/civil unrest, especially in Africa
- The rapid depletion of natural resources, such as farmland, fish, and water
- The disease AIDS, especially in sub-Saharan Africa and Asia
- High external (foreign) debt, much of which is owed to developed nations
- Poor **infrastructure,** especially poor housing, sanitation and storage facilities, education, communications, and transportation systems

Each problem deserves individual consideration (Fig. 14-3).

infrastructure The basic framework of a system of organization. For a society, this includes roads, bridges, telephones, and other basic technologies.

FIGURE 14-3 ▶ Many factors contribute to undernutrition in the developing world. Any solutions to the problem must take these factors into consideration.

▲ Poverty aggravates the problem of hunger in the developing world.

Food/Population Ratio

The world has 6.2 billion inhabitants. Population growth exceeds economic growth in much of the developing world, and as a result, poverty is increasing. This disrupts the balance in the food/population ratio, tipping it toward food shortages. If we want to ensure a decent life for a widening segment of humanity, many experts suggest that the growth in the earth's most vulnerable populations should slow. If not, by 2050 the world may have 1 to 3 billion more people than it does today—most of them in countries where the average person earns less than $2 per day. In Africa's poorest countries, nearly 65% of people live on less than $1 per day. Unless a catastrophe occurs, more than 9 of 10 infants in the next generation will be born in the poorest parts of the world.

More than three-quarters of people in the world live in developing countries, and more than half live in Asia. A United Nations report on worldwide hunger revealed that almost two-thirds of the world's undernourished live in Asia and the Pacific Rim. The world's food supplies also are not distributed equally among consumers. Gross disparities exist between developed and developing countries, among the rich and the poor within countries, and even within families (males may be fed before females).

Still, economists estimate that world food production will continue to increase more rapidly than the world population in the near future, allowing the food/population ratio to increase through the year 2020. This will come at a high cost, however, in terms of the water, fertilizer, and pesticides needed to allow for this production. Overall, in the short run, the primary problem appears not to be food production *but* distribution and use, especially in poverty-stricken areas of developing nations.

Eventually, though, food production will begin to lag behind population growth. Most good farmland in the world is already in use, and because of poor farming practices or competing land-use demands, the number of farmable acres worldwide decreases annually. For many reasons, sustainable world food output—an amount that doesn't deplete the earth's resources—is now running well behind food consumption. This discrepancy suggests that food production in less-developed countries will barely keep up with population growth and will soon lag behind.

Birth control programs, an obvious brake on population expansion, have been effective in developed countries but relatively ineffective in many developing countries that could really benefit from them. Among women, family planning and contraceptive use worldwide has increased to 60% today, up from 10% in 1969. If the United Nations, voluntary organizations, and governments had not started promoting family planning and contraceptive use, the population today might be as high as 7 or

8 billion. However, women (and men) in many developing countries are still lacking adequate access to contraceptives. Organizations such as Population Services International are trying to keep distribution costs low and make the products available to as many people as possible by subsidizing condoms and oral contraceptives to areas such as Bangladesh.

MAKING DECISIONS

Benefits of Breastfeeding

Promoting breastfeeding also contributes to the goal of birth control. Although it is not a completely reliable method of contraception, exclusively breastfeeding an infant lessens ovulation, thereby lowering the likelihood of fertilization, for an average of six months. (Women who do not breastfeed generally begin to ovulate within a month or so after giving birth.) When childbirths are more widely spaced, not only do fewer total births occur, but the mother has a longer chance to recover from pregnancy, and the infant receives feeding priority for a longer time. One possible exception to the healthful nature of breastfeeding occurs, however, when mothers are infected with the **human immunodeficiency virus (HIV).** The risk of transferring the virus through human milk is about 10%. Depending on the circumstances, this may outweigh the benefits of breastfeeding.

human immunodeficiency virus (HIV) The virus that leads to acquired immune deficiency syndrome (AIDS).

Experience with family planning programs in developing countries and historical changes in birth rates in many developed countries suggest an important conclusion: Generally, only when people have enough to eat and are financially secure do they feel confident that having fewer children will still result in enough surviving sons and/or daughters to provide for their care in later years. Increasing per capita income and improving education, especially for women in developing nations, are considered to be the most likely long-term solutions to excessive population growth. In the last few years, this effort has led to a decline in family size in Brazil, Egypt, India, and Mexico. A major concern is whether there are enough resources worldwide to raise per capita income and provide enough education to slow population growth.

CONCEPT CHECK

World food production is sufficient to meet the calorie needs of the world's population. Despite these adequate food resources, undernutrition continues to exist because of poverty, politics, and unequal food distribution. In addition, projected population growth may soon overwhelm food production. Most scientists and world leaders recommend limiting population growth, especially in developing countries where birth rates are high.

▲ Lasting gains have come slowly in the world's battle against undernutrition.

War and Political/Civil Unrest

The Millennium Summit of the United Nations pledged to "spare no effort to free our peoples from the scourge of war." Against that background stands the reality that worldwide military spending has doubled over the past 20 years. In the twentieth century, deadly weapons of war took an enormous toll on civilians living in poor, politically vulnerable, war-torn nations. Although Africa has been ravaged by economic decay and famine for years, military spending in Africa more than doubled in the 1970s and held firm through the 1990s. Less than one-half of 1% of the world's yearly production of goods and services is devoted to economic development assistance, whereas approximately 6% goes to military expenditures.

Aside from the economic impact of military spending, civil disruptions and wars are setting back the progress of the poor and contributing to massive undernutrition. All but two of the major conflicts in 2000 took place in the developing world. War-related

▶ The conflicts in the Darfur region of Sudan have led to high rates of death and undernutrition among people displaced by war.

▲ Homes and infrastructure are often damaged during times of war and political unrest.

famine affects at least 20 million people in southern and northeastern Africa. The border war between Ethiopia and neighboring Eritrea has had a tremendous negative impact on food resources. A World Bank official stated that the food shortage in Ethiopia is a problem that will persist until political changes are made. Approximately 12.4 million people in Ethiopia, Eritrea, Djibouti, Kenya, Somalia, and Zimbabwe are at risk for food shortages. Other conflicts continue between Congo (formerly Zaire) and the Republic of Congo, as well as in Angola and Sudan, where millions have been put at risk of starvation. In the capitol of war-torn Iraq, Baghdad, child malnutrition nearly doubled between 2002 and 2003. Disruptions in infrastructure from bombing and looting limit the safety of water, and as a result, health officials have observed a 250% increase in cases of diarrhea. Furthermore, health facilities needed to cope with undernutrition and dehydration have been damaged and looted throughout Baghdad and the surrounding area. Overall, most people in war-torn areas are without sufficient shelter, clothing, food, or means of obtaining them. Worldwide, this entire problem is projected to worsen over the next 15 years.

Even when food is available, political divisions may impede its distribution to the point that undernutrition will plague many people for years. Especially during emergencies, programs designed to help the poor have been undermined by unstable administration, corruption, and political influence. During such political chaos, relief agencies are often caught between warring factions and those they are trying to help. This was the case in the mid-1990s in Zaire, where Rwandan refugee camps fell under the control of a militant group. The rebels controlled the food coming into the camps and would not allow relief agencies to do their work.

During the 1960s and 1970s, the problem of undernutrition in developing countries was perceived as a technical one: how to produce enough food for the growing world population. The problem is now seen as largely political: how to achieve cooperation among and within nations, so that gains in food production and infrastructure are not wiped out by war. The best answer lies in a combination of approaches—finding technical solutions to help with the problems of chronic hunger and poverty and resolving political crises that have pushed developing nations into a state of acute hunger and chaos.

Rapid Depletion of Natural Resources

As we quickly deplete the earth's resources, population control grows increasingly critical. Agriculture production is approaching its limits in many areas worldwide. Environmentally unsustainable farming methods are undermining food production, especially in developing countries.

green revolution This refers to increases in crop yields that accompanied the introduction of new agricultural technologies in less-developed countries, beginning in the 1960s. The key technologies were high-yielding, disease-resistant strains of rice, wheat, and corn; greater use of fertilizer and water; and improved cultivation practices.

The **green revolution** was a phenomenon that began in the 1960s when crop yields rose dramatically in some countries, such as the Philippines, India, and Mexico (countries in Africa did not benefit because climates were not compatible with the crops used). The increased use of fertilizers, irrigation, and the development of superior crops through careful plant breeding made this boost in agricultural production possible. Many of the technologies associated with the green revolution have now achieved their potential. Rice yields, for example, have not increased significantly since the release of superior varieties in 1966. (The green revolution was intended as a stopgap measure until world leaders could control population growth.)

Future gains in productivity may be much harder to accomplish because of the existence of less productive farmland. Until the introduction of another superior strain of rice or other grain, developing countries will not benefit greatly from recent, more modest breakthroughs in biotechnology (see the section on use of biotechnology).

Areas of the world that remain uncultivated or ungrazed are mostly too rocky, steep, infertile, dry, wet, or inaccessible to sustain farming. Nearly all irrigation water available worldwide is being used, and groundwater supplies are becoming depleted at rapid rates in many regions. An eventual water shortage is projected to increase war and civil unrest in arid areas of the world, such as Northern Africa and the Middle East. China, which has more than 20% of the world's irrigated land, is also plagued with a growing scarcity of fresh water. In the future, billions of people will face ongoing water shortages.

The prospects of obtaining substantially more food from the oceans are also poor. In recent years, the amount of fish caught worldwide has leveled off. Fish was once considered the poor person's protein, but this is not likely to continue because farming of fish does not come close to compensating for the degree of reduction in wild fish populations.

Clearly, we can exploit the earth's resources only so far—the world population probably cannot continue to expand as it does today without the potential for serious famine and death. The Food and Agriculture Organization (FAO) of the United Nations works on this principle: "The fight to ensure that all people have enough nutritious food to eat is worthy of our greatest efforts, but it must be fought with the full recognition that it cannot be won unless agricultural, fishery, and forestry production returns to the earth as much as—or more than—it takes." Thus, if food production is to keep up with the expanding population, immediate action is needed to protect the earth's already deteriorated environment from further destruction.

Inadequate Shelter and Sanitation

When people die from undernutrition in developing countries, other factors, such as inadequate shelter and sanitation, almost always contribute. Poor sanitation along with undernutrition particularly raises the risk of infection. For example, a 1994 plague in Surat (in northwest India), which killed almost 5000 people and sparked the panicked exodus of another half a million, was linked mainly to unsanitary housing conditions.

Inadequate and deteriorating shelters threaten the lives of more than 500 million people. Many of the 15 million annual deaths of children—half of them under 5 years old—in developing countries could be prevented by improving the standards of environmental hygiene. Urban populations of some developing countries are growing at an annual rate of 5% to 7%. Such a skewed population distribution will result in more poverty. The urban explosion is the result of both high birth rates and continuing migration of people to the cities from rural areas. People go to the cities to find employment and resources the countryside can no longer provide. Worldwide, 38% of people lived in urban areas in 1975. The figure is now about 50% and is expected to reach 70% by 2050. Nine of the world's 10 largest cities will be in poor countries 20 years from now. Twelve of the 15 most polluted cities are in Asia alone.

In developing countries, the poor make up most of the urban population, and their needs for housing and community services often go beyond available governmental resources. Most of these urban poor live in overcrowded, self-made shelters, which lack a safe and adequate water supply and are only partially served by public utilities. The shantytowns and ghettos of the developing world are often worse than the rural areas the people left behind. The urban poor need cash to purchase food, so they often subsist on diets even more meager than the homegrown rural fare. Making matters worse, haphazard shelters often lack facilities to protect food from spoilage or damage by insects and rodents. This inability to protect food supplies in some developing countries leads to the loss of as much as 40% of all perishable foods.

The shift from rural to urban life takes its greatest toll on infants and children. Infants are often weaned early from the breast to infant formula, partly because the mother must find employment and partly because she may be influenced by advertisements depicting images of sophisticated, formula-feeding women. Unfortunately, because infant formulas are relatively expensive, poor parents may try to conserve the formula by either overdiluting the mixture or using too little to meet the infant's needs. The water supply may not be safe, so the prepared formula is also likely to be contaminated with bacteria. Human milk, in contrast, is much more hygienic, readily available, and nutritious. It also provides infants with immunity to some ailments.

▲ The bounty of food enjoyed in North America relies on rich agricultural resources. Many developing countries do not have such resources to employ.

▶ In Brazil, migrants displaced by multinational land developers have flooded from the north and northeast into Rio de Janeiro and São Paulo, attracted by the prospect of jobs. There they have built shantytowns next to apartment towers and affluent suburbs, but the jobs do not materialize, and urban poverty replaces rural impoverishment.

▲ Inadequate sanitation facilities and the consumption of contaminated water cause the majority of all diseases. About 1 billion people in developing countries often lack access to a safe water supply.

▶ The Group of Eight most industrialized nations is planning to forgive some external debt owed by developing countries. $40 billion has been promised; this should be able to end the external debt of 18 countries, including some in Africa and South America. The debt repayment depends on the developing country's agreement to practice good governance and to use the money saved to support health care, education, and infrastructure improvements.

Promoting breastfeeding is important when it is safe for the infant (review the earlier discussion of AIDS, HIV, and breastfeeding).

Overall, the single most effective health advantage for people, wherever they live, is a safe and convenient water supply. Inadequate sanitation and the consumption of contaminated water cause 75% of all diseases and more than one-third of deaths in developing countries. The World Health Organization (WHO) estimates that 1.1 billion people, about one-sixth of all people, have an unsafe and inadequate water supply. In addition, up to 90% of the diseases seen in developing countries may be attributed to contaminated water.

Poor sanitation, another example of inadequate infrastructure in the developing world, creates a critical public health problem. Human feces, rotting garbage, and associated insect and rodent infestations are potent sources of disease organisms commonly seen in urban areas of the developing world. Two of the most dangerous substances encountered in routine daily living are human urine and feces. The inability to dispose of the massive numbers of dead people (and dead animals) resulting from civil wars causes additional sanitation problems. In some developing countries, diarrheal diseases account for as many as one-third of all deaths in children under 5 years of age. WHO estimates that even with improvements in housing, 2 billion people in the world still lack proper sanitation facilities.

High External Debt

Since the 1970s many developing countries have become trapped in a cycle of borrowing repeatedly from foreign countries and international banks. Servicing these external debts, which now total about $2.5 trillion, has brought several countries to the verge of economic collapse. About $6 billion is owed to the United States. The external debt of Latin America represents 45% of the region's gross regional output of goods and services.

Many African nations also carry large debt burdens—currently, $350 billion. This problem is made worse by drops in prices for the raw commodities they export, higher prices for imported oil, and embezzlement of funds by high-ranking officials. To make up the difference between export income and import expenses, countries have been forced to borrow millions of dollars from international banks. Although the African debts are much smaller in absolute terms than those of Brazil, Argentina, and Mexico, for example, the burden is greater when national incomes and export earnings are considered. Nearly half the money African nations earn from exports goes to paying off the continent's multibillion-dollar debt. Much of the rest goes to fund imports of machinery, concrete, trucks, and consumer goods from developed countries. This leaves little for domestic programs, necessitating cutbacks that translate into fewer resources to counter already widespread undernutrition.

CONCEPT CHECK

War and civil strife, along with a decline in the world's natural resources, contribute to the difficulty of ending undernutrition in many developing countries. In addition, substandard housing conditions, impure water, and inadequate sanitation worldwide increase the risk for infection and disease. Infection then combines with undernutrition to compromise further the health of impoverished people. Finally, many developing countries are burdened by extremely high external debts, which severely limit their ability to implement programs to reduce undernutrition.

The Impact of AIDS Worldwide

About 40 million people around the world are infected with the human immunodeficiency virus (HIV) or have gone on to develop acquired immune deficiency syndrome (AIDS) from the infection. The male to female ratio is about 1:1 but is now increasing faster in women than in men. About 20 million people worldwide have died from AIDS.

An individual can be infected with HIV through contact with bodily fluids including blood, semen, vaginal secretions, and human milk. Thus the virus can be transmitted through sexual contact; through blood-to-blood contact; as well as from a mother to an infant during pregnancy, delivery, or breastfeeding. The virus has a very limited ability to exist outside the body.

Once infected with HIV, the individual is said to be HIV-positive. If untreated, the viral disease progresses over the next few years, and the individual develops symptoms of opportunistic infections such as diarrhea, lung disease, weight loss, and a form of cancer. Once the individual has developed these symptoms, they are said to have AIDS. Without treatment, an individual will likely die from AIDS within 4 to 5 years.

In Africa, particularly sub-Saharan countries, HIV is rampant throughout the entire population, both in men and women (Fig. 14-4). This region contains over 60% of the world's HIV-positive people. In most areas of sub-Saharan Africa, AIDS is reducing life expectancy by one-half, especially if the person also has tuberculosis. In many countries, AIDS is also creating orphans, with an estimated 12 million in Africa alone.

North America also has an AIDS problem. In the United States, it is estimated that about 1.2 million people (1 in every 280 persons) are infected with HIV, many of whom are unaware of their infections. (Reports show 1 in every 100 persons in New York City is infected with HIV.) About 530,000 people in the United States have died from the disease since it surfaced in the early 1980s, and each year about 50,000 new cases are reported. HIV affects a greater percentage of minority populations in the United States.

The face of AIDS is quickly becoming the face of a child. In 2006 there were 530,000 new cases of HIV in children under 15 years, and about 380,000 deaths of children worldwide were linked to AIDS.

Although no vaccine is available to prevent AIDS, the latest antiviral drugs can significantly slow the progression of the disease. However, there are many barriers to the use of these drugs in the developing world. For example, the newest therapies require a person to take at least three different drugs in the form of about 14 pills each day. A few missed doses can significantly reduce the effectiveness of the drugs and result in faster disease progression. Another barrier is economic: a typical drug regimen can cost approximately $14,000 per year, not including unforeseen hospital stays. Certain drug companies and governments are working to lower the cost of AIDS drugs for developing nations. Still, in most cases, the drugs will remain out of reach to those who need them. It has been suggested that developed nations should step in and cover

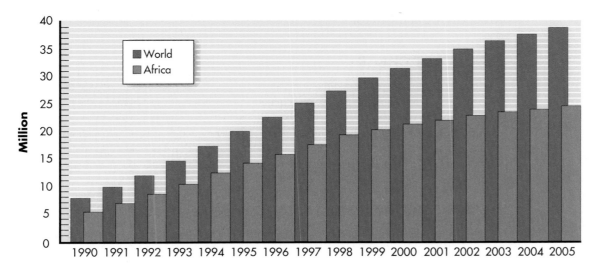

FIGURE 14-4 ▶ The number of cases of HIV has risen from around 8 million in 1990 to about 40 million today. Over 60% of people living with HIV are in sub-Saharan Africa.

Source: UNAIDS/WHO AIDS Epidemic Update, December 2006

most or all of the costs. The United Nations is spearheading an effort to raise the $8 to $10 billion needed to fight the disease.

MAKING DECISIONS

Nutrition and AIDS

Can eating a balanced diet prevent AIDS? The answer, unfortunately, is no. Healthy eating does not cure the disease, but it can help to lessen the impact of infections associated with AIDS. Poor nutritional status, such as a low status of vitamin A and vitamin E, contributes to a quicker onset of symptoms such as body wasting and fever, and a more rapid demise. This explains why daily use of a balanced vitamin and mineral supplement was shown to slow health declines in such people in one study. Overall, maintenance of nutritional status should be an integral part of the treatment for AIDS.

▲ A particularly sad consequence of AIDS in Africa is the number of AIDS orphans, children whose parents have both died of AIDS. The United Nations has estimated that there will be 20 million AIDS orphans in Africa by the year 2010.

The devastating effects of AIDS on our civilization have been rapid when measured by earth's scale of time. One study warns us that 57 countries risk major HIV outbreaks. Reported HIV cases are increasing rapidly in Africa, the Indian subcontinent, Southeast Asia, China, the Caribbean, Russia, and much of Eastern Europe. The main goal for addressing the problem of AIDS in the developing world is prevention of new cases through education regarding safer sex and the importance of clean needles, and other behavior-linked approaches. Providing AIDS drugs to pregnant women is also important. If a woman begins taking AIDS drugs such as zidovudine (AZT) by the fourteenth week of pregnancy, the risk of transferring the virus to her offspring is greatly reduced. Providing the drug immediately before birth also helps.

Behind the mind-boggling statistics on AIDS are less obvious costs to businesses, families, schools and universities, and society in general. For example, worker productivity will plummet because AIDS victims produce less and demand more, especially in the latter stages of the disease. Business productivity drops even further when relatives take time away from work and school to care for family members afflicted with AIDS. Furthermore, AIDS demands a considerable amount of family income. Hard-pressed families, who have to devote much of their income to doctors and medicines, have little left for living expenses. Other family members must struggle to keep up with daily duties because they must care for orphans left behind in the disease's wake. To learn more about AIDS, check out the website www.unaids.org.

CONCEPT CHECK

About 40 million people around the world are infected with the human immunodeficiency virus (HIV) or have gone on to develop acquired immunodeficiency syndrome (AIDS) from the infection. The virus can be transmitted through sexual contact; through blood-to-blood contact; or from a mother to a baby during pregnancy, delivery, and breastfeeding. Without treatment, an individual once infected will likely die from AIDS within 4 to 5 years. The main hope for addressing the problem of AIDS in the developing world is prevention of new cases.

Reducing Undernutrition in the Developing World

As you have probably guessed, greatly reducing undernutrition in the developing world will be complicated and will take considerable time to accomplish (Fig. 14-5). It is a common practice for the more affluent nations to supply famine areas with direct food aid. However, direct food aid is not a long-term solution. Although it reduces the number of deaths from famine, it can also reduce incentives for local production by driving down prices. In addition, the affected countries may have little or no means of transporting the food to those who need it most, and the donated foods may not be culturally acceptable.

In the short run, there is no choice—aid must be given because people are starving. Still, improving the infrastructure for poor people, especially rural people, needs to be the long-term focus. This future-minded approach is necessary because the most significant factor affecting the undernutrition of people in impoverished areas of the world is their reliance on outside sources for basic needs. Their dependence makes them constantly vulnerable.

Three basic approaches to counteract micronutrient deficiencies are suggested by the World Bank: increase diversity of the food supply; fortify specific foods with nutrients; and provide nutrient supplementation for individuals when necessary.

Development Tailored to Local Conditions Is Important. Recall that, in the past 40 years, world food supplies have grown faster than the population. Thus, the increase in undernutrition during this period has been caused by an increase in the number of people cut off from their share of this supply. Millions of farmers are losing access to resources they need to be self-reliant. There is a growing realization

FIGURE 14-5 ▶ Possible solutions to the puzzle of hunger in the developing world. Putting all the pieces together employs the action steps that contribute to meeting the overall goal.

▲ Food security is fostered by communities raising and distributing locally grown food.

CRITICAL THINKING

Stan has read about various relief efforts to help undernourished people in developing countries, especially the emergency food aid programs for famine-ravaged areas. Many of these efforts appear to be only temporary, and he wonders what long-range approaches might help alleviate the problem of undernutrition. What suggestions would you give Stan about possible long-term solutions for undernutrition in developing countries?

sustainable development Economic growth that will simultaneously reduce poverty, protect the environment, and preserve natural capital.

gender and development (GAD) approach Understanding the roles and responsibilities of both men and women in the process of sustainable development.

that unless economic opportunities can be created as part of a plan for sustainable development, rural people who own no land will flock to the overcrowded cities. In response, careful, small-scale regional development is one option.

For the most part, the solution lies in helping people meet their own needs and directing them to resources and employment opportunities, rather than giving them resources. Experience has shown that the provision of credit—along with training, food storage facilities, and marketing support—allows rural people to actively participate in their development, which will benefit their families and communities.

One U.S. program, the Peace Corps, has helped improve conditions in developing nations by providing education, distributing food and medical supplies, and building structures for local use. The aim of the Peace Corps is to help create independent, self-sustaining economies around the world.

Impoverished women are a special concern. In addition to working longer hours than men, they grow most of the food for family consumption and make up three-fourths of the labor force in the informal sector of the economy and an increasing proportion in the formal sector. Economic opportunities for women and education regarding family planning must be augmented. Of the 3 billion people in the world living on less than $2 a day, 70% are women. Moreover, among the developing world's 900 million illiterate people, women outnumber men 2 to 1. Thus, an important means of propelling nations out of poverty is to end the cycle of female neglect.

Suitable technologies for processing, preserving, marketing, and distributing nutritious local staples also need to be encouraged, so that small farmers can flourish. Education on how to use these foods to create healthful diets, such as preparing vitamin A-rich vegetables, adds further benefit. Supplementing indigenous foods with nutrients that are in short supply, such as iron, various B vitamins, zinc, and iodide, also deserves consideration. One program involves adding iron to sugar in various parts of the world. The next section examines the role of biotechnology in improving nutrient quality and other plant and animal characteristics, another possible positive step in lessening undernutrition. In addition, advances in water purification need to be employed.

Promoting extensive land ownership may also be one part of the solution. Increasing the availability of food is one of its many advantages. If food resources are concentrated among a minority of people, as often happens with unequal land ownership, food is not likely to be equally distributed unless efficient transportation systems are in place. Inequitable distribution then proves to be a difficult problem to resolve.

Raising the economic status of impoverished people by employing them is as important as expanding the food supply. If an increase in food supply is achieved without an accompanying rise in employment, there may be no long-term change in the number of undernourished people. Although food prices may fall with increased mechanization, use of fertilizers, and other modern technologies, it needs to be realized that these advances can also displace people from jobs, a result that worsens rather than helps the population.

MAKING DECISIONS

Sustainable Development and the Gender and Development (GAD) Approach

Sustainable development is economic growth that will reduce poverty while at the same time protect the environment and preserve natural capital. In its 2005 World Summit Outcome Document, the United Nations cites economic development, social development, and environmental protection as the "reinforcing pillars" of sustainable development. During the past 20 years, an understanding of the roles and responsibilities of both women and men in the community and the relationship of men and women to each other have been important components of sustainable development. The **gender and development (GAD) approach** works toward improving the status of women through the active participation of both men and women. By increasing women's access to education, information and communication technologies, economic resources, and governance, the GAD approach reduces poverty, promotes development, achieves gender equality, protects women's human rights, and eliminates violence against women.

THE ROLE OF BIOTECHNOLOGY IN EXPANDING WORLDWIDE FOOD AVAILABILITY

The ability of humans to manipulate nature has enabled us to improve the production and yield of many important foods. Traditional **biotechnology** is almost as old as agriculture. The first farmer to improve stock by selectively breeding the best bull with the best cows was implementing biotechnology in a simple sense. The first baker to use yeast to make bread rise took advantage of biotechnology.

By the 1930s, biotechnology made possible the selective breeding of better plant hybrids. As a result, corn production in the United States quickly doubled. Through similar methods, agricultural wheat was crossed with wild grasses to confer more desirable properties, such as greater yield, increased resistance to mildew and bacterial diseases, and tolerance to salt or adverse climatic conditions.

Another type of biotechnology uses hormones rather than breeding. In the last decade, Canadian salmon have been treated with a hormone that allows them to mature three times faster than normal—without changing the fish in any other way. In general terms, biotechnology can be understood as the use of living things—plants, animals, bacteria—to manufacture products.

THE NEW BIOTECHNOLOGY

The new biotechnology used in agriculture includes several methods that directly modify products. It differs from traditional methods because it more directly changes some of the genetic material (DNA) of organisms to improve characteristics. Cross-breeding plants or animals is no longer the only tool. Development of the new process, called **genetic engineering,** began in the 1970s. The field now features a wide range of cell and subcell techniques for the synthesis and placement of genetic material in organisms (Fig. 14-6).

This process of **recombinant DNA technology** allows access to a wider gene pool, and it permits faster and more accurate production of new and more useful microbial, plant, and animal species. Conventional breeding is inefficient and has inconsistent results; biotechnology uses genetic material more precisely. Scientists select the traits they want and genetically engineer or introduce the gene that produces the desired trait into plants or animals (now called a **genetically modified organism [GMO]** or **transgenic**).

biotechnology A collection of processes that involves the use of biological systems for altering and, ideally, improving the characteristics of plants, animals, and other forms of life.

genetic engineering Manipulation of the genetic makeup of any organism with recombinant DNA technology.

recombinant DNA technology A test tube technology that rearranges DNA sequences in an organism by cutting the DNA, adding or deleting a DNA sequence, and rejoining DNA molecules with a series of enzymes.

genetically modified organism (GMO) Any organism created by genetic engineering.

transgenic Organism that contains genes originally present in another organism.

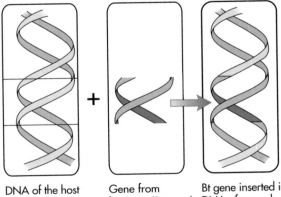

DNA of the host plant, corn.

Gene from bacteria (Bt gene) that produces a protein toxic to the European corn borer.

Bt gene inserted into DNA of corn plant. Now the corn plant is genetically modified. It makes the Bt toxin and, so, is resistant to the European corn borer.

FIGURE 14-6 ▶ Biotechnology involves various techniques for transferring foreign DNA into an organism. In this diagram, a sample of DNA is cleaved out of a larger DNA fragment and inserted into the DNA of a host cell. Thus, the host cell contains new genetic information, with the potential of providing the cell with new capabilities. For corn, this could mean resistance to the European corn borer. The corn plant is now referred to as a genetically modified organism (GMO). In another application, bacteria can be engineered to produce the human form of the hormone insulin.

▲ Both traditional plant breeding and biotechnology have produced high-yielding and disease-resistant plant varieties, such as with corn.

However, the genetic engineering does not replace conventional breeding practices; both work together.

Already, genetic engineering of agricultural products has allowed us to make use of new types of seeds, growth hormones, and microbial inoculants to stop pests and frost damage. Biotechnology is also used to develop drought-tolerant crops, as well as to detect *Listeria* and other microorganisms that cause foodborne illness. Scientists are engineering plants that grow with the use of less pesticides and new forms of potatoes that can be stored longer without preservatives. In addition, biotechnology can allow scientists to create fruits and grains with greater amounts of nutrients such as beta-carotene (e.g., "golden rice") and vitamins E and C. Researchers are also examining ways to modify the fatty-acid makeup of vegetable oils. Biotechnology is being used cautiously and conservatively, so these early benefits of the new biotechnology will strike us as only subtly different. The ultimate benefits, however, could be important if foods eaten by people in the developing world can be so enhanced.

Few consumers in the United States realize that about 40% of corn and 90% of soybeans produced in the United States have been genetically engineered to either resist certain insects, thereby reducing pesticide use, and/or survive when sprayed with herbicides that kill surrounding weeds. Some papaya plants have been genetically engineered for viral resistance.

Genetic modification of corn has received a lot of media attention. Corn can be genetically altered by inserting a gene from the bacterium *Bacillus thuringiensis*, usually referred to as the Bt gene, into the corn DNA. The gene allows the corn plant to make a protein lethal to certain caterpillars that destroy the plant. The Bt protein in the corn, however, is present in the plant in low concentrations and has no effect on humans—it is digested along with the other proteins in corn. For many years organic farmers have used the Bt bacteria as a dust on plants to destroy pests. (Dusting crops, however, does not change the DNA of the plant.)

FDA is confident that approved varieties of genetically engineered foods are safe to consume. A controversy arose over use of StarLink corn in 2000. In this case, the genetically modified corn variety was approved for animal feed but not human consumption, yet it found its way into some corn products, such as taco shells. Food manufacturers are not required to disclose the genetically modified ingredient content on food labels. FDA does not believe labeling of GMO products is needed because they pose no health risk.

Public response to use of GMO biotechnology, however, has been mixed. Even the scientific community has conflicting opinions about this technology, with supporters as convinced about the benefits as opponents are of the risks. The biggest debate in the United States surrounds the potential environmental hazards of introducing genes from one species to another. Some challengers even question the reduction in pesticide use that accompanies the cultivation of genetically modified crops. Although the use of genetically modified crops may reduce the need for environmentally harmful activities, such as spraying crops with pesticides, critics point out that seeds produced with additional insecticide potential will lead to rapid insect resistance because the insecticides are continuously emitted. Use of traditional pesticides involves prudent application, in part to avoid insect resistance. In addition, accidental release of genetically modified animals, such as fish, may go on to harm wild varieties.

Although the risks of biotechnology may appear to be momentarily negligible, they may be cumulative and therefore of concern in the long run. In addition, will allergens, such as those found in peanuts, eggs, milk, wheat, and shellfish, be added to genetically engineered foods that previously did not contain them? Evidence that this can happen has been seen in soybeans. However, FDA carefully examines all products developed using this technology and will enforce labeling of potential allergens that may be newly present in food altered by biotechnology.

The public has long been opposed to processes perceived as harmful to the environment, such as producing unnatural products. Food reserves are high in the United States, Canada, and Europe, so some question the need to increase food production. Skepticism surrounds unnatural products, as exemplified by Western

Europe's ban of hormones used in beef and milk production, and of almost all genetically modified foods.

ROLE OF THE NEW BIOTECHNOLOGY IN THE DEVELOPING WORLD

Whether applications of genetic engineering will help to significantly reduce undernutrition in the developing world remains to be seen. Unless
price cuts accompany the increased production, only landowners and sup-
pliers of biotechnology will enjoy the benefits. Small farmers may benefit
if they can afford to purchase the genetically modified seeds. This point deserves emphasis: The person who cannot afford to buy enough food today
will still face that same predicament in the future.

▲ Soybeans are a common GMO food in the marketplace.
Over 90% of the soybeans grown in the United States are
genetically modified.

As with most innovations, the more successful farmers—often those
with larger farms—will adopt the new biotechnology first. Because of
this, the present trend toward fewer and larger farms will continue in the
developing world, a movement that undermines the solution to one of the most
pressing undernutrition issues there. Furthermore, biotechnology does not promise dramatic increases in the production of most grains and cassava, the primary
food resources in developing parts of the world.

With the introduction of drought- and pest-resistant, as well as self-fertilizing
crops, agricultural biotechnology may help to lessen world hunger. Perhaps the most
promising potential of genetically modified foods today lies within the realm of plant
breeding for micronutrients. Developing countries will then have a tool to treat and
prevent selected nutrient deficiencies among their populations if they have access to
farming resources to augment the micronutrient composition of crops. In addition,
greater yields for indigenous plants, such as tomatoes that tolerate high soil salinity,
are another hopeful outcome. Biotechnology will likely be a useful tool against the
complex scourge of world undernutrition. Improved crops produced by this technology, together with political and other efforts, can contribute to success in the battle
against worldwide undernutrition.

SOME CONCLUDING THOUGHTS

The economic loss from undernutrition is staggering, and the amount of human pain
and suffering is incalculable. With all the international relief efforts and assistance
from governments and private organizations combined, we are still failing in our battle against undernutrition.

Ultimately, the depletion of world resources, the massive debt incurred by poorer
countries, the threat of danger to more prosperous countries nearby, and the toll taken
in human lives affect the world economy and well-being. The resulting instability can
go on to affect the developing world, as has been apparent in recent years. Life is not
necessarily fair, but the aim of civilization should be to make it more so. The world
has both enough food and the technical expertise to end hunger. What is lacking is the
concerted political will to do so.

CONCEPT CHECK

Overall, one important strategy to reducing undernutrition in the developing world lies in
providing sufficient employment, so that people can purchase the food their families need.
Providing access to land and other food production resources will also counteract undernutrition. Development programs must be sensitive to regional conditions to ensure that the new
technologies introduced do not intensify existing problems for the poorest people.

NUTRITION AND YOUR HEALTH
Undernutrition at Critical Life Stages

CRITICAL LIFE STAGES WHEN UNDERNUTRITION IS PARTICULARLY DEVASTATING

Prolonged undernutrition is detrimental to many aspects of human health (Fig. 14-7). It is particularly damaging during some periods of growth and old age. The United Nations Children's Fund developed a conceptual framework of malnutrition in 1990 (Fig. 14-8). According to this framework, the immediate causes of malnutrition (inadequate dietary intake and unsatisfactory health) affect individuals. The underlying causes relate to families and include inadequate access to food, inadequate care for women and children, and insufficient health services. Basic causes relate to human and economic resources and have their effect on communities and nations.

Pregnancy

Undernutrition poses the greatest health risk during pregnancy. About 500,000 women worldwide die each year from complications of pregnancy and childbirth. A pregnant woman needs extra nutrients to meet both her own needs and those of her developing offspring. Nourishing the fetus may deplete maternal stores of nutrients. Maternal iron deficiency anemia is one possible consequence (Chapter 16).

In Africa, women in their lifetimes give birth, on average, to more than six live babies. Coupled with chronic undernutrition, these high birth rates result in a 1 in 20 in chance that a woman will die from pregnancy-related causes. In contrast, North American women only face a risk of 1 death in about 8000 births from pregnancy-related causes. Pregnancy-related death is the social indicator showing the largest disparity between the developing and industrialized worlds. Smaller differences exist for literacy, life expectancy, and infant mortality.

Fetal and Infant Stages

The fetus faces major health risks from undernutrition during gestation. To support growth and development of the brain and other body tissues, a growing fetus requires a rich supply of protein, vitamins, and minerals. When these needs are not met, the infant is often born before 37 weeks of gestation, well before the ideal 40 weeks of gestation. The consequences of this preterm birth include reduced lung function and a weakened immune system. These conditions not only compromise health but also increase the likelihood of premature death. Long-term problems in growth and development can result if the infant survives. In extreme cases, low-birth-weight infants (about 5.5 pounds [2.5 kilograms] or less) face 5 to 10 times the normal risk of dying before the age of 1 year, primarily because of reduced lung development. When low birth weight is accompanied by other physical abnormalities, medical intervention can cost $200,000 or more. These costs can be met only in developed countries.

Worldwide, more than 30 million infants are born each year with low birth weight. About 7% of infants born in the United States and 6% in Canada have low birth weights. In the United States, low birth weight accounts for more than half of all infant deaths and 75% of deaths of infants younger than 1 month old. Whereas undernutrition is a major contributor to low birth weight in developing countries, the primary cause for this problem in industrialized countries is cigarette smoking. Pregnancy during the teenage years, while a girl's body is still growing, contributes to low birth weight in developing and industrialized countries alike.

The percentage of infants born with low birth weight in the United States has been increasing steadily during the past 20 years. One reason is that more twins, triplets, and higher-order multiple births are being born because of improvements

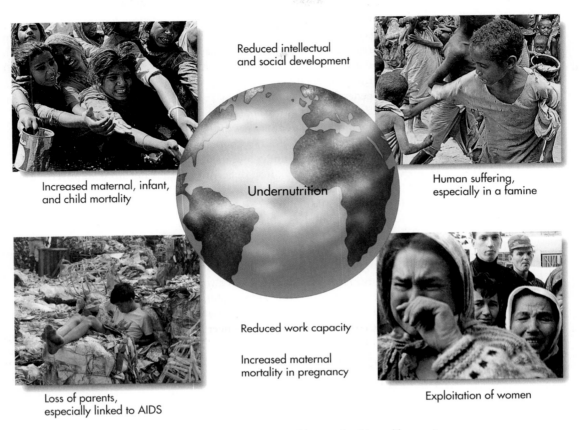

Reduced intellectual
and social development

Undernutrition

Increased maternal, infant,
and child mortality

Human suffering,
especially in a famine

Reduced work capacity

Increased maternal
mortality in pregnancy

Loss of parents,
especially linked to AIDS

Exploitation of women

FIGURE 14-7 ▶ Undernutrition affects many aspects of human health and humanity.

in medicine and fertility procedures. Rates of low birth weight also vary by race. About 13% of infants born to African-American women have low birth weights. Among Hispanics in the United States, infants of Mexican origin have the lowest rate of low birth weight (6%), while infants of Puerto Rican heritage have the highest (9%). Among Asian subgroups, low-birth-weight rates range from 5% for infants of Chinese heritage to nearly 9% for Filipino infants.

Childhood

Early childhood, when growth is rapid, is another period when undernutrition is extremely risky. The central nervous system—including the brain—continues to be vul-

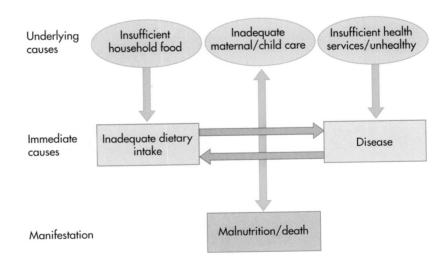

FIGURE 14-8 ▶ The UNICEF conceptual framework of the causes of malnutrition takes into account food, health, and caring practices. The causes are separated into three causes: immediate, underlying, and basic (not shown). Basic causes include human, economic, and organizational resources. The framework is used as a guide in health policy decision making.

▶ Compared to other children, homeless children suffer higher rates of many medical problems, some of which include:

- Upper respiratory tract infections
- Scabies and lice
- Tooth decay
- Ear and skin infections
- Diaper rash
- Eye infections
- Developmental delays
- Trauma-related injuries

nerable because of rapid growth through early childhood. After the preschool years, brain growth and development slow dramatically until maturity. Nutritional deprivation, especially in early infancy, can lead to permanent brain impairment. Without an effective intervention, it is projected that ongoing undernutrition could leave more than 1 billion children with mental impairment by 2020.

In general, poor children are at the greatest risk for nutritional deprivation and subsequent illness. Stunted growth is an obvious effect, seen in about one-third of children under 5 years of age worldwide. In addition, iron-deficiency anemia is much more common among low-income children than children from less deprived families. This deficiency can lead to fatigue upon exertion, reduced stamina, stunted growth, impaired motor development, and learning problems. Undernutrition in childhood can also weaken resistance to infection because immune function decreases when nutrients such as protein, vitamin A, and zinc

are low in a diet. Clearly, undernutrition and illness have a cyclical relationship. Not only does undernutrition lead to illness, but illness, particularly diarrhea and infectious diseases, worsens undernutrition. For this reason, many children in developing countries are dying from the combination of malnutrition and infection. Conversely, when missing nutrients such as vitamin A and zinc are restored to children's diets, improvements in health can be obvious.

Later Years

Older adults, especially older women living alone in poverty, are also at risk for undernutrition. Older adults in general require nutrient-dense foods, in amounts dependent on their state of health and degree of physical activity. Many of them have fixed incomes and incur significant medical costs, so food often becomes a low-priority item. In addition, depression, social isolation, and declining physical and mental health can compound the problem of undernutrition in older adults.

▶ Minimal intakes of protein and zinc limit the growth of children worldwide. About 30% of children in developing countries show evidence of poor growth rates.

CASE STUDY

Undernutrition During Childhood

Jamal traveled to the Philippines with his church group last summer. During their stay, they helped build shelters for people in a village where, a few weeks before, a storm had destroyed several houses. Jamal noticed that many of the children were very short, much shorter than the children in his neighborhood in the United States. His group worked in a remote, low-elevation area where the storm and subsequent flooding had caused the most damage. On several occasions he noticed young mothers crouched on curbs or in doorways, holding their children. These children rarely moved—they appeared pale and listless. In contrast to the children Jamal's group had met at a church in the capital city, most of the children in this village were not active and lively. One evening a nurse from the local clinic came to speak to Jamal's group. She said that many children in this area do not get enough to eat and that health problems were rampant. She considered the recent storm a blessing in disguise, hoping it would spur the Philippine government to send supplies to the village, particularly food and medicines. Jamal is shocked by such a degree of suffering. He wonders why children in the Philippines can be starving to death while many children in his hometown in the United States are overweight.

Answer the following questions, and check your responses in Appendix A.

1. Should Jamal have been surprised by widespread disease and general listlessness in the Philippine children?
2. Which nutrients are likely to be deficient in the diets of these children?
3. Which nutrient deficiencies contribute to poor growth or "stunting" of growth?
4. Which nutrient deficiencies may be causing diarrhea and illness?
5. Are these children likely to be consuming adequate calories? What effect does consumption of inadequate calories have on growth?
6. Why might the recent storm be a blessing for this small village?
7. List some reasons why the children in Jamal's neighborhood at home are more likely to be overweight

SUMMARY

1. Poverty is commonly linked to chronic or periodic undernutrition. Malnutrition can occur when the food supply is either scarce or abundant. The resulting deficiency conditions and degenerative diseases contribute to poor health.

2. Undernutrition is the most common form of malnutrition in developing countries. It results from inadequate intake, absorption, or use of nutrients or food energy. Many deficiency conditions consequently appear, and infectious diseases thrive because the immune system cannot function properly.

3. Undernutrition diminishes both physical and mental capabilities. In poor countries, this is worsened by recurrent infections, unsanitary conditions, extreme weather, inadequate shelter, and exposure to diseases.

4. In North America, famine is not seen but food insecurity and undernutrition remain problems. Soup kitchens, food stamps, the school lunch and breakfast programs, and the Special Supplemental Nutrition Program for Women, Infants, and Children (WIC) have focused on improving the nutritional health of poor and at-risk people. When adequately funded, these programs have proved effective in reducing undernutrition. The need to reduce out-of-wedlock pregnancies remains a national priority because single parents and their children are much more likely to live in poverty.

5. Multiple factors contribute to the problem of undernutrition in the developing world. In densely populated countries, food resources, as well as the means for distributing food, may be inadequate. Farming methods often encourage erosion, which deprives the soil of valuable nutrients and thereby hampers future efforts to grow food. Limited water availability hinders food production. Naturally occurring devastation from droughts, excessive rainfall, fire, crop infestation, and human causes—such as urbanization, war and civil unrest, debt, poor sanitation, and AIDS—all contribute to the major problem of undernutrition.

6. Proposed solutions to world undernutrition must consider multiple interacting factors, many thoroughly embedded in cultural traditions. Family planning efforts, for example, may not succeed until life expectancy increases. Through education, efforts should be made to upgrade farming methods, improve crops, limit pregnancies, encourage breastfeeding when it is safe to do so, and improve sanitation and hygiene.

7. Direct food aid is only a short-term solution. In what may appear to be a step backward, many experts recommend more sustainable subsistence-level farming. Small-scale industrial

development is another way to create meaningful employment and purchasing power for vast numbers of the rural poor. Various biotechnology applications may also prove beneficial.

8. The greatest risk of undernutrition occurs during critical periods of growth and development: gestation, infancy, and childhood. Low birth weight is a leading cause of infant deaths worldwide. Many

developmental problems are caused by nutritional deprivation during critical periods of brain growth. People in their later years are also at great risk.

STUDY QUESTIONS

1. Describe the difference between malnutrition and undernutrition.

2. Describe in a short paragraph any evidence of undernutrition that you saw while you were growing up, such as on television. What are/were the likely roots of these problems?

3. What do you believe are the major factors contributing to undernutrition in wealthy nations, such as the United States? What are some solutions to this problem?

4. What three points would you make to a group of seventh grade girls concern-

ing the economic perils of teen pregnancy and parenting?

5. Personal responsibility is a common theme in political circles. How does this relate to the problem of undernutrition in the United States? Does it apply to all causes of the problem?

6. Outline how war and civil unrest in developing countries have worsened problems of chronic hunger over the past few years.

7. How important is population control in addressing the problem of world

hunger now and in the future? Support your answer with three main points.

8. Why is solving the problem of undernutrition a key factor in the ability of developing countries to reach their full potential?

9. Discuss how infrastructure could influence the causes and solutions of chronic hunger in a developing nation.

10. Name three nutrients often lacking in the diets of undernourished people. What effects can be expected with each deficiency?

CHECK YOUR KNOWLEDGE

Answers to the following multiple choice questions are in Appendix A.

1. There are an estimated _____ chronically undernourished people in the world.
   a. 14 million
   b. 800 million to 1.1 billion
   c. 3 billion
   d. 6 billion

2. The number one killer of children in developing countries is
   a. xerophthalmia.
   b. iron deficiency anemia.
   c. iodide deficiency.
   d. diarrhea.

3. The human organism is particularly susceptible to the effects of undernutrition during
   a. pregnancy.
   b. infancy.
   c. childhood.
   d. All of the above.

4. A barrier to solving undernutrition in the developing world is NOT
   a. external debt.
   b. poor infrastructure.
   c. a lack of manpower.
   d. expanding population

5. Many of the child deaths each year in developing countries could be prevented if
   a. technology was improved.
   b. doctors were more specialized.
   c. mothers would learn more about nutrition.
   d. sanitation and hygiene were improved.

6. The food stamp program, revitalized by President Kennedy in the 1960s, allows
   a. low-income families to buy surplus food at government stores with government-issued Electronic Benefit Transfer cards.
   b. low-income people to purchase food, cleaning supplies, alcoholic

beverages, and anything else sold in supermarkets with Electronic Benefit Transfer cards.
   c. low-income people to turn in government-issued Electronic Benefit Transfer cards for cash to buy food.
   d. low-income people to purchase food and seeds with government-issued Electronic Benefit Transfer cards.

7. A long-term solution to world hunger is
   a. the green revolution.
   b. cash crops.
   c. jobs and self-sufficiency.
   d. government/private aid.

8. Bt corn has been genetically modified to make
   a. the bacterium *Bacillus thuringiensis*.
   b. a protein toxic to caterpillars that can destroy the corn plant.
   c. a sugar that makes the corn sweeter.
   d. a fat that makes corn oil healthier.

9. Genetically modified soybeans make up _____% of the soybeans grown in the United States.
   a. 50
   b. 75
   c. 80
   d. 90

10. FDA requires the statement "contains genetically modified ingredients" on the label of all foods containing genetically modified ingredients.
    a. True
    b. False

FURTHER READINGS

1. ADA Reports: Position of the American Dietetic Association: Agricultural and food biotechnology. *Journal of the American Dietetic Association* 106:285, 2006.

   It is the position of the American Dietetic Association that agricultural and food biotechnology techniques can enhance the quality, safety, nutritional value, and variety of food available for human consumption and increase the efficiency of food production, food processing, food distribution, and environmental and waste management.

2. ADA Reports: Position of the American Dietetic Association: Food insecurity and hunger in the United States. *Journal of the American Dietetic Association* 106:446, 2006.

   It is the position of the American Dietetic Association that systematic and sustained action is needed to bring an end to domestic food insecurity and hunger and to achieve food and nutrition security for all in the United States. Interventions are needed, including adequate funding for and increased use of food and nutrition assistance programs, the inclusion of food and nutrition education in all programs providing food and nutrition assistance, and innovative programs to promote and support the economic self-sufficiency of individuals and families, to end food insecurity and hunger in the United States.

3. ADA Reports: Position of the American Dietetic Association and Dietitians of Canada: Nutrition intervention in the care of persons with human immunodeficiency virus infection. *Journal of the American Dietetic Association* 104:1425, 2004.

   It is the position of the American Dietetic Association and Dietitians of Canada that efforts to optimize nutritional status, including medical nutrition therapy, assurance of food and nutrition security, and nutrition education, are essential components of the total health care available to people with human immunodeficiency virus infection throughout the continuum of care.

4. ADA Reports: Position of the American Dietetic Association: Assessing world hunger, malnutrition and food security. *Journal of the American Dietetic Association* 103:1046, 2003.

   It is the position of the American Dietetic Association that access to adequate amounts of safe, nutritious, and culturally appropriate foods is a fundamental human right. Still, hunger continues to be a worldwide problem of staggering proportions. In response, it is important to encourage programs and practices that combat hunger and malnutrition, increase food security, promote self-sufficiency, and are environmentally and economically sustainable.

5. ADA Reports: Position of the American Dietetic Association: Child and adolescent food and nutrition programs. *Journal of the American Dietetic Association* 103:887, 2003.

   Food programs targeted to low-income households, such as the Food Stamp Program, have gone a long way to increasing the nutrient intake of children and adolescents. It is important that these food programs are supported by adequate funding because the health of many children and adolescents is dependent upon these resources to provide sufficient nutrients to promote optimal physical, social, and cognitive growth and development.

6. Coutsoudis A: Infant feeding dilemmas created by HIV: South African experiences. *Journal of Nutrition* 135:956, 2005.

   This paper discusses the dilemma surrounding the risks and benefits of breastfeeding by an HIV-infected mother. The impact of the South African Safer Breastfeeding Programme, implemented to reduce some of the risk factors associated with HIV transmission, is reported.

7. Darton-Hill I and others: Micronutrient deficiencies and gender: Social and economic costs. *American Journal of Clinical Nutrition* 81:1198S, 2005.

   Micronutrient deficiencies, such as for vitamin A, iodine, iron, and zinc, in developing countries, lead to health problems, especially in females. Addressing these micronutrient deficiencies is important in order to improve economic status at the personal, community, and national level in developing countries.

8. Doherty T and others: A longitudinal qualitative study of infant-feeding decision making and practices among HIV-positive women in South Africa. *Journal of Nutrition* 136:2421, 2006.

   HIV-positive women face challenges regarding infant-feeding decisions. This study examined these challenges and found that successful breastfeeding resulted from a supportive home environment, a strong belief in the benefits of breastfeeding, and the ability to resist pressure to introduce other fluids.

9. Dworkin SL, Ehrhardt AA: Going beyond "ABC" to include "GEM": Critical reflections on progress in the HIV/AIDS epidemic. *American Journal of Public Health* 97:13, 2007.

   This article discusses the feminization of HIV/AIDS and the limitations of the "ABC" (abstinence, be faithful, condom use) strategy. Strategies focused on gender relation, economics, and migration (GEM) are suggested as more appropriate prevention measures.

10. Fawzi W and others: Studies of vitamins and minerals and HIV transmission and disease progression. *Journal of Nutrition* 135:938, 2005.

    Nutrient deficiencies, such as for vitamin A and vitamin E, are related to faster disease progression in HIV infections and AIDS. Daily use of a multivitamin and mineral supplement has been shown to be helpful to reduce disease progression because nutrient deficiencies are common in people with HIV infections and AIDS.

11. Gibson RS: Zinc: The missing link in combating micronutrient malnutrition in developing countries. *Proceedings of the Nutrition Society* 65:51, 2006.

    Although zinc deficiency is included as a major risk factor in the global burden of disease, zinc is still not included in the United Nations micronutrient priority list. Certain countries are at risk of zinc deficiency and should be targeted for zinc interventions. Zinc intervention strategies are discussed in this article.

12. Grandesso F and others: Mortality and malnutrition among populations living in South Darfur, Sudan. *Journal of the American Medical Association* 293:1490, 2005.

    The conflicts in the Darfur region of Sudan have led to high rates of death and undernutrition among people displaced by war. This article describes what has been seen numerous times in the last 50 years—undernutrition and related death is a typical casualty of war.

13. Hoetz PJ and others: Hookworm infection. *The New England Journal of Medicine* 351:799, 2004.

An estimated 740 million cases of hookworm infections exist in the world, primarily in the tropics and subtropics. Excellent medications are available to treat the disease, and these should be made widely available.

14. Joint United Nations Programme on HIV/AIDS (UNAIDS) and World Health Organization. AIDS epidemic update: Special report on HIV/AIDS World Health Organization: December 2006.

This UNAIDS report contains the 2006 global estimates on the scale of the AIDS pandemic. It is reported that approximately 39.5 million people were living with HIV in 2006, 2.6 million more than in 2004. It is estimated that 4.3 million adults and children became infected with HIV in 2006 (compared with 3.9 million in 2004). Forty percent of the new infections in 2006 occurred in young people aged 15-24.

15. Kalm LM, Semba RD: They starved so that others be better fed: Remembering Ancel Keys and the Minnesota experiment. *Journal of Nutrition* 135:1347, 2005.

Detailed and interesting account of the semistarvation studies conducted in the 1940's by Ancel Keys and colleagues. These experiments were conducted to better understand the effects of semistarvation that many people in World War II were experiencing, as well as to determine how best to safely refeed semistarved individuals.

16. Milman A and others: Differential improvement among countries in child stunting is associated with long-term development and specific interventions. *Journal of Nutrition* 135:1415, 2005.

Poor nutrition and health during the pre- and postnatal periods can result in the growth failure known as stunting. Factors that have reduced malnutrition and the resulting growth retardation were studied. National factors found to be most important were changes in immunization rate, safe water rate, female literacy rate, government consumption, income distribution, and the proportion of the economy devoted to agriculture. The results of this study indicate that it is possible to reduce the high prevalence of stunting by investing in specific interventions.

17. Palmer S: GE foods under the microscope. *Today's Dietitian* p. 34, May 2005.

About 70% of processed foods sold in the United States have contents that that have undergone some genetic alteration. This article explores some of the benefits and concerns regarding using this fairly recent technology in our food supply.

18. Shetty P: Achieving the goal of halving global hunger by 2015. *Proceedings of the Nutrition Society* 65:7, 2006.

This article reviews the goal of the FAO World Food Summit (WFS) and the United Nations Millennium Development Goals (MDG) to halve the numbers of the global population suffering from hunger by the year 2015. To date, the efforts have fallen short of the pace needed to achieve this goal. Developing countries are facing new challenges of hunger co-existing with new epidemics of diet-related diseases.

19. Steinbrook R: After Bangkok—Expanding the global response to AIDS. *The New England Journal of Medicine* 351:738, 2004.

The advances in treatment of AIDS have largely benefited developed countries. There is an urgent need to provide the benefits to those infected with AIDS in the developing world.

20. Yach D and others: The global burden of chronic diseases: Overcoming impediments to prevention and control. *Journal of the American Medical Association* 291:2616, 2004.

Nutrient deficiencies are common in the developing world. Such areas also experience the greatest burden of deaths from diarrhea, HIV and AIDS, and various childhood diseases. There needs be more attention to this enormous problem in the developing world.

▶ Check out the **Contemporary Nutrition ARIS site**

www.mhhe.com/wardlawcontfa1 for quizzes, flash cards, other activities, and weblinks designed to further help you learn about what you eat and why.

I. Fighting World Undernutrition on a Personal Level

If you want to do something about world and domestic undernutrition, consider the following activities. It is a noble act to try to make a difference, even if you make only one small step. As with any change in behavior, do not try to do too many things at once. Try one or two activities that represent your commitment to solving this problem.

1. Volunteer at a local soup kitchen or homeless shelter for a time (1 month, for example). What insights did you gain?

2. Coordinate the efforts of a campus organization to donate some money to a voluntary agency that does antihunger work, such as the following:

   Bread for the World
   50 F Street NW, Suite 500
   Washington, DC 20001

   Catholic Relief Services
   209 W. Fayette St.
   Baltimore, MD 21201

   Oxfam America
   226 Causeway St., 5th Floor
   Boston, MA 02114

   Second Harvest
   35 E. Wacker Dr., #2000
   Chicago, IL 60601

   CARE
   650 First Ave.
   New York, NY 10016

   EarthSave International
   PO Box 96
   New York, NY 10108

   Save the Children Foundation
   54 Wilton Rd.
   Westport, CT 06880

3. Make a contribution of nonperishable foods to the ongoing offering at a place of worship near you. If such an offering does not exist, start one.

4. Get on a food recovery program's mailing list, read its newsletters for information on upcoming fund-raisers and other activities, and become involved.

5. Participate in food drives organized by local grocery stores by contributing food or services. Food-drive organizers may need volunteers to transport the donations from the store to a food pantry. Pay special attention to events around World Food Day, October 16.

6. Point, click, and fight hunger. Internet users can find information on hunger at several sites, including the following:

   - Someone somewhere dies of hunger every 3.6 seconds. You can help stop the clock: go to www.thehungersite.com and click on Donate Free Food to send a meal to a needy someone. This site is affiliated with the UN World Food Program, which tracks the number of clicks and then sends a bill to one of its corporate or nonprofit sponsors.

   - HungerWeb, at Tufts University, offers information on hunger research, programs, mailing lists, education, and advocacy. This site contains weblinks to Internet sites run by the UN, U.S. AID, and the World Bank. http://nutrition.tufts.edu/academic/hungerweb/

   - The Food and Agriculture Organization of the United Nations has worked to alleviate poverty and hunger by promoting agricultural development, improved nutrition, and the pursuit of food security. This website will keep you up-to-date on recent issues and provides an extensive list of publications related to food security. www.fao.org

   - America's Second Harvest, the largest domestic hunger-relief organization, shows you how to help online and has information about the latest updates. www.secondharvest.org

   - Bread for the World is a nationwide Christian citizens' movement seeking justice for the world's hungry people by lobbying our nation's decision makers. www.bread.org

   - CARE is one of the world's largest private international relief and development organizations, with the goal of saving lives, building opportunities, and bringing hope to people in need. www.care.org

II. Joining the Battle Against Undernutrition

Imagine that you recently spent your summer vacation in a developing country and saw evidence of undernutrition and hunger. Then imagine that you are now asking a large corporation to support your efforts to ease hunger and suffering in this area. Develop a two-paragraph statement outlining why addressing hunger issues in this area is important. Include how you think a large corporation could assist you in your efforts.

CHAPTER 15 Safety of Food and Water

OVER 100 YEARS AGO, IN 1906, INCREASING PUBLIC PRESSURE FORCED THE PASSAGE OF THE FIRST FOOD AND DRUG ACT IN THE UNITED STATES. Federal inspection then safeguarded the public from diseased meat and generally improved food preparation standards.

Today, warnings about the safety of food and water appear everywhere. Attention has turned to more contemporary concerns, such as microbial and chemical contamination. On the one hand, we are told to eat more fruits, vegetables, fish, and poultry and to drink more water; on the other hand, we are warned that these may contain dangerous substances, so we still must ask, "How safe is our food and water?"

Scientists and health authorities agree that North Americans enjoy a relatively safe food supply, especially if foods are stored and prepared properly. Our water supply is also generally safe. Over the past 100 or so years, tremendous progress has been made to allow for this. Nonetheless, microorganisms and certain chemicals in foods still can pose a health risk. Thus, the nutritional and health benefits of food and water must be balanced against any food and water-related hazards. Chapter 15 focuses on these hazards—how real they are and how you can minimize their effect on your life. As the comic in the chapter suggests, you bear some responsibility for this—government agencies and industry can only do so much. Recall from Chapter 2 that the 2005 Dietary Guidelines for Americans encourage us to prepare and store foods safely. One goal of *Healthy People 2010* is to reduce by 50% the number of cases of foodborne illness from typical bacterial causes.

 Refresh Your Memory

As you begin your study of food safety in Chapter 15, you may want to review:

- Alternative sweeteners in Chapter 4
- The disease phenylketonuria (PKU) in Chapter 4
- Fat substitutes in Chapter 5
- Food biotechnology in Chapter 14

FOOD AND WATER SAFETY: SETTING THE STAGE

pasteurizing The process of heating food products to kill pathogenic microorganisms and reduce the total number of bacteria.

During the early stages of urbanization in North America, contaminated water and food—notably, milk—were responsible for many large outbreaks of typhoid fever, septic sore throat, scarlet fever, diphtheria, and other devastating human diseases. These experiences led to the development of processes for purifying water, treating sewage, and **pasteurizing** milk. Since that time, safe water and milk have become universally available, with only occasional problems from either.

Garfield ®   by Jim Davis

Which foods pose the greatest risk for foodborne illness? Is any food safe after being stored in the refrigerator for 6 months? Are food additives and pesticides an even greater day-to-day concern? Chapter 15 provides some answers.

The greatest health risk from food today is contamination by **viruses** and **bacteria** and, to a lesser extent, by various forms of **fungi** and **parasites**. These microorganisms can all cause **foodborne illness.** In a recent outbreak, 199 persons in 26 states were infected with *Escherichia coli* (*E. coli*) bacteria O157:H7 from fresh spinach. Of these ill persons, 102 were hospitalized, 31 developed kidney failure, and 22 were children under 5 years. Three deaths were associated with the outbreak.

Although microbial contamination is the cause of most incidents of foodborne illness, North Americans seem more concerned about health risks from chemicals in foods. In the long run, this concern has some merit. On a day-to-day basis, however, food additives cause only about 4% of all cases of foodborne illness in North America. Microbial contamination of food is by far the more important issue for our day-to-day health, so it will be discussed first. Chapter 15 will then cover chemical food safety hazards, including the use and safety of food additives, and discuss the risks of pesticides in foods.

Effects of Foodborne Illness

According to the U.S. Centers for Disease Control and Prevention, foodborne illness causes 76 million illnesses, 325,000 hospitalizations, and 5000 deaths in the United States each year. Hospital costs for foodborne illnesses are estimated at more than $3 billion per year; costs from related lost productivity are estimated at $8 billion per year. Some people are particularly susceptible to foodborne illness, including the following:

- Infants and children
- Older adults
- Those with liver disease, diabetes, HIV infection (and AIDS), or cancer
- Postsurgical patients
- Pregnant women
- People taking immunosuppressant agents (e.g., transplant patients)

It is estimated that in the United States alone about 30 million people with health problems have episodes of foodborne illness. Some bouts of foodborne illness, especially when coupled with ongoing health problems, are lengthy and lead to food allergies, seizures, blood poisoning (from **toxins** or microorganisms in the bloodstream), or other illnesses.

Foodborne illnesses often result from the unsafe handling of food at home, so we each bear some responsibility for preventing them. You can't usually tell so by taste, smell, or sight that a particular food contains harmful microorganisms, therefore, you might not even be aware that food has caused your distress. In fact, your last case of diarrhea may have been caused by foodborne illness (Table 15-1). Government agencies are at work on problems regarding food safety, but this does not substitute for individual safety efforts (Table 15-2).

Why Is Foodborne Illness So Common?

Foodborne illness is carried or transmitted to people by food. Most foodborne illnesses are transmitted through food in which microorganisms are able to grow rapidly. These foods are generally moist, rich in protein, and have a neutral or slightly acidic pH. Unfortunately, this describes many of the foods we eat every day, such as meats, eggs, and dairy products.

Our food industry tries whenever possible to increase the shelf life of food products; however, a longer shelf life allows more time for bacteria in foods to multiply. Some bacteria even grow at refrigeration temperatures. Partially cooked—and some fully cooked—products pose a particular risk because refrigerated storage may only slow, not prevent, bacterial growth. The risk of contracting foodborne illness also is high because of consumer trends. First, there is greater consumer interest in eating raw or undercooked animal products. In addition, more people receive medication that

virus The smallest known type of infectious agent, many of which cause disease in humans. A virus is essentially a piece of genetic material surrounded by a coat of protein. They do not metabolize, grow, or move by themselves. They reproduce only with the aid of a living cellular host.

bacteria Single-cell microorganisms; some produce poisonous substances, which cause illness in humans. Bacteria can be carried by water, animals, and people. They survive on skin, clothes, and hair and thrive in foods at room temperature. Some can live without oxygen and survive by means of **spore** formation.

spores Dormant reproductive cells capable of turning into adult organisms without the help of another cell. Various bacteria and fungi form spores.

fungi Simple parasitic life forms, including molds, mildews, yeasts, and mushrooms. They live on dead or decaying organic matter. Fungi can grow as single cells, like yeast, or as a multicellular colony, as seen with molds.

parasite An organism that lives in or on another organism and derives nourishment from it.

foodborne illness Sickness caused by the ingestion of food containing harmful substances.

toxins Poisonous compounds produced by an organism that can cause disease.

▼ Some restaurants that serve requested undercooked food are now warning patrons (on the menu) of the health risks of ordering such foods, particularly with undercooked eggs and meats.

TABLE 15-1 Some Examples of Cases of Foodborne Illness. We generally have a safe food supply, but there are occasional instances of foodborne illnesses, such as those listed.

Viruses

- *Norovirus:* During a Caribbean cruise, more than 380 passengers and crew members of the world's largest cruise ship, Royal Caribbean's Freedom of the Seas, were sickened by *Norovirus.* The ship, which carries 3900 passengers, was cleaned and sanitized, but one week later a second outbreak of the gastrointestinal illness afflicted 97 passengers and 11 crew members.

- *Hepatitus A:* Over 500 adults in the United States contracted hepatitis A after eating raw green onions in a Mexican restaurant. These were contaminated during growth in Mexico and not properly washed by food service workers.

Bacteria

- *Salmonella:* Unpasteurized juice products were recalled after 57 cases of *Salmonella* illness were reported in California and Colorado. Eight people became ill from *Salmonella* after consuming tiramisu, a dessert that contains raw eggs.
- *Shigella:* Six persons were reported ill from a *Shigella* infection after eating chopped, uncooked parsley served on chicken sandwiches and in coleslaw. In another incident, a cruise ship returned to port when more than 600 people developed shigellosis and one person died.
- *Listeria:* Forty-eight deaths were associated with foodborne illness caused by *Listeria* organisms in soft, Mexican-style cheeses. A listeriosis outbreak associated with undercooked hot dogs and cold cuts resulted in more than 82 illnesses and 17 deaths in 19 states.
- *E. coli:* One of the largest *E. coli* 0157:H7 outbreaks on record infected more than 1000 people in upstate New York at a county fair. The bacterium was found in infected well water. It killed a 79-year-old man and a 4-year-old girl, and it caused 10 other children to undergo kidney dialysis. Six adults and a 2-year-old child were killed after an *E. coli* outbreak from contaminated drinking water

in Canada. The bacteria entered the water supply from animal manure after flooding from a heavy storm. In northeastern Oklahoma, five children were infected with *E. coli* after consuming unpasterized apple cider. In the recent outbreak of 199 persons infected with *E. coli* from fresh spinach, *E. coli* 0157:H7 was isolated from 13 packages of fresh spinach in 10 states. At least 11 of the packages came from the same manufacturing plant on the same day.
- *C. botulinum:* A man in Arkansas developed botulism after eating stew that was cooked and then kept at room temperature for 3 days. He spent 49 days in the hospital—42 of them on mechanical ventilation.
- *Vibrio:* Since 1992, 17 people in Florida have died of *Vibrio vulnificus* infections after eating raw oysters.
- *B. cereus:* A teenage boy and his father experienced abdominal pain, vomiting, and diarrhea within 30 minutes of eating 4-day-old homemade pesto. The pesto had been reheated and left out a number of times during the 4-day period. It was apparently contaminated with *Bacillus cereus.* As a result, the boy died of liver failure.

Parasites

- *Cryptosporidium:* A group attending a dinner banquet developed diarrhea 3 to 9 days after eating green onions, the likely cause of the outbreak. Eight of 10 stool specimens obtained from the

group with foodborne illness were positive for *Cryptosporidium.* Food workers at the restaurant reported they did not consistently wash green onions before using them.

Risks from Seafood

- *Scombroid:* Four adults became ill with scombroid fish poisoning after eating tuna-spinach salad at a restaurant in Pennsylvania.
- *Ciguatera:* An outbreak of ciguatera fish poisoning involved 17 crew members of a cargo ship that caught, cooked, and ate a

barracuda in the Bahamas. All 17 men became ill with nausea, vomiting, abdominal cramps, and diarrhea within hours of eating the fish. Within 2 days, all of the men suffered from muscle pain and weakness; dizziness; and numb or itchy feet, hands, and mouth.

▲ Food contaminated in a central plant can go on to produce illness in people across the nation. In the case of juices, pasteurization is an effective method of reducing the risk of foodborne illness.

suppresses their ability to combat foodborne infectious agents. Another factor is the continuing increase in the number of older adults in the population.

The risk of illness from foodborne microorganisms increases as more of our foods are prepared in kitchens outside the home. Supermarkets have become an alternative to cooking at home by offering a variety of prepared foods from specialty meat shops, salad bars, and bakeries. With the increasing number of two-income families, more people are looking for convenient, easy-to-prepare, nutritious foods. Supermarkets offer entrées that can be served immediately or reheated. The foods are usually prepared in central kitchens or processing plants and shipped to individual stores.

This centralization of food production by the food-processing and restaurant industry enhances the risk of foodborne illness. If a food product is contaminated in a central processing plant, consumers over a wide area can suffer foodborne illness. For example, a malfunction in an ice cream plant in Minnesota resulted in 224,000 suspected cases of *Salmonella* bacterial infections, which were linked to use of con-

TABLE 15-2 Agencies Responsible for Monitoring the Food Supply in the United States

Agency Name	Responsibilities	Methods	How to Contact
United States Department of Agriculture (USDA)	• Enforces wholesomeness and quality standards for grains and produce (while in the field), meat, poultry, milk, eggs, and egg products	• Inspection • Grading • "Safe Handling Label"	www.fsis.usda.gov
Bureau of Alcohol, Tobacco, Firearms and Explosives (ATF)	• Enforces laws on alcoholic beverages	• Inspection	www.atf.treas.gov
Environmental Protection Agency (EPA)	• Regulates pesticides • Establishes water quality standards	• Approval required for all U.S. pesticides • Sets pesticide residue limits in food	www.epa.gov
Food and Drug Administration (FDA)	• Ensures safety and wholesomeness of all foods in interstate commerce (except meat, poultry, and processed egg products) • Regulates seafood • Controls product labels	• Inspection • Food sample studies • Sets standards for specific foods	www.fda.gov or call 1-800-FDA-4010
Centers for Disease Control and Prevention (CDC)	• Promotes food safety	• Responds to emergencies concerning foodborne illness • Surveys and studies environmental health problems • Directs/enforces quarantines • National programs for prevention and control of foodborne and other diseases	www.cdc.gov
National Marine Fisheries Service or NOAA Fisheries	• Domestic and international conservation and management of living marine resources	• Voluntary seafood inspection program • Can use mark to show federal inspection	www.nmfs.noaa.gov
State and local governments	• Milk safety • Monitors food industry within their borders	• Inspection of food-related establishments	Government pages of telephone book

Government agencies responsible for monitoring food safety in Canada and the specific laws followed are listed in Appendix C.

taminated ice cream mix. At least 4 people died and 700 became ill in Washington and surrounding western states after eating at a chain of fast-food restaurants. The source of the problem was undercooked hamburger contaminated with the bacterium *E. coli* 0157:H7. Restaurants generally encounter inspection by local health departments only about every 6 months. We must primarily rely on each restaurant to practice good food safety.

Greater consumption of ready-to-eat foods imported from foreign countries is still another cause of increased foodborne illness in North America. In the past, food imports were mostly raw products processed here under strict sanitation standards. Now, however, we import more ready-to-eat processed foods—such as berries from Guatemala and shellfish from Asia—some of which are contaminated. U.S. authorities are re-examining inspection procedures for these imports.

The use of antibiotics in animal feeds is also increasing the severity of cases of foodborne illness. This antibiotic use encourages bacteria to develop antibiotic-resistant

▶ One tool in the battle against foodborne illness is HACCP, or Hazard Analysis Critical Control Point. By applying the principles of HACCP, food handlers critically analyze how they approach food preparation and what conditions may exist that might allow pathogenic microorganisms to enter and thrive in the food system. Once specific hazards and critical control points (potential problems) are identified, preventive measures can be used to reduce specific sources of contamination.

irradiation A process in which **radiation** energy is applied to foods, creating compounds (free radicals) within the food that destroy cell membranes, break down DNA, link proteins together, limit enzyme activity, and alter a variety of other proteins and cell functions of microorganisms that can lead to food spoilage. This process does not make the food radioactive.

radiation Literally, energy that is emitted from a center in all directions. Various forms of radiation energy include X-rays and ultraviolet rays from the sun.

aseptic processing A method by which food and container are separately and simultaneously sterilized; it allows manufacturers to produce boxes of milk that can be stored at room temperature.

▲ This is the Radura, the international label denoting prior irradiation of the food product.

strains, those that can grow even if exposed to typical antibiotic medicines. This issue is receiving considerable attention by scientists in the field.

Finally, more cases of foodborne disease are reported now because scientists are more aware of the roles of various players in the process. Every decade the list of microorganisms suspected of causing foodborne illness lengthens. In addition, physicians are more likely to suspect foodborne contaminants as a cause of illness. Furthermore, we now know that food, besides serving as a good growth medium for some microorganisms, transmits many others as well. Seafood is receiving greater scrutiny and surveillance by FDA as a cause of foodborne illness. For more information about food safety, contact FDA's Center for Food Safety and Applied Nutrition information line at 1-888-SAFEFOOD or log on to www.FoodSafety.gov.

FOOD PRESERVATION—
PAST, PRESENT, AND FUTURE

For centuries, salt, sugar, smoke, fermentation, and drying have been used to preserve food. Ancient Romans used sulfites to disinfect wine containers and preserve wine. In the age of exploration, European adventurers traveling to the New World preserved their meat by salting it. Most preserving methods work on the principle of decreasing water content. Bacteria need abundant stores of water to grow; yeasts and molds can grow with less water, but some is still necessary. Adding sugar or salt binds water and so decreases the water available to these microbes. The process of drying evaporates off free water.

Decreasing the water content of some high-moisture foods, however, would cause them to lose essential characteristics. To preserve such foods—cucumber pickles, sauerkraut, milk (yogurt), and wine—fermentation has been a traditional alternative. Selected bacteria or yeast are used to ferment or pickle foods. The fermenting bacteria or yeast make acids and alcohol, which minimize the growth of other bacteria and yeast.

Today we can add pasteurization, sterilization, refrigeration, freezing, food **irradiation,** canning, and chemical preservation to the list of food preservation techniques. An additional method of food preservation—**aseptic processing**—simultaneously sterilizes the food and package separately before the food enters the package. Liquid foods, such as fruit juices, are especially easy to process in this manner. With aseptic packaging, boxes of sterile milk and juices can remain on supermarket shelves, free of microbial growth, for many years.

Food irradiation uses minimal doses of radiation to control pathogens such as *E. coli* 0157:H7 and *Salmonella.* The radiation energy used does not make the food radioactive. The energy essentially passes through the food, as in microwave cooking, and no radioactive residues are left behind. However, the energy is strong enough to break chemical bonds, destroy cell walls and cell membranes, break down DNA, and link proteins together. Irradiation thereby controls growth of insects, bacteria, fungi, and parasites in foods.

FDA approved the use of irradiation for raw red meat to reduce risk of *E. coli* and other infectious microorganisms. Other additions to the approved list are shell eggs and seeds. Prior to this, the only animal products so treated were pork and chicken. Irradiation also extends the shelf life of spices, dry vegetable seasonings, meats, and fresh fruits and vegetables.

Irradiated food, except for dried seasonings, must be labeled with the international food irradiation symbol, the Radura, and a statement that the product has been treated by irradiation. Foods treated in this way are safe in the opinion of FDA and many other health authorities, including the American Academy of Pediatrics. Although the demand for irradiated foods is still low in the United States, other countries, including Canada, Japan, Italy, and Mexico, all use food irradiation technology widely. Certain consumer groups continually try to block its use in the United States, claiming that irradiation diminishes the nutritional value of food and that it can lead to the formation of harmful compounds, such as carcinogens. Future research should be able to sort out this controversy, but in any case the risk is very low. Keep in mind that, even when foods, especially meats, have been irradiated, it is still important to follow basic food-safety procedures, as later contamination during food preparation is possible.

FOODBORNE ILLNESS CAUSED BY MICROORGANISMS

Most cases of foodborne illness are caused by specific viruses, bacteria, and other fungi. Prions—proteins involved in maintaining nerve cell function—can also turn infectious and lead to diseases such as mad cow disease. Bacteria specifically cause health problems either directly by invading the intestinal wall and producing an *infection* via a toxin contained in the organism, or indirectly by producing a toxin secreted into the food, which later harms us (called an *intoxication*). The main way to distinguish an infectious route from an intoxication is time: If symptoms appear in 4 hours or less, it is an intoxication.

Many types of bacteria cause foodborne illness, including *Bacillus, Campylobacter, Clostridium, Escherichia, Listeria, Vibrio, Salmonella,* and *Staphylococcus* (Table 15-3). Bacteria are everywhere: each teaspoon of soil contains about 2 billion bacteria. Luckily, only a small number of all bacteria pose a threat. Some foodborne bacteria cause infections, whereas others cause intoxications. *Salmonella,* for example causes an infection because the bacteria causes the illness. *Clostridium botulinum, Staphylococcus aureus,* and *Bacillus cereus* produce toxins and therefore cause illness from intoxication. In addition, while most strains of *E. coli* are harmless, *E. coli* O157:H7 produces a toxin that can cause severe illness, including severe bloody diarrhea and hemolytic uremic syndrome (HUS). Bacterial foodborne illnesses typically cause gastrointestinal symptoms such as vomiting, diarrhea, and abdominal cramps. *Salmonella, Listeria, E. coli* O157:H7, and *Campylobacter* are the bacterial foodborne illnesses of particular interest because they are the ones most often associated with death. *E. coli* O157:H7 has caused deaths when HUS has developed. Of the 2,500 cases of Listeriosis in the United States each year, 500 cases are fatal. Listeriosis is of particular concern for pregnant women because they are about 20 times more likely to get this infection than other healthy adults, and Listeriosis can cause spontaneous abortion or stillbirth because the *Listeria* bacteria can cross the placenta and infect the fetus.

Experts speculate that about 70% of foodborne illness cases go undiagnosed because they result from viral causes, such as Norovirus, and there is no easy way to test for these pathogens. Norovirus causes an illness commonly misdiagnosed as the "stomach flu." Norovirus infection has a sudden onset and usually a short duration of only one to two days. Noroviruses have become a problem on cruise ships. They are hardy and survive freezing, relatively high temperatures, and chlorination up to 10 ppm. A website coordinating the U.S. efforts on food safety is the www.FoodSafety.gov site mentioned earlier. Another useful website is www.homefoodsafety.org.

▲ Ground meats are a typical source of foodborne infection because bacteria on the surface of whole meats are distributed throughout the meat during grinding.

▶ A goal of *Healthy People 2010* is to reduce the number of cases of foodborne illness from *Campylobacter, E. coli, Listeria,* and *Salmonella* by 50%.

▲ Norovirus epidemics commonly occur on cruise ships. Noroviruses were originally called "Norwalk viruses" from Norwalk, Ohio, where they were first known to cause an epidemic of gastroenteritis.

CONCEPT CHECK

Viruses and bacteria pose the greatest risk for foodborne illness. In the past, the addition of sugar and salt to foods, as well as smoking and drying, were used to prevent the growth of microorganisms. Commercial processes, such as pasteurization and irradiation, offer protection from foodborne illness. Treat all raw animal products, cooked food, and raw fruits and vegetables as potential sources of foodborne illness.

TABLE 15-3 Important Microorganisms and Related Factors That Cause Foodborne Illness: Their Sources, Symptoms, and Prevention

Microorganism	Sources	Symptoms	Prevention Methods
Viruses			
Norovirus (Norwalk and Norwalk-like virus), human rotavirus	Human intestinal tract and feces. Contamination occurs: (1) when sewage is used to enrich garden/farm soil (2) by direct hand-to-food contact during the preparation of meals (3) when shellfish are harvested from waters contaminated by sewage.	Onset: 1–2 days Severe diarrhea, nausea, and vomiting. Respiratory symptoms. Usually lasts 4–5 days but may last for weeks.	• Sanitary handling of foods • Use of pure drinking water • Adequate sewage disposal • Adequate cooking of foods • Good personal hygiene
Hepatitis A virus	Fecal-oral route that contaminates food, beverages, or shellfish.	Onset: 15–50 days Anorexia, diarrhea, fever, jaundice, and fatigue. May cause liver damage and death.	• Sanitary handling of foods • Use of pure drinking water • Adequate sewage disposal • Thorough cooking of foods
Bacteria			
Campylobacter jejuni	Poultry, beef, and lamb and can contaminate meat and milk. Chief food sources are raw poultry and meat and unpasteurized milk.	Onset: 2–5 days, or longer Diarrhea, abdominal cramping, fever, and sometimes bloody stools. Lasts 2–7 days.	• Thorough cooking of foods • Sanitary handling of foods • Avoidance of unpasteurized milk
Salmonella species	Raw meats, poultry, eggs, fish, sprouts, unpasteurized milk, and products made with these items. Multiplies rapidly at room temperature. The bacteria themselves are toxic.	Onset: 1–3 days Nausea, fever, headache, abdominal cramps, diarrhea, and vomiting Can be fatal in infants, the elderly, and the sick.	• Sanitary handling of foods • Avoidance of any use of unpasteurized raw eggs or undercooked eggs • Thorough cooking of foods • Prompt refrigeration of foods
Shigella species	Transmitted via fecal-oral route and somewhat in food and water.	Onset: 1–3 days Abdominal cramps, diarrhea, fever, bloody stools	• Sanitary handling of foods
Escherichia coli (0157:H7 and other strains)	Undercooked beef, especially ground beef. Fruits, vegetables, sprouts, and yogurt are also possible sources.	Onset: 1–8 days Bloody diarrhea, abdominal cramps, kidney failure	• Thorough cooking, especially of beef • Avoidance of unpasteurized milk, untreated apple cider
Clostridium perfringens`	Meat and poultry dishes. Multiply rapidly in anaerobic conditions when foods are left for extended time at room temperature.	Onset: 8–24 hours (usually 12 hours) Abdominal pain and diarrhea Symptoms last a day or less, usually mild. Can be more serious in older or ill people.	• Sanitary handling of foods, especially meat and meat dishes, gravies, and leftovers • Thorough cooking and reheating of foods, especially leftovers • Prompt and proper refrigeration
Listeria monocytogenes	Unpasteurized milk and soft cheeses made with unpasteurized milk. Uncooked processed meats, such as hot dogs. Resists acid, heat, salt, nitrate, and refrigeration temperatures.	Onset: 9–48 hours for early symptoms;14–42 days for severe symptoms. Fever, headache, vomiting, and sometimes more severe symptoms. May be fatal.	• Thorough cooking of foods • Sanitary handling of foods • Avoidance of unpasteurized milk of particular concern during pregnancy
Staphylococcus aureus	Nasal passages and in cuts on skin. Toxin is produced when food contaminated by bacteria is left for extended time at room temperature. Meats, poultry, egg products, pose the greatest risk.	Onset: 2–6 hours Diarrhea, vomiting, nausea, and abdominal cramps, mimics flu Lasts 24–36 hours Rarely fatal	• Sanitary handling of foods • Prompt and proper refrigeration of foods • Covering cuts on skin
Clostridium botulinum	Bacteria produce toxin only in a low-acid, anaerobic environment, such as in canned green beans, mushrooms, spinach, olives, and beef. Honey may carry spores.	Onset: 12–72 hours Neurotoxic symptoms include double vision, inability to swallow, speech difficulty, and progressive paralysis of the respiratory system. OBTAIN MEDICAL HELP IMMEDIATELY. BOTULISM CAN BE FATAL.	• Use proper methods for canning low-acid foods • Avoidance of commercial cans of low-acid foods that have leaky seals or are bent, bulging, or broken • Discard if toxin is suspected (off odors are a sign)
Vibrio vulnificus	Raw seafood, especially raw oysters.	Onset: 1–7 days Diarrhea, fever, weakness, blood infection, death	• Thorough cooking of seafood

TABLE 15-3 *(continued)*

Microorganism	Sources	Symptoms	Prevention Methods
Bacteria (continued) *Vibrio cholerae*	Human carriers, infected shellfish, contaminated water and food.	Onset: 2–3 days Vomiting, severe watery diarrhea, which can lead to dehydration and cardiovascular collapse; death	• Handwashing after using the bathroom
Parasites *Trichinella spiralis*	Pork and wild game.	Onset: weeks to months Muscle weakness, fluid retention in face, fever, flulike symptoms	• Thorough cooking of pork and wild game
Anisakis	Raw fish.	Onset: 12 hours Stomach infection, severe stomach pain	• Thorough cooking of fish
Tapeworms	Raw beef, pork, and fish.	May cause abdominal discomfort, diarrhea	• Thorough cooking of all animal products • Avoidance of raw fish dishes
Cyclospora cayetanensis	Carried to food via contaminated water; Guatemalan raspberries suspected in some outbreaks.	Onset: 1–11 days Prolonged diarrhea, vomiting, muscle aches, fatigue	• Irradiation (not yet in practice)
Cryptosporidium	Contaminated water (especially by fecal material). Large outbreaks have been caused by such contamination of municipal water in Milwaukee, Wisconsin.	Onset: 1–12 days Diarrhea, vomiting, fever	• Handwashing • Consume clean or treated water • Boil water if at high risk, such as one on immune suppression drugs or who has AIDS
Toxoplasma gondii	Raw or undercooked meat, unwashed fruits and vegetables, cat feces.	Onset: 5–20 days Fever, headache, sore muscles, diarrhea (can be deadly to the fetus if pregnant mother is infected)	• Cook meats thoroughly • Wash raw fruits and vegetables • Wash hands after changing cat litter (avoid cat litter when pregnant)
Fungi Mycotoxins are a group of toxic compounds produced by molds, such as aflatoxin B-1	Found in foods relatively high in moisture. Chief food sources are beans and grains that have been stored in a moist place.	May cause liver and/or kidney disease	• Discard foods with visible mold • Proper storage of susceptible foods
Seafood-Associated Toxins Ciguatera	Large tropical fish, especially grouper, snapper, and barracuda.	Onset: generally within 6 hours Diarrhea, abdominal pain, nausea, vomiting, and nerve disorders	• Avoid grouper, amberjack, and barracuda from Caribbean waters, especially larger fish
Paralytic shellfish poisoning	Shellfish that have consumed large amounts of dinoflagellate algae (i.e., red tide).	Onset: within 4 hours Respiratory difficulty	• Observe local precautions when harvesting shellfish
Scombroid poisoning	Spoiled fish, especially tuna, mackerel, and mahi-mahi.	Onset: 1–180 minutes Facial flushing, burning sensation in the mouth, intestinal distress, and headache	• Avoid spoiled fish • Refrigerate fresh fish and use as soon as possible
Prions Proteins that help maintain nerve cells. These can turn into infectious prions, likely leading to diseases such as mad cow disease (bovine spongiform encephalopathy).	Cows, goats, and sheep harboring infectious prions. These are spread from one animal to another if certain by-products of the infected animal (e.g., brains) are used to feed other animals (this process is banned in the U.S. and Canada). Cooking does not destroy prions.	Onset: 2–30 years Dementia and psychosis, leading eventually to seizures, blindness, paralysis, and death. Once symptoms begin, death usually occurs within 1 year. At autopsy the person shows numerous holes in the brain.	• Isolated cases of mad cow disease have been confirmed in U.S. cattle, some imported from Canada. (These animals were infected before strict preventive actions were put in place in Canada.) The biggest risk is consumption of meat, from cows, goats, and sheep in Europe or Asia. FDA and USDA have banned imports of such animals from Europe. There is a possibility that the prion also may be present in foods or dietary supplements containing brain tissue from cattle.

FOOD ADDITIVES

By the time you see a food on the market shelf, it usually contains substances added to make it more palatable or increase its nutrient content or shelf life. Manufacturers also add some substances to foods to make them easier to process. Other substances may have accidentally found their way into the foods you buy. All of these extraneous substances are known as **additives,** and, although some may be beneficial, others, such as sulfites, may be harmful for some people. All purposefully added substances must be evaluated by FDA.

Why Are Food Additives Used?

Most additives are used to limit food spoilage. Common food additives serve the general function of **preservatives,** including acidic or alkaline agents, antioxidants, antimicrobial agents, curing and pickling agents, and **sequestrants.** Table 15-4 helps you to understand exactly why these are used and to learn more about the specific substances used. Food additives, such as potassium sorbate, are used to maintain the safety and acceptability of foods by retarding the growth of microbes implicated in foodborne illness.

Additives are also used to combat some enzymes that lead to undesirable changes in color and flavor in foods but don't cause anything as serious as foodborne illness. This second type of food spoilage occurs when enzymes in a food react to oxygen—for example, when apple and peach slices darken or turn rust color as they are exposed to air. Antioxidants are a type of preservative that slow the action of oxygen-requiring enzymes on food surfaces. These preservatives are not necessarily novel chemicals. They include vitamins E and C and a variety of sulfites.

Without the use of some food additives, it would be impossible to produce massive quantities of foods and safely distribute them nationwide or worldwide, as is now done. Despite consumer concerns about the safety of food additives, many have been extensively studied and proven safe when FDA guidelines for their use are followed.

Intentional versus Incidental Food Additives

Food additives are classified into two types: **intentional food additives** (directly added to foods) and **incidental food additives** (indirectly added as contaminants). Both types of agents are regulated by FDA in the United States. Currently, more than 2800 different substances are intentionally added to foods. As many as 10,000 other substances enter foods as contaminants. This includes substances that may reasonably be expected to enter food through surface contact with processing equipment or packaging materials.

The GRAS List

In 1958, all food additives used in the United States and considered safe at that time were put on a **generally recognized as safe (GRAS)** list. The U.S. Congress established the GRAS list because it believed manufacturers did not need to prove the safety of substances that had been used for a long time and were already generally recognized as safe. Since that time, FDA has been responsible for proving that a substance does not belong on the GRAS list. Substances may be added to the GRAS list if data and information about the use of the substance are known and accepted widely by qualified experts, and establish that the substance is safe under the conditions of its intended use.

Since 1958, some substances on the list have been reviewed. A few, such as cycla-mates, failed the review process and were removed from the list. The additive red dye #3 was removed because it is linked to cancer. Many chemicals on the GRAS list have not yet been rigorously tested, primarily because of expense. These chemicals have received a low priority for testing, mostly because they have long histories of use without evidence of toxicity or because their chemical characteristics do not suggest they are potential health hazards.

Are Synthetic Chemicals Always Harmful?

Nothing about a natural product makes it inherently safer than a synthetic product. Many synthetic products are laboratory copies of chemicals that also occur in nature

additives Substances added to foods, such as preservatives.

preservatives Compounds that extend the shelf life of foods by inhibiting microbial growth or minimizing the destructive effect of oxygen and metals.

sequestrants Compounds that bind free metal ions. By so doing, they reduce the ability of ions to cause rancidity in foods containing fat.

intentional food additives Additives knowingly (directly) incorporated into food products by manufacturers.

incidental food additives Additives that appear in food products indirectly, from environmental contamination of food ingredients or during the manufacturing process.

generally recognized as safe (GRAS) A list of food additives that in 1958 were considered safe for consumption. Manufacturers were allowed to continue to use these additives, without special clearance, when needed for food products. FDA bears responsibility for proving they are not safe, but can remove unsafe products from the list.

▶ Some important definitions:

toxicology	Scientific study of harmful substances
safety	Relative certainty that a substance won't cause injury
hazard	Chance that injury will result from use of a substance
toxicity	Capacity of a substance to produce injury or illness at some dosage

(see the discussion in Chapter 14 on biotechnology for some examples). Moreover, although human endeavors contribute some toxins to foods, such as synthetic pesticides and industrial chemicals, nature's poisons are often even more potent and widespread. Some cancer researchers suggest that we ingest at least 10,000 times more (by weight) natural toxins produced by plants than we do synthetic pesticide residues. (Plants produce these toxins to protect themselves from predators and disease-causing organisms.) This comparison does not make synthetic chemicals any less toxic, but it does put them in a more accurate perspective.

Consider vitamin E, often added to food to prevent rancidity of fats. This chemical is safe when used within certain limits. However, high doses have been associated with health problems, such as interfering with vitamin K activity in the body (review Chapter 8). Thus, even well-known chemicals we are comfortable using can be toxic in some circumstances and at some concentrations.

Tests of Food Additives for Safety

Food additives are tested by FDA for safety on at least two animal species, usually rats and mice. Scientists determine the highest dose of the additive that produces *no observable effects* in the animals. These doses are proportionally much higher than humans are ever exposed to. The maximum dosage that produced no observable effects is then divided by at least 100 to establish a margin of safety for human use. This 100-fold margin is used because it is assumed that we are at least 10 times more sensitive to food additives than are laboratory animals and that any one person might be 10 times more sensitive than another. This broad margin essentially ensures that the food additive in question will cause no harmful health effects in humans. In fact, many synthetic chemicals are probably less dangerous at these low doses than some of the natural compounds in common foods such as apples or celery.

One important exception applies to the schema for testing intentional food additives: If an additive is shown to cause cancer, even though only in high doses, no margin of safety is allowed. The food additive cannot be used, because it would violate the **Delaney Clause** in the 1958 Food Additives Amendment. This clause prohibits intentionally adding to foods a compound introduced after 1958 and that causes cancer at any level of exposure. Evidence for cancer could come from either laboratory animal or human studies. Few exceptions to this clause are allowed; exceptions are discussed regarding curing and pickling agents in Table 15-4.

▲ Color additives make some foods more desirable.

▶ The 100-fold margin of safety is 25 times less than that for vitamin A, when you compare the RDA for healthy women (700 micrograms) to a potentially harmful dose of vitamin A for pregnant women (3000 micrograms).

Delaney Clause A clause to the 1958 Food Additives Amendment of the Pure Food and Drug Act in the United States that prevents the intentional (direct) addition to foods of a compound shown to cause cancer in laboratory animals or humans.

TABLE 15-4 Types of Food Additives—Sources and Related Health Concerns

Food Additive Class	Attributes	Health Risks
Acidic or alkaline agents, such as citric acid, calcium lactate, and sodium hydroxide	Acids impart a tart taste to soft drinks, sherbets, and cheese spreads; inhibit mold growth; lessen discoloration and rancidity. They also reduce the risk of botulism in naturally low-acid vegetables, such as canned green beans. Alkaline agents neutralize acids produced during fermentation, and so improve flavor.	No known health risks when used properly
Alternative low-calorie sweeteners, such as saccharin, sucralose, ascesulfame potassium, aspartame, neotame, and tagatose	Sweeten foods without adding more than a few calories	Moderate use of these alternative sweeteners is considered safe (except for use of aspartame by people with the disease PKU)

▶ Sugar, salt, corn syrup, and citric acid constitute 98% of all additives (by weight) used in food processing.

(Continued)

▲ Soft drinks are typical sources of alternative sweeteners for many of us. Moderate use of these products generally poses no health risk in most people.

▶ You might wonder why, if nitrates and nitrites form chemical substances that can cause cancer, they aren't banned by the Delaney Clause. In the United States, USDA regulates the use of chemicals in meats. The laws that govern USDA regulation of foods are separate from those that govern FDA regulation. Because of this, the Delaney Clause does not apply to USDA actions. USDA sees no clear threat to public safety from the regulated use of nitrates and nitrites in meats, so no action has been taken.

TABLE 15-4 *(continued)*

Food Additive Class	Attributes	Health Risks
Anticaking agents, such as calcium silicate, magnesium stearate, and silicon dioxide	Absorb moisture to keep table salt, baking powder, or powdered sugar and powdered food products free-flowing and prevent caking and lumping	No known health risks when used properly
Antimicrobial agents, such as salt, sodium benzoate, sorbic acid, and calcium propionate	Inhibit mold and fungal growth	Salt increases the risk of developing hypertension, especially in some individuals. No known health risks from other agents when used properly
Antioxidants, such as BHA (butylated hydroxyanisole), BHT (butylated hydroxytoluene), alpha-tocopherol (vitamin E), ascorbic acid (vitamin C), and sulfites	Delay food discolorations from oxygen exposure; Reduce rancidity from the breakdown of fats; Maintain the color of luncheon meats; Prevent the formation of cancer-causing nitrosamines	Sulfites can cause an allergic reaction in about 1 in every 100 people. Symptoms include difficulty breathing, wheezing, hives, diarrhea, abdominal pain, cramps, and dizziness. Salad bars, dried fruit, and wine are typical sources of sulfites.
Color additives, such as tartrazine	Make foods more appealing	Tartrazine (FD&C yellow number 5) can cause allergic symptoms such as hives and nasal discharge in some people, especially those allergic to aspirin. FDA requires manufacturers to list all forms of synthetic colors on the labels of foods that contain them.
Curing and pickling agents, such as salt, nitrates, and nitrites	Nitrates and nitrites act as preservatives, especially to prevent the growth of *Clostridium botulinium;* often used in conjunction with salt	Salt increases the risk of developing hypertension, especially in some individuals. Nitrate and nitrite consumption from both cured foods and that found naturally in some vegetables has been associated with synthesis of nitrosamines. (An adequate vitamin C intake may reduce this synthesis.) Some nitrosamines are cancer-causing agents, particularly for the stomach, esophagus, and colon, but the risk is low. The National Cancer Institute advises consuming these foods in moderation.
Emulsifiers, such as monoglycerides and lecithins	Suspend fat in water to improve uniformity, smoothness, and body of foods, such as baked goods, ice cream, and mayonnaise	No known health risks when used properly
Fat replacements, such as Paselli SA2, Dur-Low, Oatrim, Sta-Slim 143, Stellar, and Olean	Limit calorie content of foods by reducing some of the fat content	Generally no known health risks when used properly

TABLE 15-4 *(continued)*

Food Additive Class	Attributes	Health Risks
Flavor and flavoring agents (such as natural and artificial flavors), sugar, and corn syrup	Impart more or improve flavor of foods	Sugar and corn syrup can increase risk for dental caries. Generally no known health risks for flavoring agents when used properly.
Flavor enhancers, such as monosodium glutamate (MSG) and salt	Help bring out the natural flavor of foods, such as meats	Some people (especially infants) are sensitive to the glutamate portion of MSG and after exposure experience flushing, chest pain, facial pressure, dizziness, sweating, rapid heart rate, nausea, vomiting, increase in blood pressure, and head-ache. Those so affected should look for the word glutamate on food labels, as well as isolated protein, yeast extract, bullion, and soup stock. Salt increases the risk of developing hypertension, especially in some people.
Humectants, such as glycerol, propylene glycol, and sorbitol	Retain more moisture, texture, and fresh flavor in foods such as candies, shredded coconut, and marshmallows	No known health risk when used properly
Leavening agents, such as yeast, baking powder, and baking soda	Introduce carbon dioxide into food products	No known health risk when used properly
Maturing and bleaching agents, such as bromates, peroxides, and ammonium chloride	Shorten the time needed for maturation of flour to become usable for baking products	No known health risk when used properly
Nutrient supplements, such as vitamin A, vitamin D, and potassium iodide	Enhance the nutrient content of foods such as margarine, milk, and ready-to-eat breakfast cereals	No known health risk if intake from such supplemental sources combined with other natural food sources of a nutrient does not exceed the Upper Level set for a particular nutrient (iron may be one exception; review Chapter 9)
Stabilizers and thickeners, such as pectins, gums, gelatins, and agars	Impart a smooth texture and uniform color and flavor to candies, ice cream and other frozen desserts, chocolate milk, and beverages containing alternative sweeteners. Prevent evaporation and deterioration of flavorings used in cakes, puddings, and gelatin mixes	No known health risk when used properly
Sequestrants, such as EDTA and citric acid	Bind free ions, helping preserve food quality by reducing ability of ions to cause rancidity in products containing fat	No known health risk when used properly

▲ Emulsifiers improve the texture of foods such as ice cream, baked goods, and cookies.

CRITICAL THINKING

Recognizing that Joseph is taking a nutrition class, his roommate asks him, "What is more risky: the bacteria that can be present in food or the additives listed on the label of my favorite snack cake?" How should Joseph respond? On what information should he base his conclusions?

Incidental food additives are another matter. FDA cannot ban various industrial chemicals, pesticide residues, and mold toxins from foods, even though some of these contaminants can cause cancer. These products are not purposely added to foods. FDA sets an acceptable level for these substances. An incidental substance found in a food cannot contribute to more than one cancer case during the lifetimes of 1 million people. If a higher risk exists, the amount of the compound in a food must be reduced until the guideline is met.

In general, if you consume a variety of foods in moderation, the chances of food additives jeopardizing your health are minimal. Pay attention to your body. If you suspect an intolerance or a sensitivity, consult your physician for further evaluation. Remember that in the short run, you are more likely to suffer either from foodborne illness due to poor food-handling practices that allow viral and bacterial contamination in food, or from the consumption of raw animal foods, than from consuming additives. Excess calories, saturated fat, cholesterol, *trans* fat, salt, and other potential "problem" nutrients in our diets pose the greatest long-term health risk.

Approval for a New Food Additive

Before a new food additive can be added to foods, FDA must approve its use. Besides rigorously testing an additive to establish its safety margins, manufacturers must give FDA information that (1) identifies the new additive, (2) gives its chemical composition, (3) states how it is manufactured, and (4) specifies laboratory methods used to measure its presence in the food supply at the amount of intended use.

Manufacturers must also offer proof that the additive will accomplish its intended purpose in a food, that it is safe, and that it is to be used in no higher amount than needed. Additives cannot be used to hide defective food ingredients, such as rancid oils; to deceive customers; or replace good manufacturing practices. A manufacturer must establish that the ingredient is necessary for producing a specific food product.

MAKING DECISIONS

Processed or Whole Foods?

If you are bewildered or concerned about all the additives in your diet, you can easily avoid most of them by consuming unprocessed whole foods. However, no evidence shows that this will necessarily make you healthier, nor can you avoid all additives, because some are used even on whole foods, such as with pesticides. It amounts to a personal decision. Do you have confidence that FDA and food manufacturers are adequately protecting your health and welfare, or do you want to take more personal control by minimizing your intake of compounds not naturally found in foods?

CONCEPT CHECK

Food additives are used to reduce spoilage from microbial growth, oxygen, metals, and other compounds. Additives are also used to adjust acidity, improve flavor and color, leaven, provide nutritional fortification, thicken, and emulsify food components. Additives are classified as intentional (direct; purposely added to foods), and incidental (indirect; present in foods from environmental contamination or various manufacturing practices). The amount of an additive allowed in a food is limited to one-one-hundredth of the highest amount that has no observable effect when fed to animals. The Delaney Clause allows FDA to limit intentional addition of cancer-causing compounds to food in the United States under its jurisdiction. Also set by law in the United States are the permissible amounts of carcinogens that incidentally enter foods.

▲ Depending on whether you choose fresh versus processed foods, a diet can be either essentially free of or contain food additives. For most of us, this specific concern regarding food choice is not worth worrying about.

SUBSTANCES THAT OCCUR NATURALLY IN FOODS AND CAN CAUSE ILLNESS

Foods contain a variety of naturally occurring substances that can cause illness. Here are some of the more important examples:

- *Safrole*—found in sassafras, mace, and nutmeg; causes cancer when consumed in high doses
- *Solanine*—found in potato shoots and green spots on potato skins; inhibits the action of neurotransmitters
- *Mushroom toxins*—found in some species of mushrooms such as aminita; can cause stomach upset, dizziness, hallucinations, and other neurological symptoms. The more lethal varieties can cause liver and kidney failure, coma, and even death. FDA regulates commercially grown and harvested mushrooms. These are cultivated in concrete buildings or caves. However, there are no systematic controls on individual gatherers harvesting wild species, except in Illinois and Michigan.
- *Avidin*—found in raw egg whites (cooking destroys avidin); binds the vitamin biotin in a way that prevents its absorption, so a biotin deficiency may ultimately develop over the long term
- *Thiaminase*—found in raw fish, clams, and mussels; destroys the vitamin thiamin
- *Tetrodotoxin*—found in puffer fish; causes respiratory paralysis
- *Oxalic acid*—found in spinach, strawberries, sesame seeds, and other foods; binds calcium and iron in the foods, and so limits absorption of these nutrients
- *Herbal teas* containing senna or comfrey—can cause diarrhea and liver damage

▲ When hunting wild mushrooms, know what you are looking for. Many varieties contain deadly toxins.

People have coexisted for centuries with these naturally occurring substances and have learned to avoid some of them and limit intake of others. They pose little health risk. Farmers know potatoes must be stored in the dark, so that solanine won't be synthesized. Furthermore, we've developed cooking and food-preparation methods to limit the potency of other substances, such as thiaminase. Spices are used in such small amounts that health risks don't result. Nevertheless, it's important to understand that some potentially harmful chemicals in foods occur naturally.

Is Caffeine a Cause for Concern?

Why all the controversy over a cup of coffee? Researchers have spent a great deal of time on the study of caffeine, the substance of greatest concern in the favorite beverage of many of us. So why do caffeine recommendations change from year to year?

Caffeine is a stimulant found as a natural or added ingredient in many beverages and chocolate. On average, we consume 75% of our caffeine intake as coffee, 15% as tea, 10% as soft drinks, and 2% as chocolate (Table 15-5). (For teenagers and young adults this ratio is often relatively higher for soft drinks and lower for coffee.)

Caffeine is not often consumed by itself. With the popularity of trendy coffee shops that serve everything from mocha java to flavored lattes, it is difficult to separate caffeine intake from cream, sugar, alternative sweeteners, and flavorings. So what is the conscientious coffee drinker to think? Let's explore the myths and facts of caffeine intake.

Caffeine does not accumulate in the body and is normally excreted within several hours following consumption. Caffeine can cause anxiety, increased heart rate, insomnia, increased urination (possibly resulting in dehydration), diarrhea, and gastrointestinal upset in high doses. In addition, those already suffering from ulcers may experience irritation due to increased acid production; those who have anxiety or panic attacks may find that caffeine worsens their symptoms; and those prone to heartburn may find that caffeine worsens this symptom because it relaxes sphincter muscles in the esophagus. Some people need little caffeine to feel such effects, and the dosage for children is likely even lower than that for adults.

Withdrawal symptoms are also real. Former coffee drinkers may experience head-ache, nausea, and depression for a short time after discontinuing use. These symp-toms can be expected to peak at 20 to 48 hours following the last intake of caffeine. Symptoms hold true even for those trying to quit as little as one cup of coffee per day. Slow tapering of use over a few days is recommended to avoid these problems.

Are there more serious consequences of consuming caffeine regularly? It has been hy-pothesized that caffeine consumption can lead to certain types of cancer, such as pancre-atic and bladder cancers. The association of caffeine with cancer has not been supported in recent literature. If fact, regular coffee consumption has been linked to a decreased risk of colon cancer.

Negative press has dwindled with regard to a link between cardiovascular disease and moderate coffee consumption. Heavy use does increase blood pressure for a short period of time. Coffee consumption also has been linked to increased LDL-cholesterol and triglycerides in the blood. This association was found to be caused by cafestol and kahweol, two oils in ground coffee. However, filtered and instant coffees do not contain the harmful oils. When researchers correct for tobacco use in coffee drinkers, no distinct correlation is seen between moderate use of filtered or instant coffee consumption and increased risk for cardiovascular disease. It is prudent, though, to limit the amount of coffee in general, especially from French coffee presses and from espresso as these beverages are not filtered.

Women are thought to be at higher risk for a variety of deleterious effects with caffeine consumption, including miscarriages, osteoporosis, and birth defects in their offspring. It is true that heavy caffeine use mildly increases the amount of calcium excreted in urine. For this reason, it is important that heavy coffee drinkers check their diets for adequate

▲ Coffee is a common source of caffeine for many adults.

TABLE 15-5 Caffeine Content of Common Sources

Item	Milligrams of Caffeine Typical	Range*
Coffee (8 fl oz)		
Brewed, drip method	85	65–120
Brewed, percolator	75	60–85
Decaffeinated, brewed	3	2–4
Espresso (1 fl oz serving)	40	30–50
Teas (8 fl oz)		
Brewed	40	20–90
Iced	25	9–50
Instant	28	24–31
Some soft drinks (8 fl oz)	24	20–40
"Energy drinks" such as Red Bull (8.3 fl oz)	80	0–80
Cocoa beverage (8 fl oz)	6	3–32
Chocolate milk beverage (8 fl oz)	5	2–7
Milk chocolate (1 oz)	6	1–15
Dark chocolate, semi-sweet (1 oz)	20	5–35
Baker's chocolate (1 oz)	26	26
Chocolate-flavored syrup (1 fl oz)	4	4

*For the coffee and tea products, the range varies due to brewing method, plant variety, brand of product, and so on.
Source: International Food Information Council. *Caffeine and women's health*, August 2002.

calcium sources. Some studies do show a higher likelihood for miscarriages in women consuming more than 500 milligrams of caffeine per day (about five 8 ounce cups of coffee). FDA warns women to consume caffeine in moderation (no more than the equivalent of one to two 8 ounce cups of coffee per day).

In contrast to these possibly harmful effects of caffeine consumption, many people are convinced of the benefits of a "cup of joe." Though some women testify to the idea that caffeine improves premenstrual symptoms, no study proves this theory. Some weight-loss drugs previously contained caffeine, under the assumption that it made the drugs more effective. FDA has since banned this use as it was found to be ineffective. Some newer research findings suggest caffeine may reduce the risk of developing headaches, cirrhosis of the liver, some forms of kidney stones, gallbladder stones, some nerve-related diseases, and furthermore, that it aids in blood glucose regulation. You may have heard that caffeine can improve physical performance. This has been shown in highly trained athletes; recall that use of large amounts of caffeine is banned by the NCAA (review Chapter 12). For those below professional status, though, no benefit has been shown. Also keep in mind that coffee will not "sober up" a person who is drunk.

Though the debate over caffeine will likely continue as long as North Americans drink coffee, research does not support many of the concepts previously thought of as fact. These studies are reinforcing the idea of moderation—the equivalent of about two to three 8 ounce cups of coffee per day. A prudent dose of caffeine is 200 to 300 milligrams per day. Review Table 15-5 concerning the caffeine content of typical sources.

ENVIRONMENTAL CONTAMINANTS IN FOOD

A variety of environmental contaminants can be found in foods. Aside from pesticide residues, other potential contaminants that deserve attention are listed in Table 15-6. To reduce exposure to environmental toxins present in our foods that cause disease, find out which foods pose a risk. In addition, emphasize variety and moderation in food selection. Tips provided in Tables 15-6 and 15-7 also apply to reducing exposure to environmental contaminants.

▶ Genetic alteration of foods such as corn and soybeans has created concern, especially in Europe. FDA considers genetically altered products safe if approval for human use has been granted (see Chapter 12 for details).

CONCEPT CHECK

A general program to minimize exposure to environmental contaminants includes knowing which foods pose greater risks and consuming a wide variety of foods in moderation.

Pesticides in Food

Pesticides used in food production produce both beneficial and unwanted effects. Most health authorities believe that the benefits outweigh the risks. Pesticides help ensure a safe and adequate food supply and help make foods available at reasonable cost. However, sentiment is growing nationwide that pesticides pose avoidable health risks. Consumers have come to assume that synthetic is dangerous and organic is safe. Some researchers believe this sentiment is grounded in fear and fueled by unbalanced reports. Other researchers say concern about pesticides is valid and overdue.

Most concern about pesticide residues in food appropriately focuses on chronic rather than acute toxicity because the amounts of residue present, if any, are extremely small. These low concentrations found in foods are not known to produce adverse effects in the short term, although harm has been caused by the high amounts that occasionally result from accidents or misuse. For humans, pesticides pose a danger

▶ One of the problems with pesticides is that they create new pests because they destroy the predators (spiders, wasps, and beetles) that naturally keep most plantfeeding insect populations in check. The brown plant hopper, which has plagued Indonesian rice fields, was not a serious problem before heavy pesticide use began to kill its predators in the early 1970s. In the United States, such major pests as spider mites and the cotton bollworm were merely nuisances until pesticides decimated their predators.

TABLE 15-6 Potential Environmental and Other Contaminants in Our Food Supply

Chemical Substance	Sources	Toxic Effects	Preventive Measures
Acrylamide	Fried foods rich in carbohydrate cooked at high temperatures for extended periods, such as French fries and potato chips	Potential neurotoxin and carcinogen. Known carcinogen for laboratory animals; however, studies have not clearly proven the relationship between acrylamide ingestion and the development of cancer in humans.	Limit intake of deep-fat fried foods rich in carbohydrate.
Cadmium	Plants in general if much cadmium is in the soil Clams, shellfish, tobacco smoke Occupational exposure in some cases	Kidney disease Liver disease Prostate cancer (debatable) Bone deformities Lung disease (when inhaled)	Consume a wide variety of foods, including seafood sources.
Dioxin	Trash-burning incinerators Bottom-feeding fish from the Great Lakes Animal fats from animals exposed to such contamination via water or soil	Abnormal reproduction and fetal/infant development Immune suppression Cancer (to date only clearly shown in laboratory animals)	Pay attention to warnings of dioxin risks from local fish; if risk exists, limit intake as suggested on the fishing license. Consume a variety of fish from local waters rather than mostly one specific species.
Lead	Lead-based paint chips and related dust in older homes Occupational exposure (e.g., radiator repair) Lead caps on wine bottles Fruit juices and pickled vegetables stored in galvanized or tin containers or leaded glass Some types of solder used in joining copper pipes (mostly in older homes) Mexican pottery dishes Koo Soo herbal remedies Leaded glass containers	Anemia Kidney disease Nervous system damage (tiredness and changes in behavior are symptoms) Reduced learning capacity in childhood (even from mild lead exposure)	Avoid paint chips and related dust in older homes; regular cleaning of these homes is also important (see www.hud.gov/offices/lead). Meet iron and calcium needs to reduce lead absorption. Wipe the inside and outside neck of wine bottles before use if the bottle has a lead cap. Store fruit juices and pickled vegetables in glass or plastic or waxed paper containers. Let water run 1 minute or so if off for more than 2 hours, and use only cold water for cooking; do not soften drinking water. Do not store alcoholic beverages in leaded glass containers.
Mercury	Swordfish, shark, king mackerel, and tilefish. Fresh and canned albacore tuna also is a possible source. (In contrast, the more typical light chuck tuna is very low in mercury.)	Reduced fetal/child development and birth defects; toxic to nervous system	Consume these sources no more than once per week, no more than two times per week for albacore tuna. Pregnant women should avoid these species of fish, but some albacore tuna consumption is fine. Two to three fish meals per week is appropriate for pregnant (and nursing) women if different types of fish are eaten.
Polychlorinated biphenyls (PCBs)	Fish from the Great Lakes and Hudson River Valley (e.g., coho salmon) Farmed salmon are a possible source, but less so	Cancer (to date only clearly shown in laboratory animals), as well as a potential for liver, immune, and reproductive disorders	Pay attention to warnings of PCB contamination from local fish; if risk exists, limit intake as suggested on the fishing license or on state advisories. Vary the type of fish eaten during a specific week.
Urethane	Alcoholic beverages such as sherry, bourbon, sake, and fruit brandies	Cancer (to date only clearly shown in laboratory animals)	Avoid generous amounts of typical sources.

mainly in their cumulative effects, so their threats to health are difficult to determine. However, growing evidence, including the problems of the contamination of underground water supplies and destruction of wildlife habitats, indicates that North Americans would probably be better off if we could reduce our use of pesticides. Both the U.S. federal government and many farmers are working toward that end. Chapter 14 discussed the lastest use of biotechnology to reduce pesticide use.

What Is a Pesticide?

Federal law defines a pesticide as any substance or mixture of substances intended to prevent, destroy, repel, or mitigate any pest. The built-in toxic properties of pesticides lead to the possibility that other, nontarget organisms, including humans, might also be harmed. The term *pesticide* tends to be used as a generic reference to many types of products, including insecticides, herbicides, fungicides, and rodenticides. A pesticide product may be chemical or bacterial, natural or synthetic. For agriculture, EPA allows about 10,000 pesticides to be used, containing some 300 active ingredients. About 1.2 billion pounds of pesticides are used each year in the United States, much of which is applied to agricultural crops.

Once a pesticide is applied, it can turn up in a number of unintended and unwanted places. It may be carried in the air and dust by wind currents, remain in soil attached to soil particles, be taken up by organisms in the soil, decompose to other compounds, be taken up by plant roots, enter groundwater, or invade aquatic habitats. Each is a route to the food chain; some are more direct than others.

▲ Pesticide use poses a risk-versus-benefit question. Each side has points that deserve to be considered. Rural communities, where exposure is more direct, experience the greatest short-term risk.

Why Use Pesticides?

In the United States, pests destroy nearly $20 billion of food crops yearly, despite extensive pesticide use. The primary reason for using pesticides is economic—the use of agricultural chemicals increases production and lowers the cost of food, at least in the short run. Many farmers believe that it would be impossible to stay in business without pesticides, which help protect farmers from ruinous losses.

Consumer demands also have changed over the years. At one time, we wouldn't have thought twice about buying an apple with a worm hole; we took it home, cut out the wormy part, and ate the apple. Today, consumers find worm holes less acceptable, so farmers rely more on pesticides to produce cosmetically attractive fruits and vegetables. On the practical side, pesticides can protect against the rotting and decay of fresh fruits and vegetables. This is helpful because our food distribution system doesn't usually permit consumer purchase within hours of harvest. Also, food grown without pesticides can contain naturally occurring organisms that produce carcinogens at concentrations far above current standards for pesticide residues. For example, fungicides help prevent the carcinogen aflatoxin (caused by growth of a fungus) from forming on some crops. Thus, although some pesticides may do little more than improve the appearance of food products, others help keep foods fresher and safer to eat.

Regulation of Pesticides

The responsibility for ensuring that residues of pesticides in foods are below amounts that pose a danger to health is shared by FDA, EPA, and the Food Safety and Inspection Service of USDA in the United States. Table 15-2 listed the roles of various food protection agencies. FDA is responsible for enforcing pesticide tolerances in all foods except meat, poultry, and certain egg products, which are monitored by USDA. A newly proposed pesticide is exhaustively tested, perhaps over 10 years or more, before it is approved for use. EPA must decide that the pesticide causes no unreasonable adverse effects on people and the environment and that benefits of use outweigh the risks of using it. However, there is concern about older chemicals registered before 1970, when less stringent testing conditions were permitted. EPA is now asking chemical companies to retest the old compounds using more rigorous tests. Unfortunately, inadequate funding at EPA has hampered the review of older pesticides. The slow pace of this retesting has angered the critics of pesticide use.

▲ Fruits and vegetables grown without use of pesticides are available and may bear an "organic" label (see Table 2-10 for rules regarding the use of the term "organic" on food labels). These products generally are more expensive than those grown using pesticides. Consumers need to decide if the potential benefits of the products are worth the extra cost.

When weighing whether to approve or cancel a pesticide, EPA considers how much more it would cost the farmer to use an alternative pesticide or process and whether cancellation would decrease productivity. After determining the dollar cost to the farmer, EPA then looks at costs to processors and consumers. Once a pesticide is approved for use, it must follow the margin of safety provisions required of food additives (see previous section, "Tests of Food Additives for Safety").

How Safe Are Pesticides?

Dangers from exposure to pesticides through food depend on how potent the chemical toxin is, how concentrated it is in the food, how much and how frequently it's eaten, and the consumer's resistance or susceptibility to the substance. Accumulating information links pesticide use to increased cancer rates in farm communities. For rural counties in the United States, the incidence of lymph, genital, brain, and digestive tract cancers increases with higher-than-average pesticide use. Respiratory cancer cases increase with greater insecticide use. In tests using laboratory animals, scientists have found that some of the chemicals present in pesticide residues cause birth defects, sterility, tumors, organ damage, and injury to the central nervous system. Some pesticides persist in the environment for years.

Still, some researchers argue that the cancer risk from pesticide residues is hundreds of times less than the risk from eating such common foods as peanut butter, brown mustard, and basil. Plants manufacture toxic substances to defend themselves against insects, birds, and grazing animals (including humans). When plants are stressed or damaged, they produce even more of these toxins. Because of this, many foods contain naturally occurring chemicals considered toxic, and some are even carcinogenic. Other scientists argue that if natural carcinogens are already in the food supply, then we should reduce the number of added carcinogens whenever possible. In other words, we should do what we can to decrease our overall exposure.

Tests of the Amounts of Pesticides in Foods

FDA tests thousands of raw products each year for pesticide residues. (A pesticide is considered illegal in this case if it is not approved for use on the crop in question or if the amount used exceeds the allowed tolerance.) The latest FDA studies show no residues in about 60% of samples. Less than 1% of domestic and about 3% of import samples have residues continually over tolerance. These findings continue to support previous FDA studies over the past 10 years that pesticide residues in food are generally well below EPA tolerances, and they confirm the safety of the food supply relative to pesticide residues.

Personal Action

We often take risks in our lives, but we prefer to have a choice in the matter after weighing the pros and cons. With regard to pesticides in food, however, someone else is deciding what is acceptable and what is not. Our only choice is whether to buy or avoid pesticide-containing foods. In reality, it's almost impossible to avoid pesticides entirely, because even organic produce often contains traces of pesticides, probably as the result of cross-contamination from nearby farms.

Short-term studies of the effects of pesticides on laboratory animals cannot precisely pinpoint long-term cancer risks in humans. It should be clearly understood, however, that the presence of minute traces of an environmental chemical in a food does not mean that any adverse effect will result from eating that food.

FDA and other scientific organizations believe that the hazards are comparatively low and in the short run are less dangerous than the hazards of foodborne illness created in our kitchens. We cannot avoid pesticide risks entirely, but we can limit exposure by following some simple advice (Table 15-7).

▲ FDA's yearly evaluation of a "market basket" of typical foods shows that pesticide content is minimal in most foods.

TABLE 15-7 What You Can Do to Reduce Exposure to Pesticides

FDA's sampling and testing show that pesticide residues in foods do not pose a health hazard. Nevertheless, if you want to reduce dietary exposure to pesticides, follow this advice from the Environmental Protection Agency:

- Consume a wide variety of foods, especially regarding fruits, vegetables, and fish.
- Thoroughly rinse and scrub (with a brush if possible) fruits and vegetables. Peel them, if appropriate—although some nutrients will be peeled away.
- Remove the outer leaves of leafy vegetables, such as lettuce and cabbage.
- Residues of some pesticides in animal feed concentrate in the animals' fat, so trim fat from meat, poultry, and fish; remove skin (which contains most of the fat) from poultry and fish; and discard fats and oils in broths and pan drippings.
- When fishing, throw back the big fish—the little ones have had less time to take up and concentrate pesticides and other harmful residues. In addition, pay attention to any warnings by local authorities (and on the fishing license) about the high risk for contamination in specific waters or species of fish.
- Avoid lawns, gardens, and flower beds that have recently been treated with pesticides and herbicides.

Adapted from Food and Drug Administration: Safety first: Protecting America's food supply, *FDA Consumer*, p. 26, November 1988.

▲ Rinsing fruits and vegetables under running water is advised to reduce pesticide exposure.

We can also encourage farmers to use fewer pesticides to reduce exposure to our foods and water supplies, but we'll have to settle for produce that isn't perfect in appearance or that has been grown with the aid of biotechnology (again, see Chapter 14 for details). Are you concerned enough about pesticides on food to change your shopping habits or take more political action?

OUR WATER SUPPLY: SAFETY ISSUES

It is common to see 5-gallon bottles of water being delivered to homes. Grocery store shelves are now stocked with all types of bottled waters—more than 700 brands in the United States—ranging from simple plastic jugs containing "pure spring water" to fancier, imported varieties of mineral water in glass bottles. In Europe, bottled water is an institution, as popular as soft drinks are in the United States.

It is fashionable to order a bottle of water at a restaurant or bar. Not only are people looking for alternative to alcoholic beverages and soft drinks, but they are also attracted to the perceived health value or taste of bottled water. This popularity has turned the bottled water industry into a business that rakes in more than $6 billion a year. It is debatable whether spending this much money on bottled water makes any sense.

Bottled Water

Bottled waters vary in their source, use, mineral content, and carbonation. All bottled waters must list the source of the water on the label. This source can include wells, spas, springs, geysers, and often, the public water supply. Some bottled water companies add minerals—such as calcium, magnesium, and potassium—to give the water a better taste. FDA sets definitions for terms on the label such as *artesian water, distilled water, purified water, spring water, mineral water,* and others. In essence, the source must be the same one listed on the label. Thus, for example, "spring water" must come from an underground spring. The presence of carbon dioxide gas in the water source results in carbonation. Bottled waters from these sources are said to be naturally sparkling. Other carbonated waters have had carbon dioxide added during bottling. FDA also sets high standards for purity that bottled water producers must meet.

Many people choose bottled water over tap water because they doubt the safety of their public drinking water. Some concern over municipal water supplies is warranted. For example, contamination of the public water supply by the parasite *Cryptosporidium* is possible. This parasite is usually found in lakes and rivers; the typical chlorination

▲ Bottled water is a convenient but relatively expensive source of water. In most cases, tap water is just as healthy a choice to meet our water needs.

procedures used to treat public water supplies do not kill *Cryptosporidium*. This parasite poses little risk to healthy people—other than a case of diarrhea—but it can harm people who have AIDS or other diseases that compromise function of the immune system (such as some forms of cancer therapy or organ transplant therapy). High-risk people have been advised to boil for at least 1 minute any tap water they use for cooking or drinking to ensure that the parasite is destroyed. Alternatively, individuals can purchase a water filter that screens out *Cryptosporidium* (the National Sanitation Foundation at [800] 673-8010 can provide a list of manufacturers) or use bottled water certified to be free of the parasite (contact the supplier if in doubt). Generally, distilled water or that which has undergone reverse osmosis is parasite free.

Monitoring the Safety of Your Water

Under the Safe Water Drinking Act, all public drinking water supplies are monitored for contaminants such as bacteria, various chemicals, and toxic metals (such as lead and mercury). The local municipal water department must mail the results of these tests each year to its consumers. According to the Environmental Protection Agency (EPA), the U.S. water supply ranks among the safest in the world. However, this water does sometimes fail to meet the agency's standards for contaminants such as lead and nitrates. Generally, the public will be warned about the latter, because it is dangerous to use nitrate-rich water for mixing infant formulas (Chapter 17). Some studies indicate that in one year, about one in five Americans consumes water not up to standards, especially in rural areas. These people could consider using a home water filter or bottled water. The local water department can help a person evaluate whether health risks are worth the cost of home water filters or bottled water.

As a safeguard against contamination, chlorine and ammonia are added to kill bacteria. The addition of such chemicals has raised concern that drinking water may increase rectal and bladder cancer risk, though there is no conclusive proof of such risk. If chlorine in tap water does increase cancer risk, the risk is likely extremely small (perhaps two cases of cancer in 1 million people).

If you find the taste of chlorinated tap water unpleasant or are concerned about the possible cancer risk, you can remove the chlorine from tap water by boiling it or by letting a large container filled with water stand uncovered overnight. In both cases, the chlorine will evaporate, taking its characteristic flavor with it. Alternatively, you can install a filter on the household spigot from which you obtain your water. It should be designed to remove trihalomethanes, common chlorine by-products.

Options Regarding Your Water Source

Keep in mind that by most standards, bottled water ranges from moderately expensive to expensive. In many cases, you are paying for water not much different from the water you get from your tap. If you are concerned about the safety of your tap water, you can ask the municipal water department for its most recent test results, or you can have the water tested. A local testing laboratory or state health department can be of service, as can the EPA at (800) 426-4791, if local information is not available (for example, if you have a well). This testing can point out whether there are health risks associated with your water supply. Compared with the cost of bottled water, the testing fee will be insignificant. As noted earlier in the chapter, letting cold water run for a minute or so be before taking a drink or before using it in meal preparation is a good way to limit possible lead exposure, especially if the water has been off for more than two hours. In addition, do not use hot tap water for food preparation. For more information, see the website www.epa.gov/safewater.

CONCEPT CHECK

Overall, the United States enjoys a safe water supply. However, people with poor immune status should boil water used for drinking and cooking to avoid waterborne illness. Bottled water can also be used if desired.

General Rules for Preventing Foodborne Illness

You can greatly reduce the risk of food-borne illness by following some important rules. It's a long list, because many risky habits need to be addressed.

Purchasing Food

- When shopping, select frozen foods and perishable foods, such as meat, poultry, or fish, last. Always have these products put in separate plastic bags, so that drippings don't contaminate other foods in the shopping cart. Don't let groceries sit in a warm car; this allows bacteria to grow. Get the perishable foods such as meat and egg and dairy products home and promptly refrigerate or freeze them.
- Don't buy or use food from damaged containers that leak, bulge, or are severely dented or from jars that are cracked or have loose or bulging lids. Don't taste or use food that has a foul odor or spurts liquid when the can is opened; the deadly *Clostridium botulinum* toxin may be present.
- Purchase only pasteurized milk and cheese (check the label). This is especially important for pregnant women because highly toxic bacteria and viruses that can harm the fetus thrive in unpasteurized milk.
- Purchase only the amount of produce needed for a week's time. The longer you keep fruits and vegetables, the more time is available for bacteria to grow.
- When purchasing precut produce or salads, avoid those that look slimy, brownish, or dry; these are signs of improper holding temperatures.

Preparing Food

- Thoroughly wash your hands for 20 seconds with hot, soapy water before and after handling food. This practice is especially important when handling raw meat, fish, poultry, and eggs, after using the bathroom, after playing with pets, or after changing diapers.
- Make sure counters, cutting boards, dishes, and other equipment are thoroughly sanitized and rinsed before use. Be especially careful to use hot, soapy water to wash surfaces and equipment that have come in contact with raw meat, fish, poultry, and eggs as soon as possible to remove *Salmonella* bacteria that may be present. Otherwise, bacteria on the surfaces will infect the next foods that come in contact with the surface, a process called cross-contamination. In addition, replace sponges and wash kitchen towels frequently. (Microwaving sponges for 30 to 60 seconds also helps rid them of live bacteria.)
- If possible, cut foods to be eaten raw on a clean cutting board reserved for that purpose. Then clean this cutting board using hot, soapy water. If the same board must be used for both meat and other foods, cut any potentially contaminated items, such as meat, last. After cutting the meat, wash the cutting board thoroughly.

FDA recommends cutting boards with unmarred surfaces made of easy-to-clean, non-porous materials, such as plastic, marble, or glass. If you prefer a wooden board, make sure it is made of a nonabsorbent hardwood, such as oak or maple, and has no obvious seams or cracks. Then reserve it for a specific purpose; for example, set it aside for cutting raw meat and poultry. Keep a separate wooden cutting board for chopping produce and slicing bread to prevent these products from picking up bacteria from raw meat. Many foods are served raw, so any bacteria clinging to them are not destroyed.

Furthermore, FDA recommends that all cutting boards be replaced when they become streaked with hard-to-clean grooves or cuts, which may harbor bacteria. In addition, cutting boards should be sanitized once a week in a dilute bleach solution. Flood the board with the solution, let it sit a few minutes, then rinse thoroughly.

▶ Regularly cleaning surfaces and equipment with a dilute bleach solution (1:10) is helpful in reducing the risk of cross-contamination of foods.

▶ The World Health Organization's Golden Rules for Safe Food Preparation

1. Choose foods processed for safety.
2. Cook food thoroughly.
3. Eat cooked foods immediately.
4. Store cooked foods carefully.
5. Reheat cooked foods thoroughly.
6. Avoid contact between raw and cooked foods.
7. Wash hands repeatedly.
8. Keep all kitchen surfaces meticulously clean.
9. Protect foods from insects, rodents, and other animals.
10. Use pure water.

The USDA simplified these rules into four actions as a part of their Fight BAC! Program (check out www.fightbac.org):

1. Clean. Wash hands and surfaces often.
2. Separate. Don't cross-contaminate.
3. Cook. Cook to proper temperatures.
4. Chill. Refrigerate promptly.

The 2005 Dietary Guidelines for Americans also stress the importance of these four actions.

▲ Food safety logo of USDA.

- When thawing foods, do so in the refrigerator, under cold potable running water, or in a microwave oven. Also, cook foods immediately after thawing under cold water or in the microwave. Never let frozen foods thaw unrefrigerated all day or night. Also, marinate food in the refrigerator.
- Avoid coughing or sneezing over foods, even when you're healthy. Cover cuts on hands with a sterile bandage. This helps stop *Staphylococcus* from entering food.
- Carefully wash fresh fruit and vegetables under running water to remove dirt and bacteria clinging to the surface, using a vegetable brush if the skin is to be eaten. People have become ill from *Salmonella* introduced from melons used in making a fruit salad and from oranges used for fresh-squeezed orange juice. The bacteria were on the outside of the melons and oranges.
- Completely remove moldy portions of food or don't eat the food. *When in doubt, throw the food out.* Mold growth is prevented by properly storing food at cold temperatures and using the food promptly.
- Use refrigerated ground meat and patties in 1 to 2 days and frozen meat and patties within 3 to 4 months. The 6-month interval mentioned in the comic at the beginning of this chapter is too long a time to be safe.

Cooking Food

- Cook food thoroughly using a bimetallic thermometer to check for doneness, especially for beef and fish (145°F [63°C]), pork (160°F [71°C]), and poultry (165°F [74°C]) (Fig. 15-1). Eggs should be cooked until the yolk and white are hard. Alfalfa sprouts and other types of sprouts should be cooked until they are steaming. Cooking is by far the most reliable way to destroy foodborne viruses and bacteria, such as Norovirus and toxic strains of *E. coli*. Freezing only halts viral and bacterial growth. FDA does not recommend that eggs be prepared sunny-side-up.

As noted, many restaurants now include an advisory on menus stating that an increased risk of foodborne illness is associated with eating undercooked eggs. As long as restaurants provide this warning on their menus, however, they are allowed to cook eggs to any temperature requested by the consumer. FDA warns us not to consume homemade ice cream, eggnog, and mayonnaise if made with unpasteurized, raw eggs because of the risk of *Salmonella* foodborne illness. It is safer to use eggs or egg products that have been pasteurized, which kills *Salmonella* bacteria. Overall, a good general precaution is to eat no raw animal products. USDA answers questions about the safe use of animal products (800-535-4555, 10 A.M. to 4 P.M. weekdays, Eastern time).

Seafood also poses a risk of foodborne illness, especially oysters. Properly cooked seafood should flake easily and/or be opaque or dull and firm. If it's translucent or shiny, it's not done.

- Cook stuffing separately from poultry (or wash poultry thoroughly, stuff immediately before cooking, and then transfer the stuffing to a clean bowl immediately after cooking). Make sure the stuffing reaches 165°F (74°C). *Salmonella* is the major concern with poultry.
- Once a food is cooked, consume it right away, or cool it to 41°F (5°C) within 2 hours. If it is not to be eaten immediately, in hot weather (80°F and above) make sure this cooling is done within 1 hour. Do this by separating the food into as many shallow pans as needed to provide a large surface area for cooling.

▲ Washing hands thoroughly (for at least 20 to 30 seconds) with hot water and soap should be the first step in food preparation. The 4 "F's" of food contamination are fingers, foods, feces, and flies. Handwashing especially combats the finger and fecal routes.

MEAT THERMOMETER

HACCP MIN. TEMPERATURES

Fresh ground beef, veal, lamb, and pork	155°F (68°C)
Beef, veal, lamb (roast, steaks, chops)	
Medium rare	145°F (63°C)
Medium	160°F (71°C)
Well done	170°F (77°C)
Fresh pork (roast, steaks, chops)	
Medium	160°F (71°C)
Well done	170°F (77°C)
Ham, cooked before eating	160°F (71°C)
Ham, reheat fully cooked	140°F (60°C)
Poultry	
Ground chicken, turkey	165°F (74°C)
Whole chicken, turkey	165°F (74°C)
Breasts, roasts	145°F (63°C)
Stuffing, alone or in bird	165°F (74°C)
Egg dishes, casseroles	145°F (63°C)
Leftovers, to reheat	165°F (74°C)

▲ Sushi, like all raw fish or meat dishes, is a high-risk food. For maximum protection from foodborne illness, animal foods should be cooked thoroughly before eating.

FIGURE 15-1 ▶ Minimum internal temperatures when cooking or reheating foods.

Be careful not to recontaminate cooked food by contact with raw meat or juices from hands, cutting boards, dirty utensils, or in other ways.

- Serve meat, poultry, and fish on a clean plate—never the same plate used to hold the raw product. For example, when grilling hamburgers, don't put cooked items on the same plate used to carry the raw product out to the grill.
- For outdoor cooking, cook food completely at the picnic site, with no partial cooking in advance.

Storing and Reheating Cooked Food

- Keep foods out of the "danger zone" by keeping hot foods hot and cold foods cold. Hold food below 41°F (5°C) or above 135°F (57°C). Foodborne mi-

croorganisms thrive in more moderate temperatures (60°F to 110°F [16°C to 43°C]). Some microorganisms can even grow in the refrigerator. Again, don't leave cooked or refrigerated foods, such as meats and salads, at room temperature for more than 2 hours (or 1 hour in hot

weather) because that gives microorganisms an opportunity to grow. Store dry food at 60°F to 70°F (16°C to 21°C).

- Reheat leftovers to 165°F (74°C); reheat gravy to a rolling boil to kill *Clostridium perfringens* bacteria, which may be present. Merely reheating to a good eating

▶ **Current Safe Handling Instructions Issued by USDA for Labeling Meat and Poultry Products**

This product was prepared from inspected and passed meat and/or poultry. Some food products may contain bacteria that could cause illness if the product is mishandled or cooked improperly. For your protection, follow these handling instructions.

Keep refrigerated or frozen.

Thaw in refrigerator or microwave.

Keep raw meat and poultry separate from other foods.

Wash working surfaces (including cutting boards), utensils, and hands after touching raw meat or poultry.

Cook thoroughly.

Keep hot foods hot. Refrigerate leftovers immediately or discard.

▶ **Safe Handling Instructions for Eggs**

To prevent illness from bacteria: keep eggs refrigerated, cook eggs until yolks are firm, and cook foods containing eggs thoroughly.

▶ To reduce the risk of bacteria surviving during microwave cooking,

- Cover food with glass or ceramic when possible to decrease evaporation and heat the surface.
- Stir and rotate food at least once or twice for even cooking. Then, allow microwaved food to stand, covered, after heating is completed to help cook the exterior and equalize the temperature throughout.
- Use the oven temperature probe or a meat thermometer to check that food is done. Insert it at several spots.
- If thawing meat in the microwave, use the oven's defrost setting. Ice crystals in frozen foods are not heated well by the microwave oven and can create cold spots, which later cook more slowly.

temperature isn't sufficient to kill harmful bacteria.

- Store peeled or cut-up produce, such as melon balls, in the refrigerator.
- Make sure the refrigerator stays below 41°F (5°C). Either use a refrigerator thermometer or keep it as cold as possible without freezing milk and lettuce.
- Keep leftovers in the refrigerator only for the recommended length of time (Figure 15-2).

Cross-contamination is not only a threat during food preparation; it can also become a problem during food storage. Make sure all foods, including leftovers, are contained and covered in the refrigerator to prevent drippings from uncooked and potentially hazardous foods from tainting other foods. It is a good idea to store foods likely to pose risk of foodborne illness on lower shelves of the refrigerator, beneath other foods to be eaten raw.

When in doubt, throw it out!

Food	Refrigerator Storage Time (days)
Meats	
Cooked ground beef/turkey	3-4
Deli meat	2-3
Cooked pork	3-4
Cooked poultry	3-4
Cooked beef, bison, lamb	3-4
Seafood	
Raw (e.g. sushi/sashimi)	Must consume on day of purchase
Cooked	2
Other Entrees	
Pizza	1-2
Pasta/rice	1-2
Casserole	3-4
Soups and Chili	
Chili with meat	2-3
Chili without meat	3-4
Soup/stew	3-4
Side Dishes	
Fresh salad	1-2
Fresh vegetables	1-2
Pasta or potato salad	2-3
Deviled egg	2-3
Hard boiled egg	7
Potato (any style)	3-4
Cooked vegetables	3-4
Dessert	
Cream pie	2-3
Fruit pie	2-3
Pastries	7
Cake	7
Cheesecake	7

FIGURE 15-2 ▶ Length of time to keep leftovers in the refrigerator.

CONCEPT CHECK

Thoroughly cook all meat and poultry to reduce the risk of foodborne illness from *E. coli*, and *Salmonella*. In addition, always separate raw meats and poultry products from cooked foods. To prevent foodborne intoxication from *Staphylococcus* organisms, cover cuts on hands and avoid sneezing on foods. To avoid intoxication from *Clostridium perfringens*, rapidly cool leftover foods and thoroughly reheat them. To avoid intoxication from *Clostridium botulinum*, carefully examine canned foods. Overall, don't allow cooked food to stand for more than 1 to 2 hours at room temperature. For other causes of foodborne illness, precautions already mentioned generally apply as well. In addition, thoroughly cook fish and other seafood; consume only pasteurized dairy products; wash all fruits and vegetables; and thoroughly wash your hands with soap and water before and after preparing food and after using the bathroom.

CASE STUDY

Preventing Foodborne Illness at Gatherings

Nicole attended a gathering of her co-workers on a warm Saturday in July. The theme of the party was international dining. Nicole and her husband were asked to bring an Argentinian dish, potato and beef empanadas. They followed the recipe and cooking time carefully, removing the dish from the oven at 1 P.M. and keeping it warm by wrapping the pan in a towel. They traveled in their car to the party and set the dish out on the buffet table at 3 P.M. Dinner was to be served at 4 P.M. However, the guests were enjoying themselves so much lounging around the host's pool and drinking ginger beer (also on the menu) that no one began to eat until 6 P.M. Nicole made sure she sampled the empanadas that she and her husband made, while her husband did not. She also had some salad, garlic bread, and a sweet dessert made with coconut.

The couple returned home at 11 P.M. and went to bed. At about 2 A.M., Nicole knew something was wrong. She had severe ab-

dominal pain and had to make a dash to the bathroom. She spent most of the next 3 hours in the bathroom with severe diarrhea. By dawn, the diarrhea subsided and she started to feel better. After a few cups of tea and a light breakfast, she was feeling like herself by noon.

Answer the following questions, and check your responses in Appendix A.

1. Based on her symptoms, what type of foodborne illness did Nicole contract?
2. Why is the beef the most likely vehicle for this type of foodborne illness?
3. Why is consuming food at large gatherings risky?
4. What precautions for avoiding foodborne illness were ignored by Nicole and the rest of the people at the party?
5. How could this scenario be rewritten to substanitally reduce the risk of foodborne illness?

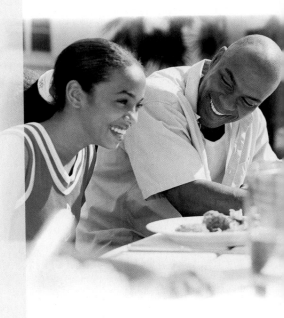

SUMMARY

1. Viruses, bacteria, and other microorganisms in food pose the greatest risk for foodborne illness. In the past, salt, sugar, smoke, fermentation, and drying were used to protect against foodborne illness. Today, careful cooking, pasteurization, keeping hot foods hot and cold foods cold, and thorough handwashing provide additional insurance.

2. Major causes of foodborne illness are Norovirus and the bacteria *Campylobacter jejuni*, *Salmonella*, *Staphylococcus aureus*, and *Clostridium perfringens*. In addition, such bacteria as *Clostridium botulinum*, *Listeria monocytogenes*, and *Escherichia coli* have been found to cause illness.

3. Food additives are used primarily to extend shelf life by preventing microbial growth and the destruction of food components by oxygen, metals, and other substances. Food additives are classified as those intentionally added to foods and those that incidentally appear in foods. An intentional additive is limited to no more than one-one-hundredth of the greatest amount that causes no

observed symptoms in animals. Under its jurisdiction in the United States, the Delaney Clause allows FDA to ban the use of any intentional food additive that causes cancer.

4. Antioxidants, such as BHA, BHT, vitamins E and C, and sulfites, prevent oxygen and enzyme destruction of food products. Emulsifiers suspend fat in water, improving the uniformity, smoothness, and body of foods such as ice cream. Common preservatives include salt, sodium benzoate, and sorbic acid, which prevent bacterial growth. Sequestrants bind metals and thus prevent spoilage of food from metal contamination. Various natural products such as natural flavors, sugar, and corn syrup, as well as artificial flavors and sweeteners, such as aspartame, improve the flavor of food.

5. Toxic substances occur naturally in a variety of foods, such as green potatoes, raw fish, mushrooms, and raw egg whites. Cooking foods limits their toxic effects in some cases; others are best to avoid altogether, such as toxic mushroom species and the green parts of potatoes.

6. A variety of environmental contaminants and pesticide residues can be found in foods. It is helpful to know which foods pose the greatest risks and act accordingly to reduce exposure, such as washing fruits and vegetables before use.

7. To protect against viruses and bacteria, cook susceptible foods thoroughly. In addition, cover cuts on the hands, do not sneeze or cough on foods, avoid contact between raw meat or poultry products and other food products, rapidly cool and thoroughly reheat leftovers, and use pasteurized dairy products. Overall, be careful when foods are in the "danger zone" (41°F to 135°F).

8. Cross-contamination commonly causes foodborne illness. It occurs particularly when bacteria on raw animal products contact foods that can support bacterial growth. Because of the risk of cross-contamination, no perishable food should be kept in the "danger zone" for more than 1 to 2 hours (depending on the environmental temperature), especially if it may have come in contact with raw animal products.

STUDY QUESTIONS

1. Identify three major classes of microorganisms responsible for foodborne illness.

2. Which types of foods are most likely to be involved in foodborne illness? Why are they targets for contamination?

3. What three trends in food purchasing and production have led to a greater number of cases of foodborne illness?

4. Why is thoroughly cooking food an important practice for reducing the risk of foodborne illness?

5. List four techniques other than thorough cooking that are important in preventing foodborne illness.

6. Define the term *food additive*, and give examples of four intentional food additives. What are their specific functions in foods? What is their relationship to the GRAS list?

7. Describe the federal process that governs the use of food additives, including the Delaney Clause.

8. Put into perspective the benefits and risks of using additives in food. Point out an easy way to reduce the consumption of food additives. Do you think this is worth the effort in terms of maintaining health? Why or why not?

9. Describe four recommendations for reducing the risk of toxicity from environmental contaminants.

10. How do various U.S. federal agencies work together to maintain the safety of food?

CHECK YOUR KNOWLEDGE

Answers to the following multiple choice questions are in Appendix A.

1. Nitrite prevents the growth of
   a. *Clostridium botulinum.*
   b. *Escherichia coli.*
   c. *Staphylococcus aureus.*
   d. yeasts.

2. Substances used to preserve foods by lowering the pH are
   a. smoke and irradiation.
   b. baking powder and soda.
   c. salt and sugar.
   d. vinegar and citric acid.

3. Food additives widely used for many years without apparent ill effects are on the _____ list.
   a. FDA   c. USDA
   b. the GRAS   d. the Delaney

4. The food-borne illness organism often associated with small cuts and boils is
   a. *Listeria.*   c. *C. botulinum.*
   b. *Staphylococcus.*   d. *Salmonella.*

5. Salmonella bacteria are usually spread via
   a. raw meats, poultry, and eggs.
   b. pickled vegetables.
   c. home-canned vegetables.
   d. raw vegetables.

6. It is unwise to thaw meats or poultry
   a. in a microwave oven.
   b. in the refrigerator.
   c. under cool running water.
   d. at room temperature.

7. Milk that can remain on supermarket shelves, free of microbial growth, for many years has been processed by which of the following methods?
   a. use of humectants
   b. using antibiotics in animal feed
   c. use of sequestrants
   d. aseptic processing

8. Those at greatest risk for food-borne illness include
   a. pregnant women.
   b. infants and children.

   c. immunosuppressed individuals.
   d. All of the above.

9. Pasteurization involves the
   a. exposure of food to high temperatures for short periods to destroy harmful microorganisms.
   b. exposure of food to heat to inactivate enzymes that cause undesirable effects in foods during storage.
   c. fortification of foods with vitamins A and D.
   d. use of irradiation to destroy certain pathogens in foods

10. Food can be kept for long periods by adding salt or sugar because these substances
    a. make the food too acidic for spoilage to occur.
    b. bind to water, thereby making it unavailable to the microorganisms.
    c. effectively kill microorganisms.
    d. dissolve the cell walls in plant foods.

FURTHER READINGS

1. Acheson DWK and Fiore AE: Preventing foodborne illness—what clinicians can do. *The New England Journal of Medicine* 350:437, 2004.

   The food supply in the United States is mostly safe, but more could be done to lessen the risk for developing foodborne illness. This article discusses strategies to do so, as well as summarizes the characteristics of the major organisms that cause foodborne illness.

2. ADA Reports: Position of the American Dietetic Association: Food and water safety. *Journal of the American Dietetic Association* 103:1203, 2003.

   It is the position of the American Dietetic Association that the public has a right to a safe food and water supply. Still, it is estimated that on an annual basis, there are 76 million cases of foodborne illness in the United States, with significant economic cost. Thus, more work needs

   to be done with regard to food safety. The safety of drinking water is a lesser concern in general for most consumers, but still deserves consideration as a potential source of illness.

3. Anderson JB and others: A camera's view of consumer food-handling behaviors. *Journal of the American Dietetic Association* 104:186, 2004.

   Improper food handling practices were common in the households studied in this survey.

Implementing the Fight BAC! Campaign recommendations, such as using a thermometer to test for doneness in meats, would improve food handling practices.

4. Atreya CD: Major foodborne illness causing viruses and current status of vaccines against the disease. *Foodborne Pathogens and Disease* 1(2):89, 2004 (Summer).

   As many as 67% of cases of foodborne illnesses are caused by viruses. Except for hepatitis A virus, no vaccines are available for the major players, but may be available in the near future. This article reviews the progress in this area.

5. Calvert GM: Health effects of pesticides. *American Family Physician* 69:1613, 2004.

   Clear cases of disease from pesticide exposure are seen from acute exposures with high amounts. The true effects of low dose, chronic exposure have been hard to quantify, but most adults have detectable pesticide levels in their blood. Thus, efforts should be made to reduce pesticide exposure when possible, especially with use in and around the house.

6. Consumers Union: Dirty birds: Even "premium" chickens harbor dangerous bacteria. *Consumer Reports* p. 20, January 2007.

   An analysis of fresh, whole chickens bought throughout the United States revealed that 83% contained Campylobacter or Salmonella, two leading causes of foodborne disease. This article describes the details of the investigation and findings.

7. Dorner B: The four most serious causes of foodborne illness. *Today's Dietitian* 5:40, April 2003.

   The CDC considers E. coli O157:H7, Salmonella enteritidis, Listeria monocytogenes, and Campylobacter jejuni the most serious causes of foodborne illness. Cases, causes, and symptoms of these illnesses are reviewed.

8. Food Safety and Inspection Service: A century of progress in food safety. *Be Food Safe* Fall:12, 2006.

   The Federal Meat Inspection Act became law in 1906. This article summarizes the 100-year history of federal inspection of meat and poultry.

9. Gerner-Smidt P and others: Invasive listeriosis in Denmark 1994-2003: A review of 299 cases with special emphasis on risk factors for mortality. *Clinical Microbiological Infections* 11:618, 2005.

   Listeria infections lead to death primarily in older people and those with underlying cases of cancer. It is therefore especially important for these people to be careful of exposure to Listeria.

10. Hillers VN and others: Consumer food-handling behaviors associated with prevention of 13 foodborne illnesses. *Journal of Food Protection* 66:1893, 2003.

    Handwashing is highly recommended by experts for the prevention of foodborne illness. The importance of not eating certain foods, such as raw seafood, is another important habit to consider. The use of a thermometer in cooking is also an important practice, as is avoidance of cross-contamination of food products.

11. How now mad cow? *Tufts University Health & Nutrition Letter* p. 4, May 2004.

    After a case of mad cow disease in the United States, the FDA expanded regulations regarding the feeding and slaughter of cattle. This goes beyond the already strict regulations put in place in 1997 to limit risk of mad cow disease. Overall, the risk of contracting mad cow disease from meat in the United States remains low. Still, one could consider avoiding ground meat products, such as hot dogs, and cow brains to further reduce risk as these are most likely to contain the agent linked to the disease.

12. McCabe-Sellers BJ, Beattie SF: Food safety: emerging trends in foodborne illness surveillance and prevention. *Journal of the American Dietetic Association* 104:1708, 2004.

    Detailed discussion of prevention of foodborne illness, such as paying attention to fresh produce as a source of the primary causative agents—viruses and bacteria. Recommendations for consumers and food handlers are given to reduce risk of foodborne illness, with proper personal hygiene being a major focus.

13. Musher DM, Musher BL: Contagious acute bacterial infections. *The New England Journal of Medicine* 351:2417, 2004.

    Detailed discussion of the viruses and bacteria associated with foodborne illness. Handwashing is one important method mentioned to reduce exposure. Use of diluted bleach solutions (1:10) on surfaces is also recommended when possible.

14. Roche SJ, Keenan MJ: Should we be eating organically grown foods? *Today's Dietitian*, p. 50, September 2003.

    Probably the most valid reason for consuming organically grown foods instead of conventionally grown foods is the protection of the environment, farmers, and wildlife from pesticide exposure. Promotion of organic foods, however, must be balanced by the observation that use of pesticides by farmers increases efficiency and is a key reason for the abundance of food available in the United States.

15. Schardt D: Get the lead out—What you don't know can hurt you. *Nutrition Action Healthletter* p. 1, March 2005.

    Reducing lead exposure as much as possible is important to protect one's health. There is evidence that hypertension, kidney disease, declines in brain function, and cataracts are linked to lead exposure. Testing your water supply for lead as outlined in the article is one inexpensive way to be alerted to a possible source. Using only cold tap water for cooking is also advised.

16. Scheier LM: The safety of beef in the United States. *Journal of the American Dietetic Association* 105:339, 2005.

    Bovine spongiform encephalopathy, better known as mad cow disease, continues to be of interest to the general public. The protocols involved in testing and keeping beef safe for the public are discussed in this article, as well as current legislation.

17. Sivapalasingam S and others: Fresh produce: A growing cause of outbreaks of foodborne illness in the United States. *Journal of Food Protection* 67:2342, 2004.

    Fresh produce such as lettuce, juices, melons, sprouts, and berries have been highlighted as sources of agents that lead to foodborne illness. Caution should be used with these items, just as one would with raw meat and dairy products.

18. U.S. Food and Drug Administration: *Food Code.* U.S. Department of Health and Human Services, Public Health Service, Food and Drug Administration: College Park, MD, 2005.

    FDA Food Code provides scientifically sound technical and legal basis for regulating the retail and food service segment of the food industry, including restaurants, grocery stores, and institutions, such as nursing homes. The Food Code serves as a model for local, state, tribal, and federal regulators to develop or update their food safety rules and to be consistent with national food regulatory policy.

19. Widdowson MA and others: Norovirus and foodborne disease, United States, 1991–2000. *Emerging Infectious Diseases* 11:95, 2005.

    The Norovirus leads to more causes of foodborne illness than any other agent. What is now needed is better surveillance for this organism so better estimates of cases can be made.

20. Yates J: Traveler's diarrhea. *American Family Physician* 71:2095, 2005.

    Millions of people who travel are affected by acute diarrhea each year. The contamination of food and water with fecal matter are the main sources of the infection. Escherichia coli, enteroaggregative E. coli, Campylobacter, Salmonella, and Shigella are common causes of traveler's diarrhea, whereas parasites and viruses are less common causes.

▶ **Check out the Contemporary Nutrition ARIS site**

www.mhhe.com/wardlawcontfa1 for quizzes, flash cards, other activities, and weblinks designed to further help you learn about issues surrounding safety of food and water.

RATE YOUR PLATE

I. Can You Spot the Improper Food Safety Practices?

In this chapter you learned that (1) foodborne illness strikes up to 76 million U.S. citizens each year and (2) about 5000 deaths each year in the United States are caused by food-borne organisms.

Carefully preparing foods to prevent foodborne illness can minimize its occurrence for most of us. Read the following excerpt and find the food safety violations that could lead to illness.

A Local Health Department Inspector Gives the Following Account of His Visit to a Local Diner

As I walked through the kitchen of the Morningside Diner, I noticed that all food handlers washed their hands thoroughly with hot, soapy water before handling the food, especially after handling raw meat, fish, poultry, or eggs. Before preparing raw foods, they also thoroughly washed the cutting boards, dishes, and other equipment. As they used their cutting boards after cutting foods, they wiped them with a damp rag and used them again to cut more food.

When preparing fresh fruits and vegetables, they washed them but were careful to leave a little dirt on for fear of washing important nutrients from the outside. The cooks generally cooked meats to an internal temperature of 180°F (82°C). However, to preserve the flavor, pork was cooked to an internal temperature of 140°F (60°C). Some cooked foods to be served later were cooled to below 41°F (5°C) within 2 hours, and foods like beef stew were cooled in shallow pans.

The diner served canned foods, even when the cans were dented. When leftovers were reheated, they were raised to an internal temperature of 130°F (55°C) and served immediately. Food handlers took great care to remove moldy portions of food. The cooks prepared stuffing separately from the poultry. The temperature of refrigerators was approximately 45°F (7°C).

1. List the violations of food safety practices that could contribute to foodborne illness.

_____

_____

_____

_____

2. If you were writing a report describing ways to correct these practices, what would you say?

_____

_____

_____

_____

_____

3. List the food safety practices that follow the general rules for preventing foodborne illness.

_____

_____

_____

_____

II. Take a Closer Look at Food Additives

Evaluate a food label of a convenience food item (e.g., frozen entree, ready-to-eat baked good) either in the supermarket or one you have available.

1. Write out the list of ingredients.

   _____

   _____

   _____

   _____

2. Identify the ingredients that you think may be food additives.

   _____

   _____

   _____

   _____

3. Based on the information available in this chapter, what are the functions of these food additives?

   _____

   _____

   _____

   _____

4. How might this food product differ without these ingredients?

   _____

   _____

   _____

   _____

CHAPTER 16 Pregnancy and Breastfeeding

PREGNANCY CAN BE A SPECIAL TIME. Exhilaration and amazement accompany parents' tremendous responsibility of helping a child develop and grow. Parents-to-be often feel an overriding desire to produce a healthy baby, which can arouse new interest in nutrition and health information. They usually want to do everything possible to maximize their chances of having a robust, lively newborn.

Despite these intentions, the infant mortality rate in North America is higher than that seen in many other industrialized nations. In Canada, about 6.1 of every 1000 infants per year die before their first birthday, while in the United States, it is 6.9. These are alarming statistics for two countries that have such a high per capita expenditure for health care compared to many other countries in the world. Comparatively, the rate of infant mortality in Sweden is roughly 3 of every 1000 infants. In addition, in the United States, about 20% of pregnant women receive inadequate prenatal care in the early months of pregnancy. Expectant teenagers are at the highest risk for this.

Producing a healthy baby is not just a matter of luck. True, some aspects of fetal and newborn health are beyond our control. Still, as the comic in this chapter suggests, conscious decisions about social, health, environmental, and nutritional factors during pregnancy significantly affect the baby's future. Choosing to breastfeed the infant adds further benefits. Let's examine how eating well during pregnancy and breastfeeding can help a baby to have a healthy start in life.

 Refresh Your Memory

As you begin your study of nutrition in pregnancy and breastfeeding in Chapter 16, you may want to review:

- Typical fortification in meal replacement bars in Chapter 1 and ready-to-eat breakfast cereals in Chapter 2
- Causes and effects of ketosis in Chapter 4
- Components of the macronutrient classes—carbohydrates, proteins, and lipids—in Chapters 4 to 6, especially omega-3 fatty aids
- Calculation of body mass index in Chapter 7
- Food sources of calcium in Chapter 10 and folate, iron, and zinc in Chapter 11

PLANNING FOR PREGNANCY

▶ *Healthy People 2010* includes a goal of increasing to 80% the number of pregnancies that begin with optimal folate status from the current estimate of 21%, in an effort to reduce the occurrence of neural tube defects.

Many practices or conditions of the mother can harm the developing fetus, so planning for pregnancy is important. The following are some potentially harmful habits that can be modified when planning to have a baby:

- Lack of enough synthetic folic acid in the diet (at least 3 months before becoming pregnant)
- Any amount of alcohol consumption

Which diet and lifestyle habits contribute to a successful pregnancy? Which are likely to be harmful? Why should a woman begin to prepare for pregnancy months before conception of her new baby? When pregnant, does the mother need to "eat for two"? Chapter 16 provides some answers.

© Rina Piccolo. Reprinted with special permission of King Features Syndicate.

- Use of certain medicines, such as aspirin and related NSAIDs (e.g., ibuprofen [Advil]), as well as typical medicines used to treat the common cold
- Use of herbal therapies
- Use of illegal drugs, such as marijuana and cocaine
- Job-related hazards and stresses
- Smoking
- Inadequate intake of other nutrients, such as too little iron, magnesium, and zinc
- Excess vitamin A intake and megadose use of other nutrient supplements
- Heavy caffeine use
- Lack of medical treatment with HIV-positive status or AIDS
- Poor control of ongoing diabetes or hypertension
- X-ray exposure, including dental X-rays

Women need to pay attention to these risks in the months before conception. This precaution is necessary because women often do not suspect they are pregnant during the first few weeks after conception and may not seek medical attention until after the first 2 to 3 months of pregnancy.

Still, even without fanfare, the child-to-be grows and develops daily. For that reason, the health and nutrition habits of a woman who is trying to become pregnant—or who has the potential to become pregnant—are particularly important. Although some aspects of fetal and newborn health are beyond the parents' control, a woman's conscious decisions about social, health, environmental, and nutritional factors affect her infant's health and future. Much research suggests that an adequate vitamin and mineral intake at least 8 weeks before conception and then during pregnancy can help prevent birth defects such as neural tube defects (review Figure 11-14 in Chapter 11). Neural tube defects especially have been linked to a folate deficiency. Recall from Chapter 11 that neural tube defects develop within 28 days after conception, and that adequate folate status before and during this part of pregnancy reduces the risk of such defects by about 70%. In addition, because about 50% of pregnancies are unplanned, all women of childbearing age should be aware of the role nutrition plays in the development of a healthy infant, both before and during pregnancy. Following a healthy diet is then important. The American College of Obstetrics and Gynecology reminds women that it is especially important to meet folate needs (400 micrograms of synthetic folic acid). This is possible if the woman makes careful dietary choices. Alternately, adding a balanced multivitamin and mineral supplement to one's diet is also appropriate for meeting this goal.

MAKING DECISIONS

Folate Supplements

Women who have previously given birth to an infant with a neural tube defect such as spina bifida should consult their physician about the need for folate supplementation; an intake of 4 milligrams of synthetic folic acid per day at least one month prior to conception is recommended, but must be taken under a physician's supervision.

PRENATAL GROWTH AND DEVELOPMENT

For 8 weeks after conception, a human **embryo** develops from a fertilized **ovum** into a **fetus.** For about another 32 weeks, the fetus continues to develop. When its body finally matures, the infant is born. Until birth, the mother nourishes it via a **placenta,** an organ that forms in her uterus to accommodate the growth and development of the fetus (Fig. 16-1). The role of the placenta is to exchange nutrients, oxygen and other gases, and waste products between the mother and the fetus.

embryo In humans, the developing offspring in utero from about the beginning of the third week to the end of the eighth week after conception.

ovum The egg cell from which a fetus eventually develops if the egg is fertilized by a sperm cell.

fetus The developing life form from about the beginning of the ninth week after conception until birth.

placenta An organ that forms in the uterus in pregnant women. Through this organ, oxygen and nutrients from the mother's blood are transferred to the fetus, and fetal wastes are removed. The placenta also releases hormones that maintain the state of pregnancy.

FIGURE 16-1 ▶ The fetus in relationship to the placenta. The placenta is the organ through which nourishment flows to the fetus.

- Amniotic fluid
- Umbilical cord (fetal circulation)
- Placenta (site of nutrient exchange and maternal circulation)
- Uterus

zygote The fertilized ovum; the cell resulting from the union of an egg cell (ovum) and sperm until it divides.

trimesters Three 13- to 14-week periods into which the normal pregnancy (the length of a normal pregnancy is about 40 weeks, measured from the first day of the woman's last menstrual period) is divided somewhat arbitrarily for purposes of discussion and analysis. Development of the offspring, however, is continuous throughout pregnancy, with no specific physiological markers demarcating the transition from one trimester to the next.

spontaneous abortion Cessation of pregnancy and expulsion of the embryo or nonviable fetus prior to 20 weeks gestation. This is the result of natural causes, such as a genetic defect or developmental problem; also called *miscarriage*.

Early Growth—The First Trimester Is a Very Critical Time

In the formation of the human organism, egg and sperm first unite, producing the **zygote** (Fig. 16-2). From this point, the reproductive process occurs very rapidly:

- Within 30 hours—zygote divides in half to form 2 cells.
- Within 4 days—cell number climbs to 128 cells.
- At 14 days—the group of cells is called an embryo.
- Within 35 days—heart is beating, embryo is 1/30 of an inch (8 millimeters) long, eyes and limb buds are clearly visible.
- At 8 weeks—the embryo is known as a fetus.
- At 13 weeks (end of first trimester)—most organs are formed, and the fetus can move.

For purposes of discussion, the duration of pregnancy—normally, 38 to 42 weeks—is commonly divided into three periods, called **trimesters.** Growth begins in the first trimester with a rapid increase in cell number. This type of growth dominates embryonic and early fetal development. The newly formed cells then begin to grow larger. Further growth is a mix of increases in cell number and cell size. By the end of 13 weeks—the first trimester—most organs are formed and the fetus can move (see Fig. 16-2).

As the embryo or fetus develops, nutritional deficiencies and other insults have the potential to impose damage or risk to organ systems. For example, adverse reactions to medications, high intakes of vitamin A, exposure to radiation, or trauma can alter or arrest the current phase of fetal development, and the effects may last a lifetime (review Fig. 16-2). The most critical time for these potential problems is during the first trimester. Most **spontaneous abortions**—premature terminations of pregnancy that occur naturally—happen at this time. About one-half or more pregnancies end in this way, often so early that a woman does not even realize she was pregnant. (An

◀ The time to begin thinking about prenatal nutrition is before becoming pregnant. This includes making sure folic acid intake is adequate (400 micrograms of synthetic folic acid per day) and that any supplemental intake of preformed vitamin A does not exceed 100% of the Daily Value (1000 micrograms RAE or 5000 IU).

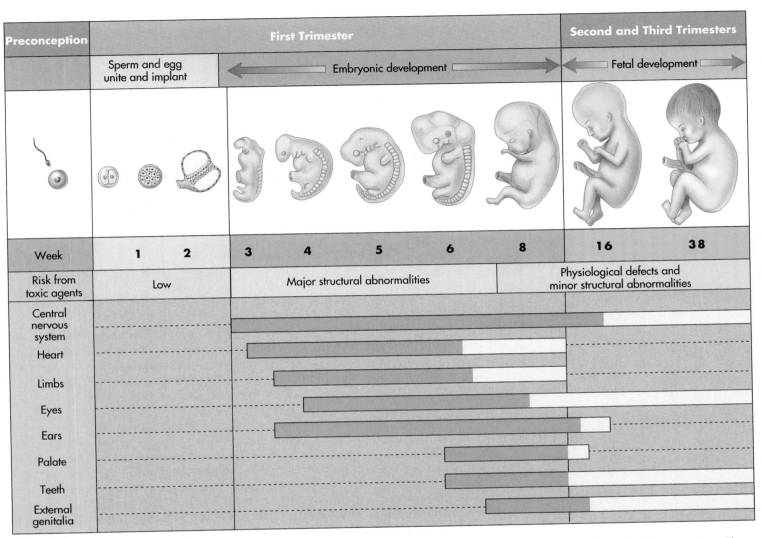

Preconception	First Trimester							Second and Third Trimesters	
	Sperm and egg unite and implant	Embryonic development						Fetal development	
Week	1	2	3	4	5	6	8	16	38
Risk from toxic agents	Low		Major structural abnormalities					Physiological defects and minor structural abnormalities	
Central nervous system									
Heart									
Limbs									
Eyes									
Ears									
Palate									
Teeth									
External genitalia									

FIGURE 16-2 ▶ Harmful effects of toxic agents during pregnancy. Vulnerable periods of fetal development are indicated with orange bars. The orange shading indicates the time of greatest risk to the organ. The most serious damage to the fetus from exposure to toxins is likely to occur during the first 8 weeks after conception, two-thirds of the way through the first trimester. As the white bars in the chart shows, however, damage to vital parts of the body—including the eyes, brain, and genitals—can also occur during the later months of pregnancy.

additional 15% to 20% are lost before normal delivery.) Early spontaneous abortions usually result from a genetic defect or fatal error in fetal development. Smoking, alcohol abuse, use of aspirin and NSAIDs, and illicit drug use raise the risk for spontaneous abortion.

A woman should avoid substances that may harm the developing fetus, especially during the first trimester. This holds true, as well, for the time when a woman is trying to become pregnant. As previously mentioned, she is unlikely to be aware of her pregnancy for at least a few weeks. In addition, the fetus develops so rapidly during the first trimester that, if an essential nutrient is not available, the fetus may be affected even before evidence of the nutrient deficiency appears in the mother.

For this reason, the quality—rather than the quantity—of one's nutritional intake is most important during the first trimester. In other words, women should consume the same amount of calories, but the foods chosen should be more nutrient dense. Although some women lose their appetite and feel nauseated during the first trimester, they should be careful to meet nutrient needs as much as possible.

▶ A healthy 1-week-old baby. At birth, a baby usually weighs about 7.5 pounds and is 20 inches long.

Although a mother's decisions, practices, and precautions during pregnancy contribute to the health of her fetus, she cannot guarantee her fetus good health because some genetic and environmental factors are beyond her control. She and others involved in the pregnancy should not hold an unrealistic illusion of total control.

Second Trimester

By the beginning of the second trimester, a fetus weighs about 1 ounce. Arms, hands, fingers, legs, feet, and toes are fully formed. The fetus has ears and begins to form tooth sockets in its jawbone. Organs continue to grow and mature, and, with a stethoscope, physicians can detect the fetus's heartbeat. Most bones are distinctly evident through the body. Eventually, the fetus begins to look more like an infant. It may suck its thumb and kick strongly enough to be felt by the mother. As was shown in Figure 16-2, the fetus can still be affected by exposure to toxins, but not to the degree seen in the first trimester.

During the second trimester, the mother's breast weight increases by approximately 30% due to the development of milk-producing cells and the deposition of 2 to 4 pounds of fat for **lactation.** This stored fat serves as a reservoir for the extra calories needed to produce breast milk.

lactation The period of milk secretion following pregnancy; typically called *breastfeeding*.

gestation The period of intrauterine development of offspring, from conception to birth; in humans, gestation lasts for about 40 weeks after the woman's previous menstrual period.

Third Trimester

By the beginning of the third trimester, a fetus weighs about 2 to 3 pounds. The third trimester is a crucial time for fetal growth. The fetus will double in length and will increase its weight by three to four times. The fetus takes higher priority than the mother with regard to iron and will deplete the stores of the mother. If the mother is not meeting her iron needs, she can be severely depleted after delivery. An infant born after about 26 weeks of **gestation** has a good chance of survival if cared for in a nursery for high-risk newborns. However, the infant will not contain the stores of minerals (mainly iron and calcium) and fat normally accumulated during the last month of gestation. This and other medical problems, such as a poor ability to suck and swallow, complicate nutritional care for preterm infants.

At 9 months, the fetus usually weighs about 7 to 9 pounds (3 to 4 kilograms) and is about 20 inches (50 centimeters) long. A soft spot on the top of the head indicates where the skull bones (fontanels) are growing together. The bones finally close by the time the baby is about 12 to 18 months of age.

▶ A goal of *Healthy People 2010* is to reduce low birth weight and preterm births by one-third.

SUCCESS IN PREGNANCY

The goal of pregnancy is to achieve optimal health for both the baby and the mother. For the mother, a successful pregnancy is one in which her physical and emotional health is protected so that she can return to her prepregnancy health status. For the infant, two widely accepted criteria are (1) a gestation period longer than 37 weeks and (2) a birth weight greater than 5.5 pounds (2.5 kilograms). Sufficient lung development, likely to have occurred by 37 weeks of gestation, is critical to the survival of a newborn. The longer the gestation, the greater the ultimate birth weight and maturation state, leading to fewer medical problems and better quality of life for the infant. Overall, a successful pregnancy is the outcome of a complex interplay between genes, various lifestyle practices, and the environment.

Infant Birthweight

Low-birth-weight (LBW) infants are those weighing less than 5.5 pounds (2.5 kilograms) at birth. Most commonly, LBW is associated with **preterm** birth. Hospital-related costs of caring for LBW newborns total more than $2 billion per year in the United States, ranging from $20,000 to $200,000 per infant. Compare this with an average hospital-related cost of $4300 for a normal delivery and an average of $800 for preventive prenatal care. Full-term and preterm infants who weigh less than the expected weight for their duration of gestation, the result of insufficient growth, are described as **small for gestational age (SGA)**. Thus, a full-term infant weighing less than 5.5 pounds at birth is SGA but not preterm, whereas a preterm infant born at 30 weeks' gestation is probably LBW without being SGA. Infants who are SGA are more likely than normal-weight infants to have medical complications, including problems with blood glucose control, temperature regulation, growth, and development in the early weeks after birth.

Prenatal Care and Counseling

Adequate prenatal care is a primary determinant of success in pregnancy. Ideally, women should receive examinations and counseling before becoming pregnant and continue regular prenatal care throughout pregnancy. If prenatal care is inadequate, delayed, or absent, untreated maternal nutritional deficiencies can deprive a developing fetus of needed nutrients. In addition, untreated health conditions, such as anemia, AIDS, hypertension, or diabetes, must be carefully addressed to minimize complications of pregnancy. Treating ongoing infections will also decrease risks of fetal damage. Without prenatal care, a woman is three times more likely to deliver an LBW baby—one who will be 40 times more likely to die during the first 4 weeks of life than a normal-birth-weight infant. Although the ideal time to start prenatal care is before conception, about 20% of women in the United States receive no prenatal care throughout the first trimester—a critical time to positively influence the outcome of pregnancy.

Food habits cannot be predicted from income, education, or lifestyle. Although some women already have good dietary habits, most can benefit from nutritional advice. All should be reminded of habits that may harm the growing fetus, such as severe dieting or fasting. By focusing on appropriate prenatal care, nutrient intake, and health habits, parents give their fetus—and later, their infant—the best chance of thriving. Overall, the chances of producing a healthy baby are maximized with education, an adequate diet, and early and consistent prenatal medical care.

Effects of Maternal Age

The age of the mother is another factor that determines pregnancy outcome. The recommended age for pregnancy is between 20 and 35 years of age. Outside that age range—at either extreme—complications may arise. Pregnant teens frequently exhibit

▲ A successful pregnancy is longer than 37 weeks and is the result of a complex interplay between genes, lifestyle practices, and the environment.

low-birth-weight (LBW) Referring to any infant weighing less than 2.5 kilograms (5.5 pounds) at birth; most commonly results from preterm birth.

preterm An infant born before 37 weeks of gestation; also referred to as *premature*.

small for gestational age (SGA) Referring to infants who weigh less than the expected weight for their length of gestation. This corresponds to less than 2.5 kilograms (5.5 pounds) in a full-term newborn. A preterm infant who is also SGA will most likely develop some medical complications.

▶ Women with acquired immune deficiency syndrome (AIDS) may pass the virus that causes this disease to the fetus during pregnancy or the birth process. About one in three infected newborns will develop AIDS symptoms and die within just a few years. Studies show that these odds of mother-infant transmission can be cut significantly if the woman begins taking the drug azidothymidine (AZT) and other related AIDS medications by the fourteenth week of pregnancy. Providing these medications just before birth is helpful as well. Thus, screening pregnant women for AIDS and treating those with AIDS using AZT are advocated by some experts.

a variety of risk factors that can complicate pregnancy and pose a risk to the fetus. For instance, teenagers are more likely than adult women to be underweight at the beginning of pregnancy and to gain too little weight during pregnancy. In addition, their bodies generally lack the maturity needed to carry a fetus safely. Sixteen percent of LBW infants are born to teenage mothers. This is true even if the mothers receive adequate prenatal care. At the other end of the spectrum, advanced maternal age poses special risks for pregnancy. The risks of LBW and preterm delivery increase modestly, but progressively, with maternal age beyond 35 years. Given close monitoring, however, a woman older than 35 years has an excellent chance of producing a healthy infant.

Closely Spaced and Multiple Births

Siblings born in succession to a mother with less than a year between birth and subsequent conception are more likely to be born with low birth weights than are those farther apart in age. The risks of low birth weight, preterm birth, or small size for gestational age are 30% to 40% higher for infants conceived less than 6 months following a birth compared to those conceived 18 to 23 months following a birth. These poor outcomes are probably linked to a lack of enough time to rebuild nutrient stores depleted by the pregnancy. Similarly, multiple births (i.e., twins) increase the risk for preterm birth.

Smoking, Medication Use, and Drug Abuse

Smoking, use of some medications, and illicit drug use during pregnancy all lead to harmful effects. Smoking is linked to preterm birth and appears to increase the risk of birth defects, sudden infant death, and childhood cancer. Problem drugs include aspirin (especially when used heavily), hormone ointments, nose drops and related "cold" medications, rectal suppositories, weight-control pills, and medications prescribed for previous illnesses. Illicit drug use is particularly harmful during pregnancy. Many chemicals in recreational drugs cross the placenta and affect the fetus, whose detoxification systems are immature. During organ development, such insults can cause malformations. Marijuana, the most common illegal drug used during the reproductive years, can result in reduced blood flow to the uterus and placenta, leading to poor fetal growth. Low birth weight and higher risk of premature delivery often are seen in infants whose mothers used marijuana during pregnancy. Cocaine use also has devastating consequences for the developing fetus.

Food Safety

▶ USDA warns pregnant women to thoroughly cook (e.g., microwave) all ready-to-eat meats, including hot dogs and cold cuts, until they are steaming to reduce risk of *Listeria* infections.

Any foodborne illness is a concern. A particularly dangerous type of foodborne illness is caused by the bacterium *Listeria monocytogenes* (review Chapter 15). Infection with this microorganism typically causes mild flulike symptoms, such as fever, headache, and vomiting, about 7 to 30 days after exposure. However, pregnant women, newborn infants, and people with depressed immune function may suffer more severe symptoms, including spontaneous abortion and serious blood infections. In these high-risk people, 25% of infections may be fatal. Unpasteurized milk, soft cheeses made from raw milk (e.g., brie, Camembert, feta, and blue cheeses), and raw cabbage can be sources of *Listeria* organisms, so it is especially important that pregnant women (and other people at high risk for infection) avoid these products. Experts advise consuming only pasteurized milk products and cooking meat, poultry, and seafood thoroughly to kill this and other foodborne organisms. It is unsafe in pregnancy to eat any raw meats or other raw animal products, uncooked hot dogs, or undercooked poultry. These food safety recommendations are included in the Dietary Guidelines for Americans discussed later in the chapter (Table 16-2 on page 568).

Nutritional Status

Is attention to good nutrition worth the effort? Yes; evidence shows that the effort is justified. Extra nutrients and calories are used for fetal growth, as well as for the changes the mother's body undergoes to accommodate the fetus. Her uterus and breasts grow, the placenta develops, her total blood volume increases, the heart and kidneys work harder, and stores of body fat increase.

Although it is difficult to predict what degree of poor nutrition will affect each pregnancy, a daily diet containing only 1000 kcal has been shown to greatly restrict fetal growth and development. Increased maternal and infant death rates seen in famine-stricken areas of Africa provide further evidence.

Genetic background can explain little of the observed differences in birth weight between developed and developing countries. Both environmental factors and nutritional factors are important. The worse the nutritional condition of the mother at the beginning of pregnancy, the more valuable a healthy prenatal diet and/or use of prenatal supplements are in improving the course and outcome of her pregnancy.

▲ In the United States, low-income pregnant women and their infants (and children) benefit from the nutritional and medical attention provided by the WIC program.

Nutrition Assistance for Low-Income Families

A low socioeconomic status is also associated with problems in pregnancy. Typical characteristics of low socioeconomic status include poverty, inadequate health care, poor health practices, lack of education, and unmarried status. In the United States about 31% of all births are to unwed mothers, many of whom are poor.

Several U.S. government programs provide high-quality health care and foods to reduce infant mortality. These are designed to alleviate the effects of poverty and insufficient education and nutrient intake. An example of such a program is the Special Supplemental Nutrition Program for Women, Infants, and Children (WIC). This program offers health assessments and vouchers for foods that supply high-quality protein, calcium, iron, and vitamins A and C to pregnant women, infants, and children (up to age 5 years) from low-income populations. The WIC program is available in all areas of the United States and has a staff trained to help women have healthy babies. More than 7 million women, infants, and young children are benefiting from this program, but many eligible pregnant women are not participating.

CONCEPT CHECK

To help ensure the optimal health of both the mother and her offspring, adequate nutrition, especially meeting folate needs from a synthetic source starting at least 3 months before pregnancy begins, is vital both before and during pregnancy. Organs and body parts in the offspring begin to develop soon after conception. The first trimester is a critical period when inadequate nutrient intake or alcohol and drug use can result in birth defects.

Infants born after 37 weeks of gestation who weigh more than 5.5 pounds (2.5 kilograms) have the fewest medical problems at birth. To reduce infant and maternal medical problems or death, the expectant mother, family, and medical care providers should take the steps necessary to allow the mother to carry the baby in her uterus for the entire 9 months, which in turn contributes to adequate growth. Good nutrition and health practices aid in this goal.

INCREASED NUTRIENT NEEDS TO SUPPORT PREGNANCY

Pregnancy is a time of increased nutrient needs. It is important to recognize the need for individual assessment and counseling of mothers-to-be, as the nutritional and health status of each woman is different. Still, there are some general principles true of most women with regard to increased nutrient needs.

▲ Pregnancy leads to increased nutrient needs for the mother. Meeting these nutrient needs is an important step toward a successful pregnancy.

▲ Many women recognize the benefits of remaining active during pregnancy. Healthcare providers typically encourage healthy, well-nourished women to engage in moderate exercise as long as increased calorie and nutrient needs are met.

Increased Calorie Needs

To support the growth and development of the fetus, pregnant women need to increase their calorie intake. Calorie needs during the first trimester are essentially the same as for the nonpregnant woman. However, during the second and third trimesters, it is necessary for a pregnant woman to consume approximately 350 to 450 kcal more per day than her prepregnancy needs (the upper end of the range is needed in the third trimester).

Rather than seeing this as an opportunity to fill up on sugary desserts or fat-filled snacks, these extra calories should be in the form of nutrient-dense foods. For example, throughout the day, about six whole-wheat crackers, 1 ounce of cheese, and ½ cup of fat-free milk would supply the extra calories (and also some calcium). Although she "eats for two," the pregnant woman must not double her normal calorie intake. The "eating for two" concept refers more appropriately to increased needs for several vitamins and minerals. Micronutrient needs are increased by up to 50% during pregnancy, whereas calorie needs during the second and third trimesters represent only about a 20% increase.

If a woman is active during her pregnancy, she may need to increase her calorie intake by even more than the estimated 350 to 450 kcal per day. Her greater body weight requires more calories for activity. While pregnancy is not the time to begin an intense fitness regimen, women can generally take part in most low- or moderate-intensity activities during pregnancy. Walking, cycling, swimming, or light aerobics for 30 minutes or more on most days of the week is generally advised and may promote an easier delivery. A few types of activities can potentially harm the fetus and should be avoided, especially those with inherent risk of falls and abdominal trauma. Examples of exercises to avoid, especially during the second and third trimesters, include downhill skiing, weightlifting, soccer, basketball, horseback riding, certain calisthenics (e.g., deep knee bends), any contact sports (e.g., hockey), and scuba diving. Many women find that they are inactive during the later months, partly because of their increased size, so an extra 350 to 450 kcal in their daily diets is usually enough.

Women with high-risk pregnancies, such as those experiencing premature labor contractions, may need to restrict their physical activity. To ensure optimal health for both herself and her infant, a pregnant woman should first consult her physician about physical activity and possible limitations.

Adequate Weight Gain

Key recommendations for weight management during pregnancy and lactation are included in the Dietary Guidelines for Americans (see Table 16-2 on page 568). Adequate weight gain for a mother is one of the best predictors of pregnancy outcome. Her diet should allow for approximately 2 to 4 pounds (0.9 to 1.8 kilograms) of weight gain during the first trimester and then a subsequent weight gain of 0.75 to 1 pound (0.3 to 0.5 kilogram) weekly during the second and third trimesters (Fig. 16-3). A healthy goal for total weight gain for a woman of normal weight (based on BMI; Table 16-1) averages about 25 to 35 pounds (11.5 to 16 kilograms). Adolescents and African-American women, who often have smaller babies, are strongly advised to aim for the greater amount. Women carrying twins should gain 35 to 45 pounds, and those carrying triplets should gain 50 pounds (23 kilograms).

For women with a low BMI, the goal increases to 28 to 40 pounds (12.5 to 18 kilograms). The goal decreases to 15 to 25 pounds (7 to 11.5 kilograms) for women at a high BMI and 15 pounds (7 kilograms) or more for an obese woman. Figure 16-3 shows why the typical recommendation begins at 25 pounds.

A weight gain of between 25 and 35 pounds for a woman starting at normal weight has repeatedly been shown to yield optimal health for both mother and fetus if gestation lasts at least 38 weeks. The weight gain should yield a birth weight of 7.5 pounds (3.5 kilograms). Although some extra weight gain during pregnancy is usually not

TABLE 16-1 Recommended Weight Gain in Pregnancy Based on Prepregnancy Body Mass Index (BMI)

Prepregnancy BMI Category	Total Weight Gain*	
	(pounds)	(kilograms)
Low (BMI less than 19.8)	28 to 40	12.5 to 18
Normal (BMI 19.8 to 25.9)	25 to 35	11.5 to 16
High (BMI 26 to 29)	15 to 25	7 to 11.5
Obese (BMI greater than 29)	15 (or more)	7 (or more)

*The listed values are for pregnancies with one fetus. Short women (less than 62 inches) should strive for gains at the lower end of the ranges. For women of normal BMI carrying twins, the range is 35 to 45 pounds (16 to 20 kilograms). Adolescents within 2 years of beginning menses and African-American women should strive for gains at the upper end of the ranges.

Reprinted with permission from *Nutrition During Pregnancy and Lactation*, Copyright 1992 by the National Academy of Sciences. Courtesy of the National Academy Press, Washington, DC.

harmful (about 5 to 10 pounds), it can set the stage for a pattern of weight gain during the child-bearing years if the mother does not return to her approximate prepregnancy weight. Overweight and obesity do contribute to complications during pregnancy. Excess maternal body weight increases risk for diabetes, hypertension, blood clots, and spontaneous abortions. For the baby, there is a greater chance of birth defects and macrosomia, in which the fetus grows larger than average in utero. Larger infants contribute to a greater need for surgical delivery (i.e., Cesarean sections) among overweight and obese mothers.

▶ During pregnancy, women in North America are more likely to gain excess weight and make poor food choices than to eat too little.

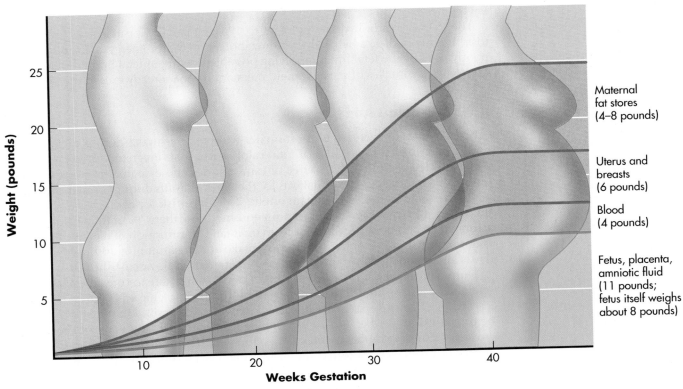

FIGURE 16-3 ▶ The components of weight gain in pregnancy. A weight gain of 25 to 35 pounds is recommended for most women. The various components total about 25 pounds.

▲ Weight gain should be carefully monitored during pregnancy.

Weight gain during pregnancy, especially in the teenage years, should generally follow the pattern in Figure 16-3. Monitoring weekly records of a pregnant woman's weight gain helps assess how much to adjust her food intake. Weight gain is a key issue in prenatal care and a concern of many mothers-to-be. Remember that inadequate weight gain can cause many problems.

If a woman deviates from the desirable pattern, she should make the appropriate adjustment. For example, if a woman begins to gain too much weight during her pregnancy, she should not lose weight to get back on track. Even if a woman gains 35 pounds in the first 7 months of pregnancy, she must still gain more during the last 2 months. She should, however, slow the increase in weight to parallel the rise on the prenatal weight gain chart. In other words, the sources of the unnecessary calories should be found and minimized. Alternately, if a woman has not gained the desired weight by a given point in pregnancy, she shouldn't gain the needed weight rapidly. Instead, she should slowly gain a little more weight than the typical pattern to meet the goal by the end of the pregnancy. A registered dietitian can help make any needed adjustments.

Increased Protein and Carbohydrate Needs

The RDA for protein increases by an additional 25 grams per day during pregnancy. A cup of milk alone contains 8 grams. Many nonpregnant women already consume protein in excess of their needs and therefore do not need to increase protein intake any further. However, all women should check to make sure they are eating enough protein and enough calories, so this protein is not used for energy needs.

The RDA for carbohydrate increases to 175 grams daily, primarily to prevent ketosis. Ketone bodies, a by-product of metabolism of fat for energy, are thought to be poorly used by the fetal brain, implying possible slowing of fetal brain development. Carbohydrate intakes of most women, pregnant or not, already exceed the RDA.

A Word About Lipids

Fat intake should increase proportionally with calorie intake during pregnancy to maintain around 20% to 30% of total calories from fat. Pregnancy is not a time for a low-fat diet, as lipids are a source of extra calories and essential fatty acids needed during pregnancy. Recommendations for the types of lipids during pregnancy are generally the same as for nonpregnant adults. To reduce risk for cardiovascular disease, the American Heart Association recommends no more than 7% of total calories from saturated fat and no more than 1% from *trans* fat. Consumption of dietary cholesterol is not required, but keeping cholesterol intake at a maximum of 300 milligrams per day is also a good goal for maintenance of maternal cardiovascular health.

During pregnancy, it is particularly important to make sure to consume adequate essential fatty acids—linoleic acid (omega-6) and alpha-linolenic acid (omega-3). As you learned in Chapter 5, essential fatty acids cannot be synthesized in the body and must be consumed in the diet. For the developing fetus, essential fatty acids are required for growth, brain development, and eye development. Recommendations are slightly increased by pregnancy: thirteen grams per day of omega-6 fatty acids and 1.4 gram per day of omega-3 fatty acids. These needs can be met by consuming 2 to 4 tablespoons per day of plant oils. Consumption of fish at least two times per week is also helpful in meeting needs for essential fatty acids in the diet. (See the "Nutrition and Your Health" section at the end of this chapter for a discussion of mercury in fish.)

Increased Vitamin Needs

Vitamin needs generally increase from prepregnancy RDAs/Adequate Intakes by up to 30% for most of the B vitamins and even greater for vitamin B-6 (45%) and folate (50%). Vitamin A needs only increase by 10%, so a specific focus on this vitamin is not needed. And remember, excess amounts of vitamin A are harmful to the developing fetus.

The extra amount of vitamin B-6 and other B vitamins (except folate) needed in the diet is easily met via wise food choices, such as a serving of a typical ready-to-eat breakfast cereal and some animal protein sources. Folate needs, however, often merit specific diet planning and possible vitamin supplementation. The synthesis of DNA, and therefore cell division, requires folate, so this nutrient is especially crucial during pregnancy. Ultimately, both fetal and maternal growth depend on an ample supply of folate. Red blood cell formation, which requires folate, increases during pregnancy. Serious folate-related anemia therefore can result if folate intake is inadequate. The RDA for folate increases during pregnancy to 600 micrograms DFE per day (review Chapter 11 for calculation of DFE). This is a critical goal in the nutritional care of a pregnant woman. Increasing folate intakes to meet 600 micrograms DFE per day for a pregnant woman can be achieved through dietary sources, a supplemental source of folic acid, or a combination of both. Choosing a diet rich in synthetic folic acid, such as from ready-to-eat breakfast cereals or meal replacement bars (look for approximately 50% to 100% of the Daily Value), is especially helpful in meeting folate needs. Recall from Chapter 11 that synthetic folic acid is much more easily absorbed than the various forms of folate found naturally in foods.

▲ Pregnancy, in particular, is not a time to self-prescribe vitamin and mineral supplements. For example, although vitamin A is a routine component of prenatal vitamins, intakes over three times the RDA for vitamin A have been shown to have toxic effects on the fetus.

Increased Mineral Needs

Mineral needs generally increase during pregnancy, especially the requirements for iodide and iron. Zinc needs also increase. (Calcium needs do not increase, but still may deserve special attention because many women have deficient intakes.)

Pregnant women need the extra iodide (total of 220 micrograms per day) for prevention of goiter. Typical iodide intakes are enough if the woman uses iodized salt. Animal proteins or a fortified ready-to-eat breakfast cereal in the diet can easily provide enough extra zinc. The extra iron (total of 27 milligrams per day) is needed to synthesize the greater amount of hemoglobin needed during pregnancy and to provide iron stores for the fetus. Women often need a supplemental source of iron, especially if they do not consume iron-fortified foods, such as highly fortified breakfast cereals containing close to 100% of the Daily Value for iron (18 milligrams). Iron supplements decrease appetite and can cause nausea and constipation, so if used, these should be taken between meals or just before going to bed. Milk, coffee, or tea should not be consumed with an iron supplement because these beverages have substances that interfere with iron absorption. Eating foods rich in vitamin C along with nonheme iron-containing foods and iron supplements helps increase iron absorption from those sources. Pregnant women who are not anemic may wait until the second trimester, when pregnancy-related nausea generally lessens, to start iron supplementation if needed.

The consequences of iron-deficiency anemia—especially during the first trimester—can be severe. Negative outcomes include preterm delivery, LBW infants, and increased risk for fetal death in the first weeks after birth.

▶ The Dietary Guidelines for Americans recommend that women who may become pregnant eat foods high in iron and consume adequate amounts of the synthetic form of folate (see Table 16-2 on page 568).

Use of Prenatal Vitamin and Mineral Supplements

Special supplements formulated for pregnancy are prescribed routinely for pregnant women by most physicians. Some are sold over the counter, while others are dispensed by prescription because of the high synthetic folic acid content (1000 micrograms),

TABLE 16-2 Key Recommendations from the Latest Dietary Guidelines for Americans, for Women of Childbearing Age who may become Pregnant, Pregnant Women, and Breastfeeding Women

Adequate Nutrients Within Calorie Needs

- *Women of childbearing age who may become pregnant.* Eat foods high in iron from animal products and/or consume iron-rich plant foods or iron-fortified foods with an enhancer of iron absorption, such as vitamin C-rich foods.

- *Women of childbearing age who may become pregnant and those in the first few months of pregnancy.* Consume an adequate amount of the synthetic form of the B vitamin folate (called folic acid) daily (from fortified foods or supplements) in addition to food forms of folate found in a varied diet.

Weight Management

- *Pregnant women.* Ensure appropriate weight gain as specified by a healthcare provider.

- *Breastfeeding women.* Moderate weight reduction is safe and does not compromise weight gain of the nursing infant.

Physical Activity

- *Pregnant women.* In the absence of medical complications, incorporate 30 minutes or more of moderate-intensity physical activity on most, if not all, days of the week. Avoid activities with a high risk of falling or abdominal trauma.

- *Breastfeeding women.* Be aware that neither acute nor regular exercise adversely affects the mother's ability to successfully breastfeed.

Alcoholic Beverages

- Alcoholic beverages should not be consumed by some individuals, including those who cannot restrict their alcohol intake, women of childbearing age who may become pregnant, pregnant and lactating women, children and adolescents, individuals taking medications that may interact with alcohol, and those with specific medical conditions.

Food Safety

- *Infants and young children, pregnant women, older adults, and those who are immunocompromised.* Do not eat or drink unpasteurized milk or any products made from unpasteurized milk, raw or partially cooked eggs or foods containing raw eggs, raw or undercooked meat and poultry, raw or undercooked fish or shellfish, unpasteurized juices, and raw sprouts.

- *Pregnant women, older adults, and those who are immunocompromised:* Only eat certain deli meats and frankfurters that have been reheated to steaming hot.

which could pose problems for others, such as older people (see Chapter 18). These supplements are high in iron (27 milligrams per pill). There is no evidence that use of such supplements causes significant health problems in pregnancy, aside perhaps from the combined amounts of supplementary and dietary vitamin A (see "Nutrition and Your Health" at the end of this chapter).

Instances when prenatal supplements may especially contribute to a successful pregnancy are with poor women, teenagers, those with a generally deficient diet, women carrying multiple fetuses, those that smoke or use alcohol or illegal drugs, and vegans. In other cases, healthy diets can provide the needed nutrients. When choosing a multivitamin, rely on brands that display the USP symbol on their label, signifying that the supplement meets the content, quality, purity, and safety standards of the U.S. Pharmacopoeia. Also, avoid megadoses of any nutrient. In particular, toxicity of vitamin A is linked with birth defects. High doses of cobalt and vitamin D are also under study for possible ill effects on pregnancy outcome. Skip supplements containing herbs, enzymes, and amino acids. Many of these ingredients have not been evaluated for safety during pregnancy or lactation and may be toxic to the fetus. Furthermore, discard supplements that are past the expiration date, as some ingredients lose potency over time.

FOOD PLAN FOR PREGNANT WOMEN

One approach to a diet that supports a successful pregnancy is based on MyPyramid. For an active 24-year-old woman, about 2200 kcal are recommended during the first trimester (the same as recommended for such a woman when not pregnant). The plan should include:

- 3 cups of calcium-rich foods from the milk group or use of calcium-fortified foods to make up for any gap between calcium intake and need
- 6 ounce-equivalents from the meat & beans group
- 3 cups from the vegetable group
- 2 cups from the fruit group
- 7 ounce-equivalents from the grain group
- 6 teaspoons of vegetable oil

MAKING DECISIONS

Cravings During Pregnancy

It is a common myth that women instinctively know what to eat during pregnancy. Cravings of the last two trimesters are often related to hormonal changes in the mother, or family traditions. Such "instinct" cannot be trusted, however, based on observations that some women crave nonfood items (called **pica**) such as laundry starch, chalk, cigarette ashes, and soil (clay). This practice can be extremely harmful to the mother and the fetus. Overall, though women may have a natural instinct to consume the right foods in pregnancy, humans are so far removed from living by instinct that relying on our cravings to meet nutrient needs is risky. Nutrition advice by experts is more reliable.

pica The practice of eating nonfood items, such as dirt, laundry starch, or clay.

Specifically, choices from the milk group should include low-fat or fat-free versions of milk, yogurt, and cheese. These foods supply extra protein, calcium, and carbohydrate, as well as other nutrients. Choices from the meat & beans group should include both animal and vegetable sources. Besides protein, these foods help provide the extra iron and zinc needed. The vegetable and fruit group choices provide a variety of vitamins and minerals. One cup from this combination should be a good vitamin C source, and 1 cup should be a green vegetable or other rich source of folate. Choices from the grain group should focus on whole-grain and enriched foods. One ounce of a whole-grain, ready-to-eat breakfast cereal significantly contributes to meeting many vitamin and mineral needs. Finally, inclusion of plant oils in the diet contributes essential fatty acids. Discretionary calories (up to about 300 kcal) can then be added to allow for weight maintenance.

In the second and third trimesters, about 2600 kcal are recommended for this woman. The plan should now include:

- 3 cups of calcium-rich foods from the milk group or use of calcium-fortified foods
- 6 ½ ounce-equivalents from the meat & beans group
- 3 ½ cups from the vegetable group
- 2 cups from the fruit group
- 8 ounce-equivalents from the grain group
- 7 teaspoons of vegetable oil

Discretionary calories (up to about 400 kcal) can then be added to allow for gradual weight gain. Table 16-3 illustrates one daily menu based on the 2600 kcal plan for pregnancy for women in the second or third trimesters. This menu meets the

▲ A salad each day provides many nutrients for the prenatal diet.

TABLE 16-3 Sample 2600 kcal Daily Menu That Meets the Nutritional Needs of Most Pregnant and Breastfeeding Women

	Vitamin B-6	Folate	Iron	Zinc	Calcium
Breakfast					
1 cup Kellogg's Smart Start cereal	✓	✓	✓	✓	✓
1 cup orange juice		✓			
1 cup fat-free milk	✓				✓
Snack					
2 tbsp peanut butter	✓	✓	✓	✓	
2 stalks of celery		✓			
1 slice whole-wheat toast		✓	✓	✓	
1 cup plain low-fat yogurt	✓				✓
½ cup strawberries					
Lunch					
2 cups spinach salad with 2 tbsp oil and vinegar dressing		✓			✓
½ tomato					
1 slice whole-wheat toast		✓	✓	✓	
1 ½ ounce provolone cheese	✓				✓
Snack					
5 whole-wheat crackers		✓	✓	✓	
1 cup grape juice					
Dinner					
3 ounces lean hamburger, broiled (with condiments)	✓		✓	✓	
½ cup baked beans	✓	✓	✓	✓	
1 hamburger bun		✓	✓		
½ sliced tomato					
1 cup cooked broccoli		✓			✓
1 tsp soft margarine					
Iced tea					
Snack					
Granola bar (2 ounces)		✓	✓	✓	
½ banana	✓				
Discretionary calories of up to 400 kcal*					

*Amount of discretionary calories will vary based on the actual food choices made within each MyPyramid group.

This diet meets nutrient needs for pregnancy and lactation. Lack of a check (✓) indicates a poor source of the nutrient. The vitamin- and mineral-fortified breakfast cereal used in this example makes an important contribution to meeting nutrient needs. Fluids can be added as desired. Total intake of fluids, such as water, should be 10 cups or so per day.

extra nutrient needs associated with pregnancy. Women who need to consume more than this—and some do for various reasons—should incorporate additional fruits, vegetables, and whole-grain breads and cereals, not poor nutrient sources such as desserts and sugared soft drinks.

Pregnant Vegetarians

Women who are either lactoovovegetarians or lactovegetarians generally do not face special difficulties in meeting their nutritional needs during pregnancy. Like nonvegetarian women, they should be concerned primarily with meeting vitamin B-6, iron, folate, and zinc needs.

On the other hand, for a vegan, careful diet planning during preconception and pregnancy is crucial to ensure sufficient protein, vitamin D (or sufficient sun exposure), vitamin B-6, iron, calcium, zinc, and especially a supplemental source of vitamin B-12. The basic vegan diet listed in Chapter 6 should be modified to include more grains, beans, nuts, and seeds to supply the necessary extra amounts of some of these nutrients. As mentioned, use of a prenatal multivitamin and mineral supplement also is generally advocated to help fill micronutrient gaps. However, although these are high in iron, this is not true for calcium (200 milligrams per pill). If iron and calcium supplements are used, they should not be taken together, to avoid possible competition for absorption.

CONCEPT CHECK

Calorie needs increase by an average of about 350 to 450 kcal per day during the second and third trimesters of pregnancy, respectively. Weight gain should be slow and steady up to a total of 25 to 35 pounds for a woman of normal weight (i.e., prepregnancy BMI of 19.8 to 25.9). Protein and certain vitamin and mineral needs increase during pregnancy. Most important to consider are vitamin B-6, folate, iron, iodide, and zinc. A pregnant woman's diet should be varied and generally follow a MyPyramid pattern. A prenatal multivitamin and mineral supplement is commonly prescribed but may not be necessary, depending on one's diet and health status. Taking too many supplements—especially vitamin A—can be hazardous to the fetus.

PHYSIOLOGICAL CHANGES OF CONCERN DURING PREGNANCY

During pregnancy, the fetus's needs for oxygen and nutrients, as well as excretion of waste products increase the burden on the mother's lungs, heart, and kidneys. Although a mother's digestive and metabolic systems work efficiently, some discomfort accompanies the changes her body undergoes to accommodate the fetus.

Heartburn, Constipation, and Hemorrhoids

Hormones (such as progesterone) produced by the placenta relax muscles in the uterus and the gastrointestinal tract. This often causes heartburn as stomach acid refluxes into the esophagus (review Chapter 3). When this occurs, the woman should avoid lying down after eating, eat less fat so that foods pass more quickly from the stomach into the small intestine, and avoid spicy foods she cannot tolerate. She should also consume most liquids between meals to decrease the volume of food in the stomach after meals, and thus relieve some of the pressure that encourages reflux. Women with more severe cases may need antacids or related medications.

Constipation often results as the intestinal muscles relax during pregnancy. It is especially likely to develop late in pregnancy, as the fetus competes with the GI tract for space in the abdominal cavity. To offset these discomforts, a woman should perform regular exercise and consume more fluid, fiber, and dried fruits, such as prunes (dried plums). The Adequate Intake for fiber in pregnancy is 28 grams, slightly more than for the nonpregnant woman. Fluid needs are 10 cups per day. These practices can help prevent constipation and a problem that frequently accompanies it, hemorrhoids. Straining during elimination can lead to hemorrhoids, more likely to occur during pregnancy because of other body changes. A re-evaluation of the need for and dose of iron supplementation also should be considered, as high iron intakes are linked to constipation.

Edema

Placental hormones cause various body tissues to retain fluid during pregnancy. Blood volume also greatly expands during pregnancy. The extra fluid normally causes some swelling (edema). There is no reason to restrict salt severely or use diuretics to limit mild edema. However, the edema may limit physical activity late in pregnancy and occasionally requires a woman to elevate her feet to control the symptoms. Overall, edema generally spells trouble only if hypertension and the appearance of extra protein in the urine accompany it (see a following section, "Pregnancy-Induced Hypertension").

Morning Sickness

About 70% to 85% of pregnant women experience nausea during the early stages of pregnancy. This nausea may be related to the increased sense of smell induced by pregnancy-related hormones circulating in the bloodstream. Although commonly called "morning sickness," pregnancy-related nausea may occur at any time and persist all day. It is often the first signal to a woman that she is pregnant. To help control mild nausea, pregnant women can try the following: avoiding nauseating foods, such as fried or greasy foods; cooking with good ventilation to dissipate nauseating smells; eating saltine crackers or dry cereal before getting out of bed; avoiding large fluid intakes early in the morning; and eating smaller, more frequent meals. The iron in prenatal supplements triggers nausea in some women, so changing the type of supplement used or postponing use until the second trimester may provide relief in some cases. If a woman thinks her prenatal supplement is related to morning sickness, she should discuss switching to another supplement with her physician.

Overall, if a food sounds good to a pregnant woman with morning sickness, whether it is broccoli, soda crackers, or lemonade, she should eat it and eat when she can, while also striving to follow her prenatal diet. The American College of Obstetricians and Gynecologists recommends the following for the prevention and treatment of nausea and vomiting of pregnancy:

- History of use of a balanced multivitamin and mineral supplement at the time of conception
- Use of megadoses of vitamin B-6 (10–25 milligrams taken 3 to 4 times a day), especially coupled with the antihistamine doxylamine (10 milligrams) with each dose
- Ginger may also be helpful (350 milligrams taken 3 times per day)

▲ A few saltine crackers upon waking or between meals can help lessen the pregnancy-related nausea.

Usually, nausea stops after the first trimester; however, in about 10% to 20% of cases, it can continue throughout the entire pregnancy. In cases of serious nausea, the preceding practices offer little relief. Excessive vomiting can cause dangerous dehydration and must be avoided. When vomiting persists (about 0.5% to 2% of pregnancies), medical attention is needed.

Anemia

To supply fetal needs, the mother's blood volume expands to approximately 150% of normal. The number of red blood cells, however, increases by only 20% to 30%, and this occurs more gradually. As a result, a pregnant woman has a lower ratio of red blood cells to total blood volume in her system. This hemodilution is known as **physiological anemia.** It is a normal response to pregnancy, rather than the result of inadequate nutrient intake. If during pregnancy, however, iron stores and/or dietary iron intake are not sufficient to meet needs, any resulting iron-deficiency anemia requires medical attention. The Dietary Guidelines for Americans recommend that women who may become pregnant eat foods high in iron (Table 16-2).

Gestational Diabetes

Hormones synthesized by the placenta decrease the efficiency of insulin. This leads to a mild increase in blood glucose, which helps supply calories to the fetus. If the rise in blood glucose becomes excessive, this leads to **gestational diabetes,** often beginning in weeks 20 to 28, particularly in women who have a family history of

physiological anemia The normal increase in blood volume in pregnancy that dilutes the concentration of red blood cells, resulting in anemia; also called *hemodilution.*

gestational diabetes A high blood glucose concentration that develops during pregnancy and returns to normal after birth; one cause is the placental production of hormones that antagonize the regulation of blood glucose by insulin.

diabetes or who are obese. Other risk factors include maternal age over 35 and gestational diabetes in a prior pregnancy. In North America, gestational diabetes develops in about 4% of pregnancies; however, it increases to 7% in the Caucasian population. Today, pregnant women often are screened for diabetes at 24 to 28 weeks by checking for elevated blood glucose concentration 1 to 2 hours after consuming 50 to 100 grams of glucose. If gestational diabetes is detected, a special diet that distributes low glycemic load carbohydrates throughout the day needs to be implemented. Sometimes insulin injections are also needed. Regular physical activity also helps control blood glucose.

The primary risk of uncontrolled diabetes during pregnancy is that the fetus can grow quite large. This is a result of the oversupply of glucose from maternal circulation coupled with an increased production of insulin by the fetus, which allows fetal tissues to take up an increased amount of building materials for growth. The mother may require a Cesarean section if the size of the fetus is not compatible with a vaginal delivery. Another threat is that the infant may have low blood glucose at birth, because of the tendency to produce extra insulin that began during gestation. Other concerns are the potential for early delivery and increased risk of birth trauma and malformations. Although gestational diabetes often disappears after the infant's birth, it increases the mother's risk of developing diabetes later in life, especially if she fails to maintain a healthy body weight. Studies show that infants of mothers with gestational diabetes may also have higher risks of developing obesity and type 2 diabetes as they grow to adulthood. For all these reasons, proper control of gestational diabetes (and any diabetes present in the mother before pregnancy) is extremely important.

Pregnancy-Induced Hypertension

Pregnancy-induced hypertension is a high-risk disorder and occurs in about 3% to 5% of pregnancies. In its mild forms, it is also known as *preeclampsia* and, in severe forms, as *eclampsia*. Early symptoms include a rise in blood pressure, excess protein in the urine, edema, changes in blood clotting, and nervous system disorders. Very severe effects, including convulsions, can occur in the second and third trimesters. If not controlled, eclampsia eventually damages the liver and kidneys, and mother and fetus may die. The populations most at risk for this disorder are women under age 17 or over age 35, overweight or obese women, and those who have had multiple-birth pregnancies. A family history of pregnancy-induced hypertension in the mother's or father's side of the family, diabetes, African-American race, and a woman's first pregnancy also raise risk. A diet inadequate in vitamin E, vitamin C, calcium, zinc, and other nutrients may also be part of the cause (conflicting research results at this time).

Pregnancy-induced hypertension resolves once the pregnancy ends, making delivery the most reliable treatment for the mother. However, because the problem often begins before the fetus is ready to be born, physicians in many cases must use treatments to prevent the worsening of the disorder. Bed rest and magnesium sulfate are the most effective treatment methods, although their effectiveness varies. Magnesium likely acts to relax blood vessels, and so leads to a fall in blood pressure. Several other treatments, such as various antiseizure and antihypertensive medications, calcium, and use of antioxidant supplements, are under study.

CRITICAL THINKING

Sandy, 4 months pregnant, has been having heartburn after meals, constipation, and difficult bowel movements. As a student of nutrition, you understand the digestive system and the role of nutrition in health. What remedies might you suggest to Sandy to relieve her problems?

pregnancy-induced hypertension A serious disorder that can include high blood pressure, kidney failure, convulsions, and even death of the mother and fetus. Although its exact cause is not known, an adequate diet (especially adequate calcium intake) and prenatal care may prevent this disorder or limit its severity. Mild cases are known as *preeclampsia*; more severe cases are called *eclampsia* (formerly called *toxemia*).

CONCEPT CHECK

Heartburn, constipation, hemorrhoids, nausea and vomiting, edema, anemia, and gestational diabetes are possible discomforts and complications of pregnancy. Changes in food habits can often ease these problems. Pregnancy-induced hypertension, with high blood pressure and kidney failure, can lead to severe complications or even death of the mother and fetus if not treated.

BREASTFEEDING

Breastfeeding the new infant further fosters his or her health, and so complements the attention given to diet during pregnancy. The American Dietetic Association and the American Academy of Pediatrics recommend breastfeeding exclusively for the first 6 months, with the continued combination of breastfeeding and infant foods until 1 year. The World Health Organization goes beyond that to recommend breastfeeding (with appropriate solid food introduction; see Chapter 17) for at least 2 years. Still, surveys show that only about 70% of North American mothers now begin to breastfeed their infants in the hospital, and at 4 and 6 months only 33% and 20%, respectively, are still breastfeeding their infants. The number falls to 18% at 1 year of age. These statistics refer to Caucasian women; minority women are even less likely to be breastfeeding at these time intervals.

Women who choose to breastfeed usually find it an enjoyable, special time in their lives and their relationship with their new infant. Although bottle feeding with an infant formula is also safe for infants, as discussed in Chapter 17, it does not equal the benefits derived from human milk in all aspects. If a woman doesn't breastfeed her child, breast weight returns to normal soon after birth.

Ability to Breastfeed

Almost all women are physically capable of breastfeeding their children (see later section "Medical Conditions Precluding Breastfeeding" for exceptions). In most cases, problems encountered in breastfeeding are due to a lack of appropriate information. Anatomical problems in breasts, such as inverted nipples, can be corrected during pregnancy. Breast size generally increases during pregnancy and is no indication of success in breastfeeding. Most women notice a dramatic increase in the size and weight of their breasts by the third or fourth day of breastfeeding. If these changes do not occur, a woman needs to speak with her physician or a lactation consultant.

Breastfed infants must be followed closely over the first days of life to ensure that feeding and weight gain are proceeding normally. Monitoring is especially important with a mother's first child, because the mother will be inexperienced with the technique of breastfeeding. Mothers and healthy infants are commonly discharged from the hospital 1 to 2 days after delivery, whereas 20 years ago they stayed in the hospital for 3 or 4 days or longer. One result of such rapid discharge is a decreased period of infant monitoring by health care professionals. Incidents have been reported of infants developing dehydration and in turn blood clots soon after hospital discharge when breastfeeding did not proceed smoothly. Careful monitoring in this first week by a physician or lactation consultant is advised.

First-time mothers who plan to breastfeed should learn as much as they can about the process early in their pregnancy. Interested women should learn the proper technique, what problems to expect, and how to respond to them. Overall, breastfeeding is a learned skill, and mothers need knowledge to breastfeed safely, especially with the first child.

Production of Human Milk

During pregnancy, cells in the breast form milk-producing cells called **lobules** (Fig. 16-4). Hormones from the placenta stimulate these changes in the breast. After birth, the mother produces more **prolactin** hormone to maintain the changes in the breast and therefore the ability to produce milk. During pregnancy, breast weight increases by about 1 to 2 pounds.

The hormone prolactin also stimulates the synthesis of milk. Infant suckling stimulates prolactin release from the pituitary gland. Milk synthesis then occurs as an infant nurses. The more the infant suckles, the more milk is produced. Because of this, even twins (and triplets) can be breastfed adequately.

▶ Many of the benefits of breastfeeding can be found in Table 16-4 on page 579 and at www.4woman.gov./Breastfeeding/index.cfm, sponsored by the U.S. Surgeon General.

▲ Breastfeeding is the preferred way to feed a young infant.

▶ *Healthy People 2010* has set a goal of 75% of women breastfeeding their infants at time of hospital discharge, 50% breastfeeding for 6 months, and 25% still breastfeeding at 1 year.

lobules Saclike structures in the breast that store milk.

prolactin A hormone secreted by the pituitary gland that stimulates the synthesis of milk in the breast.

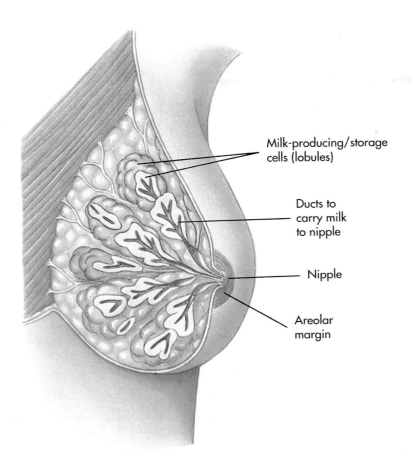

FIGURE 16-4 ▶ The anatomy of the breast. Many types of cells form a coordinated network to produce and secrete human milk.

Milk-producing/storage cells (lobules)

Ducts to carry milk to nipple

Nipple

Areolar margin

Most protein found in human milk is synthesized by breast tissue. Some proteins also enter the milk directly from the mother's bloodstream. These proteins include immune factors (e.g., antibodies) and enzymes. Fats in human milk come from both the mother's diet and those synthesized by breast tissue. The sugar galactose is synthesized in the breast, whereas glucose enters from the mother's bloodstream. Together, these sugars form lactose, the main carbohydrate in human milk.

Let-Down Reflex

An important brain-breast connection—commonly called the **let-down reflex**—is necessary for breastfeeding. The brain releases the hormone **oxytocin** to allow the breast tissues to let down (release) the milk from storage sites (Fig. 16-5). It then travels to the nipple area. A tingling sensation signals the let-down reflex shortly before milk flow begins. If the let-down reflex doesn't operate, little milk is available to the infant. The infant then gets frustrated, and this can frustrate the mother.

The let-down reflex is easily inhibited by nervous tension, a lack of confidence, and fatigue. Mothers should be especially aware of the link between tension and a weak let-down reflex. They need to find a relaxed environment where they can breastfeed.

After a few weeks, the let-down reflex becomes automatic. The mother's response can be triggered just by thinking about her infant or seeing or hearing another one cry. At first, however, the process can be a bit bewildering. A mother cannot measure the amount of milk the infant takes in, so she may fear that she is not adequately nourishing the infant.

As a general rule, a well-nourished breastfed infant should (1) have six or more wet diapers per day after the second day of life, (2) show a normal weight gain, and (3) pass at least one or two stools per day that look like lumpy mustard. In addition,

let-down reflex A reflex stimulated by infant suckling that causes the release (ejection) of milk from milk ducts in the mother's breasts; also called *milk ejection reflex*.

oxytocin A hormone secreted by the pituitary gland. It causes contraction of the musclelike cells surrounding the ducts of the breasts and the smooth muscle of the uterus.

▶ Disposable diapers can absorb so much urine that it is difficult to judge when they are wet. A strip of paper towel laid inside a disposable diaper makes a good wetness indicator. Alternatively, cloth diapers may be used for a day or two to assess whether nursing is supplying sufficient milk.

FIGURE 16-5 ▶ Let-down reflex. Suckling sets into motion the sequence of events that lead to milk let-down, the flow of milk into ducts of the breast.

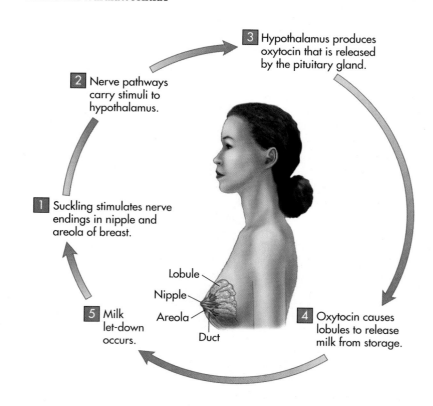

2 Nerve pathways carry stimuli to hypothalamus.

3 Hypothalamus produces oxytocin that is released by the pituitary gland.

1 Suckling stimulates nerve endings in nipple and areola of breast.

Lobule
Nipple
Areola
Duct

5 Milk let-down occurs.

4 Oxytocin causes lobules to release milk from storage.

softening of the breast during the feeding helps indicate that enough milk is being consumed. Parents who sense their infant is not consuming enough milk should consult a physician immediately because dehydration can develop rapidly.

It generally takes 2 to 3 weeks to fully establish the feeding routine: Infant and mother both feel comfortable, the milk supply meets infant demand, and initial nipple soreness disappears. Establishing the breastfeeding routine requires patience, but the rewards are great. The adjustments are easier if supplemental formula feedings are not introduced until breastfeeding is well established, after at least 3 to 4 weeks. Then it is fine if a supplemental bottle or two of infant formula per day is needed.

Nutritional Qualities of Human Milk

Human milk is different in composition from cow's milk. Unless altered, cow's milk should never be used in infant feeding until the infant is at least 12 months old. Cow's milk is too high in minerals and protein and does not contain enough carbohydrate to meet infant needs. In addition, the major protein in cow's milk is harder for an infant to digest than the major proteins in human milk. The proteins in cow's milk also may spur allergies in the infant. Finally, certain compounds in human milk presently under study show other possible benefits for the infant.

colostrum The first fluid secreted by the breast during late pregnancy and the first few days after birth. This thick fluid is rich in immune factors and protein.

Colostrum. At the end of pregnancy, the first fluid made by the human breast is **colostrum.** This thick, yellowish fluid may leak from the breast during late pregnancy and is produced in earnest for a few days to a week after birth. Colostrum contains antibodies and immune system cells, some of which pass unaltered through the infant's immature GI tract into the bloodstream. The first few months of life are the only time when we can readily absorb whole proteins across the GI tract. These immune factors and cells protect the infant from some GI tract diseases and other infectious disorders, compensating for the infant's immature immune system during the first few months of life.

One component of colostrum, the *Lactobacillus bifidus* **factor,** encourages the growth of *Lactobacillus bifidus* bacteria. These bacteria limit the growth of potentially toxic bacteria in the intestine. Overall, breastfeeding promotes the intestinal health of the breastfed infant in this way.

Mature Milk. Human milk composition gradually changes until it achieves the normal composition of mature milk several days after delivery. Human milk looks very different from cow's milk. (Table 17-1 in Chapter 17 provides a direct comparison.) Human milk is thin and almost watery in appearance and often has a slightly bluish tinge. Its nutritional qualities, however, are impressive.

Human milk's proteins form a soft, light curd in the infant's stomach and are easy to digest. Some human milk proteins bind iron, reducing the growth of iron-requiring bacteria, some of which can cause diarrhea. Still other proteins offer the important immune protection already noted.

The lipids in human breast milk are high in linoleic acid and cholesterol, needed for brain development. Breast milk also contains long-chain omega-3 fatty acids, such as docosahexaenoic acid (DHA). This polyunsaturated fatty acid is used for the synthesis of tissues in the brain and the rest of the central nervous system and in the retina of the eye.

The fat composition of human milk changes during each feeding. The consistency of milk released initially (fore milk) resembles that of skim milk. It later has a greater fat proportion, similar to whole milk. Finally, the milk released after 10 to 20 minutes (hind milk) is essentially like cream. Babies need to nurse long enough (e.g., a total of 20 or more minutes) to get the calories in the rich hind milk to be satisfied between feedings and to grow well. The overall calorie content of human milk is about the same as that of infant formulas (67 kcal per 100 milliliters).

Human milk composition also allows for adequate fluid status of the infant, provided the baby is exclusively breastfed. A question commonly asked is whether the infant needs additional water, if stressed by hot weather, diarrhea, vomiting, or fever. Providing breastfed infants with up to 4 ounces of water a day from a bottle is fine. However, greater amounts of supplemental water can lead to brain disorders, low blood sodium, and other problems. Thus, extra water should be given only with a physician's guidance.

Food Plan for Women Who Breastfeed

Nutrient needs for a breastfeeding mother change to some extent from those of the pregnant woman in the second and third trimester (see the inside cover of this book). There is a decrease in folate and iron needs and an increase in the needs for calories, vitamins A, E, and C, riboflavin, copper, chromium, iodide, manganese, selenium, and zinc. Still, these increased needs of the breastfeeding mother will be met by the general diet plan proposed for a woman in the latter stages of pregnancy. Recall that each day of this diet plan includes at least:

- 3 cups of calcium-rich foods such as from the milk group or use of calcium-fortified foods to make up for any gap between calcium intake and need
- 6 ½ ounce-equivalents from the meat & beans group
- 3 ½ cups from the vegetable group
- 2 cups from the fruit group
- 8 ounce-equivalents from the grain group
- 7 teaspoons of vegetable oil

Discretionary calories (up to about 400 kcal) can then be added to allow for weight maintenance or gradual weight loss, whichever is needed.

Table 16-3 provided a menu for such a plan. Substituting a soyburger (veggie burger) for the hamburger in that menu would make this a practical guide for a lacto-vegetarian woman as well.

Lactobacillus bifidus **factor** A protective factor secreted in the colostrum that encourages growth of beneficial bacteria in the newborn's intestines.

▲ Breastfeeding promotes the intestinal health of the breastfed infant.

▶ Most substances that the mother ingests are secreted into her milk. For this reason, she should limit intake of or avoid all alcohol and caffeine and check all medications with a pediatrician. Some mothers believe that certain foods, such as garlic and chocolate, flavor the breast milk and upset the infant. If a woman notices a connection between a food she eats and the infant's later fussiness, she could consider avoiding that food. However, she might experiment again with it later, as infants become fussy for other reasons. Some researchers, on the other hand, feel that the passage of flavors from the mother's diet into her milk affords an opportunity for the infant to learn about the flavor of the foods of its family long before solids are introduced. These researchers suspect that bottle-fed infants are missing significant sensory experiences that, until recent times in human history, were common to all infants.

▲ Eating fish at least twice a week will help breastfeeding women ensure that their infants receive important omega-3 fatty acids. It is important, however, to avoid those fish likely contaminated with mercury (listed on page 585).

▲ Human milk is tailored to meet infant nutrient needs exclusively for the first 4 to 6 months of life.

As in pregnancy, a serving of a highly fortified ready-to-eat breakfast cereal (or use of a balanced multivitamin and mineral supplement) is advised to help meet extra nutrient needs. And, as mentioned for pregnant women, breastfeeding mothers should consume fish at least twice a week (or 1 gram per day of omega-3 fatty acids from a fish oil supplement) because the omega-3 fatty acids present in fish are secreted into breast milk and are likely to be important for development of the infant's nervous system.

Milk production requires approximately 800 kcal every day. The Estimated Energy Requirement during lactation is an extra 400 to 500 kcal daily above prepregnancy recommendations. The difference between that needed for milk production and the recommended intake—about 300 kcal—should allow a gradual loss of the extra body fat accumulated during pregnancy, especially if breastfeeding is continued for 6 months or more and the woman performs some physical activity. This shows just one of the natural benefits of following pregnancy with at least several months of breastfeeding.

After giving birth, women are often eager to shed the excess "baby fat." Breastfeeding, however, is no time for crash diets. A gradual weight loss of 1 to 4 pounds per month by the nursing mother is appropriate. At significantly greater rates of weight loss—when calories are restricted to less than about 1500 kcal per day—milk output decreases. A reasonable approach for a breastfeeding mother is to eat a balanced diet that supplies at least 1800 kcal per day; has moderate fat content; and includes a variety of dairy products, fruits, vegetables, and whole grains.

To promote the best possible feeding experience for the infant, there are several other dietary factors to consider. Hydration is especially important during breastfeeding; the woman should drink fluids every time her infant nurses. Drinking about 13 cups of fluids per day encourages ample milk production. Poor health habits, such as smoking cigarettes or drinking more than two alcoholic drinks a day, can decrease milk output. (Even less alcohol can have a deleterious effect on milk output in some women.) To avoid exposure to harmful levels of mercury, precautions concerning fish likely to contain mercury should extend past pregnancy for the breastfeeding mother. Breastfeeding women also may want to avoid eating peanuts or peanut butter, as several studies have shown that peanut allergens pass into breast milk, potentially increasing the infant's risk for peanut allergy.

CONCEPT CHECK

Recognition of the importance of breastfeeding has contributed to its greater popularity. Almost all women have the ability to breastfeed. The hormone prolactin stimulates breast tissue to synthesize milk. Some components of human milk come directly from the mother's bloodstream. Infant suckling triggers a let-down reflex, which releases the milk. The more an infant nurses, the more milk is synthesized. The nutrient composition of human milk is different from that of cow's milk and changes as the infant matures. The first fluid produced, colostrum, is rich in immune factors. The diet for breastfeeding is generally similar to that for pregnancy, except for necessary additional fluids.

Breastfeeding Today

As noted, the vast majority of women are capable of breastfeeding and their infants benefit from it. The many benefits are listed in Table 16-4. Nonetheless, a woman's decision to breastfeed depends on a variety of factors, some of which may make breastfeeding impractical or undesirable for a woman. Mothers who don't want to breastfeed their infants should not feel pressured to do so. Breastfeeding provides distinct advantages, but

TABLE 16-4 Advantages of Breastfeeding

For Infant
• Bacteriologically safe
• Always fresh and ready to go
• Provides antibodies while infant's immune system is still immature, as well as substances that contribute to maturation of the immune system
• Contributes to maturation of gastrointestinal tract via *Lactobacillus bifidus* factor; decreases incidence of diarrhea and respiratory disease
• Reduces risk of food allergies and intolerances, as well as some other allergies
• Establishes habit of eating in moderation, thus decreasing possibility of obesity later in life by about 20%
• Contributes to proper development of jaws and teeth for better speech development
• Decreases ear infections
• May enhance nervous system development (by providing the fatty acid DHA) and eventual learning ability
• May reduce the risk of later developing hypertension and other chronic diseases, such as diabetes

For Mother
• Contributes to earlier recovery from pregnancy due to the action of hormones that promote a quicker return of the uterus to its prepregnancy state
• Decreases the risk of ovarian and premenopausal breast cancer
• Potential for quicker return to prepregnancy weight
• Potential for delayed ovulation and therefore reducing chances of pregnancy (short term, however)

none so great that a woman who decides to bottle feed should feel she is significantly compromising her infant.

Advantages of Breastfeeding. Just as the milk of all mammals is the perfect nutrition source for the young of that species, human milk is tailored to meet infant nutrient needs for the first 4 to 6 months of life. The possible exceptions are the relative lack of fluoride, iron, and vitamin D. Infant supplements, used under the guidance of a pediatrician, can supply these and are often recommended, especially vitamin D. The American Academy of Pediatrics recommends all breastfed infants be given 200 IU of vitamin D per day until they are consuming that much from food, such as, at least 2 cups (0.5 liters) of infant formula per day. Some sun exposure also helps in meeting vitamin D needs. Fluoride may be found in the household water supply. If it is not present in adequate amounts or the infant is not receiving tap water, a fluoride supplement should be considered and a dentist consulted. Vitamin B-12 supplements are recommended for the breastfed infant whose mother is a complete vegetarian (vegan).

Fewer Infections. Breastfeeding reduces the infant's overall risk of developing infections. This is partially because an infant can use the antibodies in human milk. Breastfed infants also have fewer ear infections (otitis media) because they do not sleep with a bottle in their mouths. Experts strongly discourage allowing any infants to

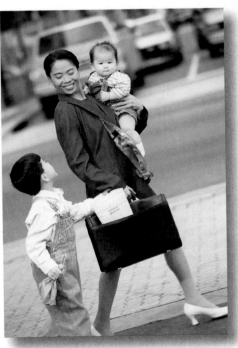

▲ Breastfeeding a baby once returning to work is possible, but requires planning.

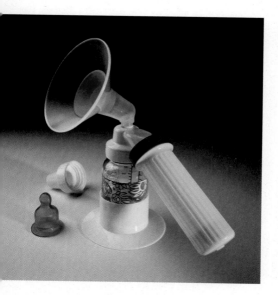

▲ Breast milk can be expressed by the mother using a manual, battery-operated (shown), or electric breast pump. The expressed milk can be stored for times when the mother is not available to breastfeed the infant.

▶ Frozen human milk should not be thawed in a microwave. The heat can destroy immune factors in the milk and create hot spots, which may scald the infant's mouth and esophagus.

sleep with a bottle in their mouths, because when that happens, milk can pool in the mouth; back up through the throat; and eventually settle in the ears, creating a growth medium for bacteria. Infant ear infections are a common problem. By avoiding these problems, parents can decrease discomfort for the infant, avoid related trips to the doctor, and prevent possible hearing loss. Tooth decay from nighttime bottles is another likely consequence of sleeping with a bottle in the mouth (see Chapter 17).

Fewer Allergies and Intolerances. Breastfeeding also reduces the chances of some allergies, especially in allergy-prone infants (see Chapter 17). The key time to attain this benefit from breastfeeding is during the first 4 to 6 months of an infant's life. A longer commitment than 4 to 6 months is best, but the first few months are most critical. Breastfeeding for even just the first few weeks is beneficial. Another benefit of breastfeeding is that infants are better able to tolerate human milk than formulas. Formulas sometimes must be switched several times until caregivers find the best one for the infant.

Convenience and Cost. Breastfeeding frees the mother from the time and expense involved in buying and preparing formula and washing bottles. Human milk is ready to go and sterile. This allows the mother to spend more time with her baby.

Possible Barriers to Breastfeeding. Widespread misinformation, the mother's need to return to a job, and social reticence serve as barriers to breastfeeding.

Misinformation. Probably the major barriers to breastfeeding are misinformation, such as the idea that one's breasts are too small, and the lack of role models. One positive note has been the widespread increase in the availability of lactation consultants over the past several years. These consultants are a valuable resource for new mothers in the adjustment to breastfeeding. If a woman is interested in breastfeeding, she should find support by talking to women who have experienced it successfully because they can be an invaluable help to the first-time mother. The first-time mother should find a friend she can call on for advice. In almost every community, a group called La Leche League offers classes in breastfeeding and advises women who have problems with it (800-LALECHE or www. lalecheleague.org). Other resources are www.breastfeeding.com, www.breastfeeding. org, and www.nal.usda.gov/wicworks.

Return to an Outside Job. Working outside the home can complicate plans to breastfeed. One possibility after a month or two of breastfeeding is for the mother to express and save her own milk. She can use a breast pump or manually express milk into a sterile plastic bottle or nursing bag (used in a disposable bottle system). Saving human milk requires careful sanitation and rapid chilling. It can be stored in the refrigerator for 3–5 days or be frozen for 3–6 months. Thawed milk should be used within 24 hours. There is a knack to learning how to express milk, but the freedom can be worth it, because it allows others to feed the infant the mother's milk. A schedule of expressing milk and using supplemental formula feedings is most successful if begun after 1 to 2 months of exclusive breastfeeding. After 1 month or so, the baby is well adapted to breastfeeding and probably feels enough emotional security and other benefits from nursing to drink both ways.

Some women can juggle both a job and breastfeeding, but others find it too cumbersome and decide to formula-feed. A compromise—balancing some breastfeedings, perhaps early morning and night, with infant formula feedings during the day—is possible. However, too many supplemental infant formula feedings decrease milk production.

Social Concerns. Another barrier for some women is embarrassment about nursing a child in public. Historically, our society has stressed modesty and has discouraged public displays of breasts—even for as good a cause as nourishing babies. In the United States, no state or territory has a law prohibiting breastfeeding. However, indecent exposure (including the exposure of women's breasts) has long been a common law or statutory offense. During the 1990s, some individual states, such as Florida and North Carolina, began to clarify the right to breastfeed and to decriminalize public breastfeeding. Since then, several other states have passed similar laws. Women who feel reluctant should be reassured that they do have social support and that breastfeeding can be done discreetly with little breast exposure.

Medical Conditions Precluding Breastfeeding. Breastfeeding may be ruled out by certain medical conditions in either the infant or mother. For example, breastfeeding may be detrimental to infants with phenylketonuria. The high concentration of phenylalanine in breast milk may overwhelm the impaired ability of these infants to metabolize this amino acid, leading to production of toxic products.

Certain medications, which pass into the milk and adversely affect the nursing infant, are best avoided while breastfeeding. In addition, a woman in North America or other developed regions of the world who has a serious chronic disease (such as tuberculosis, AIDS, or HIV-positive status) or who is being treated with chemotherapy medications should not breastfeed.

Environmental Contaminants in Human Milk. There is some legitimate concern over the levels of various environmental contaminants in human milk. However, the benefits from human milk are well established and the risks from environmental contaminants are still largely theoretical. Thus, it is probably best to continue with what has been shown to work until sufficiently strong research data contradict it. A few measures a woman could take to counteract some known contaminants are to (1) avoid freshwater fish from polluted waters; (2) carefully wash and peel fruits and vegetables; and (3) remove the fatty edges of meat, as pesticides concentrate in fat. In addition, a woman should not try to lose weight rapidly while nursing (more than ¾ to 1 pound per week) because contaminants stored in her fat tissue might then enter her bloodstream and affect her milk. If a woman questions whether her milk is safe, especially if she has lived in an area known to have a high concentration of toxic wastes or environmental pollutants, she should consult her local health department.

▶ Breastfeeding mothers should get their physician's permission before embarking on a vigorous exercise program. Breastfeeding women must also take care to drink plenty of fluids before and after workouts and should avoid exercising when fatigued.

MAKING DECISIONS

Breast Milk for Preterm Infants

There is no universal answer to whether a woman can breastfeed a preterm infant. In some cases, human milk is the most desirable form of nourishment, depending on infant weight and length of gestation. If so, it must usually be expressed from the breast and fed through a tube until the infant's sucking and swallowing reflex develops. This type of feeding demands great maternal dedication. Fortification of the milk with such nutrients as calcium, phosphorus, sodium, and protein is often necessary to match the preterm infant's rapid growth. In other cases, special feeding problems may prevent the use of human milk or necessitate supplementing it with formula. Sometimes total parenteral nutrition (intravenous feeding) is the only option. Working as a team, the pediatrician, neonatal nurses, and registered dietitian must guide the parents in this decision.

▲ If human milk is used to feed the preterm infant, fortification of the milk with certain nutrients is often needed.

CONCEPT CHECK

Human milk supplies most of an infant's nutritional needs for the first 6 months, although supplementation with vitamin D, iron, and fluoride may be needed. Breastfeeding is often more convenient than formula feeding. Compared with formula-fed infants, breastfed infants have fewer intestinal, respiratory, and ear infections and are less susceptible to some allergies and food intolerances. Despite the advantages of breastfeeding, misinformation, job responsibilities, and social reticence may dissuade a mother from breastfeeding. A combination of breastfeeding and formula feeding is possible when a mother is regularly away from the infant and is not able to express and store her milk for later use. Breastfeeding is not desirable if a mother has certain diseases or must take medication potentially harmful to the infant. The preterm infant, depending on its condition, may benefit from consuming human milk.

NUTRITION AND YOUR HEALTH
Preventing Birth Defects

Eating well for a healthy pregnancy not only supplies materials for fetal growth and development, but also helps to direct the amazing process of building a new life. Considering the complexity of the human body and its more than 20,000 genes, it's not surprising that abnormalities of structure, function, or metabolism are sometimes present at birth. Birth defects impact one of every 33 babies born in the United States. In some cases, they are so severe that a baby cannot survive or thrive. Birth defects are the presumed cause of many spontaneous abortions and are at the root of about 20% of infant deaths before one year of age. However, with medical intervention, many babies with birth defects can go on to live healthy and productive lives.

A wide range of physical or mental disabilities result from birth defects. Heart defects are present in approximately 1 of every 100 to 200 newborn babies, accounting for a large proportion of infant deaths. Cleft lip and/or cleft palate are malformations of the lip or roof of the mouth and occur in approximately 1 in 700 to 1000 births. Neural tube defects are malformations of the brain or spinal cord that occur in early stages of pregnancy, during embryonic development. Examples include spina bifida, in which all or part of the spinal cord is exposed, and anencephaly, in which some or all of the brain is missing. Babies born with spina bifida can survive to adulthood, but in many cases, have extreme disabilities. Babies born with anencephaly die soon after birth. Neural tube defects occur in 1 in 1000 births. Down syndrome, a condition in which an extra chromosome leads to mental retardation and other physical alterations, occurs in about 1 in 800 births. Other common birth defects include musculoskeletal defects, gastrointestinal defects, and metabolic disorders.

What causes a birth defect? About 15%–25% of birth defects are known to be genetic (i.e., inherited or spontaneous mutations of the genetic code). Another 10% are due to environmental influences (e.g., exposure to **teratogens**). The specific cause of the remaining 65%–75% of birth defects is unknown. Although the etiology of birth defects is multifactorial and many elements are beyond human control, good nutrition practices are an important way a mother-to-be can have a positive influence on the outcome of her pregnancy.

FOLIC ACID

During the 1980s, researchers in the United Kingdom noticed a relationship between poor dietary habits and a high rate of neural tube defects among children of impoverished women. Subsequent intervention studies demonstrated that administration of a multivitamin supplement during the periconceptional period—the months before and during early pregnancy—reduced the recurrence of these birth defects. The specific link between dietary folic acid and neural tube defects was tested and confirmed in several follow-up studies. As you learned in Chapter 11, folate plays a leading role in the synthesis of DNA and the metabolism of amino acids. The rapid cell growth of pregnancy increases needs for folate during pregnancy to 600 micrograms DFE per day. Some women, for genetic reasons, may have an even higher requirement. Adequate folic acid in the periconceptional period decreases the risk of neural tube defects by about 70% and has also been associated with decreased risk of cleft lip/palate, heart defects, and Down syndrome.

In 1998, the FDA mandated fortification of grain products to provide 140 micrograms of folic acid per 100 grams of grain consumed. In Canada, the level of fortification is 150 micrograms of folate per 100 grams of grain consumed. In general, this increases the average consumption of dietary folic acid by 100 micrograms per day. A well-planned diet can meet the RDA for folic acid, but the U.S. Public Health Service and the March of Dimes recommend that all women of childbearing age take a daily multivitamin and mineral supplement that contains 400 micrograms of folic acid. A physician may recommend prenatal vitamins or a higher dose of folic acid for some women, particularly those

teratogen A substance that may cause or increase the risk of a birth defect. Exposure to a teratogen does not always lead to a birth defect; its effects on the fetus depend on the dose, timing, and duration of exposure.

who have had a prior pregnancy complicated by a neural tube defect. The Dietary Guidelines for Americans recommend that women who may become pregnant and those in the first few months of pregnancy consume an adequate amount of the synthetic form of folate, folic acid (Table 16-2).

IODIDE

The relationship between folic acid and neural tube defects is a dramatic example of how a nutrient deficiency can negatively impact pregnancy outcome, but it is not the only nutrient of concern. Low iodide status during the first trimester of pregnancy—a critical period of brain development—may lead to cretinism. This is a congenital form of hypothyroidism that leads to diminished physical and mental development if left untreated. When the defect is identified early (by newborn screening tests), cretinism can be prevented by treatment with thyroid hormones. With use of iodized salt, however, iodide deficiencies are rare.

ANTIOXIDANTS

A case can be made for antioxidants in the prevention of birth defects as well. Free radicals are constantly generated within the body as a result of normal metabolic processes. An abundance of free radicals results in damage of cells and their DNA, which can lead to gene mutations or tissue malformations. Some research points to free radicals as a source of damage during embryo development and organogenesis, which leads to birth defects. Antioxidant systems within the body act to minimize the damage caused by free radicals, and researchers hypothesize that dietary sources of antioxidants may aid in the prevention of birth defects. At this time, there is insufficient evidence to support supplementation of individual nutrients that participate in antioxidant systems—vitamin E, vitamin C, sele-

nium, zinc, and copper—for the prevention of birth defects. However, use of a balanced multivitamin and mineral supplement while consuming a diet rich in whole grains, legumes, and a variety of fruits and vegetables will provide enough of these nutrients to meet current recommendations.

VITAMIN A

Whereas the needs for most vitamins and minerals increase by about 30% during pregnancy, the requirement for vitamin A increases by only 10%. Studies have shown teratogenic potential of vitamin A in doses as low as approximately 3000 micrograms RAE per day. This is just over three times the RDA of 770 micrograms RAE/d for pregnant adult women. Fetal abnormalities resulting from vitamin A toxicity primarily include facial and cardiac defects, but a wide range of defects have been reported. It is rare that food sources of vitamin A would lead to toxicity. Recall from Chapter 9 that preformed vitamin A is found in liver, fish, fish oils, fortified milk and yogurt, and eggs. Carotenoids, found in fruits and vegetables, are precursors of vitamin A that are converted to vitamin A in the small intestine. However, the efficiency of absorption of carotenoids decreases as intake increases. Vitamin A excesses typically arise from high-dose dietary supplements rather than food sources. Typical North American diets supply adequate vitamin A from foods, so supplemental use is not generally necessary. During pregnancy, supplemental preformed vitamin A should not exceed 3000 micrograms RAE per day (15,000 IU per day). Most multivitamins and prenatal vitamins supply less than 1500 micrograms RAE per day. A balanced diet and prudent use of dietary supplements are actions that can sidestep potential problems with vitamin A toxicity.

CAFFEINE

Caffeine has been scrutinized for its safety during pregnancy, especially for any link with rate of birth defects. Caf-

▲ Delivering a healthy baby is more than just luck. Many nutrition- and health-related practices need to be considered.

feine decreases the mother's absorption of iron and may reduce blood flow through the placenta. In addition, the fetus is unable to detoxify caffeine. In addition, as caffeine intake increases, so does the risk of delivering an LBW infant. Heavy caffeine use during pregnancy may also lead to caffeine withdrawal symptoms in the newborn. These risks are reported with caffeine intakes in excess of 500 milligrams, or the equivalent of about 5 cups of coffee per day. Moderate use of caffeine (up to the equivalent of 3 cups of coffee per day), however, is not associated with risk for birth defects. Based on current evidence, drinking no more than three cups of coffee and no more than four cups of caffeinated soft drinks per day during pregnancy, or when pregnancy is possible, is advocated. Paying attention to caffeine intake from tea, over-the-counter medicines containing caffeine, and chocolate is also important.

ASPARTAME USE

Phenylalanine, a component of the artificial sweetener, aspartame (NutraSweet® and Equal®), causes concern for some pregnant women. High amounts of phenylalanine in maternal blood disrupt fetal brain development if the mother has a disease known as *phenylketonuria* (review Chapter 4). If the mother does not have this condition, however, it is unlikely that the baby will be affected by moderate aspartame use.

For most adults, diet soft drinks are the primary source of artificial sweeteners. Of greater concern than the safety of sweeteners during pregnancy is the quality of foods and beverages consumed. A high intake of diet soft drinks may crowd out healthier beverages, such as water and low-fat milk.

OBESITY AND CHRONIC HEALTH CONDITIONS

Even before becoming pregnant, women of childbearing age should have regular medical checkups to keep an eye on any health conditions that already exist or to identify any developing health problems. In some cases, the condition itself increases risk for birth defects. Obesity, high blood pressure, and uncontrolled diabetes are common health problems known to increase the risk for birth defects, including neural tube defects. In other cases, medications used to control illnesses may pose a risk to the developing fetus. Other health issues, such as seizure disorders and metabolic disorders, could also affect fetal development. A preconception visit with a health professional can help to sort out and make plans to minimize such risks. Once a woman has become pregnant, early and regular prenatal care can aid in the success of a pregnancy.

Women with diabetes are two to three times more likely to give birth to a baby with birth defects compared to women with normal glucose metabolism. Examples of birth defects common in this group include malformations of the spine, legs, and blood vessels of the heart. Some experts speculate that the mechanism by

which diabetes increases birth defects is via excessive free radicals, which lead to oxidative damage of DNA during early gestation. Careful control of blood glucose drastically lowers risk for women with diabetes. Optimal blood glucose control can be achieved through a combination of dietary modifications and medications. Given that diabetes is on the rise among women of childbearing age, this elevated rate of birth defects has become an area of heightened awareness.

Another health condition for which maternal nutritional control is of utmost importance is PKU. Recall from Chapter 6 that PKU is an error of metabolism in which the liver lacks the ability to process phenylalanine, leading to an accumulation of this amino acid and its metabolites in body tissues. Babies born to women who have phenylketonuria that is not controlled by diet are at heightened risk for brain defects, such as microcephaly and mental retardation.

ALCOHOL

Conclusive evidence shows that repeated consumption of four or more alcoholic drinks at one sitting harms the fetus. Such binge drinking is especially perilous during the first 12 weeks of pregnancy, as this is when critical early developmental events take place in utero. Although scientists don't know whether pregnant women must totally eliminate alcohol use to avoid risk of damage to the fetus, women are advised not to drink any alcohol during pregnancy or when there is a chance pregnancy might occur—until a safe level can be established. The embryo (and, at later stages, the fetus), has no means of detoxifying alcohol.

Women with chronic alcoholism produce children with a recognizable pattern of malformations called **fetal alcohol syndrome (FAS).** A diagnosis of FAS is based mainly on poor fetal and infant growth, physical deformities (especially of facial features), and mental retardation (Fig. 16-6). The infant is frequently irritable and may develop hyperactivity and a short attention span. Limited hand-eye coordination is common. Defects in vision, hearing, and mental processing often develop over time.

Exactly how alcohol causes these defects is not known. One line of research suggests that alcohol, or products produced by the metabolism of alcohol (e.g., acetaldehyde), cause faulty movement of cells in the brain during early stages of nerve cell development or block the action of certain brain neurotransmitters. In addition, inadequate nutrient intake, reduced nutrient and oxygen transfer across the placenta, cigarette smoking commonly associated with alcohol intake, drug use, and possibly other factors contribute to the overall result.

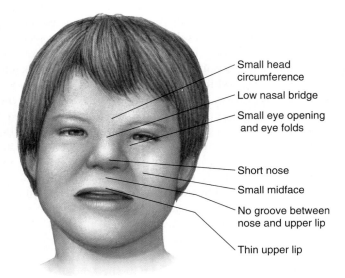

FIGURE 16-6 ▶ Fetal alcohol syndrome. The facial features shown are typical of affected children. Additional abnormalities in the brain and other internal organs accompany fetal alcohol syndrome but are not immediately apparent from simply looking at the child. Milder forms of alcohol-induced changes from a lower alcohol exposure to the fetus are known as **fetal alcohol effects.** In this case, behavior problems without physical effects, such as altered facial features, are seen.

Small head circumference

Low nasal bridge

Small eye opening and eye folds

Short nose

Small midface

No groove between nose and upper lip

Thin upper lip

The Dietary Guidelines for Americans recommend that alcoholic beverages not be consumed by pregnant and lactating women (Table 16-2). For more information about fetal alcohol syndrome visit the website www.cdc.gov/ncbddd/fas/.

ENVIRONMENTAL CONTAMINANTS

There is little evidence to link birth defects with the amounts of pesticides, herbicides, or other contaminants in foods or public water supplies in North America. However, evaluating such a link can be methodologically difficult and many would argue that regulations concerning contaminants in the food and water supply are too permissive. Thus, it seems prudent to take measures to decrease intake of pesticides and herbicides wherever possible. For fruits and vegetables, peeling, removing outer leaves, and/or thoroughly rinsing and scrubbing with a brush under running water will remove the majority of contaminants. In animal products, pesticides and other contaminants are most likely to accumulate in fatty tissues. Therefore, removing skin, discarding drippings, and trimming visible fat will decrease exposure from meat, poultry, and fish.

For fish, mercury is of particular concern because it can harm the nervous system of the fetus. Thus, FDA warns pregnant women to avoid swordfish, shark, king mackerel, and tile fish because of possible high mercury contamination. Largemouth bass are also implicated. In general, intake of other fish and shellfish should not exceed 12 ounces per week. Canned albacore tuna is a potential mercury source, so it should not be consumed in amounts exceeding 6 ounces per week. As a rule of thumb, consuming a variety of foods minimizes risk of exposure to contaminants from the food supply.

SUMMING UP

Although many risk factors for birth defects are beyond our control, a woman of childbearing potential can make some wise nutrition choices to improve her chances of having a healthy baby without birth defects. A varied and balanced diet, such as the food plan for pregnant women described in this chapter, along with a daily multivitamin and mineral supplement with 400 micrograms of folic acid will ensure adequate nutrient status. It is estimated that daily use of a multivitamin and mineral supplement containing folic acid will decrease the rate of all birth defects by 50%. Discuss use of any other dietary supplements with a physician to be sure that the fetus will not be exposed to toxic levels of vitamin A or other dangerous ingredients. Early and consistent prenatal care can help control obesity and any chronic health conditions that may complicate a pregnancy. Also, avoiding alcohol during pregnancy will eliminate any risk for fetal alcohol syndrome.

Although it seems that advice for a healthy pregnancy is always directed at the mother, fathers-to-be are not off the hook. Health is a family affair, so encouraging healthy eating habits and avoiding smoking and alcohol are important for fathers, too. Less research has been done in the area, but the genetics of the baby are certainly an outcome of both parents. Considering that spermatogenesis takes approximately 70 days, the periconceptional period is a time for good nutrition and careful lifestyle practices for the father as well.

▶ A goal of *Healthy People 2010* is 100% abstinence from alcohol, cigarettes, and illicit drugs by pregnant women.

fetal alcohol syndrome (FAS) A group of irreversible physical and mental abnormalities in the infant that result from the mother's consuming alcohol during pregnancy.

fetal alcohol effect (FAE) Hyperactivity, attention deficit disorder, poor judgment, sleep disorders, and delayed learning as a result of prenatal exposure to alcohol.

▶ Pregnant women should recognize that many cough syrups contain alcohol. Cases have been reported of infants with FAS born to mothers who consumed generous amounts of such cough syrups but no other alcoholic beverages.

▶ In North America, maternal death as a result of childbirth is uncommon—only about 11 deaths in every 100,000 live births. The infant mortality rate, however, is much higher: for each 100,000 live births, about 600 to 700 infants die within the first year. The infant death rate among African-Americans is more than double the rates among Whites and Hispanics in the United States.

CASE STUDY

Preparing for Pregnancy

Tracey and her husband have decided that they are ready to prepare for Tracey's first pregnancy. She is 25 years old, weighs 135 pounds, and is 67 inches tall. Tracey has been reading everything she can find on pregnancy because she knows that her prepregnancy health is important to the success of her pregnancy.

She knows she should avoid alcohol, especially because alcohol is potentially toxic to the growing fetus in the first weeks of pregnancy, and she could become pregnant and not know about it right away. Tracey is not a smoker, does not take any medications, and limits her coffee intake to 4 cups a day and soft drink intake to 3 colas per day. Based on her reading, she has decided to breastfeed her infant and has already inquired about childbirth classes. She has modified her diet to include some extra protein, along with more fruits and vegetables. She has also started taking an over-the-counter vitamin and mineral supplement. Tracey has always kept in good shape, and she is admittedly worried about gaining too much weight during pregnancy. Recently, she started a running program 5 days a week, and she plans to continue running throughout her pregnancy.

Answer the following questions, and check your responses in Appendix A.

1. What recommendations do you have regarding Tracey's use of dietary supplements?
2. What is Tracey doing to prevent neural tube defects? What else could she do?
3. What recommendations would you make regarding Tracey's caffeine consumption?
4. Tracey is wise to pay attention to her protein intake to prepare for pregnancy and breastfeeding. Should she include fish as a source of protein in her diet? Why or why not?
5. Constipation is a common complaint during pregnancy. What suggestions do you have to help Tracey avoid this health concern?
6. What information would you share with Tracey about appropriate weight gain during pregnancy?

SUMMARY

1. Adequate nutrition is vital during pregnancy to ensure the well-being of both the infant and mother. Poor maternal nutrition and use of some medications, especially during the first trimester, can cause birth defects. Growth restriction and altered development can also occur if these insults happen later in pregnancy.

2. Infants born preterm (before 37 weeks gestation) usually have more medical problems at and following birth than normal infants.

3. A woman typically needs an additional 350 to 450 kcal per day during the second and third trimesters of pregnancy to meet her calorie needs. A better measure of meeting energy needs is adequate weight gain. This should occur slowly, reaching a total of 25 to 35 pounds in a woman of healthy weight.

4. Protein, carbohydrate, fiber, vitamin, and mineral needs increase during pregnancy. Following a plan based on MyPyramid is recommended. A supplemental source of iron, in particular, may be needed. Folate nutriture especially should be adequate at the time of conception. Any nutrient supplement use needs to be guided by a physician, as an excess intake of vitamin A and other nutrients during pregnancy can have harmful effects on the fetus.

5. The factors that contribute to poor pregnancy outcome include inadequate health care in general and prenatal care in particular, obesity, teenage pregnancy, smoking, alcohol consumption, illicit drug use (such as cocaine), insufficient carbohydrate intake (less than 175 grams per day), heavy caffeine use, and various infections, such as *listeriosis*.

6. Pregnancy-induced hypertension, gestational diabetes, heartburn, constipation, nausea, vomiting, edema, and anemia are all possible discomforts and complications of pregnancy. Nutrition therapy can help minimize some of these problems.

7. Almost all women are able to breastfeed their infants. The nutrient composition of human milk is different from that of unaltered cow's milk and is much more desirable. Colostrum, the first fluid produced by the human breast, is rich in immune factors. Mature milk is rich in protein and in lactose. The diet plan recommended for the second and third trimesters of pregnancy is also appropriate for meeting the nutrient needs of the lactating woman, except more fluids in general should be consumed.

8. For the infant, the advantages of breastfeeding over formula feeding are numerous, including fewer intestinal, respiratory, and ear infections and fewer allergies and food intolerances. Moreover, breastfeeding is also less expensive and possibly more convenient for the mother than formula feeding. However, an infant can be adequately nourished with formula if the mother chooses not to breastfeed. Breastfeeding is not desirable if the mother has certain diseases or must take medication potentially harmful to the infant. Likewise, breastfeeding may not be advised for infants with certain medical conditions, including some preterm infants.

STUDY QUESTIONS

1. Provide three key pieces of advice for parents seeking to maximize their chances of having a healthy infant. Why did you identify those specific factors?

2. Outline current weight-gain recommendations for pregnancy. What is the basis for these recommendations?

3. Identify four key nutrients for which intake should be significantly increased during pregnancy.

4. How is the MyPyramid diet for an average woman adapted to meet the increased nutrient needs of pregnancy?

5. Why does teenage pregnancy receive so much attention these days? At what age do you think pregnancy is ideal? Why?

6. Give three reasons a woman should give serious consideration to breastfeeding her infant.

7. Describe the physiological mechanisms that stimulate milk production and release. How can knowing about these help mothers breastfeed successfully?

8. What guidelines can a woman use to determine whether her breastfed infant is receiving sufficient nourishment?

9. How should the basic food plan suitable for pregnancy be modified during breastfeeding?

10. Where can first-time mothers go for help in establishing successful breastfeeding?

CHECK YOUR KNOWLEDGE

Answers to the following multiple choice questions are in Appendix A.

1. The fetus is most susceptible to damage from nutrient deficiencies; teratogens; and use of certain medications, alcohol, and illicit drugs during
   a. the first trimester.
   b. the second trimester.
   c. the third trimester.
   d. labor and delivery.

2. An infant born at 38 weeks' gestation weighing 5.0 pounds can be described as
   a. preterm.   c. SGA.
   b. LBW.   d. LBW and SGA.

3. If a woman is 5'2" and weighs 150 pounds before becoming pregnant, how much weight should she gain during pregnancy?
   a. 28 to 40 pounds (12.5 to 18 kilograms)
   b. 25 to 35 pounds (11.5 to 16 kilograms)
   c. 15 to 25 pounds (7 to 11.5 kilograms)
   d. As little as possible.

4. Increased carbohydrate needs during pregnancy are set to
   a. prevent ketosis.
   b. alleviate nausea.
   c. prevent pregnancy-induced hypertension.
   d. supply adequate folate.

5. Which of the following is best paired with an iron supplement during pregnancy?
   a. skim milk
   b. orange juice
   c. coffee
   d. tea

6. Obesity during pregnancy is associated with higher rates of
   a. birth defects.
   b. diabetes.
   c. surgical delivery.
   d. All of the above.

7. Consuming one cup of coffee per day is associated with
   a. spontaneous abortions.
   b. LBW.

   c. birth defects.
   d. None of the above.

8. Which of the following may help to alleviate nausea during pregnancy?
   a. postponing meals until the afternoon
   b. drinking large amounts of water
   c. postponing use of iron supplements until the second trimester
   d. All of the above.

9. Which of the following conditions medically prevents a woman from breastfeeding her infant?
   a. breasts are too small
   b. infant has PKU
   c. inverted nipples
   d. None of the above.

10. Physiologically, milk production requires _____ kcals per day.
    a. 300
    b. 500
    c. 800
    d. 1000

FURTHER READINGS

1. ADA Reports: Position of the American Dietetic Association: Nutrition and lifestyle for a healthy pregnancy outcome. *Journal of the American Dietetic Association* 102:1479, 2002.

   The key components of a healthy lifestyle during pregnancy include appropriate weight gain; consumption of a variety of foods; appropriate and timely vitamin and mineral intake; avoidance of alcohol, tobacco, and other harmful substances; and safe food handling. Vitamin and mineral supplementation is appropriate for some nutrients, particularly in certain situations, such as for vegans.

2. ADA Reports: Position of the American Dietetic Association: Promoting and supporting breastfeeding. *Journal of the American Dietetic Association* 105:810, 2005.

   The American Dietetic Association strongly supports the breastfeeding of infants. This article discusses the benefits from breastfeeding that accrue to the mother and infant, as well as dietary considerations that need to be addressed, such as avoiding consumption of species of fish known to contain high amounts of mercury.

3. Allen LH: Multiple micronutrients in pregnancy and lactation: An overview. *American Journal of Clinical Nutrition* 81:1206S, 2005.

   Numerous nutrients contribute to a healthy outcome of pregnancy, including many B vitamins and iron. The author notes in many cases diet changes allow women to meet these needs, but in some cases supplementation is needed, such as for poor women. With respect to diet changes, these should begin before pregnancy so a woman has a healthy status in the first weeks while she is pregnant but still does not know this is the case.

4. Bodnar LM and others: Periconceptional multivitamin use reduces the risk of preeclampsia. *American Journal of Epidemiology* 164:470, 2006.

   In the Pregnancy Exposures and Preeclampsia Prevention Study, women who regularly consumed a multivitamin during the periconceptional period had a 45% lower risk of developing preeclampsia during their first pregnancy than those who did not consume multivitamins. The relationship between multivitamin use and disease risk was profoundly affected by prepregnancy body weight: women with BMI less than 25 benefited most from multivitamin use. The mechanism by which multivitamin use may prevent preeclampsia is not known.

5. Crowther CA and others: Effect of treatment of gestational diabetes mellitus on pregnancy outcomes. *The New England Journal of Medicine* 352:2477, 2005.

   This study found that treating gestational diabetes when it develops is important to improve the health of the mother, fetus, and ultimately the infant. Diet changes and regular blood glucose monitoring are important parts of the therapy; in some cases insulin injections are also needed to control blood glucose.

6. Field CJ: The immunological components of human milk and their effect on immune development in infants. *Journal of Nutrition* 135:1, 2005.

   Human milk contains many factors that improve immune function in the infant. This article reviews a number of these complex factors.

7. Green NS: Folic acid supplementation and prevention of birth defects. *Journal of Nutrition* 132:2356S, 2002.

   If all women began pregnancy with adequate folate status, neural tube birth defects could be decreased by up to 70%. The recommendation is for women of childbearing age to consume 400 micrograms of synthetic folic acid daily. Women who have given birth to a child with a neural tube defect should consume 4000 micrograms (4 milligrams) of synthetic folic acid per day in anticipation of a possible pregnancy.

8. Henriksen T: Nutrition and pregnancy outcome. *Nutrition Reviews* 64:S19, 2006.

   This article reviews current nutritional practices of pregnant women, which do not conform to what we know to be optimal. The increase in overweight women has been accompanied by a dramatic increase in gestational diabetes and an increase in large babies.

9. Hulsey TC and others: Maternal prepregnant body mass index and weight gain related to low birth weight in South Carolina. *Southern Medical Journal* 98:411, 2005.

   A healthy weight at conception and adequate weight gain during pregnancy contributed to a substantial reduction in low-birth-weight infants in this study. For example, women with inadequate weight gains had about a 1.5 to 2 times greater risk of delivering a low-birth-weight infant.

10. Kabiru KW, Raynor BD: Obstetric outcomes associated with increase in BMI category during pregnancy. *American Journal of Obstetrics and Gynecology* 191:928, 2004.

    Obesity in pregnant women leads to a high risk for complications in the pregnancy and so requires careful monitoring by the physician. Such potential complications in this study included gestational diabetes and the need for Cesarean deliveries.

11. Kelly, AKW: Practical exercise advice during pregnancy. *The Physician and Sports Medicine* 33(6):24, 2005.

    It is safe for pregnant women to exercise if they are experiencing uncomplicated pregnancies. The author notes that many positive effects of exercise during pregnancy are possible. Most non-weight-bearing exercises (e.g., swimming) and walking are safe for pregnant women. Women should begin with 15 minutes of exercise three times a week and progress as tolerated. The author discusses how to monitor women as they increase their physical activity.

12. King JC: Maternal obesity, metabolism, and pregnancy outcomes. *Annual Review of Nutrition* 26:271, 2006.

    Maternal obesity increases risk for complications and adverse outcomes of pregnancy, including gestational diabetes, preeclampsia, birth defects, and large-for-gestational-age births. Evidence is accumulating to support the notion that maternal obesity also negatively impacts chronic disease risk for offspring. The potential mechanisms for these relationships are discussed and practical nutrition advice, based on the 2005 Dietary Guidelines for Americans, is provided.

13. Koebnick C and others: Long-term ovo-lacto vegetarian diet impairs vitamin B-12 status in pregnant women. *Journal of Nutrition* 134:3319, 2004.

    Pregnant women consuming a long-term, predominantly vegetarian diet had an increased risk of developing a vitamin B-12 deficiency in this study. Attention to vitamin B-12 intake is thus merited in women who are vegetarians, and this needs to be done before they become pregnant.

14. Moore, VM, Davies, MJ: Diet during pregnancy, neonatal outcomes and later health. *Reproduction, Fertility, and Delivery* 17:341, 2005.

    Altering the maternal diet before and during pregnancy can induce permanent changes in the offspring birth size and adult health/life span. Consequences of inadequate maternal nutrition for the offspring depend on the specific time in gestation that they occur. The authors emphasize the importance of improving diet before a woman becomes pregnant in order to protect her health and the health of her offspring.

15. Pawley, N., Bishop, NJ: Prenatal and infant predictors of bone health: The influence of vitamin D. *American Journal of Clinical Nutrition* 80:1748S, 2004.

    Women who are vitamin D-deficient during pregnancy deliver infants with disturbed skeletal development and, in some cases, even with evidence of rickets and fractures. Populations at risk for vitamin D deficiency are those for which, for environmental, cultural, or medical reasons, exposure to sunlight is poor and the dietary intake of vitamin D is low. Especially in these cases, attention to meeting vitamin D needs is important.

16. Rosenburg, TJ and others: Maternal obesity and diabetes as risk factors for adverse pregnancy outcomes: Differences among 4 racial/ethnic groups. *American Journal of Public Health* 95:1545, 2005.

    In this large population-based study, obesity and diabetes were clearly associated with adverse pregnancy outcomes. This highlights the need for women to control these conditions as best as possible during their childbearing years to protect the health of their future infant.

17. Tamura T, Picciano MF: Folate and human reproduction. *American Journal of Clinical Nutrition* 83:993, 2006.

    Folate status is important to human reproduction due to its roles in DNA synthesis and metabolism of various amino acids. Folic acid supplementation for the prevention of megalo-blastic anemia during pregnancy and neural tube defects represents a major public health advancement. Several other areas of reproductive health are under continued study for relationships with folate status, including placental abruption, preeclampsia, spontaneous abortion, stillbirth, low birth weight, and risk for birth defects other than neural tube defects.

18. Taylor JS and others: A systematic review of the literature associating breastfeeding with type 2 diabetes and gestational diabetes. *Journal of the American College of Nutrition* 24:320, 2005.

    Breastfeeding confers health benefits to both mother and child. Breastfed infants have lower rates of obesity, type 1 diabetes, and type 2 diabetes in adulthood compared to formula-fed infants. In addition, mothers who breastfeed have improved glucose tolerance and lower risk for postpartum diabetes compared to nonlactating mothers. Studies show that mothers with diabetes are less likely to breastfeed than their nondiabetic counterparts, but the data reviewed in this article provide evidence that diabetic mothers and their babies could both benefit from breastfeeding.

19. Wagner, LK: Diagnosis and management of preeclampsia. *American Family Physician* 70:2317, 2004.

    Preeclampsia is a multisystem disorder of unknown cause. It affects about 5%–7% of pregnancies and is a significant cause of both illness and death in the mother and fetus. Management requires careful monitoring of the mother and fetus once the disorder develops. Magnesium sulfate is the major therapy used, but medications to control related hypertension may also be employed. This article reviews preeclampsia in detail.

▶ Check out the **Contemporary Nutrition ARIS site**

www.mhhe.com/wardlawcontfa1 for quizzes, flash cards, other activities, and weblinks designed to further help you learn about nutrition for pregnant and breastfeeding women.

I. Targeting Nutrients Necessary for Pregnant Women

This chapter mentioned that pregnant women may have difficulty meeting their increased needs for folate, vitamin B-6, iron, and zinc. List six foods rich in each of these nutrients next to the appropriate heading. Refer to Chapters 8 and 9 if necessary.

Nutrient	Foods	Nutrient	Foods
Folate	_____	Iron	_____
	_____		_____
	_____		_____
	_____		_____
	_____		_____
	_____		_____
Vitamin B-6	_____	Zinc	_____
	_____		_____
	_____		_____
	_____		_____
	_____		_____
	_____		_____

1. Foods rich in more than one of these nutrients would be especially valuable for pregnant women. Write on the line any foods you listed that are good sources of more than one of these critical nutrients.

   _____

2. The needs for folate, vitamin B-6, iron, and zinc increase during pregnancy. For which of these nutrients can pregnant women usually obtain adequate intakes from dietary sources?

   _____

3. Which of these nutrients are commonly taken in supplement form during pregnancy?

   _____

   _____

4. Why might it be hard for pregnant women to meet their increased needs for these nutrients from food alone?

   _____

   _____

II. Putting Your Knowledge About Nutrition and Pregnancy to Work

A college friend, Angie, tells you that she is newly pregnant. You are aware that she usually likes to eat the following foods for her meals:

Breakfast

Skips this meal, or eats a granola bar
Coffee

Lunch

Sweetened yogurt, 1 cup
Small bagel with cream cheese
Occasional piece of fruit
Regular caffeinated soda, 12 ounces

Snack

Chocolate candy bar

Dinner

2 slices of pizza, macaroni and cheese, or 2 eggs with 2 slices of toast
Seldom eats a salad or vegetable
Regular caffeinated soda, 12 ounces

Snacks

Pretzels or chips, 1 ounce
Regular caffeinated soda, 12 ounces

1. Using NutritionCalc Plus software, evaluate Angie's diet for protein, carbohydrate, folate, vitamin B-6, iron, and zinc. How does her intake compare with the recommended amounts for pregnancy?

   _____

   _____

   _____

2. Now redesign her diet and make sure that her intake meets pregnancy needs for protein, carbohydrate, folate, vitamin B-6, and zinc. (Hint: Fortified foods, such as breakfast cereal, are generally nutrient-rich foods, which can more easily help meet one's needs.) Increase the iron content as well, but it still may be below the RDA for pregnancy.

   _____

   _____

   _____

CHAPTER 17 Nutrition from Infancy Through Adolescence

CHAPTER OBJECTIVES Chapter 17 is designed to allow you to:

1. Describe the extent to which nutrition affects infant growth and physiological development.

2. Identify diet guidelines to meet the basic nutritional needs for normal growth and development for an infant and discuss some do's and don'ts associated with infant feeding.

3. List several challenges parents might face in dealing with childhood eating habits.

4. List the nutrients often found to be lacking in the diets of infants, toddlers, preschoolers, and teenagers and make recommendations to remedy the problems.

CHAPTER OUTLINE

AS HUMANS GROW THROUGH EARLY YEARS INTO YOUNG ADULTHOOD, OUR NEEDS FOR CALORIES AND NUTRIENTS CHANGE. Infants need more calories, protein, vitamins, and minerals per pound of body weight than young and older adults to support their rapid pace of growth and development. The growth rate of children is slower than that of infants, therefore children's needs and intake are proportionately less. As the chapter comic suggests, the erratic eating behaviors of young children pose major challenges for parents and other caregivers. In turn, childhood becomes an important time to establish healthful habits, including those related to food choice and physical activity.

Family behaviors exert powerful influences on the child. Thus, education designed to change children's eating behaviors must be directed simultaneously at the main caregivers. Parents and other caregivers usually determine what foods are purchased and how they are prepared. To help children adopt a lifelong healthy dietary intake, a variety of foods should be introduced at home, fast-food and sugared soft drinks should be limited to a few times per week or less, and new foods should be introduced regularly. Maintaining a healthful eating (and physical activity) pattern should continue as children grow into teenagers. In exploring all these stages of life, Chapter 17 looks at the key role nutrients play and how food choices should be tailored to meet changing needs.

Refresh Your Memory

As you begin your study of nutrition from infancy through adolescence in Chapter 17, you may want to review:

- MyPyramid and the 2005 Dietary Guidelines in Chapter 2
- The immune system in Chapter 3
- Diagnosis and treatment of type 2 diabetes in Chapter 4
- Common sources of saturated fat, cholesterol, and *trans* fat in Chapter 5
- Vegetarianism in Chapter 6
- The concept of body mass index (BMI) and the treatment of obesity, including typical medications prescribed, in Chapter 7
- Rich sources of calcium, iron, and zinc in Chapters 10 and 11
- The benefits of regular physical activity in Chapter 12
- Anorexia nervosa and other eating disorders in Chapter 13

NUTRITION AND CHILD HEALTH— AN INTRODUCTION

Current statistics describing nutrition and overall health among children and adolescents in North America have shown both positive and negative trends. On a positive note, more children are receiving vaccinations than ever before, fewer teenagers are giving birth, and the poverty rate for children has fallen considerably. In contrast to this good news, the number of children and teenagers with obesity and type 2 diabetes is rising, and physical activity in general is on the decline as more time is spent sitting in front of computer screens and television sets. Low calcium intakes are also receiving much attention, as soft drinks have replaced much of the milk that children and teenagers previously consumed on a daily basis. Fruits, vegetables, and whole grains are also often in short supply in their diets. In this chapter, we will look at these trends and their effects on nutrition and overall health of this age group.

At what age should an infant be fed solid foods? Which foods are most appropriate for those early stages of solid food introduction? Which foods should not be fed to infants? Why? Chapter 17 provides some answers.

MARVIN © Reprinted with special permission of King Features Syndicate, Inc.

INFANT GROWTH AND NUTRITION NEEDS

During infancy, attitudes toward foods and the eating process begin to take shape. If parents and other caregivers practice good nutrition and are flexible, they can lead an infant into lifelong healthful food habits. An infant that starts life in such an environment has a good chance of starting life with the nutrients needed to support brain and body growth spurts, and of developing a willingness to try new foods. However, these physical and psychological advantages alone don't guarantee that a child will thrive.

Children also need specific attention focused on them; they need to grow in a stimulating environment, and they need a sense of security. For example, children hospitalized for growth failure gain weight more quickly when more caring stimulation, such as holding and rocking the infant, accompanies needed nutrients.

The Growing Infant

All babies seem to do is eat and sleep. There's a good reason for this. An infant's birth weight doubles in the first 4 to 6 months and triples within the first year. Never again is growth so rapid. Such rapid growth requires a lot of nourishment and sleep. After the first year, growth is slower; it takes 5 more years to double the weight seen at 1 year. An infant also increases in length in the first year by 50% and then continues to gain height through the teen years. These gains are not necessarily continuous—spurts of growth alternate with plateaus. Height is essentially maximized by age 19, although increases of several inches may occur in the early twenties, especially for boys (Fig. 17-1). Head size in proportion to total height shrinks from one-fourth to one-eighth during the climb from infancy to adulthood.

The human body needs a lot more food to support growth and development than it does to merely maintain its size once growth ceases. When nutrients are missing at critical phases of this process, growth and development may slow or even stop. In countries of the developing world, about one-third of the children under 5 years of age are short and underweight for their ages. Poor nutrition—called **undernutrition**—is at the heart of the problem. This occurs to a lesser extent in North America. The undernourished children are smaller versions of nutritionally fit children. In poorer countries, when breastfeeding ceases, children are often fed a high-carbohydrate, low-protein diet. This diet supports some growth but does not allow children to attain their full genetic potential. To grow, children must consume adequate amounts of calories, protein, calcium, iron, zinc, and other nutrients.

undernutrition Failing health that results from a long-standing dietary intake that is not enough to meet nutritional needs.

Effect of Undernutrition on Growth

As with the fetus in utero, the long-term effects of nutritional problems in infancy and childhood depend on the severity, timing, and duration of the nutritional insult to cell processes.

The single best indicator of a child's nutritional status is growth, particularly weight gain in the short run and length (height) in the long run. Mild zinc deficiencies in North American children have been linked to poor growth. Improving the diets of these children then leads to improved growth. Overall, eating a poor diet as an infant or a child hampers the cell division that occurs at that critical stage. Consuming an adequate diet later usually won't compensate for lost growth, however, as the hormonal and other conditions needed for growth will not likely be present. In addition, growth ceases in girls and boys when the skeleton reaches its final size. This happens as growth plates at the ends of the bones fuse, which begins around 14 years of age in girls and 15 years of age in boys. The final stages of this process end at about 19 years of age in girls and 20 years of age in boys. Furthermore, muscles can increase in diameter later in life but their linear growth is limited by the length of the shorter bone.

For these reasons, a 15-year-old Central American girl who is 4 feet 8 inches tall cannot attain the adult height of a typical North American girl simply by eating better.

FIGURE 17-1 ▶ Growth charts for assessment of children in the growing years. The growth of a youngster is plotted to show how the charts are used in health care settings. (a) Growth charts used to assess length (height) and weight in young girls. A certain length (height) and weight correspond to a percentile value, a ranking of the person among 100 peers. This chart shows that at 36 months of age, the girl was at the 75th percentile for length and the 62nd percentile for weight. (b) Growth charts used to assess weight-for-height relationships in boys ages 2 to 20 years. Today, these charts for older children and adolescents typically use BMI for the evaluation. At 6 years of age the boy was at the 85th percentile for BMI.

Source: Developed by the National Center for Health Statistics in collaboration with the National Center for Disease Prevention and Health Promotion (2000). www.cdc.gov/growthcharts. Revised November 21, 2000.

Girls experience their peak rate of growth right before the onset of the menses. Once the time for growth ceases (in women, this is about 5 years after they start menstruating), a sufficient nutrient intake helps maintain health and weight but cannot make up for lost growth.

Assessment of Infant Growth and Development

percentile Classification of a measurement of a unit into divisions of 100 units.

Health professionals assess a child's increases in height and weight by comparing them with typical growth patterns recorded on charts (review Fig. 17-1). The charts contain **percentile** divisions, which represent the typical measurements for 90% to 96% of children. A percentile represents the rank of the person among 100 peers matched for age and gender. If a young boy, for example, is at the 90th percentile of height-for-age, he is shorter than 10% and taller than 89% of children his age. A child at the 50th percentile is considered average. Fifty children will be taller than this child; 49 will be shorter.

Individual growth charts are available for both males and females from the National Center for Health Statistics (as shown in Fig. 17-1). For ages ranging from birth to 36 months, options for growth charts include weight-for-age, length-for-age, weight-for-length, and head circumference-for-age. For males and females who are 2 to 20 years old, growth charts are available to determine weight-for-age and height-

◄ The new WHO Growth Standards for Children differ from previous standards in part because they reflect data based upon children from around the world who were raised in conditions for optimal growth and development. Go to http://www.who.int/childgrowth/en/ for more information on the WHO Child Growth Standards.

for-age; however, the preferred growth chart for children and adolescents is body mass index (BMI)-for-age. For adults, BMI has fixed cutoff points (for example, a BMI of 25 for an adult is considered overweight). As Figure 17-1 shows, this is not true for children, as BMI is both gender- and age-specific.

In 2006, the World Health Organization released a new set of growth standards for children from birth through five years of age to replace the NCHS charts currently in use. The WHO growth charts provide a way to assess the same parameters listed (e.g., height or length, weight, BMI, and head circumference) but they are based on data collected from children from various regions of the world raised under conditions for optimal growth and development: breastfed as infants, followed recommended infant and child feeding practices set forth by WHO, had adequate health care, and mothers did not use tobacco during or after pregnancy. In contrast, the NCHS growth charts are based on data from primarily Caucasian children mostly bottle-fed during infancy. The new WHO growth standards stress that breastfeeding is the biological norm for infant nutrition. Look for these new growth charts to become more widely available over the next few years.

Infants and children should have their growth assessed during regular health check-ups. It takes 1 to 3 years for the genetic potential (in terms of percentile ranking on growth charts) of infant growth to be established. By 3 years of age, a child's measurements, such as length (height)-for-age, should generally track along the established percentile. If the child's growth doesn't keep up with its length-for-age percentile, the physician needs to investigate whether a medical or nutritional problem is impeding the predicted growth. Inappropriate weight gain—too little or too much—should also be investigated.

Infants born preterm may catch up in growth in 2 to 3 years. This requires that the child move up in the percentiles. If this occurs—especially in length-for-age—it is usually no cause for alarm. On the other hand, moving up in the percentiles for weight-for-height can be disturbing if the child approaches the 80th to 90th percentiles. A child at the 85th percentile or above for BMI is considered at risk for overweight. At or above the 95th percentile, the child is considered overweight. At the 95th percentile, the diagnosis of obesity can also be established if the physical exam of the child indicates he or she is truly overfat. This is generally the case at this percentile.

▶ Children under 2 to 3 years of age are measured lying on their backs with knees unflexed, so the term *length* is used rather than *height*.

▲ Brain growth is faster in infancy than in any other stage of life. Therefore an infant's head needs to be larger in comparison to the body to allow for such growth.

▶ Children older than 2 years are less likely to experience failure to thrive because they can often get food for themselves. Younger children, for the most part, are limited to what caregivers provide.

MAKING DECISIONS

Head Circumference and Brain Development

The brain grows faster in infancy than at any other time of life. To accommodate the growth, an infant's head circumference must be very large in proportion to the rest of the body. The rapid growth stops at about 18 months of age. The rest of the body eventually grows to reach a typical proportion to head size. In early physical checkups, a health professional usually measures the head circumference as another means of assessing growth, especially brain growth. How nutritional status affects brain development and intelligence quotient (IQ) is difficult to measure because scientists have not determined how to separate the effects of nature from those of nurture. However, several studies have determined that breastfed babies have higher IQs than do babies who were fed with infant formula. At the same time, studies from Central America suggest that IQ after age 5 years relates more closely to the amount of schooling a child receives than to nutritional intake during childhood.

Adipose Tissue Growth

Since 1970, researchers have speculated that overfeeding during infancy may increase the numbers of adipose tissue cells. Today, we know that the number of adipose cells can also increase as adulthood obesity develops. Still, if calorie intake is limited during infancy to keep down the number of adipose cells, the growth of other organ systems may also be severely restricted. Special concern revolves around body growth and development, especially brain and nervous system development. In addition, most overweight infants become normal-weight preschoolers without excessive diet restrictions. For these reasons, it's unwise to greatly restrict diet, and especially fat intake in infants. After the first 12 months, fat intake can range from 30% to 40% of calorie intake for ages 1 to 3 years, and 25% to 35% of calorie intake for older children (and teenagers).

Failure to Thrive

Occasionally, an infant doesn't grow much in the first few months. Physical problems that may contribute to restricted growth range from poor oral cavity development, infections, and heart irregularities to constant diarrhea associated with intestinal problems. However, more than half the infants who fail to thrive have no apparent disease. Sometimes the cause is poor infant-parent interaction. This stems from misinformation, lack of a parent role model, too little concern about the child's welfare, or even from exerting too much control over feedings (e.g., maternal anxiety, force feeding). Poverty or food insecurity may also be at the root of infant or child undernutrition. In general, the problems arise from the parents' inexperience, rather than intentional negligence. Consequences of failure to thrive include poor physical growth, impaired mental development, and behavioral problems. When health professionals encounter an infant failing to thrive, the true causes need to be identified and then treated.

CONCEPT CHECK

Growth occurs rapidly during infancy: Birth weight doubles in about 4 to 6 months and triples within the first year. Undernutrition in childhood can irreversibly inhibit growth and maturation, so that an individual never attains his or her full genetic potential for height. Infant and child growth is assessed by tracking body weight, length (height), and head circumference over time. Body mass index (BMI) is generally used to assess weight-for-height after 2 years of age. It is not desirable for infants to become overweight, although no evidence strongly indicates that overweight infants become overweight adults. However, severe calorie restriction is not recommended for infants because it may slow the growth of organ systems. When infants do not grow properly, their failure to thrive may stem from physical disorders or inadequate care, including inappropriate feeding practices.

Infant Nutritional Needs

Infants' nutritional needs vary as they grow, and these differ from adult needs in both amount and proportion. Initially, human milk or infant formula (generally using heat-treated cow's milk as a base) supplies needed nutrients. Solid foods are not needed until around 6 months. Even after solid foods are added, the basis of an infant's diet for the first year is still human milk or infant formula. Because of the critical importance of adequate nutrition in infancy and the difficulties encountered in feeding some infants, there is more discussion in this chapter on this developmental period than on the later periods of childhood.

▲ Formula-fed infants should remain on formula until 1 year of age.

Calories. Calorie needs (based on Estimated Energy Requirements) in infancy are (89 kcal × weight of infant [kilograms]) + 75 from 0 to 3 months. From 4 to 6 months, such needs are (89 kcal × weight of infant [kilograms]) + 44; from 7 to 12 months it is (89 kcal × weight of infant [kilograms]) − 78. Based on body weight comparisons, at 6 months of age, this amounts to about 700 kcal daily and is two to four times more calories per kilogram of body weight than adults need. Infants need an easy way to get this amount of calories. Either human milk or infant formula is ideal for the first few months. Both are high in fat and supply about 640 kcal per quart of fluid (about 670 kcal per liter; Table 17-1). Later, human milk or infant formula, supplemented by solid foods, can provide even more calories and variety as well for the maturing infant.

The infant's high calorie needs are primarily driven by rapid growth and high metabolic rate. The high metabolic rate is caused in part by the ratio of the infant's body surface to its weight. More body surface allows more heat loss from the skin; the body must use extra calories to replace that heat.

Carbohydrate. Carbohydrate needs in infancy are 60 grams per day at 0 to 6 months and 95 grams per day at 7 to 12 months. These needs are based on the typical intakes of human milk by breastfed infants and their eventual use of solid foods. Both carbohydrate goals are satisfied by usual intakes of infants on a proper diet.

TABLE 17-1 Composition of Human and Cow's Milk and Infant Formulas per liter. At 3 Months of Age, Infants Typically Consume 0.75 to 1 liter of Human Milk or Formula per Day.

	Energy (kcal)	Protein (grams)	Fat (grams)	Carbohydrate (grams)	Minerals* (grams)
Milk					
Human milk	670**	11	45	70	2
Cow's milk, whole†	670	36	36	49	7
Cow's milk, fat-free†	360	36	1	51	7
Casein/Whey-Based Formulas					
Similac	680	14	36	71	3
Enfamil	670	15	37	69	3
Good Start	670	16	34	73	3
Soybean Protein-Based Formulas					
ProSobee	670	20	35	67	4
Isomil	680	16	36	68	4
Transition Formulas/Beverages‡					
Similac Toddler's Best	670	25	33	75	3
Enfamil Next Step	670	17	33	74	3
Carnation Follow-Up	670	17	27	88	3

*Calcium, phosphorus, and other minerals.

**Rough estimate; ranges from 650–700 kcal per liter.

†Not appropriate for infant feeding, based primarily on high protein and mineral content.

‡For use after 6 months of age or later (see label).

▶ Looking at Table 17-1 it is easy to see why fat-free milk products are not recommended for infants—these do not supply adequate fat and calories to meet needs. Fat-free milk (and reduced fat and whole milk as well) also would provide too much protein and minerals if it were used to meet calorie needs.

See the "Nutrition and Your Health: Food Allergies and Intolerances" at the end of this chapter.

allergy A hypersensitive immune response that occurs when immune bodies produced by us react with a protein we sense as foreign (an antigen).

Protein. Daily protein needs in infancy are about 9 grams per day for younger infants and about 14 grams per day for older infants. These needs also are based on the typical intakes of human milk by breastfed infants for 0 to 6 months, and then on the needs for growth for older infants. About half of total protein intake should come from essential (indispensable) amino acids. As with carbohydrate, protein needs are easily satisfied by either human milk or infant formula. Protein intake should not greatly exceed this standard. Excess nitrogen and minerals supplied by high-protein diets would exceed the ability of an infant's kidneys to excrete the waste products of protein metabolism, thus putting much stress on overall kidney function.

In North America, infant protein deficiency is unlikely, except in cases of mistakes in formula preparation, such as when an infant's formula is excessively diluted with water. Protein deficiency may also be induced by elimination diets used to detect food **allergies** (hypersensitivities). As foods are eliminated from the diet, infants may not be offered enough protein to compensate for the high-protein sources no longer present (see the "Nutrition and Your Health" section later in this chapter).

Fat. Infants need about 30 grams of fat per day. Essential fatty acids should make up about 15% of total fat intake (about 5 grams per day). Both recommendations are again based on the typical intakes of human milk by breastfed infants and the eventual intake of solid foods. Fats are an important part of the infant's diet because they are vital to the development of the nervous system. As a concentrated source of calories, fat also helps resolve the potential problem of the infant's high calorie needs and small stomach capacity. Again, this is not an age to greatly restrict fat intake (Fig. 17-2).

Arachidonic acid (AA) and docosahexaenoic acid (DHA) are two long-chain fatty acids that have important roles in infant development. The nervous system, especially the brain and eyes, depend on these fatty acids for proper development. During the last trimester, DHA and AA provided by the mother accumulate in the brain and retinas of the eyes in the fetus. Breastfed infants are able to continue to acquire these fatty acids from human milk, especially if their mothers are regularly eating fish. Until recently, no infant formulas sold in the United States included AA or DHA, but many brands are now available with both AA and DHA. These are particularly useful for feeding preterm infants.

Vitamins of Special Interest. As noted in Chapter 10, vitamin K is routinely given by injection to all infants at birth. Formula-fed infants receive the rest of the vitamins they need from the formula. Breastfed infants should be given a vitamin D supplement (200 IU per day) until they are weaned to infant formula and are consuming at least 500 milliliters of it per day. Breast-fed infants whose mothers are total vegetarians (vegans) should also receive vitamin B-12 in supplement form.

Minerals of Special Interest. Infants are born with some internal stores of iron. However, by the time birth weight doubles (4 to 6 months of age), iron stores are generally depleted if not otherwise part of the diet. If the mother was iron deficient during the pregnancy, these iron stores will be exhausted even sooner. As you will recall from Chapter 11, iron-deficiency anemia can lead to poor mental development in infants. Several studies indicate that iron deficiency anemia during infancy, even if corrected, has a lasting impact in terms of impaired cognition, motor development, and behavioral problems later in life. To maintain a desirable iron status, the American Academy of Pediatrics recommends that formula-fed infants should be given an iron-fortified formula from birth. Low-iron infant formulas are sometimes prescribed to treat infants with various GI tract problems but otherwise their use is discouraged. In contrast, breastfed infants at about 6 months of age need solid foods to supply extra iron. This need for iron is a major consideration

RICE

CEREAL FOR BABY

Nutrition Facts

Serving Size 1/4 cup (15g)
Servings Per Container About 15

Amount Per Serving

Calories 60

Total Fat	0.5mg
Trans Fat	0g*
Sodium	10mg
Potassium	20mg
Total Carbohydrate	12g
Dietary Fiber	0g
Sugars	0g
Protein	1g

% Daily Value	Infants 0–1	Children 1–4
Protein	4%	4%
Vitamin A	0%	0%
Vitamin C	0%	0%
Calcium	15%	10%
Iron	45%	45%
Thiamin	45%	30%
Riboflavin	45%	30%
Niacin	25%	20%
Phosphorus	10%	6%

* Intake should be as low as possible.

INGREDIENTS: RICE FLOUR, SOY OIL-LECITHIN, TRI- AND DICALCIUM PHOSPHATE, ELECTROLYTIC IRON, NIACINAMIDE, RIBOFLAVIN (VITAMIN B-2), THIAMIN (VITAMIN B-1).

Serving Size

Serving sizes for infant foods are based on the average amount eaten at one time by a child under 2 years.

Total Fat

Shows the amount of total fat in a serving of the food. Unlike adult food labels, labels on infant foods do not list calories from fat, saturated fat, or cholesterol, since infants and toddlers under 2 years need fat. Parents should not attempt to limit their infant's fat intake.

Daily Values

Food labels for infants and children under 4 years list the Daily Value percentages for protein, vitamins, and minerals. Unlike adult food labels, Daily Values for fat, cholesterol, sodium, potassium, carbohydrate, and fiber are not listed.

FIGURE 17-2 ▶ The labels on infant foods, like those on adult foods, contain a Nutrition Facts panel. However, the information provided on infant food labels differs from that on adult food labels, especially with respect to total fat, saturated fat, and cholesterol content (see Fig. 2-12 for a comparison). Some cereal brands are fortified with various other micronutrients.

in the decision to introduce solid foods. Some physicians recommend liquid iron supplements from birth or by 1 month of age for breastfed infants, especially if the infant shows evidence of iron deficiency.

To aid in tooth development, fluoride supplements are recommended for breastfed infants after 6 months of age. The same holds true for formula-fed infants if the water supply used in home formula preparation—either tap or bottled water—does not contain fluoride. Formula manufacturers use fluoride-free water in formula preparation. Parents should consult their dentist for advice on meeting their infant's fluoride needs. The American Dental Association does not recommend fluoridated bottled water for use by infants because it creates a risk for enamel fluorosis in teeth during their development before eruption through the gums.

Infants also need adequate amounts of zinc and iodide to support growth. However, when human milk and infant formula are provided in quantities to meet calorie needs, sufficient zinc and iodide are generally supplied.

▲ Supplemental fluids should be limited to 4 ounces per day unless the infant's physician prescribes a larger amount.

▶ Parents should consult a physician when choosing an appropriate infant formula. Not all formula-like products are designed for infant use. A 5-month-old girl was admitted to a hospital in Arkansas with symptoms of heart failure, rickets, inflamed blood vessels, and possible nerve damage after being fed Soy Moo (a soy beverage sold in health stores) since 3 days of age. The symptoms suggest severe vitamin deficiencies.

Water. An infant needs about 3 cups (700 to 800 milliliters) of water per day. Infants typically consume enough human milk or formula to supply this amount. In hot climates, however, supplemental water may be necessary. Furthermore, any conditions that lead to water loss—diarrhea, vomiting, fever, or too much sun—can call for supplemental water.

Infants are easily dehydrated, a condition that has serious effects if not remedied. Dehydration can result in rapid loss of kidney function, and the infant may then require hospitalization for rehydration. Special fluid-replacement formulas containing electrolytes such as sodium and potassium are available in supermarkets and pharmacies to treat dehydration. A physician should guide any use of these products.

MAKING DECISIONS

Extra Fluid for Infants

In some stores, bottled water products marketed specifically for infants may be placed alongside infant formulas and electrolyte-replacement solutions. This placement may give parents and caregivers the mistaken impression that bottled water products are an appropriate feeding supplement or substitute for fluid replacement for infants; they are not and should not be used for such purposes. It is important to remember that excessive fluid can also be harmful, especially to the brain.

Overall, it is best to limit supplemental fluids to about 4 ounces (120 milliliters) per day, unless the physician thinks that a greater need exists because of disease or other conditions. In sum, extremes in fluid intake—either too little or too much—can lead to health problems.

CONCEPT CHECK

Most nutrient needs in the first 6 months are met by human milk or infant formula. Breastfed infants need a vitamin D supplement and possibly an iron supplement; formula-fed infants and breastfed infants may need fluoride supplements after 6 months of age. Infants usually receive enough water from the human milk or infant formula they drink.

Formula Feeding for Infants

Breastfeeding was covered in detail in Chapter 16. Let's now focus on formula feeding. You'll recall that a major advantage of breastfeeding is the provision of immune protection to the infant. Overall, in areas of the world where high standards for water purity and cleanliness are common, formula feeding is a safe alternative for infants (but generally is not as beneficial as breastfeeding).

Formula Composition. Infants cannot tolerate cow's milk as such because of its high protein and mineral content. Cow's milk is perfect for the greater growth needs of calves, but not for human infants. Thus, cow's milk must be altered by formula manufacturers to be safe for infant feeding. Altered forms of cow's milk, known as infant formulas, must conform to strict federal guidelines for nutrient composition and quality. Formulas generally contain lactose and/or sucrose for carbohydrate, heat-treated proteins from cow's milk, and vegetable oils for fat (review Table 17-1). Soy protein–based formulas are available for infants who can't tolerate lactose or the types of proteins found in cow's milk. If the soybean-based formula is not tolerated, the next step is to try a predigested formula in which the proteins have been broken down into small polypeptides and amino acids. A variety of other specialized formulas also are available for specific medical conditions. In any case, it is important to use an iron-fortified formula unless a physician recommends otherwise.

Some transition formulas/beverages have been introduced for older infants and toddlers (review Table 17-1). Some of these products are intended for use after 6 months of age if the infant is consuming solid foods, whereas others are intended for use only by toddlers. These transition products are lower in fat than human milk or standard infant formulas; their iron content is higher than that of cow's milk, and their overall mineral content is generally more like that of human milk than cow's milk. According to the manufacturers, the advantages of these transition formulas/beverages over standard formulas for older infants and toddlers include reduced cost and better flavor. Parents should consult their physician with regard to the use of these products.

Formula Preparation. Some infant formulas come in ready-to-feed form. These are poured into a clean bottle and fed immediately. Room-temperature formula is acceptable for many infants. Otherwise, to warm a bottle of formula, a caregiver can run hot water over it or place it briefly in a pan of simmering water. Infant formulas should not be heated in a microwave oven because hot spots may develop, which can burn the infant's mouth and esophagus.

Powdered and concentrated fluid formula preparations are also commonly used. All utensils used in preparing formula from these preparations should be washed and thoroughly rinsed. Powdered or concentrated formulas are poured into a bottle, to which clean, cold water is added (following label directions) and then mixed. The formula is then warmed, if desired, and fed immediately to the infant. Hot water from the faucet should not be used to make formula, since it poses a risk for high lead content (see Chapter 15). Cold water poses much less risk.

Refrigerating prepared formula for 1 day is safe. However, formula left over from a feeding should be discarded because it will be contaminated by bacteria and enzymes from the infant's saliva. If well water is used, it should be boiled before making formula for at least the infant's first 3 months of life, and it should be analyzed for excessive concentration of naturally occurring nitrates, which can lead to a severe form of anemia. If nitrates are high in municipal water systems, consumers will be warned (such as in a local newspaper) not to use the water for making infant formula until the concentration falls to a safe amount. The American Dental Association does not recommend that formula be mixed with bottled nursery water, available alongside infant formula in most supermarkets, for risk of eventual tooth discoloration from high fluoride levels.

Feeding Technique

Infants swallow a lot of air as they ingest either formula or human milk, so it's important to burp an infant after either 10 minutes of feeding or 1 to 2 ounces (30 to 60 milliliters) has been consumed from a bottle and again at the end of feeding. Spitting up a bit of milk is normal at this time.

When the infant begins acting full, bottle feeding should be stopped, even if some milk is left in the bottle. Common cues that signal that an infant has had enough include turning the head away, being inattentive, falling asleep, and becoming playful. Generally, the infant's appetite is a better guide than standardized recommendations concerning feeding amounts. Breastfeeding infants usually have had enough to eat after about 20 minutes. Although it's difficult

▲ Careful attention during feeding allows the caregiver to notice the infant's signal as to when the feeding should cease.

▲ The Back to Sleep campaign advises that infants be placed on their backs for sleeping.

to tell how much milk breastfed infants are getting, they also give signs when full. By carefully observing bottle-feeding or breastfeeding infants and responding to their cues appropriately, caregivers not only can be assured that the infants' calorie needs are being met but also can foster a climate of trust and responsiveness.

Once fed, an infant should not be placed on its stomach. Placing the infant on its back is recommended by the American Academy of Pediatrics. The reason that an infant should not be placed on its stomach is because this sleeping position has been linked to sudden infant death syndrome (SIDS). The Back to Sleep campaign, started in 1994 in the United States, has reduced SIDS by 40%.

The Back to Sleep campaign, however, has led to a problem known as flattened head syndrome (clinically known as positional plagiocephaly). Infant skulls are soft and therefore can change in shape. Flattened head syndrome can occur if an excessive amount of an infant's day is spent on his or her back or against a highchair/car seat. In response to this concern, the American Academy of Pediatrics has recommended periodic repositioning of an infant's head while asleep and allowing for time on his or her stomach while awake. In addition, some infants may need to wear specially fitted helmets to correct the shape of their head.

Expanding the Infant's Mealtime Choices

By about 6 months of age, the infant is ready to start eating "table food." Initially, table foods add to—rather than replace—formula or human milk. In the first attempts to introduce solid foods, just getting the food into the infant's mouth may prove to be a challenge. By the end of the first year, though, the infant should be eating a variety of meats, vegetables, fruits, and grains so that the diet begins to resemble a balanced pattern, setting the stage for lifelong preferences and dietary habits (Table 17-2). Throughout the process of expanding the infant's mealtime choices, it is essential to allow the infant to control the situation—the caregiver must proceed slowly and respond to the infant's cues that he or she is hungry or has had enough to eat.

TABLE 17-2 Sample Daily Menu for a 1-Year-Old Child*

Breakfast 1 to 2 tbsp applesauce ¼ cup Cheerios ½ cup whole milk	**Snack** ½ ounce cheddar cheese 4 wheat crackers ½ cup whole milk
Snack ½ hard-cooked egg ½ slice wheat toast with ½ tsp margarine ½ cup orange juice	**Dinner** 1 ounce hamburger (crumbled) 1 to 2 tbsp mashed potatoes with ½ tsp margarine 1 to 2 tbsp cooked carrots (cut in strips, not coins) ½ cup whole milk
Lunch 1 ounce roasted chicken, minced 1 to 2 tbsp rice with ½ tsp margarine 1 to 2 tbsp cooked peas ½ cup whole milk	**Snack** ½ banana 2 oatmeal cookies (no raisins) ½ cup whole milk

Nutritional Analysis	
Total energy (kcal)	1100
% energy from	
Carbohydrate	40%
Protein	19%
Fat	41%

*This diet is just a start. A 1-year-old may need more or less food. In those cases, serving sizes should be adjusted. The milk can be fed by cup; some can be put into a bottle if the child has not been fully weaned from the bottle. The juice should be fed in a cup.

Recognizing the Infant's Readiness for Solid Foods. How does the caregiver know it is time to introduce solid foods? Infant size can serve as a rough indicator of readiness—reaching a weight of at least 13 pounds (6 kilograms) is a preliminary sign of readiness for solid foods. Another physiological cue is frequency of feeding, such as consuming more than 32 ounces (1 liter) of formula daily or breastfeeding more than 8 to 10 times within 24 hours. Underlying these noticeable signals are several important developmental factors:

1. *Nutritional need.* Before the infant is 6 months old, nutritional needs can generally be met with human milk and/or formula. After 6 months of age, however, many infants need the additional calories supplied by solid foods. In terms of individual nutrients, iron stores are exhausted by about 6 months of age. Either solid foods or iron supplements are then needed to supply iron if the child is breastfed or fed a low-iron or iron-free formula. (As previously mentioned, a vitamin D supplement should also be given to breastfed infants.)
2. *Physiological capabilities.* As the infant ages, the ability to digest and metabolize a wider range of food components improves. Before about 3 months of age, an infant's digestive tract cannot readily digest starch. Also, kidney function is limited until about 4 to 6 weeks of age. Until then, waste products from excessive amounts of dietary protein or minerals are difficult to excrete.
3. *Physical ability.* Three physical markers indicate that a child is ready for solid foods: (1) the disappearance of the extrusion reflex (thrusting the tongue forward and pushing food out of the mouth), (2) head and neck control, and (3) the ability to sit up with support. These usually occur around 4 to 6 months of age, but they vary with each infant.
4. *Allergy prevention.* An infant's intestinal tract is "leaky"—whole proteins can readily be absorbed from birth until 4 to 5 months of age. If the infant is exposed too early to some types of proteins—particularly those in cow's milk and egg whites—the infant may be predisposed to future allergies and other health problems, such as diabetes. For this reason, it is best to minimize the number of different types of proteins in an infant's diet, especially during the first 3 months (see the "Nutrition and Your Health" section on food allergies at the end of this chapter for details).

With these considerations in mind—nutritional need, physiological and physical readiness, and allergy prevention—the American Academy of Pediatrics recommends that solid foods not be introduced until about 6 months of age and that infants receive no unaltered cow's milk before 1 year.

▲ In the early stages of solid food introduction, these foods complement rather than replace human milk or infant formula in the diet.

 See the "Nutrition and Your Health: Food Allergies and Intolerances" at the end of this chapter.

MAKING DECISIONS

Introducing Solid Foods

Parents may believe that the early addition of solid foods will help an infant sleep through the night. Actually, this achievement is a developmental milestone, and the amount of food consumed by the infant is of little relevance to the achievement of a good night's sleep. Before 4 to 6 months of age, infants are not physically mature enough to consume much solid food. Only occasionally does a rapidly growing infant need solid foods to meet calorie and nutrient needs before 6 months of age.

Foods to Match Needs and Developmental Abilities During the First Year. If solid foods are introduced before 6 months of age, the primary goal of the food should be to meet iron needs. Therefore, the first solid foods should be iron-fortified cereals. Some pediatricians may recommend lean ground (strained) meats for more absorbable forms of iron. Rice is the best cereal to begin with because it is least likely to cause allergies.

▶ **Typical Solid Food Progression, Starting at 6 Months***

Week 1	Rice cereal
Week 2	Add strained carrots
Week 3	Add applesauce
Week 4	Add oat cereal
Week 5	Add cooked egg yolk
Week 6	Add strained chicken
Week 7	Add strained peas
Week 8	Add plums

*Extending the rice cereal step for a month or so is advised if solid food introduction begins at 4 months of age. Also, if at any point signs of allergy or intolerance develop, substitute another similar food item.

When starting solid foods, it is important to start with a teaspoon serving size of a single-ingredient food item, such as rice cereal, and increase the serving size gradually. Once the new food has been fed for about a week without ill effects, another food can be added to the infant's diet. At first, this can be another type of cereal or perhaps a cooked and strained (or mashed) vegetable, meat, fruit, or egg yolk.

Waiting about 7 days between the introduction of each new food is important because it can take that long for evidence of an allergy or intolerance to develop. Allergy symptoms to look for include diarrhea, vomiting, a rash, or wheezing. If one or more of these symptoms appear, the suspected problem food should be avoided for several weeks and then reintroduced in a small quantity. If the problem continues, a physician should be consulted.

Some foods that commonly cause an allergic response in infants are egg whites, chocolate, nuts, and cow's milk. It is best not to introduce these foods during infancy. Also, it is important to avoid introducing mixed foods until each component of the combination dish has been given separately. Otherwise, if an allergy or intolerance develops, it will be difficult to identify the offending food. Many babies outgrow food allergies during childhood.

Many strained foods for infant feeding are available at the supermarket. Single food items are more desirable than mixed dinners and desserts, which are less nutrient-dense. Most brands have no added salt, but some fruit desserts contain a lot of added sugar.

As an alternative, plain, unseasoned cooked foods—vegetables, fruits, and meats—can be ground up in an inexpensive plastic baby food grinder/mill. Another option is to puree a larger amount of food in a blender, freeze it in ice-cube portions, store in plastic bags, and defrost and warm as needed. Careful attention to cleanliness is necessary. Seasonings that may please the rest of the family should not be added to infant foods made at home. The infant doesn't notice the difference if salt, sugar, or spices are omitted. It is best to introduce infants to a variety of foods, so that at the end of the first year, the infant is consuming many foods—milk, meats, fruits, vegetables, and grains.

▲ Rice cereal is recommended as the first solid food to be fed to infants.

Self-feeding skills require coordination and can develop only if the infant is allowed to practice and experiment. By 6 to 7 months of age, the infant has learned to handle finger foods and transfer objects from one hand to the other with some dexterity. At about this time, teeth also begin to appear. Dry toast, sliced in strips, offers hours of enjoyment. By age 7 to 8 months, infants can push food around on a plate, play with a drinking cup, hold a bottle, and self-feed a cracker or a piece of toast. Through mastery of these manipulations, infants develop confidence and self-esteem. It is important that parents be patient and support these early feeding attempts, even though they appear inefficient.

At 9 to 10 months of age, the infant's desire to explore, experience, and play with foods may hinder feeding. Food is used as a means to explore the environment, and therefore feeding time is often very messy—a bowl of macaroni may end up in the child's hair. Presenting a new food on several consecutive days can aid in an infant's acceptance of that food. Caregivers need to relax and take this phase of infant development in stride. Sloppy, friendly mealtimes make for good memories. By the end of the first year, finger-feeding becomes more efficient and chewing is easier as more teeth erupt. Still, experimentation and unpredictability are to be expected.

To ease the efforts in feeding solid foods, consider the following tips:

- Use a baby-sized spoon; a small spoon with a long handle is best.
- Hold the infant comfortably on the lap, as for breastfeeding or bottle feeding, but a little more upright to ease swallowing. When in this position, the infant expects food.

- Put a small dab of food on the spoon tip and gently place it on the infant's tongue.
- Convey a calm and casual approach to the infant, who needs time to get used to food.
- Expect the infant to take only two or three bites of the first meals.

Weaning from the Breast or Bottle

Around the age of 6 months, juices can be offered in a sippy cup with a wide, flat bottom. Drinking from a cup rather than from a bottle helps prevent **early childhood caries.** If an infant drinks continuously from a bottle, the carbohydrate-rich fluid bathes the teeth, providing an ideal growth medium for bacteria adhering to the teeth. These bacteria then make acids, which dissolve tooth enamel. To avoid dental caries, infants should not be put to bed with a bottle or placed in an infant seat with a bottle propped up.

By about 10 months of age, infants are learning to self-feed and likewise to drink independently from a cup. As children drink from a cup more frequently, fewer bottle feedings and/or breastfeedings are necessary. The added mobility of crawling and walking should naturally lead to gradual weaning from the bottle or breast. Even so, getting a baby out of the bedtime-bottle habit can be difficult. Determined caregivers can either wince through a few nights of their baby's crying or slowly wean the baby away from the bottle with either a pacifier or water (for a week or so).

Dietary Guidelines for Infant Feeding

It can be difficult for new parents to make sense of nutrition goals for infants in the face of changing dietary recommendations from health authorities, cultural preferences, and outdated advice from friends and family. In response to various controversies surrounding infant feeding, the American Academy of Pediatrics has issued a number of statements concerning infant diets. The following guidelines are based on these statements:

- *Build to a variety of foods.* For the first months of life, human milk (or infant formula) is all an infant needs. (Vitamin D needs of breastfed infants is an exception.) When the infant is ready, start adding new foods, one at a time. During the first year, the goal is to teach an infant to enjoy a variety of nutritious foods. A lifetime of healthy eating habits begins with this important first step.
- *Pay attention to your infant's appetite to avoid overfeeding or underfeeding.* Feed infants when they are hungry. Never force an infant to finish an unwanted serving of food. Watch for signs that indicate hunger or fullness. This will reinforce the infant's natural capability to self-regulate food intake.
- *Infants need fat.* Although fat contributes to many adult health problems, it's an essential source of calories for growing infants. Fat also helps the nervous system develop.
- *Choose fruits, vegetables, and grains, but don't overdo high-fiber foods.* During the second half of the first year, infants are fed a variety of fruits and vegetables. However, studies show that by 1 year of age, vegetable consumption is dominated by white potatoes. Continuing to offer choices of green and yellow vegetables during infancy and the toddler years will enhance intake of important vitamins, minerals, and phytochemicals. In terms of fiber, although many adults benefit from high-fiber diets, they are not good for infants. They are bulky, filling, and often low in calories. The natural amounts of fiber and nutrients in fruits, vegetables, and grains are appropriate as part of a healthy infant diet.
- *Infants need sugars in moderation.* Sugars are an additional source of calories for active, rapidly growing infants. Foods such as human milk, fruits, and 100% juices are natural sources of sugars and other nutrients as well. Foods that contain artificial sweeteners should be avoided; they don't provide the calories growing infants

early childhood caries Tooth decay that results from formula or juice (and even human milk) bathing the teeth as the child sleeps with a bottle in his or her mouth. The upper teeth are mostly affected as the lower teeth are protected by the tongue; formerly called *nursing bottle syndrome* and *baby bottle tooth decay.*

▲ Early childhood caries. An extreme example of tooth decay probably resulting from frequently putting the child to bed with a bottle. The upper teeth have decayed almost all the way to the gum line.

▲ Early feeding attempts should be encouraged, even though they're messy.

▶ Egg whites also should not be fed to children before 1 year of age to help prevent the development of allergies.

▶ **A Summary of Infant Feeding Recommendations**

Breastfed Infants

- Breastfeed for 6 months or longer, if possible. Then introduce infant formula if and when breastfeeding declines or ceases. (Breast milk can also be pumped and placed in a bottle for later use.)
- Provide a vitamin D supplement (200 IU per day).
- Investigate the need for vitamin B-12, fluoride, and iron supplementation to prevent deficiencies.

Formula-Fed Infants

- Use infant formula for the first year of life, preferably an iron-fortified type.
- Investigate the need for a fluoride supplement if the water supply is not fluoridated.

All Infants

- Add iron-fortified cereal at about 6 months of age.
- Provide a variety of basic, soft foods after 6 months of age, advancing to a varied diet.

need. On the other hand, excessive intake of sugars, particularly from fruit-flavored drinks and soft drinks, contribute to the epidemic of childhood obesity.

- *Infants need sodium in moderation.* Sodium is a necessary mineral found naturally in almost all foods. As part of a healthy diet, infants need sodium for their bodies to work properly. However, average intakes of sodium among infants and toddlers are above the AI. Caregivers should delay introduction of cow's milk (a source of sodium for infants) until 1 year of age and refrain from offering heavily-seasoned and processed foods.
- *Choose foods containing iron, zinc, and calcium.* Infants need good sources of iron, zinc, and calcium for optimum growth in the first 2 years. These minerals are important for healthy blood, optimal growth, and strong bones. Many infant and toddler foods (e.g., cereal, crackers, and biter biscuits) are fortified with these minerals.

In essence, there is no evidence that restrictive diets during infancy have positive effects, whereas their hazards are well documented.

What Not to Feed an Infant

Following are several foods and practices to avoid when feeding an infant:

- *Honey.* This product may contain spores of *Clostridium botulinum*. The spores can eventually develop into bacteria in the stomach and lead to a foodborne illness known as *botulism*. This can be fatal, especially in children under 1 year old (see Chapter 15).
- *Excessive infant formula or human milk.* After 6 to 8 months, solid foods should play a greater role in satisfying an infant's increasing appetite. The main reason to switch is that solid foods contain considerably more bioavailable iron than do human milk and low-iron formulas. About 24 to 32 ounces (¾ to 1 liters) of human milk or formula daily is ideal after 6 months, with food supplying the rest of the infant's calorie needs.
- *Foods that tend to cause choking.* These foods include hot dogs (unless finely cut into sticks, not coin shapes), candy, whole nuts, grapes, coarsely cut meats, raw carrots, popcorn, and peanut butter. Caregivers should not allow younger children to gobble snack foods during playtime and should supervise all meals.
- *Cow's milk, especially low-fat or fat-free cow's milk.* The American Academy of Pediatrics strongly urges parents not to give children under age 2 fat-reduced, 1%, or fat-free milk. Before age 2, the amount of this milk needed for calorie needs would supply too many minerals and in turn could overwhelm the kidneys' ability to excrete the excess. The lower fat intake might also harm nervous system development. Beyond 2 years, children can drink fat-reduced, 1%, or fat-free milk, because by this age they are consuming enough solid foods to supply calorie and fat needs.
- *Feeding excessive amounts of apple or pear juice.* The fructose and sorbitol contained in these juices can lead to diarrhea because they are slowly absorbed. Also, if fruit juice or related drink products are replacing formula or milk in the diet, the infant may not be receiving adequate amounts of calcium and other minerals essential for bone growth. Studies have shown a link between excessive amounts of fruit juice and failure to thrive, GI tract complications, obesity, short stature, and poor dental health. Thus, these substances should be used sparingly. Infants over the age of 6 months can usually safely consume up to 6 ounces of juice in the course of a day, with no more than 2 to 4 ounces at a time.

Inappropriate Infant Feeding Practices

Parents and other caregivers should be aware of a variety of potential health problems related to infant nutrition, so that corrective action can be taken quickly. In some cases, such problems stem from inappropriate feeding practices and inadequate nutrient intakes, including the following:

- Diet providing insufficient iron
- Absence from the diet of an entire food group in MyPyramid as solid foods are introduced and become the main source of nutrients
- Use of cow's milk
- Premature introduction of potential allergy-causing foods, such as egg whites and nuts
- Drinking raw (unpasteurized) milk, which may be contaminated with bacteria or viruses
- Drinking goat's milk, low in folate, iron, vitamin C, and vitamin D
- Failure to begin drinking from a cup by 1 year of age
- Continuing to feed from a bottle past 18 months of age
- Intake of supplemental vitamins or minerals above 100% of the appropriate RDA or other nutrient standard
- Drinking large amounts of fruit juice after 6 months of age, especially as a substitute for infant formula or human milk. (Recall that fruit juice is not to be fed at all before 6 months of age.)

The website of the American Academy of Pediatrics (www.aap.org) can also provide useful information on these and other nutrition-related problems in infancy.

CONCEPT CHECK

Infant formulas generally contain lactose or sucrose, heat-treated proteins from cow's milk, and vegetable oil. Formulas may or may not be fortified with iron. Sanitation is important in preparing and storing formula. Solid foods should not be added to an infant's diet until the child is both ready for and needs solid food, usually at about 6 months of age. The first solid foods can be iron-fortified infant cereals, with gradual additions of other foods—one at a time each week. Some foods to avoid giving to infants in the first year are honey, cow's milk (particularly fat-reduced, 1%, or fat-free milk), foods that may cause the child to choke, and excessive amounts of fruit juice or related products (e.g., fruit drinks).

PRESCHOOL CHILDREN: NUTRITION CONCERNS

The rapid growth rate that characterizes infancy tapers off quickly during the subsequent few years. The average annual weight gain is only 4.5 to 6.6 pounds (2 to 3 kilograms), and the average annual height gain is only 3 to 4 inches (7.5 to 10 centimeters) between the ages of 2 and 5. As a toddler's growth rate tapers off, eating behavior changes. For example, the decreased growth rate leads to a decreased appetite, often called "picky eating," compared with infants.

Because of the reduced appetite of preschool children, planning a diet that meets their nutrient needs poses a challenge to caregivers. Choosing nutrient-dense foods is particularly important with children who eat relatively little. This is a good time to emphasize some whole grains, fruits, and vegetables without increasing fat and simple sugar intake. A whole-grain ready-to-eat breakfast cereal with limited fat and sugar is an excellent choice. There is no need to decrease fat or simple sugar intake severely, but fatty and sweet food choices should not overwhelm more nutritious ones.

Excessive sodium intake is a concern for preschool children as well. Caregivers can lower sodium intake by limiting salt added during cooking and at the table; cutting back on use of processed foods (e.g., luncheon meats, hot dogs); rinsing canned beans and vegetables before cooking; and encouraging consumption of fruits, vegetables, and whole grains in place of prepackaged snacks. The preschool years are the best time for a child to start a healthful pattern of living and eating, focusing on regular physical activity and nutritious foods. Parents and other caregivers are role models: If they eat a variety of foods, the children will eat a variety of foods. One possible policy is the one-bite rule: Within reason, children should take at least one bite or taste of

▲ The older infant enjoys finger-feeding.

CRITICAL THINKING

Tatiana has been breastfeeding her baby exclusively since he was born 7 months ago. When she and her husband took the baby for his checkup, they were told that he was anemic. They were surprised, because they thought that human milk contained all the nutrients the baby needed for the first year of life. How might you explain the baby's anemia?

▶ Carbohydrate requirements to supply energy for the central nervous system and prevent ketosis in childhood are 130 grams per day, the same as for adults. Protein requirements to allow for growth vary from 13 to 19 grams per day for children 1 to 3 years to 34 to 52 grams per day for older children. No specific needs for total fat intake have been set, but the diet must contain at least 5 grams per day of essential fatty acids (see the inside cover for details). The general recommendation is that total fat intake gradually fall so as to eventually fit into the recommended adult range of 20% to 35% of total calorie intake by 19 years of age.

▲ Interest in food starts early in life.

the foods presented to them. For snacks, parents should select several possibilities of acceptable choices and allow children to choose one; responsibility for food choice by the child ideally should start early.

How to Help a Child Choose Nutritious Foods

One way adults can encourage young children to eat nutritious, well-balanced meals is to serve new foods and repeat exposure to them. The dinner hour is a good time for children to experience new foods and to develop food preferences. Preschool children especially tend to be wary of new foods. One reason is that they have more taste buds, and their taste buds are more sensitive than those of adults. In addition, they have a general distrust of unfamiliar foods. If adults can be patient and persevere, children will build good food habits. It may take 8 to 10 exposures to a new food before a child finds it acceptable. Above all, the dinner table should not become a battleground, and using one food as a bribe to eat another—for example, a piece of pie for peas—is strongly discouraged.

Certain food characteristics, such as crisp textures and mild flavors, are appealing to children. Familiarity also plays an important role in food acceptance. In contrast, young children are especially wary of hot-temperature foods and tend to reject them.

Preschoolers eventually develop skill with spoons and forks and can even use dull knives. However, it's still a good idea to serve some finger foods. A goal should be to make mealtime a happy, social time to share and enjoy healthful foods.

Childhood Feeding Problems

Tensions between parents, or between parents and children, especially during mealtime, often contribute to eating problems. Getting to the root of family problems and creating a more harmonious family atmosphere are important steps toward resolving many childhood feeding problems. In addition, many parents must be educated as to what to expect of a preschool child and what food-related goals to set. Let's consider some typical complaints and concerns of parents, the causes of the problems, and suggestions for correcting them.

▶ Two-year-olds commonly prefer particular foods, but parents needn't worry about this. A child may switch from one specific food focus (often called a *jag*) to another with equal intensity (older infants may also act this way). If the caregiver continues to offer choices, the child will soon begin to eat a wider variety of foods again, and the specific food focus will disappear as suddenly as it appeared.

"My Child Won't Eat as Much or as Regularly as He Did as an Infant." This behavior is typical of preschoolers, because their growth rate slows after infancy; thus, they don't need as much food. Parents often need reminding that a 3-year-old can't be expected to eat as voraciously as an infant or to eat adult-size portions. Table 17-3 shows a general food plan, based on MyPyramid, appropriate for preschool and school-age children. Until about 5 years of age, portion sizes in the vegetables group, fruits group, and meat & beans group should be about 1 tablespoon per year of life, and can be increased as needed. The same advice does not apply to the grains or milk groups, but consuming too much milk can leave the diet short on iron. Luckily, normal-weight children have a built-in feeding mechanism, which adjusts hunger to regulate food intake at each stage of growth. If a child is developing and growing normally and the caregiver is providing a variety of healthful foods, all can be confident of the child's well-being.

A pattern of picky eating is usually just another expression of independence for children, who have a strong desire to establish a self-determined routine. Caregivers should avoid nagging, forcing, and bribing children to encourage eating. Indirectly, these tactics reinforce picky-eating behaviors due to the added attention given to them. Overall, parents should focus on offering a variety of healthy choices, allowing the child to exert some autonomy over the specific type of food and the amount eaten. A child's sudden loss of appetite, however, may be reason for concern, as a poor appetite may be a sign of underlying illness.

TABLE 17-3 Food Plans for Preschool and School-Age Children Based on MyPyramid

Food Group	Serving Size	Age 2[2]	Age 5[3]	Age 8[3]	Age 12[3, 4]
			Approximate Number of Servings[1]		
Grains	ounce	3	5	5	6–7
Vegetables	cup	1	1.5	2	2.5–3
Fruits	cup	1	1.5	1.5	2
Milk	cup	2	2	3	3
Meat & Beans	ounce	2	4	5	5.5–6
Oils	teaspoon	3	4	5	6
Discretionary calories	kcal	up to 165	up to 170	up to 130	up to 265–290

[1]Log on to www.mypyramid.gov for other ages and other physical activity levels.
[2]Based on less than 30 minutes of physical activity.
[3]Based on 30–60 minutes of physical activity.
[4]The lower amounts refer to girls.

Parents should also be reminded that food likes and dislikes change rapidly in childhood and are influenced by food temperature, appearance, texture, and taste. Sometimes children object to having foods mixed, as in stews and casseroles, even if they normally like the ingredients separately.

In addition, parents should recognize that this is an important age for children to explore the world around them. Even good eaters are sometimes more interested in exploring than eating. There's room for occasional indulgences, a skipped meal or two, or once in a while "less than ideal" choices. It's eating and lifestyle habits over the course of a month (and lifetime) that matter. Children master their eating when adults set a good example, provide opportunities to learn, give support for exploration, and limit inappropriate behavior.

"My Child Is Always Snacking, Yet She Never Finishes Her Meal." Children have small stomachs. Offering them six or so small meals succeeds better than limiting them to three meals each day. Sticking to three meals a day offers no special nutritional advantages; it's just a social custom. Snacking is fine, as long as good dental habits are practiced. When we eat isn't nearly as important as what we eat. If nutritious snacks are readily available, these are good to offer at midmorning or midafternoon when the child becomes hungry. Fruits and vegetables (fresh, frozen, or juice) and whole-grain breads and crackers are good snack choices. It is important that these snack choices be planned ahead in order to have healthy choices available. Working parents should make sure their children are provided with nutritious snacks to tide them over until dinnertime.

When a child refuses to eat, it's best not to overreact. Doing so may give the child the idea that not eating is a means of getting attention or manipulating a scene. Most children don't starve themselves to any point approaching physical harm. When children refuse to eat, have them sit at the table for a while; if they still aren't interested in eating, remove the food and wait until the next scheduled meal or snack.

"My Child Never Eats Vegetables." Children generally eat enough fruit but not an adequate amount of vegetables. Everyone dislikes certain foods. Again, the one-bite policy can be used, including vegetable servings. It takes time for a child to become enthusiastic about a new food; however, with continual exposure and a positive role model, chances are the child may even grow to like it.

▶ Choking is a very preventable hazard for young children. Some suggestions for caregivers include:

- Set a good example at the table by taking small bites and chewing foods thoroughly.
- Have children sit at the table, take their time, and focus on the food during meals and snacks.
- Avoid giving children any foods that are round, firm, sticky, or cut into large chunks. Some examples of foods to avoid are nuts, grapes, raisins, popcorn, peanut butter, and hard pieces of raw fruits or vegetables.

Children cannot and should not be forced to eat. They need to develop independence and identities separate from their parents. As stated earlier, children have to choose for themselves—a practice that should be encouraged. No one food is an essential part of a diet. Hunger is still the best means for getting a child to eat. It may be effective to feed children vegetables at the start of a meal, when they are hungriest. Offer new foods with familiar ones. A platter of raw or lightly cooked carrots, broccoli, green and red peppers, cabbage, and mushrooms eaten as a snack with friends may be accepted. A 4- or 5-year-old child can safely eat raw vegetables without fear of choking. Recall that children often are more sensitive than adults to strong flavors and odors. Nutritious dips, such as Ranch dressing, "sell" vegetables to many children. Vegetables may acquire more appeal when children help prepare them. And, as with any food, it is important to remember that children are entitled to their own likes and dislikes, too.

Do Children Need a Multivitamin and Mineral Supplement?

Major scientific groups, such as the American Dietetic Association and the American Society for Clinical Nutrition, believe that multivitamin and mineral supplements are generally unnecessary for healthy children; it's better to emphasize good foods. In fact, consuming fortified foods as well as supplements may lead to intakes above the UL for some nutrients, such as vitamin A and zinc. Fortified ready-to-eat breakfast cereals with milk are especially helpful in closing any gap between current micronutrient intake and needs, such as for vitamin E, folate, and vitamin D. Two micronutrients of particular concern are iron and zinc. These may be lacking in children's diets because they consume such small portions of rich sources, such as animal protein foods. In addition, since the 2005 Dietary Guidelines for Americans suggest that children over age 2 years follow a diet low in saturated fat and cholesterol, rich sources of iron and zinc may be lacking in their diets. To compensate, parents can search for a whole-grain breakfast cereal that the child likes that also has about 50% of the Daily Value for iron and 25% of the Daily Value for zinc. (This will supply sufficient amounts of both nutrients because the Daily Values are based on the higher needs of adults.) If that's not possible, especially for a child who is ill, has a very erratic food preference pattern or appetite, or is on a weight-loss diet, the American Academy of Pediatrics states that the child may benefit from a children's multivitamin and mineral supplement not exceeding 100% of Daily Values on the label, especially if these conditions persist. Still, as mentioned many times in this textbook, such a practice does not substitute for an otherwise healthy diet—children included.

If current childhood feeding practices are to become more healthful, the focus should be on whole-grain breads and cereals, fruits, vegetables, and low-fat milk and milk products. Children do not need to be severely restricted but, rather, should modify food habits with small changes. Some easy diet changes to begin with are bagels instead of doughnuts, fat-free frozen yogurt instead of ice cream, fat-reduced or 1% milk instead of whole milk, fruit instead of crackers and cheese for snacks, and air-popped popcorn instead of chips.

Nutritional Problems in Preschool Children

Three nutrition-related problems found in preschool children are iron-deficiency anemia, constipation, and dental caries. Proper diet can help correct or relieve these conditions. Vegetarian diets can also pose problems.

Iron-Deficiency Anemia. The best way to prevent iron-deficiency anemia in children is to provide foods that are adequate sources of iron. Iron-fortified breakfast cereals and a few ounces of lean meat are convenient means of increasing iron in

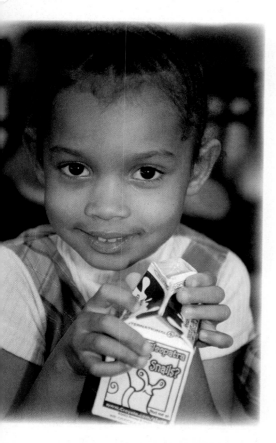

▲ Milk is a nutrient-dense source of protein, calcium, zinc, and other nutrients to support growth. It is especially challenging to meet calcium needs in childhood without regular dairy product consumption (see Chapter 10 for alternative sources of calcium).

▶ For children who follow a totally vegetarian diet, attention should also focus on protein and vitamin B-12 intake.

▶ Chapter 4 noted that it's unlikely that the use of sugar is the cause of hyperactivity or antisocial behavior in most children.

a child's diet. The high proportion of heme iron in many animal foods allows the iron to be more readily absorbed than is iron from plant foods. Consuming a vitamin C source along with the less readily absorbed iron in plants and supplements aids absorption.

Childhood iron-deficiency anemia is most likely to appear in children between the ages of 6 and 24 months. It can lead to decreases in both stamina and learning ability because the oxygen supply to cells decreases. Another effect is lowered resistance to disease. Fortunately, childhood anemia is not common today in North America, probably because of children's use of iron-fortified breakfast cereals. Also deserving of credit in the United States is the Special Supplemental Nutrition Program for Women, Infants, and Children (WIC), sponsored by the U.S. federal government. This program emphasizes the importance of iron-fortified formulas and cereals and distributes these foods—along with nutrition education—to low-income parents of infants and preschool children considered to be at nutritional risk.

Constipation. Constipation may be associated with a more serious disease, yet some young children experience constipation unrelated to any medical condition. When presented with a constipated child, a physician first has to rule out a medical cause, such as intestinal blockage. And, although the most common GI tract symptom that reflects intolerance to cow's milk is diarrhea, chronic constipation may also result. Treatment for constipation generally consists of first evacuating the bowels, generally with an enema. The promotion of regular bowel habits then follows, with laxative use as directed by the physician. Several months to years of supportive intervention may be required for effective treatment.

Dietary interventions include eating more fiber and drinking more fluids. Soy milk may also be substituted for cow's milk in the initial stages of treatment. Foods to emphasize for fiber are fruits, vegetables, whole-grain breads and cereals, and beans. The daily fiber goal for children set by the Food and Nutrition Board varies by age: 1 to 3 years, 19 grams per day; 4 to 8 years, 25 grams per day; 9 to 13 years, 31 grams per day for boys and 25 grams per day for girls. After age 13 years, typical adult recommendations are appropriate (review Chapter 4). Few children meet these goals.

Accompanying fluid recommendations are 4 cups (900 milliliters) per day for toddlers and about 5 cups (1200 milliliters) per day for older children.

Dental Caries. A proper diet goes a long way in reducing the risk for dental caries in young children. The following tips can help reduce dental problems in children:

- Begin oral hygiene when teeth start to appear.
- Seek early pediatric dental care.
- Drink fluoridated water.
- Use small amounts of fluoridated toothpaste twice daily.
- Snack in moderation.
- Have a dentist apply tooth sealants if needed.
- Avoid sticky, high-sugar snacks, especially between meals.
- If toddlers or preschoolers are chewing gum, sugarless gum is the best choice, as this has been shown to reduce the incidence of dental caries.

Vegetarianism in Childhood. Vegetarian diets can pose several risks for young children. These include the possibility of developing iron-deficiency anemia, a deficiency of vitamin B-12, and rickets from a vitamin D deficiency. During the first few years of life, children also may not consume enough calories when following a bulky vegetarian diet. But these known pitfalls are easily avoided by informed diet planning (see the "Nutrition and Your Health: Vegetarian and Plant-Based Diets

▲ Excessive fruit drink and fruit juice use is another potential problem in preschool (and later adolescent) years. The American Academy of Pediatrics recommends no more than 4 to 6 ounces per day for children 1 to 6 years (and 8 to 12 ounces per day for ages 7 to 18 years). Sweetened soft drinks should also be limited.

in Chapter 6). Diets for children who eat totally vegetarian fare should focus on protein, vitamin B-12, iron, and zinc content, with additional emphasis on vitamin D (or regular sun exposure) and calcium. Some of these dietary inadequacies can be compensated for by increasing oils, nuts, seeds, ready-to-eat breakfast cereals, and fortified soy milk in the diet.

CONCEPT CHECK

The rapid growth rate of an infant's first year slows during the toddler and preschool years (ages 1 to 5). As a child's appetite decreases, adults need to serve nutrient-dense foods and allow the child to decide how much to eat. Sudden shifts in food preferences are to be expected. Snacking is fine if attention is given to the selection of healthful foods and good dental hygiene. Although a children's multivitamin and mineral supplement is usually not needed—a plan following MyPyramid that includes a serving of fortified ready-to-eat breakfast cereal should meet nutrient needs—use of such a supplement is a reasonable practice. Children need plenty of iron-rich food to prevent iron-deficiency anemia, as well as zinc for growth. Adequate fiber and fluid help prevent constipation. Diets for children who eat totally vegetarian fare should focus on meeting needs for protein, vitamin D (or regular sun exposure), vitamin B-12, calcium, iron, and zinc.

SCHOOL-AGE CHILDREN: NUTRITION CONCERNS

The diets of many school-age students can stand general improvement, particularly with regard to fruit, vegetable, whole-grain, and dairy choices. Drinking minimal amounts of sugared soft drinks is also advised. One survey of U.S. schoolchildren revealed that on the day of the survey, 40% of the children ate no vegetables, except for potatoes or tomato sauce, and 20% ate no fruits. Another study showed that only 2% of about 3300 children 2 to 19 years old had met their recommended servings from all six MyPramid groups. In general, the nutritional concerns and goals applicable to school-age children are the same as those discussed in relation to preschoolers. However, with the added pressures of peers, health messages from the media, and an increasing desire for independence, these goals may be harder to achieve as children grow older. MyPyramid continues to be a good basis for diet planning, with an emphasis on moderating fat and sugar intake and ensuring adequate iron, zinc, and calcium intake (Fig. 17-3). The only difference is that the number of servings increases as calorie needs increase (review Table 17-3). Now let's look at several nutritional issues of particular concern during the school-age years.

Breakfast

Once children enter school, their eating patterns become more scheduled, and the consumption of regular meals—especially breakfast—becomes an important focus. A fortified ready-to-eat breakfast cereal is typically the greatest source of iron, vitamin A, and folic acid for children ages 2 to 18. Although there is controversy over the true benefit of breakfast for cognitive ability, children who eat breakfast are more likely to meet their needs for vitamins and minerals compared to children not eating breakfast. To influence morning test performance, it appears that breakfast must be eaten within a few hours of a test; the subsequent rise in blood glucose is thought to enhance performance.

Breakfast menus need not be limited to traditional fare. A little imagination can spark the interest of even the most reluctant child. Instead of conventional breakfast foods, parents can offer leftovers from dinner, such as pizza, spaghetti, soups, yogurt topped with trail mix, chili with beans, or sandwiches.

▲ Nutrition education ideally begins in the home as parents and other caregivers provide a healthy, well-balanced diet.

FIGURE 17-3 ▶ The USDA has created a version of MyPyramid for children aged 6–11. The accompanying web site (http://mypyramid.gov/kids/index.html) also features kid-friendly resources, such as an interactive MyPyramid Blast Off Game and a meal tracking worksheet, designed to encourage children to make healthier eating and activity choices. This site also contains information and resources that adults can use in educating children about proper nutrition.

Fat Intake

Diets of school-age children should include a variety of foods from each major group, not necessarily excluding any specific food because of its fat content. Overemphasis on fat-reduced diets during childhood has been linked to an increase in eating disorders and encourages an inappropriate "good food, bad food" attitude.

However, studies of dietary intake among children show that they are consuming too much saturated fat, most of which comes from whole milk, full-fat dairy products, and fatty meats. Furthermore, few children (or adults) meet recommendations to include two servings of fish per week to ensure adequate intake of omega-3 fats. Emphasizing low-fat dairy products (after age 2), offering broiled or baked fish, choosing leaner cuts of meat, trimming visible fat from meats, and removing the skin from poultry before serving foods will establish heart-healthy eating habits to last a lifetime. Snacks for children should also include only moderate fat and sugar and emphasize fruit, vegetables, whole grain and dairy choices. Ideas for healthy snacks are found in Table 17-4.

▲ Sweets should be consumed in moderation in childhood, but do not have to be avoided altogether.

CRITICAL THINKING

Tim refuses to eat breakfast before school. He doesn't like cereal, toast, or any of the other usual breakfast foods. What can Tim's parents do to ensure that he eats nutritious foods before leaving for school?

MAKING DECISIONS

Nutrition Education for Children

Children spend the majority of their waking hours in school, so it is a great place to learn about positive, healthy eating habits. A strong emphasis on nutrition in schools can help children understand why healthy diet habits will make them feel more energetic, look better, and work more efficiently. Federally-funded programs such as USDA's Team Nutrition and the CDC's National Bone Health Campaign are a good start, but more changes are needed. School foodservice outlets, including cafeterias and vending machines, must present healthier options for school children. Instruction on food preparation in home economics classes, after-school programs, or at home will help children learn to prepare healthy meals and snacks. Increased participation in physical education classes and recreational sports is more likely to improve academic performance than detract from it. However, positive nutrition influences must extend beyond the classroom to change persistent trends toward obesity and chronic diseases. Caregivers and other adult role models need to create safe opportunities for children to be active and must practice what they preach when it comes to healthy habits.

TABLE 17-4 Twenty Healthy Snack Ideas for School-Age Children

• Fruit smoothies	• Dried fruit
• Fruit salad (or cut-up fruit)	• Trail mix
• Mini-pizzas	• Bean and cheese burritos
• Yogurt with granola	• Handful of whole-grain cereal
• Pasta salad	• Hummus with veggie sticks
• Peanuts	• Applesauce
• Veggies with dip	• Low-fat microwave popcorn
• Fruit-juice popsicles	• Tuna salad with pita pocket
• Quick breads, such as banana bread	• Peanut butter and apple slices
• Cheese and whole-wheat crackers	• Hard-boiled egg

Type 2 Diabetes

Type 2 diabetes is generally thought to be an adult condition. As reviewed in the "Nutrition and Your Health" section, "Diabetes—When Blood Glucose Regulation Fails" in Chapter 4, it frequently occurs in overweight people older than 40. However, physicians have noted an alarming increase in the frequency of the disease among children (and teenagers). This is primarily due to the rise in obesity in this age group, coupled with minimal physical activity. Up to 85% of children with the disease are overweight at diagnosis. Experts are calling for screening for diabetes in at-risk children every 2 years, starting at age 10 or at the onset of puberty. Besides obesity and a sedentary lifestyle, other risk factors include having a first- or second-degree relative with the disease or belonging to a non-White population. Appropriate diet and lifestyle intervention should be implemented, along with the use of diabetes medications when necessary. A regular intake of low-glycemic-load fruits, vegetables, and whole-grain breads and cereals is especially recommended.

Overweight and Obesity

In the United States, more than 15% of school-age children are overweight or obese. The number of cases is increasing, especially in minority populations. In the short run, ridicule, embarrassment, possibly depression, and short stature linked to early puberty are the main consequences of such obesity. In the long run, significant health problems associated with obesity, such as cardiovascular disease, type 2 diabetes, and hypertension, usually will appear in adulthood. However, an increase in these health-related complications has been noted in children. Childhood obesity is a serious health threat, because about 40% of obese children (and about 80% of obese adolescents) become obese adults. Significant weight gain generally begins between ages 5 and 7, during puberty, or during the teenage years.

Research points to many potential causes of childhood obesity. Recall the nature versus nurture discussion in Chapter 7. Some infants are born with lower metabolic rates; they use calories more efficiently and in turn can more easily produce fat stores. Studies also suggest, though, that this genetic link accounts for only one-third of individual differences in body weight.

Researchers believe that, although diet is an important factor, inactivity is also a contributor to the increase in childhood obesity. Today's generation of children now glues itself to the TV for an average of 24 hours per week; many children spend another 10 hours or so playing computer and video games. The American Academy of Pediatrics recommends a limit of 14 hours of TV and video time per week for children over age 2 (no television is recommended for children younger than 2 years). In addition, excessive snacking, overreliance on fast-food restaurants, parental neglect, the media in general, lack of safe areas to play, and the abundant availability of high-calorie food choices contribute to childhood obesity. Sugared soft drinks are especially implicated.

The initial approach in treating an obese child is to assess how much physical activity he or she engages in. If a child spends much free time in sedentary activities (such as watching television or playing video games), more physical activities should be encouraged. The U.S. federal government and health professionals recommend 60 minutes or more of moderate to intense physical activity per day for children and adolescents. Learning to engage in and enjoy regular physical activity will help children not only to attain a healthy body weight but also to keep a similar body weight later in life. An increase in physical activity won't just happen; parents and other caregivers need to plan for it. Getting the family together for a brisk walk after dinner encourages healthy habits for all involved. Age-appropriate activities for elementary school-age children include walking, dancing, jumping rope, and participation in organized sports that focus on fun rather than intense competition. For middle school-age children, more complex organized sports (e.g., football and basketball) are of interest and some weight training with small weights can also be beneficial.

▲ Regular physical activity is an important part of prevention and treatment of weight problems in childhood. The goal is about 60 minutes of such activity each day. Many children do not meet this goal.

▶ To get kids involved in exercise, new physical education classes have been introduced into schools. These classes provide lifelong fitness lessons in such activities as rock climbing, in-line skating, and recreational jogging. These classes help promote activity because they take the focus away from teams and competition, which often discourage and embarrass kids who lack athletic talent.

▲ Super-sized portions of foods such as hamburgers and sugared soft drinks served to children are contributing to the obesity and type 2 diabetes epidemics they are experiencing.

menarche The onset of menstruation. Menarche usually occurs around age 13, 2 or 3 years after the first signs of puberty start to appear.

▶ Drinking soft drinks in place of milk causes many teenagers to have inadequate calcium intake. Over the last 20 years, soft drinks have been replacing milk as the preferred beverage of adolescents. Only half of school-age boys and 20% of girls meet recommendations for calcium intake. This trend has been linked to decreased bone mass and increased bone fractures in this age group.

Moderation in calorie intake is important, especially the limitation of high-calorie foods, such as sugared soft drinks and whole milk. The focus should be on more vitamin and mineral-dense foods and healthy snacks. An emphasis on appropriate portion sizes may help youth learn to curb excessive food intake. To specifically address the increased burden of overweight and obesity among minority populations, health professionals must become versed in varied cultural food preferences.

Resorting to a weight-loss diet is usually not necessary—it's best to emphasize changing habits that allow for weight maintenance. Children have an advantage over adults in dealing with obesity; their bodies can use stored energy for growth. Thus, if weight gain can be moderated, increases in height and resulting lean body tissue may reduce the percentage of body weight accounted for as stored fat, yielding a more healthful weight-to-height ratio. This is one reason it's desirable to treat obesity in childhood. Further growth can contribute to success. If weight loss is necessary in younger children, it should be gradual, about ½ to 1 pound per week. In addition, the child should be watched closely to ensure that the rate of growth continues to be normal. The child's calorie intake shouldn't be so low that gains in height diminish. In addition, medications may be prescribed under a physician's care to reduce food intake (sibutramine [Meridia]) and/or fat absorption (orlistat [Xenical]).

CONCEPT CHECK

The school-age child is advised to follow MyPyramid and especially moderate choices high in fat and simple sugars. Breakfast is an important meal to refuel the body for a new school day and to help ensure fulfilling nutrient needs for the day. Attention to regular physical activity and healthy diet should help prevent/treat childhood obesity and build a desirable lifestyle pattern for later life.

TEENAGE YEARS: NUTRITION CONCERNS

Most girls begin a rapid growth spurt between the ages of 10 and 13, and most boys experience rapid growth between the ages of 12 and 15. Nearly every organ in the body grows during these periods. Most noticeable are increases in height and weight and the development of secondary sexual characteristics. Girls usually begin menstruating (reach **menarche**) during this growth spurt, and they grow very little beyond 2 years after menarche. Early-maturing girls may begin their growth spurt as early as age 7 to 8, whereas early-maturing boys may begin growing by age 9 to 10.

During the growth spurt, girls gain about 10 inches (25 centimeters) in height, and boys gain about 12 inches (30 centimeters). Girls also tend to accumulate both lean and fat tissue, whereas boys tend to gain mostly lean tissue. This growth spurt provides about 50% of ultimate adult weight and about 15% of ultimate adult height (review Fig. 17-1).

As the growth spurt begins, teenagers begin to eat more. If teens choose nutritious food, they can take advantage of their increased hunger and easily satisfy their nutrient needs. As discussed for younger age groups, MyPyramid can provide the basis for meeting these nutrient needs (Table 17-5). Following such a plan will meet carbohydrate needs (130 grams per day) and protein needs (52 grams per day for males and 46 grams per day for females).

Nutritional Problems and Concerns of Teens

Anorexia nervosa and bulimia nervosa are nutritional concerns of the teen years, as covered in detail in Chapter 13. Other nutritional problems are more common during the teen years. A survey of high school students showed that only a little over 25% had eaten five servings of fruits and vegetables on the previous day, and they are consum-

TABLE 17-5 Food Plan for Teenagers Based on MyPyramid[1, 2]

Food Group	Serving Size	Approximate Number of Servings		
		Age 13	Age 16	Age 18
Grains	ounce	6–7	6–10	6–10
Vegetables	cup	2.5–3	2.5–3.5	2.5–3.5
Fruits	cup	2	2–2.5	2–2.5
Milk	cup	3	3	3
Meat & Beans	ounce	5.5–6	5.5–7	5.5–7
Oils	teaspoon	6	6–8	6–8
Discretionary calories	kcal	up to 265–290	up to 265–425	up to 265–425

[1]Assumes 30–60 minutes of physical activity per day. Log on to mypyramid.gov for other ages and levels of physical activity.
[2]The larger amounts refer to boys.

> A strictly vegetarian diet must be monitored for adequate energy, protein, iron, vitamin B-12, calcium, and vitamin D (the latter if sun exposure is not sufficient). These nutrients become particularly important in teenagers, as their diets are often already compromised.

ing approximately 25% more sodium than recommended. Another concern is that many teenage girls stop drinking milk, so they may not consume enough calcium to allow for maximal mineralization of bones through their early twenties. Many young women who don't consume enough calcium are likely to develop osteoporosis later.

Many teenagers are not meeting their needs for calcium. The Adequate Intake for calcium for both males and females between ages 9 and 18 years is 1300 milligrams per day, compared with only 800 milligrams per day for younger children. Three servings per day from the milk, yogurt, and cheese group are recommended for all teenagers and young adults to meet calcium needs. Figure 2-1 in Chapter 2 shows the stark contrast between milk and typical soft drinks with respect to calcium and other nutrients. If dairy products are not consumed, alternative calcium sources need to be included.

A further concern is iron deficiency. Iron-deficiency anemia sometimes appears in girls after they start menstruating (menarche) and in boys during their growth spurt. About 10% of teenagers have low iron stores or related anemia. Teens who strive to forge an identity by adopting dietary patterns unfamiliar to their families—vegetarianism, for example—may not know enough about the alternate diet pattern to keep from developing health problems, such as iron-deficiency anemia. It's important that teenagers choose good food sources of iron, such as lean meats, whole grains, and enriched cereals. Teenage girls, particularly those with heavy menstrual flows, need to eat good sources of iron (or regularly consume an iron supplement). Iron-deficiency anemia is a highly undesirable condition for a teen. It can produce increased fatigue and decreased ability to concentrate and learn. School and physical performance may suffer.

▲ An active lifestyle coupled with a healthy diet should be part of the teen years. Both habits contribute to bone development and bone strength.

MAKING DECISIONS

Nutrition and Acne

Acne is a common teen concern—about 80% of teens experience it. Although it's popularly believed that eating nuts, chocolate, and pizza can make acne worse, scientific studies have failed to show a strong link between any dietary factor and acne. Many acne medications contain analogs of vitamin A (e.g., 13-*cis* retinoic acid [Accutane]). Although these treatments can be effective, the close supervision by a physician is crucial, as vitamin A analogs can be toxic. Vitamin A itself is no help in treating acne, and excess amounts of vitamin A or related analogs taken during pregnancy can cause birth defects. Thus, girls taking these vitamin A medications should not become pregnant.

> Alcoholism is a significant health problem that may have its roots in the teen years. Smoking—another habit that compromises health—also often begins in teen years. Some of the impetus for smoking is the desire to control body weight—but this is not an advisable method.

Obesity is a growing problem among teenagers, and about 30% of obese teenagers have the metabolic syndrome (Syndrome X) discussed in Chapters 4 and 5. If a teen attains ultimate adult height and is still obese, a weight-loss regimen may be necessary. This is especially appropriate after the adolescent growth spurt. Weight loss should be gradual, perhaps 1 pound per week, and generally follow the advice in Chapter 7. Weight loss medications may also be prescribed.

Helping Teens Eat More Nutritious Foods

Teenagers face a variety of challenges. They pursue their independence, experience identity crises, seek peer acceptance, and worry about physical appearance. These factors affect food choice. Advertisers take advantage of this by pushing a vast array of products—candy, gum, soft drinks, and snacks—at the teenage market. Potato chips and French fries make up more than one-third of the vegetable servings consumed by teens. Additionally, many schools offer French fries on a regular basis, and soft drink machines can be found in school hallways and cafeterias, in turn competing with the school lunch. The increased consumption of fast-foods, sugary beverages, and snack foods crowds out nutrient-dense foods, thus limiting intake of calcium, iron, zinc, fat-soluble vitamins, and folate.

Teens often do not think about the long-term benefits of good health. They have a hard time relating today's actions to tomorrow's health outcomes. Many teenagers tend to think they can change habits later; there's no hurry.

Still, healthful teen food habits do not require giving up favorite foods. Small portions of fatty foods can complement larger portions of fat-free and reduced-fat dairy products, lean meats, vegetable proteins, fruits, vegetables, and whole-grain products. An example of this type of meal is a plain hamburger with a garden salad (minimize the amount of regular dressing or use a low-fat variety), small order of French fries or chili, and a medium diet soft drink or reduced-fat or fat-free milk.

Are Teenage Snacking Practices Harmful?

Teens often obtain one-fourth to one-third of all their calories and major nutrients from snacks. Unfortunately, studies have found just what you might expect—that teens snack mostly on potato and corn chips, cookies, candies, and ice cream. Key reasons for snacking include an opportunity to get out and socialize with friends, accessibility, hunger, and celebration of a special event. Teenagers can obtain many nutrients from snacking. Even fast-food restaurants offer some good food choices. By choosing wisely and eating in moderation, teens can eat at fast-food restaurants occasionally and still consume a very healthful diet. Snacks and fast-food restaurants themselves are not the problem; poor food choices in terms of type and quantity are.

Lack of exercise and poor dietary habits formed during teenage years often continue into adulthood and may increase risk of chronic diseases, such as cardiovascular disease, osteoporosis, and some types of cancer. Getting this message across to teenagers is an important and challenging task for parents.

▲ The teenage years are noted for snacking. With reasonable food choices, teenagers can have healthful diets.

CONCEPT CHECK

A second period of rapid growth occurs during the teen years. Girls generally start this growth spurt earlier than boys. MyPyramid can direct meal planning. Common nutritional problems in these years arise from poor food choices and include inadequate calcium intake in girls and iron-deficiency anemia. Changes occur so rapidly during these years, and in so many areas—psychological, social, and physical—it may be difficult to stress the relevance of nutrition to teenagers. Moderation in fat and sugar intake are important goals to consider when choosing snacks.

NUTRITION AND YOUR HEALTH
Food Allergies and Intolerances

Adverse reactions to foods—indicated by sneezing, coughing, nausea, vomiting, diarrhea, hives, and other rashes—are broadly classed as food allergies (also called *hypersensitivities*) or **food intolerances.** Allergies involve responses of the immune system designed to eliminate foreign proteins, called **allergens.** The symptoms experienced by susceptible people, such as rapid increase in heart rate and shortness of breath, are the result of this battle. In contrast, the symptoms of food intolerances do not result from a true allergic reaction. Rather, food intolerances are caused by an individual's inability to digest certain food components or by the direct effect of a food component or contaminant on the body. Let's examine each process, first allergies and then intolerances.

FOOD ALLERGIES: SYMPTOMS AND MECHANISM

Allergic reactions to foods are common and occur more frequently in females than males. Food allergies occur most often during infancy and young adulthood. Experts estimate that up to about 2% of adults and up to about 8% of children are allergic to certain foods (Fig. 17-4). Three types of reactions may occur after the ingestion of problem foods by susceptible people:

- *Classic*—itching, reddening skin, asthma, swelling, choking, and a runny nose
- *GI tract*—nausea, vomiting, diarrhea, intestinal gas, bloating, pain, constipation, and indigestion
- *General*—headache, skin reactions, tension and fatigue, tremors, and psychological problems

Any reaction milder than these distinct allergic ones is referred to as a **food sensitivity.**

Allergic reactions vary not only in the body system affected but also in their duration, ranging from seconds to a few days. A generalized, all-systems reaction is called **anaphylactic shock.** This severe allergic response results in low blood pressure and distress of the respiratory system and GI tract. It can be fatal. Overall, allergic reactions result in 30,000 emergency room visits and 150 to 200 deaths per year. A person who is extremely sensitive to a food may not be able to touch the food or even be in the same room where it is being cooked without reacting to it. Although any food can trigger anaphylactic shock, the most common culprits are peanuts

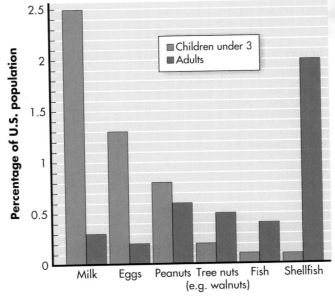

FIGURE 17-4 ▶ Types of allergies and percentage of U.S. population with those allergies.

Source: Journal of Allergy and Clinical Immunology (study done by Mount Sinai School of Medicine)

food intolerance An adverse reaction to food that does not involve an allergic reaction.

allergen A foreign protein, or antigen, that induces excess production of certain immune system antibodies; subsequent exposure to the same protein leads to allergic symptoms. Whereas all allergens are antigens, not all antigens are allergens.

food sensitivity A mild reaction to a substance in a food that might be expressed as slight itching or redness of the skin.

anaphylactic shock A severe allergic response that results in lowered blood pressure and respiratory and gastrointestinal distress. This can be fatal.

antigen Any substance that induces a state of sensitivity and/or resistance to microorganisms or toxic substances after a lag period; substance that stimulates a specific aspect of the immune system.

elimination diet A restrictive diet that systematically tests foods that may cause an allergic response by first eliminating them for 1 to 2 weeks and then adding them back, one at a time.

▶ People with a history of serious allergic reactions and those who have asthma should carry a self-administered form of epinephrine, such as EpiPen, to subside an episode of anaphylactic shock, should it occur.

▶ The American Academy of Allergy Asthma and Immunology has a 24-hour toll-free hot line (800-822-2762) to answer questions about food allergies and to help direct people to specialists who treat the problem. Free information on food allergies is available by contacting The Food Allergy & Anaphylaxis Network. The telephone number is (800-929-4040); the website is www.foodallergy.org.

▲ Eggs, wheat, milk, peanuts, tree nuts, soybeans, and seafood pose the greatest risk for food allergies in childhood.

(a legume, not a nut), tree nuts (walnuts, pecans, etc.), shellfish, milk (look for the protein casein on the label), eggs (look for the protein albumin on the label), soybeans, wheat, and fish. Other foods frequently identified with adverse reactions include meat and meat products, fruits, and cheese. For a small number of people, avoiding foods such as peanuts or shellfish is a matter of life and death. Almost all food allergies are caused by proteins in these foods that act as **antigens.**

Testing for a Food Allergy

The diagnosis of a food allergy can often be a difficult task (Table 17-6). It requires the participation of a skilled physician. The first step in determining whether a food allergy is present is to record a detailed history of symptoms, including the time from ingestion to onset of symptoms, duration of symptoms, most recent reaction, food suspected of causing a reaction, and quantity and nature of food needed to produce a reaction. A family history of allergic diseases can also help, as allergic reactions tend to run in families. A physical examination may reveal evidence of an allergy, such as skin diseases and asthma. Various diagnostic tests can rule out other conditions.

The diagnostic first step is to eliminate from the diet—for 1 to 2 weeks—all tested compounds that appear to cause allergic symptoms, plus all other foods suspected of causing an allergy based on the person's food history. The person generally starts out eating foods to which almost no one reacts, such as rice, vegetables, noncitrus fruits, and fresh meats

and poultry. If symptoms are still present, the person can more severely restrict the diet or even use special formula diets that are hypoallergenic.

Once a diet is found that causes no symptoms, called an **elimination diet,** foods can be added back one at a time. This type of food challenge is an option only when the culprit foods are known to pose no risk of anaphylactic shock in the person. Doses of ½ to 1 teaspoon (2.5 to 5 milliliters) are given at first. The amount is increased until the dose approximates usual intake. Any reintroduced food that causes significant symptoms to appear is identified as an allergen for the person.

Laboratory tests can also aid in diagnosis of food allergies. Skin testing involves pricking the skin with a small amount of purified food extract and observing any allergic response (e.g., a red eruption at the prick site). These types of tests are easy and safe, even for infants, but they may not clearly diagnose a food allergy. A positive skin-prick test merely indicates that a person has been sensitized to a food; it can't definitively identify if that food is the cause for the symptoms in question. Newer types of blood testing, however, have more diagnostic value. Blood tests estimate the blood concentration of antibodies that bind certain foodborne antigens.

Living with Food Allergies

Once potential allergens are identified, dietary modifications must be made. In some cases, small amounts of the offending food can be consumed without an observable reaction. Also, some food allergens are destroyed by

TABLE 17-6 Assessment Strategies for Food Allergies

History	Include description of symptoms, time between food ingestion and onset of symptoms, duration of symptoms, most recent allergic episode, quantity of food required to produce reaction, suspected foods, and allergic diseases in other family members.
Physical examination	Look for signs of an allergic reaction (rash, itching, intestinal bloating, etc.).
Elimination diet	Establish a diet lacking the suspected offending foods and stay on it for 1 to 2 weeks or until symptoms clear.
Food challenge	Add back small amounts of excluded foods, one at a time, as long as anaphylactic shock is not a possible consequence.
Blood test	Determine presence of antibodies in blood that bind to food antigens tested.
Skin test	Place a sample of the suspected allergen under the skin and watch for an inflammatory reaction.

heating, so cooking may eliminate the allergic response. This is effective primarily for allergies to fruits or vegetables, not for the more common allergies to milk, peanuts, or seafood. For most cases, though, complete avoidance of allergy-causing food ingredients is the safest course of action. This makes careful reading of food labels essential. As of 2006, the Food Allergen Labeling and Consumer Protection Act now requires manufacturers to clearly identify the presence of major food allergens (milk, eggs, fish, shellfish, peanuts, tree nuts, wheat, and soy) on food product labels.

A major challenge when treating a person with a food allergy is to make sure that what remains in the diet can still provide essential nutrients. The small food intake of children permits less leeway in removing offending foods that may contain numerous nutrients. A registered dietitian can help guide the diet-planning process to ensure that the remaining food choices still meet nutrient needs or to guide supplement use, if that is necessary.

About 80% of young children with food allergies outgrow them before 3 years. Parents should be made aware of this and not assume the allergy will be long-lived. Food allergies diagnosed after 3 years of age are often more long-lived, but not always. In these cases, about 33% of people outgrow their food allergies within 3 years. For others, the condition may be prolonged; some food allergies can last a lifetime, such as those for peanuts, tree nuts, and shellfish. Periodic reintroduction of offending foods can be tried every 6 to 12 months or so to see whether the allergic reaction has decreased. If no symptoms appear, tolerance to the food has developed.

Several strategies are under study to ease the dietary restrictions imposed by food allergies. One possibility includes treatment with antibodies that will increase the threshold at which an allergic response occurs. For a person with an allergy to peanuts, for example, this would alleviate some anxiety about severe reactions to trace amounts of peanuts found in foods. Vaccines are another area of research. Also, scientists are working on genetically engineered foods that do not contain common allergens.

Preventing Food Allergies

With the rising number of cases of food allergies, many new parents wonder when and how to introduce new foods during infancy and early childhood. It is evident that introducing foods other than human milk or infant formula before 4 months of age is associated with higher risk of allergic diseases. Most experts, including the American Academy of Pediatrics and the American College of Allergy, Asthma, and Immunology, advise waiting to introduce solid foods until after 6 months of age for lowest risk of food allergies.

Any food can contain a potential allergen, but certain foods have been found to have high allergenic potential: peanuts, tree nuts, eggs, cow's milk, fish, and seafood. The exact timing of introduction of these foods is a matter of debate. It is up to the health professional to advise parents individually, taking into account duration of breastfeeding and family history of food and other allergies. A consensus statement from the American College of Allergy, Asthma, and Immunology recommends waiting until 12 months of age to introduce cow's milk, 24 months of age to introduce eggs (whites), and 36 months of age to introduce peanuts, tree nuts, fish, and other seafood.

If an allergy-prone woman is pregnant or breastfeeding, many experts advise that she should avoid offending foods— such as eggs, shellfish, and peanuts—because allergens can cross the placenta during pregnancy. Allergens are also secreted via her milk. She should work with her physician and registered dietitian to make sure she still consumes an adequate diet. In addition, when food allergies are common in the family, women are advised to breastfeed their infants exclusively for 6 months. Human milk contains factors that play a role in the maturation of the small intestine. Formula-fed infants, especially those on cow's milk–based formulas, have a greater risk for developing food allergies. Breastfeeding, thus, should continue for as long as possible, preferably to 1 year.

Beyond promotion of exclusive breastfeeding for the first six months of life and delaying introduction of cow's milk until 1 year of age, other preventive practices are still speculative. Postponing introduction of other potential allergens into the infant's diet is prudent, but not proven. Likewise, although we know that allergens do cross the placenta and are secreted in human milk, there is little evidence to support avoidance of common allergens during pregnancy or breastfeeding to prevent allergies.

Food Intolerances

Food intolerances are adverse reactions to foods that do not involve allergic mechanisms. Generally, larger amounts of an offending food are required to produce the symptoms of an intolerance than to trigger allergic symptoms. Common causes of food intolerances include:

- Constituents of certain foods (e.g., red wine, tomatoes, pineapples) that have a druglike activity, causing physiological effects such as changes in blood pressure
- Certain synthetic compounds added to foods, such as sulfites, food-coloring agents, and monosodium glutamate (MSG)
- Food contaminants, including antibiotics and other chemicals used in the production of livestock and crops, as well as insect parts not removed during processing
- Toxic contaminants, which may be ingested with improperly handled and prepared foods containing *Clostridium botulinum*, *Salmonella* bacteria, or other foodborne microorganisms (see Chapter 15)
- Deficiencies in digestive enzymes, such as lactase (review Chapter 4)

Almost everyone is sensitive to one or more of these causes of food intolerance, many of which produce GI tract symptoms.

Sulfites, added to foods and beverages as antioxidants, cause flushing, spasms of the airway, and a loss of blood pressure in susceptible people. Wine, dehydrated potatoes, dried fruits, gravy, soup mixes, and restaurant salad greens commonly contain sulfites. A reaction to MSG may include an increase in blood pressure, numbness, sweating, vomiting, headache, and facial pressure. MSG is commonly found in restaurant food and many processed foods (e.g., soups). A reaction to tartrazine, a food-coloring additive, includes spasm of the airway, itching, and reddening skin. Tyramine, a derivative of the amino acid tyrosine, is commonly found in "aged" foods, such as cheeses and red wines. This natural food constituent can cause high blood pressure in people taking monoamine oxidase (MAO) inhibitor medications, which may be prescribed for clinical depression.

The basic treatment for food intolerances is to avoid specific offending components. However, total elimination often is not required because people generally are not as sensitive to compounds causing food intolerances as they are to allergens.

CASE STUDY

Undernutrition During Infancy

Damon is a 7-month-old boy who has been taken into a clinic for a routine checkup. On examination, he was found to be moderately underweight relative to his age and body length. His physician scheduled a follow-up appointment in 3 months. At the 10-month visit, Damon appeared sluggish and was now even more underweight for his age and length.

A registered dietitian interviewed Damon's 16-year-old mother to collect information on Damon's dietary intake. His intake over the previous 24 hours consisted of two bottles of infant formula, three 8-ounce bottles of Kool-Aid, and a hot dog. However, the mother was still in school, and at night she often left Damon with the neighbor, so that she could go out with friends for a few hours. Thus, she was not aware of all that he ate.

Answer the following questions, and check your responses in Appendix A.

1. Damon's mother did not specify what type of formula he takes. What questions would you ask about his formula?
2. What potential dangers await Damon if his growth continues to lag behind?
3. What foods should Damon's caregivers offer that are appropriate for his age and nutritional needs?
4. What problems might arise from consumption of sugary drinks from a bottle?
5. Does Damon need any vitamin or mineral supplements?

SUMMARY

1. Growth is rapid during infancy; birth weight doubles in 4 to 6 months, and length increases by 50% in the first year. An adequate diet, especially in terms of calories, as well as the nutrients protein and zinc, is essential to support normal growth. Undernutrition can cause irreversible changes in growth and development. Growth in infants and children can be assessed by measuring body weight, height (or length), and head circumference over time. Growth charts have been revised to include a more valid measurement for determining children's growth, body mass index (BMI).

2. Nutrient needs in the first 6 months can be met by human milk or iron-fortified infant formula. Supplementary vitamin D is needed for breastfed infants, and many infants may need supplemental iron and fluoride.

3. Infant formulas generally contain lactose or sucrose, heat-treated proteins from cow's milk, and vegetable oil. These formulas may or may not be fortified with iron. Sanitation is important when preparing and storing formula.

4. Most infants do not need solid foods before 6 months of age. Solid food should not be added to an infant's diet until the nutrients are needed, the GI tract can digest complex foods, the infant has the physical ability to control tongue thrusting, and the risk of developing food allergies has decreased.

5. The first solid foods given should be iron-fortified infant cereals or ground meats. Other single foods can be added gradually, at the rate of about one each week. Some foods to avoid giving infants in the first year include honey, cow's milk (especially fat-reduced varieties), foods with added salt or sugar, and foods that may cause choking.

6. Introducing iron-containing solid food at the appropriate time and not offering cow's milk until 1 year of age can generally prevent iron-deficiency anemia in late infancy.

7. A slower growth rate in preschool years underlies the importance of children's eating nutrient-dense foods and reducing their food serving sizes. Choosing iron-rich foods, such as lean red meats, is important at this age. Portion sizes of 1 tablespoon of each food for each year of life is a good starting point for the vegetables, fruits, and meats & beans groups of MyPyramid. Preschoolers also should be given some leeway in determining serving size and should be encouraged to try new foods.

8. Obese children and adolescents are more likely to become obese adults and, so, incur greater health risks. Parents can provide healthful food choices, and children should control portion sizes. When controlled early through diet and exercise interventions, the problem of obesity may correct itself as the child continues to grow in height.

9. During the adolescent growth spurt, both boys and girls have increased needs for iron and calcium. Inadequate calcium intake by teenage girls is a major concern because it can set the stage for the development of osteoporosis later in life. Teenagers generally should moderate their intake of high-fat and sugar-rich foods— especially snacks and fast-food, which they often consume in abundance—and perform regular physical activity.

STUDY QUESTIONS

1. List two factors that limit "catch-up" growth in adulthood when a nutrient-deficient diet has been consumed throughout childhood.

2. Describe how you would assess whether an 8-month-old infant is consuming a healthful diet.

3. Outline three key factors that help determine when to introduce solid foods into an infant's diet.

4. A 3-month-old infant is taken to a clinic with failure to thrive. What are two possible explanations?

5. List three reasons why preschoolers are noted for "picky" eating. For each, describe an appropriate parent response.

6. What three factors are likely to contribute to obesity in a typical 10-year-old child?

7. Compare the guidelines for infant feeding summarized in Chapter 15 with the 2005 Dietary Guidelines for Americans for children over age 2 and adults discussed in Chapter 2. Which guidelines are similar? Do any contradict each other? If so, why?

8. Describe three pros and cons of snacking. What is the basic advice for healthful snacking from childhood through the teenage years?

9. Which two nutrients are of particular concern in planning diets for teenagers? Why does each deserve to be singled out?

10. List three nutrients of concern for a teenage vegetarian.

CHECK YOUR KNOWLEDGE

Answers to the following multiple choice questions are in Appendix A.

1. Inadequate intake of which of the following results in poor growth?
   a. calories
   b. iron
   c. zinc
   d. All of the above.

2. Using the formulas for Estimated Energy Requirements provided in the text, an 11-month-old girl who weighs 19 pounds needs approximately _____ kcal per day.
   a. 690
   b. 810
   c. 845
   d. 930

3. Introduction of cow's milk should be delayed until 12 months of age because it
   a. contains too much fat.
   b. doesn't contain enough minerals (e.g., calcium and phosphorus) to meet infant needs.
   c. may induce a food allergy.
   d. All of the above.

4. You are trying to introduce an apple and blueberry puree to a seven-month-old infant, but she rejects it. What should you do?
   a. assume she doesn't like apples and blueberries
   b. offer the food again on another day
   c. force a spoonful into her mouth
   d. None of the above.

5. Milk is a nutrient-dense source of all of the following except
   a. protein.
   b. iron.
   c. calcium.
   d. zinc.

6. Careful diet planning is required for vegetarian children to prevent
   a. rickets.
   b. anemia.
   c. nervous system disorders.
   d. All of the above.

7. Of the following options, which is preferred to ensure adequate vitamin and mineral intake for a picky eater?
   a. consume a fortified breakfast cereal
   b. promise dessert as a reward for eating meats and vegetables
   c. use a multivitamin and mineral supplement
   d. None of the above.

8. Which of the following is advised for treatment of overweight among school-age children?
   a. eating fewer meals
   b. following a low-carbohydrate eating plan
   c. 60 minutes or more of moderate to intense physical activity
   d. avoiding dairy products

9. The prevailing dietary habits of North American teenagers contribute to all of the following except
   a. acne.
   b. high blood pressure.
   c. low bone mass.
   d. type 2 diabetes.

10. Your friend breaks out in hives and feels nauseous after eating a salad containing mango. She probably has a food
    a. sensitivity.   c. intolerance.
    b. allergy.   d. a, b, and c.

FURTHER READINGS

1. ADA Reports: Position of the American Dietetic Association: Child and adolescent food and nutrition programs. *Journal of the American Dietetic Association* 106:1467, 2006.

   It is the position of the American Dietetic Association that all children and adolescents, regardless of age, sex, socioeconomic status, racial diversity, ethnic diversity, linguistic diversity, or health status, should have access to food and nutrition programs that ensure the availability of a safe and adequate food supply that promotes optimal physical, cognitive, social, and emotional growth and development.

2. ADA Reports: Position of the American Dietetic Association: Dietary guidance for healthy children ages 2 to 11 years. *Journal of the American Dietetic Association* 104:660, 2004.

   MyPyramid combined with the Dietary Guidelines for Americans provide an appropriate blueprint for feeding children. Diets of many children are not following this advice and in turn are contributing to the nutritional problems common in childhood and later adulthood.

3. Affenito SG and others: Breakfast consumption by African-American and white adolescent girls correlates positively with calcium and fiber intake and negatively with body mass index. *Journal of the American Dietetic Association* 105:938, 2005.

   Eating breakfast on a regular basis contributes to the overall health of adolescent girls in this study. This includes helping meet calcium and fiber needs, while also contributing to weight control.

4. Bounds W and others: The relationship of dietary and lifestyle factors to bone mineral indexes in children. *Journal of the American Dietetic Association* 105:735, 2005.

   A primary influence on healthy bone mass parameters in this study was a nutritious diet—one ample in protein, phosphorus, vitamin K, magnesium, zinc, iron, and calories. Height and weight were also positively correlated to bone status.

5. Centers for Disease Control and Prevention: Physical activity levels among children ages 9–13 years—United States, 2002. *Journal of the American Medical Association* 290:1308, 2003.

   Most children do not participate in sufficient free-time physical activity, especially African-American and Hispanic children. Insufficient physical activity increases the risk for overweight and obesity and other chronic diseases. Physical activity habits that begin in childhood are likely to carry over into adulthood.

6. Council on Sports Medicine and Fitness and Council on School Health. Active healthy living: Prevention of childhood obesity through increased physical activity. *Pediatrics* 117:1834, 2006.

   In light of the increasingly sedentary lifestyles of today's youth, physical activity should be encouraged during and after school and as part of home life. Benefits of regular physical activity among children and adolescents include physical changes (e.g., improved insulin sensitivity, lowered blood pressure) and psychological improvements (e.g., increased self-esteem, less depression). Specific goals and examples of activities to promote are provided for each age group.

7. Dietz WH and Robinson TN: Overweight children and adolescents. *The New England Journal of Medicine* 352:2100, 2005.

   This article summarizes the possible diagnostic and treatment approaches for overweight children and adolescents. For the 7-year-old girl described in the article, three key recommendations were to reduce sugared-soft drink consumption and computer and television screen time, with a corresponding increase in active play.

8. Fitch C: Preventing iron deficiency in infants and toddlers. *Today's Dietitian*, p. 32, December 2004.

   The author stresses the need to prevent iron deficiency in infants and toddlers. After 4 to 6 months of age it is important to have a rich source of iron in an infant's diet, such as iron-fortified cereals. Any infant formula used should be iron fortified. Prevention of iron deficiency in toddlers includes limiting cow's milk to 3 cups per day, as it is a poor source of iron.

9. Fitzgibbon ML, Stolley M: Promoting health in an unhealthful environment: Lifestyle challenges for children and adolescents. *Journal of the American Dietetic Association* 106:518, 2006.

   This article summarizes the diet and health challenges that youth face. Youth are bombarded with conflicting messages that support the overconsumption of unhealthful foods while at the same time stigmatizing obesity and promoting dieting and unrealistic thinness.

10. Gadding SS and others: Dietary recommendations for children and adolescents: A guide for practitioners. *Pediatrics* 117:544, 2006.

    The American Heart Association recognizes that the dietary patterns of children and adolescents put them at risk for cardiovascular diseases in adulthood and even during childhood. Age-appropriate recommendations are provided for total energy intake, dietary fats, added sugars, sodium, and physical activity. In addition, this article provides practical advice for health professionals and schools for encouraging compliance with the guidelines.

11. Greer FR: Groups compare CDC, WHO growth curves. *American Academy of Pediatrics News* 27 (9):1, 2006.

    The 2006 World Health Organization (WHO) growth standards have been compared to the Centers for Disease Control and Prevention (CDC) 2000 growth reference. New recommendations for the use of growth curves in the United States more similar to the WHO growth curves are likely. Using the WHO curves for infants 0-2 years of age indicates that fewer U.S. infants would be below the 5th percentile for weight-for-age and more U.S. infants would be above the 95th percentile.

12. Hatun S and others: Vitamin D deficiency in early infancy. *Journal of Nutrition* 135:279, 2005.

    Prevention of vitamin D deficiencies in infants is essential. This includes supplementing the diet of all breastfed infants with vitamin D soon after birth.

13. Hellekson K: Report on the diagnosis, evaluation, and treatment of high blood pressure in children and adolescents. *American Family Physician* 71:1014, 2005.

    Screening for high blood pressure is an important part of regular checkups of children by the child's physician. The latest recommendations for treating high blood pressure if found includes a diet rich in vegetables, fruit, and low-fat dairy products; low in salt; and moderate in high-calorie foods and drinks. Regular physical activity is also important, as is weight loss if needed.

14. Kirk S and others: Pediatric obesity epidemic: Treatment options. *Journal of the American Dietetic Association* 105:S44, 2005.

    Reducing calorie intake and increasing energy expenditure are important for treating pediatric obesity. Medications and obesity-related surgery may also be employed. The authors stress the importance of involving the family to create a supportive environment as part of the overall therapeutic approach.

15. Koplan JP and others: Preventing childhood obesity: Health in the balance: Executive Summary. *Journal of the American Dietetic Association* 105:131, 2005.

    Preventing childhood obesity involves a healthy eating pattern and regular physical activity. The goal should be achieving and maintaining a healthy body weight. The authors note that many social factors will have to be altered to facilitate this goal, such as providing more outlets for physical activity.

16. Kranz S and others: Dietary fiber intake by American preschoolers is associated with more nutrient-dense diets. *Journal of the American Dietetic Association* 105:221, 2005.

Children in general would benefit from diets higher in fiber. Improving diet choices will allow for this, including increasing whole-grain, fruit and vegetable content. The healthier the overall diet, the greater number of fiber-rich foods.

17. Lee LA, Burks W: Food allergies: Prevalence, molecular characterization, and treatment/ prevention strategies. *Annual Review of Nutrition* 26:539, 2006.

   This article precisely defines food allergies, presents statistics regarding prevalence of various allergies, details what is known about the biological mechanisms behind food allergies, and sets forth recommendations for their treatment and prevention.

18. Monsen ER: New findings from the Feeding Infants and Toddlers Study. *Journal of the American Dietetic Association* 106:S5, 2006.

   The Gerber-sponsored Feeding Infants and Toddlers Study (FITS), covered in several articles in this issue, examined usual intakes of nutrients from foods and supplements, as well as other dietary practices, with an emphasis on dietary habits of Hispanic infants and children. Findings of the study confirm that infants and toddlers do not consume enough fruits, vegetables, or fiber, and that intakes of total kilocalories, dietary fats, and sodium are on the rise.

19. Patrick H, Nicklas TA: A review of family and social determinants of children's eating patterns and diet quality. *Journal of the American College of Nutrition* 24(2):83, 2005.

   The physical environment has a big influence on the quality of the diets of children. Adding to this is the influence of the parents. To improve the diets of children then, the authors note that many parameters must be addressed: child, parents, school, and community.

20. Wiecha JL and others: When children eat what they watch: Impact of television viewing on dietary intake in youth. *Archives of Pediatrics and Adolescent Medicine* 160:436, 2006.

   This study of children in Boston found that increased television viewing was related to increased consumption of foods advertised during that viewing and increased total calorie intake over time. Each hour increase in television viewing was associated with a general increase of 167 kcal per day.

▶ ## Check out the **Contemporary Nutrition ARIS site**

www.mhhe.com/wardlawcontfa1 for quizzes, flash cards, other activities, and weblinks designed to further help you learn about issues surrounding nutrition from infancy through adolescence.

RATE YOUR PLATE

I. Getting Young Bill to Eat

Bill is 3 years old, and his mother is worried about his eating habits. He refuses to eat vegetables, meat, and dinner in general. Some days he eats very little food. He wants to eat snacks most of the time. Mealtime is a battle because Bill says he isn't hungry, and his mother wants him to eat a sit-down lunch and dinner to make sure he gets all the nutrients he needs and to eat everything served on his plate. He drinks five or six glasses of whole milk per day because that is the one food he likes.

When his mother prepares dinner, she makes plenty of vegetables, boiling them until they are soft, hoping this will appeal to Bill. Bill's dad waits to eat his vegetables last, regularly telling the family that he eats them only because he has to. He also regularly complains about how dinner has been prepared. Bill saves his vegetables until last and usually gags when his mother orders him to eat them. Bill has been known to sit at the dinner table for an hour until the war of wills ends. Bill's mother serves casseroles and stews regularly because they are convenient. Bill likes to eat breakfast cereal, fruit, and cheese and regularly requests these foods for snacks. However, his mother tries to deny his requests, so that he will have an appetite for dinner. Bill's mother comes to you and asks you what she should do to get Bill to eat.

Analysis

1. List four mistakes Bill's parents are making that contribute to Bill's poor eating habits.

   _____

   _____

   _____

   _____

2. List four strategies they might try to promote good eating habits in Bill.

   _____

   _____

   _____

   _____

628

II. Evaluating a Teen Lunch

The following are two typical teen lunches and nutritional information for each:

	Meal 1	Meal 2	Nutrient Needs for Teens
Meal 1	**Meal 2**		
2 pieces cheese pizza	1 large hamburger sandwich with condiments		
1 milk chocolate candy bar	30 French fries		
20 fluid ounces cola	20 Fluid ounces cola		
Energy (kcal)	990	1000	Males: 3000 Females: 2200
Protein	32	20	Males: 59 Females: 44
Vitamin C (milligrams)	5	18	Both genders: 45 to 75
Vitamin A (micrograms RAE)	300	10	Males: 900 Females: 700
Iron (milligrams)	3	4	Males: 11 Females: 15
Calcium (milligrams)	545	100	Both genders: 1300

1. Keeping in mind that meals should meet about one-third of nutrient needs, what are the shortcomings and excesses of these meals (i.e., given the nutritional information, compare these meals with one-third the RDA for protein, vitamin C, vitamin A, and iron and the Adequate Intake for calcium)?

_____

_____

_____

2. How would you change these meals to improve balance and to meet the nutrient needs above? (Hint: Use NutritionCalc Plus.)

_____

_____

_____

3. Reflect on your food choices as a teenager. Do you think your meal choices were balanced and varied? Why or why not? What could you have done to improve your nutritional habits at that time?

_____

_____

_____

CHAPTER 18 Nutrition During Adulthood

CHAPTER OBJECTIVES   Chapter 18 is designed to allow you to:

1. Discuss the causes of the principal nutrition-related problems seen in adults.

2. List biological changes that occur during the aging process, and discuss how these changes affect nutrient needs of older adults.

3. Make recommendations for dietary changes in the prevention and treatment of nutritional problems in older adults.

4. List several nutritional programs available to help meet nutritional needs of older adults.

CHAPTER OUTLINE

EATING IS ONE OF OUR GREAT PLEASURES. Guided by common sense and moderation, eating well is also a means to good health. Most of us want a long, productive life, free of illness. Yet, as the comic in this chapter suggests, many people from early middle age onward suffer from obesity, cardiovascular disease, hypertension and strokes, type 2 diabetes, osteoporosis, and other chronic diseases. We can slow the development of, and in some cases even prevent, these diseases by consuming a diet that works against them. The effect of such a diet is most profitable if we begin early and continue throughout adulthood. We serve ourselves best—as individuals and as a nation—by striving to maintain vitality even in the later decades of life. This concept was first explored in Chapter 1 and is discussed again in this chapter, along with the special nutrition needs of older persons.

Keep in mind that present day-to-day health practices can significantly influence health during later life. Although genetics does play a role, as discussed in Chapter 3, many of the health problems that occur with age are not inevitable; they result from diet-related disease processes that influence physical health. Much can be learned from healthy older people whose attention to a healthy diet and physical activity—along with a little luck—keeps them active and vibrant well beyond typical retirement years. Successful aging is the goal. Age quickly or slowly—it is partly your choice.

 Refresh Your Memory

As you begin your study of adult nutrition issues in Chapter 18, you may want to review:

- Implications of the 1994 Dietary Supplement Health and Education Act in Chapter 1
- The effect of genetics on health in Chapter 3
- The various body systems covered in Chapter 3
- The sources of fiber and sugar in Chapter 4
- Definition of healthy body weight in Chapter 7
- The dietary sources of vitamin D, the various B vitamins, and calcium in Chapters 10 and 11
- Recommendations for salt intake in Chapter 8
- The benefits of regular physical activity in Chapter 12

NUTRITION AND ADULTHOOD—
AN INTRODUCTION

Health conscious adults in North America are typically doing what is within their control to achieve a healthy lifestyle, such as consuming a healthful diet, maintaining a healthy body weight, and following a regimen of regular physical activity. Coupled with avoidance of tobacco products; limitation of or adaptation to stress; adequate sleep; adequate fluid intake; maintaining friendships and optimism; lifelong learning; keeping blood cholesterol, blood glucose, and blood pressure under control; and consultation with health care professionals on a regular basis, these actions contribute to a healthful, long life. Overall, the key to maximizing health throughout

Is a decline in health inevitable as we age? Which diet and lifestyle interventions have been shown to slow (or reverse) the aging process? Which nutrition problems are typically seen in older adults? How should one compensate for these? Chapter 18 provides some answers.

life is to establish harmony among one's physical, mental, psychological, and social states (see Part I in the "Rate Your Plate" section at the end of this chapter).

Based on the needs for various nutrients set by the Food and Nutrition Board, one's adult years can be divided into four stages: ages 19 to 30, 31 to 50, 51 to 70, and beyond 70 years of age. The two intervals encompassing ages 19 through 50 can be seen as young adulthood; 51 to 70 is middle-age adulthood; and beyond 70 years of age is older adulthood. Some examples of the dynamic nutrition needs of aging are:

▲ As we age, our nutrient needs change. For example, vitamin D needs are higher for older stages of adulthood.

- *Calcium.* Needs for this bone-related mineral increase after age 50 for males and females to help counter the harmful effects of accelerated bone loss.
- *Vitamin B-12.* After age 50, one should consume foods forti-fied with vitamin B-12 or take a balanced multivitamin and mineral supplement containing vitamin B-12. Recall from Chapter 8 that about 10% to 30% of older people may have decreased absorption of food-bound vitamin B-12 in part because of reduced acid production by the stomach.
- *Vitamin D.* Compared to the amount of vitamin D needed by individuals of ages 19 to 50, needs increase by 50% for the 51 to 70 age group. Adults over age 70 need *three times more* vitamin D than they did when they were ages 19 to 50. Attention to these differing needs for vitamin D is especially important if a person does not receive regular sun exposure, such as those residing the winter months in northern United States or Canada. Experts recommend that these older adults be checked yearly for vitamin D status.

▶ Keep in mind that extending life without delaying onset of chronic disease prolongs suffering in many cases. In addition, the greater number of disabled years is costly to all North Americans. For these reasons, prolonging life without compressing the number of disabled years is called the "failure of success."

Overall, attention to healthy nutrition and overall lifestyle habits is important at all ages. Providing dietary advice for adults ages 19 to 50 years is the focus of the beginning of Chapter 18; the chapter will then look at additional recommendations for adults 51 and older.

A DIET FOR THE ADULT YEARS

One diet approach that optimizes long-term nutritional health in adulthood emphasizes low-fat and fat-free dairy products, some lean meats and fish, plant proteins, a rich variety of fruits and vegetables, and generous amounts of whole-grain breads and cereals. MyPyramid, combined with the 2005 Dietary Guidelines for Americans discussed in Chapter 2, is one blueprint for this diet.

As noted in Chapter 2, the advice provided in those two resources refers to people two years and older:

- Consume a variety of nutrient-dense foods and beverages within and among the basic food groups of MyPyramid, while choosing foods that limit the intake of saturated and *trans* fats, cholesterol, added sugars, salt, and alcohol (if used). Foods to emphasize are vegetables, fruits, legumes (beans), whole-grain breads and cereals, and fat-free or low-fat milk or equivalent milk products.
- Maintain body weight in a healthy range by balancing calorie intake from foods and beverages with calories expended. For the latter, engage in at least 30 minutes of moderate-intensity physical activity, above usual activity, at work or home on most days of the week.
- Practice safe food handling when preparing food. This includes cleaning hands, food contact surfaces, and fruits and vegetables before preparation, and cooking foods to a safe temperature to kill microorganisms.

▲ Many adults find that regular physical activity adds an important dimension to their lives. Men over 40 and women over 50 years of age should obtain physician approval before beginning a program of vigorous physical activity. This is especially important for people with evidence of cardiovascular disease, hypertension, or diabetes.

▶ Appendix C reviews diet planning guidelines issued by the Canadian government for Canadians. In addition, Chapter 1 discussed *Healthy People 2010*, a U.S. federal agenda aimed at disease prevention and health promotion.

▲ A daily serving of a whole-grain breakfast cereal provides a rich source of vitamins, minerals, and fiber and so contributes to healthy aging.

▶ Not all nutrition and health researchers agree with the blanket guidelines set by major health and science institutions, as noted in Chapter 2. Some scientists do not think that general recommendations for the public can be justified especially for salt and cholesterol. Rather, they believe that these and certain other recommendations need to be individualized.

CRITICAL THINKING

The "fountain of youth" remains a mystery. Many people believe a source exists that can stop the aging process, allowing youth to remain. However, Neil, a history student, asserts that the fountain of youth is not a place or a particular thing but, rather, a combination of diet and lifestyle. How can he justify this claim?

Beyond those general recommendations, here are a few specific nutrition tips to help promote successful aging:

- Women of childbearing age need to eat iron-rich foods, primarily to avoid developing iron-deficiency anemia. In addition, women who could become pregnant are advised to consume foods fortified with folic acid (total of 400 micrograms per day) or to take a supplement containing it, in addition to consuming folate-rich foods. Recall from Chapter 11 that this practice reduces the risk of some serious birth defects.
- Adults who seldom eat dairy products or other rich sources of calcium need a calcium supplement.
- Adults who eat no animal foods may need to take a supplement containing vitamin B-12.
- All adults could benefit from limiting their use of cured and smoked foods (see the "Nutrition and Your Health" section on cancer in this chapter), obtaining adequate fluoride to promote dental health, and drinking plenty of fluids.

Some younger adults may benefit from a balanced multivitamin and mineral supplement to meet specific nutrient needs especially if on relatively low-calorie diets (i.e., less than 1600 kcals per day). In addition, sometimes vitamins or minerals are prescribed to meet nutrient needs for various medical purposes. For example, pregnant women or those with heavy menstrual periods may be advised to take an iron supplement. Still, supplements of some nutrients, such as vitamin A and selenium, can be harmful if taken in large amounts. Foods contain many phytochemical substances that promote health, so one should use MyPyramid as a starting point when planning a diet, rather than depending mostly on supplements to meet nutrient needs.

Are Adults Following Current Dietary Recommendations?

In general, adults in North America are trying to follow many of the diet recommendations listed. Since the mid-1950s, they have consumed less saturated fat as more people substitute fat-free and low-fat milk for cream and whole milk. However, they eat more cheese, usually a concentrated form of saturated fat. Since 1963, they have eaten less butter, fewer eggs, less animal fat, and more vegetable oils and fish. These changes generally follow the recommendations to reduce the intake of saturated fat and cholesterol in favor of unsaturated fat choices. Animal breeders are raising much leaner cattle and hogs than those produced in 1950, which also helps reduce saturated fat intake.

Other aspects of the average adult diet are less promising. The latest nutrition survey of eating habits in the United States shows that the major contributors of calories to the adult diet are white bread, beef, doughnuts, cakes and cookies, soft drinks, milk, chicken, cheese, alcoholic beverages, salad dressing, mayonnaise, potatoes, and sugars/syrups/jams. If the trend in diets were truly toward decreasing sugar and saturated fat intake, and increasing fiber intake, many of these foods would not appear at the top of the list.

The overriding consideration should be quality and length of life and the impact dietary changes might have on them. Adults in general should learn more about risk factors for chronic diseases and do something about each one, when possible.

CONCEPT CHECK

A basic plan to promote health and prevent disease includes eating a healthy diet. More specifically, the 2005 Dietary Guidelines for Americans directs people to eat a variety of foods; maintain healthy weight; choose a diet low in saturated fat and cholesterol and *trans* fat; choose a diet with plenty of vegetables, fruits, legumes (beans), and whole-grain products; use sugars and salt sparingly; and drink little or no alcohol.

A CLOSER LOOK AT MIDDLE AGE AND OLDER ADULTHOOD

How long do your family members generally live? Of those who died early in adult-hood, can you pinpoint some causes? Do you plan to live longer than your parents did or will? How long will that be? Some basic statistics can help you predict this.

Life Span

Life span refers to the maximum number of years a human can live. As far as we know, this hasn't changed in recorded time. The longest human life documented to date is 122 years for a woman and 114 years for a man. One's genes play a key role in deter-mining longevity, but environment is also important. By comparison, the domestic dog has a life span of 20 years; a rat, 5 years.

Life Expectancy

Life expectancy is the time an average person born in a specific year, such as 2007, can expect to live. Life expectancy in North America is about 75 years for men and about 80 years for women, with a span of "healthy years" of about 64. Furthermore, if you survive to the age of 80, you can tack on another 7 to 10 years of life expectancy.

Worldwide, the highest average life expectancy is in Japan, 82 years for women and 76 years for men, especially on the island of Okinawa. Researchers suggest that their traditional Okinawan diet based on rice, fish, vegetable protein sources, fruits, vegetables, tea, herbs for seasonings, and small amounts of meat, as well as a generally low calorie intake (BMI remains ≈ 21), contributes to this record longevity. Alcohol and salt intake is also minimal.

Life expectancy hasn't always been this long; for primitive humans, it was about 20 to 35 years. It increased to 40 years in Medieval England and increased to 49 years by the turn of the twentieth century. During the last 80 years, life expectancy for nearly all people has increased, mainly because of changes in the principal causes of death.

In the early 1900s, infectious diseases were the first three causes of death. Vaccines and antibiotics have tremendously lowered the rate of death from these causes. The decline in infant and childhood deaths, coupled with better diets and health care, has allowed more people to age first into maturity and then into older years. Now the principal causes of death in Western societies are related to cardiovascular diseases and cancer diseases that typically surface in middle age (review Table 1-2).

Historically, the trend in the United States, Canada, and other developed na-tions has been toward an ever older population. For example, during Colonial times, half of the U.S. population was over 16 years of age. By 1990, half were over 33. By 2050, half of the U.S. population could be over 43, and approximately 20% will be 65 years and older, twice as many as reach 65 today. This age—65 years—is arbitrarily listed as a dividing line for the beginning of later life because at this age, one can currently qualify for full Social Security benefits in the United States. The time at which old age occurs, however, varies for each person, according to health and independence.

Among the older population, the group constituting those aged 85+ years is the fastest growing segment. Between 1997 and 2050, the population aged 85+ years in the United States is expected to increase from 3.4 million to 19 million. This is the first time in history North America and other Western nations will need to ac-commodate such a large population of older people. The associated expense will be enormous if a large percentage need special care because of ill health. Even more amazing, 1 million or more people in the United States alone could be over 100 years old in 2050.

life span The potential oldest age a person can reach.

life expectancy The average length of life for a given group of people born in a specific year (such as this year).

▶ Besides having other long-lived family mem-bers, people who live to 100 years generally:

- Do not smoke, nor drink heavily
- Gain little weight in adulthood
- Eat many fruits and vegetables
- Perform daily physical activity
- Challenge their minds
- Have a positive outlook
- Maintain close friendships
- Are (or were) married (especially true for men)
- Have blood lipoproteins with a large particle size

▲ Of all North Americans who have lived to age 65, more than half are now alive.

▲ A diet based on vegetables, fruits, pasta, and olive oil as a source of fat—with a small amount of alcohol in the form of red wine—contributes to the many healthy years of life of southern Italians. Their active lifestyle is an additional contributing factor.

reserve capacity The extent to which an organ can preserve essentially normal function despite decreasing cell number or cell activity.

The Graying of North America

This "graying" of North America poses some problems. Although people older than age 65 account for 13% of the U.S. population, they account for more than 25% of all prescription medications used, 40% of acute care hospital stays, and 50% of the federal health budget. Hip fractures alone cost the nation about $12 billion per year. (Regular physical activity reduces such risk.) Of older persons, 65% or more have nutrition-related problems, such as cardiovascular disease, type 2 diabetes, hypertension, and osteoporosis.

Postponing these chronic diseases for as long as possible will help control health care costs. The more independent, healthy years people live, the better life can be for them and the less they burden the health care system, which will be increasingly burdened by a growing older population. Keep in mind that aging is not a disease. Furthermore, diseases that commonly accompany old age—osteoporosis and atherosclerosis, for example—are not an inevitable part of aging. Many can be prevented or managed. Some people do die of old age, not as a direct result of disease.

What Is Aging?

One view of aging describes it as a process of slow cell death, beginning soon after fertilization. When we are young, aging is not apparent because the major metabolic activities are geared toward growth and maturation. We produce plenty of active cells to meet physiological needs. During late adolescence and adulthood, the body's major task is to maintain cells. Inevitably, though, cells age and die. Eventually, as more cells die, the body can't adjust to meet all physiological demands, and body functioning begins to decrease (Fig. 18-1). Still, organs usually retain enough **reserve capacity** that, for a long time, the body shows no outward disease. Although no symptoms appear, subclinical disease may develop, and, if the disease is allowed to progress unchecked, organ function and then body function eventually deteriorate noticeably.

The aging process is clearly illustrated by changes for many people in the function of the enzyme lactase. For some people, lactase activity in the small intestine slows during childhood. Generally, however, clear symptoms of this decline—gas and bloating after milk consumption—do not appear until adulthood. Although lactase output decreases in these cases, perhaps from birth, enough enzyme is present to digest the lactose consumed until adulthood.

FIGURE 18-1 ▶ Declines in physiological function seen with aging. The decline in many body functions is especially evident in sedentary people.

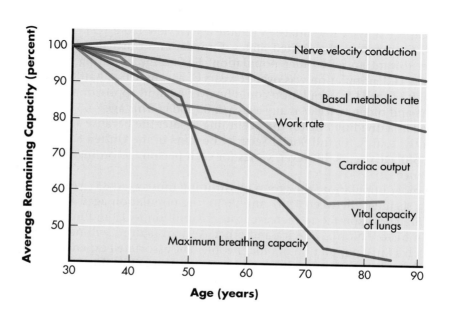

Cells age probably because of automatic cellular changes and environmental influences. Even in the most supportive of environments, cell structure and function inevitably change with time. Eventually, cells lose their ability to regenerate the internal parts they need, and they die. This predestined dying off of deteriorating cells is beneficial, as researchers have concluded it likely prevents diseases such as cancer.

Unfortunately, there are negative consequences to this natural cell progression, because as more cells in an organ system die, organ function decreases. For example, **kidney nephrons** are continually lost as we age. In some people, this loss leads to eventual kidney failure, but most of us maintain sufficient kidney cells to allow the organ to function throughout life. Again, in aging, there is first a reduction in reserve capacity. Only after the reserve capacity is exhausted does organ function noticeably decrease.

The causes of aging are still a mystery. Most likely, the physiological changes of aging are the sum of natural processes, as listed in Table 18-1, and lifestyle practices. Even very healthy people have a shortened life expectancy if they are exposed to sufficient environmental stress, such as radiation and certain chemical agents (e.g., industrial solvents). Cell aging and diseases such as cancer are aggravated by environmental

kidney nephrons The units of kidney cells that filter wastes from the bloodstream and deposit them into the urine.

glycosylation The process by which glucose attaches to (glycates) other compounds, such as proteins.

TABLE 18-1 Current Hypotheses About the Causes of Aging

Errors occur in copying the genetic blueprint (DNA).
Once sufficient errors in DNA copying accumulate, a cell can no longer synthesize the major proteins needed to function, and it therefore dies.

Connective tissue stiffens.
Parallel protein strands, found mostly in connective tissue, cross-link to each other. This decreases flexibility in key body components.

Electron-seeking compounds damage cell parts.
Electron-seeking free radicals can break down cell membranes and proteins. One way to prevent some damage from these compounds is to consume adequate amounts of vitamins E and C, selenium, and carotenoids.

Hormone function changes.
The blood concentration of many hormones, such as testosterone in men, falls during the aging process. Replacement of these and other hormones is possible, but the resulting risks and benefits are largely unknown.

Glycosylation of proteins.
Blood glucose, when chronically elevated, attaches to (glycates) various blood and body proteins. This decreases protein function and can encourage immune system attack on such altered proteins.

The immune system loses some efficiency.
The immune system is most efficient during childhood and young adulthood, but with advancing age, it is less able to recognize and counteract foreign substances, such as viruses, that enter the body. Nutrient deficiencies, particularly of protein, vitamin E, vitamin B-6, and zinc, also hamper immune function.

Autoimmunity develops.
Autoimmune reactions occur when white blood cells and other immune system components begin to attack body tissues in addition to foreign proteins. Many diseases, including some forms of arthritis, involve this autoimmune response.

Death is programmed into the cell.
Each human cell can divide only about 50 times. Once this number of divisions occurs, the cell automatically succumbs.

Excess calorie intake speeds body breakdown.
Experimentally, underfed animals, such as spiders, mice, and rats, live longer. Usual calorie intake must be reduced by about 30% to see this effect. This approach is the only proven way to substantially slow the aging process.

▲ Many older adults are healthy. The goal is to remain that way as long as possible.

▲ Older people benefit from aerobic and strength-training (resistance) exercises. Strength-training especially helps reverse some of the decline in daily function associated with the muscle loss typically seen in older adulthood.

factors, so it makes good sense to avoid such risks as excessive sunlight exposure and hazardous chemicals. Adopting diet and lifestyle practices that minimize a decline in body function in the adult years is an investment in your future health. You can obtain a free fact sheet on healthy aging from the website for the National Institute on Aging at **www.nia.nih.gov** or by calling (800) 222-2225. The first "Rate Your Plate" activity in this chapter outlines a comprehensive approach to healthful aging.

CONCEPT CHECK

Although life span has not changed, life expectancy has increased dramatically over the past century. In many societies, this means an increasing proportion of the North American population is over 65 years of age and will live for decades longer. Avoiding continually rising health care costs and maximizing satisfaction with life require postponing and minimizing chronic illness. Aging begins early in life and probably results from both automatic cellular changes and environmental influences. A healthy diet and regular physical activity can play a role in slowing such processes.

NUTRITIONAL IMPLICATIONS OF AGING

There is more variation in health status among adults over age 50 than in any other age group. This means that chronological age is not useful in predicting physical health status (physiological age). Among people age 70 and over, some are independent, healthy people, whereas others are frail and require almost total care. To predict the nutritional problems of an older person, it is necessary to know the extent of physiological change caused by aging and whether the person shows early warning signs for long-term poor nutrition. As you examine how aging affects body systems and how these changes contribute to nutritional health, note the suggested ways to lessen health risks (Table 18-2).

MAKING DECISIONS

Strength Training for Older Adults

Recommendations:

- Exercises should be performed at least two days per week.
- If weights are used, start with 1 to 2 pounds and gradually increase this amount over time.
- Perform exercises that involve the major muscle groups (e.g., arms, shoulders, chest, abdomen, back, hips, and legs) and exercises that enhance grip strength.
- Perform 8 to 15 repetitions of each exercise, then perform a second set.
- Breathe during strength exercises.
- Rest between sets.
- Avoid locking joints in arms and legs.
- Stretch after completing all exercises.
- Stop exercising if pain begins.

Source: National Institute on Aging.

Medications Influence Nutrient Needs

Medications and old age often go together. Medications can improve health and quality of life, but some of them also profoundly affect nutrient needs at all ages, including the later years. Two-thirds of older adults take prescription drugs; one-half of the older adult population regularly takes multiple prescription drugs. Many drugs affect appetite or the absorption of nutrients. Often, people must take medications for long

TABLE 18-2 Typical Physiological Changes of Aging and Recommended Diet and Lifestyle Responses

Physiological Changes	Recommended Responses
Appetite ↓	• Monitor weight and strive to eat enough to maintain healthy weight. • Use meal replacement products, such as Boost® and Ensure Plus®.
Sense of taste and smell ↓	• Vary the diet. • Experiment with herbs and spices.
Chewing ability ↓	• Work with a dentist to maximize chewing ability. • Modify food consistency as necessary. • Eat calorie-rich snacks.
Sense of thirst ↓	• Consume plenty of fluid each day. • Stay alert for evidence of dehydration (e.g., minimal output or dark-colored urine). • Dehydration can lead to many problems, especially in older adults.
Bowel function ↓	• Consume enough fiber daily, choosing primarily fruits, vegetables, and whole-grain breads and cereals. • Meet fluid needs.
Lactase production ↓	• Limit milk serving size at each use. • Substitute yogurt or cheese for milk. • Use reduced-lactose or lactose-free products. • Seek nondairy calcium sources.
Iron status ↓	• Include some lean meat and iron-fortified foods in the diet. • Ask physician to monitor blood iron status.
Liver function ↓	• Consume alcohol in moderation, if at all. • Avoid consuming excess vitamin A.
Insulin function ↓	• Maintain healthy body weight. • Perform regular physical activity.
Kidney function ↓	• If necessary, work with physician and registered dietitian to modify protein and other nutrients in diet.
Immune function ↓	• Meet nutrient needs, especially protein, vitamin E, vitamin B-6, and zinc. • Perform regular physical activity.
Lung function ↓	• Avoid tobacco products. • Perform regular physical activity.
Vision ↓	• Regularly consume sources of carotenoids, vitamin C, vitamin E, and zinc (e.g., fruits, vegetables and whole-grain breads and cereals). • Moderate total fat intake. • Wear sunglasses in sunny conditions. • Avoid tobacco products. • Perform regular physical activity (to lessen insulin resistance). • In the case of diagnosed moderate macular degeneration, talk with a physician about following a protocol of zinc, copper, vitamin E, vitamin C, and beta-carotene supplementation.
Lean tissue ↓	• Meet nutrient needs, especially protein and vitamin D. • Perform regular physical activity, including strength training.
Cardiovascular function ↓	• Use diet modifications or physician-prescribed medications to keep blood lipids and blood pressure within desirable ranges. • Stay physically active. • Achieve and maintain a healthy body weight.
Bone mass ↓	• Meet nutrient needs, especially calcium and vitamin D (regular sun exposure helps meet needs for vitamin D). • Perform regular physical activity, especially weight-bearing exercise. • Women should consider use of approved osteoporosis medications at menopause. • Remain at a healthy weight (especially avoid unneeded weight loss).
Mental function ↓	• Meet nutrient needs, especially for vitamin E, vitamin C, vitamin B-6, folate, and vitamin B-12. • Strive for lifelong learning. • Perform regular physical activity. • Obtain adequate sleep.
Fat stores ↑	• Avoid overeating. • Perform regular physical activity.

Registered dietitians, physicians, and pharmacists can help with any needed adjustments arising from these and other drug-related problems.

periods. They should make sure to work with their physician and pharmacist to co-ordinate all medications taken. Pharmacists can advise when to take drugs—with or between meals—for maximum effectiveness.

Drug-related nutritional problems include:

- Increased need for potassium when certain types of diuretics increase its excretion from the body
- Changes in appetite caused by certain antidepressant agents and antibiotics
- Increased iron needs due to blood loss from the long-term use of aspirin or aspirin-like medications

Alternative Medicine and Aging

Adults in general and older adults in particular may be interested in using various herbal remedies. Recall from Chapter 1 that these products are not evaluated by FDA for effectiveness or safety since they fall under the regulation of the 1994 Dietary Supplement Health and Education Act (DSHEA). Purity and quantity of the product in the bottle are also suspect. Table 18-3 reviews some popular herbal remedies. Note from the table that these products can pose health risks in certain people. In addition, they may be expensive, ($100 per month or more in some cases) and are not covered by health insurance plans. Use of many herbal products has declined because of expense and questionable benefits. In 2003, sales of ginseng and St. John's wort declined by 30% and 38%, respectively.

A rational approach to the use of herbal products is to use only one product at a time, keep a diary of symptoms, and check with one's physician first before discontinuing a prescribed medication. In addition, FDA advises anyone who experiences

▶ Numerous reports have documented significant health risks associated with the use of some herbal and alternative remedies, sometimes resulting in death. Studies especially implicate germander, pokeroot, sassafras, mandrake, pennyroyal, comfrey, chaparral, yohimbe, lobelia, jin bu huan, kava kava, products containing stephanie and magnolia, senna, hai gen fen, paraguay tea, kombucha tea, tung shueh (Chinese black balls), and willow bark.

TABLE 18-3 A Close Look at Some Popular Herbal Remedies

Product	Purported Effects	Side Effects	Who Should Especially Seek Physician Guidance Before Use
Black cohosh	• Mild reduction of postmenopausal symptoms (shown to be effective in some but not all women; use should not go beyond 6 months in general)	• Nausea • Fall in blood pressure	• Women who have had breast cancer • Pregnant women • Anyone taking estrogen, hypertension medications, or blood-thinning medications*
Cranberry	• Prevention or treatment of urinary tract infections (some evidence of efficacy)	• Use of concentrated tablets may increase risk of kidney stones	• People susceptible to kidney stones • Anyone taking antidepressants or prescription painkillers
Echinacea	• Stimulation of the immune system • Prevention or treatment of colds or other infections (mild effect at best)	• Nausea • Skin irritation • Allergic reactions • Minor GI tract upset • Increased urination	• Anyone with an autoimmune disease • Pre- or postsurgical patients • Anyone with allergies to daisies
Garlic	• Antibiotic properties • Slight reduction of blood cholesterol or blood pressure in some, but not all, studies	• GI tract upset (e.g., heartburn, flatulence) • Unpleasant odor	• Pre- or postsurgical patients • Perinatal women • People with a history of gallstones • Anyone taking blood-thinning medications or AIDS medications
Ginkgo biloba	• Increased circulation • Improvement of memory (especially for people with Alzheimer's disease; effect is mild at best)	• Mild headache • GI tract upset • Irritability • Reduced blood clotting • Seizures (if contaminated with toxic ginkgo seeds)	• People with bleeding disorders • Pre- or postsurgical patients • Anyone with allergies to the plant • Concurrent use of feverfew, garlic, ginseng, dong quai, or red clover • Anyone taking diabetes medications, blood-thinning medications, vitamin E supplements, antidepressants, or diuretics

This is continued from previous table.

TABLE 18-3 *(continued)*

Product	Purported Effects	Side Effects	Who Should Especially Seek Physician Guidance Before Use
Ginseng	• Increased energy • Stress relief • Decreased weakness and fatigue (efficacy largely unknown)	• Hypertension • Asthma attacks • Irregular heartbeat • Insomnia • Headache • Nervousness • GI tract upset • Reduced blood clotting • Menstrual irregularities and breast tenderness	• Anyone who takes a prescription drug should consult a physician before using • Women on hormone replacement therapy • Women who have had breast cancer • Anyone with chronic GI tract disease • Anyone with uncontrolled hypertension • Anyone taking blood-thinning medications, diabetes medications, antidepressants, or heart failure medications
St. John's wort	• Alleviation of depression (mild effect at best)	• Mild GI tract upset • Rash • Tiredness • Restlessness • Increased sensitivity to sunlight	• Anyone who takes a prescription drug • People with UV sensitivity, including that induced by medications or other treatments** • People with bipolar disorder • Anyone recovering from a graft or organ transplant • Anyone taking ritalin, caffeine, HIV medications, heart failure medications, cholesterol-lowering medications, blood-thinning medications, chemotherapy, oral contraceptives, antidepressants, antipsychotic medications, or asthma medications
Valerian	• Alleviation of restlessness and other sleeping disorders that stem from nervous conditions • Reduction of anxiety (some evidence of efficacy)	• Impaired attention • Headache • Morning grogginess • Irregular heartbeat • GI tract upset • Disagreeable odor • Withdrawal delerium	• Anyone taking central nervous system depressants*** • Anyone who drinks alcohol • People about to operate heavy machinery or drive

Pregnant or breastfeeding women, children under 2 years of age, anyone over the age of 65 years, and anyone with a chronic disease should never take supplements unless under the guidance of a physician. A concern has been raised with regard to patients who abruptly end alternative medicines at the start of hospital treatments or deny that they are involved in alternative therapy. Interactions between alternative therapies and pharmaceutical drugs can be drastic and include complications such as delirium, clotting abnormalities, and rapid heartbeat, resulting in the need for intensive care. If these patients had disclosed their treatments, many of the complications could have been prevented. Experts recommend that, if time permits, patients stop taking herbal products for about a week before a scheduled surgery or otherwise take all original supplement containers to the hospital, so that the anesthesiologist can evaluate what was taken.

*Coumadin, aspirin, Heparin, Lovenox, or Fragmin

**Sulfa medications, anti-inflammatory medications, or acid-reflux medications

***Valium, halcion, seconal

adverse side effects from an herbal remedy to contact a physician. Physicians are then encouraged to report such adverse events to FDA, state and local health departments, and consumer protection agencies.

For additional information about herbal remedies, access the following websites. These are regularly updated and cover the herbals listed in Table 18-3, as well as many others.

Alternative Medicine Foundation
www.amfoundation.org/
National Institutes of Health National Center for Complementary and Alternative Medicine (NCCAM)
nccam.nih.gov/
American Botanical Council
abc.herbalgram.org/
Complementary and Alternative Medicine Program at Stanford (CAMPS)
camps.stanford.edu/
National Institutes of Health Office of Dietary Supplements
ods.od.nih.gov/
Natural Medicines Comprehensive Database
www.naturaldatabase.com

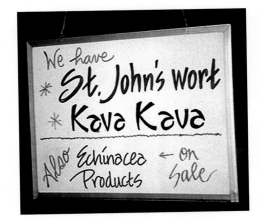

▲ Some herbal products are effective for treating specific medical problems. Follow label instructions carefully. Note potential side effects listed, as well as who should not use the product. The best advice is to only use these substances under strict supervision of a physician.

CRITICAL THINKING

Jamila went to her local pharmacy yesterday to look for a product to help her stay awake while studying. On the shelves she found a dietary supplement claiming to be a Chinese herbal remedy for sleepiness and fatigue. She thought that because a pharmacy carried the product, it should be safe and work as indicated on the label.

Is she correct in these assumptions? Are there specific risks associated with taking such herbal remedies?

▶ **Ten Warning Signs of Alzheimer's Disease**

1. Recent memory loss that affects job performance
2. Difficulty performing familiar tasks
3. Problems with language
4. Disorientation to time and place
5. Faulty or decreased judgment
6. Problems with abstract thinking
7. Tendency to misplace things
8. Changes in mood or behavior
9. Changes in personality
10. Loss of initiative

Depression in Older Adults

Depression occurs in about 12% to 30% of nursing home residents and 17% to 37% of older adults who reside outside of nursing homes. Depression—combined with isolation and loneliness as family and friends die, move away, or become less mobile—frequently contributes to apathetic eating and weight loss. Often, this becomes a downward spiral in which poor appetite produces weakness, which leads to even poorer appetite (Fig. 18-2). People living alone do not necessarily make poor food choices, but they often consume too few calories or nutrients, due in part to skipped meals. Older men are especially prone to these habits. In older adults, the resulting poor nutritional state can produce further mental confusion and increased isolation and loneliness.

If depression is left untreated, it is estimated that 15% of the cases may be fatal (suicide). Depression may signal an underlying illness and can also impair recovery from existing illnesses or injuries. For these reasons, early detection of depression is important in older adults. Depression is often treatable, but medication alone will not help those experiencing major life changes, such as the death of a spouse. Adequate social support also is essential.

MAKING DECISIONS

Alzheimer's disease

Alzheimer's disease often takes a terrible toll on the mental and eventual physical health of older people. About 4.5 million adults in the United States have the disease. In general terms, Alzheimer's disease is a type of dementia best described as a progressive brain disorder marked by an inability to remember, reason, or comprehend. The ten warning signs of Alzheimer's disease are listed in the margin. Age is the primary risk factor. Scientists propose causes, including alterations in cell development or protein production in the brain, strokes, altered composition of lipoproteins in the blood (e.g., apo E4), as well as poor blood glucose regulation (e.g., diabetes), high blood pressure, and high blood cholesterol.

Meeting needs for vitamin B-6, folate, and vitamin B-12 is especially important because elevated blood homocysteine is also a risk factor. Vitamins C and E are also important as antioxidants. For caregivers, several nutrition recommendations should be considered in meal preparation. Food intake should be monitored to ensure maintenance of a healthy weight and nutritional state. Other tips are consuming fruits and vegetables in abundance, including fish in meals twice per week, minimizing saturated and *trans* fat intake, and making sure meal habits do not pose a health risk (e.g., holding food in one's mouth or forgetting to swallow). Regular physical activity has also been shown to improve mental status in people afflicted by this disease. Four medications (e.g., donepezil [Aricept®]) have been approved to treat the disease; their effects are modest at best.

Preventive measures for Alzheimer's disease focus on maintaining brain activity through lifelong learning. Experimental therapies include regular use of ibuprofen. Studies cast doubt on other popular approaches, such as megadose vitamin E use. To find out more about Alzheimer's disease, you can go to the website for the Alzheimer's Association at www.alz.org, or call (800) 272-3900. You can also call the Alzheimer's Disease Education and Referral Center of the National Institute of Aging at (800) 438-4380.

CONCEPT CHECK

Nutritional problems common to aging adults relate to both the process of chronic diseases and the normal decrease in organ function that occurs with time. These organ systems and functions can decrease as we age: appetite; sense of taste, smell, thirst, hearing, and sight; digestion and absorption; liver, gallbladder, pancreatic, kidney, lung, and heart function; and the immune system. In addition, bone mass and muscle mass gradually decrease, the latter largely because of a deficient diet and inactivity. Appropriate dietary changes and regular physical activity can often help reduce the impact of these results of aging.

Social isolation; perhaps spouse has died.

Loses interest in food: diet deteriorates.

Poor diet leads to weakness; this increases a feeling of isolation and abandonment.

Further isolation can then decrease desire for self-care.

Health declines visibly; weakness remains.

Self-care is seriously hampered.

FIGURE 18-2 ▶ The decline of health often seen in older adults. A small change leads to a chain of events or "domino effect" that results in poor health. This decline needs to be prevented whenever possible.

NUTRITION IMPLICATIONS OF ALCOHOL CONSUMPTION

Given the wide spectrum of alcohol use and abuse, knowledge of alcohol consumption and its relationship to overall health is essential to the study of nutrition. Alcoholic beverages contain the chemical form of alcohol known as **ethanol**. Although not a nutrient *per se*, alcohol is a source of calories (about 7 kcal per gram) for approximately half of adults, constituting about 3% of total calories in the average North American diet (Table 18-4).

Moderate consumption of alcohol by a person of legal age is an acceptable practice and even has some health benefits. However, only about half of alcohol consumed is done so in moderation. Nearly 14 million people in the United States suffer from

ethanol Chemical term for the form of alcohol found in alcoholic beverages.

TABLE 18-4 Alcohol, Carbohydrate, and Calorie Content of Alcoholic Beverages*

Beverage	Amount (fluid ounces)	Alcohol (grams)	Carbohydrates (grams)	Calories (kcal)
Beer				
Regular	12.0	13	13	146
Light	12.0	11	5	99
Distilled Spirits				
Gin, rum, vodka, bourbon, whiskey (80 proof), brandy, cognac	1.5	14	—	96
Wine				
Red	5	14	2	102
White	5	14	1	100
Dessert, sweet	5	23	17	225
Rosé	5	14	2	100
Mixed Drinks				
Manhattan	3.0	26	3	191
Martini	3.0	27	—	189
Bourbon and soda	3.0	11	—	78
Whiskey sour	3.0	14	113	144

*There is little to no fat or protein contribution to calorie content.

Source: USDA.

▲ One standard drink is universally defined as one 12-oz bottle of beer or wine cooler, one 5-ounce glass of wine, 3 ounces of sherry or liqueur, or 1.5 ounces of 80-proof distilled spirits.

▲ Of all the alcohol sources, red wine in moderation is often singled out as the best choice because of the added bonus of the many phytochemicals present (e.g., resveratrol). These are leached out from the grape skins as the red wine is fermented. Dark beer is also a source of phytochemicals.

▶ Alcohol proof represents twice the volume of alcohol in percentage terms. Thus, 80 proof vodka is 40% alcohol.

alcohol dehydrogenase An enzyme used in alcohol (ethanol) metabolism that converts alcohol into acetaldehyde.

acetaldehyde dehydrogenase An enzyme used in ethanol metabolism that eventually converts acetaldehyde into carbon dioxide and water.

alcoholism, and another 31.9 million engage in binge drinking. Alcohol by far is the most commonly abused drug.

How Alcoholic Beverages are Produced

The basis of alcohol production is fermentation, a process by which microorganisms break down simple sugars (e.g., glucose or maltose) to alcohol, carbon dioxide, and water in the absence of oxygen. High-carbohydrate foods especially encourage the growth of yeast, the microorganism responsible for alcohol production. Wine is formed by the fermentation of grape or other fruit juices. Beer is made from malted cereal grain. Distilled spirits (e.g., vodka, gin, whiskey) are made from any number of fruits, vegetables, and grains. Production temperatures, the composition of the food used for fermentation, and aging techniques determine the characteristics of the product.

Absorption and Metabolism of Alcohol

Alcohol requires no digestion. It is absorbed rapidly from the GI tract by diffusion, making it the most efficiently absorbed of all calorie sources. Once absorbed, alcohol is freely distributed into all the fluid compartments within the body. About 1% to 3% of alcohol is excreted via urine and about 1% to 5% evaporates via the breath, the basis for the breathalyzer test. Most alcohol (90% to 98%), however, is metabolized. The liver is the primary site for alcohol metabolism, and some may also be metabolized by the cells lining the stomach. The main pathway of alcohol metabolism involves the enzymes **alcohol dehydrogenase** and **acetaldehyde dehydrogenase**. Alcohol cannot be stored in the body, so it takes absolute priority over other energy sources for metabolism.

As a person's alcohol consumption exceeds the body's capacity to metabolize it, blood alcohol concentration rises, the brain is exposed to alcohol, and symptoms of intoxication appear (see Table 18-5). Absorption and metabolism of alcohol depend on numerous factors: gender, race, body size, physical condition, meal composition,

TABLE 18-5 Blood Alcohol Concentration and Symptoms

Concentration*	Sporadic Drinker	Chronic Drinker	Hours for Alcohol to Be Metabolized**
50 (party high) (0.05%)	Congenial euphoria; decreased tension; noticeable impairment in driving and coordination	No observable effect	2–3
75 (0.075%)	Gregarious	Often no effect	3–4
80 to 100 (0.08%–0.1%)	Uncoordinated; 0.08% is legally drunk (as in drunk driving) in the United States and Canada.	Minimal signs	4–6
125–150 (0.125%–0.15%)	Unrestrained behavior; episodic uncontrolled behavior	Pleasurable euphoria or beginning of uncoordination	6–10
200–250 (0.2%–0.25%)	Alertness lost; lethargic	Effort is required to maintain emotional and motor control	10–24
300–350 (0.3%–0.35%)	Stupor to coma	Drowsy and slow	10–24
>500 (>0.5%)	Some will die	Coma	>24

*Milligrams of alcohol per 100 milliliters of blood.

**For a social drinker, alcohol metabolism is somewhat faster in chronic alcohol abusers.

Modified from Wyngaarder JB, Smith LH: *Cecil Textbook of Medicine*, fourth edition, Philadelphia, 1988, WB Saunders. Used with permission.

rate of gastric emptying, the alcohol content of the beverage, use of certain drugs, chronic alcohol abuse, and even how much sleep one has had. Women absorb and metabolize alcohol differently than men. The amount of alcohol metabolized by the cells lining the stomach is greater in men than in women. Women also have less body water in which to dilute the alcohol than do men. Overall, women develop alcohol-related ailments, such as cirrhosis of the liver, more rapidly than men do with the same alcohol-consumption habits.

Benefits of Moderate Alcohol Use

When used in moderation, alcohol is linked to several health benefits. Benefits of alcohol use are associated with specific intakes of about one drink per day for men and slightly less than one for women. Socialization and relaxation are among the intangible benefits of moderate alcohol use by people of legal drinking age. In terms of physiological benefits, moderate drinkers experience lower risk of developing cardiovascular diseases and type 2 diabetes. Previous consumers of alcohol no longer experience the benefits of alcohol when consumption ceases. See Table 18-6 for additional benefits of alcohol consumption.

Risks of Alcohol Abuse

Despite the few benefits of regular, moderate use, the risks of **alcohol abuse** are more numerous and harmful. Although it is one of the most preventable health problems, excessive consumption of alcohol contributes significantly to 5 of the 10 leading causes of death in North America: heart failure, certain forms of cancer, **cirrhosis** of the liver, motor vehicle and other accidents, and suicides (review Table 18-6 for additional health risks). In the United States, about $185 billion is spent annually in terms of lost productivity, premature deaths, direct treatment expenses, and legal fees associated with alcoholism. Overall, alcohol abuse typically reduces a person's life expectancy by 15 years.

Alcoholic beverages have little nutritional value and, thus, nutrient deficiencies are a common result of alcoholism. The protein and vitamin content is extremely low, except in beer, where it is marginal. Iron content varies from drink to drink, with red wine ranking especially high in iron. Typical deficiencies seen in alcoholism arise mostly from poor nutrient intakes, but increased urinary losses and fat malabsorption (linked to poor pancreatic function) are also to blame. Vitamins most susceptible to depletion in alcoholism include vitamins A, D, E, and K; thiamin; niacin; folate; vitamin B-6 and B-12; and vitamin C. Mineral deficiencies of calcium, phosphorus, potassium, magnesium, zinc, and iron are possible. On the other hand, vitamin and mineral toxicity is also of concern. Damage to the GI tract and liver, as well as high levels of some minerals in alcoholic beverages, may lead to toxicity of vitamin A, iron, lead, or cobalt. In nutritional treatment of alcoholism, the immediate aim is eliminating alcohol intake, followed by replenishment of nutrient stores.

Alcohol dependence is the most common psychiatric disorder, affecting 13% of the North American population. Studies suggest that about 40% of a person's risk for developing alcoholism comes from genetic factors, although the gene or genes have not been identified. Therefore, people with a family history of alcoholism, particularly children of alcoholics, should be especially aware of their alcohol consumption.

Early diagnosis of **alcoholism** can prevent multiple health problems and save millions in health care costs. Asking a person about the quantity and frequency of alcohol consumption is an important means of detecting abuse and dependence (see the margin note on the CAGE questionnaire on p. 647). Alcoholics may exhibit some or all of the following criteria:

- Physiologic dependence on alcohol with evidence of withdrawal symptoms when intake is interrupted
- Tolerance to the effects of alcohol, prompting greater alcohol intake to achieve the desired effect

▲ There is no such thing as controlled drinking once a person has alcoholism. Total abstinence is mandatory for recovery.

alcohol abuse Excessive alcohol consumption that leads to severe alcohol-related health and other problems, such as recurrent sickness, inability to fulfill major obligations, use in hazardous situations (e.g., driving), related legal problems, or use despite social and interpersonal difficulties.

cirrhosis A loss of functioning liver cells, which are replaced by nonfunctioning connective tissue. Any substance that poisons liver cells can lead to cirrhosis. The most common cause is a chronic, excessive alcohol intake. Exposure to certain industrial chemicals also can lead to cirrhosis.

alcohol dependence The person experiences repeated alcohol-related difficulties, such as an inability to control use, spending a great deal of time associated with alcohol use, continued use of alcohol despite physical or psychological consequences, persistent desire or unsuccessful efforts to cut down or control alcohol use, and withdrawal symptoms. Tolerance is also seen.

alcoholism As defined by the American Medical Association, an illness characterized by significant impairment directly related to persistent and excessive use of alcohol.

CRITICAL THINKING

For many people, drinking and smoking go hand-in-hand. What risks and diseases could correlate with the combination of these behaviors?

TABLE 18-6 A Summary of Benefits and Risks of Alcohol Use

	Moderate Use*	Alcohol Abuse**
Coronary heart disease	Decreased risk of death in those at high risk for coronary heart disease-related death, primarily by increasing HDL-cholesterol in some people, decreasing blood clotting, and relaxing blood vessels	Heart rhythm disturbances, heart muscle damage, increased blood triglycerides, and increased blood clotting
Hypertension and stroke	Mild decrease in blood pressure; less ischemic stroke in people with normal blood pressure	Increased blood pressure (hypertension); more ischemic and hemorrhagic stroke
Peripheral vascular disease	Decreased risk due to reduced blood clotting	No benefit
Blood glucose regulation and type 2 diabetes	Decreased risk of developing type 2 diabetes; decreased risk of death from cardiovascular disease	Hypoglycemia; reduced insulin sensitivity; damage to pancreas (site of insulin production)
Bone and joint health	Some increase in bone mineral content in women, linked to estrogen output	Loss of active bone-forming cells and eventual osteoporosis (many nutrient deficiencies also contribute to this problem); increased risk of gout
Brain function	Enhanced brain function and decreased risk of dementia by increasing blood circulation in the brain	Brain tissue damage and decreased memory
Skeletal muscle health	No benefit	Skeletal muscle damage
Cancer	No benefit	Increased risk of oral, esophageal, stomach, liver, lung, colorectal, and breast cancer, to name a few (especially if the diet is deficient in the vitamin folate)
Liver function	No benefit	Fat infiltration and eventual liver cirrhosis, especially if a person is also infected with hepatitis C; iron toxicity
GI tract disease	Decreased risk of certain bacterial infections in the stomach	Inflammation of the stomach (and pancreas); absorptive cell damage leading to malabsorption of nutrients
Immune system function	No benefit	Reduced function and increased infections
Nervous system function	No benefit	Loss of nerve sensation and nervous system control of muscles
Sleep disturbances	Some relaxation	Fragmented sleep patterns; worsens sleep apnea
Impotence and decreased libido	No benefit	Contributes to the problem in both men and women
Drug overdose	No benefit	Contributes to the problem, especially in combination with sedatives
Obesity	No benefit	Increased abdominal fat deposition, contributes to weight gain as calories from alcoholic beverages quickly add up
Nutrient intake	May supply some B vitamins and iron	Leads to numerous nutrient deficiencies: protein, vitamins, and minerals
Alcoholism	No benefit. Due to risk for birth defects, even moderate alcohol use is not advised during pregnancy (see Chapter 16)	Increased risk of developing alcoholism, including the teenage and young adult years
Fetal health	No benefit	Variety of toxic effects on the fetus when alcohol is consumed by pregnant women (see Chapter 16)
Socialization and relaxation	Provides some benefit to socialization and leads to relaxation by increasing brain neurotransmitter activity	Contributes to violent behavior and agitation
Traffic deaths and other violent deaths	No benefit	Contributes to both traffic death and violent death

*About one drink per day for men and slightly less than one for women.

**The risks from alcohol abuse begin at an intake of more than two to three drinks per day for men or one to two drinks per day for women and all adults age 65 and older. Binge drinking (more than four drinks in a row for women or more than five drinks for men) can be especially harmful.

- Evidence of alcohol-associated illnesses such as alcoholic liver disease or irreversible brain damage exhibited by memory loss, inability to concentrate, and decline in intellectual functions
- Continued drinking in defiance of strong medical and social contraindications and disruptions in normal life
- Depression, blackouts, and impairment in social and occupational functioning

Other signs of alcoholism include: alcohol odor on the breath; flushed face and reddened skin; and nervous system disorders, such as tremors. Unexplained work absences, frequent accidents, and falls or injuries of vague origin are possible signs of alcoholism. Laboratory evidence (e.g., impaired liver function, enlarged red blood cells, and elevated triglycerides) are also helpful for diagnosis of alcoholism.

Older adults are uniquely vulnerable to alcoholism, perhaps due to an abundance of free time, social events involving drinking, loneliness, or depression. Common symptoms of alcoholism—trembling hands, slurred speech, sleep problems, memory loss, and unsteady gait—can be easily overlooked as signs of old age. Slower alcohol metabolism and decreased body water allow older adults to become intoxicated from a smaller amount of alcohol than their younger counterparts. As well, even small amounts of alcohol can react negatively with various medications used by older persons. The adverse health effects of drinking may be amplified in older adults, so people over the age of 65 should limit alcohol consumption to no more than one drink per day.

Once a diagnosis of alcohol abuse or dependence is established, a physician can arrange appropriate treatment and counseling for the person and family. Treatment of alcoholism often includes the use of certain medications, counseling, and social support. Total abstinence must be the ultimate objective. Alcoholics Anonymous (AA) or other reputable therapy programs can support alcoholics and their families as they recover from this devastating disease.

▶ The CAGE questionnaire is used to identify alcohol abuse. More than one positive response suggests an alcohol problem.

C: Have you ever felt you ought to *cut* down on drinking?

A: Have people *annoyed* you by criticizing your drinking?

G: Have you ever felt bad or *guilty* about your drinking?

E: Have you ever had a drink first thing in the morning to steady your nerves or get rid of a hangover (*eye-opener*)?

▶ Ethnicity plays an important role in both the probability of and health risks associated with alcohol dependency and abuse. Native Americans suffer the highest rates of unintentional injuries, suicide, homicide, and domestic abuse related to alcohol use. African-American alcoholics are at greater risk than other racial groups for tuberculosis, hepatitis C, HIV/AIDS, and other infectious diseases. Hispanic Americans are at particular risk for cirrhosis-related death.

MAKING DECISIONS

Liver Cirrhosis

Alcohol is most damaging to the liver. Cirrhosis develops in up to 20% of cases of alcoholism and is the second leading reason for liver transplants, affecting about 2 million people in the United States. This chronic and usually relentlessly progressive disease is characterized by fatty infiltration of the liver. Fatty liver occurs in response to increased synthesis of fat and decreased use of it for energy by the liver. Eventually, the enlarged fat deposits choke off the blood supply, depriving the liver cells of oxygen and nutrients. Liver cells can accumulate so much fat that they burst and die and are replaced by connective (scar) tissue. At this stage, the liver is deemed cirrhotic. Early stages of alcoholic liver injury are reversible, but advanced stages are not. Once a person has cirrhosis, there is a 50% chance of death within 4 years, a far worse prognosis than many forms of cancer. While no specific level of alcohol consumption guarantees cirrhosis, some evidence suggests that damage is caused by a dose as low as 40 grams per day for men (3 beers) and 20 grams per day for women (1½ beers).

▲ Alcohol is particularly damaging to the liver. Pictured are (a) healthy liver, (b) liver with cirrhosis. There is no cure for this disease except a liver transplant.

Guidance Regarding Alcohol Use

No government agencies recommend drinking alcohol. The 2005 Dietary Guidelines for Americans provides the following advice regarding use of alcoholic beverages:

- Those who choose to drink alcoholic beverages should do so sensibly and in moderation—defined as the consumption of up to one drink per day for women and older adults and up to two drinks per day for men.
- Alcoholic beverages should not be consumed by some individuals, including those who cannot restrict their alcohol intake, women of childbearing age who may become pregnant, pregnant and lactating women, children and adolescents,

▲ The limit for alcohol intake for older adults is one drink per day.

▶ *Healthy People 2010* set an important goal regarding alcohol use: Reduce by 25% the proportion of adults who exceed the guidelines for appropriate alcohol use (currently, 73% of those who consume alcohol).

▶ To learn more about alcoholism, visit these websites:

National Institute on Alcohol Abuse and Alcoholism; www.niaaa.nih.gov

American Society of Addiction Medicine; asam.org

American Self-Help Clearinghouse; mentalhelp.net/selfhelp.

individuals taking medications that can interact with alcohol, and those with specific medical conditions.

- Alcoholic beverages should be avoided by individuals engaging in activities that require attention, skill, or coordination, such as driving or operating machinery.

As the understanding of the relationship between drinking alcohol and health grows, registered dietitians and other health professionals can promote healthy lifestyles—not by encouraging indiscriminate drinking, but rather by reassuring adults that moderate alcohol consumption may have beneficial health outcomes.

CONCEPT CHECK

Alcohol is not an essential nutrient, but does supply calories for the body. It requires no digestion, and alcohol metabolism takes precedence over metabolism of the other energy-yielding nutrients. Alcohol is primarily metabolized in the liver by alcohol dehydrogenase and acetaldehyde dehydrogenase. A number of individual factors, such as gender, race, and body composition, determine how a person reacts to alcohol. Despite modest benefits of moderate alcohol use, alcoholism interferes with all aspects of family, professional, and social life. Excessive alcohol use increases the risk of hypertension, strokes, heart damage, birth defects, inflammation of the pancreas, brain damage, and malnutrition, to name a few. Treatment of alcoholism often includes the use of certain medications, counseling, and social support.

NUTRIENT NEEDS IN MIDDLE AGE AND OLDER ADULTHOOD

The latest RDAs and related standards for nutrients and calories include categories for both men and women 51 to 70 years of age and more than 70 years of age. Macronutrient needs do not change from young adults' needs, but needs for some micronutrients do. In addition, because the lifestyle of an active older person can differ considerably from that of a nursing home resident, establishing nutrient needs during these wide age ranges is problematic.

A well-planned diet that follows MyPyramid can meet all nutrient needs for healthy older people within about 1600 to 1800 kcal, except for probably vitamin D and vitamin B-12. Meeting the vitamin B-12 standard is aided by use of fortified foods, such as ready-to-eat breakfast cereals. The use of a balanced multivitamin and mineral supplement is especially helpful for meeting vitamin D needs if the person does not receive regular sun exposure. Any supplement used should be low in or free of iron, as it may have a pro-oxidant effect. Many nutrition experts recommend a daily balanced multivitamin and mineral supplement for older adults, especially for those 70 years of age and older. If rich calcium sources advised by MyPyramid are not consumed, the person would also need a calcium supplement, as typical multivitamin and mineral supplements contain little calcium (about 200 milligrams). Providing more calcium than that would greatly increase the pill size.

MAKING DECISIONS

Iron Needs of Older Adults

Postmenopausal women have iron needs that are the same as men, as they no longer lose iron in menstruation. Recall from Chapter 9 that men should not take a supplement containing iron unless they have evidence of iron-deficiency anemia, as they consume enough iron from foods and it can easily accumulate to toxic amounts in the body. This advice now applies to women, as they experience minimal iron loss in the postmenopausal state.

▶ Sodium needs for older adults are 1200 to 1300 milligrams per day. Older adults routinely consume at least this much sodium. Potassium needs are 4700 milligrams per day. Many older adults do not meet this goal.

Planning a Diet for People in Their Later Years

Recommended dietary practices for later years would be to increase the diet's nutrient density and to make sure fiber and fluid intake is adequate. In addition, some protein should come from lean meats to help meet protein, vitamin B-6, vitamin B-12, and zinc needs.

Singles of all ages face logistical problems with food: Purchasing, preparing, storing, and using food with minimal waste are challenging. Economy packages of meats and vegetables are normally too large to be useful for a single person. Many singles live in small dwellings, some without kitchens and freezers. Creating a diet to accommodate a limited budget and facilities and a single appetite requires special considerations. Following are some practical suggestions for diet planning for singles:

- If one owns a freezer, cook large amounts, divide into portions, and freeze.
- Buy only what one uses; small containers may be expensive, but letting food spoil is also costly.
- Ask the grocer to break open a family-sized package of wrapped meat or fresh vegetables and separate it into smaller units.
- Buy only several pieces of fruit—perhaps a ripe one, a medium-ripe one, and an unripe one—so that the fruit can be eaten over a period of several days.
- Keep a box of dry milk handy to add nutrients to recipes for baked foods and other foods for which this addition is acceptable.

Table 18-7 provides even more ideas.

Nutritional deficiencies and protein-calorie undernutrition have been identified among some aging populations, particularly those in nursing homes or long-term

▲ Great attention to food safety is also important for older adults. Chapter 15 provides advice on this topic, such as washing one's hands and work surface before preparing food.

▶ To learn about meal programs for senior citizens in your area, call the *Administration on Aging's Elder Care Locator*, (800) 677-1116. For general information on programs for older persons, visit the following websites: *National Institute on Aging*, www.nia.nih.gov; *American Geriatrics Society*, www.americangeriatrics.org/; and *Administration on Aging*, www.aoa.gov.

TABLE 18-7 Guidelines for Healthful Eating in Later Years

- Eat regularly; small, frequent meals may be best. Use nutrient-dense foods as a basis for menus.

- Use labor-saving devices and some convenience foods, but try to incorporate some fresh foods into daily menus.

- Try new foods, new seasonings, and new ways of preparing foods. Use canned goods in moderation or choose those low in sodium.

- Keep easy-to-prepare foods on hand for times when you feel tired.

- Have a treat occasionally, perhaps an expensive cut of meat or a favorite fresh fruit.

- Eat in a well-lit or sunny area; serve meals attractively; use foods with different flavors, colors, shapes, textures, and smells.

- Arrange kitchen and eating area so that food preparation and clean-up are easier.

- Eat with friends, relatives, or at a senior center when possible.

- Share cooking responsibilities with a neighbor.

- Use community resources for help in shopping and other daily care needs.

- Stay physically active.

- If possible, take a walk before eating to stimulate appetite.

- When necessary, chop, grind, or blend hard-to-chew foods. Softer, protein-rich foods (e.g., shredded meats, eggs) can be substituted for meat when poor dental function limits normal food intake. Prepare soups, stews, cooked whole-grain cereals, and casseroles.

- If your dexterity is limited, cut the food ahead of time, use utensils with deep sides or handles, and obtain more specialized utensils if needed.

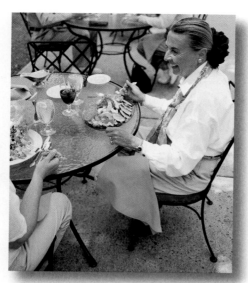

▲ As we age, some nutrient needs increase, whereas overall calorie needs decrease. Nutrient density is of utmost importance.

care facilities and those hospitalized. These nutritional problems increase the risk for many diseases, including bed sores (pressure ulcers), and compromise recovery from illness and surgery. Friends, relatives, and health care personnel should look for poor nutrient intake in all older people, including those who live in nursing home settings. Family members have a unique opportunity to make sure nutrient needs are met by looking for weight maintenance based on regular, healthful meal patterns. If problems arise in consuming a healthful diet, registered dietitians can offer professional and personalized advice.

Overall, good nutrition benefits older adults in many ways. Meeting nutrient needs delays the onset of some diseases; improves the management of some existing diseases; hastens recovery from many illnesses; increases mental, physical, and social well-being; and often decreases the need for and length of hospitalization.

Obtaining enough food may be difficult for some older persons, especially if they are unable to drive and relatives do not live close enough to help with cooking or shopping. For an older person, a request for help may be equated to a loss of independence. Pride, or fear of being victimized by those they hire, may stand in the way of much-needed help. In these cases, friends can be a big help. Special transportation arrangements may also be available through a local transit company or taxi service.

Many eligible older people are missing meals and are poorly nourished because they don't know of available programs to help them. Irregular meal patterns and weight loss, often caused by difficulties in preparing food, are warning signs that undernutrition may be developing. An effort should be made to identify poorly nourished people and inform them of community services.

COMMUNITY NUTRITION SERVICES FOR OLDER PEOPLE

hospice care A facility offering care that emphasizes comfort and dignity in death.

▶ **Determine:**
- **D**isease
- **E**ating poorly
- **T**ooth loss or mouth pain
- **E**conomic hardship
- **R**educed social contact and interaction
- **M**ultiple medications
- **I**nvoluntary weight loss or gain
- **N**eed for assistance with self-care
- **E**lder at an advanced age

Health care advice and services for older people can come from clinics, private practitioners, hospitals, and health maintenance organizations. Home health care agencies, adult day-care programs, adult overnight-care programs, and **hospice care** (for the terminally ill) can provide daily care.

The Nutrition Screening Initiative, a nutrition checklist for health care workers, family members, and older persons, can be used as a tool to increase health and nutrition awareness and to plan related education of older persons (Fig. 18-3). The Nutrition Screening Initiative uses the acronym "DETERMINE" (see margin) to help identify older people whose health needs require extra attention.

Nutrition programs for those age 60 and over in the United States include congregate meal programs, which provide lunch at a central location, and home-delivered meals (often known as Meals on Wheels if sponsored by the local private or public agencies). About 2.6 million older adults are served each year. About half of the meals use the home-delivered method.

The U.S. federal government sets specific standards for home-delivered meals and for those served in congregate feeding centers. The meals are designed to provide one-third of RDA/AI. The social aspect often improves appetite and general outlook on life.

Still, congregate meal programs generally provide one meal a day (some provide more) and usually just 5 days per week. Another problem with home-delivered meals is that the one or two meals delivered may never be eaten, and, if not eaten on delivery and left at room temperature, they may become unsafe to eat later. Thus, these programs can help older adults but probably don't meet all their nutritional needs.

In addition to congregate and home-delivered meals, federal commodity distribution is available in some areas of the United States to low-income older people.

A Nutrition Test for Older Adults

Here's a nutrition check for anyone over age 65. Circle the number of points for each statement that applies. Then compute the total and check it against the nutritional score.

Points	
2	1. The person has a chronic illness or current condition that has changed the kind or amount of food eaten.
3	2. The person eats fewer than two full meals per day.
2	3. The person eats few fruits, vegetables, or milk products.
2	4. The person drinks 3 or more servings of beer, liquor, or wine almost every day.
2	5. The person has tooth or mouth problems that make eating difficult.
4	6. The person does not have enough money for food.
1	7. The person eats alone most of the time.
1	8. The person takes three or more different prescription or over-the-counter drugs each day.
2	9. The person has unintentionally lost or gained 10 pounds within the last 6 months.
2	10. The person cannot always shop, cook, or feed himself or herself.
Total	

Nutritional score:

0–2: Good. Recheck in 6 months.

3–5: Marginal. A local agency on aging has information about nutrition programs for the elderly. The National Association of Area Agencies on Aging can assist in finding help; call (800) 677-1116. Recheck in 6 months.

6 or more: High risk. A doctor should review this test and suggest how to improve nutritional health.

FIGURE 18-3 ▶ A nutrition checklist for older adults.

Reprinted with permission by the Nutrition Screening Initiative, a project of the American Academy of Family Physicians, the American Dietetic Association, and the National Council on Aging, Inc., and funded in part by a grant from Ross Products Division, Abbott Laboratories.

▲ Help is available in most communities to assist older adults in daily tasks. This, in turn, helps older adults meet nutrient needs.

Food stamps can benefit older people whose incomes are below the poverty level (see Chapter 14 for details on these programs). Food cooperatives and a variety of clubs and religious and social organizations provide additional aid.

CONCEPT CHECK

Specific nutrient requirements for older adults are only now being extensively studied. Diet plans should be modified for decreased physical abilities, the presence of drug-nutrient interactions, possible depression, and economic constraints. Particular attention should be paid to the opportunity for sun exposure and intake of the vitamins D, B-6, E, folate, and B-12, as well as the minerals calcium and zinc and fiber. A nutrient-dense diet helps meet these needs. Carefully planned multivitamin and mineral supplement use can also help, especially for adults 70 years of age and older. In the United States, many nutrition services—such as congregate and home-delivered meals—are available to help the aging population obtain a healthful diet.

Cancer is the second leading cause of death for North American adults. It is further estimated that more than 1500 people die each day of cancer in the United States. Cancer-related expenses exceed $100 billion each year. The top four cancers, causing more than 50% of cancer deaths, are lung, colorectal, breast, and prostate cancers. Of those, lung cancer in female smokers is the only form increasing on a yearly basis.

Cancer is many diseases; these differ in the types of cells affected and, in some cases, in the factors contributing to cancer development (Fig. 18-4). For example, the factors leading to skin cancer differ from those leading to breast cancer. Similarly, the treatments for the different types of cancer often vary.

Cancer essentially represents abnormal and uncontrollable division of cells that results from mutations in DNA. This initiates the cancer process. The cells then go through a variety of steps (called promotion and progression). A cancer cell is the result. Without effective treatment, cancer then typically leads to death. Most cancers take the form of tumors, although not all tumors are cancers. A **tumor** is spontaneous new tissue growth that serves no physiological purpose. It can be **benign,** like a wart, or **malignant,** like most lung cancers. The terms *malignant tumor* and *malignant neoplasm* are synonymous with cancer.

Whereas benign tumors are only dangerous if their presence interferes with normal body functions, malignant (cancerous) tumors are capable of invading surrounding structures, including blood vessels, the lymph system, and nervous tissue. Cancer can also spread, or **metastasize,** to distant sites via the blood and lymphatic circulation, thereby producing invasive tumors in almost any part of the body. Metastasis then makes the cancer much more difficult to treat. That cancer can spread explains why early detection of cancer is so important. Cancers that can be diagnosed in the early stages are those in the colon, breast, and cervix.

Both genetics and lifestyle are potent forces that influence the risk for developing cancer. A genetic predisposition is especially important in development of colon cancer, some types of breast cancer (e.g., mutated BRCA1 or BRCA2 gene) and prostate cancer (35%, 27%, and 42%, respectively). About 30 cancer-susceptibility genes have been identified. However, experts estimate that only 1% to 5% of most cancers can be explained by the inheritance of a cancer gene. Overall, lifestyle is also a critical factor in most forms of cancer, as evidenced by the variation in cancer rates from country to country. In fact, diet likely accounts for 30% to 40% or more of all cancers.

Although we have little control over our genetic risks for cancer, we can exert a great deal of authority when making decisions about lifestyle risks, especially with regard to smoking, alcohol abuse, physical activity, and nutrient intake (food choice). It is well established that one-third of all

▲ Cruciferous vegetables such as cabbage and cauliflower are rich in cancer-preventing phytochemicals.

tumor Mass of cells; may be cancerous (malignant) or noncancerous (benign).

benign Noncancerous; tumors that do not spread.

malignant Malicious; in reference to a tumor, the property of spreading locally and to distant sites.

metastasize The spreading of disease from one part of the body to another, even to parts of the body that are remote from the site of the original tumor. Cancer cells can spread via blood vessels, the lymphatic system, or direct growth of the tumor.

Estimated % of Cancer Deaths for 2004		
Male		Female
<1%	Brain	2%
4%	Esophagus and stomach	<1%
32%	Lung	25%
	Breast	15%
3%	Liver	<1%
5%	Pancreas	6%
9%	Leukemia and lymphomas	9%
10%	Colon and rectum	10%
6%	Urinary	
	Ovary	6%
10%	Prostate	
	Uterus and cervix	3%
25%	All others (e.g., oral and skin) (e.g., oral, skin, and bladder)	24%

FIGURE 18-4 ▶ Cancer is many diseases. Numerous types of cells and organs are its target. About one-third of all cancers arise from smoking (primarily lung cancer).

cancers in North America are due directly to tobacco use. About half of the cancers of the mouth, pharynx, and larynx are associated with heavy use of alcohol. A combination of alcohol use and smoking increases cancer risks even higher.

A CLOSER LOOK AT DIET AND CANCER

Some food constituents may contribute to cancer development, whereas others have a protective effect (Table 18-8). First the association between fat/calorie intake and cancer risk is discussed, and then some of the food constituents that may reduce the risk for cancer are presented.

Contribution of Calorie and Fat Intakes to Cancer Risk

An excess calorie intake, leading eventually to obesity, is related to all major forms of cancer, except of lung cancer. This is the

main diet-cancer risk factor. This includes cancer of the breast (especially in post-menopausal women), pancreas, kidney, gallbladder, colon, **endometrium**, and prostate gland. The link probably occurs between adipose tissue and the synthesis of estrogen. High concentrations of circulating estrogen in the blood over time promote cancer. Excess insulin output resulting from an obese, insulin-resistant state is also implicated.

The National Cancer Institute (NCI) also believes there is sufficient evidence for a link between dietary fat and cancer to encourage North Americans to reduce fat intake. It recommends initially decreasing dietary fat to about 30% of total calorie intake and eventually to 20% or less of total calories if the person is at high risk and can follow such a dietary pattern.

Some scientists, however, believe that the NCI has overreacted to the fat and cancer issue. Although epidemiological

endometrium The membrane that lines the inside of the uterus. It increases in thickness during the menstrual cycle until ovulation occurs. The surface layers are shed during menstruation if conception does not take place.

TABLE 18-8 Some Food Constituents Suspected of Having a Role in Cancer

Constituent	Dietary Sources	Action
Possibly Protective*		
Vitamin A	Liver, fortified milk, fruits, vegetables	Encourages normal cell development.
Vitamin D	Fortified milk	Increases production of a protein that suppresses cell growth, such as in the colon.
Vitamin E	Whole grains, vegetable oils, green leafy vegetables	Prevents formation of nitrosamines; general antioxidant properties.
Vitamin C	Fruits, vegetables	Can block conversion of nitrites and nitrates to potent carcinogens; likely has general antioxidant properties.
Folate	Fruits, vegetables, whole grains	Encourages normal cell development; especially reduces the risk of colon cancer.
Selenium	Meats, whole grains	Part of antioxidant system that inhibits tumor growth and kills developing cancer cells.
Carotenoids, such as lycopene	Fruits, vegetables	Likely act as antioxidants; some of these possibly influence cell metabolism. Lycopene in particular may reduce the risk of prostate cancer.
Indoles, phenols, and other phytochemical substances	Vegetables, especially cabbage, cauliflower, broccoli, brussels sprouts, garlic, onions, tea	May reduce cancer in the stomach and other organs.
Calcium	Milk products, green vegetables	Slows cell division in the colon, binds bile acids and free fatty acids, thus reducing colon cancer risk.
Omega-3 fatty acids	Cold-water fish, such as salmon and tuna	May inhibit tumor growth.
Soy products	Tofu, soy milk, tempeh, soy nuts	Phytic acid present possibly binds carcinogens in the intestinal tract; the genistein component possibly reduces growth and metastasis of malignant cells.
Conjugated linoleic acid	Milk products, meats	May inhibit tumor development and act as an antioxidant.
Fiber-rich foods	Fruits, vegetables, whole-grain breads and cereals, beans, nuts	Colon and rectal cancer risk may be decreased by accelerating intestinal transit of binding carcinogens such that they are excreted.
Possibly Carcinogenic		
Excessive calorie intake	All macronutrients can contribute	Excess fat mass leading to obesity; linked to increased synthesis of estrogen and other sex hormones, which in excess may themselves increase the risk for cancer. Resulting excess insulin output from creation of an insulin-resistant state is also implicated.
Total fat	Meats, high-fat milk and milk products, animal fats and vegetable oils	The strongest evidence is for excessive saturated and polyunsaturated fat intake. Saturated fat is linked to an increased risk of prostate cancer.
High glycemic load carbohydrates	Cookies, cakes, sugared soft drinks, candy	Insulin surges associated with these foods may increase tumor growth, such as in the colon.
Alcohol	Beer, wine, liquor	Contributes to cancers of the throat, liver, bladder, breast, and colon (especially if the person does not consume enough folate).
Nitrites, nitrates	Cured meats, especially ham, bacon, and sausages	Under very high temperatures will bind to amino acid derivatives to form nitrosamines, potent carcinogens.
Multi-ring compounds: Aflatoxin	Formed when mold is present on peanuts or grains	May alter DNA structure and inhibit its ability to properly respond to physiologic controls; aflatoxin in particular is linked to liver cancer.
Benzo(a)pyrene and other heterocyclic amines	Charcoal-broiled foods, especially meats	Linked to stomach and colon cancer. To limit this risk, trim fat from meat before cooking, cut barbecuing time by partially cooking meat (such as in a microwave oven), and don't consume blackened parts.

*Many of the actions listed for these possibly protective agents are speculative and have been verified only by experimental animal studies. The best evidence supports obtaining these nutrients and other food constituents from foods. The U.S. Preventive Services Task Force (USPSTF) supports this statement, noting there is no clear evidence that nutrient supplements provide the same benefits.

evidence does link fat and certain forms of cancer, the evidence is not strong. A stronger link exists between cancer and total calories in the diet. In animal experiments, restricting total calorie intake to about 70% of usual intake results in about a 40% reduction in tumor development, regardless of the amount of fat in the diet. Calorie restriction is the most effective technique for preventing cancer in laboratory animals.

Unfortunately, it is difficult for humans to reduce dietary calories to 70% of usual intake. So while the data obtained from laboratory animal studies are interesting, nutritionists do not see any practical way to make recommendations on the basis of these studies. In addition, once cancer is present, calorie restriction is no longer helpful.

Cancer-Inhibiting Food Constituents

Many single nutrients may have cancer-inhibiting properties. These anticarcinogens include antioxidants and certain phytochemicals (review Table 18-8).

The antioxidant activity of vitamin C and vitamin E helps to prevent formation of **nitrosamines** in the GI tract, thus preventing formation of a potent carcinogen. Vitamin E also helps protect unsaturated fatty acids from damage by free radicals. Overall, carotenoids, vitamin E, vitamin C, and selenium function as or contribute to antioxidant protection for the body. Some of these antioxidant systems help prevent DNA mutations by electron-seeking compounds, the main way that cancer develops in the first place.

In addition, phytochemicals from fruits and vegetables, and even tea, block cancer development in some types of cells. Numerous studies suggest that fruit and vegetable intake reduces the risk of nearly all types of cancer. These foods are normally rich in carotenoids, vitamin C, and vitamin E. Adequate vitamin D intake is suspected of reducing breast, colon, prostate, and other forms of cancer. Calcium is also linked to a decreased risk for developing colon cancer. In sum, a diet that follows MyPyramid, so that fruits, vegetables, whole grains, low-fat and fat-free dairy products, and some plant oils are eaten daily, is aimed at cancer prevention. It is likely that all of these foods have a "cocktail" effect, and that no one particular food can make as strong a claim.

THE BOTTOM LINE

A variety of dietary changes will reduce your risk for cancer. Start by making sure that your diet is moderate in calorie and fat content and that you consume many fruits and vegetables, whole-grain breads and cereals, beans, some fish, and low-fat or fat-free milk products. In addition, remain physically active; avoid obesity; consume alcohol in moderation (if at all); and limit intake of animal fat and salt-cured, smoked, and nitrate-cured foods.

Remember also that if a cancer is left untreated, it can spread quickly throughout the body. When this happens, it is much more likely to lead to death. Thus early detection is critical. Aids to early detection include the following warning signs (acronym is CAUTION):

- A change in bowel or bladder habits
- A sore that does not heal
- Unusual bleeding or discharge
- A thickening or lump in the breast or elsewhere
- Indigestion or difficulty in swallowing
- An obvious change in a wart or mole
- A nagging cough or hoarseness
  Unexplained weight loss is an additional warning sign.

There are still other ways to detect cancer early. Colonoscopy examinations for middle-age and older adults, PSA (prostate-specific antigen) tests for middle-age and older men, and Papanicolaou tests (Pap smears) and regular breast examinations (and mammograms starting about age 40) for women are recommended by the American Cancer Society. Finally, to learn still more about cancer, review these sources of credible cancer information on the Internet:

American Cancer Society
www.cancer.org
National Cancer Institute
www.cancer.gov
Oncolink
cancer.med.upenn.edu
Harvard University Center for Cancer
    Prevention
www.yourdiseaserisk.harvard.edu

nitrosamine A carcinogen formed from nitrates and breakdown products of amino acids; can lead to stomach cancer.

▶ **American Institute for Cancer Research Diet and Health Guidelines for Cancer Prevention**

1. Choose a diet rich in a variety of plant-based foods.
2. Eat plenty of vegetables and fruits.
3. Maintain a healthy weight and be physically active.
4. Drink alcohol only in moderation, if at all.
5. Select foods low in fat and salt.
6. Prepare and store food safely.

And always remember ...

Do not use tobacco in any form.

CASE STUDY

Dietary Assistance for an Older Adult

Frances is a 78-year-old woman who suffers from macular degeneration, osteoporosis, and arthritis. Since her husband died a year ago, she has moved from their family house to a small one-bedroom apartment. Her eyesight is progressively getting worse, making it hard to go to the grocery store or even to cook (for fear of burning herself). She is often lonely; her only son lives 1 hour away and works two jobs, but he visits her as often as he can. Frances has lost her appetite and, as a result, often skips meals during the week. She has resorted to eating mostly cold foods, simple to prepare but seriously limiting diet variety and palatability in her diet. She is slowly losing weight as a result of her dietary changes and loss of appetite.

Her typical diet usually consists of a breakfast that may include 1 slice of wheat toast with margarine, honey, and cinnamon, and 1 cup of hot tea. If she has lunch, she normally has ½ can of peaches, half of a turkey and cheese sandwich, and ½ glass of water. For dinner, she might have half of a tuna fish sandwich made with mayonnaise and 1 cup of iced tea. She usually includes one or two cookies at bedtime.

Answer the following questons, and check your responses in Appendix A.

1. What nutrients are likely to be inadequate in her current diet?
2. What potential effects will Frances' poor dietary pattern have on her health status?
3. Which physiological changes of aging will add to the effects of her poor diet (review Table 18-2)?
4. What services are available in the community that could help Frances improve her diet and possibly increase her appetite?
5. What other convenience foods could be included in her diet to make it more healthful and more varied?

SUMMARY

1. Most scientists agree upon diet recommendations for the general public, including those provided by MyPyramid and the 2005 Dietary Guidelines for Americans. Such authorities recommend that individuals eat a variety of foods; balance the food eaten with physical activity to maintain or improve weight; choose a diet with plenty of grain products, vegetables, and fruits; choose a diet low in saturated fat, *trans* fat, and cholesterol; limit sugars and salt; and moderate or avoid alcoholic beverage intake. Regular physical activity is also important as is safe food preparation. In addition, recommendations to reduce cancer risk also emphasize moderation in the use of cured and smoked meats.

2. Although maximum life span hasn't changed, life expectancy has increased dramatically over the past century. For many societies, this means that an increasing proportion of the population is over 65 years of age. As health care costs rise, the goal of delaying disease becomes ever important.

3. Aging begins before birth. Cell aging probably results from automatic cellular changes and environmental influences, such as DNA damage. Add to this list damage caused by electron-seeking free-radical compounds, high blood glucose, hormonal changes, and alterations in the immune system as possible causes.

4. Nutritional problems of older adults are related to the presence of chronic diseases and to the normal decreases in organ function that occur with time. These include loss of teeth, lessened sensitivity to taste and smell, changes in GI tract function, and deterioration in cardiovascular and bone health. Although disease affects nutritional state, the reverse is also true. Undernutrition adversely affects immune function, allowing for infection.

5. Scientists are only now beginning extensive study of specific nutrient needs for older people. Diet plans should be based on a nutrient-dense approach and individualized for existing health problems, decreased physical abilities, presence of drug-nutrient interactions, possible depression, and economic constraints. Specific nutrients, such as protein, vitamin D, vitamin B-6, folate, vitamin B-12, zinc, and calcium, along with fiber and fluid, often deserve special attention in diet planning. A balanced multivitamin and mineral supplement can be used to help meet needs, especially for adults age 70 years and older.

6. Health care workers and family members should use available options for the procurement of food for older adults, especially for those who are nutritionally compromised. Most communities have congregate or home-delivered meal systems, food stamps, and other provisions for those who qualify.

7. Alcohol use is a complex issue becaue it involves psychological, social, economic, health, legal, and family issues. Alcohol is metabolized in the liver and other tissues. The benefits of alcohol use are associated with low to moderate alcohol consumption. These benefits include the pleasurable and social aspects of alcohol use, a reduction in various forms of cardiovascular disease, increase in insulin sensitivity, and protection against some harmful stomach bacteria. Alcohol as the potential to worsen health as well. Excessive consumption of alcohol contributes significantly to 5 of the 10 leading causes of death in North America. Alcohol increases the risk of developing certain forms of heart damage, inflammation of the pancreas, GI tract damage, vitamin and mineral deficiencies, cirrhosis of the liver, certain forms of cancer, hypertension, and hemmorhagic stroke—to name a few. If alcohol is consumed, it should be consumed in moderation with meals. Women are advised to drink no more than one drink per day, as are adults 65 years and older; men are advised to limit intake to two drinks a day.

STUDY QUESTIONS

1. List three important points made by the 2005 Dietary Guidelines for Americans for the general population and give an example of why each one may be difficult for older adults to implement. What are some suggestions for overcoming these barriers?

2. What is the difference between life span and life expectancy?

3. List five general guidelines for cancer prevention.

4. Describe two hypotheses proposed to explain the causes of aging, and note evidence for each in your daily life experiences.

5. List four organ systems that can decline in function in later years, along with a diet/lifestyle response to help cope with the decline.

6. Defend the recommendation for regular physical activity during older adulthood, including some resistance activity (weight training).

7. How might the nutritional needs of older people differ from those of younger people? How are their needs similar? Be specific.

8. What three resources in a community are widely available to aid older adults in maintaining nutritional health?

9. Describe some warning signs of depression and note a possible nutritional implication as this problem advances.

10. List four warning signs of undernutrition in older people that are part of the acronym DETERMINE. Briefly justify the inclusion of each.

CHECK YOUR KNOWLEDGE

Answers to the following multiple choice questions are in Appendix A.

1. Among the older population of the United States, the age of the fastest growing segment is _____ years.
   a. 65
   b. 74
   c. 79
   d. 85+

2. The two key terms for adequate adult nutrition are
   a. varied and minimum amounts.
   b. colorful foods and abundance.
   c. varied and moderate amounts.
   d. similar and adequate.

3. The reason the incidence of obesity increases with age is that
   a. the basal metabolic rate decreases with age.
   b. physical activity often decreases with age.
   c. energy intake exceeds energy expenditure.
   d. All of the above.

4. The immune system becomes less efficient with age, so it is especially important to consume adequate _____ and _____, nutrients that contribute to immune function.
   a. vitamin A, vitamin B-6
   b. protein, zinc
   c. zinc, iodide
   d. vitamin A, vitamin K

5. Which of the following does not describe a physiological change of aging?
   a. decreases in digestion and absorption capacity
   b. reduction in lean body mass
   c. lower basal metabolism
   d. increase in taste sensitivity

6. To maintain optimal nutritional status and healthy weight, the diet of an older person should have a _____ nutrient density and be _____ in energy content.
   a. low, high
   b. low, low
   c. high, moderate
   d. high, high

7. Nutrition programs such as congregate meals or home-delivered meals provide which of the following?
   a. an improved nutritional status
   b. a social atmosphere
   c. an economical meal for low-income elderly
   d. All of the above.

8. During aging, the needs for vitamins and minerals
   a. continually fluctuate.
   b. greatly decrease.
   c. somewhat increase in some cases.
   d. greatly increase.

9. Alcohol is digested in the
   a. stomach.
   b. small intestine.
   c. liver.
   d. None of the above; alcohol requires no digestion.

10. Alcohol is most damaging to the
    a. brain cells because alcohol can be used as an energy source even before glucose.
    b. kidney cells because this is where alcohol is excreted.
    c. cells of the gastrointestinal tract because they are in direct contact with ingested alcohol.
    d. liver cells where alcohol is metabolized.

FURTHER READINGS

1. ADA Reports: Position of the American Dietetic Association: Nutrition across the spectrum of aging. *Journal of the American Dietetic Association* 105:616, 2005.

   Behaviors such as a healthful diet, being physically active, and not using tobacco in any form are three keys to healthful aging. The American Dietetic Association supports these practices, as well as encourages older adults to seek medical and nutritional care to treat ongoing health problems, such as diabetes and hypertension.

2. Birrer RB, Vermuri SP: Depression in later life: A diagnostic and therapeutic challenge. *American Family Physician* 69:2375, 2004.

   Depression is a common problem in older adulthood. It needs to be addressed as it raises the risk for suicide. Diagnosis and treatment of depression are reviewed in detail in this article.

3. Brannon CA: Perimenopause: Nutritional management. *Today's Dietitian* 8(10):10, 2006.

   For most women, perimenopause begins in the mid-40s to early 50s. The most significant change during perimenopause is fluctuating levels of estrogen and progesterone. This article reviews several nutrition-related symptoms of this stage of the female life cycle and offers suggestions of several functional foods that contain components that may decrease these unpleasant symptoms.

4. Byers T and others: American Cancer Society guidelines on nutrition and physical activity for cancer prevention: Reducing the risk of cancer with healthy food choices and physical activity. *CA: Cancer Journal for Clinicians* 52:92, 2002.

   A diet low in red and processed meats and rich in fruits, vegetables, and whole grains is advocated as a strategy for reducing cancer risk. Regular physical activity is also important to include.

5. Cancer-fighting foods. *Mayo Clinic Health Letter* 22(12):1, 2004.

   There are many foods, particularly plant-based foods, that might help lower the risk of certain cancers. Unlike individual supplements, foods offer a unique mix of vitamins and minerals, multiple phytochemicals, fiber and—not least of all—the pleasure of eating.

6. Dickerson LM, Gibson MV: Management of hypertension in older persons. *American Family Physician* 71:469, 2005.

   Hypertension is a too common result of the aging process, especially elevated systolic blood pressure. The authors suggest older people try to combat this trend by following a healthy diet low in sodium and alcohol (if consumed), as well as performing regular physical activity. Typical medications used to treat hypertension in the population are also reviewed.

7. DiMaria-Ghalili RA, Amella E: Nutrition in older adults. *American Journal of Nursing* 105(3): 40, 2005.

   Malnutrition in older persons is important to prevent, as it is a bigger risk than overweight to the health of this population. Risk factors that contribute to this state of malnutrition include a poor diet, as well as limited income, isolation, chronic illness, and various physiological changes that result from aging. These in turn can be addressed by appropriate lifestyle interventions reviewed in the article.

8. Getting smart about Alzheimer's. *Tufts University Health & Nutrition Letter* 23(3):1, 2005.

   As many as 4.5 million Americans suffer from Alzheimer's disease. Consuming a diet rich in brightly colored fruits and vegetables contains many phytochemicals that may prevent the disease. Consuming fish on a regular basis is also important, as well as avoiding obesity, exercising regularly, and keeping mentally active. Meeting B vitamin needs is also crucial, as many contribute to brain health, such as niacin.

9. Heilbronn JK, Ravussin E: Calorie restriction and aging: Review of the literature and implications for studies in humans. *American Journal of Clinical Nutrition* 78:361, 2003.

   Calorie restriction has been long known to extend the life span and retard related chronic diseases of rats, mice, fish, flies, and other species. This may be due to a reduction in metabolic rate and oxidative stress, improved insulin sensitivity, and altered nervous system and hormonal activities. Trials are underway to test whether prolonged caloric restriction increases life span or retards the aging process in humans.

10. Litchford MD: Declining nutritional status in older adults. *Today's Dietitian*, p.12, July 2004.

    The most common causes of declining nutritional status in older adults are poor food choices, failing cognitive status, oral health problems, loss of appetite, and dehydration. Implementing an action plan to treat these problems is important; a registered dietitian can help develop such a plan.

11. Liu RH: Potential synergy of phytochemicals in cancer prevention: Mechanism of action. *Journal of Nutrition* 134:347S, 2004.

    No single antioxidant can replace the combination of natural phytochemicals in fruits and vegetables to achieve the health benefits. Antioxidants or bioactive compounds are best acquired through whole-food consumption, not from dietary supplements. Consumption of 5–10 servings daily of a wide variety of fruits and vegetables is an appropriate strategy for significantly reducing the risk of chronic diseases, such as cancer, and to meet nutrient requirements for optimum health.

12. Manini TM and others: Daily activity energy expenditure and mortality among older adults. *Journal of the American Medical Association* 296:171, 2006.

    Energy expended in free-living activity by healthy older adults (aged 70–82 years) was strongly associated with lower risk of mortality. This study of 302 high-functioning, community-dwelling older adults suggests that any activity may increase survival.

13. Moeller SM and others: Overall adherence to the Dietary Guidelines for Americans is associated with reduced prevalence of early age-related nuclear lens opacities in women. *Journal of Nutrition* 134:1812, 2004.

    A high-quality diet, such as one that follows the Dietary Guidelines for Americans, was shown to prevent or delay the development of lens opacities (i.e., cataracts) in women in this study. Implementing all the recommendations was more helpful than following one or two in isolation, such as just consuming a diet rich in fruits and whole grains.

14. Mozaffarian D and others: Cereal, fruit, and vegetable fiber intake and the risk of

cardiovascular disease in elderly individuals. *Journal of the American Medical Association* 289:1659, 2003.

An adequate cereal fiber intake by older adults is associated with a lower risk of developing cardiovascular disease. This study supports the typical recommendation for older adults to increase consumption of fiber, such as from whole-grain cereals.

15. Newton KM and others: Treatment of vasomotor symptoms of menopause with black cohosh, multibotanicals, soy, hormone therapy, or placebo: A randomized trial. *Annals of Internal Medicine* 145:869, 2006.

Herbal supplements are frequently used to treat vasomotor symptoms of menopause (e.g., hot flashes), so this 1-year randomized study was conducted. Herbal supplements and hormone therapy were compared to a placebo in 351 women, age 45 to 55 years, in menopausal transition or postmenopausal with two or more vasomotor symptoms per day. Vasomotor symptoms or symptom intensity did not differ between the herbal interventions, including black cohosh, or placebo except for those receiving a multibotanical plus soy supplement whose symptoms were worse than with the placebo. Hormone therapy (estrogen with or without progesterone) did result in a decrease in vasomotor symptoms compared to the placebo.

16. Petersen RC and others: Vitamin E and donepezil for the treatment of mild cognitive impairment. *The New England Journal of Medicine* 352:2379, 2005.

Megadose vitamin E therapy did not slow development of mild cognitive impairment in this study. This result questions earlier studies that showed a modest, but short-lived effect of such therapy. The medication donepezil was somewhat effective, but even this therapy only led to a modest benefit.

17. Staying well—at your age. *Consumer Reports on Health* 17(9):1, 2005.

A detailed plan of health promotion and disease prevention as one ages is presented in the article. This includes dietary recommendations (e.g., meeting calorie, calcium, iron, and vitamin D needs), as well as a plan for aerobic and strength-training physical activities, and appropriate medical screening tests for each decade of adult life.

18. Trichopoulou A and others: Modified Mediterranean diet and survival: EPIC-elderly prospective cohort study. *British Medical Journal* 330:991, 2005.

A diet characterized by high intakes of vegetables, legumes, fruits, cereals, and unsaturated fats; moderate amounts of fish and alcohol; and low-to-moderate amounts of dairy products and meats lessened the risk of developing cardiovascular disease in people in this study. Total mortality was also reduced, especially so in people who closely adhered to this diet pattern.

19. Tucker KL and others: The combination of high fruit and vegetable and low saturated fat intakes is more protective against mortality in aging men than is either alone: The Baltimore longitudinal study of aging. *Journal of Nutrition* 135: 556, 2005.

A diet rich in fruits and vegetables and low in saturated fat intakes reduced mortality in aging men in this study. Putting all three recommendations into practice was especially helpful in this regard.

20. Willett WC: Diet and cancer: An evolving picture. *Journal of the American Medical Association* 293(2):233, 2005.

The relation between red meat consumption and colorectal cancer may not be conclusive, but prudence would suggest that red meat, and processed meats in particular, should be eaten sparingly to minimize risk. When this advice is combined with other healthful diet and lifestyle factors, it appears that approximately 70% of colon cancer can be avoided.

▶ Check out the **Contemporary Nutrition ARIS site**
www.mhhe.com/wardlawcontfa1 for quizzes, flash cards, other activities, and weblinks designed to further help you learn about nutrient needs in adulthood.

RATE YOUR PLATE

I. Am I Aging Healthfully?

Take Control of Your Aging by Dr. William B. Malarkey (Wooster Book Co., Wooster OH, 1999) includes a plan that incorporates various diet and lifestyle factors associated with successful aging. Indicate the degree to which you are following such a plan (or alternatively fill this out with a parent or another older relative in mind).

Physical: Do you eat a well-balanced diet, exercise on a regular basis, remain free of illness, abstain from smoking, refrain from drinking alcohol excessively, and experience refreshing sleep?

_____

_____

_____

Intellectual: Are you analytical, do you read regularly, do you learn new things each day, do you engage your mental ability at work (or at school), and do you often reflect on your life?

_____

_____

_____

Emotional: Are you at peace, do you like who you are, are you optimistic, and do you laugh and relax regularly?

_____

_____

_____

Relational: Are you a good listener, do you feel supported by friends, do you attend social functions, do you talk with family members often, and do you feel close to coworkers (or fellow students)?

_____

_____

_____

Spiritual: Do you appreciate nature, give to or serve others, meditate or seek religious worship, and feel life has meaning?

_____

_____

_____

The more of these factors that you include in your life, the more well-rounded your plan is for maintaining overall health. Any one of the five areas in which you are not achieving success should show you characteristics to work on in the future.

II. Helping Older Adults Eat Better

During their lifetimes, most people usually eat meals with families or loved ones. As people reach their older ages, many of them are faced with living and eating alone. In a study of the diets of 4400 older adults in the United States, one man in every five living alone and over age 55 ate poorly. One of four women between the ages of 55 and 64 years followed a low-quality diet. These poor diets can contribute to deteriorating mental and physical health. Consider the following example of the living situation of an older adult.

Neal, a 70-year-old man, lives alone in a home in a local suburban area. His wife died 1 year ago. He doesn't have many friends; his wife was his primary confidante. His neighbors across the street and next door are friendly, and Neal used to help them with yard projects in his spare time. Neal's health has been good, but he has had trouble with his teeth recently. His diet has been poor, and in the past 3 months his physical and mental vigor have deteriorated. He has been slowly lapsing into a depression and, so, keeps the shades drawn and rarely leaves his house. Neal keeps very little food in the house because his wife did most of the cooking and shopping, and he just isn't that interested in food.

If you were one of Neal's relatives and learned of Neal's situation, what six things could you do or suggest to help improve his nutritional status and mental outlook? Look back into this chapter to get some ideas.

1. _____
2. _____
3. _____
4. _____
5. _____
6. _____

CASE STUDY SOLUTIONS

Chapter 1: Eating Habits in College

1. The most positive aspect of Andy's diet is that it contains good sources of protein from animal products also rich in zinc and iron. Alternating his hamburger and fries for lunch with pizza or tacos is a move in the right direction.

2. a. On the downside, Andy's diet is low in dairy products, fruits, and vegetables. This will result in a low intake of calcium, several of the vitamins and the phytochemical (plant-based) substances discussed in Chapter 1. His diet is also low in fiber because fast-food restaurants primarily use refined grain products, rather than whole-grain products and have few fruit and vegetable choices on the menu. Most of the beverages are soft drinks loaded with sugar. Many menu items, especially fries and chicken nuggets, are high in fat.

   b. Most super-sized options apply to foods rich in fat (French fries) and sugar (soft drinks) resulting in excessive amounts of these two components.

   c. He could choose a low-fat granola bar instead of the candy bar for breakfast, or he could take the time to eat a bowl of whole-grain breakfast cereal with low-fat or fat-free milk to increase fiber and calcium (in the latter case) intake. Overall, Andy could improve his intake of fruits, vegetables, and dairy products by focusing on variety in food choice and balance among the food groups.

   d. Andy could alternate between tacos and bean burritos to gain the benefits of plant proteins in a diet. When choosing pizza, he can replace high-fat toppings (e.g., pepperoni), with veggies (e.g., green peppers and onions). Many sub shops and delis offer several low-fat sandwiches, emphasizing lean meats such as turkey and vegetable toppings. For his beverages, Andy could order milk at least half of the time at his restaurant visits and substitute diet soft drinks for the regular variety. This would help moderate his sugar intake.

Chapter 2: Dietary Supplements

1. Brenda should be cautious about taking any supplement, especially one advertised as a "recent breakthrough." As you have read, dietary supplements are not closely regulated by FDA.

2. A general statement such as "increases energy" would be considered a structure/function claim and therefore does not require prior approval by FDA with regard to product labeling.

3. FDA will not have evaluated either the safety or effectiveness of such a product and even harmful dietary supplements are difficult for FDA to recall.

4. There is a chance that the supplement, if effective, would contain little or none of the purported active ingredients.

5. Unfortunately, Brenda will find out all of this the hard way and will be out $60.

6. Brenda's hard-earned money would be better spent on a medical checkup at the Student Health Center. Consumers need to be cautious about nutrition information, especially regarding dietary supplements marketed as cure-alls and breakthroughs. Let the buyer beware!

Chapter 3: Gastroesophageal Reflux Disease

1. Overeating at mealtimes appears to bring on Caitlin's regular bouts of heartburn. Other factors that encourage relaxation of the sphincter and/or irritate the esophagus are smoking; being overweight; and consumption of chili powder, onions, garlic, peppermint, caffeine, alcohol, and chocolate.
2. Typical dietary advice includes consuming smaller, more frequent meals low in fat, not overeating at mealtimes, waiting about 2 hours after meals before lying down, and elevating the head of the bed about 6 inches (review Table 3-4). These recommendations reduce the risk of stomach contents forcing their way back up the esophagus. Other helpful advice includes stopping smoking if practiced, losing excess weight if overweight, and limiting the intake of the items listed in the solution to question 1.
3. If dietary advice does not control symptoms, the primary medication used to control GERD inhibits acid production in the stomach (see earlier discussion on the proton pump inhibitors such as omeprazole [Prilosec] also used to treat peptic ulcers). If this and other medical therapy fails to control the problem, surgery to strengthen the lower esophageal sphincter is possible.
4. Caitlin's GERD can be treated, but most likely will be a lifelong condition. Even surgery will generally not cure the problem. Lifetime diet and lifestyle management, and most likely medications, will still be needed to manage the problem.
5. Lifelong management of GERD is important because long-standing GERD increases the risk of esophageal cancer.

Chapter 4: Problems with Milk Intake

1. Myeshia suspected that she was sensitive to milk because she developed bloating and gas when she consumed milk during one meal.
2. The disaccharide, lactose, is the most likely cause of Myeshia's symptoms.
3. When the enzyme lactase is missing or in short supply in the small intestine, undigested lactose travels to the large intestine and is fermented by bacteria there. The fermentation of lactose by bacteria produces abdominal gas, bloating, and pain. Diarrhea can also occur because the presence of lactose in the colon draws water from the blood vessels into the large intestine.
4. Lactose maldigestion is a normal pattern of physiology that often begins to develop at about ages 3 to 5 years in populations that do not rely on milk and other dairy foods as a main food source. When significant symptoms develop after lactose intake it is then called lactose intolerance.
5. The primary form of lactose maldigestion is estimated to occur in about 75% of the world's population. Most lactose maldigesters are African-Americans (like Myeshia), Asian-Americans, and Latino/Hispanic Americans. The occurrence of lactose maldigestion also increases as people age.
6. The active bacteria cultures in yogurt digest the lactose when these bacteria are broken apart in the small intestine and release their lactase.
7. Many products, such as low-lactose milk and lactase pills, are available to enable lactose maldigesters to tolerate milk.
8. Many lactose maldigesters can consume moderate amounts of lactose with minimal or no intestinal discomfort because of the eventual lactose breakdown by bacteria in the large intestine.
9. In North America and Western Europe, milk and other dairy products are important sources of calcium and vitamin D. These are important for maintaining bone health.
10. Secondary lactose maldigestion occurs when a condition (e.g., long-standing diarrhea from a viral infection), results in a significant decline in lactase production.

Chapter 5: Planning a Heart-Healthy Diet

1. Jackie's approach to lowering blood cholesterol does not incorporate the best choices. She has excluded a great deal of fat in her diet, perhaps more than necessary, and has failed to include some key food groups that have cholesterol-lowering components.
2. Lowering fat as drastically as she has is not really necessary, especially for a physically active 21-year-old female.
3. Jackie could allow a more liberal amount of fat in her diet by including more monounsaturated fats. Canola oil and olive oil, as well as fats found in nuts and avocados are rich sources of monounsaturated fats. These fats do not increase blood cholesterol. In addition she should include good sources of omega-3 fatty acids such as fatty fish, walnuts, flaxseeds, or soybean oil. One option is to use a canola oil-and-vinegar dressing on her salad, rather than lemon juice.
4. She has excluded a great deal of fat in her diet by merely replacing it with refined carbohydrates.
5. To make a shift to a more heart-healthy diet, Jackie would need to include at least 2 cups of fruit and 3 cups of vegetables a day, along with more whole-grain products. She should use whole-wheat bread instead of white bread for her sandwiches and eat a breakfast cereal that has at least 3 grams of fiber per serving.
6. Taking a brisk walk each morning is an excellent way to guarantee at least 30 minutes of activity on most days of the week. Exercise has been shown to increase concentration of HDL-cholesterol in the blood and decrease risk of cardiovascular disease.

Chapter 6: Planning a Vegetarian Diet

1. Studies show that the incidence of and the death rates from some chronic diseases, such as certain cardiovascular diseases, hypertension, many forms of cancer, type 2 diabetes, and obesity, are lower for vegetarians than for nonvegetarians.
2. Many components of a healthy vegetarian diet—whole grains, nuts, soy products, beans, 2 to 4 servings of fruits, and 3 to 5 servings of vegetables per day—are missing. With so few fruits and vegetables, his diet is also low in the many phytochemicals under study for numerous health benefits.
3. Protein appears to be low in the diet because Jordan has not replaced meat with a good plant source of protein. Vitamin B-12, iron, and zinc are also missing from the foods he is choosing. His diet seems to be adequate in calcium and riboflavin because he is including dairy products (milkshake and cheese).
4. Some of Jordan's food choices are high in fat (Danish pastry, milkshake, cookies) and sugar (fruit punch).
5. A healthy vegetarian diet includes whole grains, nuts, soy products, beans, 2 to 4 servings of fruits, and 3 to 5 servings of vegetables per day. It is apparent that he has not yet learned to implement the concept of complementary proteins, so the quality of protein in his diet is low. Meals that combine legumes or vegetables with grains or nuts (see Figure 6-13) will provide the needed amounts of all amino acids.

Chapter 7: Choosing a Weight-Loss Program

1. Joe's weight has been climbing, so he has been experiencing positive energy balance.
2. When Joe is not working, his activity level is low. His time watching TV and studying does not use much energy. Joe should try to find time for physical activity after work and on weekends.
3. Balancing calorie intake with energy expenditure is the main key to weight loss and weight maintenance. Changes that Joe could make to his diet include a decrease in high-fat and -calorie items in his take-out meals. He should include more fruits,

vegetables, and whole grains in his meals. A whole-grain cereal with fruit would be a healthy and convenient substitute for his pastry for breakfast. A grilled chicken sandwich or a taco salad would be a nutritious change for lunch. Grilled chicken or chili with a baked potato or salad would be healthier choices for dinner. Table 7-3 includes many ideas for food substitutions that will lower calories.

4. Joe will be wasting his money if he buys the product seen in the infomercial. Unfortunately, regulation of the supplement industry is woefully lacking. In the future, if there is a meaningful breakthrough in weight loss and weight control, health authorities such as the Surgeon General's Office or the National Institutes of Health will make North Americans aware of that fact.

5. The characteristics of a sound weight-loss diet are shown in Figure 7-13. These characteristics include a slow and steady rate of loss, flexibility relative to your habits and tastes, nutritional adequacy, behavior modification, physical activity, and maintenance of overall health.

Chapter 8

1. The American Heart Association defines a blood pressure below 120/80 as normal, up to 140/90 as pre-hypertension, and above 140/90 as hypertension. Greg's blood pressure of 135/88 falls into the pre-hypertension range. His goal should be to reduce his blood pressure to 120/80 or lower.

2. Lifestyle factors mentioned in the case study that may have contributed to Greg's elevated blood pressure include lack of exercise, stress, excess weight, and poor diet (including low intakes of fruits, vegetables, whole grains, and low-fat dairy products and high intake of saturated fat, cholesterol, and sodium). To lower his blood pressure, Greg could start an exercise program with the goal of exercising at least 30 minutes per day on most days of the week. In terms of diet, Greg could start the day with a whole-grain breakfast cereal, skim milk, and a piece of fruit; include more fruits, vegetables, whole grains, and low-fat dairy product; and decrease his sodium intake by using fewer prepared and processed foods. Restaurant foods and frozen dinners are usually high in sodium. Dietary and exercise changes will likely help Greg shed excess pounds. Stress reduction techniques also may help lower his blood pressure.

3. The AI for sodium for an adult is 1500 mg/d. Considering Greg's heavy reliance upon prepared and processed foods, his sodium intake probably exceeds the AI, as does the sodium intake of most North Americans.

4. Excess sodium may increase blood pressure by causing the kidneys to conserve water, thus increasing blood volume. This places stress on the heart, blood vessels, and kidneys. Only about 10% to 15% of the adult population is sodium-sensitive, so efforts to lower the sodium content of Greg's diet may not affect his blood pressure. Other micronutrients that impact blood pressure include calcium, potassium, magnesium, and vitamin C. Diets high in these micronutrients decrease blood pressure.

5. By controlling hypertension, Greg will reduce his risk for several chronic health problems, including cardiovascular disease, kidney disease, stroke, and vision problems.

Chapter 9: Choosing a Dietary Supplement

1. The maintenance dose of two to three tablets per day poses no risk per se because this dose of Nutramega does not exceed the Upper Tolerable Intake levels for vitamin A, vitamin C, zinc, or selenium.

2. a. **VitaminA**

    33% (0.33) times the DV of 1000 micrograms RAE equals 330 micrograms RAE per tablet. Sixteen tablets would yield 5280 micrograms RAE. The UL is 3000 micrograms RAE for preformed vitamin A. Seventy-five percent of the vitamin A is preformed vitamin A, so this yields 3960 micrograms RAE of preformed vitamin A ($5280 \times 0.75 = 3960$), or 1.3 times the UL ($3960/3000 = 1.3$).

b. **Vitamin C**

Seven hundred percent of the DV of 60 milligrams equals 420 milligrams per tablet. Sixteen tablets would yield 6720 milligrams. The UL is 2000 milligrams. This would then yield 3.4 times the UL (6720/2000 = 3.4).

c. **Zinc**

Fifty percent of the DV of 15 milligrams equals 7.5 milligrams per tablet. Sixteen tablets would yield 120 milligrams. The UL is 40 milligrams. This would then yield 3 times the UL (120/40 = 3).

d. **Selenium**

Ten percent of the DV of 70 micrograms equals 7 micrograms per tablet. Sixteen tablets would yield 112 micrograms. This is less than the UL of 400 micrograms.

e. The suggested use of Nutramega "at the first sign of feeling ill" poses some health risks for Amy. Taking two to three tablets every 3 hours would mean taking at least 16 tablets per day. This dosage would provide an intake of vitamin A, vitamin C, and zinc well in excess of the Upper Levels for these nutrients.

3. Nutramega is expensive compared to the cost of the typical multivitamin and mineral supplement (a 1-month supply would cost about $2 compared to about $50 for Nutramega).

4. Overall, Amy is smart to be concerned about meeting her nutrient needs, but the stress she is under does not increase nutrient needs.

5. A healthy diet as suggested by MyPyramid should be Amy's primary focus. Taking a balanced multivitamin and mineral supplement is also a reasonable practice.

Chapter 10: Giving Up Milk

1. Factors contributing to her potential risk of osteoporosis include a poor dietary intake of calcium and vitamin D. Her diet is also low in protein, an important nutrient for the synthesis of connective tissue important in the skeletal system.

2. Ashley is increasing her chances of developing osteoporosis later in life because of her current high-risk lifestyle. Her new smoking habit and her low level of daily physical activity increase her risk of developing osteoporosis.

3. Ashley should rethink her rationale for avoiding milk. Fat-free milk is low in calories and provides much calcium. Dairy products such as milk do not lead to weight gain per se. There are even some studies suggesting that a regular intake of dairy products rich in calcium may aid in weight loss when on an otherwise calorie-restricted diet.

4. Ashley needs to find some reliable sources of calcium and vitamin D. These could include calcium-fortified juices, calcium-fortified bread and snack bars, and calcium-fortified chewable chocolate candies. Tofu (made with calcium) is another potential source, as well as calcium-fortified soy milk. Tofu and soy milk are also good sources of high-quality plant protein. Meeting the AI of 1000 milligrams per day for her age would not be that hard if she were to make an effort to use these calcium-rich foods and/or incorporate other rich sources.

5. To decrease her risk of osteoporosis and several other chronic diseases, Ashley should also stop smoking. In addition, including at least 30 minutes of physical activity on most days of the week will decrease her risk of osteoporosis and help her maintain a healthy weight.

Chapter 11

1. Iron is part of hemoglobin, the protein in red blood cells that transports oxygen from the lungs to the body's cells and also returns carbon dioxide to the lungs for excretion. At age 60, Anita is postmenopausal, so monthly losses of blood are not depleting her iron stores. Good sources of iron include ready-to-eat breakfast cereals, beans, and meats. Anita's food choices probably do supply

adequate iron, but she could increase absorption of iron by consuming iron-containing foods with a source of vitamin C, such as orange juice.

2. Vitamin B-6 is involved in the synthesis of hemoglobin, and a lack of vitamin B-6 may lead to microcytic hypochromic anemia. Vitamin B-6 is widely available in the typical North American diet and is found in ready-to-eat breakfast cereals, animal products, dairy products, fruits, and vegetables. Given Anita's healthy food choices, it is not likely that vitamin B-6 deficiency is the reason for her anemia.

3. Folate is involved in the maturation of red blood cells, leading to megaloblastic (large cell) anemia. Immature red blood cells are less efficient at carrying oxygen. Food sources of folate include green, leafy vegetables; organ meats; and beans. Given Anita's healthy food choices, it is not likely that folate deficiency is the reason for her anemia.

4. Vitamin B-12 is involved in the metabolism of folate, so a lack of vitamin B-12 may lead to megaloblastic anemia (described previously). Vitamin B-12 is naturally found in foods of animal origin, including meats and dairy products, and is also added to ready-to-eat breakfast cereals. With aging, many adults produce insufficient stomach acid and intrinsic factor, required for vitamin B-12 absorption. Thus, even though Anita's diet may appear adequate in vitamin B-12, her absorption of the vitamin may be low. Consuming a synthetic source of vitamin B-12, which does not require intrinsic factor for absorption, may improve her vitamin B-12 status. Fortified breakfast cereals or multivitamin supplements are typical sources of synthetic vitamin B-12.

5. Anita should talk with her health care provider to determine the cause and severity of her anemia. If Anita does have iron-deficiency anemia, the cause needs to be diagnosed. For a postmenopausal woman, a possible cause could be bleeding in the gastrointestinal tract, which could be serious if left untreated. Dietary changes, such as consuming vitamin C to enhance iron absorption, can improve the health of her red blood cells and prevent future deficiencies, but in many cases, supplementation is necessary. A synthetic source of vitamin B-12 will overcome any absorption problems if this is the source of her anemia.

Chapter 12: Planning a Training Diet

1. Michael is correct in following a high-carbohydrate diet.
2. In his effort to minimize his fat intake, he is probably not consuming enough calories, protein, iron, and calcium to support his training routine. He has fallen into the bagel, pasta, and pretzel routine that sports nutritionists warn is not conducive to peak performance. Low protein, iron, and overall calories may contribute to fatigue.
3. Michael's performance would improve if he also had a high-protein source at each meal. He could include milk with breakfast and possibly some low-fat yogurt or low-fat cheese at lunch. He should have a carbohydrate/protein snack before his workout, such as half a sandwich with fruit and some water. The sandwich and fruit will help provide him with fuel to support his vigorous training. In the evenings, he could substitute oil and vinegar dressing for the fat-free dressing on his salad and cheese and crackers for the pretzels to improve protein intake.
4. During his workouts, he could consume a sports drink to meet fluid needs and supply some carbohydrate, or he could consume water, along with a few fig cookies or other high-carbohydrate food.
5. Overall, it is important for Michael to fuel his body before, during, and after workouts.

Chapter 13: Eating Disorders—Steps to Recovery

1. Sarah has the characteristics to be diagnosed with anorexia nervosa.
2. Sarah's disordered eating habits began when she became self-conscious about her body when her peers teased her about being overweight. She began exercising each day and

was successful at losing weight. Her disordered eating then began with restricting her food intake more. She enjoyed the self-control she had over her body.

3. Sarah has the following physical symptoms of anorexia nervosa: she refuses to maintain a healthy weight-for-height, is at a weight below 85% of that expected, has a distorted view of her appearance, and has had no menstrual periods for over 3 consecutive months.

4. Her treatment would most likely consist of moderate bed rest to promote weight gain and an intake of 1000 to 1600 kcal initially, then increased by increments of about 100 to 200 kcal every few days until an acceptable rate of weight gain is achieved. The goal is to achieve a body weight that is at least 90% of an expected weight for her height, such as a BMI of at least 19.

5. Several nutrient deficiencies are likely in this case. Deficiencies of calcium and iron are probably most likely. The physician would likely prescribe a multivitamin and mineral supplement, along with an additional supplement of calcium as needed to make sure intake is in the range of 1200 to 1500 milligrams per day. Additional iron may be needed if Sarah is anemic. This overall practice will correct vitamin and mineral deficiencies that exist. The calcium in particular will contribute to bone maintenance.

6. Sarah would need to be hospitalized initially, due to her low BMI of 13.8.

7. A team of health professionals, most likely consisting of a physician, registered dietitian, and psychologist, would provide therapy. Sarah's cooperation would be the most important element for therapy to be successful. She needs to realize that she has a problem and that she needs help. She must be willing to accept the assistance these professionals are willing to offer. The team, especially the psychologist, may use cognitive behavior therapy to help Sarah improve her self-image.

8. Sarah's outlook for recovery is not good unless she realizes she has a problem. Even if she is willing to accept the therapy and counseling, a relapse is likely to occur. Only 50% of anorexia nervosa patients have been found to recover fully from the disease. Sarah's disordered eating habits have been in place for about 6 years, so her problem is deep-rooted. The chances of recovery are greater if a vigorous treatment program is reinforced with close follow-up.

Chapter 14: Undernutrition During Childhood

1. Jamal should not be surprised that the children in the village were often sick and listless. The living conditions and recent natural disaster have added to the already poor conditions in this village. We know that children are especially susceptible to the effects of poverty and undernutrition.

2. Based on the reports that the children do not get enough to eat and on the outward signs of the children's health, protein, vitamin A, iron, iodide, and zinc are likely to be deficient in the diets of these children.

3. Protein, vitamin A, iron, iodide, and zinc deficiencies contribute to poor growth and stunting because of their essential functions in the body. One or more of these deficiencies is likely present in many children in the village.

4. Protein, vitamin A, iron, iodide, and zinc deficiencies may also contribute to depressed immune function, which can cause diarrhea and illness. These deficiencies are particularly risky in children.

5. The diets of these children are most likely also marginal in caloric content. A low-calorie intake during childhood will further depress the growth and overall health compromised by the protein and micronutrient deficiencies. Recall from Chapter 6 that protein-calorie malnutrition (PCM) is a form of undernutrition caused by an extremely deficient intake of calories or protein and generally is accompanied by an illness.

6. The recent storm will hopefully cause the Philippine government to send food and medicines to the village, which will be a short-term solution to some of their nutrition and health needs.

7. Poverty and undernutrition occur at much lower rates in the United States and other developed countries. Childhood nutrition concerns in developed countries are more likely to be the increasing incidence of overweight and obesity. As we discussed in Chapter 7, maintaining a healthy weight requires the proper balance of calories in and calories out. In Chapter 17 we will learn that overweight children are becoming more common because the typical number of calories they consume per day has increased at the same time that calorie expenditure in physical activity has decreased.

Chapter 15: Preventing Foodborne Illnesses at Gatherings

1. Nicole likely contracted *Clostridium perfringens*, based on the fact that she had diarrhea but did not vomit and the symptoms occurred about 8 hours after consuming the contaminated food (review Table 15-3).
2. Spores of *Clostridium perfringens* are typically present in meat. Thorough cooking will kill any of the live bacteria present, but the product may still contain spores. These can later develop into bacteria if the food is kept in a warm setting for a few hours. The beef in the empanadas was likely the bearer of the spores, and they likely germinated and produced a toxin as the beef sat in the car and on the buffet table.
3. Consuming food at large gatherings is risky for several reasons. First, foods for these events are typically cooked ahead of time and not consumed right away. Unfortunately, the foods end up remaining in the "danger zone" between 41°F and 135°F. Hot foods should be kept hot and cold foods cold. Unfortunately, proper refrigeration or heating equipment is not always available at these events. In addition, many people handle foods and serving utensils at large gatherings. It is important for anyone handling food or serving utensils to thoroughly wash their hands before and after handling food and to avoid coughing or sneezing over foods. Also, when returning to the "buffet" table, always use a clean plate to avoid cross-contamination. Finally, the focus at these events is usually on having fun and socializing and not on food safety.
4. The main precaution that was ignored was keeping the food out of the "danger zone." Overall, it is risky to leave perishable items such as meat, fish, poultry, eggs, and dairy products at room temperature for more than 1 to 2 hours.
5. Ideally, the cooked food should have remained at room temperature for no longer than 1 hour. Thus, soon after Nicole and her husband took it out of the oven, it should have been separated into a few smaller pans to speed cooling and then refrigerated because they knew it was not going to be served within 1 to 2 hours. Before leaving, they could have recombined the dish into one clean pan. Once they arrived at the party, the dish should have been refrigerated again, and then thoroughly reheated when it was time to eat.

Chapter 16: Preparing for Pregnancy

1. Tracey's use of an over-the-counter vitamin and mineral supplement provides ample synthetic folic acid and can help fill some gaps between dietary intakes and requirements for various nutrients. Still, she should discuss this supplement use with her physician and would eventually benefit more from a prenatal supplement, as this will have more iron than the over-the-counter supplement. She should be sure not to exceed 100% of the Daily Value for preformed vitamin A because toxicities of this vitamin could cause birth defects. Tracey is wise to avoid use of herbal supplements during pregnancy unless her physician approves of them.

2. Folate deficiency is known to be linked to neural tube defects. The synthetic folic acid in Tracey's vitamin and mineral supplement is well absorbed and will certainly help to meet her needs for this nutrient. Consuming more fruits and vegetables—especially green leafy vegetables—is also a wise choice. A fortified, ready-to-eat breakfast cereal also contributes to vitamins and mineral intake. Her physician may recommend a prenatal supplement instead of the over-the-counter supplement.

3. Many experts would say that she is consuming too much caffeine and would be wise to cut down coffee and caffeine-containing soft drinks to a total of three servings or fewer per day.

4. If Tracey likes fish, she could include two servings of fish per week in her diet plan for pregnancy and breastfeeding. Fish are a good source of protein and also supply healthy fats, including omega-3 fatty acids, linked to brain and eye development in the fetus. However, Tracey should avoid some types of fish that may have high mercury content, which can harm the nervous system of the developing fetus. Fish that typically have high levels of mercury include swordfish, shark, king mackerel, tile fish, largemouth bass, and canned albacore tuna.

5. The additional fruits and vegetables Tracey is consuming will provide some fiber to help prevent constipation. Other ideas to increase her fiber intake include consuming a variety of whole grains and incorporating beans and legumes into her diet plan. Tracey should also increase her fluid intake and be sure to maintain regular exercise, such as walking.

6. Tracey expressed concern about her weight gain during pregnancy. Research clearly shows that adequate weight gain during pregnancy is critical for growth and development of the fetus. Inadequate weight gain contributes to risk for delivering a low-birth-weight or small-for-gestational-age baby. On the other hand, excessive weight gain during pregnancy can present problems as well. Excessive weight gain may promote long-term health problems and complicate the pregnancy with gestational diabetes or large-for-gestational age babies. At her pre-pregnancy weight and height, Tracey's BMI (21 kg/m^2) is within the normal range, so she should aim to gain 25–35 pounds during the entire pregnancy. During the second and third trimesters, consuming an extra 350–450 kilocalories per day of nutrient-dense foods will help her to meet this goal. Regular, moderate exercise is also recommended throughout pregnancy. However, pregnancy is not a time to begin a vigorous exercise routine. Walking or riding a stationary bike are good activities to regulate weight gain. Tracey should be reassured that her choice to breastfeed her baby will help her to lose those extra pounds after the baby is born.

Chapter 17: Undernutrition During Infancy

1. Ask if the formula is iron-fortified. Also, verify that Damon's caregivers are appropriately preparing his formula—adding the correct amount of powder or concentrated liquid to water. Be sure that Damon's caregivers plan to continue giving him formula until 1 year of age.

2. The scenario described puts Damon at risk for failure to thrive, likely due to his caregiver's lack of knowledge about appropriate infant feeding practices. His diet is probably lacking in total calories as well as calcium, iron, and zinc. Inadequacies may lead to stunted growth, cognitive problems, behavioral problems, and weak bones.

3. In addition to an iron-fortified infant formula, Damon should be eating fortified infant cereals, pureed fruits, vegetables, and meats, and even some table foods that are soft and cut into small pieces. After six months of age, solid foods help to meet increased nutrient demands. Processed foods, such as the hot dog described in the scenario, are usually high in sodium, fat, or sugars. These are not ideal for meeting Damon's nutritional needs. Allowing Damon to self-feed to some extent will help him to develop motor skills and build confidence. Potentially allergenic

foods, such as seafood, egg whites, cow's milk, peanuts, and tree nuts, should not be offered until Damon is older.

4. Infants should not be drinking sugary beverages such as colas or fruit-flavored drinks, as these items lack the nutrient density essential to meeting Damon's needs. His caregivers should provide him no more than 4 to 6 ounces of 100% fruit juice. To prevent early childhood caries and develop self-feeding skills, Damon should be learning to drink from a cup rather than a bottle.

5. The combination of an appropriately-prepared, iron-fortified infant formula and a variety of solid foods should provide Damon all the nutrients he needs. However, if he is anemic, he may need an iron supplement.

Chapter 18: Dietary Assistance for an Older Adult

1. Frances' typical diet is low in many nutrients, including protein, calcium, iron, zinc, and vitamins B-12 and D.

2. Her poor diet will cause a more rapid decline in her lean tissue and bone mass, as well as decrease her iron status, vision, and mental function.

3. Physiological changes that will exacerbate the effects of her poor diet include increases in fat stores and decreases in her appetite; sense of taste, smell and thirst; chewing ability; bowel function; lactase production; iron status; liver, kidney, lung, cardiovascular and immune function; vision; lean tissue; bone mass; and mental function. Review Table 18-2 for the recommended responses to these changes.

4. Frances could contact a local government office that offers congregate meal programs at a central location. She could inquire about location and availability of transportation to the site. This would give her social contact with other older persons, probably an important element missing in her life. This could help alleviate her loneliness. She could also request Meals on Wheels (if available) to provide one hot meal per day. One hot meal per day prepared for her may be what she needs to help stimulate her appetite. She could also have groceries delivered to her home if her budget could withstand the extra cost.

5. Other convenience foods that could be added to her diet include milk; assorted nuts; peanut butter; breakfast cereals; canned chicken or deli meats; yogurt; sliced cheese; cottage cheese; calcium-fortified orange juice; canned or frozen fruits and vegetables; and some fresh fruits and vegetables that do not require preparation, such as prewashed lettuce and bananas. A further possibility is a nutrition bar or a liquid nutritional supplement, such as a can of Ensure® Plus. The resulting increase in her nutrient intake would help prevent disease in the future and increase her sense of well-being.

CHECK YOUR KNOWLEDGE ANSWERS

Chapter 1	Chapter 2	Chapter 3	Chapter 4
1. b	1. a	1. b	1. b
2. d	2. c	2. a	2. c
3. c	3. d	3. d	3. a
4. e	4. d	4. d	4. b
5. a	5. b	5. c	5. a
6. c	6. b	6. c	6. e
7. c	7. b	7. d	7. b
8. b	8. d	8. d	8. b
9. c	9. d	9. a	9. c
10. b	10. c	10. b	10. a

Chapter 5	Chapter 6	Chapter 7	Chapter 8
1. d	1. b	1. b	1. a
2. a	2. c	2. d	2. d
3. c	3. b	3. d	3. d
4. b	4. c	4. b	4. a
5. a	5. b	5. a	5. c
6. a	6. b	6. c	6. b
7. c	7. c	7. b	7. d
8. c	8. c	8. c	8. c
9. b	9. d	9. b	9. b
10. c	10. c	10. c	10. d

Chapter 9	Chapter 10	Chapter 11	Chapter 12
1. b	1. b	1. d	1. b
2. a	2. a	2. b	2. d
3. a	3. b	3. d	3. c
4. b	4. c	4. b	4. d
5. d	5. c	5. b	5. d
6. c	6. c	6. b	6. d
7. d	7. b	7. a	7. c
8. a	8. c	8. d	8. d
9. b	9. b	9. b	9. b
10. c	10. d	10. a	10. a

Chapter 13	Chapter 14	Chapter 15	Chapter 16
1. d	1. b	1. a	1. a
2. c	2. d	2. d	2. d
3. a	3. d	3. b	3. c
4. c	4. c	4. b	4. a
5. a	5. d	5. a	5. b
6. d	6. d	6. d	6. d
7. c	7. c	7. d	7. d
8. e	8. b	8. d	8. c
9. b	9. d	9. a	9. b
10. c	10. b	10. b	10. c

Chapter 17

1. d
2. a
3. c
4. b
5. b
6. d
7. a
8. c
9. a
10. b

Chapter 18

1. d
2. c
3. d
4. b
5. d
6. c
7. d
8. c
9. d
10. d

The Daily Values Used on Food Labels in the United States, with a Comparison to the Latest RDAs and Other Nutrient Standards*

Dietary Constituent	Unit of Measure	Current Daily Values for People Over 4 Years of Age	RDA or Other Current Dietary Standard	
			Males 19 Years Old	Females 19 Years Old
Total Fat[†]	g	<65	—	—
Saturated fatty acids[†]	"	<20	—	—
Protein[†]	"	50	56	46
Cholesterol[§]	mg	<300	—	—
Carbohydrate[†]	g	300	130	130
Fiber	"	25	38	25
Vitamin A	µg Retinol activity equivalents	1000	900	700
Vitamin D	International units	400	200	200
Vitamin E	"	30	22–33	22–33
Vitamin K	µg	80	120	90
Vitamin C	mg	60	90	75
Folate	µg	400	400	400
Thiamin	mg	1.5	1.20	1.10
Riboflavin	"	1.7	1.30	1.10
Niacin	"	20	16	14
Vitamin B-6	"	2	1.30	1.30
Vitamin B-12	µg	6	2.40	2.40
Biotin	mg	0.3	0.03	0.03
Pantothenic acid	"	10	5	5
Calcium	"	1000	1000	1000
Phosphorus	"	1000	700	700
Iodide	µg	150	150	150
Iron	mg	18	8	18
Magnesium	"	400	400	310
Copper	"	2	0.9	0.9
Zinc	"	15	11	8
Sodium[‡]	"	<2400	1500	1500
Potassium[‡]	"	3500	4700	4700
Chloride[‡]	"	3400	2300	2300
Manganese	"	2	2.3	1.8
Selenium	µg	70	55	55
Chromium	"	120	35	25
Molybdenum	"	75	45	45

Abbreviations: g = gram, mg = milligram, µg = microgram

*Daily Values are generally set at the highest nutrient recommendation in a specific age and gender category. Many Daily Values exceed current nutrient standards. This is in part because aspects of the Daily Values were originally developed in the early 1970s using estimates of nutrient needs published in 1968. The Daily Values have yet to be updated to reflect the current state of knowledge.

[†]These Daily Values are based on a 2000 kcal diet, instead of RDAs, with a caloric distribution of 30% from fat (and one-third of this total from saturated fat), 60% from carbohydrate, and 10% from protein.

[‡]The considerably higher Daily Values for sodium and chloride are there to allow for more diet flexibility, but the extra amounts are not needed to maintain health.

[§]Based on recommendations of U.S. federal agencies.

APPENDIX C Dietary Advice for Canadians

Recommended Nutrient Intake (RNI)
The Canadian version of RDA published in 1990.

▶ Excellent World Wide Web resources for Canadians are Health Canada (www.hc-sc.gc.ca), Dietitians of Canada (www.dietitians.ca), and the Institute of Nutrition, Metabolism, and Diabetes (www.cihr-irsc.gc.ca).

▶ A downloadable copy of *Canada's Food Guide* is available at http://www.hc-sc.gc.ca/fn-an/food-guide-ailment/index_e.html.

The information in this appendix includes advice on dietary patterns, as well as regulations that apply to food labeling. Previous **Recommended Nutrient Intakes (RNIs)** for nutrients have been replaced by the Dietary Reference Intakes (DRIs) that apply to Canadian and U.S. citizens. These are listed on the inside cover. Both Canadian and American scientists worked on the various DRI committees, coming up with a set of harmonized Dietary Reference Intakes for both countries.

SUMMARY OF THE NUTRITION RECOMMENDATIONS FOR CANADIANS

The Canadian federal department responsible for helping Canadians maintain and improve their health is Health Canada. The Office of Nutrition Policy and Promotion is within the Health Products and Food Branch of Health Canada and focuses on nutrition. Health Canada's National Dietary Guidance programs have been in existence since the 1930s and have always relied on scientific and other related evidence. Since 1977, a pattern of eating that meets nutrient needs and reduces the risk of chronic diseases has been promoted. In the 1990s, dietary guidance included *Canada's Guidelines for Healthy Eating* and *Food Guide to Healthy Eating* as well as *Nutrition for a Healthy Pregnancy* and *Nutrition for Healthy Term Infants*. The *Recommended Nutrient Intake* (RNI), a Canadian version of the RDA, was published in 1990.

In 1995, the U.S. Institutes of Medicine (IOM) brought together Canadian and American scientists to work on various committees, which came up with a set of harmonized Dietary Reference Intakes for both countries. The DRIs replaced the previous RNIs and a new set of recommendations (EAR, AI, RDA, UL) similar to those in the United States were adopted in Canada. This led to a review and subsequent revision of *Canada's Food Guide to Healthy Eating* and *Guidelines for Healthy Eating*.

The revised *Canada's Food Guide* (Fig. C-1) was released in early 2007. The basic message to Canadians is to "Eat Well" with *Canada's Food Guide*. Learning more about *Canada's Food Guide* will help Canadians know how much food they need, what types of foods are better for them, and the importance of physical activity in their day.

In addition, if Canadians have the amount and type of food recommended and follow the tips included in *Canada's Food Guide,* this will help them:

- Meet their needs for vitamins, minerals, and other nutrients.
- Reduce their risk of obesity, type 2 diabetes, heart disease, certain types of cancer, and osteoporosis.
- Contribute to their overall health and vitality.

Canada's Food Guide places foods into four groups: vegetables and fruits; grain products; milk and alternatives; and meat and alternatives. *Canada's Food Guide* also includes information on the recommended number of Food Guide Servings per day, examples of what is one Food Guide Serving and how to make each Food Guide Serving count within each food group (Fig. C-2) and at each meal (Fig. C-3). Recommendations are also included about the types and amounts of oils and fats to consume, along with guidance to enjoy a variety of foods and to satisfy your thirst with water. Similar to the MyPyramid recommendations, *Canada's Food Guide* emphasizes the combination of eating well and being active every day (Fig. C-4). The new Canadian Nutrition Facts label is also highlighted in *Canada's Food Guide* with the message to "Read the label." Finally, specific nutrition advice for different ages and stages is included (Fig. C-5). Another similarity to the U.S. MyPyramid is the availability of "My Food Guide", a web-based interactive tool that will help you personalize the information found in *Canada's Food Guide.* Check out "My Food Guide" at http://www.hc-sc.gc.ca/fn-an/food-guide-aliment/myguide-monguide/index_e.html.

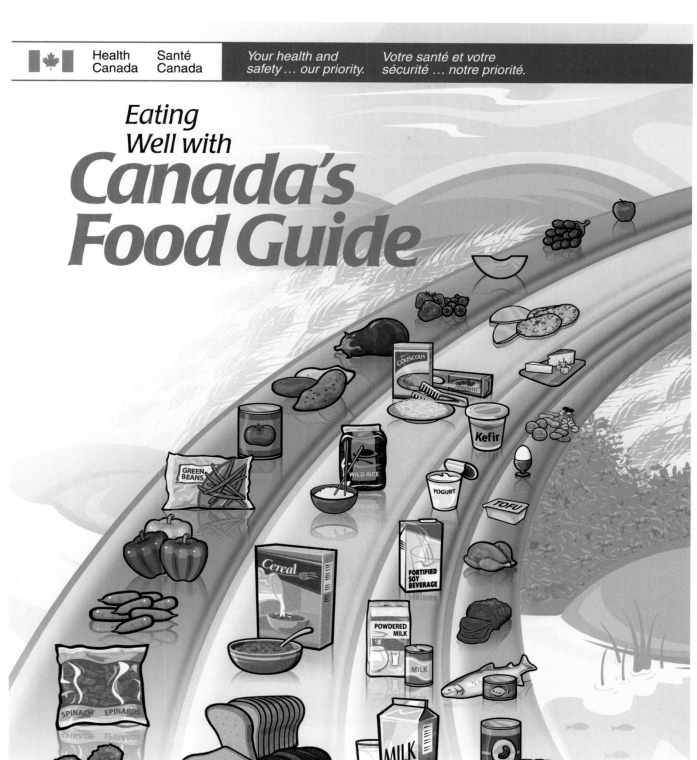

FIGURE C-1 ▶ Eating Well with Canada's Food Guide.

Recommended Number of Food Guide Servings per Day

	Children			Teens		Adults			
Age in Years	2-3	4-8	9-13	14-18		19-50		51+	
Sex	Girls and Boys			Females	Males	Females	Males	Females	Males
Vegetables and Fruit	4	5	6	7	8	7-8	8-10	7	7
Grain Products	3	4	6	6	7	6-7	8	6	7
Milk and Alternatives	2	2	3-4	3-4	3-4	2	2	3	3
Meat and Alternatives	1	1	1-2	2	3	2	3	2	3

The chart above shows how many Food Guide Servings you need from each of the four food groups every day.

Having the amount and type of food recommended and following the tips in *Canada's Food Guide* will help:

• Meet your needs for vitamins, minerals and other nutrients.
• Reduce your risk of obesity, type 2 diabetes, heart disease, certain types of cancer and osteoporosis.
• Contribute to your overall health and vitality.

FIGURE C-2 ▶ Information about Food Guide Servings from *Canada' Food Guide*.

What is One Food Guide Serving?
Look at the examples below.

Fresh, frozen or canned vegetables
125 mL (½ cup)

Leafy vegetables
Cooked: 125 mL (½ cup)
Raw: 250 mL (1 cup)

Fresh, frozen or canned fruits
1 fruit or 125 mL (½ cup)

100% Juice
125 mL (½ cup)

Bread
1 slice (35 g)

Bagel
½ bagel (45 g)

Flat breads
½ pita or ½ tortilla (35 g)

Cooked rice, bulgur or quinoa
125 mL (½ cup)

Cereal
Cold: 30 g
Hot: 175 mL (¾ cup)

Cooked pasta or couscous
125 mL (½ cup)

Milk or powdered milk (reconstituted)
250 mL (1 cup)

Canned milk (evaporated)
125 mL (½ cup)

Fortified soy beverage
250 mL (1 cup)

Yogurt
175 g
(¾ cup)

Kefir
175 g
(¾ cup)

Cheese
50 g (1 ½ oz.)

Cooked fish, shellfish, poultry, lean meat
75 g (2 ½ oz.)/125 mL (½ cup)

Cooked legumes
175 mL (¾ cup)

Tofu
150 g or
175 mL (¾ cup)

Eggs
2 eggs

Peanut or nut butters
30 mL (2 Tbsp)

Shelled nuts and seeds
60 mL (¼ cup)

Oils and Fats

- Include a small amount – 30 to 45 mL (2 to 3 Tbsp) – of unsaturated fat each day. This includes oil used for cooking, salad dressings, margarine and mayonnaise.
- Use vegetable oils such as canola, olive and soybean.
- Choose soft margarines that are low in saturated and trans fats.
- Limit butter, hard margarine, lard and shortening.

FIGURE C-2 ▶ *(continued)*

Make each Food Guide Serving count...
wherever you are – at home, at school, at work or when eating out!

▸ **Eat at least one dark green and one orange vegetable each day.**
- Go for dark green vegetables such as broccoli, romaine lettuce and spinach.
- Go for orange vegetables such as carrots, sweet potatoes and winter squash.

▸ **Choose vegetables and fruit prepared with little or no added fat, sugar or salt.**
- Enjoy vegetables steamed, baked or stir-fried instead of deep-fried.

▸ **Have vegetables and fruit more often than juice.**

▸ **Make at least half of your grain products whole grain each day.**
- Eat a variety of whole grains such as barley, brown rice, oats, quinoa and wild rice.
- Enjoy whole grain breads, oatmeal or whole wheat pasta.

▸ **Choose grain products that are lower in fat, sugar or salt.**
- Compare the Nutrition Facts table on labels to make wise choices.
- Enjoy the true taste of grain products. When adding sauces or spreads, use small amounts.

▸ **Drink skim, 1%, or 2% milk each day.**
- Have 500 mL (2 cups) of milk every day for adequate vitamin D.
- Drink fortified soy beverages if you do not drink milk.

▸ **Select lower fat milk alternatives.**
- Compare the Nutrition Facts table on yogurts or cheeses to make wise choices.

▸ **Have meat alternatives such as beans, lentils and tofu often.**

▸ **Eat at least two Food Guide Servings of fish each week.***
- Choose fish such as char, herring, mackerel, salmon, sardines and trout.

▸ **Select lean meat and alternatives prepared with little or no added fat or salt.**
- Trim the visible fat from meats. Remove the skin on poultry.
- Use cooking methods such as roasting, baking or poaching that require little or no added fat.
- If you eat luncheon meats, sausages or prepackaged meats, choose those lower in salt (sodium) and fat.

Enjoy a variety of foods from the four food groups.

Satisfy your thirst with water!

Drink water regularly. It's a calorie-free way to quench your thirst. Drink more water in hot weather or when you are very active.

* Health Canada provides advice for limiting exposure to mercury from certain types of fish. Refer to www.healthcanada.gc.ca for the latest information.

FIGURE C-2 ▸ *(continued)*

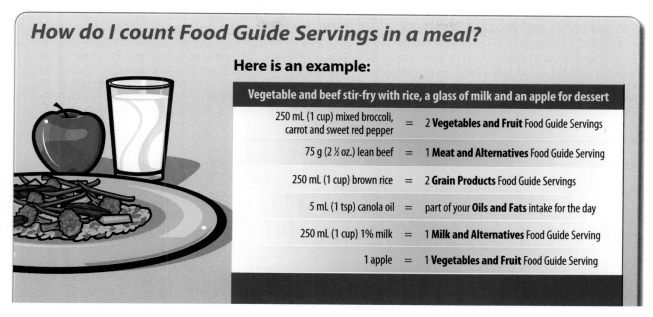

How do I count Food Guide Servings in a meal?

Here is an example:

Vegetable and beef stir-fry with rice, a glass of milk and an apple for dessert

250 mL (1 cup) mixed broccoli, carrot and sweet red pepper	=	2 **Vegetables and Fruit** Food Guide Servings
75 g (2 ½ oz.) lean beef	=	1 **Meat and Alternatives** Food Guide Serving
250 mL (1 cup) brown rice	=	2 **Grain Products** Food Guide Servings
5 mL (1 tsp) canola oil	=	part of your **Oils and Fats** intake for the day
250 mL (1 cup) 1% milk	=	1 **Milk and Alternatives** Food Guide Serving
1 apple	=	1 **Vegetables and Fruit** Food Guide Serving

FIGURE C-3 ▶ How to count Food Guide Servings in a meal.

Nutrition Labels

New labeling requirements were published on January 1, 2003. The new regulations require most food labels to carry a mandatory Nutrition Facts table listing Calories and 13 key nutrients.

How to Read the Canadian Nutrition Label

The Regulations provide for the optional declaration of the number of Calories both from fat and from saturates plus *trans*. Recommendations on the % of Calories from fat apply to the total diet rather than to an individual food. Therefore, inclusion of the % of Calories from fat in the Nutrition Facts table may be confusing and is not permitted.

The Nutrition Facts table provides information on saturated and *trans* fatty acids, shown to raise serum cholesterol levels. The declaration of the other groups of fatty acids, monounsaturates, omega-3, and omega-6 polyunsaturates, is optional unless claims are made, in which case all three must be declared.

Potassium is not included as a mandatory nutrient of the Nutrition Facts table because it is not considered to be a nutrient of general public health importance. The declaration of potassium, however, is mandatory when a claim is made for the sodium or salt content of a food that contains an added potassium salt.

Daily Value is a comparison standard comprised of
(a) vitamin or mineral amounts referred to in the definition of a recommended daily intake for that vitamin or mineral
(b) nutrient amounts referred to in the definition of reference standard for that nutrient

Nutrition Facts
Per 1 cup (264g)

Amount	% Daily Value
Calories 260	
Fat 13g	20%
Saturated Fat 3g + *Trans* Fat 2g	25%
Cholesterol 30mg	
Sodium 660mg	28%
Carbohydrate 31g	10%
Fibre 0g	0%
Sugars 5g	
Protein 5g	
Vitamin A 4%	Vitamin C 2%
Calcium 15%	Iron 4%

g = gram
mg = milligram

Serving size is stipulated for various foods.

The amount of vitamins and minerals is expressed as a percentage of the Daily Value per serving of stated size.

Eat well and be active today and every day!

The benefits of eating well and being active include:

- Better overall health.
- Lower risk of disease.
- A healthy body weight.
- Feeling and looking better.
- More energy.
- Stronger muscles and bones.

Be active

To be active every day is a step towards better health and a healthy body weight.

Canada's Physical Activity Guide recommends building 30 to 60 minutes of moderate physical activity into daily life for adults and at least 90 minutes a day for children and youth. You don't have to do it all at once. Add it up in periods of at least 10 minutes at a time for adults and five minutes at a time for children and youth.

Start slowly and build up.

Eat well

Another important step towards better health and a healthy body weight is to follow *Canada's Food Guide* by:

- Eating the recommended amount and type of food each day.
- Limiting foods and beverages high in calories, fat, sugar or salt (sodium) such as cakes and pastries, chocolate and candies, cookies and granola bars, doughnuts and muffins, ice cream and frozen desserts, french fries, potato chips, nachos and other salty snacks, alcohol, fruit flavoured drinks, soft drinks, sports and energy drinks, and sweetened hot or cold drinks.

Read the label

- Compare the Nutrition Facts table on food labels to choose products that contain less fat, saturated fat, trans fat, sugar and sodium.
- Keep in mind that the calories and nutrients listed are for the amount of food found at the top of the Nutrition Facts table.

Limit trans fat

When a Nutrition Facts table is not available, ask for nutrition information to choose foods lower in trans and saturated fats.

Nutrition Facts
Per 0 mL (0 g)

Amount	% Daily Value
Calories 0	
Fat 0 g	0 %
Saturates 0 g	0 %
+ Trans 0 g	
Cholesterol 0 mg	
Sodium 0 mg	0 %
Carbohydrate 0 g	0 %
Fibre 0 g	0 %
Sugars 0 g	
Protein 0 g	

Vitamin A	0 %	Vitamin C	0 %
Calcium	0 %	Iron	0 %

Take a step today...

✓ Have breakfast every day. It may help control your hunger later in the day.

✓ Walk wherever you can — get off the bus early, use the stairs.

✓ Benefit from eating vegetables and fruit at all meals and as snacks.

✓ Spend less time being inactive such as watching TV or playing computer games.

✓ Request nutrition information about menu items when eating out to help you make healthier choices.

✓ Enjoy eating with family and friends!

✓ Take time to eat and savour every bite!

For more information, interactive tools, or additional copies visit Canada's Food Guide on-line at:
www.healthcanada.gc.ca/foodguide

or contact:

Publications
Health Canada
Ottawa, Ontario K1A 0K9
E-Mail: publications@hc-sc.gc.ca
Tel.: 1-866-225-0709
Fax: (613) 941-5366
TTY: 1-800-267-1245

Également disponible en français sous le titre : Bien manger avec le Guide alimentaire canadien

This publication can be made available on request on diskette, large print, audio-cassette and braille.

FIGURE C-4 ▶ Recommendations to eat well and be active from *Canada's Food Guide.*

Advice for different ages and stages...

Children	Women of childbearing age	Men and women over 50
Following *Canada's Food Guide* helps children grow and thrive. Young children have small appetites and need calories for growth and development. • Serve small nutritious meals and snacks each day. • Do not restrict nutritious foods because of their fat content. Offer a variety of foods from the four food groups. • Most of all... be a good role model.	All women who could become pregnant and those who are pregnant or breastfeeding need a multivitamin containing **folic acid** every day. Pregnant women need to ensure that their multivitamin also contains **iron**. A health care professional can help you find the multivitamin that's right for you. Pregnant and breastfeeding women need more calories. Include an extra 2 to 3 Food Guide Servings each day. **Here are two examples:** • Have fruit and yogurt for a snack, or • Have an extra slice of toast at breakfast and an extra glass of milk at supper.	The need for **vitamin D** increases after the age of 50. In addition to following *Canada's Food Guide*, everyone over the age of 50 should take a daily vitamin D supplement of 10 µg (400 IU).

FIGURE C-5 ▶ Advice for different ages and stages from *Canada's Food Guide*.

The new regulations make nutrition labeling mandatory on most food labels using a new format. The regulations also update requirements for nutrient content claims and permit, for the first time in Canada, diet-related health claims for foods.

Templates for Canadian "Nutrition Facts" Tables

Bilingual Label

Nutrition Facts
Valeur nutritive
Per 125 mL (87 g) / 0par 125 mL (87 g)

Amount Teneur	% Daily Value % valeur quotidienne
Calories / Calories 80	
Fat / Lipids 0.5 g	**1** %
Saturated / saturés 0 g + *Trans* / trans 0 g	**0** %
Cholesterol / Cholestérol 0 mg	
Sodium / Sodium 0 mg	**0** %
Carbohydrate / Glucides 18 g	**6** %
Fibre / Fibres 2 g	**8** %
Sugars / Sucres 2 g	
Protein / Protéines 3 g	
Vitamin A / Vitamine A	2 %
Vitamin C / Vitamine C	10 %
Calcium / Calcium	0 %
Iron / Fer	2 %

English Label

Nutrition Facts
Per 125 mL (87 g)

Amount	% Daily Value
Calories 80	
Fat 0.5 g	**1** %
Saturated 0 g + *Trans* 0 g	**0** %
Cholesterol 0 mg	
Sodium 0 mg	**0** %
Carbohydrate 18 g	**6** %
Fibre 2 g	**8** %
Sugars 2 g	
Protein 3 g	
Vitamin A 2 %	Vitamin C 10 %
Calcium 0 %	Iron 2 %

French Label

Valeur nutritive
par 125 mL (87 g)

Teneur	% valeur quotidienne
Calories 80	
Lipids 0,5 g	**1** %
saturés 0 g + trans 0 g	**0** %
Cholestérol 0 mg	
Sodium 0 mg	**0** %
Glucides 18 g	**6** %
Fibres 2 g	**8** %
Sucres 2 g	
Protéines 3 g	
Vitamine A 2 %	Vitamine C 10 %
Calcium 0 %	Fer 2 %

g = gram
mg = milligram

New Canadian Nutrition Facts Label for Children Under Two Years of Age

Nutrition Facts
Per 1 jar (126 mL)

	Amount
Calories	110
Fat	0g
Sodium	10 mg
Carbohydrate	27g
Fibre	4g
Sugars	18g
Protein	0g

% Daily Value

Vitamin A 6%	Vitamin C 45%
Calcium 2%	Iron 2%

g = gram
mg = milligram

Recommended Daily Intakes and Reference Standards

The following are the Recommended Daily Intakes and Reference Standards used on Nutrition Labels for persons 2 years of age and older.*†‡

Dietary Constituent	Amount	Dietary Constituent	Amount
Fat	**65 g**	Folacin	220 µg
The sum of saturated fatty acids and *trans* fatty acids	**20 g**	Vitamin B$_{12}$	2 µg
Cholesterol	**300 mg**	Pantothenic acid or pantothenate	7 mg
Carbohydrate	**300 g**	Vitamin K	**80 mg**
Fibre	**25 g**	Biotin	**30 µg**
Sodium	**2400 mg**	Calcium	1100 mg
Chloride	**3400 µg**	Phosphorus	1100 mg
Potassium	**3500 mg**	Magnesium	250 mg
Vitamin A	1000 RE	Iron	14 mg
Vitamin D	5 µg	Zinc	9 mg
Vitamin E	10 mg	Iodide	160 µg
Vitamin C	60 mg	Selenium	**50 µg**
Thiamin, thiamine or vitamin B$_1$	1.3 mg	Copper	**2 mg**
Riboflavin or vitamin B$_2$	1.6 mg	Manganese	**2 mg**
Niacin	23 NE	Chromium	**120 µg**
Vitamin B$_6$	1.8 mg	Molybdenum	**75 µg**

*RE = retinol equivalents

†NE = niacin equivalents

‡Together these constitute the Daily Values used on the Canadian Nutrition Facts Label. Reference Standards are bolded.

Approved Nutrient Content Claims for Canada

The following is a sample of approved nutrient content claims for food labels (for the complete list of regulations see the website http://canadagazette.gc.ca/partII/2003/20030101/html/sor11-e.html).

Energy

- *Free of energy:* The food provides less than 5 Calories or 21 kilojoules per reference amount and serving of stated size.
- *Low in energy:* The food provides 40 Calories or 167 kilojoules or less per reference amount and serving of stated size.
- *Reduced in energy:* The food is processed, formulated, reformulated, or otherwise modified so that it provides at least 25% less energy per reference amount of a similar food.
- *Lower in energy:* The food provides at least 25% less energy per reference amount of a similar food.

- *Source of energy:* The food provides at least 100 Calories or 420 kilojoules per reference amount and serving of stated size.
- *More energy:* The food provides at least 25% more energy, totalling at least 100 more Calories or 420 more kilojoules per reference amount of a similar food.

Protein

- *Low in protein:* The food contains no more than 1 gram of protein per 100 grams of the food.
- *Source of protein:* The food has a protein rating of 20 or more, as deter-

mined by official method FO-1, *Determination of Protein Rating,* October 15, 1981, (*a*) per reasonable daily intake; or (*b*) per 30 grams combined with 125 milliliters of milk, if the food is a breakfast cereal.

- *Excellent source of protein:* The food has a protein rating of 40 or more, as determined by official method FO-1, *Determination of Protein Rating,* October 15, 1981, (*a*) per reasonable daily intake; or (*b*) per 30 grams combined with 125 milliliters of milk, if the food is a breakfast cereal.
- *More protein:* The food (*a*) has a protein rating of 20 or more, as determined by official method

FO-1, *Determination of Protein Rating*, October 15, 1981, (i) per reasonable daily intake, or (ii) per 30 grams combined with 125 milliliters of milk, if the food is a breakfast cereal; and (*b*) contains at least 25% more protein, totalling at least 7 grams more, per reasonable daily intake compared to the reference food of the same food group or the similar reference food.

Fat

- *Free of fat:* The food contains less than 0.5 grams of fat per reference amount and serving of stated size.
- *Low in fat:* The food contains 3 grams or less of fat per reference amount and serving of stated size and, if the reference amount is 30 grams or 30 milliliters or less, per 50 grams.
- *Reduced in fat:* The food is processed, formulated, reformulated, or otherwise modified so that it contains at least 25% less fat than the reference amount of a similar food.
- *Lower in fat:* The food contains at least 25% less fat per reference amount of the food, than the reference amount of the reference food of the same food group.
- *100% fat-free:* The food (*a*) contains less than 0.5 grams of fat per 100 grams; (*b*) contains no added fat.
- *No added fat:* The food contains no added fats or oils set out in Division 9, or added butter or ghee, or ingredients that contain added fats or oils, or butter or ghee.
- *Free of saturated fatty acids:* The food contains less than 0.2 grams saturated fatty acids and less than 0.2 grams *trans* fatty acids per reference amount and serving of stated size.
- *Low in saturated fatty acids:* (1) The food contains 2 grams or less of saturated fatty acids and *trans* fatty acids combined per reference amount and serving of stated size. (2) The food provides 15% or less energy from the sum of saturated fatty acids and *trans* fatty acids.

- *Reduced in saturated fatty acids:* The food is processed, formulated, reformulated, or otherwise modified without increasing the content of *trans* fatty acids, so that it contains at least 25% less saturated fatty acids per reference amount of the food than the reference amount of the similar reference food.
- *Lower in saturated fatty acids:* The food contains at least 25% less saturated fatty acids and the content of *trans* fatty acids is not higher per reference amount of the food, than the reference amount of the reference food of the same food group.
- *Free of trans fatty acids:* The food contains less than 0.2 grams of *trans* fatty acids per reference amount and serving of stated size.
- *Reduced in trans fatty acids:* The food is processed, formulated, reformulated, or otherwise modified without increasing the content of saturated fatty acids, so that it contains at least 25% less *trans* fatty acids per reference amount of the food than the reference amount of the similar reference food.
- *Lower in trans fatty acids:* The food contains at least 25% less *trans* fatty acids and the content of saturated fatty acids is not higher per reference amount of the food compared to the reference amount of a similar food.
- *Source of omega-3 polyunsaturated fatty acids:* The food contains 0.3 grams or more of omega-3 polyunsaturated fatty acids per reference amount and serving of stated size.
- *Source of omega-6 polyunsaturated fatty acids:* The food contains 2 grams or more of omega-6 polyunsaturated fatty acids per reference amount and serving of stated size.

Cholesterol

- *Free of cholesterol:* The food contains less than 2 milligrams of cholesterol per reference amount and serving of stated size.
- *Low in cholesterol:* The food contains 20 milligrams or less of cholesterol per reference amount and serving of

stated size (if the reference amount is 30 grams or 30 milliliters or less, per 50 grams).
- *Reduced in cholesterol:* The food is processed, formulated, reformulated, or otherwise modified so that it contains at least 25% less cholesterol per reference amount of a similar food.
- *Lower in cholesterol:* The food contains at least 25% less cholesterol per reference amount of a similar food.

Sodium or Salt

- *Free of sodium or salt:* The food contains less than 5 milligrams of sodium per reference amount and serving of stated size.
- *Low in sodium or salt:* The food contains 140 milligrams or less of sodium per reference amount and serving of stated size.
- *Reduced in sodium or salt:* The food is processed, formulated, reformulated, or otherwise modified so that it contains at least 25% less sodium per reference amount of a similar food.
- *Lower in sodium or salt:* The food contains at least 25% less sodium per reference amount of the food.
- *No added sodium or salt:* The food contains no added salt, other sodium salts, or ingredients that contain sodium that functionally substitute for added salt.
- *Lightly salted:* The food contains at least 50% less added sodium than the sodium added to a similar reference food.

Sugars

- *Free of sugars:* The food contains less than 0.5 milligrams of sugars per reference amount and serving of stated size.
- *Reduced in sugars:* The food is processed, formulated, reformulated, or otherwise modified so that it contains at least 25% less sugars, totalling at least 5 grams less, per reference amount of the food.
- *Lower in sugars:* The food contains at least 25% less sugars, totalling at least 5 grams less, per reference amount of the food.

- *No added sugars:* The food contains no added sugars, no ingredients containing added sugars or ingredients that contain sugars that functionally substitute for added sugars.

Fibre

- *Source of fibre:* The food contains 2 grams or more (*a*) of fibre per reference amount and serving of stated size, if no fibre or fibre source is identified in the statement or claim; or (*b*) of each identified fibre or fibre from an identified fibre source per reference amount and serving of stated size, if a fibre or fibre source is identified in the statement or claim.
- *High source of fibre:* The food contains 4 grams or more (*a*) of fibre per reference amount and serving of stated size, if no fibre or fibre source is identified in the statement or claim; or (*b*) of each identified fibre or fibre from an identified fibre source per reference amount and serving of stated size, if a fibre or fibre source is identified in the statement or claim.
- *Very high source of fibre:* The food contains 6 grams or more (*a*) of fibre per reference amount and serving of stated size, if no fibre or fibre source is identified in the statement

or claim; or (*b*) of each identified fibre or fibre from an identified fibre source per reference amount and serving of stated size, if a fibre or fibre source is identified in the statement or claim.
- *More fibre:* The food contains at least 25% more fibre, totalling at least 1 gram more, if no fibre or fibre source is identified in the statement or claim, or at least 25% more of an identified fibre or fibre from an identified fibre source, totalling at least 1 gram more, if a fibre or fibre source is identified in the statement or claim compared to reference amount of a similar food.

Light and Lean

- *Light in energy or fat:* The food meets the conditions set out for the subject "reduced in energy" or "reduced in fat."
- *Lean:* The food (*a*) is meat or poultry that has not been ground, a marine or fresh water animal or a product of any of these; and (*b*) contains 10% or less fat.
- *Extra lean:* The food (*a*) is meat or poultry that has not been ground, a marine or fresh water animal or a product of any of these; and (*b*) contains 7.5% or less fat.

Approved Health Claims for Nutrition Labels

If a manufacturer follows specific guidelines addressing both the nutrients noted in the claim as well as guidelines pertaining to other nutrients in a food, the following health claims can be made.
- A healthy diet containing foods high in potassium and low in sodium may reduce the risk of high blood pressure, a risk factor for stroke and heart disease.
- A healthy diet with adequate calcium and vitamin D, and regular physical activity, help to achieve strong bones and may reduce the risk of osteoporosis.
- A healthy diet low in saturated and *trans* fats may reduce the risk of heart disease.
- A healthy diet rich in a variety of vegetables and fruit may help reduce the risk of some types of cancer.
- Foods very low in starch and fermentable sugars can make the following health claims:
  - Won't cause cavities;
  - Does not promote tooth decay;
  - Does not promote dental caries; or is
  - Non-cariogenic.

THE EXCHANGE SYSTEM

Exchange System A system for classifying foods into numerous lists based on the foods' macronutrient composition and establishing serving sizes, so that one serving of each food on a list contains the same amount of carbohydrate, protein, fat, and calorie content.

exchange The serving size of a food on a specific exchange list.

The **Exchange System** is a valuable tool for roughly estimating the calorie, protein, carbohydrate, and fat content of a food or meal. This tool organizes many details of the nutrient composition of foods into a manageable framework. By using the Exchange System, you can plan daily menus to fall roughly within specific percentages of macronutrients without having to look up or memorize the nutrient values of numerous foods, so the time you spend now becoming familiar with the Exchange System will pay off in the future.

In the Exchange System, individual foods are placed into three broad groups: carbohydrate, meat and meat substitutes, and fat. Within these groups are lists that contain foods of similar macronutrient composition: various types of milk, fruit, vegetables, starch, other carbohydrates, meat and meat substitutes, and fat. These lists are designed so that, when the proper serving size is observed, each food on a list provides about the same amount of carbohydrate, protein, fat, and calories. This equality allows the exchange of foods on each list, hence the term *Exchange System*.

The Exchange System was originally developed for planning diabetic diets. Diabetes is easier to control if the person's diet has about the same composition day after day. If a certain number of **exchanges** from each of the various lists is eaten each day, that regularity is easier to achieve. However, because the Exchange System provides a quick way to estimate the calorie, carbohydrate, protein, and fat content in any food or meal, it is a valuable menu-planning tool for people without diabetes, as well.

Becoming Familiar with the Exchange System

To use the Exchange System, you must know which foods are on each list and the serving sizes for each food.

Table D-1 gives the serving sizes for foods on each exchange list, as well as the carbohydrate, protein, fat, and calorie content per exchange. The meat and milk lists are divided into subclasses, which vary in fat content and, hence, in the amount of calories they provide. Foods on the meat and fat lists contain essentially no carbohydrate; those on the fruit and fat lists lack appreciable amounts of protein; and those on the vegetable, fruit, and other carbohydrates lists contain essentially no fat. You need to study Table D-1 and Figure D-1 to become familiar with the exchange lists, the sizes of the exchanges (that is, serving sizes) on each list, and the amounts of carbohydrate, protein, fat, and calories per exchange.

Before you can turn a group of exchanges into a daily meal plan, you must be aware of which foods are on each exchange list (Figure D-1). The entire U.S. Exchange System (2003) is presented in Appendix D, which you should consult frequently while exploring the system to discover its various peculiarities. For example, the starch list includes not only bread, dry cereal, cooked cereal, rice, and pasta, but also baked beans, corn on the cob, and potatoes. These foods are not identical to those composing the bread, cereal, rice, and pasta group in MyPyramid. The Exchange System is not concerned with the origin of a food, whether animal or vegetable. It is primarily concerned with the macronutrients carbohydrate, protein, and fat in each food on a specific list. For example, the carbohydrate composition of potatoes resembles that of bread more than that of broccoli, although potatoes are vegetables. In addition, several foods on the meat and meat substitutes list are not meats. The list of other carbohydrates includes jam, angel food cake, fat-free frozen yogurt, and foods such as frosted cake that count as both other carbohydrate exchanges and fat exchanges. Bacon appears in the fat list, rather than the high-fat meat category.

TABLE D-1 Nutrient Composition of Exchange System Lists (2003 Edition)

Groups/Lists	Household Measures*	Carbohydrate (g)	Protein (g)	Fat (g)	Energy (kcal)
Carbohydrate Group					
Starch	1 slice, ¾ cup raw, or ½ cup cooked	15	3	1 or less†	80
Fruit	1 small/medium piece	15	—	—	60
Milk	1 cup				
Fat-free/very low-fat		12	8	0–3†	90
Reduced-fat		12	8	5	120
Whole		12	8	8	150
Other carbohydrates	Varies	15	Varies	Varies	Varies
Nonstarchy vegetables	1 cup raw or ½ cup cooked	5	2	—	25
Meat and Meat Substitutes Group	1 ounce				
Very lean		—	7	0–1	35
Lean		—	7	3	55
Medium-fat		—	7	5	75
High-fat		—	7	8	100
Fat Group	1 teaspoon	—	—	5	45

*An estimate; see exchange lists for actual amounts.
†Calculated as 1 gram for purposes of calorie contribution.

Reproduction of the exchange lists in whole or in part, without permission of The American Dietetic Association or the American Diabetes Association, Inc. is a violation of federal law. This material has been modified from *Exchange Lists for Meal Planning,* which is the basis of a meal planning system designed by a committee of the American Diabetes Association and The American Dietetic Association. While designed primarily for people with diabetes and others who must follow special diets, the exchange lists are based on principles of good nutrition that apply to everyone. © 2003 by the American Diabetes Association and the American Dietetic Association.

Starch exchange choices

Meat and meat substitutes exchange choices

Vegetable exchange choices

Fruit exchange choices

Milk exchange choices

Fat exchange choices

FIGURE D-1 ▶ Foods arranged according to the Exchange System lists.

TABLE D-2 Possible Exchange Patterns That Yield 55% of Calories as Carbohydrate, 30% as Fat, and 15% as Protein

Exchange List	1200*	1600*	2000	kcal/Day 2400	2800	3200	3600
Milk (reduced-fat)	2	2	2	2	2	2	2
Vegetable	3	3	3	4	4	4	4
Fruit	3	4	5	6	8	9	9
Starch	5	8	11	13	15	18	21
Meat (lean)	4	4	4	5	6	7	8
Fat	2	4	6	8	10	11	13

This is just one set of options. More meat could be included if less milk were used, for example.

*Calorie intakes of 1200 and 1600 kcal contain 20% of calories as protein and 50% of calories as carbohydrate to allow for greater flexibility in diet planning.

Free foods (essentially calorie-free) include bouillon, diet soda, coffee, tea, dill pickles, and vinegar, as well as herbs and spices. Most vegetables, such as cabbage, celery, mushrooms, lettuce, and zucchini, also can be considered free foods; their minimal energy contribution need not count in the calculations when they are eaten in moderation (1 to 2 servings per meal or snack).

Using the Exchange System to Develop Daily Menus

Now let's use the Exchange System to plan a 1-day menu. Let's target a calorie content of 2000 kcal, with 55% derived from carbohydrates (1100 kcal), 15% from protein (300 kcal), and 30% from fat (600 kcal). This can be translated into 2 reduced-fat milk exchanges, 3 vegetable exchanges, 5 fruit exchanges, 11 starch exchanges, 4 lean meat exchanges, and 6 fat exchanges (Table D-2). This is only one of many possible combinations; the Exchange System offers great flexibility.

Table D-3 arbitrarily separates these exchanges into breakfast, lunch, dinner, and a snack. Breakfast includes 1 reduced-fat milk exchange, 2 fruit exchanges, 2 starch exchanges, and 1 fat exchange. This total corresponds to ¾ cup of a ready-to-eat breakfast cereal, 1 cup of reduced-fat milk, 1 slice of bread with 1 teaspoon margarine, and 1 cup of orange juice.

Lunch consists of 2 fat exchanges, 4 starch exchanges, 1 vegetable exchange, 1 reduced-fat milk exchange, and 2 fruit exchanges. This translates into one slice of bacon with 1 teaspoon mayonnaise on two slices of bread, with tomato—in other words, a bacon and tomato sandwich. You can also add lettuce to the sandwich. This can be considered a free vegetable choice. Add to this meal a 9-inch banana (1 exchange = 1 small banana), 1 cup of reduced-fat milk, and 6 graham crackers (2½ inches by 2½ inches). Later add a snack of ¾ ounce of pretzels for another starch exchange.

Dinner consists of 4 lean meat exchanges, 1 fruit exchange, 2 vegetable exchanges, 1 fat exchange, and 2 starch exchanges. This total corresponds to a 4-ounce broiled steak (meat only, no bone), 1 medium baked potato (1 exchange = 1 small baked potato) with 1 teaspoon of margarine, 1 cup of broccoli, and 1 kiwi fruit. Coffee (if desired) is not counted, because it contains no appreciable calories.

Finally, we have a snack containing 2 starch exchanges and 2 fat exchanges. This translates into 1 bagel with 2 tablespoons of regular cream cheese.

This 1-day menu is only one of many possible with the exchange lists. Apple juice could replace the orange juice; two apples could be exchanged for the banana. The choices are endless. An exchange diet is much easier to plan if you use individual foods, as was done here; however, the Exchange System tables list some combination foods to help you. Using combination foods, such as pizza or lasagna, however, makes it more difficult to calculate the number of exchanges in a serving. For instance, lasagna typically has meat exchanges, vegetable exchanges, and starch

TABLE D-3 Sample 1-Day 2000-kcal Menu Based on the Exchange System Plan*

Breakfast	
1 reduced-fat milk exchange	1 cup reduced-fat milk (some on cereal)
2 fruit exchanges	1 cup orange juice
2 starch exchanges	¾ cup ready-to-eat breakfast cereal, 1 piece whole-wheat toast
1 fat exchange	1 teaspoon soft margarine on toast
Lunch	
4 starch exchanges	2 slices whole-wheat bread, 6 graham crackers (2½ inches by 2½ inches)
2 fat exchanges	1 slice bacon, 1 teaspoon mayonnaise
1 vegetable exchange	1 sliced tomato
2 fruit exchanges	1 banana (9 inches)
1 reduced-fat milk exchange	1 cup reduced-fat milk
Snack	
1 starch exchange	¾ ounce pretzels
Dinner	
4 lean meat exchanges	4 ounces lean steak (well trimmed)
2 starch exchanges	1 medium baked potato
1 fat exchange	1 tsp soft margarine
2 vegetable exchanges	1 cup cooked broccoli
1 fruit exchange	1 kiwi fruit
	Coffee (if desired)
Snack	
2 starch exchanges	1 bagel
2 fat exchanges	2 tablespoons regular cream cheese

*The target plan was a 2000 kcal intake, with 55% of calories from carbohydrate, 15% from protein, and 30% from fat. Computer analysis indicates that this menu yielded 2040 kcal, with 53% of calories from carbohydrate, 16% from protein, and 31% from fat—in close agreement with the targeted goals.

exchanges. With practice, you will be able to tackle such complex foods (Fig. D-2). For now, using individual foods makes learning the Exchange System much easier. Finally, you might want to prove to yourself that the food choices listed in Table D-3 really meet the Exchange plan. This demonstration will give you practice turning exchanges into food servings.

EXCHANGE SYSTEM LISTS

MILK EXCHANGE LIST**

Fat-Free and Low-Fat Milk

(12 g carbohydrate, 8 g protein, 0–3 g fat, 90 kcal)

1 cup	fat-free, ½%, and 1% milk, and buttermilk
⅓ cup	powdered (fat-free dry, before adding liquid)
½ cup	canned, evaporated fat-free milk
1 cup	buttermilk made from fat-free or low-fat milk
1 cup	soy milk (low-fat or fat-free)
⅔ cup (6 oz)	yogurt made from fat-free milk (plain, unflavored)
⅔ cup (6 oz)	yogurt, fat-free, flavored, sweetened with nonnutritive sweetener and fructose

*The exchange lists are the basis of a meal planning system designed by a committee of the American Diabetes Association and the American Dietetic Association. While designed primarily for people with diabetes and others who must follow special diets, the exchange lists are based on principles of good nutrition that apply to everyone. © 2003 by the American Diabetes Association and the American Dietetic Association.

**g = gram

FIGURE D-2 ▶ Record the Exchange System pattern you have chosen in the left-hand column. Then distribute the exchanges throughout the day, noting the food to be used and the serving size.

Exchange List	Total Exchanges to be Consumed Daily	Exchanges Consumed at Each Meal		
		Breakfast	Lunch	Dinner
MILK				
VEGETABLE				
FRUIT				
STARCH				
MEAT AND SUBSTITUTES				
FAT				

Reduced-Fat Milk

(12 g carbohydrate, 8 g protein, 5 g fat, 120 kcal)

1 cup	2% milk
1 cup	soy milk
¾ cup	yogurt plain, low-fat (added milk solids)
1 cup	sweet acidophilus milk

Whole Milk

(12 g carbohydrate, 8 g protein, 8 g fat, 150 kcal)

1 cup	whole milk
½ cup	evaporated whole milk
1 cup	goat's milk
1 cup	kefir
1 cup	yogurt, plain (made from whole milk)

VEGETABLE EXCHANGE LIST

(5 g carbohydrate, 2 g protein, 0 g fat, 25 kcal)
1 vegetable exchange equals:
½ cup cooked vegetables or vegetable juice
1 cup raw vegetables

artichoke	cucumber	peppers (all varieties)
artichoke hearts	eggplant	radishes
asparagus	green onions or scallions	salad greens (all varieties)
beans (green, wax, Italian)	greens (e.g., collard)	sauerkraut
bean sprouts	kohlrabi	spinach
beets	leeks	squash (summer)
broccoli	mixed vegetables (without corn, peas, or pasta)	tomato (fresh, canned, sauce)
brussels sprouts		tomato/vegetable juice
cabbage	mushrooms	turnips
carrots	okra	water chestnuts
cauliflower	onions	watercress
celery	pea pods	zucchini

FRUIT EXCHANGE LIST

Fruit

(15 g carbohydrate, 0 g protein, 0 g fat, 60 kcal)
1 fruit exchange equals:

1 (4 oz)	apple, unpeeled (small)	1 (4 oz)	peach, fresh (medium)
4 rings	apple, dried	½ cup	peaches, canned
½ cup	applesauce (unsweetened)	1 (4 oz)	pear, fresh
4 (5½ oz)	apricots, fresh	½ cup	pear, canned
8 halves	apricots, dried	¾ cup	pineapple, fresh
½ cup	apricots, canned	½ cup	pineapple, canned
1 (4 oz)	banana (small)	2 (5 oz)	plums (small)
¾ cup	blackberries	½ cup	plums, canned
¾ cup	blueberries	3	plums dried (prunes)
⅓ melon (11 oz)	cantaloupe (small)	2 tbsp	raisins
1 cup cubes	cantaloupe	1 cup	raspberries
12 (3 oz)	cherries	1¼ cup	strawberries (raw, whole)
½ cup	cherries, canned	2 (8 oz)	tangerines (small)
3	dates	1 slice (13½ oz)	watermelon (or 1¼ cups cubes)
2 (3½ oz)	figs, fresh (large)		
1½	figs, dried		
½ cup	fruit cocktail	**Fruit Juice**	
½ (11 oz)	grapefruit (large)		
¾ cup	grapefruit sections, canned	½ cup	apple juice/cider
17 (3 oz)	grapes (small)	⅓ cup	cranberry juice cocktail
1 slice (10 oz)	honeydew melon (or 1 cup cubes)	1 cup	cranberry juice cocktail, reduced-calorie
1 (3½ oz)	kiwi	⅓ cup	fruit juice blends, 100% juice
¾ cup	mandarin orange sections	⅓ cup	grape juice
½ (5½ oz)	mango (or ½ cup)	½ cup	grapefruit juice
1 (5 oz)	nectarine (small)	½ cup	orange juice
1 (6½ oz)	orange (small)	½ cup	pineapple juice
½ (8 oz)	papaya (or 1 cup cubes)	⅓ cup	prune juice

STARCH EXCHANGE LIST

(15 g carbohydrate, 3 g protein, 0–1 g fat, 80 kcal)
1 starch exchange equals:

Bread

¼ (1 oz)	bagel
2 slices (1½ oz)	bread, reduced-calorie
1 slice (1 oz)	bread, white, whole-wheat, pumpernickel, or rye
4 (⅔ oz)	bread sticks, crisp, 4 inch × ½ inch
½	English muffin
½ (1 oz)	hot dog or hamburger bun
¼	naan, 8 inch × 2 inch
1	pancake, 4 inch across × ¼ inch thick
½	pita, 6 inches across
1 slice (1 oz)	raisin bread, unfrosted
1 (1 oz)	roll, plain (small)
1	tortilla, corn, 6 inches across
1	tortilla, flour, 6 inches across
⅓	tortilla, flour, 10 inches across
1	waffle, 4 inches square or across, reduced-fat

Cereals and Grains

½ cup	bran cereal
½ cup	bulgur
½ cup	cereal, cooked
¾ cup	cereal, unsweetened, ready-to-eat
3 tbsp	cornmeal (dry)
⅓ cup	couscous
3 tbsp	flour (dry)
¼ cup	granola, low-fat
¼ cup	Grape-Nuts®
½ cup	grits
½ cup	kasha
⅓ cup	millet
¼ cup	muesli
½ cup	oats
⅓ cup	pasta
1½ cups	puffed cereal
⅓ cup	rice, white or brown
½ cup	Shredded Wheat
½ cup	sugar-frosted cereal
3 tbsp	wheat germ

Starchy Vegetables

⅓ cup	baked beans
½ cup	corn
½ (5 oz)	corn on the cob (large)
1 cup	mixed vegetables with corn, peas, or pasta
½ cup	peas, green
½ cup	plantain
½ cup or ½ medium (3 oz)	potato, boiled
¼ large (3 oz)	potato, baked with skin
½ cup	potato, mashed
1 cup	squash, winter (acorn, butternut, pumpkin)
½ cup	yam, sweet potato, plain

Crackers and Snacks

8	animal crackers
3	graham crackers, 2½-inch square
¾ oz	matzoh
4 slices	melba toast
24	oyster crackers
3 cups	popcorn (popped, no fat added or low-fat microwave)
¾ oz	pretzels
2	rice cakes, 4 inches across
6	saltine-type crackers
15–20 (¾ oz)	snack chips, fat-free (tortilla, potato)
2–5 (¾ oz)	whole-wheat crackers, no fat added

Dried Beans, Peas, and Lentils

(Counts as 1 starch exchange plus 1 very lean meat exchange)

½ cup	beans and peas (garbanzo, pinto, kidney, white, split, black-eyed)
½ cup	lentils
⅔ cup	lima beans
3 tbsp	miso

Starchy Foods Prepared with Fat

(Counts as 1 starch exchange, plus 1 fat exchange)

1	biscuit, 2½ inches across
½ cup	chow mein noodles
1 piece (2 oz)	corn bread, 2-inch cube
6	crackers, round butter type
1 cup	croutons
1 cup (2 oz)	French-fried potatoes (oven-baked) (see also the fast-foods list)
¼ cup	granola
⅓ cup	hummus
⅕ (1 oz)	muffin, 5 oz
3 cups	popcorn, microwaved
3	sandwich crackers, cheese or peanut butter filling

9–13 (3/4 oz)	snack chips (potato, tortilla)	1
1/3 cup	stuffing, bread (prepared)	4–6 (1 oz)
2	taco shells, 6 inches across	

waffle, 4-inch square or across	
whole-wheat crackers, fat added	

OTHER CARBOHYDRATES EXCHANGE LIST

One exchange equals 15 g carbohydrate, or 1 starch, or 1 fruit, or 1 milk.

Exchanges per Serving

1/12 cake (about 2 oz)	angel food cake, unfrosted	2 carbohydrates
2-inch square (about 1 oz)	brownie, unfrosted (small)	1 carbohydrate, 1 fat
2-inch square (about 1 oz)	cake, unfrosted	1 carbohydrate, 1 fat
2-inch square (about 2 oz)	cake, frosted	2 carbohydrates, 1 fat
2	cookies, fat-free (small)	1 carbohydrate
2 (about 2/3 oz)	cookies or sandwich cookies with creme filling (small)	1 carbohydrate, 1 fat
1/4 cup	cranberry sauce, jellied	1½ carbohydrates
1 (about 2 oz)	cupcake, frosted (small)	2 carbohydrates, 1 fat
1 (1½ oz)	doughnut, plain cake (medium)	1½ carbohydrates, 2 fats
3¾ inches across (2 oz)	doughnuts, glazed	2 carbohydrates, 2 fats
1 bar (1⅓ oz)	Energy, sport, or breakfast bar	2 carbohydrates, 1 fat
1 bar (2 oz)	Energy, sport, or breakfast bar	3 carbohydrates, 1 fat
½ cup (3½ oz)	fruit cobbler	3 carbohydrates, 1 fat
1 bar (3 oz)	fruit juice bars, frozen, 100% juice	1 carbohydrate
1 roll (¾ oz)	fruit snacks, chewy (puréed fruit concentrate)	1 carbohydrate
1½ tbsp	fruit spread, 100% fruit	1 carbohydrate
½ cup	gelatin, regular	1 carbohydrate
3	gingersnaps	1 carbohydrate
1 bar (1 oz)	granola or snack bar (regular and low-fat)	1½ carbohydrates
1 tbsp	honey	1 carbohydrate
½ cup	ice cream, low-fat	1½ carbohydrates
½ cup	ice cream	1 carbohydrate, 2 fats
½ cup	ice cream, light	1 carbohydrate, 1 fat
½ cup	ice cream, fat-free, no sugar added	1 carbohydrate
1 tbsp	jam or jelly, regular	1 carbohydrate
1 cup	milk, chocolate, whole	2 carbohydrates, 1 fat
1/6 pie	pie, fruit, 2 crusts (8 inches across)	3 carbohydrates, 2 fats
1/8 pie	pie, pumpkin or custard (8 inches across)	2 carbohydrates, 2 fats
½ cup	pudding, regular (made with reduced-fat milk)	2 carbohydrates
½ cup	pudding, sugar-free (made with fat-free milk)	1 carbohydrate
1 can (10–11 oz)	reduced-calorie meal replacement (shake)	1½ carbohydrates, 0–1 fat
1 cup	rice milk, low-fat or fat-free, plain	1 carbohydrate
1 cup	rice milk, low-fat, flavored	1½ carbohydrates
1/4 cup	salad dressing, fat-free	1 carbohydrate
½ cup	sherbet, sorbet	2 carbohydrates
½ cup	spaghetti or pasta sauce, canned	1 carbohydrate, 1 fat
1 cup (8 oz)	sports drinks	1 carbohydrate
1 tbsp	sugar	1 carbohydrate
1 (2½ oz)	sweet roll or Danish	2½ carbohydrates, 2 fats
2 tbsp	syrup, light	1 carbohydrate
1 tbsp	syrup, regular	1 carbohydrate
5	vanilla wafers	1 carbohydrate, 1 fat
1/3 cup	yogurt, frozen, fat-free	1 carbohydrate
1 cup	yogurt, low-fat with fruit	3 carbohydrates, 0–1 fat

MEAT AND MEAT SUBSTITUTES EXCHANGE LIST

Very Lean Meat and Substitutes List

(0 g carbohydrate, 7 g protein, 0–1 g fat, and 35 kcal)
One very lean meat exchange equals:

Poultry

1 oz	chicken or turkey (white meat, no skin), Cornish hen (no skin)

Fish

1 oz	fresh or frozen cod, flounder, haddock, halibut, trout; tuna, fresh or canned in water

Shellfish

1 oz	clams, crab, lobster, scallops, shrimp, imitation shellfish

Game

1 oz	duck or pheasant (no skin), venison, buffalo, ostrich

Cheese with 1 g or less fat per oz

¼ cup	fat-free or low-fat cottage cheese
1 oz	fat-free cheese

Other

1 oz	processed sandwich meats with 1 g or less fat per oz, such as deli thin, shaved meats, chipped beef, turkey, ham
¼ cup	egg substitute, plain
2	egg whites
1 oz	hot dogs with 1 g or less fat per oz
1 oz	kidney (high in cholesterol)
1 oz	sausage with 1 g or less fat per oz

Counts as one very lean meat and one starch exchange:

½ cup	dried beans, peas, lentils (cooked)

Lean Meat and Substitutes List

(0 g carbohydrate, 7 g protein, 3 g fat, and 55 kcal)
One lean meat exchange equals:

Beef

1 oz	USDA Select or Choice grades of lean beef trimmed of fat, such as round, sirloin, and flank steak; tenderloin; roast (rib, chuck, rump); steak (T-bone, porterhouse, cubed), ground round

Pork

1 oz	lean pork, such as fresh ham; canned, cured, or boiled ham; Canadian bacon; tenderloin, center loin chop

Lamb

1 oz	roast, chop, leg

Veal

1 oz	lean chop, roast

Poultry

1 oz	chicken, turkey (dark meat, no skin), chicken white meat (with skin), domestic duck or goose (well drained of fat, no skin)

Fish

1 oz	herring (uncreamed or smoked)
6	oysters (medium)
1 oz	salmon (fresh or canned), catfish
2	sardines (canned, medium)
1 oz	tuna (canned in oil, drained)

Game

1 oz	goose (no skin), rabbit

Cheese

¼ cup	4.5%–fat cottage cheese
2 tbsp	grated Parmesan
1 oz	cheeses with 3 g or less fat per oz

Other

1½ oz	hot dogs with 3 g or less fat per oz
1 oz	processed sandwich meat with 3 g or less fat per oz, such as turkey pastrami or kielbasa
1 oz	liver, heart (high in cholesterol)

Medium-Fat Meat and Substitutes List

(0 g carbohydrate, 7 g protein, 5 g fat, and 75 kcal)
One medium-fat meat exchange equals:

Beef

1 oz	most beef products (ground beef; meatloaf; corned beef; short ribs; prime grades of meat trimmed of fat, such as prime rib)

Pork

1 oz	top loin, chop, Boston butt, cutlet

Lamb

1 oz	rib roast, ground

Veal

1 oz	cutlet (ground or cubed, unbreaded)

Poultry

1 oz	chicken dark meat (with skin), ground turkey or ground chicken, fried chicken (with skin)

	Fish
1 oz	any fried fish product

Cheese (with 5 g or less fat per oz)

1 oz	feta
1 oz	mozzarella
¼ cup (2 oz)	ricotta

	Other
1	egg (high in cholesterol, limit to 3 per week)
1 oz	sausage with 5 g or less fat per oz
¼ cup	tempeh
4 oz (½ cup)	tofu

High-Fat Meat and Substitutes List

(0 g carbohydrate, 7 g protein, 8 g fat, and 100 kcal)
One high-fat meat exchange equals:

	Pork
1 oz	spareribs, ground pork, pork sausage

Cheese

1 oz	all regular cheeses, such as American, cheddar, Monterey Jack, Swiss

	Other
1 oz	processed sandwich meats with 8 g or less fat per oz, such as bologna, pimento loaf, salami
1 oz	sausage, such as bratwurst, Italian, knockwurst, Polish, smoked
1	hot dog (turkey or chicken) (10 per pound)
3 slices	bacon (20 slices per pound)

Counts as one high-fat meat plus one fat exchange:

1	hot dog (beef, pork, or combination) (10 per pound)

FAT EXCHANGE LIST

Monounsaturated Fats List

(5 g fat and 45 kcal)
One exchange equals:

2 tbsp (1 oz)	avocado (medium)
1 tsp	oil (canola, olive, peanut)
	olives:
8	ripe, black (large)
10	green, stuffed (large)
6 nuts	almonds, cashews

6 nuts	mixed (50% peanuts)
10 nuts	peanuts
4 halves	pecans
½ tbsp	peanut butter, smooth or crunchy
1 tbsp	sesame seeds
2 tsp	tahini or sesame paste

Polyunsaturated Fats List

(5 g fat and 45 kcal)
One exchange equals:

	margarine:
1 tsp	stick, tub, or squeeze
1 tbsp	lower-fat (30% to 50% vegetable oil)
	mayonnaise:
1 tsp	regular
1 tbsp	reduced-fat
4 halves	nuts, walnuts, English
1 tsp	oil (corn, safflower, soybean)

	salad dressing:
1 tbsp	regular
2 tbsp	reduced-fat
	Miracle Whip Salad Dressing®:
2 tsp	regular
1 tbsp	reduced-fat
1 tbsp	seeds: pumpkin, sunflower

Saturated Fats List

(5 g fat and 45 kcal)
One exchange equals:

1 slice	bacon, cooked (20 slices per pound)
1 tsp	bacon, grease

	butter:
1 tsp	stick
2 tsp	whipped
1 tbsp	reduced-fat

2 tbsp (½ oz)	chitterlings, boiled		sour cream:
	cream cheese:	2 tbsp	regular
1 tbsp (½ oz)	regular	3 tbsp	reduced-fat
2 tbsp (1 oz)	reduced-fat		
1 tsp	shortening or lard		

FREE FOODS LIST

A *free food* is any food or drink that contains less than 20 kcal or less than 5 g of carbohydrate per serving. Foods with a serving size listed should be limited to three servings per day. Foods listed without a serving size can be eaten as often as you like.

Fat-Free or Reduced-Fat Foods

1 tbsp (½ oz)	cream cheese, fat-free	1 tbsp	salad dressing, fat-free nonstick cooking
1 tbsp	creamers, nondairy, liquid		spray
2 tsp	creamers, nondairy, powdered	1 tbsp	salad dressing, fat-free or low-fat, Italian
1 tbsp	mayonnaise, fat-free	2 tbsp	salad dressing, fat-free, Italian
1 tsp	mayonnaise, reduced-fat	1 tbsp	sour cream, fat-free, reduced-fat
4 tbsp	margarine, fat-free	1 tbsp	whipped topping, regular
1 tsp	margarine, reduced-fat	2 tbsp	whipped topping, light or fat-free
1 tbsp	Miracle Whip®, fat-free		
1 tsp	Miracle Whip®, reduced-fat nonstick cooking spray		

Sugar-Free Foods

1 candy	candy, hard, sugar-free; gelatin dessert, sugar-free; gelatin, unflavored; gum, sugar-free	2 tsp	jam or jelly, light sugar substitutes*
		2 tbsp	syrup, sugar-free

Drinks

	bouillon, broth, consommé		coffee
	bouillon or broth, low-sodium		diet soft drinks, sugar-free
	carbonated or mineral water		drink mixes, sugar-free
	club soda		tea
1 tbsp	cocoa powder, unsweetened		tonic water, sugar-free

Condiments

1 tbsp	catsup	2 slices	pickles, sweet (bread and butter)
	horseradish	¾ oz	pickles, sweet (gherkin)
	lemon juice	¼ cup	salsa
	lime juice	1 tbsp	soy sauce, regular or light
	mustard	1 tbsp	taco sauce
1 tbsp	pickle relish		vinegar
1½	pickles, dill (medium)	2 tbsp	yogurt

*Sugar substitutes, alternatives, or replacements approved by Food and Drug Administration (FDA) are safe to use. Common brand names include:

Equal® (aspartame)

Splenda® (sucralose)

Sprinkle Sweet® (saccharin)

Sweet One® (acesulfame K)

Sweet-10® (saccharin)

Sugar Twin® (saccharin)

Sweet 'N Low® (saccharin)

Seasonings

flavoring extracts
garlic
herbs, fresh or dried
pimento

spices
Tabasco® or hot pepper sauce
wine, used in cooking
Worcestershire sauce

COMBINATION FOODS LIST

	Entrées	Exchanges per Serving
1 cup (8 oz)	tuna noodle casserole, lasagna, spaghetti with meatballs, chili with beans, macaroni and cheese	2 carbohydrates, 2 medium-fat meats
2 cups (16 oz)	chow mein (without noodles or rice)	1 carbohydrate, 2 lean meats
½ cup (3½ oz)	tuna or chicken salad	½ carbohydrate, 2 lean meats, 1 fat
	Frozen Entrées and Meals	
generally 14–17 oz	dinner-type meal	3 carbohydrates, 3 medium-fat meats, 3 fats
3 oz	meatless burger, soy-based	½ carbohydrate, 2 lean meats
3 oz	meatless burger, vegetable and starch-based	1 carbohydrate, 1 lean meat
¼ of 12-inch (6 oz)	pizza, cheese, thin crust	2 carbohydrates, 2 medium-fat meats, 1 fat
¼ of 12-inch (6 oz)	pizza, meat topping, thin crust	2 carbohydrates, 2 medium-fat meats, 2 fats
1 (7 oz)	pot pie	2½ carbohydrates, 1 medium-fat meat, 3 fats
8–11 oz	entrée or meal with less than 340 kcal	2–3 carbohydrates, 1–2 lean meats
	Soups	
1 cup	bean	1 carbohydrate, 1 very lean meat
1 cup (8 oz)	cream (made with water)	1 carbohydrate, 1 fat
6 oz prepared	instant	1 carbohydrate
8 oz prepared	instant with beans/lentils	2½ carbohydrates, 1 very lean meat
½ cup (4 oz)	split pea (made with water)	1 carbohydrate
1 cup (8 oz)	tomato (made with water)	1 carbohydrate
1 cup (8 oz)	vegetable beef, chicken noodle, or other broth-type	1 carbohydrate

Fast-Foods

		Exchanges per Serving
1 (5–7 oz)	burritos with beef	3 carbohydrates, 1 medium-fat meat, 1 fat
6	chicken nuggets	1 carbohydrate, 2 medium-fat meats, 1 fat
1 each	chicken breast and wing, breaded and fried	1 carbohydrate, 4 medium-fat meats, 2 fats
1	chicken sandwich, grilled	2 carbohydrates, 3 very lean meats
6 (5 oz)	chicken wings, hot	1 carbohydrate, 3 medium-fat meats, 4 fats
1	fish sandwich/tartar sauce	3 carbohydrates, 1 medium-fat meat, 3 fats
1 medium serving (5 oz)	French fries	4 carbohydrates, 4 fats
1	hamburger (regular)	2 carbohydrates, 2 medium-fat meats
1	hamburger (large)	2 carbohydrates, 3 medium-fat meats, 1 fat
1	hot dog with bun	1 carbohydrate, 1 high-fat meat, 1 fat
1	individual pan pizza	5 carbohydrates, 3 medium-fat meats, 3 fats
¼ 12-inch (about 6 oz)	pizza, cheese, thin crust	2½ carbohydrates, 2 medium-fat meats
¼ 12-inch (about 6 oz)	pizza, meat, thin crust	2½ carbohydrates, 2 medium-fat meats, 1 fat
1 (5 oz)	soft-serve cone (small)	2½ carbohydrates, 1 fat
1 sub (6 inches)	submarine sandwich	3 carbohydrates, 1 vegetable, 2 medium-fat meats, 1 fat
1 (3–3½ oz)	taco, hard or soft shell	1 carbohydrate, 1 medium-fat meat, 1 fat

APPENDIX E Dietary Intake and Energy Expenditure Assessment

Although it may seem overwhelming at first, it is easy to track the foods you eat. One tip is to record foods and beverages consumed as soon as possible after consumption.

1. **Fill in the food record form that follows.** Appendix E contains a blank copy (see the completed example in Table E-1). Then, to estimate the nutrient values of the foods you are eating, consult food labels and use the NutritionCalc Plus software (CD or online) available with this book. If these resources do not have the serving size you need, adjust the value. If you drink ½ cup of orange juice, for example, but a table has values only for 1 cup, halve all values before you record them. Then, consider pooling all the same food to save time; if you drink a cup of 1% milk three times throughout the day, enter your milk consumption only once as 3 cups. As you record your intake for use on the nutrient analysis form that follows, consider the following tips:
   - Measure and record the amounts of foods eaten in portion sizes of cups, teaspoons, tablespoons, ounces, slices, or inches (or convert metric units to these units).
   - Record brand names of all food products, such as "Quick Quaker Oats."
   - Measure and record all those little extras, such as gravies, salad dressings, taco sauces, pickles, jelly, sugar, catsup, and margarine.
   - For beverages
     — List the type of milk, such as whole, fat-free, 1%, evaporated, chocolate, or reconstituted dry.
     — Indicate whether fruit juice is fresh, frozen, or canned.
     — Indicate type for other beverages, such as fruit drink, fruit-flavored drink, Kool-Aid, and hot chocolate made with water or milk.
   - For fruits
     —Indicate whether fresh, frozen, dried, or canned.
     —If whole, record number eaten and size with approximate measurements (such as 1 apple—3 in. in diameter).
     —Indicate whether processed in water, light syrup, or heavy syrup.
   - For vegetables
     — Indicate whether fresh, frozen, dried, or canned.
     — Record as portion of cup, teaspoon, or tablespoon, or as pieces (such as carrot sticks—4 in. long, ½ in. thick).
     — Record preparation method.
   - For cereals
     — Record cooked cereals in portions of tablespoon or cup (a level measurement after cooking).
     — Record dry cereal in level portions of tablespoon or cup.
     — If margarine, milk, sugar, fruit, or something else is added, measure and record amount and type.
   - For breads
     — Indicate whether whole wheat, rye, white, and so on.
     — Measure and record number and size of portion (biscuit—2 in. across, 1 in. thick; slice of homemade rye bread—3 in. by 4 in., ¼ in. thick).
     — Sandwiches: list all ingredients (lettuce, mayonnaise, tomato, and so on).

700

- For meat, fish, poultry, and cheese
  — Give size (length, width, thickness) in inches or weight in ounces after cooking for meat, fish, and poultry (such as cooked hamburger patty— 3 in. across, ½ in. thick).
  — Give size (length, width, thickness) in inches or weight in ounces for cheese.
  — Record measurements only for the cooked, edible part—without bone or fat left on the plate.
  — Describe how meat, poultry, or fish was prepared.
- For eggs
  — Record as soft or hard cooked, fried, scrambled, poached, or omelet.
  — If milk, butter, or drippings are used, specify types and amount.
- For desserts
  — List commercial brand or "homemade" or "bakery" under brand.
  — Purchased candies, cookies, and cakes: specify kind and size.
  — Measure and record portion size of cakes, pies, and cookies by specifying thickness, diameter, and width or length, depending on the item.

TABLE E-1 One Day's Food Record—This Activity Can Help You Understand More About Your Food Habits

Time	Minutes Spent Eating	M or S*	H† (0–3)	Activity While Eating	Place of Eating	Food and Quantity	Others Present	Reason for Choice
7:10 a.m.	15	M	2	Standing, fixing lunch	Kitchen	Orange juice, 1 cup Crispix, 1 cup Reduced-fat milk, ½ cup Sugar, 2 tsp Black coffee	—	Health Habit Health Taste Habit
10:00 a.m.	4	S	1	Sitting, taking notes	Classroom	Diet cola, 12 oz	Class	Weight control
12:15 p.m.	40	M	2	Sitting, talking	Student union	Chicken sandwich with lettuce and mayonnaise (3 oz chicken, 2 slices of bread, 2 tsp mayonnaise) Pear, 1 Reduced-fat milk, 1 cup	Friends	Taste Health Health
2:30 p.m.	10	S	1	Sitting, studying	Library	Regular cola, 12 oz	Friend	Hunger
6:30 p.m.	35	M	3	Sitting, talking	Kitchen	Pork chop, 1 Baked potato, 1 Margarine, 2 tbsp Lettuce and tomato salad Ranch dressing, 2 tbsp Peas, ½ cup Whole milk, 1 cup Cherry pie, 1 piece Iced tea, 12 oz	Boyfriend	Convenience Health Taste Health Taste Health Habit Taste Health
9:10 p.m.	10	S	2	Sitting, studying	Living room	Apple, 1 Glass mineral water, 1	—	Weight control Weight control

*M or S: Meal or snack
†H: Degree of hunger (0 = none; 3 = maximum)

Time	Minutes Spent Eating	M or S*	H† (0–3)	Activity While Eating	Place of Eating	Food and Quantity	Others Present	Reason for Choice

*M or S: Meal or snack

†H: Degree of hunger (0 = none; 3 = maximum)

II. **Now complete the nutrient analysis form as shown, using your food record.** A blank copy of this form for your use is on pages 705 and 706. NutritionCalc Plus will create such a table for you if you enter all food eaten.

Nutrient Analysis Form (Sample)

Name	Quantity	kcal	Protein (g)	Carbohydrates (g)	Fiber (g)	Total fat (g)	Monounsaturated fat (g)	Polyunsaturated fat (g)	Saturated fat (g)	Cholesterol (g)	Calcium (mg)	Iron (mg)
Egg bagel, 3.5-in. diameter	1 ea.	180	7.45	34.7	0.748	1.00	0.286	0.400	0.171	44.0	20.0	2.10
Jelly	1 tbsp	49.0	0.018	12.7	—	0.018	0.005	0.005	0.005	—	2.00	0.120
Orange juice, prepared fresh or frozen	1½ cup	165	2.52	40.2	1.49	0.210	0.037	0.045	0.025	—	33.0	0.411
Cheeseburger, McDonald's	2 ea.	636	30.2	57.0	0.460	32.0	12.2	2.18	13.3	80.0	338	5.68
French fries, McDonald's	1 order	220	3.00	26.1	4.19	11.5	4.37	0.570	4.61	8.57	9.10	0.605
Cola beverage, regular	1½ cup	151	—	38.5	—	—	—	—	—	—	9.00	0.120
Pork loin chop, broiled, lean	4 oz	261	36.2	—	—	11.9	5.35	1.43	4.09	112	5.67	1.04
Baked potato with skin	1 ea.	220	4.65	51.0	3.90	0.200	0.004	0.087	0.052	—	20.0	2.75
Peas, frozen, cooked	½ cup	63.0	4.12	11.4	3.61	0.220	0.019	0.103	0.039	—	19.0	1.25
Margarine, regular or soft, 80% fat	20 g	143	0.160	0.100	—	16.1	5.70	6.92	2.76	—	5.29	—
Iceberg lettuce, chopped	2 cup	14.6	1.13	2.34	1.68	0.212	0.008	0.112	0.028	—	21.2	0.560
French dressing	2 oz	300	0.318	3.63	0.431	32.0	14.2	12.4	4.94	—	7.10	0.227
Reduced-fat (i.e., 2%) milk	1 cup	121	8.12	11.7	—	4.78	1.35	0.170	2.92	22.0	297	0.120
Graham crackers	2 ea.	60.0	1.04	10.8	1.40	1.46	0.600	0.400	0.400	—	6.00	0.367
Totals		2584	99.0	300	17.9	112	44.1	24.8	33.4	266	792	15.4
RDA or related nutrient standard*		2900	58	130	38						1000	8
% of nutrient needs		89	170	230	47						79	193

Abbreviations: g = grams, mg = milligrams, μg = micrograms

*Values from inside cover. The values listed are for a male age 19 years. The number of kcal is a rough estimate. It is better to base energy needs on actual energy output.

†In RAE units. Table values generally are in RE units because the food values have not been updated to reflect the latest vitamin A standards. RAE equals SRE for foods with preformed vitamin A, such as for the pork chop, but RAE are only about half the RE listed for foods with provitamin A carotenoids, such as for the peas (see Chapter 9 for details).

‡Amounts refer to actual folate content, rather than dietary folate equivalents (DFE). This difference is important to consider if the food contains added synthetic folic acid as part of enrichment or fortification. Any such folic acid is absorbed about twice as much as the folate present naturally in foods. So the total contribution of folate in the food in comparison to human needs will be greater than if all the folate was naturally in the food product. Nutrient analysis tables have yet to be updated to reflect the dietary folate equivalents of products (see Chapter 11 for more details).

Nutrient Analysis Form (Sample) cont'd

Magnesium (mg)	Phosphorus (mg)	Potassium (mg)	Sodium (mg)	Zinc (mg)	Vitamin A (RE)	Vitamin C (mg)	Vitamin E (mg)	Thiamin (mg)	Riboflavin (mg)	Niacin (mg)	Vitamin B-6 (mg)	Folate (µg)	Vitamin B-12 (µg)
18.0	61.0	65.0	300	0.612	7.00	—	1.80	2.58	0.197	2.40	0.030	16.3	0.065
0.720	1.00	16.0	4.00	—	0.200	0.710	0.016	0.002	0.005	0.036	0.005	2.00	—
36.0	60.0	711	3.00	0.192	28.5	145	0.714	0.300	0.060	0.750	0.165	163	
45.8	410	314	1460	5.20	134	4.10	0.560	0.600	0.480	8.66	0.230	42.0	1.82
26.7	101	564	109	0.320	5.00	12.5	0.203	0.122	0.020	2.26	0.218	19.0	0.027
3.00	46.0	4.00	15.0	0.049	—	—	—	—	—	—	—	—	—
34.0	277	476	88.2	2.54	3.15	0.454	0.405	1.30	0.350	6.28	0.535	6.77	0.839
55.0	115	844	16.0	0.650	—	26.1	0.100	0.216	0.067	3.32	0.701	22.2	—
23.0	72.0	134	70.0	0.750	53.4	7.90	0.400	0.226	0.140	1.18	0.090	46.9	—
0.467	4.06	7.54	216	0.041	199	0.028	2.19	0.002	0.006	0.004	0.002	0.211	0.017
10.1	22.4	177	10.1	0.246	37.0	4.36	0.120	0.052	0.034	0.210	0.044	62.8	—
5.81	3.63	7.03	666	0.045	0.023	—	15.9	—	—	—	0.006	—	—
33.0	232	377	122	0.963	140	2.32	0.080	0.095	0.403	0.210	0.105	12.0	0.888
6.00	20.0	36.0	86.0	0.113	—	—	—	0.020	0.030	0.600	0.011	1.80	—
298	1425	3732	3165	11.7	607	204	22.5	5.52	1.79	25.9	2.14	395	3.65
400	700	4700	1500	11	900†	90	15	1.2	1.3	16	1.3	400‡	2.4
75	204	80	210	106	67	226	150	450	138	162	160	99	152

Nutrient Analysis Form

Name	Quantity	kcal	Protein (g)	Carbohydrates (g)	Fiber (g)	Total fat (g)	Monounsaturated fat (g)	Polyunsaturated fat (g)	Saturated fat (g)	Cholesterol (g)	Calcium (mg)	Iron (mg)
Totals												
RDA or related nutrient standard*												
% of nutrient needs												

*Values from inside cover. The number of kcals is a rough estimate. It is better to base energy needs on actual energy output.

†Use RAE values, even though food table is based on RE units.

‡Use DFE values, even though the food table is based on total folate content, irrespective of natural or synthetic source.

Nutrient Analysis Form cont'd

Magnesium (mg)	Phosphorous (mg)	Potassium (mg)	Sodium (mg)	Zinc (mg)	Vitamin A (RE)	Vitamin C (mg)	Vitamin E (mg)	Thiamin (mg)	Riboflavin (mg)	Niacin (mg)	Vitamin B-6 (mg)	Folate (μg)	Vitamin B-12 (μg)

III. Complete the following table as you summarize your dietary intake.

Percentage of kcal from Protein, Fat, Carbohydrate, and Alcohol

Intake

Protein (P): ____g/day × 4 kcal per gram = (P)____kcal per day
Fat (F): ____g/day × 9 kcal per gram = (F)____kcal per day
Carbohydrate (C): ____g/day × 4 kcal per gram = (C)____kcal per day
Alcohol (A): = (A)____kcal per day*
Total kcal (T)/day = (T)____kcal per day

Percentage of kcal from protein:
$\frac{(P)}{(T)} \times 100 =$ ____%

Percentage of kcal from fat:
$\frac{(F)}{(T)} \times 100 =$ ____%

Percentage of kcal from carbohydrate:
$\frac{(C)}{(T)} \times 100 =$ ____%

Percentage of kcal from alcohol:
$\frac{(A)}{(T)} \times 100 =$ ____%

Note: The four percentages can total 99, 100, or 101, depending on the way in which figures were rounded off earlier.

*To calculate how many kcal in a beverage are from alcohol, first look up the beverage in Appendix J. Then determine how many kcal are from carbohydrate (multiply carbohydrate grams times 4), fat (fat grams times 9), and protein (protein grams times 4). The remaining kcal are from alcohol.

IV. Use the table on the following page to again record your food intake for one day, placing each food item in the correct category of MyPyramid, with the correct number of servings (see Chapter 2). A food such as toast with soft margarine contributes to two categories—namely, to the grains group and to the oils group. You can expect that many food choices will contribute to more than one group. Indicate the number of servings from MyPyramid that each food yields.

Indicate the Number of Servings from MyPyramid That Each Food Yields

Food or Beverage	Amount Eaten	Milk	Meat & Beans	Fruits	Vegetables	Grains	Oils
Group totals							
Recommended servings from www.mypyramid.gov							
Overages/Shortages in numbers of servings							

V. **Evaluation.** Are there weaknesses suggested in your nutrient intake that correspond to missing servings in MyPyramid? Consider adjusting your food choices to meet MyPyramid recommendations to improve your nutrient intake.

VI. **For the same day you keep your food record, also keep a 24-hour record of your activities.** Include sleeping, sitting, and walking, as well as the obvious forms of exercise. Calculate your energy expenditure for these activities using Table 7-4 in Chapter 7 or the diet analysis software available with this book. Try to substitute a similar activity if your particular activity is not listed. Calculate the total kcal you used for the day (total for column 3). Following is an example of an activity record. A blank form follows for your use. Ask your professor whether you are to turn in the form or the activity printout from NutritionCalc Plus.

Weight (kg)*: 70 kg

Activity	Time (Minutes): Convert to Hours	Energy Cost		
		Column 1 kcal/kg/hr (from Table 7-4)	Column 2 (Column 1 × Time)	Column 3 (Column 2 × Weight in kg)
Brisk walking	(60 min) 1 hr	4.4	(× 1) = 4.4	(× 70) = 308

*lb/2.2

Weight (kg)*:

Activity	Time (Minutes): Convert to Hours	Energy Cost		
		Column 1 kcal/kg/hr (from Table 7-4)	Column 2 (Column 1 × Time)	Column 3 (Column 2 × Weight in kg)

Total kcal used (from adding all of column 3)
*lb/2.2

AMINO ACIDS

Histidine (His)
(essential)

Tryptophan (Trp)
(essential)

Glycine (Gly)

Methionine (Met)
(essential)

Leucine (Leu)
(essential)

Alanine (Ala)

Arginine (Arg)
(essential in infancy)

Lysine (Lys)
(essential)

Proline (Pro)

Glutamic Acid (Glu)

Aspartic Acid (Asp)

Serine (Ser)

Phenylalanine (Phe)
(essential)

Isoleucine (Ile)
(essential)

Tyrosine (Tyr)

Glutamine (Gln)

Asparagine (Asn)

Threonine (Thr)
(essential)

Valine (Val)
(essential)

Cysteine (Cys)

VITAMINS

Vitamin A: retinol

Beta-carotene

Vitamin E

Vitamin K

7-dehydrocholesterol

Carbon #25

Carbon #1

1,25-dihydroxy-vitamin D₃ (calcitriol)

Carbon #25

Carbon #1

Active vitamin D (calcitriol) and its precursor 7-dehydrocholesterol

Thiamin

Nicotinic acid   Nicotinamide

Niacin (nicotinic acid and nicotinamide)

Riboflavin

Pyridoxine   Pyridoxal   Pyridoxamine

Vitamin B-6 (a general name for three compounds—pyridoxine, pyridoxal, and pyridoxamine)

Biotin

Pantothenic acid

Folate (folic acid form)

Vitamin C (ascorbic acid)

Vitamin B-12 (cyanocobalamin) The arrows in this diagram indicate that the spare electrons on the nitrogens are attracted to the cobalt atom.

Ketone Bodies

$$CH_3 - \overset{\displaystyle O}{\overset{\|}{C}} - CH_2 - \overset{\displaystyle O}{\overset{\|}{C}} - OH$$

Acetoacetic Acid

CO_2

$$CH_3 - \overset{\displaystyle O}{\overset{\|}{C}} - CH_3$$

Acetone

$2H^+$

$$CH_3 - \overset{\displaystyle OH}{\overset{\|}{CH}} - CH_2 - \overset{\displaystyle O}{\overset{\|}{C}} - OH$$

ß-Hydroxybutyric Acid

Triphosphate

OH
|
HO — P = O
|
O
|
HO — P = O
|
O
|
HO — P = O
|
O
|

Point of cleavage to yield
ADP and energy release

NH_2

Adenine

Ribose
(a sugar)

CH_2

OH   OH

Adenosine Triphosphate
(ATP)

1983 Metropolitan Life Insurance Company Height-Weight Table*†

Women					Men				
Height		Frame			Height		Frame		
Ft.	In.	Small	Medium	Large	Ft.	In.	Small	Medium	Large
4	10	102–111	109–121	118–131	5	2	128–134	131–141	138–150
4	11	103–113	111–123	120–134	5	3	130–136	133–143	140–153
5	0	104–115	113–126	122–137	5	4	132–138	135–145	142–156
5	1	106–118	115–129	125–140	5	5	134–140	137–148	144–160
5	2	108–121	118–132	128–143	5	6	136–142	139–151	146–164
5	3	111–124	121–135	131–147	5	7	138–145	142–154	149–168
5	4	114–127	124–138	134–151	5	8	140–148	145–157	152–172
5	5	117–130	127–141	137–155	5	9	142–151	148–160	155–176
5	6	120–133	130–144	140–159	5	10	144–154	151–163	158–180
5	7	123–136	133–147	143–163	5	11	146–157	154–166	161–184
5	8	126–139	136–150	146–167	6	0	149–160	157–170	164–188
5	9	129–142	139–153	149–170	6	1	152–164	160–174	168–192
5	10	132–145	142–156	152–173	6	2	155–168	164–178	172–197
5	11	135–148	145–159	155–176	6	3	158–172	167–182	176–202
6	0	138–151	148–162	158–179	6	4	162–176	171–187	181–207

*Based on a weight-height mortality study conducted by the Society of Actuaries and the Association of Life Insurance Medical Directors of America, Metropolitan Life Insurance Medical Directors of America, Metropolitan Life Insurance Company, revised 1983.

†Weights in pounds (lb) at ages 25 to 59 based on lowest mortality. Height includes 1-in. heel. Weight for women includes 3 lb for indoor clothing. Weight for men includes 5 lb for indoor clothing.

Reprinted courtesy of Metropolitan Life Insurance Company, *Statistical Bulletin*.

Permission granted courtesy of Metropolitan Life Insurance Company, *Statistical Bulletin*.

USING THE METROPOLITAN LIFE INSURANCE TABLE TO ESTIMATE HEALTHY WEIGHT

The Metropolitan Life Insurance table is a common method for estimating healthy weight. The table lists, for any height, the weight that is associated with a maximum life span. The table does not tell the healthiest weight for a living person; it lists the weight associated with longevity.

There are many criticisms of this table. These stem from the inclusion of some people and the exclusion of others. For example, only policyholders of life insurance are included. In addition, smokers are included, but anyone over the age of 60 is excluded. Weight is only measured at the time of purchase of insurance, and there is no follow-up. All of these factors contribute to the fact that this table is to be used only as a rough screening tool; not meeting the exact recommendations should not be cause for alarm.

To diagnose overweight or obesity using the table, calculate the percentage of the Metropolitan Life Insurance table weight. Use the midpoint of a weight range for a specific height.

Equation: $\dfrac{(\text{Current wt.} - \text{wt. from table})}{\text{Weight from table}} \times 100$

Example:

$$\frac{140 - 120}{120} \times 100 = 17\% \text{ over standard}$$

Overweight can be defined as weighing at least 10% more than the weight listed on the table. Determination of obesity is 20% more than that listed on the table. Moreover, this measure of obesity comes in degrees. Whereas mild obesity carries little health risk, severe obesity raises overall health risk twelvefold.

Degrees of Obesity	
% Over Healthy Body Weight	**Form of Obesity**
20–40%	Mild
41–99%	Moderate
100%+	Severe

DETERMINING FRAME SIZE

Method 1

Height is recorded without shoes.

Wrist circumference is measured just beyond (toward the hand) the bony (styloid) process at the wrist joint on the right arm, using a tape measure.

The following formula is used:

$$r = \frac{\text{Height (cm)}}{\text{Wrist circumference (cm)}}$$

Frame size can be determined as follows:[†]

Males	Females
$r > 10.4$ small	$r > 11$ small
$r = 9.6–10.4$ medium	$r = 10.1–11$ medium
$r < 9.6$ large	$r < 10.1$ large

[†]From Grant JP: *Handbook of Total Parenteral Nutrition*. Philadelphia: WB Saunders, 1980.

Method 2

The person's right arm is extended forward, perpendicular to the body, with the arm bent so the angle at the elbow forms 90 degrees, with the fingers pointing up and the palm turned away from the body. The greatest breadth across the elbow joint is measured with a sliding caliper along the axis of the upper arm, on the two prominent bones on either side of the elbow. This is recorded as the elbow breadth. The following tables give elbow breadth measurements for medium-framed men and women of various heights. Measurements lower than those listed indicate a small frame size; higher measurements indicate a large frame size.[‡]

Men		Women	
Height in 1″ Heels	**Elbow Breadth**	**Height in 1″ Heels**	**Elbow Breadth**
5′2″–5′3″	2½–2⅞″	4′10″–4′11″	2¼–2½″
5′4″–5′7″	2⅝–2⅞″	5′0″–5′3″	2¼–2½″
5′8″–5′11″	2¾–3″	5′4″–5′7″	2⅜–2⅝″
6′0″–6′3″	2¾–3¼″	5′8″–5′11″	2⅜–2⅝″
6′4″ and over	2⅞–3¾″	6′0″ and over	2½–2¾″

[‡]From Metropolitan Life Insurance Co., 1983.

Consider the following reliable sources of food and nutrition information:

Journals That Regularly Cover Nutrition Topics

American Family Physician*
American Journal of Clinical Nutrition
American Journal of Epidemiology
American Journal of Medicine
American Journal of Nursing
American Journal of Obstetrics and
    Gynecology
American Journal of Physiology
American Journal of Public Health
American Scientist
Annals of Internal Medicine
Annual Review of Medicine
Annual Review of Nutrition
Archives of Disease in Childhood
Archives of Internal Medicine
British Journal of Nutrition
BMJ (British Medical Journal)
Canadian Journal of Dietetic Practice and
    Research
Cancer
Cancer Research

Circulation
Diabetes
Diabetes Care
Disease-a-Month
FASEB Journal
FDA Consumer*
Food and Chemical Toxicology
Food Engineering
Food Technology
Gastroenterology
Geriatrics
Gut
Journal of the American College of
    Nutrition*
Journal of the American Dietetic
    Association*
Journal of the American Geriatrics Society
JAMA (Journal of the American Medical
    Association)
Journal of Applied Physiology
Journal of Clinical Investigation
Journal of Food Science

JNCI (Journal of the National Cancer
    Institute)
Journal of Nutrition
Journal of Nutrition Education and
    Behavior*
Journal of Nutrition for the Elderly
Journal of Pediatrics
Lancet
Mayo Clinic Proceedings
Medicine & Science in Sports & Exercise
Nature
The New England Journal of Medicine
Nutrition
Nutrition Reviews
Nutrition Today*
Pediatrics
The Physician and Sports Medicine
Postgraduate Medicine*
Proceedings of the Nutrition Society
Science
Science News*
Scientific American*

The majority of these journals are available in college and university libraries or in a specialty library on campus, such as one designated for health services or home economics. As indicated, a few journals will be filed under their abbreviations, rather than the first word in their full name. A reference librarian can help you locate any of these sources. The journals with an asterisk (*) are ones you may find especially interesting and useful because of the number of nutrition articles presented each month or the less technical nature of the presentation.

Magazines for the Consumer That Cover Nutrition Topics

Better Homes and Gardens
Good Housekeeping

Health
Men's Health

Parents
Self

Textbooks and Other Sources for Advanced Study of Nutrition Topics

Brody T: Nutritional biochemistry. 2nd ed. San Diego: Academic Press, 1999.
Groff JL, Gropper SS: Advanced human nutrition and metabolism. 4th ed. Belmont, CA: Wadsworth, 2004.
Bowman BA, Russell RM: Present knowledge in nutrition. Vol. I and II. 9th ed.

Washington DC: International Life Sciences Institute, 2006.
Mahan LK, Escott-Stump S: Krause's food, nutrition, and diet therapy. 11th ed. Philadelphia: W.B. Saunders, 2003.
Murray RK and others: Harper's illustrated biochemistry. 27th ed. New York: McGraw-Hill, 2006.

Schils ME, Olson JA, Shike M, Ross AC: Modern nutrition in health and disease. 10th ed. Philadelphia: Lippincott, Williams & Wilkins, 2005.
Stipanuk MH: Biochemical, physiological, & molecular aspects of human nutrition. 2nd ed. Philadelphia: W.B. Saunders, 2006.

Newsletters That Cover Nutrition Issues on a Regular Basis

American Institute for Cancer Research e.Newsletter
American Institute for Cancer Research
www.aicr.org

Consumer Health Digest
National Council Against Health Fraud
www.ncahf.org

Dairy Council Digest
National Dairy Council
www.nationaldairycouncil.org

Diabetes E-News Now (and others)
American Diabetes Association
www.diabetes.org

Environmental Nutrition
www.environmentalnutrition.com

Harvard Health Letter (and others)
Harvard Medical School
www.health.harvard.edu/newsletters

Health and Nutrition Letter
Tufts University
www.healthletter.tufts.edu

In-Touch
Heinz Infant Nutrition Institute
www.hini.org

Nutrition Action Healthletter
Center for Science in the Public Interest
www.cspinet.org

Nutrition Close-Up
Egg Nutrition Center
www.enc-online.org

House Call
Mayo Clinic
www.mayoclinic.com

Soy Connection
United Soybean Board
www.talksoy.com

U-Mail: Everyday Nutrition Solutions You Can Use
National Cattlemen's Beef Association
www.beefnutrition.org

Wellness Letter
University of California at Berkeley
www.wellnessletter.com

Professional Organizations

American Academy of Pediatrics
141 Northwest Point Boulevard
Elk Grove Village, IL 60007-1098
www.aap.org

American Cancer Society
1599 Clifton Road, NE
Atlanta, GA 30329
www.cancer.org

American College of Sports Medicine
PO Box 1440
Indianapolis, IN 46206-1440
www.acsm.org

American Dental Association
211 East Chicago Avenue
Chicago, IL 60611-2678
www.ada.org

American Diabetes Association
1701 North Beauregard Street
Alexandria, VA 22311
www.diabetes.org

American Dietetic Association
120 South Riverside Plaza #2000
Chicago, IL 60606-6995
www.eatright.org

American Geriatrics Society
350 Fifth Avenue #801
New York, NY 10118
www.americangeriatrics.org

American Heart Association
7272 Greenville Avenue
Dallas, TX 75231
www.americanheart.org

American Medical Association
515 North State Street
Chicago, IL 60610
www.ama-assn.org

American Public Health Association
800 I Street, NW
Washington, DC 20001
www.apha.org

American Society for Nutrition
9650 Rockville Pike #L-4500
Bethesda, MD 20814
http://www.asnutrition.org/

Canadian Council of Food and Nutrition
3800 Steeles Avenue West, #301A
Woodbridge, Ontario L4L 4G9
http://www.ccfn.ca/

Canadian Diabetes Association
1400-522 University Avenue
Toronto, ON M5G 2R5
www.diabetes.ca

Canadian Society for Nutritional Sciences
Department of Nutritional Sciences
University of Toronto
150 College Street
Toronto, ON M5S 3E2
www.nutritionalsciences.ca

Dietitians of Canada
480 University Avenue #604
Toronto, ON M5G 1V2
www.dietitians.ca

Environmental Working Group
1436 U Street, NW #100
Washington, DC 20009
www.ewg.org

Food and Nutrition Board
Institute of Medicine
The National Academies
500 Fifth Street, NW
Washington, DC 20001
www.iom.edu/CMS/3788.aspx

Institute of Food Technologists
525 West Van Buren #1000
Chicago, IL 60607
www.ift.org

National Council on Aging
1901 L Street, NW, 4th floor
Washington, DC 20036
www.ncoa.org

National Osteoporosis Foundation
1232 22nd Street, NW
Washington, DC 20037-1292
www.nof.org

Society for Nutrition Education
7150 Winton Drive #300
Indianapolis, IN 46268
www.sne.org

Professional Organizations with a Commitment to Nutrition Issues

Bread for the World Institute
50 F Street, NW #500
Washington, DC 20001
www.bread.org

Food Research and Action Center
1875 Connecticut Avenue, NW #540
Washington, DC 20009
www.frac.org

Institute for Food and Development Policy
398 60th Street
Oakland, CA 94618
www.foodfirst.org

La Leche League International
PO Box 4079
Schaumburg, IL 60168-4079
www.lalecheleague.org

March of Dimes
1275 Mamaroneck Avenue
White Plains, NY 10605
www.marchofdimes.com

National Council Against Health Fraud
119 Foster Street
Peabody, MA 01960
www.ncahf.org

National WIC Association
2001 S Street, NW #580
Washington, DC 20009
www.nwica.org

Overeaters Anonymous
PO Box 44020
Rio Rancho, NM 87174-4020
www.oa.org

Oxfam America
226 Causeway Street, 5th floor
Boston, MA 02114
www.oxfamamerica.org

Local Resources for Advice on Nutrition Issues

Registered dietitians (RDs or in Canada also RDNs) in health care, city, county, or state agencies, as well as in private practice
Cooperative extension agents in county extension offices
Nutrition faculty affiliated with departments of food and nutrition, home economics, and dietetics

Government Agencies Concerned with Nutrition Issues or That Distribute Nutrition Information

United States

Agricultural Research Service
United States Department of Agriculture
Jamie L. Whitten Building
1400 Independence Avenue, SW
Washington, DC 20250
www.ars.usda.gov

Federal Citizen Information Center
1800 F Street, NW #G-142 (XCC)
Washington, DC 20405
www.pueblo.gsa.gov

Food and Drug Administration
5600 Fishers Lane
Rockville, Maryland 20857
www.fda.gov

Food Safety & Inspection Service
United States Department of Agriculture
331-E Jamie L. Whitten Building
1400 Independence Avenue, SW
Washington, DC 20250
www.fsis.usda.gov

MyPyramid
USDA Center for Nutrition Policy and Promotion
3101 Park Center Drive #1034
Alexandria, VA 22302-1594
www.mypyramid.gov

National Agricultural Library
Abraham Lincoln Building
10301 Baltimore Avenue
Beltsville, MD 20705-2351
www.nal.usda.gov

National Cancer Institute
6116 Executive Boulevard #3036A
Bethesda, MD 20892-8322
www.cancer.gov

National Center for Health Statistics
3311 Toledo Road
Hyattsville, MD 20782
www.cdc.gov/nchs

National Heart, Lung, and Blood Institute
31 Center Drive, MSC 2486
Building 31, Room 5A48
Bethesda, MD 20892
www.nhlbi.nih.gov

National Institute on Aging
31 Center Drive, MSC 2292
Building 31, Room 5C27
Bethesda, MD 20892
www.nia.nih.gov

U.S. Government Printing Office
732 North Capitol Street, NW
Washington, DC 20401
www.gpo.gov

Canada

Canadian Food Inspection Agency
59 Camelot Drive
Ottawa, Ontario K1A 0Y9
www.inspection.gc.ca

Health Canada
Brooke Claxton Building, Tunney's Pasture
Postal Locator: 0906C
Ottawa, Ontario K1A 0K9
www.hc-sc.gc.ca

United Nations

Food and Agriculture Organization
Liaison Office with North America
2175 K Street, NW #300
Washington, DC 20437-0001
www.fao.org

World Health Organization
Regional Office for the Americas
525 23rd Street, NW
Washington, DC 20037
www.who.int

Trade Organizations and Companies That Distribute Nutrition Information

American Institute of Baking
1213 Bakers Way
PO Box 3999
Manhattan, Kansas 66505-3999
www.aibonline.org

American Meat Institute
1150 Connecticut Avenue, NW, 12th floor
Washington, DC 20036
www.meatami.com

Beech-Nut Nutrition
100 South Fourth Street #1010
St. Louis, MO 63102
www.beech-nut.com

Campbell Soup Company
1 Campbell Place
Camden, NJ 08103-1701
www.campbellsoup.com

Dannon Company
100 Hillside Avenue, 3rd Floor
White Plains, NY 10603
www.dannon.com

Del Monte Foods
One Market Plaza
PO Box 193575
San Francisco, CA 94119-3575
www.delmonte.com

DSM Nutritional Products
45 Waterview Boulevard
Parsippany, NJ 07054-1298
www.nutraaccess.com

General Mills/Pillsbury
PO Box 9452
Minneapolis, MN 55440
www.generalmills.com

Gerber Products Company
445 State Street
Fremont, MI 49413
www.gerber.com

H.J. Heinz
90 Sheppard Avenue East #400
Toronto, ON M2N 7K5
www.heinzbaby.com

Idaho Potato Commission
661 South Rivershore Lane
Eagle, ID 83616
www.idahopotatoes.com

Kellogg Company
One Kellogg Square
Battle Creek, MI 49016
www.kelloggs.com/us/

Kraft Foods Global
Three Lakes Drive
Northfield, IL 60093
www.kraftfoods.com

Mead Johnson Nutritionals
2400 West Lloyd Expressway
Evansville, IN 47721-0001
www.meadjohnson.com

National Dairy Council
10255 West Higgins Road #900
Rosemont, IL 60018
www.nationaldairycouncil.org

NutraSweet Company
222 Merchandise Mart Plaza
Chicago, IL 60654
www.nutrasweet.com

Ross Product Division
Abbott Laboratories
625 Cleveland Avenue
Columbus, OH 43216
www.ross.com

Sunkist Growers
14130 Riverside Drive
Sherman Oaks, CA 91423
www.sunkist.com

METRIC-ENGLISH CONVERSIONS

Length

English (USA)	Metric
inch (in)	= 2.54 cm, 25.4 mm
foot (ft)	= 0.30 m, 30.48 cm
yard (yd)	= 0.91 m, 91.4 cm
mile (statute) (5280 ft)	= 1.61 km, 1609 m
mile (nautical) (6077 ft, 1.15 statute mi)	= 1.85 km, 1850 m

Metric	English (USA)
millimeter (mm)	= 0.039 in (thickness of a dime)
centimeter (cm)	= 0.39 in
meter (m)	= 3.28 ft, 39.37 in
kilometer (km)	= 0.62 mi, 1091 yd, 3273 ft

Weight

English (USA)	Metric
grain	= 64.80 mg
ounce (oz)	= 28.35 g
pound (lb)	= 453.60 g, 0.45 kg
ton (short—2000 lb)	= 0.91 metric ton (907 kg)

Metric	English (USA)
milligram (mg)	= 0.002 grain (0.000035 oz)
gram (g)	= 0.04 oz ($^1/_{28}$ of an oz)
kilogram (kg)	= 35.27 oz, 2.20 lb
metric ton (1000 kg)	= 1.10 tons

Volume

English (USA)	Metric
cubic inch	= 16.39 cc
cubic foot	= 0.03 m^3
cubic yard	= 0.765 m^3
teaspoon (tsp)	= 5 ml
tablespoon (tbsp)	= 15 ml
fluid ounce	= 0.03 liter (30 ml)*
cup (c)	= 237 ml
pint (pt)	= 0.47 liter
quart (qt)	= 0.95 liter
gallon (gal)	= 3.79 liters

Metric	English (USA)
milliliter (ml)	= 0.03 oz
liter (L)	= 2.12 pt
liter	= 1.06 qt
liter	= 0.27 gal

1 liter ÷ 1000 = 1 milliliter or 1 cubic centimeter (10^{-3} liter)
1 liter ÷ 1,000,000 = 1 microliter (10^{-6} liter)
*Note: 1 ml = 1 cc

METRIC AND OTHER COMMON UNITS

Unit/Abbreviation	Other Equivalent Measure
milligram/mg	$^1/_{1000}$ of a gram
microgram/µg	$^1/_{1,000,000}$ of a gram
deciliter/dl	$^1/_{10}$ of a liter (about ½ cup)
milliliter/ml	$^1/_{1000}$ of a liter (5 ml is about 1 tsp)
International Unit/IU	Crude measure of vitamin activity generally based on growth rate seen in animals

FAHRENHEIT-CELSIUS CONVERSION SCALE

To convert temperature scales:
Fahrenheit to Celsius °C = (°F − 32) × 5/9
Celsius to Fahrenheit °F = 9/5 (°C) + 32

HOUSEHOLD UNITS

3 teaspoons	= 1 tablespoon
4 tablespoons	= ¼ cup
5$^1/_3$ tablespoons	= $^1/_3$ cup
8 tablespoons	= ½ cup
10$^2/_3$ tablespoons	= $^2/_3$ cup
16 tablespoons	= 1 cup
1 tablespoon	= ½ fluid ounce
1 cup	= 8 fluid ounces
1 cup	= ½ pint
2 cups	= 1 pint
4 cups	= 1 quart
2 pints	= 1 quart
4 quarts	= 1 gallon

GLOSSARY Medical Terminology to Aid in the Study of Nutrition

absorption The process by which substances are taken up from the GI tract and enter the bloodstream or the lymph.

absorptive cells The intestinal cells that line the villi; these cells participate in nutrient absorption.

acetaldehyde dehydrogenase An enzyme used in ethanol metabolism that eventually converts acetaldehyde into carbon dioxide and water.

acquired immune deficiency syndrome (AIDS) A disorder in which a virus (human immunodeficiency virus [HIV]) infects specific types of immune system cells. This leaves the person with reduced immune function and, in turn, defenseless against numerous infectious agents; typically contributes to the person's death.

additives Substances added to foods, such as preservatives.

adenosine diphosphate (ADP) A breakdown product of ATP. ADP is synthesized into ATP using energy from foodstuffs and a phosphate group (abbreviated Pi).

adenosine triphosphate (ATP) The main energy currency for cells. ATP energy is used to promote ion pumping, enzyme activity, and muscular contraction.

adipose tissue A group of fat storing cells.

adjustable gastric banding A restrictive procedure in which the opening from the esophagus to the stomach is reduced by a hollow gastric band.

aerobic Requiring oxygen.

air displacement A method for estimating body composition that makes use of the volume of space taken up by a body inside a small chamber.

alcohol Ethyl alcohol or ethanol (CH_3CH_2OH) is the compound in alcoholic beverages.

alcohol abuse Excessive alcohol consumption that leads to severe alcohol-related health and other problems, such as recurrent sickness, inability to fulfill major obligations, use in hazardous situations (e.g., driving), related legal problems, or use despite social and interpersonal difficulties.

alcohol dehydrogenase An enzyme used in alcohol (ethanol) metabolism that converts alcohol into acetaldehyde.

alcohol dependence The person experiences repeated alcohol-related difficulties, such as an inability to control use, spending a great deal of time associated with alcohol use, continued use of alcohol despite physical or psychological consequences, persistent desire or unsuccessful efforts to cut down or control alcohol use, and withdrawal symptoms. Tolerance is also seen.

alcoholism As defined by the American Medical Association, an illness characterized by significant impairment directly related to persistent and excessive use of alcohol.

aldosterone A hormone, produced by the adrenal glands, that acts on the kidneys to conserve sodium (and therefore water).

allergen A foreign protein, or antigen, that induces excess production of certain immune system antibodies; subsequent exposure to the same protein leads to allergic symptoms. Whereas all allergens are antigens, not all antigens are allergens.

allergy A hypersensitive immune response that occurs when immune bodies produced by us react with a protein we sense as foreign (an antigen).

alpha-linolenic acid An essential omega-3 fatty acid with 18 carbons and three double bonds.

amino acid The building block for proteins containing a central carbon atom with nitrogen and other atoms attached.

amphetamine A group of medications that induce stimulation of the central nervous system and have other effects in the body. Abuse is linked to physical and psychological dependence.

amylase Starch-digesting enzyme produced by the salivary glands and pancreas.

amylopectin A digestible branched-chain type of starch composed of glucose units.

amylose A digestible straight-chain type of starch composed of glucose units.

anaerobic Not requiring oxygen.

anal sphincters A group of two sphincters (inner and outer) that help control expulsion of feces from the body.

anaphylactic shock A severe allergic response that results in lowered blood pressure and respiratory and gastrointestinal distress. This can be fatal.

anemia A decreased oxygen-carrying capacity of the blood. This can be caused by many factors, such as iron deficiency or blood loss.

animal model Study of disease in animals that duplicates human disease. This can be used to understand more about human disease.

anorexia nervosa An eating disorder involving a psychological loss or denial of appetite, followed by self-starvation; related in part to a distorted body image and to various social pressures commonly associated with puberty.

anthropometric assessment Measurement of body weight and the lengths, circumferences, and thicknesses of parts of the body.

antibody Blood protein (immunoglobulin) that binds foreign proteins found in the body. This helps to prevent and control infections.

antidiuretic hormone A hormone secreted by the pituitary gland when blood volume is low. It causes the kidneys to decrease water excretion, which increases blood volume.

antigen Any substance that induces a state of sensitivity and/or resistance to microorganisms or toxic substances after a lag period; foreign substance that stimulates a specific aspect of the immune system.

antioxidant A substance that has the ability to prevent or repair the damage caused by oxidation.

anus Last portion of the GI tract; serves as an outlet for that organ.

appetite The primarily psychological (external) influences that encourage us to find and eat food, often in the absence of obvious hunger.

arachidonic acid An omega-6 fatty acid made from linoleic acid with 20 carbon atoms and 4 carbon-carbon double bonds.

artery A blood vessel that carries blood away from the heart.

aseptic processing A method by which food and container are separately and simultaneously sterilized; it allows manufacturers to produce boxes of milk that can be stored at room temperature.

atherosclerosis A buildup of fatty material (plaque) in the arteries, including those surrounding the heart.

atom Smallest combining unit of an element, such as iron or calcium. Atoms consist of protons, neutrons, and electrons.

bacteria Single-cell microorganisms; some produce poisonous substances, which cause illness in humans. Bacteria can be carried by water, animals, and people. They survive on skin, clothes, and hair and thrive in foods at room temperature. Some can live without oxygen and survive by means of **spore** formation.

bariatrics The medical specialty focusing on the treatment of obesity.

basal metabolism The minimal amount of calories the body uses to support itself in a fasting state when resting (e.g., 12 hours for both) and awake in a warm, quiet environment. It amounts to roughly 1 kcal per kilogram per hour for men and 0.9 kcal per kilogram per hour for women; these values are often referred to as *basal metabolic rate (BMR)*.

benign Noncancerous; tumors that do not spread.

beriberi The thiamin deficiency disorder characterized by muscle weakness, loss of appetite, nerve degeneration, and sometimes edema.

BHA, BHT Butylated hydroxyanisole and butylated hydroxytoluene—two common synthetic antioxidants added to foods.

bile A liver secretion stored in the gallbladder and released through the common bile duct into the first segment of the small intestine. It is essential for the digestion and absorption of fat.

binge-eating disorder An eating disorder characterized by recurrent binge eating and feelings of loss of control over eating that have lasted at least 6 months. Binge episodes can be triggered by frustration, anger, depression, anxiety, permission to eat forbidden foods, and excessive hunger.

bioavailability The degree to which an ingested nutrient is absorbed and thus is available to the body.

biochemical assessment Measurement of biochemical functions (e.g., concentrations of nutrient by-products or enzyme activities in the blood or urine) related to a nutrient's function.

bioelectrical impedance The method to estimate total body fat that uses a low-energy electrical current. The more fat storage a person has, the more impedance (resistance) to electrical flow will be exhibited.

biotechnology A collection of processes that involves the use of biological systems for altering and, ideally, improving the characteristics of plants, animals, and other forms of life.

bisphosphonates Drugs that bind minerals and prevent osteoclast breakdown of bone. Examples are alendronate (Fosamax) and risedronate (Actonel).

body mass index (BMI) Weight (in kilograms) divided by height (in meters) squared; a value of 25 and above indicates overweight and a value of 30 and above indicates obesity.

bolus A moistened mass of food swallowed from the oral cavity into the pharynx.

bomb colorimeter An instrument used to determine the calorie content of a food.

bond A linkage between two atoms formed by the sharing of electrons, or attractions.

bone remodeling The chemical process by which bone is broken down and replaced by new bone.

branched-chain amino acids Amino acids with a branching carbon backbone; these are leucine, isoleucine, and valine. All are essential amino acids.

brown adipose tissue A specialized form of adipose tissue that produces large amounts of heat by metabolizing energy-yielding nutrients without synthesizing much useful energy for the body. The unused energy is released as heat.

buffer Compounds that function to take up or release hydrogen ions thereby causing a fluid to resist changes in pH.

bulimia nervosa An eating disorder in which large quantities of food are eaten at one time (binge eating) and then purged from the body by vomiting, or misuse of laxatives, diuretics, or

enemas. Alternate means to counteract the binge behavior are fasting and excessive exercise.

capillary A microscopic blood vessel that connects the smallest arteries and veins; site of nutrient, oxygen, and waste exchange between body cells and the blood.

capillary bed Network of one-cell thick vessels that create a junction between arterial and venous circulation. It is here that gas and nutrient exchange occurs between body cells and the blood.

carbohydrate A compound containing carbon, hydrogen, and oxygen atoms. Most are known as *sugars*, *starches*, and *fibers*.

carbohydrate loading A process in which a high carbohydrate intake is consumed for 6 days before an athletic event while tapering exercise duration in an attempt to increase muscle glycogen stores.

carbon skeleton Amino acid structure that remains after the amino group ($-NH_2$) has been removed.

cardiovascular system The body system consisting of the heart, blood vessels, and blood. This system transports nutrients, waste products, gases, and hormones throughout the body and plays an important role in immune responses and regulation of body temperature.

carotenoids Pigment materials that range in color from yellow to orange to red; three of the carotenoids are converted into Vitamin A. Many are antioxidants.

case-control study Individuals who have the condition in question, such as lung cancer, are compared with individuals who do not have the condition.

cell The structural basis of plant and animal organization. In animals it is bounded by a cell membrane. Cells contain both genetic material and systems for synthesizing energy-yielding compounds. Cells have the ability to take up compounds from and excrete compounds into their surroundings.

cell nucleus An organelle bound by its own double membrane and containing chromosomes, the genetic information for cell protein synthesis and cell replication.

cell-mediated immunity A process in which certain white blood cells come in contact with the invading cells to destroy them.

cellulose An undigestible nonfermentable straight-chain polysaccharide made of glucose molecules.

cerebrovascular accident (CVA) Death of part of the brain tissue due typically to a blood clot. Also termed a *stroke*.

chain-breaking Breaking the link between two or more behaviors that encourage overeating, such as snacking while watching television.

chemical reaction An interaction between two chemicals that changes both chemicals.

cholecystokinin (CCK) A hormone that participates in enzyme release from the pancreas,

bile release from the gallbladder, and hunger regulation.

cholesterol A waxy lipid found in all body cells. It has a structure containing multiple chemical rings that is found only in foods that contain animal products.

chlorosis In traditional medical terminology, a form of iron-deficiency anemia characterized by pale or greenish skin, weakness, fatigue, and shortness of breath. In modern medical literature, chlorosis is termed hypochromic anemia.

chromosome A single, large DNA molecule and its associated proteins; contains many genes to store and transmit genetic information.

chylomicron Lipoprotein made of dietary fats surrounded by a shell of cholesterol, phospholipids, and protein. Chylomicrons are formed in the absorptive cells of the small intestine after fat absorption and travel through the lymphatic system to the bloodstream.

chyme A mixture of stomach secretions and partially digested food.

cirrhosis A loss of functioning liver cells, which are replaced by nonfunctioning connective tissue. Any substance that poisons liver cells can lead to cirrhosis. The most common cause is a chronic, excessive alcohol intake. Exposure to certain industrial chemicals also can lead to cirrhosis.

***cis* fatty acid** A form of an unsaturated fatty acid that has the hydrogens lying on the same side of the carbon-carbon double bond.

clinical assessment Examination of general appearance of skin, eyes, and tongue; evidence of rapid hair loss; sense of touch; and ability to cough and walk.

coenzyme A compound that combines with an inactive enzyme to form a catalytically active form. In this manner, coenzymes aid in enzyme function.

cofactor A mineral or other substance that binds to a specific region on a protein, such as an enzyme, and is necessary for the protein's function.

cognitive behavior therapy Psychological therapy in which the person's assumptions about dieting, body weight, and related issues are confronted. New ways of thinking are explored and then practiced by the person. In this way, an individual can learn new ways to control disordered eating behaviors and related life stress.

cognitive restructuring Changing one's frame of mind regarding eating—for example, instead of using a difficult day as an excuse to overeat, substituting other pleasures for rewards, such as a relaxing walk with a friend.

colostrum The first fluid secreted by the breast during late pregnancy and the first few days after birth. This thick fluid is rich in immune factors and protein.

complementary proteins Two food protein sources that make up for each other's inadequate supply of specific essential amino acids; together they yield a sufficient amount of all nine and, so provide high-quality (complete) protein for the diet.

compound A group of different types of atoms bonded together in definite proportion.

connective tissue Protein tissue that holds different structures in the body together. Some structures are made up of connective tissue—notably, tendons and cartilage. Connective tissue also forms part of bone and the nonmuscular structures of arteries and veins.

constipation A condition characterized by infrequent bowel movements.

contingency management Forming a plan of action to respond to a situation in which overeating is likely, such as when snacks are within arm's reach at a party.

control group Participants in an experiment who are not given the treatment being tested.

cortical bone The compact or dense bone found on the outer surfaces of bone.

creatine An organic (i.e., carbon-containing) molecule in muscle cells that serves as a part of a high-energy compound (termed creatine phosphate or phosphocreatine) capable of synthesizing ATP from ADP.

cretinism The stunting of body growth and poor development in the offspring that result from inadequate maternal intake of iodide during pregnancy.

cytoplasm The fluid and organelles (except the nucleus) in a cell.

dehydration Inadequate intake of water to replace losses.

Delaney Clause A clause to the 1958 Food Additives Amendment of the Pure Food and Drug Act in the United States that prevents the intentional (direct) addition to foods of a compound shown to cause cancer in laboratory animals or humans.

dementia A general loss or decrease in mental function.

denaturation Alteration of a protein's three-dimensional structure, usually because of treatment by heat, enzymes, acid or alkaline solutions, or agitation.

dental caries Erosions in the surface of a tooth caused by acids made by bacteria as they metabolize sugars.

deoxyribonucleic acid (DNA) The site of hereditary information in cells; DNA directs the synthesis of cell proteins.

diastolic blood pressure The pressure in the arterial blood vessels when the heart is between beats.

dietary assessment Estimation of typical food choices relying mostly on the recounting of one's usual intake or a record of one's previous days' intake.

dietary fiber Fiber found in food.

Dietary Guidelines for Americans General goals for nutrient intakes and diet composition set by the USDA and the U.S. Department of Health and Human Services.

digestion The process by which large ingested molecules are mechanically and chemically broken down to produce basic nutrients that can be absorbed across the wall of the GI tract.

digestive system The body system consisting of the gastrointestinal tract and accessory structures such as the liver, gallbladder, and pancreas. This system performs the mechanical and chemical processes of digestion, absorption of nutrients, and elimination of wastes.

diglyceride A breakdown product of a triglyceride consisting of two fatty acids bonded to a glycerol backbone.

direct calorimetry A method of determining a body's energy use by measuring heat released from the body. An insulated chamber is usually used.

discretionary calories The calories allowed in a diet after the person has met overall nutrition needs. This generally small amount of calories gives individuals the flexibility to consume some foods and beverages that may contain alcohol (e.g., beer and wine), added sugars (e.g., soft drinks, candy, and desserts), or added fats that are part of moderate- or high-fat foods (e.g., many snack foods).

disordered eating Mild and short-term changes in eating patterns that occur in relation to a stressful event, an illness, or a desire to modify one's diet for a variety of health and personal appearance reasons.

diuretic A substance that increases urinary fluid excretion.

diverticula Pouches that protrude through the exterior wall of the large intestine.

diverticulitis An inflammation of the diverticula caused by acids produced by bacterial metabolism inside the diverticula.

diverticulosis The condition of having many diverticula in the large intestine.

docosahexaenoic acid (DHA) An omega-3 fatty acid with 22 carbons and six carbon-carbon double bonds. It is present in large amounts in fatty fish and is slowly synthesized in the body from alpha-linolenic acid. DHA is especially present in the retina and brain.

double-blind study An experimental design in which neither the participants nor the researchers are aware of each participant's assignment (test or placebo) or the outcome of the study until it is completed. An independent third party holds the code and the data until the study has been completed.

duel energy X-ray absorptiometry (DEXA) A scientific tool used to measure bone mineral density.

early childhood caries Tooth decay that results from formula or juice (and even human milk) bathing the teeth as the child sleeps with a bottle in his or her mouth. The upper teeth are mostly affected as the lower teeth are protected by the tongue; formerly called *nursing bottle syndrome* and *baby bottle tooth decay*.

eating disorder Severe alterations in eating patterns linked to physiological changes. The alterations are associated with food restriction, binge eating, purging, and fluctuations in weight. They also involve a number of emotional and cognitive changes that affect the way a person perceives and experiences his or her body.

economic assessment Estimation of the ability of the person to purchase, transport, and cook food. The person's weekly budget for food purchases is also a key factor to consider.

edema The buildup of excess fluid in extracellular spaces.

eicosapentaenoic acid (EPA) An omega-3 fatty acid with 20 carbons and five carbon-carbon double bonds. It is present in large amounts in fatty fish and is slowly synthesized in the body from alpha-linolenic acid.

electrolytes Minerals that separate into positively or negatively charged ions in water. They are able to transmit an electrical current.

element A substance that cannot be separated into simpler substances by chemical processes. Common elements in nutrition include carbon, oxygen, hydrogen, nitrogen, calcium, phosphorus, and iron.

elimination diet A restrictive diet that systematically tests foods that may cause an allergic response by first eliminating them for 1 to 2 weeks and then adding them back, one at a time.

embryo In humans, the developing offspring in utero from about the beginning of the third week to the end of the eighth week after conception.

emulsifier A compound that can suspend fat in water by isolating individual fat droplets, using a shell of water molecules or other substances to prevent the fat from coalescing.

endocrine gland A hormone-producing gland.

endocrine system The body system consisting of the various glands and the hormones these glands secrete. This system has major regulatory functions in the body, such as reproduction and cell metabolism.

endometrium The membrane that lines the inside of the uterus. It increases in thickness during the menstrual cycle until ovulation occurs. The surface layers are shed during menstruation if conception does not take place.

endoplasmic reticulum (ER) An organelle in the cytoplasm composed of a network of canals running through the cytoplasm. Part of the endoplasmic reticulum contains ribosomes.

endorphins Natural body tranquilizers that may be involved in the feeding response and function in pain reduction.

energy balance The state in which energy intake, in the form of food and beverages, matches the energy expended, primarily through basal metabolism and physical activity.

energy density A comparison of the calorie (kcal) content of a food with the weight of the food. An energy-dense food is high in calories but weighs very little (e.g., potato chips), whereas a food low in energy density has few calories but weighs a lot, such as an orange.

enterohepatic circulation A continual recycling of compounds between the small intestine and the liver; bile acids are one example of a recycled compound.

enzyme A compound that speeds the rate of a chemical reaction but is not altered by the reaction. Almost all enzymes are proteins (some are made of genetic material).

epidemiology The study of how disease rates vary among different population groups.

epiglottis The flap that folds down over the trachea during swallowing.

epinephrine A hormone also known as *adrenaline*; it is released by the adrenal glands (located on each kidney) at times of stress and various nerve endings in the body. It acts to increase glycogen breakdown in the liver, among other functions.

epithelial cells The cells that line the outside of the body and the inside of all external passages within it, such as the GI tract.

epithelial tissue The surface cells that line the outside of the body and all external passages within it.

ergogenic Work-producing. An ergogenic aid is a mechanical, nutritional, psychological, pharmacological, or physiological substance or treatment intended to directly improve exercise performance.

erythrocyte Mature red blood cell. They have no nucleus and a life span of about 120 days; they contain hemoglobin, which transports oxygen and carbon dioxide.

erythropoietin A hormone secreted mostly by the kidneys that enhances red blood cell synthesis and stimulates red blood cell release from bone marrow.

esophagus A tube in the GI tract that connects the pharynx with the stomach.

essential amino acids The amino acids that cannot be synthesized by humans in sufficient amounts or at all and therefore must be included in the diet; there are nine essential amino acids. These are also called *indispensable amino acids*.

essential fatty acids Fatty acids that must be supplied by the diet to maintain health. Currently, only linoleic acid and alpha-linolenic acid are classified as essential.

ethanol Chemical term for the form of alcohol found in alcoholic beverages.

extracellular fluid Fluid found outside the cells; it represents about one-third of all body fluid.

extracellular space The space outside cells; represents one-third of body fluid.

famine An extreme shortage of food, which leads to massive starvation in a population; often associated with crop failures, war, and political unrest.

fasting hypoglycemia Low blood glucose that follows about a day of fasting.

fat-soluble vitamins Vitamins that dissolve in fat and such substances as ether and benzene but not readily in water. These vitamins are A, D, E, and K.

fatty acid Major part of most lipids; primarily composed of a chain of carbons flanked by hydrogen.

female athlete triad A condition characterized by disordered eating, lack of menstrual periods (amenorrhea), and osteoporosis.

fermentation The conversion of carbohydrates to alcohols, acids, and carbon dioxide without the use of oxygen.

fetal alcohol effect (FAE) Hyperactivity, attention deficit disorder, poor judgment, sleep disorders, and delayed learning as a result of prenatal exposure to alcohol.

fetal alcohol syndrome (FAS) A group of irreversible physical and mental abnormalities in the infant that result from the mother's consuming alcohol during pregnancy.

fetus The developing human life form from 8 weeks after conception until birth.

fiber Substances in plant foods not digested by the processes that take place in the human stomach or small intestine. These add bulk to feces. Fiber naturally found in foods is also called *dietary fiber*.

fluorosis Discoloration of tooth enamel sometimes accompanied with pitting due to consuming a large amount of fluoride for an excessive period.

food insecurity A condition of anxiety regarding running out of either food or money to buy more food.

food intolerance An adverse reaction to food that does not involve an allergic reaction.

food sensitivity A mild reaction to a substance in a food that might be expressed as slight itching or redness of the skin.

foodborne illness Sickness caused by the ingestion of food containing harmful substances.

free radical An unstable atom with an unpaired electron in its outermost shell.

fructose A six-carbon monosaccharide that usually exists in a ring form; found in fruits and honey; also known as *fruit sugar*.

fruitarian A person who primarily eats fruits, nuts, honey, and vegetable oils.

functional fiber Fiber added to foods that has been shown to provide health benefits.

functional foods Foods that have health benefits beyond basic nutrition.

fungi Simple parasitic life forms, including molds, mildews, yeasts, and mushrooms. They live on dead or decaying organic matter. Fungi can grow as single cells, like yeast, or as a multicellular colony, as seen with molds.

galactose A six-carbon monosaccharide that usually exists in a ring form; closely related to glucose.

gallbladder An organ attached to the underside of the liver; site of bile storage, concentration, and eventual secretion.

gastrointestinal (GI) tract The main sites in the body used for digestion and absorption of nutrients. It consists of the mouth, esophagus, stomach, small intestine, large intestine, rectum, and anus. Also called the *digestive tract*.

gastroplasty Gastric bypass surgery performed on the stomach to limit its volume to approximately 30 milliliters. Also referred to as *stomach stapling*.

gender and development (GAD) approach Understanding the roles and responsibilities of both men and women in the process of sustainable development.

gene A specific segment on a chromosome. Genes provide the blueprint for the production of cell proteins.

gene expression Use of DNA information on a gene to produce a protein. Thought to be a major determination of cell development.

generally recognized as safe (GRAS) A list of food additives that in 1958 were considered safe for consumption. Manufacturers were allowed to continue to use these additives, without special clearance, when needed for food products. FDA bears responsibility for proving they are not safe, but can remove unsafe products from the list.

genetic engineering Manipulation of the genetic makeup of any organism with recombinant DNA technology.

genetically modified organism (GMO) Any organism created by genetic engineering.

gestation The period of intrauterine development of offspring, from conception to birth; in humans, gestation lasts for about 40 weeks after the woman's previous menstrual period.

gestational diabetes A high blood glucose concentration that develops during pregnancy and returns to normal after birth; one cause is the placental production of hormones that antagonize the regulation of blood glucose by insulin.

ghrelin A hormone made by the stomach that increases the desire to eat.

glucagon A hormone made by the pancreas that stimulates the breakdown of glycogen in the liver into glucose; this ends up increasing blood glucose. Glucagon also performs other functions.

glucose A six-carbon monosaccharide that usually exists in a ring form; found as such in blood, and in table sugar bonded to fructose; also known as *dextrose*.

glycemic index (GI) The blood glucose response of a given food, compared to a standard (typically, glucose or white bread). Glycemic index is influenced by starch structure; fiber content; food processing; physical structure; and macronutrients in the meal, such as fat.

glycemic load (GL) The amount of carbohydrate in a serving of food multiplied by the glycemic index of that carbohydrate. The result is then divided by 100.

glycerol A three-carbon alcohol used to form triglycerides.

glycogen A carbohydrate made of multiple units of glucose with a highly branched structure. It is the storage form of glucose in humans and is synthesized (and stored) in the liver and muscles.

glycosylation The process by which glucose attaches to (glycates) other compounds, such as proteins.

goiter An enlargement of the thyroid gland; this is often caused by insufficient iodide in the diet.

Golgi complex The cell organelle near the nucleus that processes newly synthesized protein for secretion or distribution to other organelles.

green revolution This refers to increases in crop yields that accompanied the introduction of new agricultural technologies in less-developed countries, beginning in the 1960s. The key technologies were high-yielding, disease-resistant strains of rice, wheat, and corn; greater use of fertilizer and water; and improved cultivation practices.

gruels A thin mixture of grains or legumes in milk or water.

gums A viscous fiber containing chains of galactose, glucuronic acid, and other monosaccharides; characteristically found in exudates from plant stems.

hard water Water that contains high levels of calcium and magnesium.

heart attack Rapid fall in heart function caused by reduced blood flow through the heart's blood vessels. Often part of the heart dies in the process. Technically called a *myocardial infarction*.

heat cramps A frequent complication of heat exhaustion. They usually occur in people who have experienced large sweat losses from exercising for several hours in a hot climate and have consumed a large volume of water. The cramps occur in skeletal muscles and consist of contractions for 1 to 3 minutes at a time.

heat exhaustion The first stage of heat-related illness that occurs because of depletion of blood volume from fluid loss by the body. This increases body temperature and can lead to headache, dizziness, muscle weakness, and visual disturbances, among other effects.

heatstroke Heatstroke can occur when internal body temperature reaches 104°F. Sweating generally ceases if left untreated, and blood circulation is greatly reduced. Nervous system damage may ensue, and death is likely. Often the skin of individuals who suffer heatstroke is hot and dry.

hematocrit The percentage of blood made up of red blood cells.

heme iron Iron provided from animal tissues in the form of hemoglobin and myoglobin. Approximately 40% of the iron in meat is heme iron; it is readily absorbed.

hemicellulose An nonfermentable fiber containing xylose, galactose, glucose, and other monosaccharides bonded together.

hemochromatosis A disorder of iron metabolism characterized by increased iron absorption and deposition in the liver and heart. This eventually poisons the cells in those organs.

homocysteine An amino acid that arises from the metabolism of methionine. Adequate levels of vitamin B-6, folate, and vitamin B-12 are required for its metabolism. Elevated levels are associated with an increased risk of cardiovascular disease.

hemoglobin The iron-containing part of the red blood cell that carries oxygen to the cells and carbon dioxide away from the cells. The heme iron portion is also responsible for the red color of blood.

hemorrhagic stroke Damage to part of the brain resulting from rupture of a blood vessel and subsequent bleeding within or over the internal surface of the brain.

hemorrhoid A pronounced swelling of a large vein, particularly veins found in the anal region.

high-density lipoprotein (HDL) The lipoprotein in the blood that picks up cholesterol from dying cells and other sources and transfers it to the other lipoproteins in the bloodstream, as well as directly to the liver; low HDL increases the risk for cardiovascular disease.

high-quality (complete) proteins Dietary proteins that contain ample amounts of all nine essential amino acids.

histamine A breakdown product of the amino acid histidine that stimulates acid secretion by the stomach and has other effects on the body, such as contraction of smooth muscles, increased nasal secretions, relaxation of blood vessels, and changes in relaxation of airways.

homocysteine An amino acid not used in protein synthesis, but instead arises during metabolism of the amino acid methionine. Homocysteine is likely toxic to many cells, such as those lining the blood vessels.

hormone A compound secreted into the bloodstream by one type of cell that acts to control the function of another type of cell. For example, certain cells in the pancreas produce insulin, which in turn acts on muscle and other types of cells to promote uptake of nutrients from the blood.

hospice care A facility offering care that emphasizes comfort and dignity in death.

human immunodeficiency virus (HIV) The virus that leads to acquired immune deficiency syndrome (AIDS).

hunger The primarily physiological (internal) drive to find and eat food, mostly regulated by innate cues to eating.

hydrogenation The addition of hydrogen to a carbon-carbon double bond, producing a single carbon-carbon bond with two hydrogens attached to each carbon. Hydrogenation of unsaturated fatty acids in a vegetable oil increases its hardness, so this process is used to convert liquid oils into more solid fats, used in making margarine and shortening. *Trans* fatty acids are a by-product of hydrogenation of vegetable oils.

hyperglycemia High blood glucose, above 125 milligrams per 100 milliliters of blood.

hypertension High blood pressure. The pressure inside the blood vessels exceeds 140/90 millimeters of mercury.

hypoglycemia Low blood glucose, below 40 to 50 milligrams per 100 milliliters of blood.

hyponatremia Dangerously low blood sodium level.

hypothalamus A region at the base of the brain that contains cells that play a role in the regulation of hunger, respiration, body temperature, and other body functions.

hypotheses Tentative explanations by a scientist to explain a phenomenon.

identical twins Two offspring that develop from a single ovum and sperm and, consequently, have the same genetic makeup.

ileocecal sphincter The ring of smooth muscle between the end of the small intestine and the large intestine.

immune system The body system consisting of white blood cells, lymph glands and vessels, and various other body tissues. The immune system provides defense against foreign invaders, primarily due to the action of various types of white blood cells.

immunoglobulins Proteins found in the blood that bind to specific antigens; also called antibodies. The five major classes of immunoglobulins play different roles in antibody-mediated immunity.

incidental food additives Additives that appear in food products indirectly, from environmental contamination of food ingredients or during the manufacturing process.

indirect calorimetry A method to measure energy use by the body by measuring oxygen uptake. Formulas are then used to convert this gas exchange value into energy use.

infrastructure The basic framework of a system of organization. For a society, this includes roads, bridges, telephones, and other basic technologies.

inorganic Any substance lacking carbon atoms bonded to hydrogen atoms in the chemical structure.

insulin A hormone produced by the pancreas. Among other processes, insulin increases the synthesis of glycogen in the liver and the movement of glucose from the bloodstream into body cells.

intentional food additives Additives knowingly (directly) incorporated into food products by manufacturers.

intracellular fluid Fluid contained within a cell; it represents about two-thirds of body fluid.

intrinsic factor A proteinlike compound produced by the stomach that enhances vitamin B-12 absorption in the ileum.

ion A positively or negatively charged atom.

irradiation A process in which **radiation** energy is applied to foods, creating compounds (free radicals) within the food that destroy cell membranes, break down DNA, link proteins together, limit enzyme activity, and alter a variety of other proteins and cell functions of microorganisms that can lead to food spoilage. This process does not make the food radioactive.

ketone bodies Partial breakdown products of fat that contain three or four carbons.

ketosis The condition of having a high concentration of ketone bodies and related breakdown products in the bloodstream and tissues.

kidney nephrons The units of kidney cells that filter wastes from the bloodstream and deposit them into the urine.

kwashiorkor A disease occurring primarily in young children who have an existing disease and consume a marginal amount of calories and insufficient protein in relation to needs. The child generally suffers from infections and exhibits edema, poor growth, weakness, and an increased susceptibility to further illness.

kyphosis Abnormally increased bending of the spine.

lactase An enzyme made by absorptive cells of the small intestine; this enzyme digests lactose to glucose and galactose.

lactation The period of milk secretion following pregnancy; typically called *breastfeeding*.

lactic acid A three-carbon acid formed during anaerobic cell metabolism; a partial breakdown product of glucose; also called *lactate*.

Lactobacillus bifidus **factor** A protective factor secreted in the colostrum that encourages growth of beneficial bacteria in the newborn's intestines.

lactoovovegetarian A person who consumes plant products, dairy products, and eggs.

lactose Glucose bonded to galactose; also known as *milk sugar*.

lactose intolerance A condition in which symptoms such as abdominal gas and bloating appear as a result of severe lactose maldigestion.

lactose maldigestion (primary and secondary) Primary lactose maldigestion occurs when production of the enzyme lactase declines for no apparent reason. Secondary lactose maldigestion occurs when a specific cause, such as long-standing diarrhea, results in a decline in lactase production. When significant symptoms develop after lactose intake, it is then called lactose intolerance.

lactovegetarian A person who consumes plant products and dairy products.

lanugo Down-like hair that appears after a person has lost much body fat through semi-starvation. The hair stands erect and traps air, acting as insulation for the body to compensate for the relative lack of body fat, which usually functions as insulation.

laxative A medication or other substance that stimulates evacuation of the intestinal tract.

lean body mass Body weight minus fat storage weight equals lean body mass. This includes organs such as the brain, muscles, and liver, as well as bone and blood and other body fluids.

lecithin A group of phospholipid compounds that are major components of cell membranes.

leptin A hormone made by adipose tissue in proportion to total fat stores in the body that influences long-term regulation of fat mass. Leptin also influences reproductive functions, as well as other body processes, such as release of the hormone insulin.

let-down reflex A reflex stimulated by infant suckling that causes the release (ejection) of milk from milk ducts in the mother's breasts; also called *milk ejection reflex*.

life expectancy The average length of life for a given group of people born in a specific year (such as this year).

life span The potential oldest age a person can reach.

lignins An nonfermentable fiber made up of a multiringed alcohol (noncarbohydrate) structure.

limiting amino acid The essential amino acid in lowest concentration in a food or diet relative to body needs.

linoleic acid An essential omega-6 fatty acid with 18 carbons and two double bonds.

lipase Fat-digesting enzyme produced by the salivary glands, stomach, and pancreas.

lipid A compound containing much carbon and hydrogen, little oxygen, and sometimes other atoms. Lipids dissolve in ether or benzene, but not in water, and include fats, oils, and cholesterol.

lipoprotein A compound found in the bloodstream containing a core of lipids with a shell composed of protein, phospholipid, and cholesterol.

lipoprotein lipase An enzyme attached to the cells that form the inner lining of blood vessels; it breaks down triglycerides into free fatty acids and glycerol.

lobules Saclike structures in the breast that store milk.

long-chain fatty acid A fatty acid that contains 12 or more carbons.

low birth weight (LBW) Referring to any infant weighing less than 2.5 kilograms (5.5 pounds) at birth; most commonly results from preterm birth.

low-density lipoprotein (LDL) The lipoprotein in the blood containing primarily cholesterol; elevated LDL is strongly linked to cardiovascular disease risk.

lower esophageal sphincter A circular muscle that constricts the opening of the esophagus to the stomach. Also called the *gastroesophageal sphincter*.

lower-body obesity The type of obesity in which fat storage is primarily located in the buttocks and thigh area. Also known as *gynoid* or *gynecoid obesity*.

lower-quality (incomplete) proteins Dietary proteins that are low in or lack one or more essential amino acids.

lymph A clear fluid that flows through lymph vessels; carries most forms of fat after their absorption by the small intestine.

lymphatic system A system of vessels and lymph that accepts fluid surrounding cells and large particles, such as products of fat absorption. Lymph eventually passes into the bloodstream from the lymphatic system.

lysosome A cellular organelle that contains digestive enzymes for use inside the cell for turnover of cell parts.

lysozyme An enzyme produced by a variety of cells; it can destroy bacteria by rupturing their cell membranes.

macrocytic anemia Anemia characterized by the presence of abnormally large red blood cells.

macronutrient A nutrient needed in gram quantities in a diet.

major mineral A mineral vital to health; required in amounts greater than 100 milligrams per day.

malignant Malicious; in reference to a tumor, the property of spreading locally and to distant sites.

malnutrition Failing health that results from long-standing dietary practices that do not coincide with nutritional needs.

maltase An enzyme made by absorptive cells of the small intestine; this enzyme digests maltose to two glucoses.

maltose Glucose bonded to glucose.

marasmus A disease resulting from consuming a grossly insufficient amount of protein and calories; one of the diseases classed as protein-calorie malnutrition. Victims have little or no fat stores, little muscle mass, and poor strength. Death from infections is common.

megadose Intake of a nutrient beyond estimates of needs to prevent a deficiency or what would be found in a balanced diet; two to 10 times human needs is a starting point for such a dosage.

megaloblast A large, immature red blood cell that results from the inability of the cell to divide normally.

menarche The onset of menstruation. Menarche usually occurs around age 13, 2 or 3 years after the first signs of puberty start to appear.

menopause The cessation of the menstrual cycle in women, usually beginning at about 50 years of age.

metabolic syndrome A condition in which a person has poor blood glucose regulation, hypertension, increased blood tri-glycerides, and other health problems. This condition is usually accompanied by obesity, lack of physical activity, and a diet high in refined carbohydrates. Also called Syndrome X.

metabolic water When carbohydrates, lipids, and proteins are used as an energy source, carbon dioxide and water are formed as a by-product.

metabolism Chemical processes in the body by which energy is provided in useful forms and vital activities are sustained.

metastasize The spreading of disease from one part of the body to another, even to parts of the body that are remote from the site of the original tumor. Cancer cells can spread via blood vessels, the lymphatic system, or direct growth of the tumor.

micronutrient A nutrient needed in milligram or microgram quantities in a diet.

microorganism Bacteria, virus, or other organism invisible to the naked eye, some of which cause diseases. Also called *microbes*.

mineral Element used in the body to promote chemical reactions and to form body structures.

mitochondria The main sites of energy production in a cell. They also contain the pathway for oxidizing fat for fuel, among other metabolic pathways.

monoglyceride A breakdown product of a tri-glyceride consisting of one fatty acid attached to a glycerol backbone.

monounsaturated fatty acid A fatty acid containing one carbon-carbon double bond.

motility Generally, the ability to move spontaneously. It also refers to movement of food through the GI tract.

mucilages A viscous fiber consisting of chains of galactose, mannose, and other monosaccharides; characteristically found in seaweed.

mucus A thick fluid secreted by many cells throughout the body. It contains a compound that has both carbohydrate and protein parts. It acts as a lubricant and means of protection for cells.

muscle tissue A type of tissue adapted to contract to cause movement.

myelin sheath A lipid and protein combination (lipoprotein) that covers nerve fibers.

myocardial infarction Death of part of the heart muscle. Also termed *heart attack*.

myoglobin Iron-containing protein that binds oxygen in muscle tissue.

negative energy balance The state in which energy intake is less than energy expended, resulting in weight loss.

negative protein balance A state in which protein intake is less than related protein losses, such as often seen during acute illness.

nervous system The body system consisting of the brain, spinal cord, nerves, and sensory receptors. This system detects sensations, directs movements, and controls physiological and intellectual functions.

nervous tissue Tissue composed of highly branched, elongated cells, which transport nerve impulses from one part of the body to another.

neural tube defects A defect in the formation of the neural tube occurring during early fetal development. This type of defect results in various nervous system disorders, such as spina bifida. Folate deficiency in the pregnant woman increases the risk that the fetus will develop this disorder.

neuron The structural and functional unit of the nervous system. Consists of a cell body, dendrites, and an axon.

neuropeptide Y A chemical substance made in the hypothalamus that stimulates food intake. The hormone leptin inhibits neuropeptide Y production.

neurotransmitter A compound made by a nerve cell that allows for communication between it and other cells.

night blindness A vitamin A-deficiency disorder that results in loss of the ability to see under low-light conditions.

night eating syndrome Eating a lot of food in the late evening and nocturnal awakenings with ingestion of food.

nitrosamine A carcinogen formed from nitrates and breakdown products of amino acids; can lead to stomach cancer.

nonessential amino acids Amino acids that can be synthesized by a healthy body in sufficient amounts; there are 11 nonessential amino acids. These are also called *dispensable amino acids*.

nonfermentable fiber A fiber that is not easily metabolized by intestinal bacteria.

nonheme iron Iron provided from plant sources and animal tissues other than in the forms of hemoglobin and myoglobin. Nonheme iron is less efficiently absorbed than heme iron; absorption is closely dependent on body needs.

norepinephrine A neurotransmitter from nerve endings and and a hormone from the adrenal gland. It is released in times of stress and is involved in hunger regulation, blood glucose regulation, and other body processes.

NSAIDs Nonsteroidal anti-inflamatory drugs; includes aspirin, ibuprofen (Advil®), and naproxen (Aleve®).

nutrient density The ratio derived by dividing a food's nutrient content by its calorie content. When its contribution to our need for that nutrient exceeds its contribution to our calorie need, the food is considered to have a favorable nutrient density.

nutrients Chemical substances in food that contribute to health, many of which are essential parts of a diet. Nutrients nourish us by pro-

viding calories to fulfill energy needs, materials for building body parts, and factors to regulate necessary chemical processes in the body.

nutritional state The nutritional health of a person as determined by anthropometric measurements (height, weight, circumferences, and so on), biochemical measurements of nutrients or their by-products in blood and urine, a clinical (physical) examination, a dietary analysis, and economic evaluation; also called *nutritional status*.

oleic acid An omega-9 fatty acid with 18 carbons and one double bond.

omega-3 (ω-3) fatty acid An unsaturated fatty acid with the first double bond on the third carbon from the methyl end ($-CH_3$).

omega-6 (ω-6) fatty acid An unsaturated fatty acid with the first double bond on the sixth carbon from the methyl end ($-CH_3$).

organ A group of tissues designed to perform a specific function—for example, the heart, which contains muscle tissue, nerve tissue, and so on.

organ system A collection of organs that work together to perform an overall function.

organelles Compartments, particles, or filaments that perform specialized functions within a cell.

organic Any substance that contains carbon atoms bonded to hydrogen atoms in the chemical structure.

osmosis The passage of water through a membrane from a less concentrated compartment to a more concentrated compartment.

osteoblast Bone cells that initiate the synthesis of new bone.

osteoclast Bone cells that breakdown bone and subsequently release bone minerals into the blood.

osteocyte Osteoblast embedded into the bone matrix.

osteomalacia Adult form of rickets. The bones have low mineral density and subsequently are at risk for fracture.

osteopenia A bone disease defined by low mineral density.

osteoporosis The presence of a stress-induced fracture or a T-score of −2.5 or lower. The bones are porous and fragile due to low mineral density.

overnutrition A state in which nutritional intake greatly exceeds the body's needs.

ovum The egg cell from which a fetus eventually develops if the egg is fertilized by a sperm cell.

oxalic acid An organic acid found in spinach, rhubarb, and other leafy green vegetables that can depress the absorption of certain minerals present in the food, such as calcium.

oxidize In the most basic sense, the loss of an electron or gain of an oxygen by a chemical substance. This change typically alters the shape and/or function of the substance.

oxytocin A hormone secreted by the pituitary gland. It causes contraction of the musclelike cells surrounding the ducts of the breasts and the smooth muscle of the uterus.

parasite An organism that lives in or on another organism and derives nourishment from it.

parathyroid hormone (PTH) A hormone made by the parathyroid gland that increases synthesis of the active form of vitamin D. This hormone works with vitamin D to increase blood levels of calcium.

pasteurizing The process of heating food products to kill pathogenic microorganisms and reduce the total number of bacteria.

pectin A viscous fiber containing chains of galacturonic acid and other monosaccharides; characteristically found between plant cell walls.

pepsin A protein-digesting enzyme produced by the stomach.

peptide bond A chemical bond formed between amino acids in a protein.

percentile Classification of a measurement of a unit into divisions of 100 units.

periosteum A specialized connective tissue covering all bones and having bone-forming potentialities.

peristalsis A coordinated muscular contraction used to propel food down the gastrointestinal tract.

pernicious anemia The anemia that results from a lack of vitamin B-12 absorption; it is pernicious because of associated nerve degeneration that can result in eventual paralysis and death.

peroxisome A cell organelle that destroys toxic products within the cell.

pH A measure of the concentration of hydrogen ions. A pH below 7.0 is acidic.

phagocytosis A process in which a cell forms an indentation, and particles or fluids entering the indentation are then engulfed by the cell.

pharynx The organ of the digestive tract and respiratory tract located at the back of the oral and nasal cavities, commonly known as the throat.

phosphocreatine (PCr) A high-energy compound that can be used to re-form ATP. It is used primarily during bursts of activity, such as lifting and jumping.

phospholipid Any of a class of fat-related substances that contain phosphorus, fatty acids, and a nitrogen-containing component. Phospholipids are an essential part of every cell.

photosynthesis Process by which plants use energy from the sun to synthesize energy-yielding compounds, such as glucose.

physical fitness The ability to perform moderate to vigorous activity without undue fatigue.

physiological anemia The normal increase in blood volume in pregnancy that dilutes the concentration of red blood cells, resulting in anemia; also called *hemodilution*.

phytic acid (phytate) A constituent of plant fiber that chemically binds minerals and prevents their absorption.

phytochemicals Chemicals found in plants that have health protective actions.

pica The practice of eating nonfood items, such as dirt, laundry starch, or clay.

placebo Generally a fake medicine used to disguise the treatments given to the participants in an experiment.

placenta An organ that forms in the uterus in pregnant women. Through this organ, oxygen and nutrients from the mother's blood are transferred to the fetus, and fetal wastes are removed. The placenta also releases hormones that maintain the state of pregnancy.

plaque A cholesterol-rich substance deposited in the blood vessels; it contains various white blood cells, smooth muscle cells, various proteins, cholesterol and other lipids, and eventually calcium.

plasma The fluid, extracellular portion of blood.

platelets A protoplasmic disc smaller than a red blood cell that promotes coagulation.

polypeptide A group of amino acids bonded together, from 50 to 2000 or more.

polysaccharides Carbohydrates containing many glucose units, from 10 to 1000 or more.

polyunsaturated fatty acid A fatty acid containing two or more carbon-carbon double bonds.

pool The amount of a nutrient stored within the body that can be mobilized when needed.

portal circulation The portion of the circulatory system that uses a large vein (portal vein) to carry nutrient-rich blood from capillaries in the intestines and portions of the stomach to the liver.

positive energy balance The state in which energy intake is greater than energy expended, generally resulting in weight gain.

positive protein balance A state in which protein intake exceeds related protein losses, as is needed during times of growth.

pregnancy-induced hypertension A serious disorder that can include high blood pressure, kidney failure, convulsions, and even death of the mother and fetus. Although its exact cause is not known, an adequate diet (especially adequate calcium intake) and prenatal care may prevent this disorder or limit its severity. Mild cases are known as *preeclampsia*; more severe cases are called *eclampsia* (formerly called *toxemia*).

premenstrual syndrome (PMS) A disorder found in some women a few days before a menstrual period begins. It is characterized by depression, anxiety, headache, bloating, and mood swings. Severe cases are termed premenstrual dysphoric disorder (PDD).

preservatives Compounds that extend the shelf life of foods by inhibiting microbial growth or minimizing the destructive effect of oxygen and metals.

preterm An infant born before 37 weeks of gestation; also referred to as *premature*.

prolactin A hormone secreted by the pituitary gland that stimulates the synthesis of milk in the breast.

prooxidant A nutrient that promotes oxidation and oxidative cell and tissue damage.

prostate gland A solid, chestnut-shaped organ surrounding the first part of the urinary tract in the male. The prostate gland secretes substances into the semen.

protease Protein-digesting enzyme produced by the stomach, small intestine, and pancreas.

protein Food and body components made of amino acids; proteins contain carbon, hydrogen, oxygen, nitrogen, and sometimes other atoms, in a specific configuration. Proteins contain the form of nitrogen most easily used by the human body.

protein equilibrium A state in which protein intake is equal to related protein losses; the person is said to be in protein balance.

protein turnover The process by which cells break down old proteins and resynthesize new proteins. In this way the cell will have the proteins it needs to function at that time.

protein-calorie malnutrition (PCM) A condition resulting from regularly consuming insufficient amounts of calories and protein. The deficiency eventually results in body wasting, primarily of lean tissue, and an increased susceptibility to infections.

proton pump inhibitor A medication that inhibits the ability of gastric cells to secrete hydrogen ions. Low doses of this class of medications are also available without prescription (e.g., omeprazole [Prilosec®]).

provitamin A substance that can be converted into vitamin A.

pyloric sphincter The ring of smooth muscle between the stomach and the small intestine.

pyruvic acid A three-carbon compound formed during glucose metabolism; also called *pyruvate*.

radiation Literally, energy that is emitted from a center in all directions. Various forms of radiation energy include X-rays and ultraviolet rays from the sun.

rancid Containing products of decomposed fatty acids that have an unpleasant flavor and odor.

reactive hypoglycemia Low blood glucose that follows a meal high in simple sugars, with corresponding symptoms of irritability, headache, nervousness, sweating, and confusion; also called *postprandial hypoglycemia*.

receptor A site in a cell at which compounds (such as hormones) bind. Cells that contain receptors for a specific compound are partially controlled by that compound.

recombinant DNA technology A test tube technology that rearranges DNA sequences in an organism by cutting the DNA, adding or deleting a DNA sequence, and rejoining DNA molecules with a series of enzymes.

rectum Terminal portion of the large intestine.

registered dietitian (R.D.) A person who has completed a baccalaureate degree program approved by the American Dietetic Association, performed at least 900 hours of supervised professional practice, and passed a registration examination.

relapse prevention A series of strategies used to help prevent and cope with weight-control lapses, such as recognizing high-risk situations and deciding beforehand on appropriate responses.

reserve capacity The extent to which an organ can preserve essentially normal function despite decreasing cell number or cell activity.

resting metabolism The amount of calories the body uses when the person has not eaten in 4 hours and is resting (e.g., 15 to 30 minutes) and awake in a warm, quiet environment. It is roughly 6% higher than basal metabolism due to the less strict criteria for the test; often referred to as *resting metabolic rate (RMR)*.

retina A light-sensitive lining in the back of the eye. It contains retinal.

retinoids Chemical forms of preformed vitamin A; one source is animal foods.

ribonucleic acid (RNA) The single-stranded nucleic acid involved in the transcription of genetic information and translation of that information into protein structure.

ribosomes Cytoplasmic particles that mediate the linking together of amino acids to form proteins; may exist freely in the cytoplasm or attached to endoplasmic reticulum.

rickets The vitamin D deficiency disease observed in infants and children. Mineral content of the bones is markedly reduced.

salivary amylase A starch-digesting enzyme produced by salivary glands.

satiety State in which there is no longer a desire to eat; a feeling of satisfaction.

saturated fatty acid A fatty acid containing no carbon-carbon double bonds.

scavenger cells Specific form of white blood cells that can bury themselves in the artery wall and accumulate LDL. As these cells take up LDL, they contribute to the development of atherosclerosis.

scurvy The deficiency disease that results after a few weeks to months of consuming a diet that lacks vitamin C; pinpoint sites of bleeding on the skin are an early sign.

secretory vesicles Membrane-bound vesicles produced by the Golgi apparatus; contains protein and other compounds to be secreted by the cell.

self-monitoring Tracking foods eaten and conditions affecting eating; actions are usually recorded in a diary, along with location, time,

and state of mind. This is a tool to help people understand more about their eating habits.

semiessential amino acids Amino acids that, when consumed, spare the need to use an essential amino acid for their synthesis. Tyrosine in the diet, for example, spares the need to use phenylalanine for tyrosine synthesis. Also called *conditionally essential amino acids.*

sequestrants Compounds that bind free metal ions. By so doing, they reduce the ability of ions to cause rancidity in foods containing fat.

serotonin A neurotransmitter synthesized from the amino acid tryptophan that affects mood (sense of calmness), behavior, and appetite, and induces sleep.

set point Often refers to the close regulation of body weight. It is not known what cells control this set point or how it functions in weight regulation. There is evidence, however, that mechanisms exist that help regulate weight.

sickle cell disease (sickle cell anemia) An illness that results from a malformation of the red blood cell because of an incorrect structure in part of its hemoglobin protein chains. The disease can lead to episodes of severe bone and joint pain, abdominal plain, headache, convulsions, paralysis, and even death.

small for gestational age (SGA) Referring to infants who weigh less than the expected weight for their length of gestation. This corresponds to less than 2.5 kilograms (5.5 pounds) in a full-term newborn. A preterm infant who is also SGA will most likely develop some medical complications.

soft water Water that contains a high level of sodium.

solvent A liquid substance in which other substances dissolve.

spontaneous abortion Cessation of pregnancy and expulsion of the embryo or nonviable fetus prior to 20 weeks gestation. This is the result of natural causes, such as a genetic defect or developmental problem; also called *miscarriage.*

spores Dormant reproductive cells capable of turning into adult organisms without the help of another cell. Various bacteria and fungi form spores.

starch A carbohydrate made of multiple units of glucose attached together in a form the body can digest; also known as *complex carbohydrate.*

sterol A compound containing a multi-ring (steroid) structure and a hydroxyl group (–OH). Cholesterol is a typical example.

stimulus control Altering the environment to minimize the stimuli for eating—for example, removing foods from sight and storing them in kitchen cabinets.

stress fracture A fracture that occurs from repeated jarring of a bone. Common sites include bones of the foot.

stroke A decrease or loss in blood flow to the brain that results from a blood clot or other

change in arteries in the brain. This in turn causes the death of brain tissue. Also called a *cerebrovascular accident.*

subclinical Stage of a disease or disorder not severe enough to produce symptoms that can be detected or diagnosed.

sucrase An enzyme made by absorptive cells of the small intestine; this enzyme digests sucrose to glucose and fructose.

sucrose Fructose bonded to glucose; table sugar.

sugar A simple carbohydrate with the chemical composition $(CH_2O)_n$. The basic unit of all sugars is glucose, a six-carbon ring structure. The primary sugar in the diet is sucrose, which is made up of glucose and fructose.

sustainable development Economic growth that will simultaneously reduce poverty, protect the environment, and preserve natural capital.

symptom A change in health status noted by the person with the problem, such as stomach pain.

synapse The space between one neuron and another neuron (or cell).

systolic blood pressure The pressure in the arterial blood vessels associated with the pumping of blood from the heart.

teratogen A substance that may cause or increase the risk of a birth defect. Exposure to a teratogen does not always lead to a birth defect; its effects on the fetus depend on the dose, timing, and duration of exposure.

theory An explanation for a phenomenon that has numerous lines of evidence to support it.

thermic effect of food (TEF) The increase in metabolism that occurs during the digestion, absorption, and metabolism of energy-yielding nutrients. This represents 5% to 10% of calories consumed.

thermogenesis This term encompasses the ability of humans to regulate body temperature within narrow limits (thermoregulation). Two visible examples of thermogenesis are fidgeting and shivering when cold.

thyroid hormones Hormones produced by the thyroid gland that among their functions increase the rate of overall metabolism in the body.

tissues Collections of cells adapted to perform a specific function.

tocopherols The chemical name for some forms of vitamin E. The alpha form is the most potent.

total fiber Combination of dietary fiber and functional fiber in a food. Also just called *fiber.*

total parenteral nutrition The intravenous feeding of all necessary nutrients, including the most basic forms of protein, carbohydrates, lipids, vitamins, minerals, and electrolytes.

toxins Poisonous compounds produced by an organism that can cause disease.

trace mineral A mineral vital to health; required in the diet in amounts less than 100 milligrams per day.

***trans* fatty acid** A form of an unsaturated fatty acid, usually a monounsaturated one when found in food, in which the hydrogens on both carbons forming the double bond lie on opposite sides of that bond, rather than on the same side, as in most natural fats. Stick margarine, shortenings, and deep fat-fried foods in general are rich sources.

transcription Information on DNA needed to make a protein is copied onto RNA.

transgenic Organism that contains genes originally present in another organism.

translation The information contained in RNA is used to determine the amino acids in a protein.

triglyceride The major form of lipid in the body and in food. It is composed of three fatty acids bonded to glycerol, an alcohol.

trimesters Three 13- to 14-week periods into which the normal pregnancy (the length of a normal pregnancy is about 40 weeks, measured from the first day of the woman's last menstrual period) is divided somewhat arbitrarily for purposes of discussion and analysis. Development of the offspring, however, is continuous throughout pregnancy, with no specific physiological markers demarcating the transition from one trimester to the next.

trypsin A protein-digesting enzyme secreted by the pancreas to act in the small intestine.

tumor Mass of cells; may be cancerous (malignant) or noncancerous (benign).

type 1 diabetes A form of diabetes prone to ketosis and that requires insulin therapy.

type I osteoporosis Porous trabecular bone characterized by rapid bone demineralization following menopause.

type 2 diabetes A form of diabetes characterized by insulin resistance and often associated with obesity. Insulin therapy can be used but is often not required.

type II Osteoporosis Porous trabecular and cortical bone observed in men and women after the age of 60.

ulcer Erosion of the tissue lining, usually in the stomach (gastric ulcer) or the upper small intestine (duodenal ulcer). As a group these are generally referred to as *peptic ulcers.*

ultratrace mineral A mineral present in the been shown to be essential to human health.

umami A brothy, meaty, savory flavor in some foods. Monosodium glutamate enhances this flavor when added to foods.

undernutrition Failing health that results from a long-standing dietary intake that is not enough to meet nutritional needs.

underwater weighing A method of estimating total body fat by weighing the individual on a standard scale and then weighing him or her again submerged in water. The difference between the two weights is used to estimate total body volume.

underweight A body mass index below 18.5. The cutoff is less precise than for obesity because this condition has been less studied.

unsaturated fatty acid A fatty acid containing one or more carbon-carbon double bonds.

upper-body obesity The type of obesity in which fat is stored primarily in the abdominal area; defined as a waist circumference more than 40 inches (102 centimeters) in men and more than 35 inches (89 centimeters) in women; closely associated with a high risk for cardiovascular disease, hypertension, and type 2 diabetes. Also known as *android obesity.*

urea Nitrogen-containing waste product of protein metabolism; major source of nitrogen

$$O$$
$$||$$

in the urine, chemically NH_2-C-NH_2.

ureter Tube that transports urine from the kidney to the urinary bladder.

urethra Tube that transports urine from the urinary bladder to the outside of the body.

urinary system The body system consisting of the kidneys, urinary bladder, and the ducts that carry urine. This system removes waste products from the circulatory system and regulates blood acid-base balance, overall chemical balance, and water balance in the body.

vegan A person who eats only plant foods.

vein A blood vessel that carries blood to the heart.

very-low-calorie diet (VLCD) Known also as *protein-sparing modified fast (PSMF),* this diet allows a person 400 to 800 kcal per day, often in liquid form. Of this, 120 to 480 kcal is car-

bohydrate, and the rest is mostly high-quality protein.

very-low-density lipoprotein (VLDL) The lipoprotein created in the liver that carries cholesterol and lipids that have been taken up or newly synthesized by the liver.

villi (singular, villus) (singular, **villus**) The fingerlike protrusions into the small intestine that participate in digestion and absorption of food.

virus The smallest known type of infectious agent, many of which cause disease in humans. A virus is essentially a piece of genetic material surrounded by a coat of protein. They do not metabolize, grow, or move by themselves. They reproduce only with the aid of a living cellular host.

viscous fiber A fiber that is readily fermented by bacteria in the large intestine.

vitamin Compound needed in very small amounts in the diet to help regulate and support chemical reactions and processes in the body

water The universal solvent; chemically, H_2O. The body is composed of about 60% water. Water (fluid) needs are about 9 (women) or 13 (men) cups per day; needs are greater if one exercises heavily.

water-soluble vitamins Vitamins that dissolve in water. These vitamins are the B vitamins and vitamin C.

white blood cells One of the formed elements of the circulating blood system; also called *leukocytes.* White blood cells are able to squeeze through intracellular spaces and migrate. They phagocytize bacteria, fungi, and viruses, as well as detoxify proteins that may result from allergic reactions, cellular injury, and other immune system cells.

whole grains Grains containing the entire seed of the plant, including the bran, germ, and endosperm (starchy interior). Examples are whole wheat and brown rice.

xerophthalmia Hardening of the cornea and drying of the surface of the eye, which can result in blindness.

zoochemicals Chemicals found in animal products that have health protective actions.

zygote The fertilized ovum; the cell resulting from the union of an egg cell (ovum) and sperm until it divides.

PHOTO CREDITS

Design Elements

Part 1(apple), 2(peaches), 3(peas): C Squared Studios/ Getty Images; 4(banana): © Stockdisc/PunchStock; 5(broccoli), 6(pear): C Squared Studios/Getty Images; "Nutritions and your Health" (tomatoes): Cole Group/ Getty Images; "Study Questions" (young girl): © SW Productions/Brand X Pictures/Getty Images; "Check Your Knowledge" (young guy): Doug Menuez/Getty Images; "Rate your Plate" (salad): © Photodisc

Chapter 1

Opener: © Photodisc/Getty Images; p. 5: © Photodisc website; p. 6: Digital Vision/Getty Images; Table 1-3 (bread, potatoe, apples, oil, steak, eggs, beans): © Corbis/ Vol. 83; (water): © PhotoDisc/Vol. 30; (orange juice): © John A. Rizzo/Getty Images; (broccoli, strawberry): © Corbis/Vol. 83; (lettuce): © Corbis/RF website; (milk): © Corbis/Vol. 83; (cereal): © Corbis/RF website; (banana): © Corbis/Vol. 83; (tofu): © Photodisc/OS49; (salmon): © Corbis/Vol. 83; (nuts): © PhotoDisc/OS49; 10: © Royalty Free/Corbis; 11: Reproduction with permission. © Culinary Hearts Kitchen, 1982; p. 12: © Corbis/ Vol. 83; Fig 1-1(potatoe): The McGraw-Hill Companies, Inc./Christopher Kerrigan, photographer; (steak): RF Comstock Images; (smiling man): RF/Getty Images; (smiling woman): RF/Getty Images; p. 15: © Corbis/ Vol. 4; p. 16: Steve Cole/ Getty Images; p. 17(top): RF/ Getty Images; (bottom): Healthy People 2010 Cover U.S. Department of Health and Human Services, Healthy People 2010. 2nd Edition. With Understanding and Improving Health and Objectives for Improving Health. 2 Volumes. Washington, DC: U.S. Government Printing Office, November 2000; p. 18: © Ohio State University Communications Photo Service; p. 19: © Digital Vision/ PunchStock; Fig 1-4: © Corbis/Vol. 115; p. 22: © Corbis/Vol. 4; p. 23 (pizza): James Darell/Getty Images; p. 24: Steve Mason/Getty Images; p. 25: © PhotoAlto/PunchStock; p. 26: © Burke/Triolo Productions/Getty Images; p. 27: © Corbis/Vol. 589

Chapter 2

Opener (man): The McGraw-Hill Companies, Inc./ John Flournoy, photographer; p. 34: The McGraw-Hill Companies, Inc./Ken Karp, photographer; p. 35: Courtesy of U.S. Rice Federation; p. 36: © Comstock/ PunchStock; p. 38: Steve Allen/Getty Images; p. 39: © Photodisc/Vol. 67; p. 40: The McGraw-Hill Companies, Inc./Lars A. Niki, photographer; Fig 2-3 (Anthropometric): The McGraw-Hill Companies, Inc./Lars A. Niki, photographer; (Biochemical): © Photodisc/Vol. 29; (Clinical): © Photodisc website; (Dietary): © Corbis/Vol. 102; (Economic): © Comstock/ PunchStock; p. 43: © Corbis/Vol. 154; p. 44: Steve Cole/Getty Images; Fig 2-7 (yo-yo): © Corbis/RF website; (baseball), (tennis ball): © PhotoDisc/OS25; (golf ball): © Corbis/Vol. 127; (dice): Digital Vision/Getty Images; (playing cards): Photodisc Collection/Getty Images; p. 48(top): Karl Weatherly/Getty Images; (bottom): Getty Images/Jonelle Weaver; p. 49(top): Mitch Hrdlicka/Getty Images; (middle): Getty Images; (bottom): C Squared Studios/Getty Images; p. 50: © PhotoDisc/Vol. 67; p. 52 (top): RF Getty Images; (middle): Dynamic Graphics/JupiterImages; (bottom): RF Getty Images; p. 53(top & middle): RF Getty Images; (bottom): © Bananastock; p. 54(top & middle): RF Getty Images; (bottom): RF/Corbis;

p. 55(top): © Peter Cade/Getty Images; (bottom): © Comstock PunchStock; p. 56: © The Ohio State University Communications Photo Service, Jodi Miller; p. 57: © Corbis/Vol. 130; p. 61: RF/Getty Images; p. 62: © Ryan McVay/Getty Images; p. 64: © PhotoDisc/ Vol. 110; p. 67: © The McGraw-Hill Companies, Inc./ Andrew Resek, photographer; p. 70: © Corbis/Vol. 275; p. 71: © Royalty Free/Corbis

Chapter 3

Opener: © Royalty Free/Corbis; p. 81: Dynamic Graphics/JupiterImages; p. 83: © Corbis/Cdrphoto; p. 87: © Photodisc; p. 97: © Mitch Hrdlicka/Getty Images; p. 100: © Corbis/Vol. 40; p. 105: © PhotoDisc/ Vol. 83; p. 106: Royalty Free/Corbis; p. 107: © Corbis/ Vol. 40; Fig 3-20b: © J. James/Photo Researchers, Inc.; p. 111: © Gordon Wardlaw; p. 112: C Squared Studios/ Getty Images; p. 113: © Gladden Willis, M.D./Visuals Unlimited; p. 114: © Stockdisc/Becky Denzin

Chapter 4

Opener: The McGraw-Hill Companies, Inc./Andrew Resek, photographer; p. 123: © PhotoDisc/OS49; p. 125: © Photolink/Getty Images; p. 129: © Comstock/ PunchStock; p. 130: © Corbis/Vol. 83; p. 131 (top): Courtesy of The Sugar Association, Inc., Washington, D.C.; (middle): Ryan McVay/Getty Images; p. 133(top): The McGraw-Hill Companies, Inc./Andrew Resek, photographer; (bottom): Burke/Triolo Productions/Getty Images; p. 135: © PhotoDisc/Vol. 49; p. 136: Beano TM is a registered trademark of AkPharma Inc.; p. 139: Royalty Free/Corbis; p. 140: Triolo Productions/Getty Images; p. 142(top): John A. Rizzo/RF Getty Images; (bottom): Nancy R. Cohen/Getty Images; p. 143: Getty Images; p. 144: Nancy R. Cohen/RF Getty Images; p. 147: C Squared Studios/RF Getty Images; p. 150: © Stockdisc/PunchStock; p. 151: Ryan McVay/RF Getty Images; p. 152: Dyanamic Graphics/JupiterImages; p. 154: © Getty Images/Eyewire

Chapter 5

Opener: McVay/Getty Images; p. 165: © Greg Kidd and Joanne Scott; p. 169: © PhotoDisc/Vol. 12; p. 170: © PhotoDisc/OS49; p. 172: © PhotoDisc/Vol. 02; p. 173: © PhotoDisc/Vol. 4; p. 174: C Squared Studios/ Getty Images; p. 175: © Saffola Quality Foods, Inc.; p. 176(top): © Corbis/Vol. 4; (bottom): Burke/Triolo Productions/Getty Images; p. 182: Courtesy National Fisheries Institute; p. 183: Jack Star/PhotoLink/Getty Images; p. 184: SW Productions/Getty Images; p. 187: National Cancer Institute; p. 188: Digital Vision/Getty Images; p. 189: RF/Getty Images; p. 190(top): Royalty Free/Corbis; (bottom): John A. Rizzo/Getty Images; p. 191(Left): © image100/PunchStock; p. 192: © The McGraw-Hill Companies, Inc./Photo by Eric Misko, Elite Images Photography; p. 193: © The McGraw-Hill Companies, Inc./Gary He, photographer; p. 195: © The McGraw-Hill Higher Education, Inc./Jill Braaten, photographer; p. 196: trbfoto/Brand X Pictures/Jupiterimages

Chapter 6

Opener: © Royalty Free/Corbis; p. 206: RF/Getty Images; p. 207: Corbis/PictureQuest; p. 208: © PhotoDisc; Fig 6-3a: © Bill Longcore/SPL/Photo

Researchers; b: © Bill Longcore/SPL/Photo Researchers; p. 211: John A. Rizzo/Getty Images; p. 213: © Corbis/ Vol. 130; p. 215: Dynamic Graphics/JupiterImages; Fig 6-11a: © Photodisc; b: Stockbyte/Punchstock Images; c: Dynamic Graphics/JupiterImages; p. 220: © The Ohio State University Communcations Photo Service; Fig 6-12(left): © Kevin Fleming/Corbis; (right): Peter Turnley/Corbis; p. 222: © Dr. Parvinder Sethi; p. 223(left): Images/Jonelle Weaver; p. 224: Courtesy of Walnut Marketing Board; p. 225: © Getty Images/ Vol. 49; p. 226: © Greg Kidd and Joanne Scott; p. 227: Getty Images/Jonelle Weaver; p. 228: Image Source/ JupiterImages; p. 233: Ryan McVay/Getty Images

Chapter 7

Opener: Duncan Smith/Getty Images; p. 239: © Mitch Hrdlicka/Getty Images; p. 241: © Corbis/Vol. 130; Fig 7-4: © Samuel Ashfield/FPL/Photo Researchers, Inc.; p. 243: Steve Mason/Getty Images; p. 245: TRBfoto/Getty Images; Fig 7-7: © Rick O'Quihn University of Georgia; Fig 7-8: Courtesy of Life Measurement Instruments; Fig 7-9: © Diana Linsley/Linsley Photographics; Fig 7-10: © Gordon Wardlaw; Fig 7-11: DEXA; p. 249: © Corbis/ RF website; p. 251(top): © The Ohio State University Communications Photo Service, Jodi Miller; (bottom): Jack Hollingsworth/Getty Images; p. 252: Getty Images/ SW Productions; p. 253: © PhotoDisc/Getty Images/ Vol. 190; Fig 7-14(1): © Digital Vision; (2): Ryan McVay/Getty Images; (3): JupiterImages; p. 254 & 255: © PhotoDisc/Vol. 76; p. 256 & 258: PhotoDisc/Vol. 20; p. 260: © Royalty Free/Corbis/Vol. 306; p. 261: Dynamic Graphics/JupiterImages; p. 265: Keith Brofsky/Getty Images; p. 269: Ernie Friedlander/Cole Group/Getty Images; p. 270: Ryan McVay/Getty Images

Overview of the Micronutrients

Opener p. 280: © Stockbyte/PunchStock; p. 282: Photodisc Collection/Getty Images

Chapter 8

Opener: © Photodisc Collection/Getty Images; p. 303: © PhotoDisc; p. 306: Comstock Images/PictureQuest; p. 307: © Corbis/Vol. 43; p. 309: Getty Images; p. 311: © Stockdisc/PunchStock; p. 312: © Corbis/Vol. 43; p. 314(left): © PhotoDisc/Vol. 40; (right): Melnychuk/ Getty Images; p. 315 & 316: Ryan McVay/Getty Images; p. 320: Hoby Finn/Getty Images

Chapter 9

Opener: © Brand X Pictures/Jupiterimages; p. 327: © Greg Kidd & Joanne Scott; Fig 9-7 & 9-11: "A Color Atlas and Text of Nutritional Disorders" by Dr. Donald D. McLaren/Mosby-Woolfe Europe, Ltd.; p. 335: Keith Ovregaard/Cole Group/Getty Images; p. 338: Sanchez/ Cole Group/ Getty Images; Fig 9-15a & b: National Eye Institute, National Institutes of Health; p. 339: Duncan Smith/Getty Images; p. 343: Adam Crowley/Getty Images; (bottom): © Image Source/PunchStock

Chapter 10

Opener: Getty Images; p. 351: MHHE Image Library; p. 353: Yoav Levy/Phototake; p. 360: The McGraw-Hill Companies, Inc./Andrew Resek, photographer; p. 361: Getty Images/Jonelle Weaver; p. 364: © Corbis/Vol. 43; p. 365: © Royalty Free/Corbis; Fig 10-16: © Jeffrey L. Rotman/Corbis; p. 369(left): Dex Image/Getty Images; (right): The McGraw-Hill Companies, Inc./ John Thoeming, photographer; p. 370: © Royalty Free/Corbis; p. 373: © Paul Casamassimi, DDS, MS; p. 374: © PhotoDisc/Vol. 02; p. 375: © Royalty Free/Corbis

Chapter 11

Opener: Menuez/Getty Images; p. 383: © PhotoDisc/OS49; p. 385: D. Fischer and Pl. Lyose/Cole Group/Getty Images; Fig 11-5 & 11-7: © "A Color Atlas and Text of Nutritional Disorders" by Dr. Donald D. McLaren/Mosby-Woolfe Europe, Ltd.; p. 389: Images/Jonelle Weaver; p. 391: © Corbis/Vol. 130; Fig 11-13(top): Abbey/Photo Researchers, Inc.; (bottom): Biophoto Associates/SPL/Photo Researchers, Inc.; p. 396: © Photodisc/PunchStock; p. 399: Royalty Free/Corbis; p. 400: David Buffington/Getty Images; p. 401: © Corbis/RF website; Fig 11-20: Doug Menuez/Getty Images; p. 405: © "A Color Atlas and Text of Nutritional Disorders" by Dr. Donald D. McLaren/Mosby-Woolfe Europe, Ltd.; p. 406: © Corbis/RF website; p. 407: Photo courtesy of Almond Board of California; p. 409: © Corbis/Royalty Free; p. 410: Courtesy National Cattlemen's Beef Associations; p. 411: © Royalty Free/Corbis; p. 412: Keith Brofsky/Getty Images; p. 414: © The Ohio State University Communications Photo Service, Jodi Miller; p. 415: C Squared Studios/Getty Images; p. 418(top): Courtesy of Fishery Products International, Danver, MA; (bottom): © Stockbyte/PunchStock

Chapter 12

Opener: © Getty Images; p. 427: JupiterImages; Table 12-1(left): Karl Weatherly/Getty Images; (middle, right): JupiterImages; p. 429: © Getty Images/Vol. 67/Duncan Smith; p. 431: © PhotoDisc/Sports Metaphors; p. 432: Royalty Free/Corbis; p. 434: JupiterImages; p. 435: © Corbis/Vol. 20; p. 436: James Mulligan; p. 437: © Corbis/RF website; p. 440: Royalty Free/Corbis; p. 441: © Gordon Wardlaw; p. 442: RF/Corbis; p. 443: © PhotoDisc/Vol. 51; p. 444: © Corbis/Vol. 103; p. 446: John A. Rizzo/Getty Images; p. 447: © Getty Images/Vol. 1/Photolink; p. 448: © PhotoDisc/Vol. 51; p. 452: © Corbis/Vol. 20; p. 453: Royalty Free/Corbis; p. 456(bottom): JupiterImages

Chapter 13

Opener: © Corbis/Vol. 75; p. 465: The McGraw-Hill Companies, Inc./Lars A. Niki, photographer; p. 466: © PhotoDisc website; p. 467: © Royalty Free/Corbis; p. 468: Mark Andersen/Getty Images; p. 469: Ryan McVay/Getty Images; p. 470: © PhotoDisc website; p. 473: © Tom Stewart Photography/Corbis; p. 474: © PhotoDisc website; Fig 13-2: © PhotoDisc/EP047; Fig 13-3: © Paul Casamassimo, DDS, MS; p. 477: Royalty Free/Corbis; p. 478: PhotoDisc website; p. 479: Jack Star/PhotoLink/Getty Images; p. 480: © BananaStock/PunchStock; p. 481: © Photodisc/Vol. 45; p. 481: The McGraw-Hill Companies, Inc./Lars A. Niki, photographer; p. 482: © PhotoDisc website; p. 483(left): © PhotoDisc/Vol. 95; p. 484: © Corbis/RF website; p. 485: BananaStock/PunchStock; p. 485: © Digital Vision/PunchStock

Chapter 14

Opener: Dr. Parvinder Sethi; p. 492: Corbis/RF website; p. 497: USDA photo by Peter Manzelli; p. 499: © Royalty Free/Corbis; p. 500: © PhotoDisc/Vol. 25; p. 502: © The McGraw-Hill Companies, Inc./Barry Barker, photographer; p. 503: © Getty Images/Digital Vision; p. 504: © The McGraw-Hill Companies, Inc./Barry Barker, photographer; p. 505(top, bottom): © The Ohio State University Communications Photo Service; p. 506: © Corbis/RF website; p. 508: © Corbis/Vol. 25; p. 510: MHHE Image Library; p. 512: © Corbis/Vol. 609; p. 513: © The Ohio State University Communications Photo Service, Jodi Miller; Fig 14-7(reaching for food): © Corbis/RF website; (others): AP Wide World Photos; p. 516: © Corbis/RF website; p. 517: John Wang/Getty Images

Chapter 15

Opener: Creatas Images/JupiterImages; p. 525: Royalty Free/Corbis; p. 526: © The Ohio State University Communications Photo Service; p. 529(top): John A. Rizzo/Getty Images; (bottom): Royalty Free/Corbis; p. 533: Bob Montesclaros/Cole Group/Getty Images; p. 534: © Corbis/Vol. 83; p. 535: © Corbis/Vol. 192; p. 536: Rob Melnychuk/Getty Images; p. 537: © The Ohio State University Communications Photo Service; p. 538(top): © Corbis/Vol. 43; (bottom): John A. Rizzo/Getty Images; p. 541: © The Ohio State University Communications Photo Service; p. 542(top): © PhotoDisc website; (bottom): © Corbis/Vol. 49; p. 543: Royalty Free/Corbis; p. 544: © Corbis/Vol. 83; p. 546(top): USDA; (bottom): © Gregg Wolff; p. 547: © PhotoDisc/Vol. 48; p. 549: © PhotoDisc/Vol. 58; p. 552(bottom): Jess Alford/Getty Images; p. 553: Digital Vision/Getty Images

Chapter 16

Opener: © Royalty Free/Corbis; p. 558: David Buffington/Getty Images; p. 560: © Gordon Wardlaw, photographer Greg Wolff; p. 561: © Corbis/PunchStock; p. 563(both): USDA; p. 564: Keith Brofsky/Getty Images; p. 566: Smith/Getty Images; p. 567: Collection/Getty Images; p. 570: © Corbis/RF website; p. 572: © Corbis/Vol. 83; p. 574: Getty Images; p. 577: Scott T. Baxter/Getty Images; p. 578(top): © PhotoDisc/Vol. 192; (bottom): Andersen Ross/Getty Images; p. 579: © PhotoDisc/EP039; p. 580: Spike Mafford/Getty Images; p. 581: © Corbis/Vol. 52; p. 583: USDA; p. 586: Doug Menuez/Getty Images; p. 591: Andersen Ross/Getty Images

Chapter 17

Opener: Comstock/Febienne Dudognon; p. 597: © PhotoDisc/Vol. 113; p. 598: © Corbis/Vol. 135; p. 602: © Corbis/Vol. 9; p. 603: © PhotoDisc/Vol. 58; p. 604: Corbis/PictureQuest; p. 605: © Corbis/Vol. 26; p. 606: © PhotoDisc/Vol. 113; p. 607: © Paul Casamassimo, DDS, MS; p. 608: © Corbis/Vol. 9; p. 609: © Corbis/Vol. 552; p. 610: © Joanne Scott; p. 612: USDA Photo by Ken Hammond; p. 613: © Creatas/PunchStock; p. 614: Jim Arbogast/Getty Images; p. 616: © Corbis/Vol. 552; p. 617: © Greg Kidd and Joanne Scott; p. 618: © Corbis/RF website; p. 619: © PhotoDisc/Vol. 95; p. 620: © Corbis/Vol. 124; p. 622: © Greg Kidd & Joanne Scott; p. 624: © PhotoDisc/Vol. 61; p. 628: The McGraw-Hill Companies, Inc./Jill Braaten, photographer

Chapter 18

Opener: Dynamic Graphics/JupiterImages; p. 633(top): © Digital Vision/PunchStock; (bottom): © PhotoDisc Vol. 15; p. 634: Hrdlicka/Getty Images; p. 635: © Corbis/RF website; p. 636: © Corbis/Vol. 36; p. 637: © Corbis/RF website; p. 638: Royalty Free/Corbis; p. 641: © Gordon Wardlaw; p. 643: © Corbis/Vol. 192; p. 644: © PhotoDisc/Vol. 20; p. 645: © PhotoDisc website; p. 647(both): Arthur Glauberman/Photo Researchers, Inc.; p. 648: © Photodisc/Vol. 48; p. 649 & 650: © RF/Corbis; p. 651: © PhotoDisc/Vol. 58; p. 652: © PhotoDisc/OS49; p. 656: © PhotoDisc website; p. 660: © RF/Corbis; p. 661: © PhotoDisc/SS45

Appendix

(Grapes): © Burke Triolo Productions/Getty Images; Figure D-1(all): © Greg Kidd & Joanne Scott

INDEX

A

AA (Alcoholics Anonymous), 647
Abortion, spontaneous, 558
Absorption, 94, 95
  active, 101
  of carbohydrates, 135–36
  of cholesterol, fiber and, 142
  of lipids, 178
  of minerals, 288, 291
  of proteins, 213–14
  of vitamins, 285–86
Absorptive cells, 101
Accidents, alcohol use and abuse and, 646
Accutane (13-*cis*-retinoic acid), 335, 619
Acesulfame-K, 133
Acetaldehyde dehydrogenase, 644
Acid, in stomach, 97
Acid-base balance, 299–300
  proteins and, 215
Acid groups, in fatty acids, 163
Acidic agents, as food additives, 533
Acne treatment, 335, 619
Acquired immunodeficiency syndrome. *See* HIV/AIDS
Acrylamide, in foods, 540
Active absorption, 101
Active lifestyle, 46
Activity. *See* Athletes; Endurance exercise; Physical activity
Additives. *See* Food additives
Adenosine diphosphate (ADP), 430, 431
Adenosine triphosphate (ATP), 84, 434
  chemical structure of, 714
  production of, 430–33
Adequate Intakes (AIs), 57, 59
ADH (antidiuretic hormone), 303
ADHD (attention-deficit hyperactive disorder), sugar intake and, 145
Adipose cells, 180
Adipose tissue, 20, 21
  brown, 241
  growth of, 598
Adjustable gastric banding, 263, 264
Adolescents, 618–20
  eating disorders in. *See* Anorexia nervosa; Binge-eating disorder; Bulimia nervosa; Eating disorders
  growth spurt in, 618
  helping to eat more nutritious foods, 620
  iron-deficiency anemia in, 619
  nutritional problems and concerns of, 618–19
  snacking by, 620
  vegetarian diets for, 619
ADP (adenosine diphosphate), 430, 431
Adrenal glands, 92
Adrenaline (epinephrine), 90, 92, 138
Adulthood, 631–56
  cancer and, 652–56
  diet for, 633–34

middle and older. *See* Middle and older adulthood
Advanced glycation end products, 149, 150
Aerobic metabolism, 83
Aerobic workout, 429–30
Aflatoxin, cancer and, 654
African Americans
  alcohol dependency in, 647
  bone mass of, 647
  hypertension among, 313, 314
  sickle cell disease in, 209
Age. *See also* Adolescents; Children; Infants; Middle and older adulthood; Preschool children; School-age children
  maternal, pregnancy outcome and, 561–62
Aging
  of North American population, 636–38
  nutritional implications of, 638–42
  theories of, 637–38
Agriculture and Agrifood Canada, 16
AHA. *See* American Heart Association (AHA)
AI(s) (Adequate Intakes), 57, 59
AIDS. *See* HIV/AIDS
Air displacement, for body fat estimation, 246, 247
Alanine, chemical structure of, 710
Alcohol (ethanol), 13, 643–48. *See also* Alcohol abuse; Alcoholism
  absorption and metabolism of, 644–45
  cancer and, 654
  on college campuses, 24–25
  in diabetes, 151–52
  Dietary Guidelines key recommendations for, 54
  fetal health and, 584, 646
  guidance regarding use of, 647–48
  hypertension and, 314, 315
  moderate use of, benefits of, 645
  during pregnancy, 568, 584–85
  production of alcoholic beverages and, 644
  proof of, 644
  thiamine and, 386
  while breastfeeding, 577
Alcohol(s), sugar, 131–32
Alcohol abuse, 645–47. *See also* Alcoholism
  CAGE questionnaire and, 647
  risks of, 645–47
Alcohol dehydrogenase, 644
Alcohol dependence, 645
Alcoholics Anonymous (AA), 647
Alcoholism, 646
  adolescent roots of, 619
  diagnosis of, 645
  fetal alcohol syndrome and, 584
  in older adults, 645–47
Alcohol poisoning, signs and symptoms of, 25
Aldosterone, 303
Alkaline agents, as food additives, 533
Allergens, 621
Allergies. *See* Food allergies

All-or-none principle, 212
Alpha-carotene, 341
Alpha-linolenic acid, 165, 566
Alternative medicine, 640–41
Alternative sweeteners, 132–33
  as food additives, 533
Alzheimer's disease, 642
American Academy of Allergy and Immunology, 622
American Dietetic Association
  recommendations regarding diet and health, 56
American Heart Association (AHA)
  fat intake guidelines of, 187, 189
soy protein recommendation by, 224
Amino acids, 10, 205–7. *See also* Protein(s)
  branched-chain, 205, 451
  chemical structure of, 710
  essential (indispensable), 206
  limiting, 206
  nonessential (dispensable), 205, 206
  pool of, 217
  semiessential (conditionally essential), 207
  supplementing, 220
  in vegan diets, 226
Amphetamines, 261
Amylases, 97, 134–35
Amylopectin, 125
Amylose, 125
Anabolic steroids, 452
Anaerobic metabolism, 83
Anal sphincters, 103
Anaphylactic shock, 621
Android obesity, 248–49
Anemia
  blood loss causing, 494
  iron-deficiency. *See* Iron-deficiency anemia
  megaloblastic (macrocytic), 401, 495
  pernicious, 399
  physiological, 572
  during pregnancy, 572
  sickle cell, 209
  sports, 442
Animal fats, 170
Animal models, 61
Anisakis, 531
Anorexia nervosa, 465–74, 485
  early warning signs of, 469–70
  physical effects of, 469, 470–71
  thoughts of woman with, 483–84
  treatment of, 472–73
  typical person with, 469
Anthropometric assessment, 41, 42
Antibodies, 93

Physical fitness, 426
    designing programs for, 428–30
    guidelines for achieving and maintaining, 428–30
    nutrition related to, 426–28
Physicians' Weight Loss Center, 260
Physiological anemia, 572
Phytates, calcium absorption and, 361
Phytic acid (phytate), 288, 411
Phytochemicals, 35, 324, 340–41
    cancer prevention and, 224–25
    functions of, 341
    heart health and, 224
Pica, 569
Pickling agents, 534
Picky eating, in preschool children, 610–12
Piles. See Hemorrhoids
Pinocytosis, 101
Pints, 721
Pituitary gland, 92
PKU. See Phenylketonuria (PKU)
Placebo effect, 61
Placenta, 458, 557
Plant(s)
    carbohydrate formation by, 123
    proteins from, 212–13
Plant oils, 170, 224
Plaque, atherosclerotic, 191
Plasma, 87, 408
Plasma membrane, 81–83, 185–86
Platelets, 408
PMS (premenstrual syndrome), vitamin B-6 and, 393
Political unrest, in developing world, 503–4
Polychlorinated biphenyls (PCBs), in foods, 540
Polycystic ovary syndrome (PCOS), eating disorders and, 482
Polypeptides, 208
Polysaccharides, 7, 125
Polyunsaturated fatty acids, 163
Pool of amino acids, 217
Population, in developing world, ratio of food to, 502–3
Portal circulation, 87
Portal vein, 87
Portion size, 35–36. See also Serving sizes
Positive energy balance, 237, 238
Positive protein balance, 218
Potassium, 309–10
    deficiency of, 289
    Dietary Guidelines key recommendations for, 54
    dietary standards for, 675
    functions of, 289
    needs for, 289, 309–10, 675, 685
    sources of, 289, 309–10
    Upper Level/toxicity of, 289, 310
Pounds, 15, 721
Poverty
    possible solutions to, 500–501
    undernutrition and, 499–500
Prebiotics, 103
Preeclampsia, 573
Pregnancy, 556–73
    first trimester of, 558–60
    food allergies and, 623
    food plan for, 569–71

food safety during, 562, 568
HIV/AIDS during, 561
increased nutrient needs in, 563–69
nutritional status and, 563
outcome of, factors affecting, 561–63
physiological changes during, 571–73
planning for, 556–57, 586
prenatal care and counseling in, 561
second trimester of, 560
successful, definition of, 561–63
teenage, 561–62
third trimester of, 560
toxic agents during, 559, 562
undernutrition during, 514
vegetarian diet during, 570–71
Pregnancy-induced hypertension, 573
Premenstrual syndrome (PMS), vitamin B-6 and, 393
Prenatal care, inadequate, 561
Prenatal growth and development, 557–60. See also Pregnancy
    undernutrition during, 514–15
Preschool children, 609–14
    feeding problems with, 610–12
    helping to choose foods, 610
    nutritional problems in, 612–14
    nutritional supplements for, 612
Preservatives, 174, 528
Preterm infants, 222, 561
    breastfeeding, 581
    growth and development of, 596
Prevacid (lansoprazole), 110
Prilosec (omeprazole), 110
Prions, 531
Pritikin Diet, 268
Probiotics, 103
Professional organizations, 718–19
Prolactin, 574
Proline, chemical structure of, 710
Prooxidants, 324
Prostate cancer, 107, 652
Prostate gland, 339
Proteases, 97
Protein(s), 7, 8, 9, 10, 203–29. See also Amino acids
    absorption of, 213–14
    acid-base balance and, 215
    athletes' needs for, 441–42
    Canadian nutrient content claims for, 685–86
    carbohydrate sources from, 210
    celiac disease and, 113
    complementary, 212
    definition of, 7
    denaturation of, 209–10
    dietary standards for, 675
    diets high in, 220–21
    digestion of, 213, 214
    as energy source, 137, 216–17
    enzyme synthesis and, 216
    fluid balance and, 215, 216
    in foods, 210–13
    as fuel source for endurance exercise, 435–36
    glucose formation and, 216, 217
    high-quality (complete), 211
    hormone synthesis and, 216

    immune function and, 216
    increased need for, during pregnancy, 566
    infants' need for, 600
    lower-quality (incomplete), 211
    needs for, 217–19, 675
    organization of, 209
    plant sources of, 212–13
    satiety and, 217
    synthesis of, 207–8
    turnover of, 215
Protein balance, 218
Protein-calorie malnutrition (PCM), 221–22
Protein-energy malnutrition (PEM), 221–22
Protein equilibrium, 218
Protein sparing diet, 137
Protein-sparing modified fasts (PSMFs), 262
Protein turnover, 215
Proton pump inhibitors, 110, 111
Provitamin A. See Carotenoids
Prozac. See Fluoxetine (Prozac)
PSMFs (protein-sparing modified fasts), 262
Psychotherapy
for anorexia nervosa, 473
for bulimia nervosa, 476
PTCA (percutaneous transluminal coronary angioplasty), 195
PTH (parathyroid hormone), vitamin D and, 366
Purging, in bulimia nervosa, 466
Pyloric sphincter, 99
Pyridoxal, chemical structure of, 712
Pyridoxamine, chemical structure of, 712
Pyridoxine. See also Vitamin B-6
    chemical structure of, 712
Pyruvic acid, 432

Q

Quackery, in popular diets, 269
Quarts, 15, 721

R

Radiation, for food preservation, 528–29
RAEs (retinol activity equivalent), 335
Rancidity, of fats, 174, 184
Ranitidine (Zantac), 110
Rating of Perceived Exertion (RPE) scale, 430
Raw sugar, 131
RDAS (Recommended Dietary Allowances), 57–58, 59
Reactive hypoglycemia, 152
Receptors, 92
Recombinant DNA technology, 511
Recommended Dietary Allowances (RDAs), 57–58, 59
Recommended Nutrient Intakes (RNIs), 676
Rectum, 103
Red blood cells, 394
Reduced-fat foods, 172
Reduction, 323–24
Registered dietitians, 70
Reheating food, 547
Relapse prevention, for weight control, 259
Reproduction. See also Pregnancy
    vitamin A and, 335
Reproductive system, 85

Reserve capacity, 636
Respiratory system, 85
Resting metabolism, 239
Restricted-carbohydrate diets, 267, 268
Retina, 333
Retin-A (tretinoin), 335
13-*cis*-Retinoic acid (Accutane), 335, 619
Retinoids, 337
Retinol activity equivalents (RAEs), 335
Riboflavin
    chemical structure of, 712
    deficiency of, 284, 386, 403
    dietary standards for, 675
    in energy metabolism, 386–87
    functions of, 284, 386, 403
    needs for, 284, 387, 403, 675, 685
    sources of, 284, 387, 403
    Upper Level/toxicity of, 284, 403
    in vegan diets, 226
Ribonucleic acid. *See* RNA (ribonucleic acid)
Ribosomes, 83
Rickets, 281, 367, 495
Rimonabant, 261
Risk factors
    for cardiovascular disease, 193–94
    definition of, 5, 194
RNA (ribonucleic acid), 83
    messenger, 208
    transfer, 208
RNIs (Recommended Nutrient Intakes), 676
Roux-en-Y gastric bypass, 263, 264
RPE (Rating of Perceived Exertion) scale, 430

S

Saccharin, 132
Safety
    definition of, 532
    of food. *See* Food safety
    of water, 543–44
Safrole, 537
St. John's wort, 641
Saliva, 96, 97
Salivary amylase, 96, 97
Salmonella species, 526, 530
Sanitation, inadequate, in developing world,
        505–6
Satiety, 20, 21
    fats and, 172
    proteins and, 217
Satiety center, 20
Saturated fatty acids, 8, 163
    dietary standards for, 675
    needs for, 675, 685
Scavenger cells, 181
School-age children, 614–18
    diabetes in, 617
    food choices for, 614–16
    overweight and obesity in, 617–18
School Breakfast Program, 498, 499
Scientific method, 59–62
Scombroid poisoning, 526, 531
Scurvy, 59–60, 281, 330, 495
Seafood, risks from, 526
Secretin, 97
Sedentary lifestyle, 46

Selective estrogen receptor modulators (SERMs),
        for osteoporosis, 357
Selenium, 341–43
    cancer prevention by, 654
    deficiency of, 290
    dietary standards for, 675
    functions of, 290
    needs for, 290, 342, 675
    sources of, 290, 342
    Upper Level/toxicity of, 290, 342
Self-feeding skills, 608
Self-help groups
    for anorexia nervosa, 473
    for binge-eating disorder, 478
Self-monitoring, for weight control, 259
Semiessential amino acids, 207
Semistarvation, 495–96
Seniors. *See* Middle and older adulthood
Sequestrants, as food additives, 535
Serine, chemical structure of, 710
SERMs (selective estrogen receptor modulators),
        for osteoporosis, 357
Serotonin, 20, 21
Serum, 87
Serving sizes, 46, 47. *See also* Portion size
    food labeling and, 64
Set-point theory of weight, 251
SGA (small for gestational age) infants, 561
Shellfish, risks of, 526, 531
Shelter, inadequate, in developing world, 505–6
Shigella species, 526, 530
Sibutramine (Meridia), 261
Sickle cell disease (sickle cell anemia), 209
SIDS (sudden infant death syndrome), Back to
        Sleep campaign to prevent, 604
Silicon, bone health and, 374
Simple sugars, 7, 123–25
Simvastatin/ezetimibe (Vytorin), 195
Skeletal system, 85. *See also* Bone; Osteoporosis
Skin, immune function of, 93
Skinfold measurements, 247
Sleep, alcohol use and abuse and, 646
Small for gestational age (SGA) infants, 561
Small intestine, 100–102
Smoking
    adolescent roots of, 619
    cardiovascular disease related to, 193
    during pregnancy, 562
    vitamin C needs and, 331
Snacks
    in adolescence, 620
    in childhood, 611
Social barriers, to breastfeeding, 580–81
Social support, for weight control, 259
Socioeconomic status
    pregnancy outcome and, 563
    undernutrition and, 499–500
Sodium, 306–8
    Canadian nutrient content claims for, 686
    deficiency of, 289
    Dietary Guidelines key recommendations
        for, 54
    dietary standards for, 675
    functions of, 289, 306–7
    needs for, 289, 307, 675, 685
    older adults' needs for, 648

sources of, 289, 307–8
    Upper Level/toxicity of, 289, 308
Sodium bicarbonate, as ergogenic aid, 451
Sodium pump, 299
Soft water, 305–6
Solanine, 537
Solid foods, introducing to infants, 604–7
Soluble fiber, 126, 127, 136
Solvents, 300
Sorbitol, limiting, for infants, 608
South Beach diet, 268
Soy products
    allergy to, 213
    cancer prevention by, 654
    health benefits of, 225
Special Supplemental Nutrition Program for
        Women, Infants, and Children (WIC),
        498, 499, 563, 613
Specific immune function, 93
Splenda (sucralose), 132–33
Spontaneous abortions, 558
Sports anemia, 442
Sports drinks, 26, 445
Spot reducing, 434
Stabilizers, as food additives, 535
Staphylococcus aureus, 530
Starch(es), 7, 123, 125–26
    digestion of, 134–35
Starch derivatives, as fat replacement, 173
Statins, 195
Sterols, 163, 167
Stevia, 133
Stimulus control, for weight control, 259
Stomach, 99
Stomach stapling, 263, 264
Storing food, 547
Stress fractures, 443
Stroke, 6, 191
    alcohol use and abuse and, 646
    hemorrhagic, 183
    prevention of, 194
Students. *See* College, eating well in
Subclinical, definition of, 39
Substance abuse, during pregnancy, 562
Sucralfate (Carafate), 110
Sucralose (Splenda), 132–33
Sucrase, 135
Sucrose, 124, 125
Sudden infant death syndrome (SIDS), Back to
        Sleep campaign to prevent, 604
Sugar(s), 123–25, 130–31
    attention-deficit hyperactive disorder and,
        145
    blood. *See* Blood glucose
    brown, 131
    Canadian nutrient content claims for, 686–87
    dental caries and, 146
    disaccharides, 124–25
    fruit. *See* Fructose
    monosaccharides, 123–24, 125
    reducing intake of, 145, 147
    simple, 7, 123–25
    table, 124, 125
    turbinado (raw), 131
Sugar alcohols, 131–32
Sugar Busters diet, 268

Dietary Reference Intakes (DRIs): Recommended Intakes for Individuals, Vitamins

Food and Nutrition Board, Institute of Medicine, National Academies

Life Stage Group	Vitamin A (µg/d)[a]	Vitamin C (mg/d)	Vitamin D (µg/d)[b,c]	Vitamin E (mg/d)[d]	Vitamin K (µg/d)	Thiamin (mg/d)	Riboflavin (mg/d)	Niacin (mg/d)[e]	Vitamin B6 (mg/d)	Folate (µg/d)[f]	Vitamin B-12 (µg/d)	Pantothenic Acid (mg/d)	Biotin (µg/d)	Choline (mg/d)[g]
Infants														
0–6 mo	400*	40*	5*	4*	2.0*	0.2*	0.3*	2*	0.1*	65*	0.4*	1.7*	5*	125*
7–12 mo	500*	50*	5*	5*	2.5*	0.3*	0.4*	4*	0.3*	80*	0.5*	1.8*	6*	150*
Children														
1–3 y	300	15	5*	6	30*	0.5	0.5	6	0.5	150	0.9	2*	8*	200*
4–8 y	400	25	5*	7	55*	0.6	0.6	8	0.6	200	1.2	3*	12*	250*
Males														
9–13 y	600	45	5*	11	60*	0.9	0.9	12	1.0	300	1.8	4*	20*	375*
14–18 y	900	75	5*	15	75*	1.2	1.3	16	1.3	400	2.4	5*	25*	550*
19–30 y	900	90	5*	15	120*	1.2	1.3	16	1.3	400	2.4	5*	30*	550*
31–50 y	900	90	5*	15	120*	1.2	1.3	16	1.3	400	2.4	5*	30*	550*
51–70 y	900	90	10*	15	120*	1.2	1.3	16	1.7	400	2.4[h]	5*	30*	550*
>70 y	900	90	15*	15	120*	1.2	1.3	16	1.7	400	2.4[h]	5*	30*	550*
Females														
9–13 y	600	45	5*	11	60*	0.9	0.9	12	1.0	300	1.8	4*	20*	375*
14–18 y	700	65	5*	15	75*	1.0	1.0	14	1.2	400[i]	2.4	5*	25*	400*
19–30 y	700	75	5*	15	90*	1.1	1.1	14	1.3	400[i]	2.4	5*	30*	425*
31–50 y	700	75	5*	15	90*	1.1	1.1	14	1.3	400[i]	2.4	5*	30*	425*
51–70 y	700	75	10*	15	90*	1.1	1.1	14	1.5	400	2.4[h]	5*	30*	425*
>70 y	700	75	15*	15	90*	1.1	1.1	14	1.5	400	2.4[h]	5*	30*	425*
Pregnancy														
≤18 y	750	80	5*	15	75*	1.4	1.4	18	1.9	600[j]	2.6	6*	30*	450*
19–30 y	770	85	5*	15	90*	1.4	1.4	18	1.9	600[j]	2.6	6*	30*	450*
31–50 y	770	85	5*	15	90*	1.4	1.4	18	1.9	600[j]	2.6	6*	30*	450*
Lactation														
≤18 y	1,200	115	5*	19	75*	1.4	1.6	17	2.0	500	2.8	7*	35*	550*
19–30 y	1,300	120	5*	19	90*	1.4	1.6	17	2.0	500	2.8	7*	35*	550*
31–50 y	1,300	120	5*	19	90*	1.4	1.6	17	2.0	500	2.8	7*	35*	550*

mg = milligram, mg = microgram

NOTE: This table (taken from the DRI reports, see www.nap.edu) presents Recommended Dietary Allowances (RDAs) in **bold type** and Adequate Intakes (AIs) in ordinary type followed by an asterisk (*). RDAs and AIs may both be used as goals for individual intake. RDAs are set to meet the needs of almost all (97 to 98 percent) individuals in a group. For healthy breastfed infants, the AI is the mean intake. The AI for other life stage and gender groups is believed to cover needs of all individuals in the group, but lack of data or uncertainty in the data prevent being able to specify with confidence the percentage of individuals covered by this intake.

[a] As retinol activity equivalents (RAEs). 1 RAE = 1 µg retinol, 12 µg β-carotene, 24 µg α-carotene, or 24 µg β-cryptoxanthin. To calculate RAEs from REs of provitamin A carotenoids in foods, divide the REs by 2. For preformed vitamin A in foods or supplements and for provitamin A carotenoids in supplements, 1 RE = 1 RAE.

[b] cholecalciferol. 1 µg cholecalciferol = 40 IU vitamin D.

[c] In the absence of adequate exposure to sunlight.

[d] As α-tocopherol. α-Tocopherol includes RRR-α-tocopherol, the only form of α-tocopherol that occurs naturally in foods, and the 2R-stereoisomeric forms of α-tocopherol (RRR-, RSR-, RRS-, and RSS-α-tocopherol) that occur in fortified foods and supplements. It does not include the 2S-stereoisomeric forms of α-tocopherol (SRR-, SSR-, SRS-, and SSS-α-tocopherol), also found in fortified foods and supplements.

[e] As niacin equivalents (NE). 1 mg of niacin = 60 mg of tryptophan; 0–6 months = preformed niacin (not NE).

[f] As dietary folate equivalents (DFE). 1 DFE = 1 µg food folate = 0.6 µg of folic acid from fortified food or as a supplement consumed with food = 0.5 µg of a supplement taken on an empty stomach.

[g] Although AIs have been set for choline, there are few data to assess whether a dietary supply of choline is needed at all stages of the life cycle, and it may be that the choline requirement can be met by endogenous synthesis at some of these stages.

[h] Because 10 to 30 percent of older people may malabsorb food-bound B-12, it is advisable for those older than 50 years to meet their RDA mainly by consuming foods fortified with B-12 or a supplement containing B-12.

[i] In view of evidence linking folate intake with neural tube defects in the fetus, it is recommended that all women capable of becoming pregnant consume 400 µg from supplements or fortified foods in addition to intake of food folate from a varied diet.

[j] It is assumed that women will continue consuming 400 µg from supplements or fortified food until their pregnancy is confirmed and they enter prenatal care, which ordinarily occurs after the end of the periconceptional period—the critical time for formation of the neural tube.

Adapted from the Dietary Reference Intakes series, National Academies Press. Copyright 1997, 1998, 2000, 2001, by the National Academy of Sciences. The full reports are available from the National Academies

Dietary Reference Intakes (DRIs): Recommended Intakes for Individuals, Elements

Food and Nutrition Board, Institute of Medicine, National Academies

Life Stage Group	Calcium (mg/d)	Chromium (µg/d)	Copper (µg/d)	Fluoride (mg/d)	Iodine (µg/d)	Iron (mg/d)	Magnesium (mg/d)	Manganese (mg/d)	Molybdenum (µg/d)	Phosphorus (mg/d)	Selenium (µg/d)	Zinc (mg/d)
Infants												
0–6 mo	210*	0.2*	200*	0.01*	110*	0.27*	30*	0.003*	2*	100*	15*	2*
7–12 mo	270*	5.5*	220*	0.5*	130*	11	75*	0.6*	3*	275*	20*	3
Children												
1–3 y	500*	11*	340	0.7*	90	7	80	1.2*	17	460	20	3
4–8 y	800*	15*	440	1*	90	10	130	1.5*	22	500	30	5
Males												
9–13 y	1,300*	25*	700	2*	120	8	240	1.9*	34	1,250	40	8
14–18 y	1,300*	35*	890	3*	150	11	410	2.2*	43	1,250	55	11
19–30 y	1,000*	35*	900	4*	150	8	400	2.3*	45	700	55	11
31–50 y	1,000*	35*	900	4*	150	8	420	2.3*	45	700	55	11
51–70 y	1,200*	30*	900	4*	150	8	420	2.3*	45	700	55	11
>70 y	1,200*	30*	900	4*	150	8	420	2.3*	45	700	55	11
Females												
9–13 y	1,300*	21*	700	2*	120	8	240	1.6*	34	1,250	40	8
14–18 y	1,300*	24*	890	3*	150	15	360	1.6*	43	1,250	55	9
19–30 y	1,000*	25*	900	3*	150	18	310	1.8*	45	700	55	8
31–50 y	1,000*	25*	900	3*	150	18	320	1.8*	45	700	55	8
51–70 y	1,200*	20*	900	3*	150	8	320	1.8*	45	700	55	8
>70 y	1,200*	20*	900	3*	150	8	320	1.8*	45	700	55	8
Pregnancy												
≤18 y	1,300*	29*	1,000	3*	220	27	400	2.0*	50	1,250	60	12
19–30 y	1,000*	30*	1,000	3*	220	27	350	2.0*	50	700	60	11
31–50 y	1,000*	30*	1,000	3*	220	27	360	2.0*	50	700	60	11
Lactation												
≤18 y	1,300*	44*	1,300	3*	290	10	360	2.6*	50	1,250	70	13
19–30 y	1,000*	45*	1,300	3*	290	9	310	2.6*	50	700	70	12
31–50 y	1,000*	45*	1,300	3*	290	9	320	2.6*	50	700	70	12

NOTE: This table presents Recommended Dietary Allowances (RDAs) in **bold type** and Adequate Intakes (AIs) in ordinary type followed by an asterisk (*). RDAs and AIs may both be used as goals for individual intake. RDAs are set to meet the needs of almost all (97 to 98 percent) individuals in a group. For healthy breastfed infants, the AI is the mean intake. The AI for other life stage and gender groups is believed to cover needs of all individuals in the group, but lack of data or uncertainty in the data prevent being able to specify with confidence the percentage of individuals covered by this intake.

SOURCES: Dietary Reference Intakes for Calcium, Phosphorus, Magnesium, Vitamin D, and Fluoride (1997); Dietary Reference Intakes for Thiamin, Riboflavin, Niacin, Vitamin B-6, Folate, Vitamin B-12, Pantothenic Acid, Biotin, and Choline (1998); Dietary Reference Intakes for Vitamin C, Vitamin E, Selenium, and Carotenoids (2000); and Dietary Reference Intakes for Vitamin A, Vitamin K, Arsenic, Boron, Chromium, Copper, Iodine, Iron, Manganese, Molybdenum, Nickel, Silicon, Vanadium, and Zinc (2001). These reports may be accessed via www.nap.edu.

Adapted from the Dietary Reference Intake series, National Academies Press. Copyright 1997, 1998, 2000, 2001, by the National Academy of Sciences. The full reports are available from the National Academies Press at www.nap.edu.

Dietary Reference Intakes (DRIs): Recommended Intakes for Individuals, Macronutrients
Food and Nutrition Board, Institute of Medicine, National Academies

Life Stage Group	Carbohydrate (g/d)	Total Fiber (g/d)	Fat (g/d)	Linoleic Acid (g/d)	α-Linolenic Acid (g/d)	Protein[a] (g/d)
Infants						
0–6 mo	60*	ND	31*	4.4*	0.5*	9.1*
7–12 mo	95*	ND	30*	4.6*	0.5*	**13.5**
Children						
1–3 y	**130**	19*	ND[b]	7*	0.7*	**13**
4–8 y	**130**	25*	ND	10*	0.9*	**19**
Males						
9–13 y	**130**	31*	ND	12*	1.2*	**34**
14–18 y	**130**	38*	ND	16*	1.6*	**52**
19–30 y	**130**	38*	ND	17*	1.6*	**56**
31–50 y	**130**	38*	ND	17*	1.6*	**56**
51–70 y	**130**	30*	ND	14*	1.6*	**56**
>70 y	**130**	30*	ND	14*	1.6*	**56**
Females						
9–13 y	**130**	26*	ND	10*	1.0*	**34**
14–18 y	**130**	26*	ND	11*	1.1*	**46**
19–30 y	**130**	25*	ND	12*	1.1*	**46**
31–50 y	**130**	25*	ND	12*	1.1*	**46**
51–70 y	**130**	21*	ND	11*	1.1*	**46**
>70 y	**130**	21*	ND	11*	1.1*	**46**
Pregnancy						
14–18 y	**175**	28*	ND	13*	1.4*	**71**
19–30 y	**175**	28*	ND	13*	1.4*	**71**
31–50 y	**175**	28*	ND	13*	1.4*	**71**
Lactation						
14–18 y	**210**	29*	ND	13*	1.3*	**71**
19–30 y	**210**	29*	ND	13*	1.3*	**71**
31–50 y	**210**	29*	ND	13*	1.3*	**71**

NOTE: This table presents Recommended Dietary Allowances (RDAs) in **bold type** and Adequate Intakes (AIs) in ordinary type followed by an asterisk (*). RDAs and AIs may both be used as goals for individual intake. RDAs are set to meet the needs of almost all (97 to 98 percent) individuals in a group. For healthy breastfed infants, the AI is the mean intake. The AI for other life stage and gender groups is believed to cover needs of all individuals in the group, but lack of data or uncertainty in the data prevent being able to specify with confidence the percentage of individuals covered by this intake.

[a]Based on 0.8g protein/kg body weight for reference body weight.

[b]ND = not determinable at this time

SOURCES: Dietary Reference Intakes for Energy, Carbohydrate, Fiber, Fat, Fatty Acids, Cholesterol, Protein, and Amino Acids (2002). This report may be accessed via www.nap.edu.

Adapted from the Dietary Reference Intake series, National Academies Press. Copyright 1997, 1998, 2000, 2001, by the National Academy of Sciences. The full reports are available from the National Academies Press at www.nap.edu.

Dietary Reference Intakes (DRIs): Recommended Intakes for Individuals, Electrolytes and Water
Food and Nutrition Board, Institute of Medicine, National Academies

Life Stage Group	Sodium (mg/d)	Potassium (mg/d)	Chloride (mg/d)	Water (L/d)
Infants				
0–6 mo	120*	400*	180*	0.7*
7–12 mo	370*	700*	570*	0.8*
Children				
1–3 y	1,000*	3,000*	1,500*	1.3*
4–8 y	1,200*	3,800*	1,900*	1.7*
Males				
9–13 y	1,500*	4,500*	2,300*	2.4*
14–18 y	1,500*	4,700*	2,300*	3.3*
19–30 y	1,500*	4,700*	2,300*	3.7*
31–50 y	1,500*	4,700*	2,300*	3.7*
51–70 y	1,300*	4,700*	2,000*	3.7*
> 70 y	1,200*	4,700*	1,800*	3.7*
Females				
9–13 y	1,500*	4,500*	2,300*	2.1*
14–18 y	1,500*	4,700*	2,300*	2.3*
19–30 y	1,500*	4,700*	2,300*	2.7*
31–50 y	1,500*	4,700*	2,300*	2.7*
51–70 y	1,300*	4,700*	2,000*	2.7*
> 70 y	1,200*	4,700*	1,800*	2.7*
Pregnancy				
14–18 y	1,500*	4,700*	2,300*	3.0*
19–50 y	1,500*	4,700*	2,300*	3.0*
Lactation				
14–18 y	1,500*	5,100*	2,300*	3.8*
19–50 y	1,500*	5,100*	2,300*	3.8*

NOTE: The table is adapted from the DRI reports. See www.nap.edu. Adequate Intakes (AIs) are followed by an asterisk (*). These may be used as a goal for individual intake. For healthy breastfed infants, the AI is the average intake. The AI for other life stage and gender groups is believed to cover the needs of all individuals in the group, but lack of data prevent being able to specify with confidence the percentage of individuals covered by this intake; therefore, no Recommended Dietary Allowance (RDA) was set.

SOURCE: *Dietary Reference Intakes for Water, Potassium, Sodium, Chloride, and Sulfate.* This report may be accessed via www.nap.edu.

Acceptable Macronutrient Distribution Ranges

Macronutrient	Range (percent of energy)		
	Children, 1–3 y	Children, 4–18 y	Adults
Fat	30–40	25–35	20–35
omega-6 polyunsaturated fats (linoleic acid)	5–10	5–10	5–10
omega-3 polyunsaturated fats[a] (α-linolenic acid)	0.6–1.2	0.6–1.2	0.6–1.2
Carbohydrate	45–65	45–65	45–65
Protein	5–20	10–30	10–35

[a]Approximately 10% of the total can come from longer-chain n-3 fatty acids.
SOURCE: *Dietary Reference Intakes for Energy, Carbohydrate, Fiber, Fat, Fatty Acids, Cholesterol, Protein, and Amino Acids (2002).* The report may be accessed via www.nap.edu.

Dietary Reference Intakes (DRIs): Tolerable Upper Intake Levels (UL[a]), Vitamins
Food and Nutrition Board, Institute of Medicine, National Academies

Life Stage Group	Vitamin A (µg/d)[b]	Vitamin C (mg/d)	Vitamin D (µg/d)	Vitamin E (mg/d)[c,d]	Vitamin K	Thiamin	Riboflavin	Niacin (mg/d)[d]	Vitamin B-6 (mg/d)	Folate (µg/d)[d]	Vitamin B-12	Pantothenic Acid	Biotin	Choline (g/d)	Carotenoids[e]
Infants															
0–6 mo	600	ND	25	ND	ND	ND	ND	ND	ND	ND	ND	ND	ND	ND	ND
7–12 mo	600	ND	25	ND	ND	ND	ND	ND	ND	ND	ND	ND	ND	ND	ND
Children															
1–3 y	600	400	50	200	ND	ND	ND	10	30	300	ND	ND	ND	1.0	ND
4–8 y	900	650	50	300	ND	ND	ND	15	40	400	ND	ND	ND	1.0	ND
Males, Females															
9–13 y	1,700	1,200	50	600	ND	ND	ND	20	60	600	ND	ND	ND	2.0	ND
14–18 y	2,800	1,800	50	800	ND	ND	ND	30	80	800	ND	ND	ND	3.0	ND
19–70 y	3,000	2,000	50	1,000	ND	ND	ND	35	100	1,000	ND	ND	ND	3.5	ND
> 70 y	3,000	2,000	50	1,000	ND	ND	ND	35	100	1,000	ND	ND	ND	3.5	ND
Pregnancy															
≤18 y	2,800	1,800	50	800	ND	ND	ND	30	80	800	ND	ND	ND	3.0	ND
19–50 y	3,000	2,000	50	1,000	ND	ND	ND	35	100	1,000	ND	ND	ND	3.5	ND
Lactation															
≤18 y	2,800	1,800	50	800	ND	ND	ND	30	80	800	ND	ND	ND	3.0	ND
19–50 y	3,000	2,000	50	1,000	ND	ND	ND	35	100	1,000	ND	ND	ND	3.5	ND

[a]UL = The maximum level of daily nutrient intake likely to pose no risk of adverse effects. Unless otherwise specified, the UL represents total intake from food, water, and supplements. Due to lack of suitable data, ULs could not be established for vitamin K, thiamin, riboflavin, vitamin B-12, pantothenic acid, biotin, or carotenoids. In the absence of ULs, extra caution may be warranted in consuming levels above recommended intakes.

[b]As preformed vitamin A only.

[c]As α-tocopherol; applies to any form of supplemental α-tocopherol.

[d]The ULs for vitamin E, niacin, and folate apply to synthetic forms obtained from supplements, fortified foods, or a combination of the two.

[e]β-Carotene supplements are advised only to serve as a provitamin A source for individuals at risk of vitamin A deficiency.

[f]ND = Not determinable due to lack of data of adverse effects in this age group and concern with regard to lack of ability to handle excess amounts. Source of intake should be from food only to prevent high levels of intake.

SOURCES: Dietary Reference Intakes for Calcium, Phosphorus, Magnesium, Vitamin D, and Fluoride (1997); Dietary Reference Intakes for Thiamin, Riboflavin, Niacin, Vitamin B-6, Folate, Vitamin B-12, Pantothenic Acid, Biotin, and Choline (1998); Dietary Reference Intakes for Vitamin C, Vitamin E, Selenium, and Carotenoids (2000); and Dietary Reference Intakes for Vitamin A, Vitamin K, Arsenic, Boron, Chromium, Copper, Iodine, Iron, Manganese, Molybdenum, Nickel, Silicon, Vanadium, and Zinc (2001). These reports may be accessed via www.nap.edu.

Adapted from the Dietary Reference Intakes series, National Academies Press. Copyright 1997, 1998, 2000, 2001, by the National Academy of Sciences. The full reports are available from the National Academies Press at www.nap.edu.